MILITARY PREVENTIVE MEDICINE:
MOBILIZATION AND DEPLOYMENT
VOLUME 1

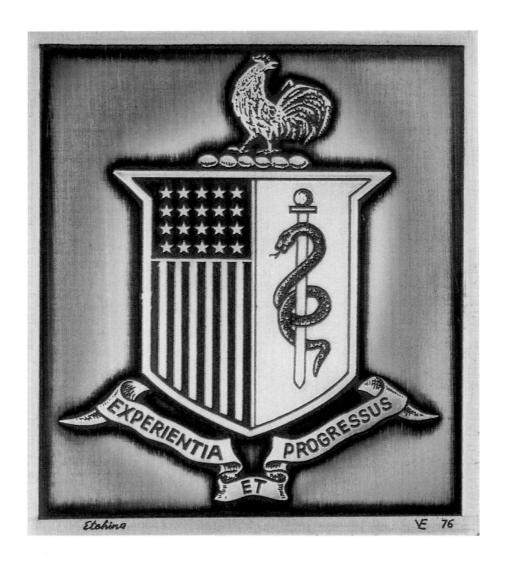

The Coat of Arms
1818
Medical Department of the Army

A 1976 etching by Vassil Ekimov of an
original color print that appeared in
The Military Surgeon, Vol XLI, No 2, 1917

The first line of medical defense in wartime is the combat medic. Although in ancient times medics carried the caduceus into battle to signify the neutral, humanitarian nature of their tasks, they have never been immune to the perils of war. They have made the highest sacrifices to save the lives of others, and their dedication to the wounded soldier is the foundation of military medical care.

Textbooks of Military Medicine

Published by the

Office of The Surgeon General
Department of the Army, United States of America

Editor in Chief and Director
Dave E. Lounsbury, MD, FACP
Colonel, MC, US Army
Borden Institute
Assistant Professor of Medicine
F. Edward Hébert School of Medicine
Uniformed Services University of the Health Sciences

Military Medical Editor
Ronald F. Bellamy, MD
Colonel, US Army, Retired
Borden Institute
Associate Professor of Military Medicine
Associate Professor of Surgery
F. Edward Hébert School of Medicine
Uniformed Services University of the Health Sciences

Editor in Chief Emeritus
Russ Zajtchuk, MD
Brigadier General, US Army, Retired
Former Commanding General
US Army Medical Research and Materiel Command
Professor of Surgery
F. Edward Hébert School of Medicine
Uniformed Services University of the Health Sciences
Bethesda, Maryland

ISBN 0-16-050500-3

9 780160 505003

The TMM Series

Published Textbooks

Medical Consequences of Nuclear Warfare (1989)

Conventional Warfare: Ballistic, Blast, and Burn Injuries (1991)

Occupational Health: The Soldier and the Industrial Base (1993)

Military Dermatology (1994)

Military Psychiatry: Preparing in Peace for War (1994)

Anesthesia and Perioperative Care of the Combat Casualty (1995)

War Psychiatry (1995)

Medical Aspects of Chemical and Biological Warfare (1997)

Rehabilitation of the Injured Soldier, Volume 1 (1998)

Rehabilitation of the Injured Soldier, Volume 2 (1999)

Medical Aspects of Harsh Environments, Volume 1 (2002)

Medical Aspects of Harsh Environments, Volume 2 (2002)

Ophthalmic Care of the Combat Casualty (2003)

Military Preventive Medicine: Mobilization and Deployment, Volume 1 (2003)

Upcoming Textbooks

Medical Aspects of Harsh Environments, Volume 3 (2003)

Military Preventive Medicine: Mobilization and Deployment, Volume 2 (2003)

Military Medical Ethics, Volume 1 (2003)

Military Medical Ethics, Volume 2 (2003)

Combat Injuries to the Head

Combat Injuries to the Extremities

Surgery for Victims of Conflict

Military Medicine in Peace and War

Recruit Medicine

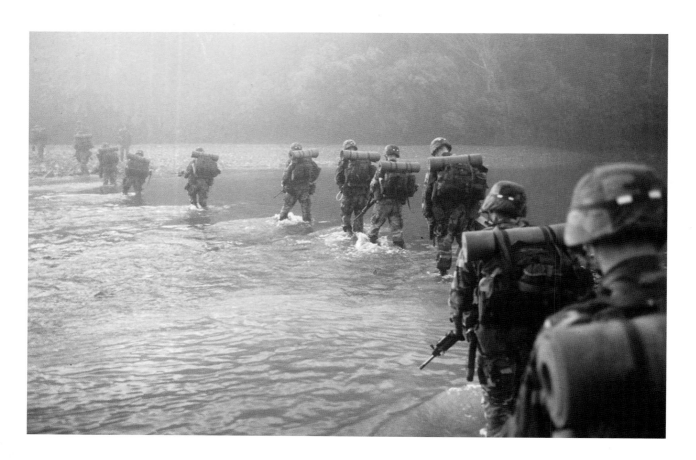

Deploying a healthy force at any time to any part of the world requires comprehensive and coordinated preventive medicine services. The challenges and the achievements of military preventive medicine in the US Armed Forces are embodied by these soldiers crossing a river in Haiti in 1995. They represent a carefully screened cadre of young Americans who enter military service and benefit from a scientifically sound program to reduce the threat of infectious diseases and injuries during basic training and deployment. When deployed to a harsh environment such as this one, they are prepared for potential hazardous exposures—infectious diseases, climatic extremes, chemical and nuclear exposures, and mental stressors—by military preventive medicine professionals. Military medical research and development provides their commanders with effective countermeasures. Their health is monitored to detect events that threaten individual health and operational effectiveness both in the field and in garrison. Military preventive medicine has always been a fundamental factor for ensuring operational success, but as US military doctrine shifts to emphasize rapid and relatively smaller deployments of forces accompanied by small medical elements, the preventive medicine mission takes on a new urgency.

Department of Defense photograph. DoD Joint Combat Camera Center Reference Number -SPT-95-000922. Photographer: SPC Kyle Davis, US Army

MILITARY PREVENTIVE MEDICINE
MOBILIZATION AND DEPLOYMENT
Volume 1

Specialty Editor

PATRICK W. KELLEY
Colonel, MC, U.S. Army

Borden Institute
Walter Reed Army Medical Center
Washington, D. C.

Office of The Surgeon General
United States Army
Falls Church, Virginia

United States Army Medical Department Center and School
Fort Sam Houston, Texas

United States Army Medical Research and Materiel Command
Fort Detrick, Frederick, Maryland

Uniformed Services University of the Health Sciences
Bethesda, Maryland

2003

Editorial Staff: Lorraine B. Davis
                       Senior Production Manager

                       Douglas A. Wise
                       Senior Layout Editor

                       Bruce G. Maston
                       Desktop Publishing Editor

                       Andy C. Szul
                       Desktop Publishing Editor

Kathleen A. Huycke
Technical Editor

This volume was prepared for military medical educational use. The focus of the information is to foster discussion that may form the basis of doctrine and policy. The opinions or assertions contained herein are the private views of the authors and are not to be construed as official or as reflecting the views of the Department of the Army or the Department of Defense.

Dosage Selection:

The authors and publisher have made every effort to ensure the accuracy of dosages cited herein. However, it is the responsibility of every practitioner to consult appropriate information sources to ascertain correct dosages for each clinical situation, especially for new or unfamiliar drugs and procedures. The authors, editors, publisher, and the Department of Defense cannot be held responsible for any errors found in this book.

Use of Trade or Brand Names:

Use of trade or brand names in this publication is for illustrative purposes only and does not imply endorsement by the Department of Defense.

Neutral Language:

Unless this publication states otherwise, masculine nouns and pronouns do not refer exclusively to men.

Published by the Office of The Surgeon General at TMM Publications
Borden Institute
Walter Reed Army Medical Center
Washington, DC 20307-5001

Library of Congress Cataloging-in-Publication Data

Military preventive medicine : mobilization and deployment / specialty editor, Patrick W. Kelley.
        p. ; cm. -- (Textbooks of military medicine)
    Includes bibliographical references and index.
    1. Medicine, Military. 2. Medicine, Preventive. 3. Military hygiene. I. Kelley, Patrick W. II. United States. Dept. of the Army. Office of the Surgeon General. III. Series.
    [DNLM: 1. Military Medicine. 2. Preventive Medicine. UH 600 M6444 2003]
    RC971.M64 2003
    616.9'8023--dc21
                                                                                    2003048099

PRINTED IN THE UNITED STATES OF AMERICA

10, 09, 08, 07, 06, 05, 04, 03   5 4 3 2 1

Contents

Contributors

DAVID ARDAY, MD, MPH
Medical Epidemiologist, Office of Clinical Standards and Quality, Health Care Financing Administration, 7500 Security Boulevard, Baltimore, MD 21244

THOMAS J. BALKIN, PhD
Research Psychologist, Chief, Department of Neurobiology and Behavior, Division of Neuropsychiatry, Walter Reed Army Institute of Research, Silver Spring, MD 20910–7500

PAUL L. BARROWS, DVM, PhD
Colonel, Veterinary Corps, US Army (Ret); l56 Crazy Cross Road, Wimberly, TX 78676

GREGORY BELENKY, MD
Colonel, Medical Corps, US Army; Director, Division of Neuropsychiatry, Walter Reed Army Institute of Research, Silver Spring, MD 20910–7500

KENT BRADLEY, MD, MPH
Lieutenant Colonel, Medical Corps, US Army; 7th Infantry Division Surgeon, Fort Carson, CO 80913

LAUREL BROADHURST, MD, MPH
Staff Physician, Weaverville Family Medicine Associates, 117 Hillcrest Drive, Weaverville, NC 28782

RICHARD BROADHURST, MD, MPH
Colonel, Medical Corps, North Carolina Army Guard, Commander, Company C, 161st Area Support Medical Battalion, Weaverville, NC 28782

STEPHANIE BRODINE, MD
Captain, Medical Corps, US Navy (Ret); Professor and Head, Division of Epidemiology and Biostatistics, Graduate School of Public Health, San Diego State University, San Diego, CA 92184

JOANNE BROWN, DVM
Colonel, Veterinary Corps, US Army (Ret); Rt 2, Box 152B, Monticello, FL 32344

DORIS BROWNE, MD, MPH
Colonel, Medical Corps, US Army (Ret); President and Chief Executive Officer, Browne and Associates, Inc. Washington, DC 21702

JOHN F. BRUNDAGE, MD, MPH
Colonel, Medical Corps US Army (Ret); Epidemiologist, Henry M. Jackson Foundation for the Advancement of Military Medicine, Army Medical Surveillance Activity, US Army Center for Health Promotion and Preventive Medicine, Aberdeen Proving Ground, MD

A.P.C.C. HOPPERUS BUMA, MD
Commander, Medical Branch, Royal Netherlands Army; Head of Naval Medical Training; PO Box 1010 (MCP 24D), 1201 DA Hilversum, The Netherlands

ROBERT E. BURR, MD
Director of Endocrine Education, Division of Endocrinology, Bayside Medical Center, 3300 Main Street, Suite 3A, Springfield, MA 01199

LESTER C. CAUDLE III, MD, MTM&H
Lieutenant Colonel, Medical Corps, US Army; Office of The Surgeon General, 5111 Leesburg Pike, Falls Church, VA 22041–3206

DALE A. CARROLL, MD, MPH
Colonel, Medical Corps, US Army (Ret); Senior Vice President, Medical Affairs and Performance Improvement, Rockingham Memorial Hospital, 235 Cantrell, Harrisburg, VA 22801

KATHRYN L. CLARK, MD, MPH
Infectious Disease Analyst, Armed Forces Medical Intelligence Center, Fort Detrick, Frederick, MD 21702–5004

BRIAN J. COMMONS, MSPH, MS
Colonel, Medical Service, US Army; US Army Center for Health Promotion and Preventive Medicine, Europe, CMR 402, APO AP 09180

CARLOS A. COMPERATORE, PhD
Research Psychologist, US Coast Guard Research and Development Center, Niantic, CT 06357

DAVID N. COWAN, PhD, MPH
Lieutenant Colonel, Medical Service, US Army; Special Projects Officer, Division of Preventive Medicine, Walter Reed Army Institute of Research, Silver Spring, MD 20910–7500

STEPHEN C. CRAIG, DO, MTM&H
Colonel, Medical Corps, US Army; Chief, Preventive Medicine Service, Keller Army Community Hospital, West Point, NY 10996

PATRICIA A. DEUSTER, PhD, MPH
Human Performance Laboratory, Department of Military and Emergency Medicine, Uniformed Services University of the Health Sciences, 4301 Jones Bridge Road, Bethesda, MD 20814

EDWARD M. EITZEN, Jr., MD, MPH
Colonel, Medical Corps, US Army; Commander, US Army Medical Research Institute of Infectious Diseases, Fort Detrick, Frederick, MD 21702–5011

RALPH L. ERICKSON, MD, DrPH
Lieutenant Colonel, Medical Corps, US Army; Chief, Preventive Medicine Service, Landstuhl Regional Medical Center, APO AE 09180

VICKY L. FOGELMAN, DVM, MPH
Colonel, Biomedical Science, US Air Force; Academic Director, International Health Program, US Air Force Radiobiology Research Institute, 8901 Wisconsin Avenue, Bethesda, MD 20889–5603

JEFFREY M. GAMBEL, MD, MPH, MSW
Lieutenant Colonel, Medical Corps, US Army; Staff Physiatrist, Walter Reed Army Medical Center, Washington, DC 20307-5001

W. DAVID GOOLSBY, DVM, MPH
Lieutenant, Veterinary Corps, US Army (Ret); 1247 Shadowwood Drive, Spartanburg, SC 29301

HARRY GREER, MD
Captain, Medical Corps, US Navy; Instructor, Defense Medical Readiness Training Institute, Fort Sam Houston, TX

JEFFREY D. GUNZENHAUSER, MD, MPH
Colonel, Medical Corps, US Army; Preventive Medicine Staff Officer, Office of The Surgeon General, 5109 Leesburg Pike, Suite 684, Falls Church, VA 22041

RAJ K. GUPTA, PhD
Colonel, Medical Service, US Army; Research Area Director, Research Plans and Programs, US Army Medical Research and Development Command, Fort Detrick, Frederick, MD 21702–5012

PAUL S. HAMMER, MD
Commander, Medical Corps, US Navy; Staff Psychiatrist, Mental Health Department, Naval Medical Center, San Diego, CA 92136

ROSE MARIE HENDRIX, DO, MPH
Medical Director, Santa Cruz County Health Clinic, 1080 Emeline, Santa Cruz, CA 95060

CHARLES R. HOWSARE, MD
Medical Director, Healthforce, 210 W. Holmes Avenue, Altoona, PA 16602

BRUCE H. JONES, MD, MPH
Colonel, Medical Corps, US Army (Ret); Division of Unintentional Injury Prevention/National Center for Injury Prevention and Control, Centers for Disease Control and Prevention, 4770 Buford Highway, Atlanta, GA 30341–3724

LISA KEEP, MD, MPH
Lieutenant Colonel, Medical Corps, US Army; Residency Director, General Preventive Medicine Residency, Walter Reed Army Institute of Research, Silver Spring, MD 20190–7500

MARGOT R. KRAUSS, MD, MPH
Colonel, Medical Corps, US Army; Deputy Director, Division of Preventive Medicine, Walter Reed Army Institute of Research, Silver Spring, MD 20910–7500

DAVID M. LAM, MD, MPH
Colonel, Medical Corps, US Army (Ret); Associate Professor, University of Maryland School of Medicine, National Study Center for Trauma and Emergency Medical Systems, and US Army Telemedicine and Advanced Technology Research Center, PSC 79, Box 145, APO AE 09714

ROBERT LANDRY, MS
Colonel, Medical Service, US Army; Headquarters and Headquarters Company, 18th Medical Command, Unit 15281, APO AP 96205–0054

PHILLIP G. LAWYER, PhD
Colonel, Medical Service, US Army; Department of Preventive Medicine and Biometrics, Division of Tropical Public Health, Uniformed Services University of the Health Sciences, 4301 Jones Bridge Road, Bethesda, MD 20814

CRAIG H. LLEWELLYN, MD, MPH
Colonel, Medical Corps, US Army (Ret); Professor of Military Medicine, Professor of Preventive Medicine and Biometrics, Professor of Surgery, Director, Center for Disaster and Humanitarian Assistance Medicine (CDHAM), Uniformed Services University of the Health Sciences, 4301 Jones Bridge Road, Bethesda, MD 20814–4799

K. MILLS McNEILL, MD, MPH, PhD
Colonel, Medical Corps, US Army (Ret); Medical Director for Bioterrorism Preparedness, Office of Epidemiology, Mississippi State Department of Health, 570 E. Woodrow Wilson, PO Box 1700, Jackson, MS 39215-1700

RAMY A. MAHMOUD, MD, MPH
Lieutenant Colonel, Medical Corps, US Army Reserve; Group Director, Janssen Research Foundation, 1125 Trenton–Harbourton Road, PO Box 200, Room A11010, Titusville, NJ 08560–0200

LAUREL A. MAY, MD, MPH
Commander, Medical Corps, US Navy; Epidemiologist, Naval Medical Clinic, 480 Central Avenue, Pearl Harbor, HI 96860–4908

ROY D. MILLER, PhD
Department of Preventive Medicine and Biometrics, Uniformed Services University of the Health Sciences; 4301 Jones Bridge Road, Bethesda, MD 20814–4799

GEORGE E. MOORE, DVM
Colonel, Veterinary Corps, US Army; Chief, Department of Veterinary Sciences, Army Medical Department Center and School, Building 2840, Suite 248, 2250 Stanley Road, Fort Sam Houston, TX 78234–6145

LELAND JED MORRISON, MD
Captain, Medical Corps, US Navy (Ret); Chief Physician Naval Forces, United Arab Forces

DOUG OHLIN, PhD
Hearing Conservation Program, Occupational and Environmental Medicine, US Army Center for Health Promotion and Preventive Medicine, 5158 Blackhawk Road, Aberdeen Proving Ground, MD 21010

RELFORD E. PATTERSON, MD, MPH
Colonel, Medical Corps, US Army (Ret); Medical Director, General Motors Corporation Truck Group Assembly Plant, 2122 Broenig Highway, Baltimore, MD 21224

JULIE A. PAVLIN, MD, MPH
Lieutenant Colonel, Medical Corps, US Army; Chief, Department of Field Studies, Division of Preventive Medicine, Walter Reed Army Institute of Research, Silver Spring, MD 20910–7500

BRUNO P. PETRUCCELLI, MD, MPH
Lieutenant Colonel, Medical Corps, US Army; Director, Epidemiology and Disease Surveillance, US Army Center for Health Promotion and Preventive Medicine, 5158 Blackhawk Road, Aberdeen Proving Ground, MD 21010–5403

WILLIAM A. RICE, MD, MPH
Lieutenant Colonel, Medical Corps, US Army; currently, Division Surgeon, 1st Armored Division, Germany; formerly, Center for Health Promotion and Preventive Medicine, Europe, APO AE 09180

LEON L. ROBERT, JR., PhD
Lieutenant Colonel, Medical Service, US Army; Department of Preventive Medicine and Biometrics, Division of Tropical Public Health, Uniformed Services University of the Health Sciences, 4301 Jones Bridge Road, Bethesda, MD 20814

WELFORD C. ROBERTS, PhD
Department of Preventive Medicine and Biometrics, Uniformed Services University of the Health Sciences, 4301 Jones Bridge Road, Bethesda, MD 20814–4799

ANDREW F. ROCCA, MD
Lieutenant Commander, Medical Corps, US Navy; Senior Resident, Department of Orthopedics, National Naval Medical Center, Bethesda, MD 20889-5600

BERNARD A. SCHIEFER, MS
Colonel, Medical Service, US Army (Ret); 7238 Ford Street, Mission, TX 78572–8946

RICHARD A. SHAFFER, PhD, MPH
Lieutenant Commander, Medical Service Corps, US Navy; Head, Operational Readiness Research Program, Naval Health Research Center, PO Box 85122, San Diego, CA 92186–5122

FREDERICK R. SIDELL, MD
Chemical Casualty Consultant, Bel Air, MD 21014

ANITA SINGH, PhD, RD
Food and Nutrition Service, US Department of Agriculture, 3101 Park Center Drive, Alexandria, VA 22302

RICHARD W. SMERZ, MD, MPH
Colonel, Medical Corps, US Army (Ret)

PAUL D. SMITH, DO, MPH
Lieutenant Colonel, Medical Corps, US Army; Occupational Environmental Medicine Staff Officer, Proponency Officer for Preventive Medicine, Office of The Surgeon General, 5109 Leesburg Pike, Falls Church, VA 22041–3258

STEVE SMITH, MD, MPH
Site Medical Director, Umatilla Chemical Agent Demilitarization Facility, Umatilla Chemical Depot, 78068 Ordnance Road, Hermiston, OR 97838

BONNIE L. SMOAK, MD, PhD, MPH
Colonel, Medical Corps, US Army; Director, Division of Tropical Public Health, Department of Preventive Medicine and Biometrics, Uniformed Services University of the Health Sciences, 4301 Jones Bridge Road, Bethesda, MD 20814–4799

HENRY P. STIKES, MD, MPH
Colonel, Medical Corps, US Army (Ret); Commander, Lawrence Joel US Army Health Clinic, 1701 Hardee Avenue, SW, Fort McPherson, GA 30330–1062

JAMES W. STOKES, MD
Colonel, Medical Corps, US Army; Combat Stress Control Program Officer, Behavioral Health Division, Health Policy and Services, US Army Medical Command, 2050 Worth Road, Fort Sam Houston, TX 78234–6010

RICHARD THOMAS, MD, MPH
Captain, Medical Corps, US Navy; Naval Environmental Health Center, 2510 Walmer Avenue, Norfolk, VA 23513–2617

RANDALL THOMPSON, DVM
Major, Veterinary Corps, US Army; 18th Medical Command, Unit 15252, APO AP 96205–0025

NANCY JO WESENSTEN, PhD
Research Psychologist; Department of Neurobiology and Behavior, Division of Neuropsychiatry, Walter Reed Army Institute of Research, Silver Spring, MD 20910–7500

RICHARD WILLIAMS, MD
Captain, Medical Corps, US Navy; Chief Clinical Consultant, Armed Forces Medical Intelligence Center, Fort Detrick, Frederick, MD 21702–7581

BENJAMIN G. WITHERS, MD, MPH
Colonel, Medical Corps, US Army; Command Surgeon, US Army Materiel Command, 5001 Eisenhower Avenue, Alexandria VA 22333–0001

JAMES WRIGHT, MD
Colonel, Medical Corps, US Air Force (Ret); Occupational Medicine Physician, Concentra Medical Centers, 400 East Quincy, San Antonio, TX 78235

JAMES V. WRITER, MPH
Environmental Monitoring Team, US Department of Agriculture Animal and Plant Health Inspection Service, 4700 River Road, Riverdale, MD 20737

STEVEN YEVICH, MD, MPH
Colonel, Medical Corps, US Army (Ret); Director, VA National Center for Health Promotion and Disease Prevention, 3000 Croasdaile Drive, Durham, NC 27707

Foreword

It has been over 60 years since George Dunham wrote the last major US textbook on military preventive medicine. Both then and now, the mission of military preventive medicine has been to preserve the fighting strength through population-based methods of disease and injury avoidance. A comparison, however, of the tables of contents of Dunham's textbook and this one, *Military Preventive Medicine: Mobilization and Deployment*, illustrates that the scope of military preventive medicine has grown tremendously. This reflects changes in US warfighting doctrine, the expansion of the US military's role in operations other than war, the emergence of new disease and injury threats, and the changing demographics of our warfighters.

US military doctrine is increasingly focused on rapid deployment of lighter units that (1) are more widely dispersed on the battle space and (2) achieve advantages through information, tactical, and strategic dominance. Future military engagements will often evolve rapidly and put a premium on conserving scarce, highly trained, human resources. Central to the conservation of human resources are the needs for knowledgeable leadership, an understanding of the lessons of past conflicts, and systematic estimates of the medical threat prior to exposure; this new volume in the *Textbooks of Military Medicine* series reflects these needs. In a force drawn from a finite pool of volunteers, it is critical to have balanced accession standards and to do minimal damage while realistically training recruits. The growing interest of women in military service has not only increased the pool of much-needed talent but has also necessitated that approaches to prevention of training injuries and health maintenance be reevaluated to ensure that they reflect the needs of all service members.

Unlike 50 years ago, our forces are now expected to be able to move within hours from the US to the battlefield and arrive ready to fight. Although warfare is obviously dangerous, the risk of disease and nonbattle injury on the battlefield has often been underappreciated—along with the potential of countermeasures to mitigate that risk. This morbidity is appreciated increasingly as not just physical but also psychological. In Dunham's era, war-associated syndromes, nuclear and biological warfare, and emerging infections such as drug-resistant malaria, hepatitis C, and acquired immunodeficiency syndrome were not the threats that they are today. The requirement to conduct continuous surveillance for disease and nonbattle injury before, during, and after deployment speaks to the high investment that our military has in each service member and of their individual importance to military success.

In the post–Cold War era, the US military has been called on increasingly to assist with operations other than war including not only peacekeeping operations but also humanitarian assistance operations. In many of these operations, military preventive medicine is at the tip of the spear. Thus it is critical that all military medical personnel have an appreciation for the challenges posed by natural and manmade disasters, by large numbers of displaced persons, and for the different roles we may be called on to fill.

Military Preventive Medicine: Mobilization and Deployment reflects the evolution of preventive medicine in the military from its traditional focus on field hygiene and infectious disease control to encompassing the wide range of threats and scenarios associated with modern military service. There are many lessons to be learned from the textbook's emphasis on history and the military relevance of the conditions covered. However, the essence of this volume, like the practice of military preventive medicine, is timeless: our nation's greatness is reflected in our comprehensive care of those who serve. Preventive medicine of the highest quality is just recognition for their sacrifices and those of their families and communities. It is also a cornerstone to our military readiness. I hope that this textbook will help illuminate the path for those dedicated to pursuing that vision.

Lieutenant General James B. Peake
The Surgeon General
US Army

Washington, DC
September 2003

Preface

Force health protection, although often a loosely defined focus of military medical departments in the past, has in the aftermath of the Persian Gulf War received especially explicit, thorough, and vigorous emphasis within the US Department of Defense. The overall US national military strategy at the turn of the millennium is to "shape, prepare, and respond" to potential national security threats around the world. As is noted in the Department of Defense's *Doctrine for Health Service Support in Joint Operations*, force health protection has three corresponding functions: to shape a healthy and fit force, to prevent casualties through proper preparation of personnel, and to respond to casualties when they occur. Preventive Medicine is inherently central to developing a healthy and fit force and in keeping the force healthy through mobilization and deployment—even into the postdeployment phase. This is more critical than ever in light of a shrinking medical footprint and the need to provide immediate casualty care on the modern, rapidly mobile battlefield. Even once casualties occur, Preventive Medicine has an important tertiary prevention role that must be vigorously pursued if service members are to be successfully rehabilitated and avoid having their relatively manageable physical or mental problems evolve into long-term disabilities.

Force health protection is not only beneficial to the individual but also essential to unit readiness and performance. Contemporary military operations, whether in training, on the battlefield, or in the conduct of operations other than war, place units under the threat of an ever-widening array of biological, physical, and mental stressors. The mitigation of these requires military Preventive Medicine professionals to be familiar with a broad array of disciplines and to provide cohesive leadership and sound advice up and down the chain of command. This textbook aims to provide enabling insights with respect to these scientific, administrative, and leadership challenges.

The challenges of military Preventive Medicine are becoming ever more complex but are also very old. The solutions in many cases are well documented but often forgotten. In 1827, John Macculloch wrote prophetically that

> it would seem, as if fatal, that the wisdom and experience of one generation should be forgotten by the next, that peace should extirpate the knowledge that had been gained in war.[1]

In 2003, *Preventive Medicine: Mobilization and Deployment* emphasizes these often-forgotten lessons of the past and it also provides a comprehensive approach to protecting the force in the current context of the US military's global security mission. We, as military medical professionals, must understand this approach to be well prepared for responding to this mission in a focused, competent, and compassionate manner. Our great nation and its sons and daughters who volunteer to take on its most arduous burdens have ever-rising expectations of military Preventive Medicine. At their peril, we ignore the lessons at our fingertips.

Dave Ed. Lounsbury, MD
Colonel, Medical Corps, US Army
Director, Borden Institute, and
Editor in Chief, Textbooks of Military Medicine

Washington, DC
September 2003

1. Macculloch J. *Malaria: An essay on the production and propagation of this poison and on the nature and localities of the places by which it is produced: With an enumeration of the diseases caused by it, and to the means of preventing or diminishing them, both at home and in the naval and military service.* London, England: Longman & Co; 1827.

The current medical system to support the U.S. Army at war is a continuum from the forward line of troops through the continental United States; it serves as a primary source of trained replacements during the early stages of a major conflict. The system is designed to optimize the return to duty of the maximum number of trained combat soldiers at the lowest possible echelon. Far-forward stabilization helps to maintain the physiology of injured soldiers who are unlikely to return to duty and allows for their rapid evacuation from the battlefield without needless sacrifice of life or function.

MILITARY PREVENTIVE MEDICINE: MOBILIZATION AND DEPLOYMENT
Volume 1

Section 1: A Historic Perspective on the Principles of Military Preventive Medicine

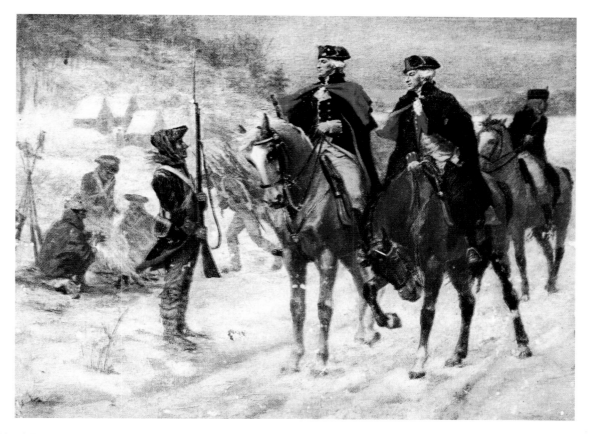

John Ward Dunsmore   *Washington and Lafayette at Valley Forge*   1907

Many of the medical challenges of deployment have not changed in the centuries since Washington and Lafayette rode out among the soldiers at Valley Forge. Personnel still have to be protected from the elements, they still need safe food and water, they still need properly located latrines, and they still must be given means to protect themselves from disease and insects. General Washington's innovations, such as army-wide smallpox vaccinations, strict camp hygiene (instituted by Baron von Steuben), and command emphasis on preventive medicine measures, make him a hero of modern military preventive medicine.

Art: Courtesy of Brown & Bigelow, St. Paul, Minnesota.

Chapter 1

PREVENTIVE MEDICINE AND COMMAND AUTHORITY—LEVITICUS TO SCHWARZKOPF

CRAIG H. LLEWELLYN, MD, MPH

C. H. Llewellyn; Colonel, Medical Corps, US Army, (Retired); Professor of Military Medicine; Professor of Preventive Medicine and Biometrics; Professor of Surgery; Director, Center for Disaster and Humanitarian Assistance Medicine (CDHAM), Uniformed Services University of the Health Sciences, 4301 Jones Bridge Road, Bethesda, MD 20814-4799

INTRODUCTION

Throughout history under a variety of titles—cleanliness, field hygiene, environmental sanitation, preventive medicine, force protection—activities and programs have been developed to maintain the health and operational performance of military forces and to prevent disease, injury, and disability. Legters and Llewellyn describe military medicine as "a unique brand of occupational medicine, one that deals with the prevention and treatment of diseases and injuries resulting from work in military occupations and operational environments."[1(p1141)] Bayne-Jones notes that through the performance of inspectorial, advisory, and regulatory duties, military preventive medicine is concerned with the administration of the entire military force, thus having a scope that exceeds all other elements of the military medical departments.[2] Military preventive medicine is therefore the central function of military medicine. Unlike casualty management of individual patients, military preventive medicine is intimately involved with military commanders, staffs, and units on a continuous basis.

The promotion and preservation of health and the prevention of illness and injury can rarely be accomplished solely through medical channels. Responsibility for the health and welfare of the members of a military unit falls on the commander, as dictated by federal law and military regulation. Law and regulation are the basis for command authority and military preventive medicine through which unit commanders can influence the health of their commands and thus gain command of health.

An understanding of these seemingly simple relationships among military preventive medicine, military medicine, and command authority and responsibility has been the essential foundation for successful preventive medicine activities throughout military history and continues to be so today. Equally important are the relationships between unit commanders and their staffs and the military preventive medicine personnel advising and supporting them. This chapter will explore the historical basis for these relationships and the generic lessons that may be learned and applied in the current and future practice of military preventive medicine.

LEVITICUS AND THE PREVENTIVE MEDICINE PARADIGM

The Book of Leviticus

As Commander-in-Chief of the Continental Army during the American Revolutionary War, General George Washington published a general order on "The Means of Preserving Health" (Figure 1-1) in which he referred to Moses as "the wisest General that ever lived" and quoted elements of the Mosaic Sanitary Code from the Old Testament. This echoed similar references by the leading military physicians of the 18th century, such as Pringle,[3] Brocklesby,[4] and Munro[5] in England and Rush[6] and Tilton[7] in the United States, and presaged Wood's book *Moses, the Founder of Preventive Medicine*.[8] Each of the above authors recognized that the book of Leviticus is probably the earliest textbook of preventive medicine.

In his "Notes on the History of Military Medicine," Garrison[9] analyzes Leviticus, chapters 8 through 15, and identifies several functions of the Levites, or Jewish priests, whom he defined as hygienic police. Their functions included regulating diet, food sources, water, and personal and sexual hygiene; recognizing and investigating disease; quarantining diseased persons and purifying contaminated articles and structures; educating the community on these topics; advising leaders on the community's hygiene; and conducting a census of the community. In addition, these priests accompanied the army into the field and into battle, providing guidance on all aspects of camp sanitation and the health of the force.

The priests of Israel, while having wide-ranging responsibilities to the leaders and members of the community they served, are not identified as having responsibilities for treating the sick or injured. Thus began a separation of those responsible for the health and well-being of the group from those who provided treatment in an attempt to restore health.

The Paradigm

From the five books of Moses found in the Old Testament, a broad picture of preventive functions emerges that has continuing relevance for military preventive medicine. The nation, religion, and army of Israel were inseparable during the 40 years in the wilderness, and the activities of the priests, the hygienic police, were intimately involved with all three. The priests' functions can be broadly charac-

INSTRUCTIONS for SOLDIERS in the Service of the
UNITED STATES, concerning the Means of preserving HEALTH
Of CLEANLINESS

It is extremely difficult to persuade Soldiers that Cleanliness is absolutely necessary to the Health of an Army. They can hardly believe that in a military State it becomes one of the *Necessaries of Life.* They are either too careless to pay Attention to this Subject, or they deceive themselves by reasoning from Cases, that are by no Means similar. Hitherto they have enjoyed a good State of Health, tho' they paid little or no Attention to such Punctilios; hence they conclude, that, tho' in the Army, they shall continue to enjoy an equal Degree of Health, under the like Degree of Negligence: Such reasoning has proved fatal to thousands. They do not consider the prodigious Difference there is in the Circumstances of five or six People, who live by themselves on a Farm, and of thirty or forty thousand Men, who live together in a Camp. The former chiefly subsist on vegetable Food; they lodge warm and dry, and they breathe in pure Air, which is not contaminated by noxious Vapours: The latter in general subsist too much on animal Food; they sleep frequently on cold and damp Beds, and they breathe foul Air, that is constantly injured by the very Breath of a Multitude; and is frequently rendered much more dangerous by the Stench and Exhalations that arise from putrid Bodies. The Air is injured, as I have just said by the Breath of a Multitude and the perspirable Matter that comes through the Pores of the Skin helps to extend the Disorder. But the Blood and Offals of Cattle that are killed near the Camp, with the different animal Substances that are daily thrown there by the Soldiers themselves, must soon fill the Air with a pestilential Smell, unless they are immediately removed or covered sufficiently deep. When the Soldier pours out Water, in which Flesh has been boiled; when in a peevish Mood he throws away Part of his Ration, because it is too much roasted, or because it is not roasted enough; or even when he throws away Bones that are not well picked; he seldom considers that such Things must soon become putrid, and that he is sowing the Seeds of Disease and Death for himself or his Companions. The Soldier should burn his Meat rather than throw it away: History informs us that great Armies have followed this Rule. Soldiers are not supposed to be acquainted with the Art of preserving Health; they are little versed in Books; but, to the Honour of American Soldiers, it is allowed that no men in Christendom of the same Occupation are so well acquainted with their Bibles: Let them, once more, read the History and Travels of the Children of Israel while they continued in the Wilderness, under the Conduct of Moses; and let them consider at the same Time that they are reading the History of a great Army, that continued forty Years in their different Camps under the Guidance and Regulations of the wisest General that ever lived, for he was inspired. In the History of these People, the Soldier must admire the singular Attention that was paid to the Rules of Cleanliness. They were obliged to wash their Hands two or three Times a Day. Foul Garments were counted abominable; every Thing that was polluted or dirty was absolutely forbidden; and such Persons as had Sores or Diseases in their Skin were turned out of the Camp*. The utmost Pains were taken to Keep the Air in which they breathed, free from Infection. They were commanded, to have *a Place without the Camp, whither they should* go, and *have a Paddle with which they should dig,* so that *when they went abroad to ease themselves, they might turn back and cover that which came from them†.*

Besides these general Regulations, it is also necessary for the Preservation of Health, that every Soldier be particularly attentive to his own Person. The Straw on which he sleeps should be frequently dried; and he should never spread it on damp Ground, when he can get Hurdles, Bark, Boards, Leaves, or any other dry Substance to put under it. A Soldier should change his Shirt and Stockings once every two or three Days: Though his Stock of Linen is small, a Shirt is soon washed. Little Attention is due to the Colour, provided it be clean. Women are never wanting in a Camp for such Offices. A Man is seldom aware of the Quantity of noxious Matter that comes through his own Skin and is deposited on his Shirt; but if he takes up a Shirt that has been worn a few Days by another Person, he is frequently offended by the disagreeable Smell.

These are some of the reasons why CLEANLINESS of every kind is necessary towards preserving Health in an Army: They are Reasons which every Soldier may understand; but should he neglect to regulate himself accordingly, the Regimental Surgeon will doubtless attend to the Neglect, and his Officers will see that he does his Duty. For every Soldier by his Neglect not only endangers his own Life, but the Lives of his Companions. Nature, or the God of Nature, has commanded, that men who live in Camps should be cleanly: Whoever proves too obstinate, or too slothful to obey this Command, may expect to be punished with Death, or suffer under some dangerous Disease.

W.

Numb. 5. i.   †Deut. 23 xii.

Fig. 1-1. The text of General George Washington's broadside: Instructions for Soldiers in the Service of the United States Concerning the Means of Preserving Health: Of Cleanliness. Source: Bayne-Jones S. *The Evolution of Preventive Medicine in the United States Army, 1607–1939.* Washington, DC: Office of the Surgeon General, Department of the Army; 1968: 190–191.

terized as advisory, educational, inspectorial, investigational, and interventional. Focus was placed equally on individual and community behavior in attempting to prevent and control threats from disease, the natural environment, and food and water. In the absence of scientifically grounded medical knowledge, these efforts were based on pragmatic, experiential, or ritualistic actions. Elements of these practices can be found later in the successful military medicine that supported the Roman legions. A strong case can be made for these five functions—advice to leaders, education of unit members, inspection to ensure compliance, investigation of noncompliance, and intervention to protect the group—as the continuing core functions of military preventive medicine.

COMMAND AUTHORITY AND PREVENTIVE MEDICINE IN AMERICAN MILITARY HISTORY

The Revolutionary War

During the 18th century, two outstanding English surgeons general, Sir John Pringle[3] and Dr. Richard Brocklesby,[4] drew on their own extensive experience and that of van Swieten[10] in Austria, among others, to publish several books on military hygiene and the preservation of the health of troops. The doctrine and practices described were known to George Washington from his service in the colonial militia alongside regular British troops during the French and Indian Wars. Many of the American physicians who provided the medical leadership during the Revolutionary War had received their medical degrees from Edinburgh, read Brocklesby's and van Swieten's books and knew Sir John Pringle personally. Thus from the beginnings of the republic, both the commander in chief and the leading physicians who served with him shared a view of the importance of preserving the health of troops and the fundamental responsibility of command at all levels to accomplish this mission by relying on sound medical advice.

In his writings, Pringle addressed the officers as well as the physicians because of his conviction that the maintenance of the health of troops is the responsibility of command and, therefore, line officers. In addition, he noted that prevention cannot be based on anything that a soldier can avoid but must be governed by regulations and orders he is required to obey. Each of Pringle's themes appeared in the publications of the leading American physicians during the Revolution. Dr. John Jones[11] specifically referred to Pringle, and Dr. Benjamin Rush, in *Directions for Preserving the Health of Soldiers*, addressed his book equally to Army line officers and to physicians, while clearly stating that the health of troops is a command responsibility.[6] In a letter they wrote to President John Adams, Rush and then-retired General Washington described the relationship of the physician general to the commander-in-chief as having the closeness of a family member; the physician general was an essential element of the Army staff who should be aware of and concur with all orders and plans for the Army.[2]

Recognition of the role of command authority in preventive medicine is seen in many of Washington's letters and general orders but is nowhere more clearly indicated than in his decision in 1777 to order the inoculation of the entire Army against smallpox, describing it as "the greatest enemy to the Continental Army."[2(p52)] This decision was based on the recommendation of his Physician in Chief, Dr. John Morgan. Many historians point to the subsequently smallpox-free condition of the Continental Army as a major contribution to winning the war.

Also of importance was the work of Baron von Steuben, first Inspector General of the Continental Army, who wrote and published, with Congressional approval, *Regulations for the Order and Discipline of Troops of the United States*[12] in 1779. This document contained many directions for the preservation of health and prevention of disease. Congressional approval made these legal regulations that required compliance and execution by all officers.

By the end of the American Revolutionary War, then, nearly all the basic concerns of preventive medicine had been identified and, in many cases, made mandatory by the commander in chief and the Congress:[2(184–185)]

- Responsibility of command for the health of troops
- Medical officers as advisors to line officers
- Discipline
- Personal hygiene
- Diet and nutrition
- Clothing and shoes
- Threats from extreme heat, cold, fatigue, and wetness
- Morale building and recreation
- Health education
- Immunization
- Environmental hygiene
  - Location and design of campsites and

shelters
- ○ Avoidance of crowding
- ○ Sanitation of camps
- ○ Disposal of excreta and waste
- ○ Protection of water supplies
- Reduction of disease-transmitting human contacts
- Rudimentary medical intelligence

Further progress depended on developments in the biological and medical sciences during the late 19th century and throughout the 20th century.

The Civil War

The relationship between command and military preventive medicine during this period was strongly influenced by the abysmal sanitation and disease experience of the Mexican War (1846–1848) and more directly by the British and French experience in the Crimea (1854–1856). Press reports made these experiences common knowledge. In Britain, the government responded by establishing the Royal Sanitary Commission. This body was composed of leading civilians who exerted enormous influence directly on commanders and their chief medical officers, forcing the former to pay more attention to medical advice. Equally important among the commission's work were the establishment of the specialty of Army Health in the British Army; the publication of a new British Army regulation giving medical officers the power to advise commanders on all matters pertaining to the health of troops; the establishment of the Royal Army Medical School in 1860, with specific courses of instruction in military hygiene; and the publication of the sanitary history of the Crimean War, the first medical war history published by a government. Thus, at the outbreak of the American Civil War, knowledge of these experiences and accomplishments was available and exerted a significant influence in the United States on government officials, military leaders both medical and nonmedical, and the general population.[2(p89–92)]

The incompetence of the US Army Medical Department in the earliest days of the war led President Lincoln to follow the British model and appoint the United States Sanitary Commission. The Commission's initially circumscribed inspectorial and advisory powers rapidly expanded to true operational agency status, with the authority to conduct preventive services for the Army and authorization to communicate directly with the Surgeon General, medical officers, commanders of troops at all levels, the Secretary of War, and the President. As evidence of its power, the Commission played a major role in Congressional legislation directing the reorganization of the Medical Department and forcefully influencing the appointment of Lieutenant William A. Hammond as Surgeon General and Surgeon Jonathan Letterman as Medical Director for the Army of the Potomac.[2(p102–104)]

Among the myriad activities of the Commission, several stand out. First was capturing the attention of command, from the commander in chief down to divisions in the field, concerning its responsibilities for the health of troops. Second was establishing the highly efficient Camp Inspection Service, with a heavy emphasis on sanitation and hygiene. Third was publishing material by distinguished physicians and surgeons to educate both medical and nonmedical officers with such titles as "Military Hygiene and Therapeutics," "Rules for Preserving the Health of Soldiers," "Control and Prevention of Infectious Diseases," "Quinine as a Prophylactic against Malarious Diseases," and "Scurvy."[2(p104)] Each of these topics was recognized as requiring medical advice and command action. These publications introduced a new model for health education and set the standard for several decades.

Perhaps the most important action influenced by the Commission was the appointment of LT Hammond as Surgeon General in 1862. Enormously talented, he attracted and appointed equally able medical officers, such as Letterman, John Shaw Billings, and Joseph Janvier Woodward, each of whom had proven ability to work well with field commanders. Hammond doubled the number of medical inspectors supervising sanitary matters, established the Army Medical Museum for educational purposes, compiled and issued the pamphlets of the Sanitary Commission, and established a comprehensive system of sanitary reports.

The command-directed and then Congressionally dictated inoculation of troops against smallpox during the Revolutionary War continued during the Civil War. A major medical innovation during the Civil War was the official introduction of quinine sulphate as prophylaxis for malaria. Recommended by the US Sanitary Commission and enthusiastically promoted by Hammond, oral quinine prophylaxis (given daily as a whiskey bitters drink) was mandated by the command (Figure 1-2) and enforced by line officers. The alcohol content reportedly made this a troop favorite.

During the Civil War, the initial chaos of mobilization was replaced by a military establishment within which commanders were made to take responsibil-

Headquarters, Army of the Mississippi,
Iuxa, August 25th, 1862.

**GENERAL ORDERS,
NO. 117.**

The season for billious and intermittent fevers in this region and climate is at hand. The Medical Officers of this Army will, therefore, take the most prompt and efficacious measures to counteract the effects of malaria on our troops. To this end, their attention is again called to the Circular of the Medical Director of the Department, dated, July 13th, 1862. In addition to which, the following directions will be strictly carried out, viz:

1st. All working parties will invariably be supplied with rations of bitters, prepared as prescribed below, and to be given twice a day to the individuals of each party under the direction of a commissioned officer in quantities not to exceed half a gill at a time.

2nd. All guides and scouting-parties out at night, will, likewise, have administered to them, under the direction of a Medical officer, a half-ration of bitters. It will be given to them between Retreat and Tattoo.

3rd. The bitters to be issued, will be made, as follows:

    96 grains of Sulp. Quinia,
    100 "   "Cinchinoa,

to each gallon of whisky; or, for each barrel of 40 gallons:

    8 ounces of quinine,
    13 "   "Sulp. Cinchinoa;

this will make about thirteen hundred full rations.

4th. Medical Directors of Divisions will make prompt requisitions for the necessary supplies to carry this Order into effect.

5th. Division, brigade and detachment commanders will see to the execution of this order, and direct the issues under it to be accurately stated in the weekly Sanitary and Inspection Report.

BY ORDER OF GENERAL ROSECHANS.
H.G. KENNETH,
Lieut.-Col and Chief of Staff

[OFFICIAL]

Fig. 1-2. Army of the Mississippi's General Order No. 117 concerning the use of quinine bitters for the prevention of malaria. Source: US Archives

ity for the health of troops and to accept the advice of both the US Sanitary Commission and their own military physicians. In spite of the fact that there was still no scientific basis for preventive medicine interventions and that disease remained the major cause of morbidity and mortality in the military, great improvements had been made. As reported by Duncan,[13] this experience was significantly better than that recorded during the Mexican War or by the French in the Crimea, as is shown in Table 1-1.

TABLE 1-1

DEATHS FROM DISEASE AND BATTLE DEATHS IN PRINCIPAL WARS, FOREIGN ARMIES AND U.S. ARMY, 1846-1945

War	Date	Deaths from Disease	Deaths from Battle injuries and wounds[*]	Ratio of deaths from disease to deaths from battle injuries and wounds
Mexican War (United States)[†]	25 Apr 1846-5 Jul 1848	11,155	1,721	6.48:1
Crimean War (French)	1854-1856	70,000	7,500	9.33:1
Civil War (North)	15 Apr 1861-1 Aug 1865	199,720[‡]	138,154	1.45:1
Danish War	1864			
German		310	738	0.42:1
Danish		820	1,446	0.57:1
German War (German)	1866	5,219	4,008	1.30:1
Franco-Prussian War (German)	1870-1871	14,904	17,225	0.86:1
Russo-Turkish War	1877-1878	80,000	20,000	4.00:1
Sino-Japanese War (Japanese)	1894-1895	15,850	1,311	12.09:1
Spanish-American War	1 May 1898-31 Aug 1898	1,939	369	5.25:1
Philippine Insurrection	Feb 1899-Dec 1902	4,356	1,061	4.11:1
Boer War (British)	1899-1901	11,377	6,425	1.77:1
War in Southwest Africa (German)	1904-1907	689	802	0.86:1
Russo-Japanese War	1904-1905			
Japanese		21,802	58,257	0.37:1
Russian, less Port Arthur		18,830	23,008	0.82:1
World War I	1 Apr 1917-31 Dec 1918			
Total United States Army		51,447	50,510[§]	1.02:1
American Expeditionary Forces		16,951	50,105[§]	0.34:1
World War II	7 Dec 1941-31 Dec 1945			
Total United States Army		15,779	234,874	0.07:1
United States Army in Europe		1,779	135,576	0.01:1

[*]Includes deaths due to disease or nonbattle injury while captured or missing in action
[†]Data are derived in part from *Historical Register and Dictionary of the United States Army, 1789-1903*. Vol 2. Washington, DC: Government Printing Office;1903: 282, and are somewhat understated
[‡]Includes disease deaths among the relatively small number of volunteers remaining in federal service subsequent to 1 Aug 1865
[§]Includes gas casualties
Source: *Communicable Diseases Transmitted Chiefly through Respiratory and Alimentary Tracts*. Vol 4. In: *Preventive Medicine in World War II*. Washington, DC: US Army Medical Department, Office of the Surgeon General; 1958: 11.

World War I

The US military entered World War I better prepared from the preventive medicine standpoint than at any other time in its history. Several factors produced this situation. The medical debacle of the Spanish–American War, with typhoid fever outbreaks at many military camps causing extraordinary morbidity and mortality, focused attention on these problems and led to governmental attention in the post-war period. This resulted in Congressional legislation to reorganize the Army Medical Department and empower it by giving it direct communication with the newly established Chief of Staff and General Staff Corps.

More importantly, the emergence of medical microbiology, the growth of diagnostic laboratory capabilities, and the expanding understanding of vector-borne diseases (eg, malaria, yellow fever) and disease causation in general provided the tools needed for scientific military preventive medicine. The success of the Army Medical School and the Army Medical Research Board in Cuba, Puerto Rico, and the Philippines led to the development of an extraordinarily competent and experienced cadre of military physicians. These physicians earned national and international respect for their medical research, thus greatly enhancing the status of military medicine and demonstrating to line officers the potential contributions of military preventive medicine. New immunizations (eg, typhoid fever vaccine) and field hygiene innovations (eg, chlorination of water using the Lyster bag) from the Army Medical School were matched by the publication of outstanding manuals and textbooks of military preventive medicine by Munson,[14] Ashburn,[15] Havard,[16] Vedder,[17] and Dunham.[18]

Against this background, most of the US Army had developed significant field experience during annual maneuvers beginning in 1910 and culminating in the 1916 expedition into Mexico led by General Pershing. Troop hygiene and health were excellent during the latter part of this period due to the experience gained by commanders and their supporting medical officers. So when the United States entered the war in 1917, the operational experience of the past 7 years and the bioscientific and medical knowledge base developed over the preceding 3 decades produced a highly competent and ready force. The commanders who went to Europe shared General Pershing's view of the commander's responsibility for troop health and the essential role of sound medical advice and technical expertise. The Medical Department benefited not only from the field experience and intimate staff relationships of the preceding 7 years but also from the experiences of allied British and French forces during the first 3 years of the war in Europe.

General Pershing set the tone for his expeditionary force by placing his chief surgeon and a small group of medical officers on his general staff. This intimate involvement of medical officers in all staff actions and operational planning provided the essential foundation for command responsibility and support for preventive medicine activities throughout the American Expeditionary Forces. Sanitary inspections by medical officers, first established by Surgeon General Lovell in 1818 and vigorously employed by Surgeon General Hammond in the Civil War, were reintroduced. The model for activities of sanitary inspectors had been developed during field exercises and the expedition into Mexico. It was now implemented throughout the US Army in the United States and Europe with exceptional results—the health of the American Expeditionary Forces was as good as that of troops in the United States.

Perhaps the most important outcome of this period was the official recognition that the activities of military preventive medicine extend well beyond the limits of the Medical Department and are, in fact, concerned with the administration of the whole Army. This valuable lesson had been and continues to be difficult to learn and retain when the mission of military medicine seems to focus solely on the hospital-based care of sick troops and combat casualties. Military physicians are often the first to forget this fundamental point and thus contribute to the misunderstanding and ignorance of their line officer colleagues.

Between the World Wars

The 2 decades preceding World War II saw enormous advances in microbiology and medical science in general. Many of these emanated from ongoing research at the Army Medical School and the overseas medical research boards. Perhaps more important was the broadening of epidemiology as a discipline in both civilian and military preventive medicine. From focusing almost solely on infectious disease and its causative agents, epidemiology expanded to encompass noncommunicable diseases, with the recognition that host, environmental, occupational, cultural, and social factors are influential elements in health and disease. This broadened scope fit the increasingly broad scope of military operations and supporting activities as new technologies were rapidly introduced into the servicemembers' environment.

Preventive medicine and public health educational resources, such as schools, courses, and institutes, increased rapidly during this period. Impressive also was the publication of many notable textbooks for practitioners of preventive medicine and the revisions of military preventive medicine texts. Atabrine was introduced and tested as a quinine substitute for prophylaxis and treatment of malaria. During this same time, sulforamides were shown to cure and prevent many bacterial infections, thus expanding the concept of chemoprophylaxis.

World War II

The volumes published by the Army Medical Department covering preventive medicine in World War II are a rich source of information on the fundamental principles of military preventive medicine, which endure in spite of changes in the biomedical sciences. They should be read by anyone seeking to become or claiming to be a specialist in military preventive medicine. From them come two major examples of command authority and preventive medicine—one successful and one not.

The successful example involves the control of malaria in the Pacific theater of operations. Malaria was incapacitating the US Army with attack rates of 1,781 per 1,000 on Guadalcanal and 4,000 per 1,000 at Milne Bay. This led General MacArthur to comment "This will be a long war if for every division facing the enemy I must count on a second division in hospital with malaria and a third division convalescing...."[19(p2)] General MacArthur recognized not only the threat to his forces but also the need to change the attitude of his subordinate commanders. This attitude was exemplified by a general officer with 40% of his troops incapacitated with malaria who said playing with mosquitoes in wartime was a waste of time while he was busy preparing to fight. MacArthur grasped the basic concepts: (a) command from highest to lowest levels must be educated about malaria and its prevention and understand that command authority must be used to enforce malaria discipline; (b) there must be a highly trained and competent malaria control organization operating with the full support and authority of the chain of command; and (c) malaria control supplies, equipment, and personnel must have a high priority for transportation ordered by the command. MacArthur realized that technical competence and advice of medical specialists was

essential, but command must recognize its responsibility and use its authority to accomplish this mission. The medical establishment acting alone will fail. Recognition and application of these principles greatly reduced the strategic medical threat from malaria in this theater.

Cold injury has been recognized as a substantial threat to troops, at least since the time of Napoleon, and was even described in the armies of Alexander the Great. The World War II volume entitled *Cold Injury—Ground Type*[20] provides lasting lessons on this strategic medical threat, successful prevention strategies, and painful examples of failures such as occurred during the winter of 1944–1945 in Western Europe. The threat had been recognized by operational and medical staffs in 1943, but plans for educating and training commanders and troops in foot care were not implemented. While the planners recognized that cold weather uniforms and footwear were essential to prevent a disaster, only inadequate amounts of marginally acceptable items were procured.

The price paid was 90,000 cold injury casualties, with a preponderance among combat infantrymen—the equivalent of losing seven divisions of riflemen at a time when no replacements were available. General Patton described the situation: "The most serious menace confronting us today is not the German Army, which we have practically destroyed, but the weather which, if we do not exert ourselves, may well destroy us through the incidence of trench foot."[20(p168)]

The knowledge was available and the threat had been recognized, but neither the commanders nor their staffs had been energized. This was partially due to a failure in the relationships between commanders and their Chief Surgeons and medical staffs. It was also attributable to the attitude engendered by the seeming total collapse of the German forces and the rapid Allied advances that raised hopes for a German surrender and an end to the war before cold weather arrived. General Bradley wrote after the war that in September he responded to a crisis in supply and transport by deliberately bypassing winter clothing in favor of ammunition and gasoline.[21] The command gambled and lost. There is no evidence that the medical staff estimated or presented the possible casualty numbers before this apparently uncalculated risk was taken.

The Korean War

The Korean War is notable in that medical officers recognized the threats posed by infectious disease, such as malaria, and the environmental extremes of the Korean winters. Drawing on the recent lessons of World War II, malaria discipline was successful, with commanders actively involved at all levels.

In contrast, the first year in Korea saw a repetition of command ignoring medical advice about cold injury, leading to devastating effects on improperly clothed, shod, and trained troops.[22] After the experience of the first chaotic year, the military made significant improvements in the prevention of cold injury in such areas as command and medical planning training, provision of appropriate uniforms, and enforcement of foot care down to the individual level. In spite of these advances, the tactical situation frequently overcame the best prevention efforts, again taking a toll primarily on riflemen in forward exposed areas.

The Vietnam War

During the 12 years between Korea and the introduction of large US units into the Republic of South Vietnam in 1965, many experienced preventive medicine officers left active duty, taking with them hard-earned expertise. In addition, chloroquine-resistant falciparum malaria emerged, requiring renewed attention to basic malaria discipline. Prophylaxis now required chloroquine–primaquine on a weekly basis and Dapsone taken daily, thus increasing the requirement for command supervision of compliance. Preventive medicine assets supported command supervision through urine testing of randomly selected field units to confirm the presence of prophylactic drug metabolites.[23]

A highly significant example of command attention to preserving the health of soldiers can be found in the experience of the 9th Infantry Division commanded by Major General Julian Ewell. Operating in the inundated Mekong Delta area, troops were continuously exposed to environmental conditions leading to bacterial and fungal skin infections and warm-water immersion foot. General Ewell documented staggering losses from these conditions among his riflemen—in some cases, reducing company strength by 50%.[24]

COL Alfred Allen in *Skin Diseases in Vietnam, 1965–72*[25] documents the comprehensive preventive medicine program of field research, field surveillance, training, and education brought to bear in response to Ewell's request for assistance. Appropriate prophylaxis and treatment helped, but the major impact was achieved by gathering and presenting data related to the most significant problem—warm-water immersion foot. The data showed that prevention depended on restricting field operations to 48 hours of troop exposure, followed by a 24-hour drying period. General Ewell implemented this policy through a command directive, holding subordinate commanders at each level responsible for its vigorous implementation. In response, the rates of "paddy foot" and troop losses declined significantly.

Operations Desert Shield and Desert Storm

The deployment of US Central Command forces to the Saudi Arabian desert under the command of General Norman Schwarzkopf raised the specter of previous military operations in the same locale, which were associated with large servicemember losses because of disease and environmental conditions.[26] Schwarzkopf's force sustained the lowest disease and nonbattle injury rates seen in US forces during the 20th century (Figure 1-3).

This success was due in considerable measure to the willingness of commanders at all levels to include in their deployment and campaign plans the important medical threats and command policies based on sound medical advice to control their impact. Well-prepared military preventive medicine officers established essential surveillance activities down to the battalion level to monitor preventable disease. This allowed them to respond rapidly with appropriate recommendations and essential interventions to control identified breakdowns and outbreaks.

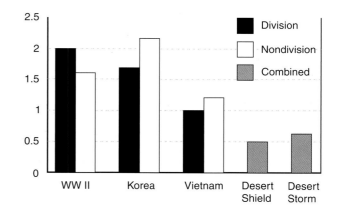

Fig. 1-3. Disease and nonbattle injury rates in World War II, Korea, Vietnam, Desert Shield, and Desert Storm, showing the particularly low rates in Operations Desert Shield and Storm (number of hospital admissions/1,000 soldiers/d). Source: Briefing slides, Office of the Surgeon General, US Army, Washington, DC, 1992.

The success of these activities led to the Joint Chiefs of Staff requirement that surveillance for preventable disease at the small-unit level be implemented in all future deployments of US forces.[27] Preventive medicine activities during the subsequent deployment of US forces to Somalia followed this model of command recognition of responsibility for preserving the health of servicemembers. The message reproduced in Figure 1-4 demonstrates the concern and attention of the Somalia Task Force commander to these issues. Again, command policies, preventive medicine advice and surveillance, and rapid investigation and intervention when outbreaks occurred successfully preserved the fighting strength.

```
ADMINISTRATIVE MESSAGE

PRIORITY

P 08I621Z DEC 92 ZYB PSN 277700S23

FM CJIF SOMALIA//J-4/MED//

TO USCINCCENT MACDILL AFB FL//CCSG
CG FIRST FSSG// G-1//              CG FIRST MARDIV//G-1//
CG THIRD MAW//G-1//               FIRST SRI GROUP//S-1//

INFO BUMED WASHINGTON DC//JJJ//   CMC WASHINGTON DC//MED//
COMMARFURPAC//G4/MED//

BT
UNCLAS      //N06200//

MSGID/GENADMIN/CG  I  MEF  G4  MED//
SUBJ/COMMAND RESPONSIBILITIES IN MAINTAINING TROOP HEALTH//
RMKS/1.    THE MEDICAL THREAT IN OPERATION PROVIDE HOPE IS
AMONG THE HIGHEST EVER FACED BY US FORCES, PROBABLY MUCH GREATER
THAN IN THE VIETNAM CONFLICT. THE PREVENTION OF FORCE DEGRAD-
ING ILLNESS IS A COMMAND RESPONSIBILITY.
2.    PREVENTIVE MEDICINE PERSONNEL HAVE PROVIDED VERY SPECIFIC
RECOMMENDATIONS WHICH WILL PRESERVE COMBAT READINESS BY KEEP-
ING PERSONNEL HEALTHY. IT IS UP TO INDIVIDUAL COMMANDERS TO
IMPLEMENT THESE RECOMMENDATIONS IN THE MOST AGGRESSIVE MANNER.
3.    SPECIFICALLY, UNIT COMMANDERS ARE RESPONSIBLE TO INSURE
THE FOLLOWING:
   A.    ALL PERSONNEL ARE TO EXERCISE COMPLETE MALARIA AND
MOSQUITO DISCIPLINE, INCLUDING KEEPING SLEEVES DOWN AT ALL
TIMES, PROPER USE OF DEET INSECT REPELLENT ON ALL EXPOSED SKIN,
AND THE FULLEST USE OF BEDNETS. PERMETHRINE SPRAY SHOULD BE
ISSUED, AND ALL UNIFORMS AND BEDNETS SHOULD BE TREATED.
   B.    MALARIA MEDICATION WILL BE TAKEN AS PRESCRIBED, AND
MONITORED BY UNIT COMMAND STRUCTURE. IF MEFLOQUINE IS USED, IT
WILL BE TAKEN ON SUNDAYS BY ALL UNITS. IF DOXYCYLINE IS USED,
IT WILL BE TAKEN WITH THE MORNING MEAL BY ALL UNITS. ACCOUNT-
ABILITY IS REQUIRED.
   C.    HAND WASHING AFTER USE OF LATRINE AND BEFORE MEALS
IS REQUIRED. UNIT LEADERS WILL INSURE THAT ALL TROOPS UNDER-
STAND AND COMPLY WITH THIS REQUIREMENT. HAND-WASHING STATIONS
ARE TO BE PROVIDED AT THE EARLIEST POSSIBLE TIME. WHEN CHOW
HALLS ARE ESTABLISHED, NO TROOP WILL BE PERMITTED TO ENTER
WITHOUT WASHING HANDS. ENFORCEMENT IS REQUIRED.
   D.    ABSOLUTELY NO FOOD, WATER, OR ICE WILL BE CONSUMED
FROM THE LOCAL ECONOMY. FAILURE TO COMPLY WITH THIS RESTRICTION
CARRIES THE HIGH POTENTIAL OF EPIDEMIC DIARRHEA AND HEPATITIS.
UNIT COMMANDERS SHOULD INSURE THAT ALL TROOPS UNDERSTAND THE
TREMENDOUS THREAT ASSOCIATED WITH EATING FROM THE ECONOMY.
```

(**Fig. 1-4** *continues*)

```
      E.   COMMANDERS WILL INSURE THAT HUMAN WASTE IS HANDLED
IN STRICT ACCORDANCE WITH PREVENTIVE MEDICINE RECOMMENDATIONS,
SPECIFICALLY, LATRINES ARE TO BE CONSTRUCTED AND MAINTAINED IN
FLY-PROOF CONDITION, TO PREVENT FLY CONTACT WITH HUMAN FECES
AND SUBSEQUENT DIARRHEA EPIDEMICS
      F.   WHEN CHOW HALLS ARE ESTABLISHED, THEY ARE TO BE
OPERATED IN FULL ACCORDANCE WITH PREVENTIVE MEDICINE RECOMMEN-
DATIONS. AN IMPROPERLY RUN CHOW HALL CAN RESULT IN EPIDEMIC
DIARRHEA. THE PRIORITY ON "GETTING A HOT MEAL TO THE TROOP"
SHOULD AT NO TIME OVERRIDE PROPER PROCEDURES IN CHOW PREPARA-
TION. INATTENTION IN THIS AREA HAS RESULTED IN MASSIVE EPI-
DEMIC DIARRHEA IN PAST OPERATIONS.
      G.   COMMANDERS WILL INSURE THAT HEAT INJURIES ARE PRE-
VENTED BY ALLOWING A PERIOD OF ACCLIMATIZATION, ADJUSTING WORK
SCHEDULES TO AVOID THE HOTTEST PARTS OF THE DAY, AND ENFORCING
AGGRESSIVE WATER DRINKING (UP TO 1 CANTEEN PER HOUR).
      H.   HIV AND AIDS ARE EXTREMELY COMMON IN EAST AFRICA,
INCLUDING SOMALIA. PROSTITUTES ARE REPORTED TO BE 50% OR MORE
HIV INFECTED. COMMAND CLIMATE SHOULD ACTIVELY DISCOURAGE ANY
SEXUAL CONTACT WITH LOCAL PERSONNEL THROUGH POSITIVE LEADER-
SHIP AND EDUCATION.
4.    PREVENTIVE MEDICINE PERSONNEL ARE AVAILABLE FOR UNIT
TRAINING. ALL TROOPS ARE TO BE THOROUGHLY BRIEFED AS EARLY AS
POSSIBLE IN THE EXERCISE, AND RE-BRIEFED AS NEEDED.
5.    DISEASE AND INJURY TREND WILL BE AGGRESSIVELY MONITORED
THEATER-WIDE TO IDENTIFY PROBLEMS IMMEDIATELY AND TAKE CORREC-
TIVE ACTION. ACCURATE DISEASE REPORTING IS A HIGH INTEREST
ITEM.
B/
```

Fig. 1-4. The text of the Joint Task Force Somalia commander's administrative message outlining the responsibilities of unit commanders in maintaining their troops' health. Source: Commander Joint Task Force Somalia. *Command Responsibilities in Maintaining Troop Health*. Washington, DC: US Central Command; December 1992.

THE PREVENTIVE MEDICINE CONCEPT FOR COMMANDERS

The Commander's Principal Staff and Operational Planning

The preceding review presents a deceptively simple picture that intentionally ignores the major obstacles to preventive medicine and command interaction. It is imperative to identify these issues, which originate both from commanders and their staffs and from the military preventive medicine personnel advising and supporting them.

Prevention activities lack the glamour and immediacy of saving the lives of combat casualties. Prevention is focused on potential threats, requires considerable investment of resources (eg, money, personnel, supplies, equipment, time), and involves modifications of behavior by units and individuals. And if prevention is successful, nothing happens. In this situation, the command emphasis required for successful prevention programs may easily be replaced by command resistance.

Commanders and their principal staff officers—chief of staff, G/J1 Personnel, G/J2 Intelligence, G/J3 Operations, G/J4 Logistics—may be ignorant of the historical impact of medical threats. They may not have been exposed earlier in their careers to military medical officers with competence in and understanding of military preventive medicine. Common attitudes of staff are reflected in the statements "If it ain't broke, don't fix it" and "Come back when there is a clear need or problem, Doc." Of course by the time it is "broke" or the need is clear, it is too late for prevention. Other attitudes focus on the dangers of death or dismemberment in combat and ridicule efforts to maintain health and prevent disease. Another negative attitude is reflected in using operational security (OPSEC or the "need to know") considerations to avoid sharing essential mission information and intelligence with medical staff sections. Commanders foster these attitudes and exacerbate the obstacles to successful preventive medicine programs if they do not provide emphasis and support for these activities through both personal and corporate behavior.

Commanders can make preventive medicine a part of their daily personal behavior and a consistently high-ranked item on the list of things they vigorously check on. From a corporate standpoint, commanders can make clear to their senior staff and subordinate commanders the importance they attach to having preventive medicine involvement in all aspects of operational planning and mission execution. The commander's model should include centralized planning and decentralized execution, with priority for resources given to combat units. Subordinate commanders must be given adequate resources so they can make prevention work. Good data gathering systems are required to enable the commander to constantly check up on this area and to have a basis for rewarding success and punishing failure.

As important as these command-centered problems are the barriers to successful preventive medicine from within the medical staff. Preventive medicine is the reverse of the usual clinical medicine paradigm where the individual patient goes or is taken to the provider of care. In preventive medicine, the provider and the intervention must go to the "patient," who in this case is the military unit. Some medical personnel, while they have excellent clinical skills, have only the most rudimentary understanding of preventive medicine in general and of military preventive medicine in particular. This lack of understanding may be matched by a similarly abysmal lack of knowledge of or experience in nonmedical military matters, such as military planning, the operational environment, and the functioning of military organizations.

Medical staff sections must establish strong relationships with all nonmedical principal staff well before planning for a major military operation starts. The medical personnel must be able to recognize the essential elements of the operational plan options being developed. They can then provide information early in the planning process regarding possible medical threats and estimates of their impact on the force and mission accomplishment. Military preventive medicine officers must participate in the planning process by proactively coordinating with the Personnel, Intelligence, Operations, and Logistics staff sections; they must not remain confined with the Medical Staff section. They must bring to bear knowledge of the history of successes and failures in military preventive medicine and a detailed technical knowledge of all the elements of the multi-disciplinary preventive medicine team.

The point must be clearly made that no war has been won because one side had the superior medical treatment and casualty care capability, but throughout military history, battles and entire campaigns have been lost because of the impact of preventable disease. Preventive medicine also has a role in reducing other types of medical threats. Of equal importance is the education of commanders and staff officers, both nonmedical and medical, that preventive medicine plays a major, officially recognized role in health hazard assessment of weapons systems; transportation platforms; toxicity of fuels, propellants, and obscurants; and changes in operational doctrine that cause potential decrements in servicemember performance (eg, continuous operations). A similar role for preventive medicine is also defined within force protection programs, which have become a major focus during post–Cold War military deployments and operations.

Recognition of the staff and command context within which preventive medicine activities affect a specific operational plan is as important as skill in and technical knowledge of preventive medicine and military operational planning. During a recent multinational military exercise in the United States, the medical threat from the tick vector of Lyme disease was identified. One allied force ordered permethrin for treating field uniforms after arrival in the United States. The G4 (Logistics) executed the order, which was delivered exactly on time and rapidly distributed to the allied force. However, there had been no coordination with the G3 (Operations) and G1 (Personnel) staff sections, and thus no time was allowed in the exercise schedule for training troops in the use of permethrin, nor was there time or a suitable area for application. Very few troops accomplished even partial treatment of one of their three field uniforms. A high percentage of the force sustained tick bites, and more than 24 cases of Lyme disease were diagnosed.[28] Even with recognition of the threat and appropriate procurement and distribution, prevention may fail if the actual implementation is not completely coordinated with each staff section, integrated into the operational plan, and understood by commanders and leaders at all levels.

The Medical Threat Estimate

The fundamental planning tool for medical staffs in general and preventive medicine officers in particular is the medical threat estimate. Appropriate analysis and development of the medical threat estimate provide the basis for interaction with the principle staff sections as the operational plan is developed.

All staff planning activity, including medical, fundamentally starts with the commander's mission statement and the operational options being considered by the staff to accomplish this mission. For each option considered, there should be an estimate of supportability from each staff section. For the medical staff, this begins with the generic elements of the medical threat, as documented in Joint Publication 4-02, *Doctrine for Health Service Support in Joint Operations, 1994*.[29] These elements, as shown in Exhibit 1-1, are used in making an assessment of medical threats that potentially apply to the specific operational setting and are a composite of ongoing or potential enemy action and environmental conditions that could reduce the operational effectiveness of military units.

The medical threat assessment is then applied to each of the operational planning options under consideration. An estimate is made of the potential threat to the health of the force and mission accomplishment: first, if policies and programs are not implemented for maximum reduction and control of these threats and, second, if policies and programs are given appropriate resources, integrated into the operational plan, and supported by command at all levels. This medical threat estimate must be developed in close consultation with each principle staff section, and cost-benefit estimates should be made before the estimate is presented to command as part of the decision package. This process is outlined in Exhibit 1-2.

An essential element of both the medical threat assessment and the medical threat estimate is the absolute requirement for consistent and accurate medical reporting, sick-call surveillance, and rapid investigation of any breakdowns in program execution or outbreaks of disease. All of this must be accomplished within all units of the command, reaching down to the battalion or company level. Routine hospital reports will not accomplish this goal.

Only by having these tools at hand can the commander make informed choices during the planning process based on a sound estimate of the medical threats, the policies and programs to counter the threats, and the data gathering requirements for monitoring and rewarding success and identifying and correcting failure.

EXHIBIT 1-1

THE MEDICAL THREAT: GENERIC ELEMENTS TO CONSIDER IN REGULAR OPERATIONS AND OPERATIONS OTHER THAN WAR

Elements of Regular Military Operations

- Infectious disease
- Extremes of environment
- Conventional munitions
- Biological weapons
- Chemical weapons
- Directed energy weapons
- Blast effect weapons
- Flame and incendiary weapons
- Mobilization, deployment, and battle stress
- Nuclear weapons

Elements of Operations Other Than War

- Medical threats to the indigenous population
- General stability of the country (eg, social, political, economic, security), within which the operation is conducted
- Specific type of military operation
- Scenarios for use of force
- Application of Geneva Convention protection
- Logistical support, host-nation infrastructure, and other support considerations

Adapted from: *Doctrine for Health Service Support in Joint Operations.* Joint Staff: Washington, DC; 15 November 1994: A-1 through A-7. Joint Publication 4-02.

EXHIBIT 1-2

THE MEDICAL THREAT ESTIMATE PROCESS

---

1. Identify the medical threat categories that apply to the military operation being planned.

2. Assess within these medical threat categories, the specific threats that may be encountered. Rank these within each threat category (eg, disease, environmental) by probable time of occurrence (before, early in, during, or after deployment). This results in a prioritized medical threat assessment.

3. Apply this medical threat assessment to each of the operational planning options. Estimate the potential impact on the force and mission accomplishment in both the absence and presence of appropriate command policies, programs, and resource commitments for threat reduction. This is the medical threat estimate; it provides the command with decision-making information regarding operational plan options and costs for threat reduction.

Source: *Medical Threat Estimate*. Bethesda, Md: Department of Military and Emergency Medicine and Department of Preventive Medicine and Biometrics, Uniformed Services University of the Health Sciences; 1995. PMO580.

SUMMARY

The core functions of military preventive medicine have remained constant from the book of Leviticus to the present. So too has the inescapable relationship between preventive medicine and command authority. Obstacles exist to the successful development of these relationships, from both the nonmedical and the medical points of view, but they can be overcome. The medical threat estimate can be used as a tool and a process for integrating preventive medicine into the military planning process. This chapter and the rest of this text are dedicated to assisting military preventive medicine officers in their efforts to support the commanders, who are responsible for the health of their commands, by providing them the means to gain command of health.

REFERENCES

1. Legters LJ, Llewellyn CH. Military medicine. In: Last JM, Wallace FB, eds. *Maxcy-Rosenau-Last Public Health and Preventive Medicine*. 13th ed. Norwalk, Conn: Appleton & Lange; 1992: Chap 71.

2. Bayne-Jones S. *The Evolution of Preventive Medicine in the United States Army, 1607–1939*. Washington, DC: Office of the Surgeon General, Department of the Army; 1968.

3. Pringle J. *Observations on the Diseases of the Army in Camp and Garrison*. London: A. Millar, D. Wilson, T. Payne;1752.

4. Brocklesby R. *Oeconomical and Medical Observations, in Two Parts, from the Year 1758 to the Year 1763, Inclusive. Tending to the Improvement of Military Hospitals and to the Cure of Camp Diseases Incident to Soldiers*. London: T. Becket and P.A. DeHoudt; 1764.

5. Munro D. *An Account of the Diseases Which Were Most Frequent in the British Military Hospitals in Germany from 1761 to 1763*. London: A. Millar, D. Wilson, T. Durham, and T. Payne; 1764.

6. Rush B. *Directions for Preserving the Health of Soldiers. Recommended to the Consideration of the Officers of the Army of the United States. Published by Order of the Board of War*. Lancaster: John Dunlap; 1778.

7. Tilton J. *Economical Observations on Military Hospitals; and the Prevention and Cure of Diseases Incident to an Army*. Wilmington, Del: J. Wilson; 1813.

8. Wood P. *Moses, the Founder of Preventive Medicine*. New York: The Macmillan Co; 1920.

9. Garrison FH. *Notes on the History of Military Medicine*. Washington, DC: Association of Military Surgeons, 1922. Reprinted from: *Mil Surg*. 1921–1922, Vols 49–51.

10. van Swietan G. *A Short Account of the Most Common Diseases Incident to Armies.* 2nd ed. London: T. Becket and P.A. DeHonde; 1767.

11. Jones J. *Plain Concise Practical Remarks on the Treatment of Wounds and Fracture.* Philadelphia: R. Bell; 1776.

12. von Steuben F. *US Inspector General's Office: Regulations for the Order and Discipline of the Troops of the United States.* Part I. Philadelphia: Stuver and Cest; 1779.

13. Duncan LC. The comparative mortality of disease and battle casualties in the historic wars of the world. *J Mil Serv Inst US.* 1914;54:140–177.

14. Munson EL. *The Theory and Practice of Military Hygiene.* New York: William Wood and Co; 1901.

15. Ashburn PM. *The Elements of Military Hygiene: Especially Arranged for Officers and Men of the Line.* 2nd ed. Boston: Houghton Mifflin Co; 1915.

16. Havard V. *Manual of Military Hygiene for the Military Services of the United States.* New York: William Wood and Co; 1917.

17. Vedder EB. *Sanitation for Medical Officers. Medical War Manual No. 1. Authorized by the Secretary of War and Under the Supervision of the Surgeon-General and the Council of National Defense.* 2nd ed. Philadelphia: Lea & Febiger; 1918.

18. Dunham GC. *Military Preventive Medicine.* 3rd ed. Carlisle Barracks, Penn: Medical Field Service School; 1938.

19. Hoff EC, ed. *Communicable Diseases: Malaria.* Vol 6. In: *Preventive Medicine in World War II.* Washington, DC: Office of the Surgeon General, Department of the Army; 1963.

20. Whayne TF, DeBakey ME. *Cold Injury, Ground Type.* Washington, DC: Office of the Surgeon General, Department of the Army; 1958.

21. Bradley ON. *A Soldier's Story.* New York: Henry Holland Co; 1951.

22. Cowdrey AE. *The Medic's War.* In: *United States Army in the Korean War.* Washington, DC: Center of Military History, US Army; 1987.

23. Neel S. *Medical Support of the U.S. Army in Vietnam 1965–1970.* In: *Vietnam Studies.* Washington, DC: Center of Military History, Department of the Army; 1973.

24. Ewell JJ, Hunt IA. *Sharpening the Combat Edge.* In: *Vietnam Studies.* Washington, DC: Center of Military History, Department of the Army; 1974.

25. Allen AM. *Skin Diseases in Vietnam, 1965–72.* Vol 1. In: *Internal Medicine in Vietnam.* Washington, DC: Office of the Surgeon General and Center of Military History, US Army; 1977.

26. Scales RH. *Certain Victory. The U.S. Army in the Gulf War.* Brassey's: Washington, DC; 1994: 80, 121.

27. Department of Defense. *Joint Medical Surveillance.* Washington, DC: DoD; 1997. DoD Directive 6490.2.

28. Royal Army Medical Corps Preventive Medicine presentation. Presented at: Royal Society of Medicine United Services Section Meeting; 1996; London.

29. Joint Chiefs of Staff. *Doctrine for Health Service Support in Joint Operations.* Joint Staff: Washington, DC; 15 November 1994. Joint Publication 4-02.

Chapter 2

THE HISTORICAL IMPACT OF PREVENTIVE MEDICINE IN WAR

BENJAMIN G. WITHERS, MD, MPH; AND STEPHEN C. CRAIG, DO, MTM&H

B. G. Withers; Colonel, Medical Corps, US Army; Command Surgeon, US Army Materiel Command, 5001 Eisenhower Ave., Alexandria VA 22333-0001

S. C. Craig; Colonel, Medical Corps, US Army; Chief, Preventive Medicine Service, Keller Army Community Hospital, West Point, NY 10996

INTRODUCTION

A corps of Medical officers was not established solely for the purpose of attending the wounded and sick; the proper treatment of these sufferers is certainly a matter of very great importance, and is an imperative duty, but the labors of Medical officers cover a more extended field. The *leading idea*, which should be constantly kept in view, is to strengthen the hands of the Commanding General by keeping his army in the most vigorous health, thus rendering it, in the highest degree, efficient for enduring fatigue and privation, and for fighting.[1p100] [emphasis added]

> —*Jonathan Letterman, 1866*
> *Medical Director, Army of the Potomac*

Jonathan Letterman was best known for his operational and administrative contributions, such as his system of field hospitals and his reorganization of medical services.[2,3] Yet, in his mind, the *leading idea*, as he put it, was prevention.

Letterman's emphasis was (and is) appropriate on at least two counts. First, disease and nonbattle injury (DNBI) historically caused more deaths than battle injury (BI) until World War II, with few exceptions.[4,5] Table 2-1 illustrates this point using US Army war experience. Note that this relationship became less pronounced with time until, during World War II, BI deaths exceeded DNBI deaths. This crossover from DNBI to BI, resulting largely from advances in both preventive and curative medicine,[6] does not mean that DNBI has become less of a concern. When one studies morbidity (by considering hospital admissions) as opposed to mortality, it is clear that DNBI causes more combat ineffectiveness than BI, even during periods of sustained fighting (Figure 2-1). From 1941 to 1945, 95% of all Army admissions (16,941,081 of 17,664,641) were due to DNBI. During the Korean War, DNBI accounted for 82% of admissions (365,375 of 443,163, includes those hospitalized and excused from duty).[4] The second point in support of Letterman's emphasis is that DNBI is largely preventable, whereas BI is less amenable to prevention.

TABLE 2-1

US ARMY DEATHS FROM DISEASE AND NONBATTLE INJURY VS BATTLE INJURY, MEXICAN WAR THROUGH PERSIAN GULF WAR.[*]

War	Number Serving[†]	BI	DNBI	DNBI:BI
Mexican War[‡§]	78,718	1,733	11,550	6.7
Civil War (Union)[§]	2,128,948	138,154	221,374	1.6
Spanish American War[§]	280,564	369	2,061	5.6
World War I	4,057,101	50,510	55,868	1.1
World War II	11,260,000	234,874	83,400	0.35
Korean War	2,834,000	27,709	2,452	0.09
Vietnam War	4,368,000	30,922	7,273	0.24
Persian Gulf War[¥]	246,682	98	105	1.1

[*]Historically, DNBI has caused more deaths than BI. This relationship became less pronounced with time. Since World War II, BI deaths have generally exceeded DNBI deaths.
[†]Total number in Army during conflict (See notes for Mexican and Persian Gulf Wars.)
[‡]Predominately Army force; contains unknown number of sailors and Marines
[§]Based on incomplete records
[¥]Includes only Army troops deployed on Operation Desert Storm
BI: battle injuries
DNBI: disease and nonbattle injuries
Sources: (1) *The World Almanac 1996.* Mahwah, NJ: World Almanac Books, Funk & Wagnalls Corporation; 1996: 166. (2) Data from the Department of Defense, Directorate for Information, Operations, and Reports, Statistical Information Analysis Division, Washington, DC, July 1997. Prepared by Judith Bowles.

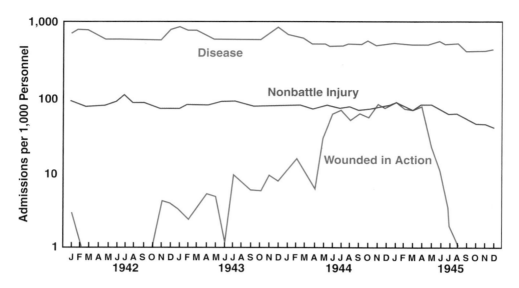

Fig. 2-1. US Army hospital admissions by type, 1942–1945. These data, which indicate *morbidity* as opposed to *mortality*, reveal that DNBI causes significant combat ineffectiveness, even during periods of sustained fighting. Footnote: Rates expressed as admissions per 1,000 average strength per year. Adapted from: Reister FA, ed. *Medical Statistics in World War II.* Washington, DC: Office of The Surgeon General, US Department of the Army; 1975: page facing title page. Prepared by Judith Bowles.

Throughout history, some commanders have taken care to reduce DNBI while others have not. This chapter presents historical examples that illustrate the impact of preventive medicine on warfighting. The goal is to instill in medical and line officers alike an appreciation of the critical importance of preventive medicine efforts during war.

These eight vignettes—four that demonstrate the problems associated with ignoring preventive medicine and four that illustrate the benefits of prevention—cover a variety of threats: environmental, communicable, and vector-borne. All are drawn from the 20th century to take advantage of its better science, data, and reporting.

THE COSTS OF IGNORING PREVENTIVE MEDICINE PRINCIPLES

Typhoid Fever in British Troops During the Second Boer War

Setting

Field Marshall Lord Frederick Roberts took command of British forces in South Africa (Figure 2-2) in January 1900 in an effort to reverse Britain's fortunes in the field and defeat the Boers.[7] To relieve the sieges of Ladysmith, Kimberley, and Mafeking and to stop rebellion in the Cape Colony, Roberts planned to seize the republican capitals of Bloemfontein, in the Orange Free State, and Praetoria, in the Transvaal.[8] Between 11 February and 13 March, Roberts' forces marched east from the Western Railway Station on the Modder River, heading for Bloemfontein. This drive, along with General Sir Redvers Bullers' push against Lady-

smith in Natal, caused the Boers to retreat, giving up Ladysmith, Kimberley, and Bloemfontein. Hopes ran high that the war would end quickly.[7] Unfortunately, the British bivouacked downstream when they surrounded the typhoid-infected Boer garrison at Paardeberg. The British force's sole source of water, the Modder River, was saturated with Boer refuse.[9] When Roberts seized Bloemfontein, his main supply line was 750 miles long. His march to the capital had exhausted his supply of rations, horses, and equipment of all kinds. And while the British forces awaited supplies, typhoid fever joined their ranks.[7]

Health Issues

Field Marshall Roberts encountered four major health issues during his campaign: troop immuni-

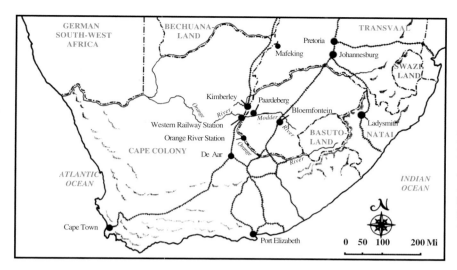

Fig. 2-2. South Africa, circa 1900. Rail lines are shown by hatched solid lines. Field Marshal Lord Roberts began his flank march to Bloemfontein from Western Railway Station on 11 February 1900 with an army corps of 40,000 men and 100 guns. By the time he reached the Free State capital, his troops were weary, poorly supplied, and becoming ill with typhoid fever. Adapted with permission from: Pagaard S. Disease and the British Army in South Africa, 1899–1900. *Mil Affairs.* 1986;Apr:71.

zation, sanitation measures, water supply and sanitation, and general medical support (Figures 2-3 and 2-4). Each was mishandled and compounded the effects of the other three.

Typhoid fever was a recognized threat to soldiers in the tropics before the South African deployment.[9] Sir Almroth Wright's anti–typhoid fever inoculation appeared promising from results obtained from troops in India and Egypt,[10,11] but vaccine side effects and uncertain efficacy precluded compulsory inoculation of the army.[11] Voluntary inoculation was permitted by the War Office in the fall of 1897.[10] Inoculation was offered to troops en route to South Africa, but less than 5% of the total force received the vaccine.[7] Using 5% as an estimate, only 1,700 of Roberts' 34,000 soldiers were inoculated.

Field sanitation had been dismissed as a "fad" and sanitary officers as "useless"[12p529] by the Commander-in-Chief, Lord Wolseley, in 1886. Those holding this viewpoint overruled a suggestion by a member of Parliament in October 1899 to create a special sanitary commission for the South African campaign. Roberts' only guidance in field sanitation came from the meager training his medical officers had received.[9]

Roberts was handicapped from the beginning of the campaign by his inability to supply his army with enough clean drinking water. There were insufficient numbers of the standard wooden barrel water carts, and their design kept them from following troops over rough terrain. In addition, the insides of these carts and individual canteens were squalid and quickly covered with mold. As one colonel reported later: "Probably nothing harbours germs and disease more than our present type of wooden barrel water cart."[7p242]

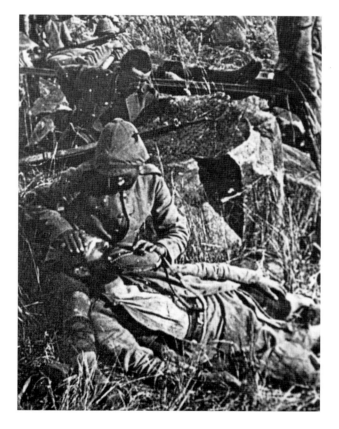

Fig. 2-3. British soldiers receiving first aid, South Africa, circa 1900. Command-directed water rationing proved intolerable to soldiers in the South African heat. Many soldiers filled their water bottles directly from the typhoid-laced Modder River and ignored orders to boil water before drinking. Reproduced with permission from: Pakenham T. *The Boer War.* New York: Random House, 1979: between pages 234–235. Published in Great Britain by Wiedenfeld and Nicolson.

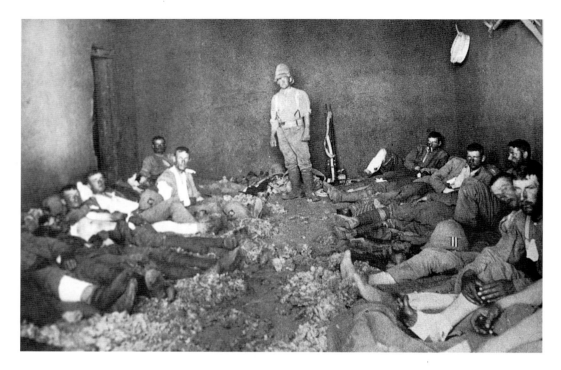

Fig. 2-4. British dressing station on the Modder River, South Africa, circa 1900. Filthy, inadequate treatment facilities such as this were the only accommodations available for many sick troops. Reproduced with permission from: Pakenham T. *The Boer War*. New York: Random House, 1979: between pages 234–235. Published in Great Britain by Wiedenfeld and Nicolson.

From the beginning of the war, the Royal Army Medical Corps had been inadequate for the needs of the large force deployed. In March 1900, there were only 800 physicians to care for the 207,000 British troops in South Africa. Roberts began his march with 10 small hospital units and ten bearer companies. These medical assets could only accommodate 4% of his army, or 1,360 patients, simultaneously.[7] After 4 weeks of campaigning and combat, medical provisions were low and, with his long supply line, it would take time to restock them.

Roberts' Actions

Roberts recognized his water problems early. He rationed his soldiers to half a water bottle per day and ordered from India 2,000 water carriers with goat and ox skin waterbags.[7,13] Standing orders to boil water existed but were often ignored because of lack of fuel and the soldiers' dislike of the "insipid taste."[7p242]

As early as February 1900, Roberts was aware of the typhoid fever problem in hospitals along the Modder River. He visited hospitals at De Aar and Orange River Station, finding them "as bad as he feared."[13p404] There were not nearly enough orderlies or nurses to deal with the situation. He re-

sponded by sending for 20 additional nurses but later changed this figure to 50 for all of South Africa. Roberts had no confidence in his Surgeon-General, W. D. Wilson, and commented that Wilson "does not seem to have any idea of what is required"[13p404]; however, Roberts did not relieve him.

Roberts' medical problems were compounded by "Boer daring" and "British military negligence"[9p74] when the enemy seized the waterworks at Sanna's Post on 1 April. Bloemfontein wells, of doubtful cleanliness at any time, were the British Army's only source of water until Sanna's Post was retaken 3 weeks later. This situation set the stage for a second typhoid fever epidemic, which erupted during the second week of May.[9]

Roberts failed to act promptly during the early stages of the initial epidemic. It was not until late April 1900 that he requested 300 orderlies and 30 doctors from England.[13]

Results

Roberts' unrealistic water ration for soldiers who required at least a quart and a half per hour, compounded by his inability to provide clean water in sufficient quantities, led to thirsty soldiers obtaining water from any source available and drinking it directly. On 23 March, 10 days after the British entered Bloemfontein, the first typhoid fever epidemic had 1,000 soldiers in the hospital. By 1 June, the second epidemic had increased this number almost 4-fold. Roberts' medical staff, supplies, and facilities were overwhelmed. Two general military hospitals, Numbers 8 and 9, and three private hospitals were not enough to treat all the cases. Public buildings, schools, and convents received the overflow.[7,14]

Doctors, nurses, and supplies were rushed to South Africa but not before word of the epidemic and its mismanagement had caught the attention of the British public and Parliament. Despite Roberts' attempt to explain the situation by stating that "...a certain amount of suffering is inseparable from the rapid advance of a large army in the enemy's country, when railway communication has been destroyed...,"[7p246] a royal commission was convened to investigate. While patients and civilian physicians proclaimed universal medical mismanagement, the officers and nurses of the Royal Army Medical Corps closed ranks, declaring that things were really not that bad. The royal commission sided with those in uniform, saying that overall the campaign

> '...has not been one where it can properly be said that the medical and hospital arrangements have broken down.... [There was] no general or widespread neglect of patients, or indifference to suffering.'[7p248] The commission's report gave only passing notice to sanitation and made no mention of immunization, concluding 'we do not consider that the great outbreak of enteric fever, or any considerable part of it, was due to preventable causes.'[9p75]

Impact

Roberts lost his momentum at Bloemfontein. Hamstrung by a long logistics train, his drive to Praetoria was delayed while he waited on supplies, horses, and men. Cape Town was reinforcing his army from one end while typhoid fever was depleting it from the other. He could not even be sure his reinforcements were healthy as they traveled the same road to Bloemfontein that he had weeks earlier.[7] When Roberts marched out of the city on 3 May bound for Praetoria, he found an enemy rejuvenated by a new leader, Christian deWet, and ready to continue the war.[7,13]

The typhoid epidemic also caused the medical world to reevaluate the efficacy of anti–typhoid fe-

ver inoculation. From June to November 1900 and February to March 1901, Dr. Dodgson compared the incidence of typhoid fever among the uninoculated and inoculated noncommissioned officers and men at General Hospital Number 8. In the 110 uninoculated, he found an incidence rate of 40/100. In the 21 inoculated, it was 24/100. Although his numbers were small and his data collected as the epidemic was burning out, Dodgson was struck by the magnitude of disease among the inoculated. He concluded that "Unless some system of prevention can be devised which will give better results than this, it is difficult to see that it can be of very great use."[15p251] Dodgson also reviewed a number of military hospitals across South Africa and determined that "there is little to distinguish the inoculated from the uninoculated cases, as regards death-rate, severity of disease, the incidence and severity of complications, the differences being so small as to easily come within the errors of observation."[15p254]

Anti–typhoid fever inoculation was discontinued after the war. It was not resumed until 1904, again on a voluntary basis, after a reevaluation of inoculation data from British forces in South Africa and repeated immunogenicity studies proved its value.[10,11]

Conclusion

Due to a lack of command emphasis on known preventive measures, the British army in South Africa suffered a medical disaster. Inadequate planning, along with inappropriate immunization and sanitation procedures, fostered two typhoid fever epidemics. The epidemics delayed the British drive to Praetoria, caused needless suffering for British soldiers, and produced a public scandal for the Royal Army Medical Corps.

British Experience with Malaria in Salonika, Greece, During World War I

Setting

Early in the 20th century, expanding colonialism and nationalism lead to tension across Europe. Alliances that were established to regain some sense of security only served to divide Europe into two armed camps: the Triple Alliance of Germany, Austria, and Italy and the Triple Entente of France, Russia, and Britain. The brittle and unstable peace was shattered with the assassination of Austro-Hungarian Archduke Ferdinand on 28 June 1914. World War I began on 4 August.[16]

By the beginning of 1915, the war had come to an operational stalemate. Opposing forces on the

Western Front had settled into fixed fortifications, linked by a maze of trenches and separated by an expanse of desolate land. The tedium of trench warfare, highlighted by artillery bombardment and the occasional battle, became the order of the day.[16] Independently, British and French strategists determined that a thrust through the Balkans, an area undefended by the Triple Alliance, would be the key to breaking the stalemate. British supporters of the plan, led by Lloyd George, Chancellor of the Exchequer, proposed an attempt to unite the Balkans against Turkey and to relieve pressure on the Russians, while at the same time aiding the Serbs struggling with Austria. A complicated series of events involving British and French military dissent, chaotic Greek politics, and Winston Churchill's plea for naval intervention in the Dardanelles delayed a decision on the Balkans and produced the debacle at Gallipoli. Finally, the Secretary of State for War, Field Marshal Lord Kitchener, and the French government reluctantly agreed to deploy troops. On 5 October 1915, elements of the British 10th Division and the French 156th Division disembarked at Salonika (now Thessaloniki), Greece.[16,17]

Health Issues

The malaria threat in the Balkans was known to the British. Arriving after the malarial season, British medical authorities had time to reconnoiter the terrain and plan an anti-malaria campaign for 1916.

The British originally camped in an area that was "a continuous series of hills and valleys"[18p227] south of Lake Langaza, east of the Galiko River, and west of Salonika along the Monastir Road. The malaria

vectors *Anopheles superpictus* and *A maculipennis* held the high and low ground, respectively. After a wet winter and spring, large numbers of these mosquitoes, well fed on the malarious population of the region, would be ready to infect nonimmune British troops with *Plasmodium vivax* and *P falciparum*.[18]

Preventive measures in the British armamentarium consisted of prophylactic medication, insect repellents, mosquito destruction, and other personal protective measures. Quinine prophylaxis was not a panacea (Figure 2-5). Insect repellent development was in its infancy; the repellents on hand were ineffective and were considered a waste of money. Therefore, the plan to reduce the mosquito threat and thereby the incidence of malaria was based on mosquito destruction and personal protective measures.[19]

In the spring of 1916, mosquito destruction was implemented by anti-malaria squads organic to corps and divisional units. The squads destroyed adult mosquitoes; destroyed ova, larvae, and pupae using disinfectants; applied oil to standing water; and drained breeding sites (Figure 2-6). Collective and personal protective measures included appropriate camp placement, screening and bed netting, and clothing (eg, head nets, gauntlet gloves, flapped shorts [Figure 2-7]).[19]

Military Actions, 1916

In late May 1916, Bulgarian infantry invaded Greece and took up positions in the Rupel Pass northeast of Lake Butkova. From this vantage point, the Bulgarians threatened the Struma Valley. French General and theater commander Maurice Sarrail

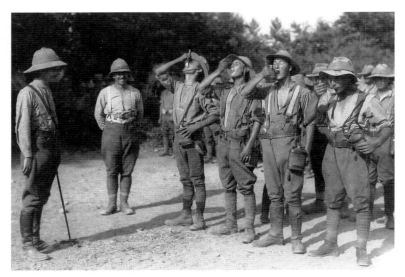

Fig. 2-5. "Quinine Parade." British soldiers in Macedonia taking quinine—under supervision—as prophylaxis against malaria, circa 1916. The use of quinine prophylaxis had been debated before the war, but no consensus on its value had been reached. Official histories state that quinine was "extensively used," but of 129 medical officers surveyed during the war, only 11% thought it had value while 75% reported it had very little or no value.
Source: McPherson WG, Horrocks WH, Beveridge WWO, eds. *Medical Services: Hygiene of the War*. Vol 2. In: *History of the Great War*. London: His Majesty's Stationery Office; 1923: 212–219. The quotation is from page 216. Photograph reproduced from: McPherson WG, Mitchell TJ, eds. *Medical Services: General History*. Vol 4. In: *History of the Great War*. London: His Majesty's Stationery Office; 1924: 106.

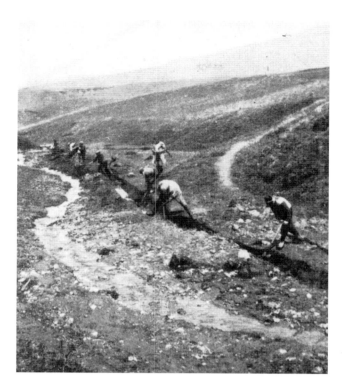

Fig. 2-6. A British work party improving drainage ditches in Macedonia, north of Salonika, during World War I in the effort to eliminate mosquito breeding sites. This was part of a larger plan to prevent malaria.
Reproduced from: McPherson WG, Horrocks WH, Beveridge WWO, eds. *Medical Services: Hygiene of the War.* Vol 2. In: *History of the Great War.* London: His Majesty's Stationery Office; 1923: 231.

directed British General George F. Milne to move his forces forward to occupy the entire Struma Valley and a line from Lake Butkova to Lake Doiran and then west to the Vardar River north of Smol.[17,18]

Sarrail was anxious for an offensive but met continued resistance to the idea from the British. In July, Sarrail informed Milne that he would attack the Bulgarians with or without British support. Milne cleared his troops from Sarrail's line of advance, moving them into the southern Struma River valley.[17]

These unanticipated moves, coming at the beginning of the malaria season, put British forces in a highly malarious area with no antimosquito preparation.[18] Working parties began mosquito destruction activities in this new area, but they "were never very satisfactory, owing to the vast amount of water and the changing courses of the streams, which constantly formed new pools."[20p288] In addition, bed nets, although recognized by General Milne to be "as important as the rifle,"[20p7] were constantly in short supply.[19] Likewise, screens for huts and tents

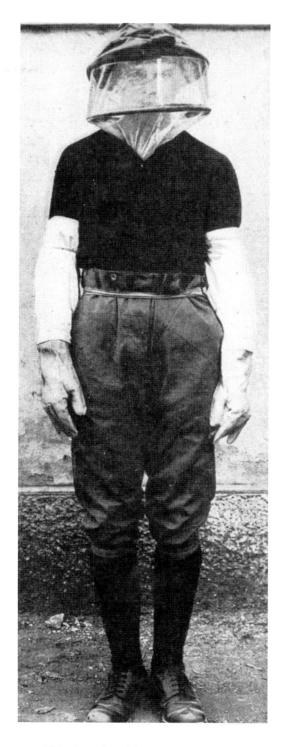

Fig. 2-7. This British soldier is wearing the complete personal protective kit issued by his command, including head net, gauntlets, and flapped shorts. The flaps folded down to cover the knees and then were inserted into puttees. Reproduced from: McPherson WG, Horrocks WH, Beveridge WWO, eds. *Medical Services: Hygiene of the War.* Vol 2. In: *History of the Great War.* London: His Majesty's Stationery Office; 1923: 220.

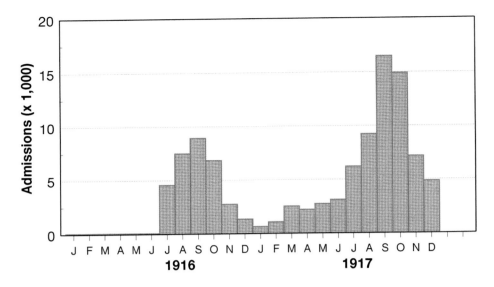

Fig. 2-8. Malaria incidence by month in the British Salonika force, 1916–1917. The rapid increase in malaria cases in 1916 came after the British had moved into positions in the Struma Valley. Relapsing and recrudescing cases are noted throughout the winter and early spring of 1916-1917. These cases provided a nidus of infection for the following year and contributed to the greater incidence of malaria in the late summer of 1917. Adapted from data on pages 108-109 in: McPherson WG, Mitchell TJ, eds. *Medical Services: General History.* Vol 4. In: *History of the Great War.* London: His Majesty's Stationery Office; 1924: 108-109. Prepared by Judith Bowles.

were pushed to the end of the logistics train in favor of what was felt to be more essential equipment.[20]

Results

Once in their new positions, British soldiers began to contract malaria at an alarming rate, despite regular dosing with quinine. By the end of July, the 10th Division was suffering 100 to 150 malaria casualties per day. A number of units with critically low troop strengths were combined to maintain combat effectiveness.[17,20] From 1 May to 31 October 1916, the malaria hospital admission rate was 237/1,000 strength, but many more soldiers were treated at field ambulances and in their unit areas. A total of 30,000 cases were recorded for 1916 (Figure 2-8). While most cases were caused by *P vivax*, enough were caused by *P falciparum* to generate a mortality rate of 1%.[18]

Blood smear examinations, performed during the winter of 1916–1917 on soldiers not then manifesting malaria, demonstrated that asymptomatic cases existed. From November 1916 to April 1917, admissions from relapsing (*P vivax*) and recrudescent (*P falciparum*) disease occurred at a rate of 57/1,000 strength. This reservoir of infected soldiers, along with the native population, would provide the nidus for the next malaria season.[18]

Military Actions, 1917

In April and May of 1917, Allied forces launched a poorly coordinated offensive against the Bulgarian Army. Casualties were high and little was gained. To suppress Allied operations in Macedonia, the Germans increased submarine activity in the Mediterranean, thus slowing the flow of supplies and halting hospital ship operations completely.[20,21] Demoralized, the Allies in Salonika resumed a defensive posture. Milne, fully aware the malaria season was now upon him, withdrew his troops from the Struma valley, continued the anti-mosquito campaign, and waited for bed nets.[17,21]

As summer gave way to autumn in 1917, it became apparent to the British high command that operations on the Balkan front were having no impact on the outcome of the war. Furthermore, British operations in Palestine needed immediate reinforcement. Units were transferred to Palestine and Egypt, and, in 1918, to the Western Front.[17,21]

Results

Although the British evacuation probably reduced primary malaria cases, the rate of admissions between May and October 1917 was 278/1,000 strength, exceeding that of the previous year. By the end of 1917, another 70,000 admissions had been recorded (see Figure 2-8). Due to improved treatment and ground evacuation, the mortality rate dropped to 0.37%.[18]

With the termination of hospital ship evacuation, a population of some 15,000 chronic malaria cases was created,[21] which ambulated from hospitals to convalescent stations "with an occasional day or two of light duty."[21p58] Sir Ronald Ross was dispatched to the area in December, and through his recommendations, a troop evacuation and exchange program was initiated.[21] Large-scale evacuation of sick troops to England and France began in January 1918.[19]

Impact on Operations

Malaria incapacitated entire battalions of the British Expeditionary Force from the late spring of 1916 to the close of the war.[17,19,20] By the end of 1916, 17% of British troops had infected, and by the end of 1917 this figure had risen to 39%.[18] Allied disunity underlay the failed 1917 spring offensive; however, malaria contributed through its effects on the endurance and efficiency of the soldiers involved.[18,20]

As they retired from the Balkan front en route to France, some units left a trail of debilitated soldiers along the way. Other units made it to the Western Front, only to have recurrent disease keep them from entering the line. These troops required special treatment and rest, burdening medical and supply operations, but they finally did return to duty.[21]

Conclusion

On their arrival in Salonika, the British used their experience and knowledge to counter the malaria threat. Their failure in this endeavor resulted from operational, medical, and supply decisions that, to some extent, were beyond the control of the local commander, medical staff, and quartermaster.

First, Milne was directed by Sarrail to reposition British forces in a highly malarious area before antimosquito measures could be implemented. Shortly thereafter, Milne was forced, by pressure from London to keep Britain in a defensive posture, to shift his forces again in the same malarious region. These unexpected moves during the height of mosquito season kept Milne's anti-mosquito squads from establishing effective vector control, resulting in intense exposure of long duration.

Second, the prophylactic use of quinine was not the standard of care. Historical accounts state that quinine was used extensively; however, it is difficult to believe that many prophylactic doses were given, with the majority of medical officers perceiving it to have no preventive efficacy, the ever-increasing numbers requiring treatment, and the slow rate of resupply.[19] Additionally, quinine has no effect on the exoerythrocytic stages of malaria. *P vivax*, which accounted for the vast majority of cases, has an obligatory exoerythrocytic stage during its life-cycle and thus can produce relapse if treatment consists only of a blood, not a tissue, schizonticide.

Third, without effective insect repellents, personal protective measures consisted of mechanical barriers. The most effective of these, the bed net, was continually in short supply because of enemy submarine interference with shipping operations, and, more importantly, because of its low priority with commanders and logisticians at all levels. If bed nets had had higher priority and had enough of them accompanied the initial deployment, then resupply difficulties would have had less impact.

Historian Cyril Falls concluded:

> Had it from the first been possible to decide that in Macedonia protection from malaria was, after food and ammunition, the very first necessity, it is reasonable to suppose that the Salonika Army might have been kept at a higher standard of strength and efficiency, that a certain number of lives might have been saved, and that many thousands of men might have been spared ill health after the war.[20p288]

Cold Injury in the US Army during World War II

Setting

In heavy fog on 11 May 1943, the US 7th Infantry Division made an amphibious assault on Attu Island, Alaska, (Figure 2-9), westernmost island in the Aleutian chain.[22,23] Landing at Holtz Bay in the north and Massacre Bay in the south, the Americans met light resistance until they pushed inland.[22,24] The 2,500 Japanese defenders had strongly fortified the mountainous terrain. Heavy artillery and automatic weapon fire, along with semi-frozen mud, rain, and fog, stopped the US advance.[23,24] The "bewildered 7th, ill-led, badly trained, and having its first experience in combat, went to pieces."[23p500] The Division commander was relieved of command, and 4,300 more troops landed to bolster the 11,000 already engaged. The Japanese, their food and ammunition dwindling, launched suicide attacks on 29 and 30 May, concluding the debacle and ending their occupation of North America.[22,24]

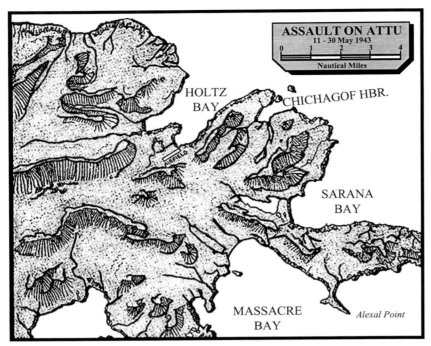

Fig. 2-9. Attu Island, Alaska, 1943. Adapted from: Morrison SE. Aleutians, Gilberts, and Marshalls, June 1942-April 1944. In: *History of United States Naval Operations in World War II.* Vol 7. Boston: Little, Brown & Co; 1951: 45.

Health Issues

At the end of the First World War, the US Army had considerable knowledge and experience in cold weather campaigning on the Great Plains during the Indian Wars and in Europe during World War I.[22,25–29] Between the world wars, the army forgot about cold injuries and their impact on troops in the field. Colonel George Dunham's *Military Preventive Medicine,* published in 1940, did not have a word on cold injuries. The *Medical Department Soldier's Handbook* (TM 8-220), 1941, failed to include trench foot, and *The Guide to Therapy for Medical Officers* (TM 8-210), 1942, not only excluded trench foot but also advised troops to lace shoes snugly, thereby decreasing circulation. American forces went to war poorly indoctrinated on cold injuries and inadequately clothed to operate in such environments.[25] The hierarchy in line, medical, and logistics commands failed to learn the lessons of history, lessons replete with cold disasters and valid preventive measures.

Contributory Actions and Inactions

The reasons for this environmentally induced disaster can be found at major and local command levels. Before the war, the army failed to develop functional cold weather protective clothing for general troop issue.[22,25,30] During the planning phase of the Attu Campaign, the Quartermaster Corps recommended the use of special clothing and footgear, but commanders did not heed this advice.[22] Troops went ashore on Attu without properly insulated and windproofed and waterproofed clothing. The more comfortable but less protective leather boot was employed instead of the shoepac, a warmer, commercially made boot with a moccasin-style rubber foot and a leather top.[22,25,30,31] Commanders and soldiers were poorly trained and ill equipped to live and fight in cold, wet climates. Foot hygiene was not enforced. Soldiers did not change wet boots and socks for days and frequently discarded wet clothing rather than dry it out. In addition, the logistics system failed in that sleeping bags were not issued for the first 4 to 5 nights after landing.[22,25,30]

Impact on Army Operations

In 22 days of combat, the 7th Infantry Division sustained 3,829 casualties of which 1,200 (31%) were due to the cold.[22] Cold injury and wounded-in-action rates (Table 2-2) were virtually the same. Although this initial experience with cold injury in combat demonstrated the necessity of proper equipment and clothing, the importance of soldier training regarding foot care, and the importance of command responsibility in enforcing foot care discipline, it did not generate rapid corrective procedures.[25] During the Italian Campaign in the winter of 1943–1944, the 5th US Army sustained 5,752 cases of trench foot, with an admission rate of 54/1,000 average strength. The ratio of trench foot to nonfatal battle

TABLE 2-2

BATTLE CASUALTIES AND ADMISSIONS FOR DISEASE AND NONBATTLE INJURY, ALLIED TROOPS, ATTU CAMPAIGN, 11 MAY THROUGH 1 JUNE 1943.

Cause	Number	Rate[*]
Battle casualties		
Killed in action	549	1.6
Wounded in action	1,148	3.4
Nonbattle admissions		
Disease	614	1.8
Nonbattle injury	1,518	4.5
Cold injury	(1,200)[1]	(3.6)[†]
Other	(318)[1]	(0.9)[†]
All causes	3,829	11.4

[*]Rate expressed as number per day per 1,000 average strength
[†]Figures in parentheses are subtotals
Source: Whayne TF, DeBakey ME. *Ground Injury, Cold Type.* Washington, DC: Office of The Surgeon General, Department of the Army; 1958: 85.

injury was 1:5 (Table 2-3).[22] Additionally, clothing was still inadequate and in short supply, troops lived on cold rations, and few had received cold weather training before deployment.[25,30]

Cold weather indoctrination and training improved during the summer of 1944. Field commands were apprised of training materials and directed to provide appropriate training and enforce foot hygiene. During the Italian Campaign of 1944–1945, woolen socks and hot rations were supplied and foot hygiene was enforced. Improved shoepacs reached the front by October 1944; however, there was resistance among soldiers to using them because of sizing difficulties and lack of training.[25,30] When the 5th Army Quartermaster realized that 80% of cold casualties in Italy were not wearing shoepacs, he developed and implemented training on the supply and use of winter clothing.[25] The trench foot admission rate dropped to 20/1,000 average strength during the winter of 1944–1945, demonstrating the success of preventive efforts.[22]

The US experience with cold environments in the Aleutians and Italy did not translate into adequate prevention in the European Theater during the war's last winter. The European Command expanded rapidly after June 1944 and planned for a quick victory as the 3rd Army drove through France. The Theater Quartermaster General downgraded the priority of winter clothing, ignoring the Italy experience and preventive medicine advice to the contrary. Poor planning and delayed requisitions resulted in soldiers fighting through the severe winter of 1944–1945 inadequately clothed and shod.[22,25,30] The Theater Adjutant General disapproved a preventive medicine publication to edu-

TABLE 2-3

CASES OF TRENCH FOOT (HOSPITALIZED AND GIVEN QUARTERS) AND OF BATTLE INJURIES AND WOUNDS, BY MONTH, FIFTH US ARMY, NOVEMBER 1943 THROUGH APRIL 1944.

Month and year	Trench foot Cases	Trench foot Rate[*]	Battle injuries and wounds Cases	Battle injuries and wounds Rate[*]	Ratio of trench foot to battle injuries and wounds
1943					
November	371	24	3,897	249	1:11
December	1,265	69	5,020	274	1:4
1944					
January	1,490	96	4,496	289	1:3
February	1,805	108	8,378	500	1:5
March	779	35	3,685	167	1:5
April	42	2	2,126	121	1:51
Total	5,752	54	27,602	261	1:5

[*]Rate expressed as number per annum per 1,000 average strength
Adapted from Whayne TF, DeBakey ME. *Ground Injury, Cold Type.* Washington, DC: Office of The Surgeon General, Department of the Army; 1958: 103.

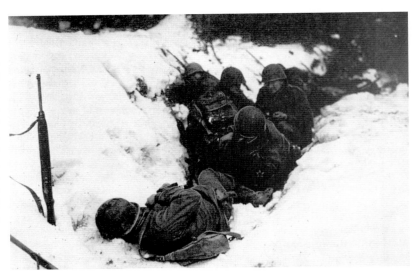

Fig. 2-10. Infantrymen from the 9th Regiment, 2d Division, 1st US Army take cover from German artillery during the Battle of the Bulge. An unusually heavy snowfall and intense cold accompanied the German offensive in December 1944. These conditions made combat operations difficult, strained an already overworked logistics system, and induced an epidemic of cold injuries among US troops.Reproduced from: Whayne TF, DeBakey ME. *Ground Injury, Cold Type.* Washington, DC: Office of The Surgeon General, Department of the Army; 1958: 137.

cate commanders on general foot care because the subject was covered in existing manuals. Not until late November did the Command Surgeon provide official guidance on this issue. By that time, the 3rd Army, advancing on Metz, had sustained over 6,200 cold injuries. Not uncommonly, units lost 10% to 15% of their strength. In the first 4 days of the Lorraine Campaign in November 1944, the 328th Infantry Regiment evacuated 500 cold casualties and was rendered combat ineffective.[22,25] In mid-December, the Germans launched a counteroffen-

sive, the Battle of the Bulge (Figure 2-10). Heavy fighting in extreme cold generated a second epidemic of cold injuries in US forces.[22]

There were 46,107 hospital admissions for cold injuries in the European Theater between October 1944 and April 1945.[25] (The figures for the 5th US Army are in Table 2-4.) Fifty percent of these cold casualties, roughly equivalent to one and a half infantry divisions, occurred during November and December 1944.[22] The magnitude of these casualties stimulated action at the general-staff level. Cold

TABLE 2-4

CASES OF TRENCH FOOT (HOSPITALIZED AND GIVEN QUARTERS) AND OF BATTLE INJURIES AND WOUNDS, BY MONTH, 5TH US ARMY, OCTOBER 1944 THROUGH MARCH 1945.

Month and year	Trench foot		Battle injuries and wounds		Ratio of trench foot to battle injuries and wounds
	Cases	Rate[*]	Cases	Rate[*]	
1944					
October	258	24	8,404	783	1:33
November	274	25	2,046	188	1:7
December	305	22	1,274	90	1:4
1945					
January	309	26	561	48	1:2
February	324	25	1,966	154	1:6
March	102	6	1,613	97	1:16
Total	1,572	20	15,864	206	1:10

[*]Rate expressed as number per annum per 1,000 average strength
Adapted from Whayne TF, DeBakey ME. *Ground Injury, Cold Type.* Washington, DC: Office of The Surgeon General, Department of the Army; 1958: 1034.

injury prevention received a high priority during planning for the invasion of Japan. Medical personnel taught soldiers the importance of foot hygiene, proper footgear, and nutrition. The Quartermaster Corps geared up to provision the invasion force for cold weather operations. And most importantly, commanders were made responsible for cold injuries among their troops.[25]

Conclusion

The Aleutian Island campaign clearly demonstrated the US Army's unpreparedness for cold weather operations. The European campaigns illustrate how difficult it can be to correct such deficiencies in a large field army. During World War II, the Army only gradually relearned the value of planning, training, logistics, and awareness (both command and medical) in cold weather operations.

Heat Injury in the US Persian Gulf Command During World War II

Setting

Before the US entered World War II, American leaders realized that helping enemies of the Axis powers was, in effect, self defense. This notion led to the Lend–Lease Act of 1941. Ultimately, the US and its allies established five major transportation lines that by war's end had funneled 17.5 million tons of mostly American and British supplies to the Soviet Union.[32] Through most of the war, the US allocated 20% of its production to Lend–Lease, with substantial shipments occurring during 1943 and 1944.[33]

The Persian corridor, one of the five major Lend–Lease routes to the Soviet Union, extended from the headwaters of the Persian Gulf through northern Iran. Development of this primarily British–US effort began in 1941. Allied logistics efforts here were critical in thwarting Axis designs on the Suez Canal and the oil fields of Iran, Iraq, and the Caucasus.[32,34]

Supply was the main business of the US Persian Gulf Command, which came to number 30,000 soldiers.[32] The command primarily operated truck and rail routes between the Persian Gulf ports of Basra, Khorramshahr, and Bandar Shahpur and the northern Iranian terminals of Kazvin and Tehran (Figures 2-11 and 2-12).[32–34] From 1941 to 1945, the Persian Gulf Command handled 3.9 million tons of supplies—enough to sustain 60 combat divisions—with 90% going to the Soviet Union.[32]

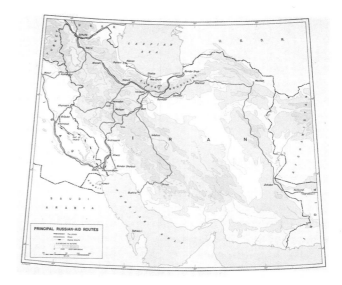

Fig. 2-11. The principal transportation routes and terminals of the Persian corridor, World War II. The red lines are roads and the hatched solid lines are railroads. The US Persian Gulf Command operated truck and rail routes between Persian Gulf ports and northern Iranian terminals, with most of the supplies going to the Soviet Union. Reproduced from Motter THV. *The Persian Corridor and Aid to Russia. United States Army in World War II, The Middle East Theater.* Washington, DC: Office of The Chief of Military History; 1952: inside back cover.

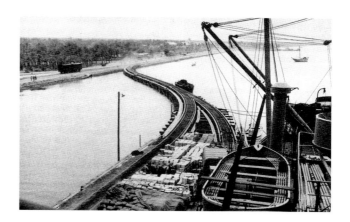

Fig. 2-12. Liberty ship with supplies bound for the Soviet Union at the port of Khorramshahr, Iran, WW II. The Persian corridor began at the ports of Basra, Khorramshahr, and Bandar Shahpur in the headwaters of the Persian Gulf, and the coastal port of Bushire. Here, supplies were downloaded from ships, such as the one pictured, for the journey north via truck, rail, or barge. Reproduced from: Coakley RW, Leighton RM. Global logistics and strategy, 1943–1945. *United States Army in World War II, The War Department.* Washington, DC: Office of the Chief of Military History; 1968: 677.

Health Issues

While the Persian Gulf Command did not engage in combat, the environment was enemy enough, as the region is one of the hottest in the world. Gulf coastal areas are warm and moist, with outside daytime temperatures in the summer averaging 32°C to 46°C (90°F–115°F) in the shade and humidity reaching 90%. Inland is the Iranian desert, where the climate is hotter and very dry, with temperatures ranging from 38°C to 54°C (100°F–130°F). Temperatures climb even higher inside vehicles, buildings, rail cars, and tents. The mountainous areas of Iran, such as in the vicinity of Tehran, have a more pleasant climate (Figure 2-13).[35,36]

The common scheme for classifying heat injuries, which includes heat stroke, heat exhaustion, and heat cramps, was used during World War II. Additionally, miliaria (heat rash) caused extensive morbidity and sometimes resulted in hospitalization.

During World War I, the incidence of heat injury admissions in the US Army was 1.0/1,000 soldiers per year.[35] During 1940, heat injury admissions occurred at the rate of 0.5/1,000 per year.[36] For the war years (1942–1945), there were 35,398 heat injury admissions, each lasting an average of 5.3 days, producing a rate of 1.38/1,000 per year. There were 238 deaths. Overall, however, heat injury was a relatively minor problem in World War II, except in hot regions.[35]

Preventive Actions Taken and Missed

When the US entered World War II, it had not fought a major war in hot climates in nearly 40 years, and many experienced officers had left the army since World War I. Furthermore, basic science knowledge of heat stress physiology was lacking. There were misconceptions concerning hot environments. The need for exogenous salt was misapplied and overemphasized. Many believed that drinking water while working in the heat was harmful. And there was the concept of "water discipline," which held that men could be "trained" to require less water while working in the heat. While these misconceptions played some role in heat casualties, the main problem was that many known and practical principles of heat injury management were simply not followed early in the war.[35–37]

When the Middle East Theater was formed and planning begun in late 1941, there was a paucity of medical intelligence available to the command surgeon. Medical planning occurred but focused more on hospitalization and communicable disease than on heat injury prevention.[34]

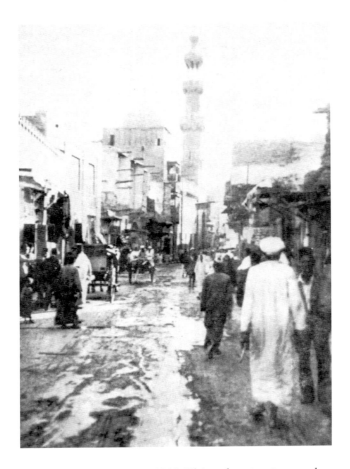

Fig. 2-13. Tehran, Iran, 1943. This calm street scene belies the activity of the US Persian Gulf Command. With its network of roads and rail lines, Tehran figured prominently in the command's mission and served as the location for its headquarters. Impressive amounts of supplies were shipped from the ports north through Tehran before moving east, west, and north, en route to the Soviet Union. Reproduced from: Sams CF. The Middle East countries. In: Hoff EC, ed. *Civil Affairs/Military Government Public Health Activities.* Vol 8. In: *Preventive Medicine in World War II.* Washington, DC: Office of The Surgeon General, US Department of the Army; 1976: 226.

Thus, when the Persian Gulf Command became operational, several problems existed—in addition to its location—that predisposed its soldiers to heat injury. Officers were inexperienced, and training for operations in hot environments was lacking. Medical planning was inadequate, as were knowledge and equipment for treating heat casualties. Preventive medicine concerns were often subordinated to logistical considerations or discarded. More specifically, operations, including desert convoys, were routinely conducted in the heat of the day. No respite was available as quarters lacked fans, evaporative coolers, or air conditioners. Night crews especially got little rest in the relentless heat of the day.[35]

Results

Heat injury was a serious problem for the Persian Gulf Command during the summers of 1942 and 1943. Indeed, this command suffered more heat-related morbidity than any other during the war. What makes this remarkable is the fact that the command *never engaged in combat operations.*[34–36]

During the first 7 months of operations, from June to December 1942, heat trauma was the second leading cause of admission (behind enteritis) to the Army hospital at Ahwaz, and heat stroke accounted for 11.7% of all admissions. The problem peaked in June 1943, when heat trauma incidence from all causes, including those hospitalized and treated as outpatients, reached 296/1,000 per year command-wide, with 8 heat-related deaths.[35] Medical treatment of heat casualties sometimes added to the problem, as initially there were no cool areas for recovering patients. Mild cases, when sent to hot wards without observation, sometimes became severe casualties within hours.[35]

Little was written specifically addressing the impact of heat trauma on the Persian Gulf Command's operations, but it was significant. No unit can suffer morbidity like that described without experiencing a decrement in effectiveness.

Conclusion

This story illustrates the advantage of operational experience in an environment, and the absolute necessity of proper planning and enforcement of preventive medicine measures. Heat injury took an unnecessarily large toll on the Persian Gulf Command during 1942 and 1943. The command, however, did eventually take specific actions to counter the heat problem: it controlled work schedules, curtailed routine operations between 1200 and 1700 hours, upgraded and cooled living quarters, and set up air-conditioned heat-casualty treatment centers at strategically located hospitals.[35,36] As a result of these measures and the knowledge gained by experience, heat-related morbidity declined sharply in 1944. The incidence of heat trauma fell from a high of 296/1,000 per year in June 1943 to 49/1,000 per year in July 1944, and then to 41/1,000 per year in August 1945. This is remarkable when one considers that a record tonnage of supplies was moved in 1944 and that the summer was just as hot as that of 1943.[35]

Because of anticipated and actual operations in desert and tropical environments, World War II spurred much hot-environment research. A team led by Dr. E. F. Adolph, working under contract for the Office of Scientific Research and Development, conducted research in various US deserts from 1942 through 1945, significantly increasing our understanding of human physiology in hot environments.[37] Applied studies were conducted at the Armored Medical Research Laboratory, Fort Knox, Ky.[35] The Army Medical Department remains actively involved in hot environment research at the US Army Research Institute of Environmental Medicine at Natick, Mass.[38,39]

Some 50 years later, from 1990 to 1991, the US military again deployed to the Persian Gulf region but in even larger numbers (696,000 personnel).[40] The Persian Gulf War involved combat as well. This time, however, command awareness was high, and preventive medicine measures were published and enforced. As a result, US forces suffered minimally from the effects of heat. While the majority of forces were deployed during the cooler months, it is still remarkable that no deaths were attributed to heat injury.[41]

The more one knows about an adversary, the less threatening it becomes, hence the importance of medical intelligence. Adolph makes this point poetically in the preface to his classic text.

> Once the desert environment is understood, it loses its mystery. The great, open desert soon grows to be a friendly place with an ever-changing beauty of shifting color and shadow…Especially at night is the desert serene and friendly; the stars stud the sky, or the landscape is flooded with moonlight.[37p vii]

THE BENEFITS OF PREVENTION

The US Army Yellow Fever Commission in Cuba, 1900–1901

Setting

The issue of Cuban independence from Spain and the US role in negotiating Spanish withdrawal from Cuba had been a thorny problem since 1895. By late April 1898, tensions had increased to a fever pitch, and President McKinley requested a declaration of war against Spain. A hastily mobilized army, commanded by Major General William R. Shafter, landed at Daiquiri, Cuba, on 22 June. Shafter realized that he had to subdue the Spaniards before yellow fever and malaria incapacitated his forces. He drove obliquely from Daiquiri to Santiago de

Cuba, forcing the capitulation of the Spanish garrison on 16 July. US forces accomplished their mission but not before tropical diseases began to decimate their ranks. With a US military government and army of occupation established on Cuba, commanders engaged a more dreaded enemy.[42]

Health Issues

During the war, US troops suffered "severely from yellow fever and other tropical diseases."[43p4] One priority of the US military government was to eradicate yellow fever from Havana. This would help maintain the health of the occupying force and, the authorities hoped, preclude the introduction of yellow fever epidemics into the US.[43]

Medical authorities agreed that because yellow fever was a filth disease, appropriate sanitation in cities such as Havana would eliminate the problem. With this in mind, Major William C. Gorgas, Chief Surgeon for the city of Havana, began an intense cleaning program for Havana and other Cuban cities.[43,44] These efforts reduced the cases of typhoid fever and dysentery, and the general death rate declined, but yellow fever remained unabated.[43–45] Epidemics broke out in Havana and other Cuban cities in 1899 and 1900, fueled by nonimmune from the United States and a growing number of Spanish immigrants attracted by the economic opportunities of the newly stable political situation.[42,43,46] Frustration mounted, along with yellow fever cases, as the year 1900 progressed. Major General Leonard Wood, the new governor-general and a physician himself, appointed Gorgas Chief Sanitary Officer of Havana, continued to fund the cleaning efforts, and prodded Army Surgeon General George Sternberg to appoint a special medical commission to investigate the etiology of yellow fever.[47] Whether in reaction to Wood's urging, to discussions with Major Walter Reed, or to criticism of his management of the typhoid fever epidemic in the mobilization camps, Sternberg ordered the creation of a medical board, The Second Havana Yellow Fever Commission, to convene at Columbia Barracks, Quemados, Cuba. This board was to investigate "acute infectious diseases prevalent on the island of Cuba" and "give special attention to questions relating to the etiology and prevention of yellow fever."[48]

Actions of the Yellow Fever Commission

Reed presided over the board, which consisted of himself and Drs. James Carroll, Jesse Lazear, and Aristides Agramonte (Figure 2-14).[48,49] Reed and Carroll were intimately familiar with the prevalent theory that the *Bacillus icteroides* of Dr. Giuseppe Sanarelli was the yellow fever agent. They had done much to disprove it, although had not conclusively done so.[50] In late June 1900, the Board initiated bacteriological studies using blood from yellow fever patients and blood and organs from deceased victims, in an effort to isolate *B icteroides*. These studies yielded negative results.[48]

When the Board arrived in Cuba, a yellow fever epidemic was in progress at Quemados, making it a compelling and convenient subject for immediate investigation.[48] During the last week of July 1900, a yellow fever epidemic occurred in the military barracks at Pinar del Rio. This epidemic was misdiagnosed as pernicious malarial fever and no disinfection of fomites occurred. The Board noted that this omission of fomite disinfection did not increase the number of cases, nor did any of the nonimmunes who slept in beds of the sick or handled contaminated clothes become ill. This agreed with earlier observations that nonimmunes who cared for yellow fever patients or came in contact with them during early convalescence did not contract the disease. Reed knew of Dr. Carlos Finlay's old and unproven theory that yellow fever was transmitted by the *Aedes aegypti* mosquito and Dr. Henry R. Carter's recent studies concerning the time interval between primary and secondary infection. In addition, he observed the seasonal nature of both yellow fever and malaria and felt it reasonable that yellow fever might require a special agent for its transmission.[46] Reed may not have regarded Finlay's theory any more highly than Sternberg or Gorgas did. But when considered in conjunction with Carter's observations, seasonal variations, and the noncontagious nature of the epidemic at Pinar del Rio, he considered the idea of an intermediate host as a possibility. Reed obtained mosquito eggs from Finlay for cultivation and redirected the focus of the Board toward disease transmission.[48]

In early August, Reed was temporarily recalled to Washington. He directed the Board to begin experiments on human subjects. Lazear and several others failed to become ill after being bitten in mid-August.[44,48] On 27 August, Carroll allowed himself to be bitten by a mosquito that had fed on a yellow fever patient 12 days before. Three days later he was gravely ill. Carroll admitted to being in infected areas just before being bitten, however. To definitely prove what they now suspected, Lazear and Agramonte needed a nonimmune volunteer who

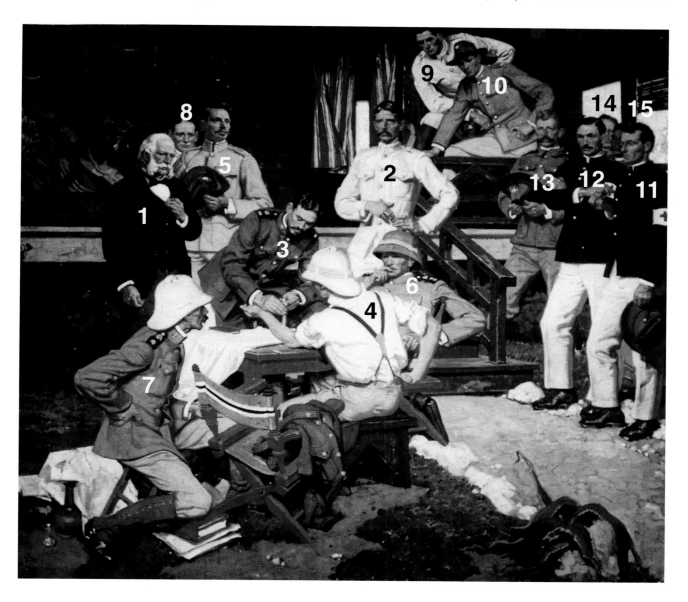

Key: (1) Dr. Carlos Finlay, Cuban physician who originated the theory of mosquito transmission of yellow fever; (2) Major Walter Reed, President of the Yellow Fever Board; (3) Dr. Jesse W. Lazear, Yellow Fever Board member; (4) Dr. James Carroll, Yellow Fever Board member; (5) Dr. Aristides Agramonte, Yellow Fever Board member; (6) Major General Leonard Wood, Governor-General of Cuba; (7) Major Jefferson R. Kean, Chief Surgeon, Dept. of Western Cuba; (8) Lieutenant Albert E. Truby, Commander, Columbia Barracks Post Hospital; (9) Dr. Roger P. Ames, clinician; (10) Dr. Robert P. Cooke, Contract Surgeon and experimental volunteer; (11) Private John R. Kissinger, Hospital Corps, experimental volunteer; (12) John J. Moran, Acting Steward, Hospital Corps, experimental volunteer; (13) Private Warren G. Jernegan, Hospital Corps, experimental volunteer; (14) an American, representative of eleven additional volunteers; (15) a Spanish immigrant, representative of four additional volunteers. Data source: *Conquerors of Yellow Fever*, American Medical Association, Copyright 1941.

Fig. 2-14. "Conquerors of Yellow Fever," by Dean Cornwell, 1941. With Major Walter Reed and Dr. Carlos Finlay among the spectators, Dr. Lazear inoculates Dr. Carroll with an infected mosquito on August 27, 1900. This experiment indicated that the mosquito was the carrier of yellow fever. The painting includes portraits of many of the men whose combined efforts made this great achievement possible. Reproduced with permission of Wyeth-Ayerst Laboratories.

had not been out of camp. On 31 August 1900, Private William H. Dean of B Troop, 7th Cavalry, stated that he met the requirements and offered his arm. Five days later Dean became the first proven case of yellow fever experimentally produced by infected mosquitoes.[48,49] Convinced that mosquitoes transmitted yellow fever, the Board ceased further human experimentation.[49] Carroll and Dean survived, but, regrettably, Lazear was accidentally bitten in mid-September and died on the 25th.[44]

Reed returned to Cuba the first week in October to find a devastated Board and a depressed medical staff at Columbia Barracks.[44] Studying Lazear's notes, he became convinced that Finlay had been correct but felt the theory must be proven beyond a shadow of a doubt. He produced a preliminary report of the Board's results and persuaded Wood to fund an "experimental sanitary station"[46p204] where controlled experiments could be conducted to exclude any other sources of infection.[44,46,51]

Reed designed and oversaw construction of the experimental station, composed of tents and frame buildings, which was named Camp Lazear (Figure 2-15). The "Infected Clothing Building" was sealed to prevent ventilation, while the "Infected Mosquito Building" was constructed for ventilation and divided into two living areas by a wire screen partition.[44]

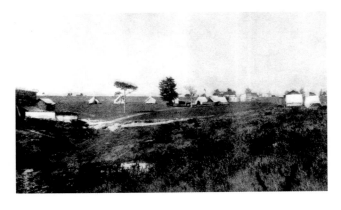

Fig. 2-15. Camp Lazear. The experimental sanitary station near Quemados, Cuba, 1900. At this unimposing camp, the Reed Board, assisted by the staff of the Columbia Barracks Post Hospital, conducted the experiments that established the *Aedes aegypti* mosquito as a vector of yellow fever. Major William Gorgas implemented practical anti-mosquito measures in Havana that virtually eliminated yellow fever from the Cuban capital, thereby confirming the Board's results. Reproduced courtesy of the Historical Collections, Health Sciences Library, University of Virginia.

The Board would now attempt to infect nonimmunes by three methods: (1) bites from infected mosquitoes, (2) exposure to fomites contaminated with discharges from yellow fever patients, and (3) injection of blood from confirmed yellow fever cases. Between 8 December 1900 and 10 February 1901, the Board fed mosquitoes, infected 10 to 57 days previously, on 13 nonimmune volunteers. This produced 10 yellow fever cases. Five nonimmunes were injected with blood from these experimentally induced cases, producing 4 additional cases. In the "Infected Mosquito Building," those in contact with infected mosquitoes contracted the disease while controls on the opposite side of the screen remained healthy. No cases resulted from intimate contact with clothing, towels, and bed linens soiled by yellow fever patients.[46]

Results

The Board concluded that the yellow fever agent was transmitted by the *Stegomyia fasciata* (*A aegypti*) mosquito, that the agent required approximately 12 days incubation in the intermediate host, that the mosquito remained infectious for at least 57 days, and that the theory of propagation by filth was a myth.[46]

Gorgas acted on the Board's conclusions immediately. In Havana, yellow fever patients were quarantined, and, through the use of wire screening, uninfected mosquitoes were kept at bay. "Stegomyia Squads" controlled the mosquito population by screening or oiling cisterns and water barrels and fumigating patients and nearby houses with sulfur or pyrethrum. These control measures dramatically reduced yellow fever cases and deaths (Figure 2-16).[43,52]

Impact on Operations

The operational importance of the Board's work was 2-fold. First, field commanders no longer needed to continuously shift bivouac sites in an effort to avoid yellow fever. Rather, they and their surgeons implemented vector control procedures in camp.[53] Second, it provided medical researchers with a starting point for isolating the yellow fever agent, ultimately leading to vaccine development. This vaccine was first administered to US Army soldiers in 1941.[54]

Conclusion

The outcomes of the Spanish-American War and the Philippine Insurrection rapidly increased US influence in areas where the endemicity of a vari-

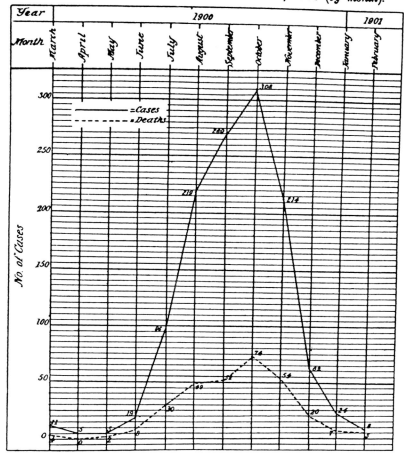

CHART II.

Cases and Deaths from Yellow Fever in the City of Havana, for the Epidemic year, March 1, 1900, to March 1, 1901 (by month).

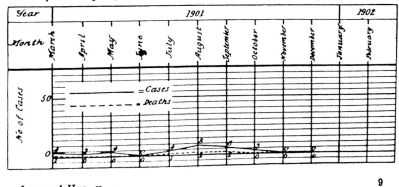

CHART III.

Cases and Deaths from Yellow Fever in the City of Havana, for the Epidemic year, March 1, 1901, to March 1, 1902 (by month).

Journ. of Hyg. II

9

Fig. 2-16. Walter Reed's graphs of yellow fever cases and deaths in Havana for the years beginning March 1, 1900 (top) and 1901 (bottom), showing the dramatic reductions that resulted from the work of the Yellow Fever Commission. Reproduced with permission from: Reed W. Recent researches concerning the etiology, propagation, and prevention of yellow fever, by the United States Army Commission. *J Hyg.* 1902;2(2);117.

ety of diseases provided an abundance of research material. The Army Medical Department took full advantage of these opportunities. Scientific medical research in the Army, which included the Typhoid Fever Board in 1898 and the Yellow Fever Commission, expanded and developed in these tropical areas, becoming a valuable asset not only to the Army but also to medicine as a whole.

Lieutenant General William Slim in the China–Burma–India Theater, World War II

Setting

British Lieutenant General William Slim (Figure 2-17) provides one of the finest examples of the application of preventive medicine to war. In the China—Burma–India (CBI) theater of World War II, he faced enormous challenges. From January to May 1942,

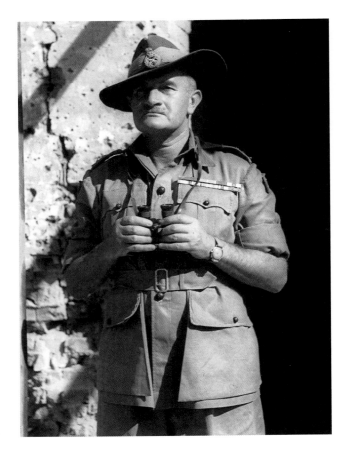

Fig. 2-17. Lieutenant General William Slim, Commander-in-Chief, 14th Army, World War II. Slim was knighted during the war for his brilliant conduct of the China–Burma–India campaign. Reproduced courtesy of the Imperial War Museum, London, England.

the Japanese 15th Army invaded Burma, driving out the combined British, Burmese, Indian, and Chinese forces. The British Army retreated north through Mandalay and west into India. Slim took over the I Burma Corps during the retreat in March 1942. In October 1943, he assumed command of the British 14th Army. Made up primarily of English and Indian forces, the army was demoralized and in poor health. His task was to retake Burma from the Japanese (Figure 2-18).[55–61]

Health Issues

Many diseases thrive among armies in tropical environments when the public health infrastructure is absent. The CBI theater was extremely harsh and unhealthy.[62,63] The main disease threats were malaria, dysentery, nonbloody diarrhea, various skin diseases, and scrub typhus. In the hot, humid environment of the CBI theater, skin diseases—particularly fungal infections and immersion foot—were hard to control. With no effective drug therapy, scrub typhus caused significant mortality. In 1943, the year Slim assumed command of the 14th Army, allied forces in the CBI theater were in bad shape. The force-wide incidence of malaria was 491/1,000 per year; the incidence of dysentery was 48/1,000 per year.[64] Hepatitis A incidence was 18/1,000 per year, having risen from 0.7/1,000 per year in 1938.[65]

Slim's Actions

Slim dealt deliberately with the army's poor health. He assessed the situation, developed and implemented a medical plan, and enforced it.

Shortly after Slim took over the 14th Army, he *assessed the health of his command*. He was amazed at what he found. On an annualized basis, 84% of his soldiers got malaria, and rates were even higher in forward units. His DNBI evacuation rate was 12/1,000 per day, 120 times greater than his BI evacuation rate. Slim concluded that "...in a matter of months at this rate my army would have melted away. Indeed, it was doing so under my eyes."[55p177] With the help of his surgeons, he formulated a list of medical threats and problems. After the initial assessment, he conducted ongoing medical surveillance, following key health indicators such as hospital admission rates. In this way he kept abreast of the health of the Army.[55]

Slim *developed and implemented a medical plan* that emphasized four points: research, forward treatment, air evacuation, and prevention. He assembled teams of scientists and physicians to conduct field

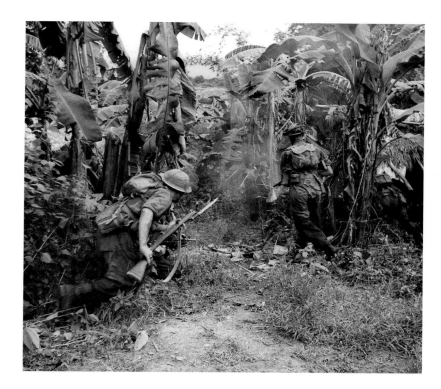

Fig. 2-18. British troops fighting in Burma jungle, World War II. Combat was fierce and difficult in the dense jungles of the China–Burma–India theater. Moreover, the hot, humid environment made many diseases hard to control. Reproduced courtesy of the Imperial War Museum, London, England.

research and apply this knowledge to prevention and treatment. He emphasized forward treatment instead of evacuation to India, establishing malaria forward-treatment units and forward surgical teams just miles behind the lines. He employed aircraft for medical evacuation. Air evacuation to India was faster and better tolerated by the seriously wounded, particularly given the heat, humidity, and tortuous road system of the CBI theater. His most important initiative was to raise "medical discipline," the British term for field hygiene and sanitation. Slim had concluded that "…prevention was better than cure. We had to stop men going sick, or, if they went sick, from staying sick."[55p178] Slim issued orders regarding various personal and collective preventive measures, such as not bathing after dark and taking anti-malarial medicine under supervision.[55,66]

Finally, Slim *enforced* his medical plan. He had relatively little trouble getting his research, forward treatment, and air evacuation initiatives going, but medical discipline was—and remains—a problem requiring frequent command emphasis. Slim spent most afternoons visiting his troops. While his main purpose was to encourage them by his presence and brief talks from the hood of his jeep, he paid close attention to their hygiene and sanitation, thereby forcing his leaders to give priority to preventive measures. He was tough in this regard, to the point of relieving commanders who tolerated poor medical discipline. Concerning the taking of the anti-malarial drug mepacrine (atabrine), for example, Slim wrote

> I, therefore, had surprise checks of whole units, every man being examined [by a blood test]. If the overall result was less than ninety-five per cent positive I sacked the commanding officer. I only had to sack three; by then the rest had got my meaning.[55p180]

Results

Slim observed that

> Slowly, but with increasing rapidity, as all of us, commanders, doctors, regimental officers, staff officers, and N.C.O.s, united in the drive against sickness, results began to appear.[55p180]

The results were dramatic, comparing 1943 to 1945. The DNBI evacuation rate dropped from 12/1,000 per day to 1/1,000 per day. Not only did the incidence of malaria, the major contributor to DNBI, decrease, but with forward treatment, time lost per case dropped from 5 months to 3 weeks.[55]

Impact on Operations

Confident in the health of his army, Slim was able to pursue combat operations during the monsoon season, when the disease threat peaked. Though Slim denied this, some thought he purposefully chose disease-ridden areas to engage the Japanese to take tactical advantage of his superior preventive medicine.[55,66]

During 1944, the 14th retook northwest Burma. From January to May 1945, the Allies pushed south to regain the remainder. With the occupation of Rangoon on 2 May 1945, Japanese resistance effectively ended.[55–61]

Conclusion

William Slim was one of the truly superb generals of World War II. Under arduous conditions, he took aggressive action that restored the health of his command and earned him an honored place in the history of military medicine. The success of the 14th Army in the field owed greatly to its good health and to the vision and leadership of General Slim.[63]

Slim recognized the central truth that the commander is responsible for the health of his command, with the medical officer as the primary advisor. This is his legacy to military medicine. His classic statement on this topic bears repeating: "Good doctors are no use without good discipline. More than half the battle against disease is fought, not by the doctors, but by the regimental officers."[55p180]

Meningococcal Disease in the US Army Training Base

Setting

In considering the application of preventive medicine to war, it is common to think of actions at or near the front. This bias toward the theater of operations overlooks many less noticeable but equally important efforts, such as mobilization and training, that occur in the zone of the interior (the continental United States). The story of meningococcal disease in the US Army training base is unlike the others treated in this chapter. Efforts to control this problem involved many different workers

pursuing various lines of effort at numerous locations over several decades.

US military trainee populations are generally representative of the young adult populations from which they come. Recruits are mustered at training posts and trained for several weeks. Environmental factors in camp that predispose recruits for meningococcal disease include crowded living conditions, poorly ventilated barracks, rigorous training schedules, exposure to the elements, and sleep deprivation. While the US military always has recruits in training, the number swells in wartime.

Health Issues in the Early Twentieth Century

Infection with *Neisseria meningitidis* can produce a wide range of results, including asymptomatic nasopharyngeal carriage, local infection (eg, pharyngitis and pneumonia), and invasive disease (eg, disseminated meningococcemia and meningitis). Meningococcal disease is endemic in the US population, causing 1 to 3 cases per 100,000 population per year.[67] The petechial rash (Figure 2-19) often seen with invasive disease is classic.[68]

Meningitis has been a problem in the US Army during past wars, including the War of 1812, the Mexican–American War, and the Civil War; how-

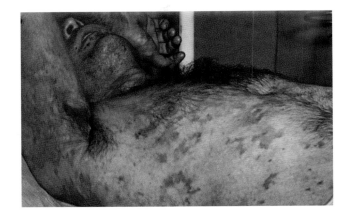

Fig. 2-19. A classic petechial rash in a patient with fulminant meningococcal disease. Other signs and symptoms include fever, headache, nausea, vomiting, and neck stiffness. Meningitis has historically been a problem in US military training camps during periods of mobilization. The disease is still formidable; even with early diagnosis, modern therapy, and life support, the case-fatality rate is 5% to 15%. Reproduced from: Daniels WB. Meningococcal infections. In: Havens PW, ed. *Infectious Diseases.* Vol 2. In: *Internal Medicine in World War II.* Washington, DC: Office of The Surgeon General, US Department of the Army; 1963: 254.

ever, exact diagnoses could not be established until the turn of the 20th century, when bacteriologic methods had developed sufficiently.[69,70] The disease is most common at recruit training camps, where organisms from various locales are shared.

During World War I from April to October of 1917, over 1 million American men were mobilized and trained at 39 different camps, most of which had meningitis epidemics. In January 1918, the annualized incidence rose to a peak of 459/100,000 enlisted men in the continental United States. By war's end, the overall annualized meningitis admission rate for the Army was 141/100,000 men. While the incidence was moderate, the case fatality rate (CFR) was not. The standard treatment was intrathecal injection of polyvalent antimeningococcal serum. Despite this treatment, there were 2,279 deaths in 5,839 cases for a CFR of 39%.[69,70]

Actions Taken and Results Achieved

During the 20th century, US wartime mobilization has always led to epidemic meningococcal disease, with the exception of the Korean and Persian Gulf Wars. These epidemics have prompted actions leading to advances in prevention and treatment.

During the World War I era, there was no effective prevention for meningococcal disease. Military doctors at several recruit camps studied various aspects of the problem, such as demographics, carriage, and transmission. Some attempted, unsuccessfully, to control transmission by methods such as isolation and treatment of cases and contacts. Glover noted a relation between crowding and carriage rate and between carriage rate and incidence, leading to the notion of increasing living space as a means of prevention.[70] Herrick, an Army physician at Camp Jackson, South Carolina, who studied 265 patients, recognized the importance of early diagnosis and treatment. His work led to the creation of special surveillance wards for acute respiratory disease patients, an effective practice still in use today.[69,71] While these pioneer physicians were unable to control the disease, they made practical advances and contributions to the understanding of meningococcal pathophysiology and epidemiology. With the war's end, though, the problem waned.

The era of effective antimicrobial therapy began in the mid 1930s when sulfonamide drugs were introduced.[70] Their efficacy against meningococcal infection was soon proven.[72] The CFR dropped dramatically but remained significant.

Antimicrobial therapy had little effect on incidence, however, and when mobilization for World War II began, there was cause for concern. In June 1941, the newly formed Board for the Investigation and Control of Influenza and Other Epidemic Diseases in the Army (later chartered as The Armed Forces Epidemiological Board [AFEB]) established the Commission on Meningococcal Meningitis to study the incidence, treatment, and prevention of cerebrospinal meningitis.[73] Ultimately under the direction of Dr. John J. Phair and drawing on both military and civilian scientists, this commission conducted extensive research into the epidemiology of meningococcal disease. The commission concluded that the most effective way to decrease incidence was to eradicate carriage. This theory underlay the concept of mass antimicrobial prophylaxis.

The anticipated epidemic of meningococcal meningitis began in December 1942 and rose to a peak in March 1943, when incidence reached 290/100,000 troops per year in the Army. This epidemic accounted for half of the 13,922 cases that occurred during World War II. Based on the work of the Commission on Meningococcal Meningitis, the Army Surgeon General responded in September 1943 to the epidemic by directing sulfadiazine prophylaxis for concentrated troops, including those in training camps. This practice successfully controlled the epidemic. By war's end, 559 deaths were attributed to meningococcal disease, yielding a CFR of 4.0% and making it the second leading cause of infectious disease mortality, behind tuberculosis.[71,74]

After World War II, Aycock and Mueller reviewed meningococcal carriage and incidence studies conducted during the war years. They made several key observations, notably that military epidemics occur only in concert with civilian epidemics and therefore mirror US trends (Figure 2-20). This and other observations caused them to deemphasize factors such as carriage, rate of spread, and environment in favor of individual susceptibility factors. This theory underlay the concept of immuno-prophylaxis for definitive prevention.[71,75]

During the Korean War buildup, meningococcal disease epidemics did not occur in either the general US or trainee populations. Sulfadiazine prophylaxis controlled meningococcal activity at low levels. In fact, this grace period would last nearly 2 decades. Inevitably, antibiotic resistance developed. Meningitis became a serious problem at Fort Ord, Calif, beginning in 1960, 1 year after the rate in the surrounding county began increasing. The number of cases grew steadily, with the first death occurring in 1963. During 1964 there were 108 cases at Fort Ord. With public anxiety and pressure running high, recruit training was temporarily suspended

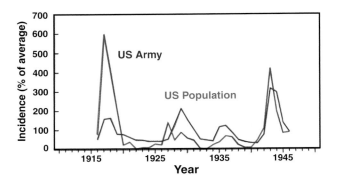

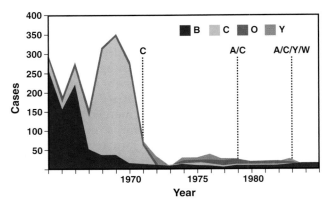

Fig. 2-20. Meningococcal meningitis incidence trends in the [continental] U.S. Army (blue line) and in the general U.S. population (red line), 1916–1946. For both groups, average incidence for the entire period is defined as 100% to facilitate direct comparison on the same graph. The actual Army incidence was approximately 7-fold higher than that of the US population. Note that military epidemics historically occur only in concert with civilian epidemics and so mirror US trends. Adapted from: Phair JJ. Meningococcal meningitis. In: Hoff EC, ed. *Communicable Diseases Transmitted Chiefly Through Respiratory and Alimentary Tracts.* Vol 4. In: *Preventive Medicine in World War II.* Washington, DC: Office of The Surgeon General, US Department of the Army; 1958: 203. Prepared by Judith Bowles.

Fig. 2-21. Cases of meningococcal disease in U.S. Army personnel, 1964–1984. Vertical lines indicate introduction of group-specific vaccines. "Group O" indicates not grouped or grouped other than B, C, or Y. The Army's vaccine development program produced dramatic results. Adapted with permission from: Brundage JF, Zollinger WD. Evolution of meningococcal disease epidemiology in the US Army. In: Vedros NA, ed. *Evolution of Meningococcal Disease.* Vol 1. Boca Raton, Fla, CRC Press; 1987: 11. Prepared by Judith Bowles.

at Fort Ord in late 1964.[76,77] Ultimately, widespread sulfadiazine resistance rendered routine prophylaxis useless and the policy was discontinued. Without effective control measures and with the Vietnam War in full swing, meningococcal disease incidence in the Army increased to a high of 350 cases and 38 deaths in 1969.[71,78]

With emphasis on meningococcal meningitis renewed by wartime mobilization, the Army Medical Department sought a definitive solution to this problem. Research efforts intensified, centered at the Walter Reed Army Institute of Research (WRAIR), and led by Dr. Malcolm Artenstein. Goldschneider, Gotschlich, and colleagues investigated the safety and immunogenicity of group A, B, and C *N meningitis* polysaccharides in humans. The WRAIR team developed a group C polysaccharide vaccine and began field testing in 1969 at Army training centers. Full-scale immunization of all Army recruits began in October 1971, albeit after the epidemic had peaked. Vaccines against groups A, Y, and W-135 were developed and tested by WRAIR during the 1970s. By late 1982, all recruits were immunized with the tetravalent meningococcal vaccine.[71,78–91]

The Army's vaccine development program produced dramatic results. Since 1973, meningococcal disease has been well controlled in the US military training base (Figure 2-21). Moreover, for the first time since statistics have been kept, meningococcal disease incidence in the trainee population has become dissociated from that in the general US popu-

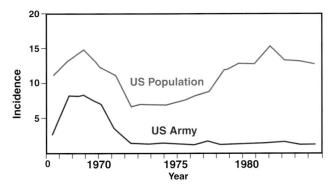

Fig. 2-22. Meningococcal disease incidence rates for the general US population (top line, cases/1 million per year) and the US Army (bottom line, cases/10,000 per year), 1967–1984. This conclusively illustrates the effectiveness of the Army's meningococcal vaccine program. Compare with Figure 2.20. Adapted with permission from: Brundage JF, Zollinger WD. Evolution of meningococcal disease epidemiology in the US Army. In: Vedros NA, ed. *Evolution of Meningococcal Disease.* Vol 1. Boca Raton, Fla, CRC Press; 1987: 13. Prepared by Judith Bowles.

lation (Figure 2-22). The effectiveness of the tetravalent vaccine is further shown by the virtual absence of groups A, C, Y, and W-135 disease in soldiers, though it still occurs in the general US population.[71]

Impact

Today, the US military training base operates with almost complete freedom from the once onerous burden of meningococcal disease. While sporadic cases occur,[92,93] they are generally due to group B, for which there is not yet an effective vaccine.[94]

Conclusion

The effort to control meningococcal disease involved a great number of people over many years, demonstrating the interplay of epidemiology, basic science, and clinical investigation in prevention. Contributions came from the general scientific community, with the Army Medical Department carrying the effort forward during mobilization periods.

The meningococcal story illustrates the great potential of immunization, as opposed to other strategies, in preventing disease in military and other populations. Short of disease eradication, an effective vaccine is generally the best possible solution, especially for military personnel.

As successful as this story seems, it is not yet over. Because of the continued difficulty in developing an effective group B vaccine, today's trainees are still at risk for meningococcal infection, particularly if a group B epidemic in the general population were to occur coincident with a military buildup. Diagnosis and treatment continue to pose a challenge; the CFR remains formidable at 5% to 15%.[68] The claim of victory must await either a total coverage vaccine or disease eradication. Lieutenant Colonel J. D. Bartley, an Army physician who studied meningococcal meningitis in the recruits at Fort Dix from 1968 to 1970, had these words to say about overconfidence:

> … the solution to the meningococcal problem seemed at hand once before, when SDZ [sulfadiazine] was introduced. Nature does not accept conquest lightly and may once again emerge the victor from apparent defeat.[78p379]

Skin Disease in the US 9th Infantry Division, Republic of Vietnam

Setting

During the summer of 1968, the US 9th Infantry Division, commanded by Major General Julian J.

Ewell, moved from its sector near Saigon to the Mekong (Nine Dragon) River delta area. Having fought in the January 1968 Tet and May 1968 Mini-Tet offensives, the 9th was in a suboptimal state of combat effectiveness due to a variety of administrative and operational factors, including unit organization, static mission, high operational tempo, and recent losses.[95,96]

Known as the "Mouth of the Dragon," the Mekong delta region is low, flat, hot, and wet. The ground averages only 2 m above sea level, with the main relief features being dikes that rise a meter or so above the rice paddies. Average daily temperatures range from a low of 24°C (75°F) to a high of 32°C (90°F), with little seasonal variation. During the rainy season, up to 90% of the area is covered by water.[95,97]

To deny the enemy respite that is so critical to guerrilla forces, the 9th employed the constant pressure concept. This tactic was highly effective in weakening the Viet Cong but demanded much field time of American units as well. Rifle companies typically spent two thirds of their time in the field, often remaining there for 5 or more continuous days. While armored personnel carriers were useful during the dry season (November through March), vehicular traffic was difficult if not impossible during the rainy season (May through October). As the dikes were often booby trapped, the infantry had to walk in the flooded paddies to maintain constant pressure (Figure 2-23).[95]

Health Issues

During French operations in Indochina from 1945 to 1954, skin disease had caused considerable morbidity and manpower degradation.[98] With an incidence of 42 admissions per 1,000 troops per year (average experience over 9 years),[99] dermatological disease was the leading cause of hospitalization. Fungal and staphylococcal infections were the most common diagnoses.[97]

During the American experience in Vietnam from 1965 to 1972, dermatological complaints were the most frequent cause of outpatient presentation, accounting for 12.2% of all visits.[97,100] Given the conditions in the Mekong delta area, it is not surprising that skin problems were even more significant in the 9th Infantry. For the 1-year period from July 1968 through June 1969, skin disease accounted for 47% of all disease and injury, including battle injury, in maneuver battalions.[95]

Typically, one third of the men went on sick call after an operation in the delta, the majority with

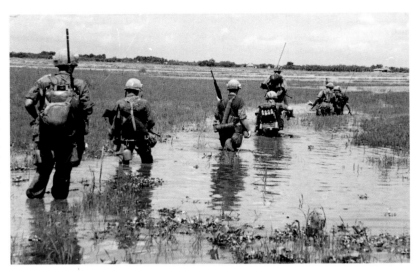

Fig. 2-23. Combat patrol entering rice paddy, Mekong River delta, Vietnam. Mission demands sent rifle companies of the 9th Infantry Division into the field, often for 5 or more continuous days. The infantrymen normally had to walk in the flooded paddies. The constant exposure to wet conditions made skin disease a major problem. Official US Army photo, Walter Reed Army Institute of Research, Silver Spring, Md.

skin complaints. The three main problems were pyoderma (bacterial infection, usually streptococcal), dermatophytosis (fungal infection), and immersion foot (tropical type).[95,97,101] Most were given light duty or quarters for an average of 4 days, but many received permanent restrictions from field duty.[97] By March 1968, many 164-man rifle companies were taking only 65 to 70 men to the field on combat operations.[95]

The epidemic of dermatological disease in the 9th occurred in part because, with only four trained US military dermatologists in-country, there was insufficient knowledge at the battalion level of prevention, diagnosis, and treatment of skin disease. The reason the epidemic went largely unnoticed was administrative. Neither medical nor personnel reports listed the number of men on restricted duty, thus neither indicated the problem.[95]

At the same time, the local population was noted to have no significant skin problems.[101,102] The rice farmers went barefoot or wore sandals in the paddies by day and allowed their feet to dry at night.[103]

A Series of Actions and Results

Dermatological disease caused great concern outside the 9th Infantry Division as well. In May 1967, the AFEB Commission on Cutaneous Diseases offered to send an expert team of dermatological consultants to Vietnam to study the problem. Noting the steady rise of dermatological disease, the US Army, Vietnam (USARV) Surgeon invited the AFEB consultants.

The team, consisting of Dr. Harvey Blank, Dr. Nardo Zaias, and Mr. David Taplin, arrived in October 1967 and spent several weeks visiting soldiers in the field, in clinics, and in hospitals. They brought a field laboratory with culture capability, which proved very useful. The team defined the various causes of dermatological morbidity and made several practical recommendations, which were implemented in USARV Medical Service Regulation 40-29 (10 January 1968).[97,100] The team submitted its final report on 24 May 1968.[73]

From November 1968 through February 1969, a field dermatology research team from WRAIR, headed by Captain Alfred M. Allen, studied dermatological conditions in soldiers and Vietnamese civilians in the 9th Division area. Its findings were similar to those of the AFEB team.[97,101,102] These and many other scientific efforts contributed significantly to the understanding of dermatological disease in Vietnam.[104-114]

In the 9th Infantry Division, Major General Ewell took several actions to address the problems. First, he defined the manpower status. Ewell's Chief of Staff, Colonel Ira A. Hunt, assembled a group of captains and majors and applied operations research techniques to problems the division faced.[115] With a goal of optimizing the number of infantrymen in the field, the group developed a "paddy strength report" that provided details on those not present for combat operations—details the morning report was missing. Through this, Ewell saw that as many as half of the men in the rifle companies were nonavailable due to skin disease.[95]

Surprised and alarmed, Ewell pursued two actions simultaneously. He sent unfit infantrymen with duty limitations to other units with garrison duty in dry areas, exchanging them for healthy soldiers. More importantly, he commissioned Operation Safe Step.[95]

Operation Safe Step was a medical research pro-

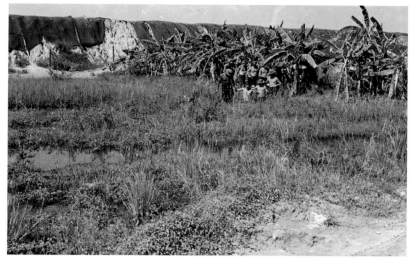

Fig. 2-24. Soldier volunteers in test paddy at Dong Tam, Vietnam during Operation Safe Step. This paddy, in a rear area, was used to test disease incidence, clothing, and various protective measures under simulated combat conditions. Small groups of soldier volunteers were rotated in and out of Dong Tam. Official US Army photo, Walter Reed Army Institute of Research Silver Spring, Md.

gram designed to control and minimize foot problems. This three-pronged effort tested various types of footgear, several protective skin ointments, and skin disease in volunteers exposed to paddy water over varying lengths of time. Two successive division surgeons, Lieutenant Colonels Travis L. Blackwell and Archibald W. McFadden, directed Operation Safe Step, in consultation with Colonel William A. Akers, US Army Medical Research Unit, Presidio of San Francisco (later Letterman Army Institute of Research). A test center was established at Dong Tam, where field trials were conducted in actual rice paddies, and used soldier volunteers (Figure 2-24) to test ointments provided by Colonel Akers and experimental footgear provided by the US Army Natick Research Laboratories. Captain Allen's field dermatology research team assisted as well. Operation Safe Step's findings encompassed etiology, prevention, treatment, and equipment and served as the basis for many decisions and policies.[95,97,104,105] McFadden also assembled data that suggested a time course relation between paddy water exposure and incidence of pyoderma, dermatophytosis, and immersion foot (Figure 2-25).[104]

Convinced by the findings, Ewell altered division tactical procedure to accommodate the health of his soldiers. On 28 October 1968, he issued an order limiting operations in paddies to 48 hours (unless pinned down by the enemy), followed by a 24-hour drying period.[95,97] With this strong command interest and the onset of the dry season, time lost to skin disease in rifle battalions dropped from well over 3,000 man-days per month to nearly 1,000 man-days per month.[97]

On a larger scale, the US Army in Vietnam fared better than the French. Over 99% of all American skin cases were handled as outpatients. Dermatological hospitalization, with incidence ranging from 19 to 33 admissions per 1,000 troops per year during the period 1965 to 1972, accounted for 7.4% of the 619,121 Army hospital admissions during the war. Skin disease was the third leading cause of hospitalization, behind diarrheal disease (12.5%) and respiratory infection (11.6%), and just ahead of malaria (7.3%).[97,116]

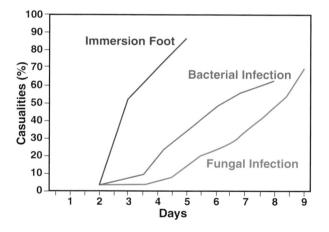

Fig. 2-25. Temporal relation between exposure to paddy water and incidence of debilitating pyoderma, dermatophytosis, and immersion foot in infantrymen. This figure was developed from data (Division Weekly Dermatology Sick Call Report Summaries, May 1968 to August 1969, and other) collected by Lieutenant Colonel Archibald W. McFadden, 9th Infantry Division Surgeon. Paddy foot: a warm water immersion foot syndrome variant. *Mil Med.* 1974;139:611. Prepared by Judith Bowles. Adapted with permission from *Military Medicine: The Official Journal of AMSUS.* Akers WA.

Impact

The knowledge gained by the AFEB, the Army Medical Department, and the 9th Infantry Division staff was translated into actions that significantly affected company-level operations. Paddy strength—the number of infantrymen available for combat operations—rose from 65 to 120 men per rifle company, enabling these units to operate effectively. While other administrative efficiencies contributed, Ewell and Hunt wrote, "This medical research effort [Operation Safe Step] proved to be the most important single factor in increasing the paddy strength of the 9th Division."[95p23]

Conclusion

The story of the 9th Infantry underscores at least three preventive medicine themes. First, surveillance data is invaluable, both in identifying problems and in pointing toward solutions. Second, medical research is not only possible but can be extremely useful, *even when units are deployed.* Finally, command emphasis is central to prevention of disease and nonbattle injury. Without it, other seemingly more pressing issues will inevitably preoccupy the junior leaders and soldiers. Like Lieutenant General Sir William Slim, Major General Ewell was an astute leader who exploited preventive medicine, as he put it, to "sharpen the combat edge."[95]

SUMMARY

While the main purpose of this chapter is to illustrate the impact of preventive medicine in war, it is possible to draw from these eight stories at least four major conclusions concerning the practice of preventive medicine in war.

There is no substitute for preparation. Consider the problems of the British in South Africa and the Americans on Attu Island, caused in part by inadequate preparation. Medical planning should begin not with force size, casualty estimates, and hospital bed projections but with medical intelligence, medical threat analysis, and preventive medicine planning.

Medical surveillance must be conducted. With an ongoing medical surveillance system, commanders and medical managers can rapidly identify medical threats and devise appropriate countermeasures. Without it they are blind to the threats until they become obvious. Generals Slim and Ewell made excellent use of medical surveillance.

Field research is often invaluable during operations. It is shortsighted to believe that field research is not important or cost-effective during wartime, even at the operational level. Many of the stories discussed in this chapter illustrate this point: the work of the Yellow Fever Commission in Cuba, the nearly complete conquest of meningococcal disease in the US training base, Adolph's desert research during World War II, and the various dermatological research efforts conducted by the US Army in Vietnam.

Preventive medicine plans need solid command support to succeed. Without continued and strong command emphasis, *including enforcement,* the tedious, mundane, and often distasteful soldier-level tasks so critical to preventive medicine will go undone. Slim's tough enforcement and dramatic results demonstrate this principle. Unfortunately, this most important lesson is perhaps most easily forgotten, because, indeed, the individual preventive medicine measures are often tedious, mundane, and distasteful.

Returning to the impact of preventive medicine in war, the examples presented here illustrate the price paid by commanders who do not pay attention to Jonathan Letterman's *leading idea,* and the rewards that accrue to those who do. Leaders who properly apply preventive medicine significantly increase their combat strength. Those who ignore it forgo this advantage at the least. At the most, when battle conditions or nature turn against them, they suffer terrible consequences.

There are many more examples that could be cited. On the negative side are Napoleon's losses to cold injury in Russia,[117,118] Hitler's making the same mistake over a century later,[119–121] and Rommel's lack of attention to field sanitation in North Africa.[122–125] On the positive side are Washington's concern for variolation and field sanitation in the Continental Army,[2,126,127] the British Army's successes with "shell shock" during World War I,[128,129] and MacArthur's actions against malaria in the Southwest Pacific in World War II.[130]

In the press of war, when tactical and operational concerns close in, men sometimes become shortsighted. The responsibility for a military force's health is shared. Commanders—who bear the ultimate responsibility—should not forget Letterman's leading idea.[1,131,132] And their medical officers should not let them.[133]

Those who cannot remember the past are condemned to repeat it.[134p284]

George Santayana (1863–1952)

REFERENCES

1. Letterman J. *Medical Recollections of the Army of the Potomac.* New York: D. Appleton & Co; 1866.

2. Bayne-Jones S. *The Evolution of Preventive Medicine in the United States Army, 1607–1939.* Washington, DC: Office of the Surgeon General, US Department of the Army; 1968: 31–33, 97–110.

3. Joy RJT. Jonathan Letterman of Jefferson. *Topic: Journal of Liberal Arts.* July 1983(Supplement):26–38.

4. James JJ, Frelin AJ, Jeffery RJ. Disease and nonbattle injury rates and military medicine. *Med Bull US Army, Europe.* 1982;39(8):17–27.

5. Garfield RM, Neugut AI. Epidemiologic analysis of warfare. *JAMA.* 1991;266:688–692.

6. Cook EL, Gordon JE. Accidental trauma. In: Hoff EC, ed. *Personal Health Measures and Immunization.* Vol 3. In: Coates JB Jr, ed. *Preventive Medicine in World War II.* Washington, DC: Office of the Surgeon General, US Department of the Army; 1955: Chap 7.

7. Farwell B. *The Great Anglo-Boer War.* New York: WW Norton & Co; 1990: 146–265.

8. Barthorpe M. *The Anglo-Boer Wars: The British and the Afrikaners, 1815–1902.* New York: Blandford Press; 1987: 100.

9. Pagaard SA. Disease and the British Army in South Africa, 1899–1900. *Mil Affairs.* 1986;50(2):71–76.

10. Leishman WB. The progress of anti-typhoid inoculation in the army. *J R Army Med Corps.* 1907;8:463–471.

11. Cope Z. *Almroth Wright: Founder of modern vaccine-therapy.* London: Thomas Nelson & Sons, Ltd; 1966: 19–30.

12. Sanitary officers in the field. *BMJ.* 1901;1(2 Mar):529–530.

13. Pakenham T. *The Boer War.* New York: Random House; 1979: 403–404, 417.

14. Conan-Doyle A. The epidemic of enteric fever at Bloemfontein. *BMJ.* 1900;2(7 Jul):49–50.

15. Bruce D. Analysis of the results of Professor Wright's method of anti-typhoid inoculation. *J R Army Med Corps.* 1905; 4:244–255.

16. Falls C. *The Great War.* New York: Putnam Pub Co; 1959. Reprinted by Easton Press, Norwalk, Conn; 1987: 22–31, 103.

17. Palmer A. *The Gardeners of Salonika.* New York: Simon and Schuster; 1965: 11–36, 66–67, 143–147.

18. McPherson WG, Herringham WP, Elliott TR, Balfour A, eds. *Medical Services: Diseases of the War.* In: *History of the Great War.* London: His Majesty's Stationery Office; 1923: 227–242.

19. McPherson WG, Horrocks WH, Beveridge WWO, eds. *Medical Services: Hygiene of the War.* Vol 2. In: *History of the Great War.* London: His Majesty's Stationery Office; 1923: 212–219.

20. Falls C. *Military Operations Macedonia: From the Outbreak of the War to the Spring of 1917.* Vol 1. In: *History of the Great War.* London: His Majesty's Stationery Office; 1933: 144, 288, 290.

21. Falls C. *Military Operations Macedonia: From the Spring of 1917 to the End of the War.* Vol 2. In: *History of the Great War.* London: His Majesty's Stationery Office; 1935: 4, 5, 58, 94, 95, 294.

22. Whayne TF, DeBakey ME. *Cold Injury, Ground Type.* Washington, DC: Office of the Surgeon General, Department of the Army; 1958: 48, 83–106, 127–142.

23. Hart BHL. *History of the Second World War.* New York: GP Putnam & Sons; 1971.

24. Bateson C. *War with Japan*. Ann Arbor: Michigan State University Press; 1968: 271.

25. Yaglou CP, Hawley WL. Disabilities due to environmental and climatic factors: cold injury. *Special Fields*. Vol 9. In: *Preventive Medicine in World War II*. Washington, DC: Office of The Surgeon General, US Department of the Army; 1969: Chap 4, Part 2.

26. Munson EL. *The Theory and Practice of Military Hygiene*. New York: William Wood Co; 1901:912-922.

27. Havard V. *Manual of Military Hygiene for the Military Services of the United States*. New York: William Wood Co; 1917: 712-718.

28. Vaughn PB. Local cold injury–menace to military operations: a review. *Mil Med*. 1980;145(3):305–311.

29. Medical and Casualty Statistics, Part 2. Vol 15. In: *The Medical Department of the US Army in the World War*. Washington, DC: Government Printing Office; 1925: 106, 146, 234.

30. Hoff EC, ed. *Personal Health Measures and Immunization*. Vol 3. In: *Preventive Medicine in World War II*. Washington, DC: Office of The Surgeon General, US Department of the Army; 1955: 63–70.

31. Risch E. *The Quartermaster Corps: Organization, Supply, and Services*. Vol 1. In: *The Technical Services*. Washington, DC: Office of the Chief of Military History, Department of the Army; 1953: 106.

32. Motter THV. *The Persian Corridor and Aid to Russia*. In: *The Middle East Theater*. In: *United States Army in World War II*. Washington, DC: Office of the Chief of Military History, US Department of the Army; 1952: 3–7.

33. Coakley RW, Leighton RM. *Global Logistics and Strategy, 1943–1945*. In: *The War Department*. In: *United States Army in World War II*. Washington, DC: Office of the Chief of Military History, US Army; 1968: 627.

34. Sams CF. The Middle East countries. In: Hoff EC, ed. *Civil Affairs/Military Government Public Health Activities*. Vol 8. In: *Preventive Medicine in World War II*. Washington, DC: Office of The Surgeon General US Department of the Army; 1976: Chap 7.

35. Yaglou CP, Hawley WL. Disabilities due to environmental and climatic factors: heat injury. *Special Fields*. Vol 9. In: *Preventive Medicine in World War II*. Washington, DC: Office of The Surgeon General, US Department of the Army; 1969: Chap 4, Part 1.

36. Whayne TF. History of Heat Trauma as a War Experience (lecture to Medical Service Officer Basic Course, 9 June 1951). Notes, Medical Service Company, Vol 2. Washington, DC: Army Medical Service Graduate School, Walter Reed Army Medical Center; 1951: Section 5, 1–38.

37. Adolph EF and Associates. *Physiology of Man in the Desert*. New York: Interscience Publishers; 1947.

38. Malamud N, Haymaker W, Custer RP. Heat stroke. *Mil Surg*. 1946;99:397–449.

39. Fregly MJ, Blatteis CM, eds. Environmental Physiology. In: *Handbook of Physiology*. Vol 1. New York: Oxford University Press; 1996: Section 4.

40. Dove M. Defense Manpower Data Center, Seaside, Calif. Personal communication, 1997.

41. Writer JV, DeFraites RF, Brundage JF. Comparative mortality among US military personnel in the Persian Gulf region and worldwide during operations desert shield and desert storm. *JAMA*. 1996;275:118–121.

42. Trask DF. *The War with Spain in 1898*. New York: Macmillan Pub Co; 1981: 1, 51–57, 162, 206, 315–326.

43. Gorgas WC. *Sanitation in Panama*. New York: D. Appleton & Co; 1915: 4–6, 50–73.

44. Truby AE. *Memoir of Walter Reed: The Yellow Fever Episode*. New York: Paul B. Hoeber, Inc; 1943: 26–42, 94–141.

45. Gorgas M, Hendrick BJ. *William Crawford Gorgas: His Life and Work.* New York: Doubleday, Page, & Co; 1924: 87, 88.

46. Reed W. The propagation of yellow fever observations based on recent researches. *Med Rec.* 1901;60(6):201–209.

47. Hagedorn H. *Leonard Wood: A Biography.* Vol 1. New York: Harper & Bros; 1931: 281.

48. Reed W, Carroll J, Agramonte A, Lazear J. The etiology of yellow fever: a preliminary note. *Philadelphia Medl J.* 1900;6(17):790–796.

49. Bean WB. *Walter Reed: A Biography.* Charlottesville, Va: University of Virginia Press; 1982: 95–134.

50. Reed W, Carroll J. A comparative study of the biological characteristics and pathogenesis of *Bacillus X* (Sternberg), *Bacillus icteroides* (Sanarelli), and the hog-cholera bacillus (Salmon and Smith). *J Exp Med.* 1900;5(3):215–270.

51. Kean JR. Walter Reed, dedication of his birthplace. *Mil Surg.* 1928;62(3):293–304.

52. Reed W. Recent researches concerning the etiology, propagation, and prevention of yellow fever, by the United States Army Commission. *J Hyg.* 1902;2(2):101–119.

53. Craig CF. The importance to the army of diseases transmitted by mosquitoes and methods for their prevention. *Mil Surg.* 1910;26(3):292–308.

54. Bayne-Jones S. Yellow fever. In: Hoff EC, ed. *Communicable Diseases.* Vol 7. In: *Preventive Medicine in World War II.* Washington, DC: Office of The Surgeon General, US Department of the Army; 1986: Chap 13.

55. Slim W. *Defeat Into Victory.* London: Cassell and Company, Ltd; 1956: 167–180, 345, 354.

56. Esposito VJ, ed. *The West Point Atlas of American Wars.* Vol 2. New York: Praeger; 1959: 127, 151.

57. Addington LH. *The Patterns of War Since the Eighteenth Century.* Bloomington, Ind: Indiana University Press; 1984: 195–206.

58. Evans G. *Slim as Military Commander.* Princeton: D. Van Nostrand Company, Inc; 1969.

59. Calvert M. *Slim.* New York: Ballantine Books; 1973.

60. Matthews GF. *The Re-conquest of Burma, 1943–1945.* Aldershot, England: Gale & Polden; 1966.

61. Great Britain, Central Office of Information. *The Campaign in Burma.* London: His Majesty's Stationery Office; 1946.

62. Mason P. *A Matter of Honor.* London: Trinity Press; 1974: 492, 510.

63. Stone JH, ed. *Crisis Fleeting.* Washington, DC: Department of the Army; 1969: 97–98.

64. Raina BL, ed. Preventive medicine. In: *Official History of the Indian Armed Forces in the Second World War 1939–45, Medical Services.* Vol 4. Kanpur, India: Combined Inter-Service Historical Section, India & Pakistan; 1961: 437.

65. Crew FAE, ed. *Administration. History of the Second World War: The Army Medical Services.* Vol 2. London: Her Majesty's Stationery Office; 1955: 186.

66. Lewin R. *Slim: The Standardbearer.* London: Leo Cooper Ltd; 1976.

67. Fraser DW, Broome CV, Wenger JD. Meningococcal meningitis. In: Diseases spread by close personal contact. In: Last JM, Wallace RB, eds. *Maxcy-Rosenau-Last Public Health & Preventive Medicine.* 13th ed. Norwalk, Conn: Appleton & Lange; 1992: Chap 7.

68. Benenson AS, ed. *Control of Communicable Diseases Manual.* 16th ed. Washington, DC: American Public Health Association; 1995: 303.

69. Simmons MC, Michie HC. Cerebrospinal meningitis. In: Siler JF, ed. *Communicable and Other Diseases*. Vol 9. In: *The Medical Department of the United States Army in the World War*. Washington, DC: Office of The Surgeon General, US Department of the Army; 1928: Chap 4.

70. Phair JJ. Meningococcal meningitis. In: Hoff EC, ed. *Communicable Diseases Transmitted Chiefly Through Respiratory and Alimentary Tracts*. Vol 4. In: *Preventive Medicine in World War II*. Washington, DC: Office of The Surgeon General, US Department of the Army; 1958: Chap 11.

71. Brundage JF, Zollinger WD. Evolution of meningococcal disease epidemiology in the U.S. Army. In: Vedros NA, ed. *Evolution of Meningococcal Disease*. Vol 1. Boca Raton, Fla, CRC Press; 1987: Chap 2.

72. Dingle JH, Thomas L, Morton AR. Treatment of meningococcic meningitis and meningococcemia with sulfadiazine. *JAMA*. 1941;116:2666–2668.

73. Woodward TE. *The Armed Forces Epidemiological Board: Its First Fifty Years*. Washington, DC: The Borden Institute, Office of The Surgeon General, US Department of the Army; 1990: 21–27, 350.

74. Daniels WB. Meningococcal infections. In: Havens PW, ed. *Infectious Diseases*. Vol 2. In: *Internal Medicine in World War II*. Washington, DC: Office of The Surgeon General, US Department of the Army; 1963: Chap 9.

75. Aycock WL, Mueller JH. Meningococcus carrier rates and meningitis incidence. *Bacteriol Rev*. 1950;14:115–160.

76. Woodward TE, ed. *The Armed Forces Epidemiological Board: The Histories of the Commissions*. Washington, DC: The Borden Institute, Office of The Surgeon General, US Department of the Army; 1994: 26–27.

77. Gauld JR, Nitz RE, Hunter DH, Rust JH, Gauld RL. Epidemiology of meningococcal meningitis at Fort Ord. *Am J Epidemiol*. 1965;82:56–72.

78. Bartley JD. Natural history of meningococcal disease in basic training at Fort Dix, N.J. *Mil Med*. 1972;137(10):373–380.

79. Goldschneider I, Gotschlich EC, Artenstein MS. Human immunity to the meningococcus, I: the role of humoral antibodies. *J Exp Med*. 1969;129(suppl 6):1307–1326.

80. Goldschneider I, Gotschlich EC, Artenstein MS. Human immunity to the meningococcus, II: development of natural immunity. *J Exp Med*. 1969;129(suppl 6):1327–1348.

81. Gotschlich EC, Liu TY, Artenstein MS. Human immunity to the meningococcus, III: preparation and immunochemical properties of group A, group B, and group C meningococcal polysaccharides. *J Exp Med*. 1969;129(suppl 6):1349–1365.

82. Gotschlich EC, Goldschneider I, Artenstein MS. Human immunity to the meningococcus, IV: immunogenicity of group A and group C meningococcal polysaccharides in human volunteers. *J Exp Med*. 1969;129(suppl 6):1367–1384.

83. Gotschlich EC, Goldschneider I, Artenstein MS. Human immunity to the meningococcus, V: the effects of immunization with meningococcal group C polysaccharide on the carrier state. *J Exp Med*. 1969;129(suppl 6):1385–1395.

84. Artenstein MS, Gold R. Current status of prophylaxis of meningococcal disease. *Mil Med*. 1970;135:735–739.

85. Artenstein MS, Gold R, Zimmerly JG, Wyle FA, Schneider H, Harkins C. Prevention of meningococcal disease by group C polysaccharide vaccine. *N Eng J Med*. 1970;282:417–420.

86. Artenstein MS, Schneider H, Tingley MD. Meningococcal infections, I: prevalence of serogroups causing disease in US Army personnel in 1964–70. *Bull WHO*. 1971;45:275–278.

87. Gold R, Artenstein MS. Meningococcal infections, II: field trial of group C meningococcal polysaccharide vaccine in 1969–1970. *Bull WHO*. 1971;45:279–282.

88. Artenstein MS, Branche WC, Zimmerly JG, Cohen RL, Tramont EC, Kasper DL, et al. Meningococcal infections, III: studies of group A polysaccharide vaccines. *Bull WHO*. 1971;45:283–286.

89. Artenstein MS. Meningococcal infections, IV: stability of group A and group C polysaccharide vaccines. *Bull WHO.* 1971;45:287–290.

90. Artenstein MS. Meningococcal infections, V: duration of polysaccharide-vaccine-induced antibody. *Bull WHO.* 1971;45:291–293.

91. Artenstein MS, Gold R, Winter PE, Smith CD. Immunoprophylaxis of meningococcal infection. *Mil Med.* 1974;139:91–95.

92. Lednar WM, Brundage JF, Boslego JW, Brandt BL, Miller RN. An outbreak of meningococcal disease in trainees at Fort Benning. Report of the Epidemiology Consultant Service to the Office of the Surgeon General, US Department of the Army. Washington, DC: Walter Reed Army Institute of Research; 1984.

93. Kelley PW, Brundage JF, Brandt BL, Miller RN. An outbreak of meningococcal disease in trainees at Fort McClellan. Report of the Epidemiology Consultant Service to the Office of the Surgeon General, US Department of the Army. Washington, DC: Walter Reed Army Institute of Research; 1984.

94. Legters LJ, Llewellyn CH. Military medicine. In: Last JM, Wallace RB, eds. *Maxcy-Rosenau-Last Public Health & Preventive Medicine.* 13th ed. Norwalk, Conn, Appleton & Lange; 1992: Chap 71.

95. Ewell JJ, Hunt IA. *Sharpening the Combat Edge.* Washington, DC: Department of the Army; 1974.

96. Elsberg J, ed. *American Military History.* Washington, DC: Center of Military History, US Army; 1989: Chap 28.

97. Allen AM. *Skin Diseases in Vietnam, 1965–72.* Vol 1. In: Ognibene AJ, ed. *Internal Medicine in Vietnam.* Washington, DC: Medical Department, US Army, Office of The Surgeon General, and Center of Military History; 1989: 8, 22–42, 108, 149–151.

98. Blanc FCJ, Armengaud M. The general medical causes of morbidity and mortality in an expeditionary force in tropical zones. *Rev Internat Serv Sante Armees.* 1959;32(Oct):515–533.

99. *General Medicine and Infectious Diseases.* Vol 2. In: Ognibene AJ and Barrett O, eds. *Internal Medicine in Vietnam.* Washington, DC: Medical Department, US Army, Office of The Surgeon General, and Center of Military History; 1982: 11.

100. James WD, ed. *Military Dermatology.* Washington, DC: Medical Department, US Army, Office of The Surgeon General; 1994: 3–4, 57–59.

101. Allen AM, Taplin D, Lowy JA, Twigg L. Skin infections in Vietnam. *Mil Med.* 1972;137:295–301.

102. Allen AM, Taplin D. Epidemic *Trichophyton mentagrophytes* infections in servicemen. *JAMA.* 1973;226:864–867.

103. Ewell JJ. Personal communication, 1996.

104. Akers WA. Paddy foot: a warm water immersion foot syndrome variant, part I: the natural disease, epidemiology. *Mil Med.* 1974;139:605–612.

105. Akers WA. Paddy foot: a warm water immersion foot syndrome variant, part II: field experiments, correlation. *Mi Med.* 1974;139:613–618.

106. Taplin D, Zaias N, Blank H. The role of temperature in tropical immersion foot syndrome. *JAMA.* 1967;202:546–549.

107. Rietschel RL, Allen AM. A method for studying the effects of protracted water exposure on human skin. *Mil Med.* 1976;141:778–780.

108. Taplin D, Zaias N. Tropical immersion foot syndrome. *Mil Med.* 1966;131:814–818.

109. Allen AM, Taplin D. Tropical immersion foot. *Lancet.* 1973;2(839):1185–1189.

110. McMillan MR, Hurwitz RM. Tropical bacterial pyoderma in Vietnam: an improved therapeutic regimen. *JAMA.* 1969;210:1734–1736.

111. Douglas JS, Eby CS. Silicone for immersion foot prophylaxis: where and how much to use. *Mil Med.* 1972;137:386–387.

112. Gilbert DN, Greenberg JH. Vietnam: preventive medicine orientation. *Mil Med.* 1967;132:769–790.

113. Allen AM, Taplin D, Twigg L. Cutaneous streptococcal infections in Vietnam. *Arch Dermatol.* 1971;104:271–280.

114. Sulzberger MB, Akers WA. Impact of skin diseases on military operations. *Arch Dermatol.* 1969;100(6):702.

115. Hunt IA. Personal communication, 1996.

116. Neel S. *Medical Support of the U.S. Army in Vietnam 1965–1970.* Washington, DC: Department of the Army; 1973: 36, 43–44.

117. Dible JH. *Napoleon's Surgeon.* London: Heinemann Medical; 1970.

118. Comite d'Histoire du Service de Sante. *Histoire de la Medecine aux Armees.* Vol 2. In: *De la Revolution francaise au conflit mondial de 1914.* Paris: Charles-Lavauzelle; 1984.

119. Clark A. *Barbarossa, The Russian-German Conflict, 1941–45.* New York: William Morrow and Company; 1965.

120. Jacobsen HA, Rohwer J, eds; Fitzgerald E trans. *Decisive Battles of World War II: the German View.* London: Andre Deutsch Ltd; 1965.

121. *The German Campaign in Russia, Planning and Operations (1940–1942).* Washington DC: US Army Center of Military History; 1988. Publication 104–21, facsimile edition.

122. Rommel E; Hart BHL, ed. *The Rommel Papers.* New York: Harcourt, Brace and Company; 1953.

123. Toppe A; Heitman H, ed. *Desert Warfare: German Experience in World War II.* Heidelberg, Germany: US Army European Command Historical Division; 1952.

124. Bellamy RF, Llewellyn CH. Preventable casualties: Rommel's flaw, Slim's edge. *Army.* 1990;40:52–56.

125. Gear HS. Hygiene aspects of the El Alamein victory, 1942. *BMJ.* 1944;March 18:383–387.

126. Blanco RL. *Physician of the American Revolution: Jonathan Potts.* New York: Garland STMP Press; 1979.

127. Freeman DS. *Leader of the Revolution.* In: *George Washington: A Biography.* Vol 4. New York: Charles Scribner's Sons; 1951: Chap 14.

128. Neurasthenia and war neuroses. In: *Medical Services, Diseases of the War.* Vol. 2. In: Macpherson WG, Herringham WP, Elliot TR, Balfour A, eds. *History of the Great War.* London: His Majesty's Stationery Office, 1923: 1–67.

129. Merskey H. Shellshock. In: Berrios GE, Freeman H, eds. *150 Years of British Psychiatry, 1841–1991.* London: Gaskell; 1991: 245–267.

130. Hart TA, Hardenbergh WA. The Southwest Pacific area. In: Coates JB, ed. *Communicable Diseases, Malaria.* Vol 6. In: *Preventive Medicine in World War II.* Washington, DC: Office of The Surgeon General, US Department of the Army; 1963: 513–580.

131. Withers BG, Erickson RL. Good doctors are not enough. *Mil Rev.* 1994;March:57–63.

132. Withers BG. Slim, Rommel, and preventive medicine. *Infantry.* 1995;85:21–22.

133. Withers BG, Erickson RL, Petruccelli BP, Hanson RK, Kadlec RP. Preventing disease and non-battle injury in deployed units. *Mil Med*. 1994;159:39–43.

134. Santayana G. *The Life of Reason or the Phases of Human Progress*. New York: Charles Scribner's Sons; 1920.

Chapter 3

THE HISTORIC ROLE OF MILITARY PREVENTIVE MEDICINE AND PUBLIC HEALTH IN US ARMIES OF OCCUPATION AND MILITARY GOVERNMENT

RALPH LOREN ERICKSON, MD, DrPH

R.L. Erickson; Lieutenant Colonel, Medical Corps, US Army; Chief, Preventive Medicine Service, Landstuhl Regional Medical Center, APO AE 09180

INTRODUCTION

Military preventive medicine personnel are well known for their vital service rendered before and during wartime operations (see chapter 2, The Historical Impact of Preventive Medicine in War), but they have also played a critical role following the defeat of the United States' adversaries. With the signing of armistices and treaties in the aftermath of wars, the United States has frequently found itself in control of foreign territories, necessitating at times the formal establishment of short-term military governments over the people of those lands.[1–3] Under such conditions, military commanders and governors have become responsible not only for the health and welfare of their troops, but also for the well-being of thousands, even millions of civilians. Within this context, the civilian counterpart to military preventive medicine—public health—has been recognized as an "integral and essential function"[4(pxiii)] of civil affairs and military government.[4,5] The pre-

ventive medicine and public health initiatives of US military governments (or the lack thereof) have historically been directly linked to the good (or poor) health of US occupying forces.[6,7] In fact, the case was made strongly at the close of World War II that since they are identical in their aims, "preventive medicine for troops and public health for civilians who become wards of the army" should become combined into one organization.[8(p5)] In addition to fulfilling humanitarian requirements and international law obligations, the establishment or restoration and preservation of civilian public health infrastructure following war has been found to enhance the legitimacy of and local support for the occupying force.[9,10] While not an exhaustive review of the subject, this chapter will discuss the evolving role of preventive medicine and public health in military government following four of the United States' major wars.

THE MEXICAN WAR

The United States' first large-scale experience with military government is traced to General Winfield Scott and his declaration of martial law in Tampico, Vera Cruz, Puebla, and Mexico City during and at the conclusion of the Mexican War (1846–1848).[11] The public relations success of his administration was rooted in firm but fair regulations, which ultimately encouraged the people to oppose the Mexican president, General Santa Anna.[1] Unfortunately, from a preventive medicine and public health standpoint, General Scott's military government was rather impotent in the face of rampant disease in these communities and among his own troops.

Vera Cruz, the primary port city on the Gulf of Mexico occupied by Scott's troops, was well known as an extremely unhealthy place. Backing onto a large stagnant swamp, the city had been so wracked for centuries by malaria, yellow fever, and dysentery that the Spanish could hardly maintain a garrison there. Lieutenant (later General) Isaac Stevens wrote:

> Vera Cruz is a miserable, dirty place; the streets are full of filth....The filth and nastiness are almost beyond belief, our authorities are now making every effort to clean the city.[12(p443)]

Colonel Hitchcock, the Army's inspector general, wrote in his diary: "Have moved my tent to the

suburbs, in preference to being in the city, which is very offensive and soon become sickly."[12(p443)] (Interestingly, one of the American officers who contracted yellow fever at Vera Cruz, Lieutenant Josiah Gorgas, was the father of William Crawford Gorgas, whose public health successes are discussed later in this chapter.[13]) Mexico City, which was entered by US forces on September 14, 1847, was also described as "exceedingly filthy,"[14(p298)] with human excrement on the open street. Sewage and adjacent bodies of water made ideal breeding sites for mosquitoes.[12]

At the encouragement of his medical advisors (particularly Surgeon General Thomas Lawson), General Scott directed that the following public health actions be taken in the towns and cities he controlled: the restoration of water supplies and sanitary facilities, the removal of waste and debris, the burial of dead bodies, and the inspection of food.[15] It is not at all clear what impact these efforts had on the health of the civilian populace and the occupying troops. General Scott's army suffered terribly while in Mexico, with an annual disease death rate of more than 10%. The physicians accompanying the US Army at this time had little idea how to prevent or control the epidemics of malaria, yellow fever, and dysentery, which would ultimately kill more than 2,600 US soldiers. In addition to lacking the requisite knowledge about the underlying causes and transmission of these diseases, the physicians also held no rank or authority within the army they served.[12] After the signing of the Treaty of Guadalupe Hidalgo (February 2, 1848) and the election of a new Mexican government, US forces withdrew from Mexico City in June 1848, thus ending the United States' first foray into military government with its accompanying public health responsibilities.[15]

THE SPANISH–AMERICAN WAR

Although martial law was declared in certain US cities during the American Civil War (eg, New Orleans[15]), the military did not engage again in large-scale military government with its requisite civil public health activities until after the Spanish–American War. In the Treaty of Paris, signed December 10, 1898, Spain renounced its claim to Cuba, ceded Guam and Puerto Rico, and transferred sovereignty over the Philippines (for $20 million) to the United States. Under the newly established military governments of these conquered territories, military physicians and sanitarians would take the lead in bringing these new US possessions up to 20th century public health standards to help the inhabitants and protect the US soldiers and sailors stationed there.

Impoverished and disease-ridden, these tropical lands presented enormous public health challenges to the occupying forces. Unlike their military predecessors at the end of the Mexican War, however, the military medical professionals of this era knew much more about the microbial origin of infectious disease. Typhoid fever and cholera, for example, were known to be waterborne and transmitted in human excreta. Public health reformers and veterans of the US sanitation movement had seen mortality rates drop dramatically in major US cities with the installation of city sewers and the provision of safe drinking water. Military medical boards commissioned to investigate tropical diseases in these occupied territories would further advance this new "science" of preventive medicine, especially in understanding the transmission and control of lethal diseases such as yellow fever.[16]

Cuba

With the Spanish Caribbean Fleet destroyed, the city of Santiago, Cuba, surrendered to General William Shafter on July 17, 1898. Brigadier General Leonard Wood, United States Volunteers, Commander of the Department of Santiago, reported from the newly captured city that

> the conditions in and about the City of Santiago were serious in the extreme. [People] were dying at the rate of 180 per day. The city was full of sick

people, there being hardly a house which did not contain one or more persons suffering from disease. The water main, which had been partially destroyed during the siege, had not been placed in complete repair, and there was a great shortage of water.[17(p171)]

General Wood ordered an immediate sanitary cleanup of the city. In the first 2 months alone, more than 1,100 animal and human bodies and 200 loads of trash per day were removed from the streets of the city. His people also started work on preparing a modern sewage system for the city. The mortality rate within the city dropped by 64% in the first 3 weeks of the cleanup(. Ironically, at this same time the "victorious" V Corps, rendered ineffective by yellow fever and malaria, was being shipped home, soon to be replaced by fresh troops. The addition of new, "non-immune" troops from the United States for occupation duty promised real problems for US military leaders. A smallpox epidemic that struck Santiago in the fall of 1898 was met with vigor by General Wood, who dispatched his 100 sanitary workers to disinfect buildings while his medical officers immunized 30,000 people[17,18] (Figure 3-1).

Sanitary conditions were bad throughout Cuba. Parts of Havana, in particular, were said to resemble "an outdoor cesspool" due the numerous dead animals, ubiquitous garbage, and open sewers.[19] From the city of Trinidad, Major Lewis Balch, Brigade Surgeon, US Volunteers, made the following recommendations:

> To insure the health of the troops in this province, necessary sanitary work should be done quickly….The camps are near towns. Disease is to be feared from these towns, not from the country or mountainous districts. It is therefore, just as necessary that sanitary measures for prevention, the cleaning of streets, garbage collection, disinfection, reports of contagious disease, its location and character, the isolation of infected persons or things, and such like measures be taken, as it is to have camps pitched in healthy localities and properly policed….[17(p167)]

He went on to suggest that an engineer and a medical officer familiar with sanitation issues decide the necessary steps. His recommendations were put into action.

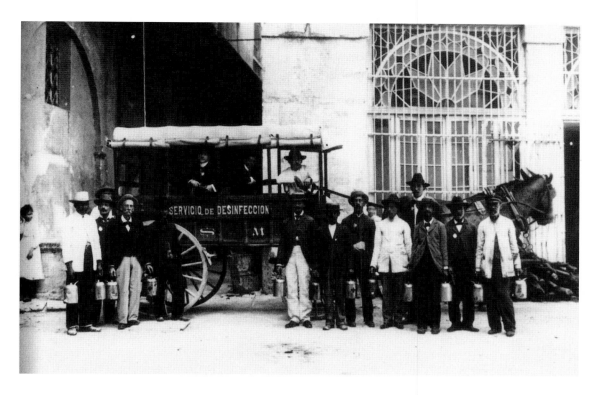

Fig. 3-1. The sanitary cleanup of Cuba under General Leonard Wood and the breakthrough discoveries of the Walter Reed Yellow Fever Commission resulted in a transformation of the island from its "cesspool" reputation to a place safe and healthy for both civilians and US troops. Pictured here is a team of public health workers responsible for disinfecting homes and public buildings. Photograph: Courtesy of the National Museum of Health and Medicine, Armed Forces Institute of Pathology, Catalog No. NCP 1734.

Military medical historian Mary Gillett has observed that the Army really had no choice but to clean up the civilian towns:

> The proximity of troops to Cuban communities made the problems involved in preventing disease among the troops and in the civilian community interdependent. Because local authorities in the impoverished nation did not have the resources needed to conduct a thorough cleanup and disinfection of Cuban towns, "reclaiming towns from their present unsanitary condition" became the responsibility of the military government of the island.[20(p232)]

Once he took over as the Military Governor of all of Cuba in December 1899, General Wood provided renewed vigor to an island-wide sanitation campaign begun by his predecessor, General Brooke. Not having to gather public support as the sanitation reformers had to in the United States, the military commanders of the different administrative departments of Cuba mounted their campaigns with military precision. However, those who incor-

rectly believed yellow fever to be a "filth disease" were dumbfounded when the disease struck the "disinfected" island in mid-1899. Through 1900, the yellow fever epidemic would claim 300 lives from both the civilian and military populations of the island, prompting Army Surgeon General George Sternberg to appoint what would be called the Yellow Fever Commission, chaired by Major Walter Reed.[15,21,22]

By 1901 the commission confirmed Carlos Findlay's theory that the disease was transmitted by mosquito and not by filth or fomites.[23,24] Armed with this information, General Wood gave his full support to Major Gorgas' anti–yellow fever campaign, which would focus primarily on eliminating the *Aedes aegypti* mosquito.[15,24,25] In addition, steps were taken to isolate yellow fever patients from mosquitoes to prevent any further transmission. Within 3 months, yellow fever had disappeared from Havana.[23,24] A similar campaign against *Anopheles* mosquitoes was subsequently mounted and given credit for reducing Havana's malaria rate 75% by 1902, the year the United States ended its occupation of Cuba.[16,17,25,26] As the US occupation ended, General Wood appointed Cuban civilians to run the government and named a five-member board of public health for the island. Major Gorgas remained in Cuba as the "District Surgeon for troops."[20(p250)] Following civil unrest, US forces again governed the island from 1906 through 1910 during which time sanitation and public health programs again became the responsibility of the US military.[27–31]

Puerto Rico

Health conditions in Puerto Rico in 1898 were comparable with those of Cuba. The US Army's sanitary cleanup of the island included disinfecting homes, rehabilitating the city's water system, and immunizing more than 800,000 citizens against smallpox, which was epidemic at the time. Major John van R. Hoff established a board of health in 1899 to oversee public health for the island and to write its first sanitary code.[17,32] A major hurricane hit the island on August 8, 1899, destroying many buildings, including barracks and hospitals. The devastating impact on the island's agricultural economy placed many at risk for starvation and led to a million-dollar relief program run by the military: "From Sept 16, 1899, to Jan 22, 1900, the average number of destitute people fed each day was reported as 182,195."[21(p189)] It was during this relief program that Lieutenant Bailey K. Ashford discovered that all of the inhabitants were severely anemic. Later he would reach near-hero status for leading an island-wide campaign to eradicate hookworm, the cause of the anemia.[33–35] Military government in Puerto Rico formally ended in 1900 with the election of a civilian government, yet US military involvement in Puerto Rican public health matters would continue until after World War II.[36]

The Philippines

Commodore George Dewey led a US naval squadron into Manila Bay on May 1, 1898, and quickly destroyed the anchored Spanish fleet. By August 1898, US soldiers occupied the city of Manila. The sanitary conditions found by US troops in the towns and villages of the Philippines were described as "execrable." "Filth of all kinds underlay and surround the houses, and the hogs were the only scavengers."[21(p98)] Sources of drinking water, commonly shallow wells, were highly contaminated. The city of Manila, in particular, got its drinking water from the Pasig River, in which 20,000 inhabitants bathed, defecated, and dumped dead bodies. Years of poverty, overcrowding, and malnutrition favored the spread of numerous infectious diseases. Spanish records from before the US occupation revealed a death rate some 50% above that of major US cities.[37] A large US troop presence was necessary, though, because after years of fighting the Spanish, Filipino guerrillas now challenged their new colonial master, the United States.[38]

Within the first month of occupation (September 1898), the military government formally organized a Municipal and Marine Board of Health for the Manila area. This board, which established a set of sanitary and quarantine regulations, was composed of six US Army Medical Corps officers (active members) and two Filipino doctors (honorary members). The board divided the city into 10 districts, with a Filipino physician assigned to each one.[39] Individuals from the community were then trained and made responsible for conducting regular house-to-house sanitary inspections and levying fines on those who violated sanitary regulations.[23] Colonel Charles R. Greenleaf reported that by 1900 this Board of Health had

> …made great progress in cleaning the streets of the city, in removing filth that has been accumulating for years, and in regulating, to a certain extent, the purity of the food supply; it has practically stamped out smallpox by forcible vaccination and revaccination, where it was necessary, and has held in check the progress of bubonic plague.[21(p99)]

Within 1 year, 2 million homes were inspected or reinspected.[23]

During the Philippine cholera epidemic of 1902 to 1904, the Board of Health closed all of the city's shallow wells, digging new ones to a depth of 700 to 1,000 ft. In an effort to protect the river, some public latrines and laundries were established along the Pasig. The sale of fruits and vegetables that could be eaten raw was prohibited, and the entire city was placed under quarantine. Unfortunately, these public health efforts did not reach beyond the city into the rural provinces. During this 2-year epidemic, cholera claimed at least 109,461 lives, 305 of whom were US soldiers.[40]

Two military tropical disease boards for research operated out of the city of Manila from 1899 to 1902 and 1906 to 1914, primarily studying dysentery, dengue, plague, beri beri, cholera, and yaws.[41] Epizootics of rinderpest and surra decimated the islands' livestock in the first few years of occupation, killing 90% of cattle and water buffalo and 60% to

75% of horses and ponies. A serum development and immunization campaign mounted by the Tropical Disease Board dropped the death rate of large animals to just 3% by 1903, perhaps saving the economy of the Philippines.[42–44]

After 1904, the Board of Health was replaced by the Bureau of Health with a US Public Health Service doctor as director.[39] Thereafter, the military's role in public health diminished as civilian responsibility increased.

WORLD WAR I

Less than 20 years later and under very different circumstances, US military preventive medicine personnel would play a key role in the occupation of a defeated Germany.[45] In compliance with the terms of the armistice signed on November 11, 1918, Germany turned over to Allied armies all occupied regions, Alsace-Lorraine, the west bank of the Rhine (the Rhineland), and the bridgeheads of Mainz and Coblenz. The newly formed, 8-division, 260,000-man US 3rd Army occupied and governed parts of the Luxembourg and the Rhineland from Trier to Coblenz.[46]

Having just 3 weeks to prepare for this mission, the 3rd Army was fortunate in that it faced a generally cooperative population of nearly 1 million. No destruction had preceded the occupation, and there were no serious shortages of civilian supplies. At the request of General Pershing, civilian officials continued to serve in their original capacities.[15] US Army medical officers (generally division surgeons) were given supervisory and disease reporting responsibilities for the administrative districts (*Kreise*) that corresponded to their division's geographic location. In addition to evaluating the general conditions of sanitation within each *Kreis*, a US Army sanitary officer from the Office of Civil Affairs specifically supervised each civilian district health officer (*Kreisarzt*) in the performance of his duty.[16]

The considerable movement of people during and after the war, coupled with a lack of laboratory supplies, had hurt the German government's established anti–typhoid fever program. Interested in reviving this disease-control effort, US medical personnel conducted a bacteriological survey to determine the carrier rate in the civilian population. German physicians and medical laboratories were also surveyed concerning the incidence of disease in the zone of occupation.[47] During the winter of 1918 to 1919, a seriously contaminated well led to an outbreak of typhoid fever in the town of Brück. When the *Kreisarzt* appeared to be unable (or unwilling) to stop public use of this well, US authorities took charge and shut down the well and removed its pump. This was followed by a US-sponsored typhoid fever vaccination program for the community. A similar typhoid fever outbreak in the town

of Altenahr required the same interventions, with the local *Kreisarzt* being fired and replaced by a competent German physician.[48]

German-speaking US Army nurses took the lead in the city of Trier, visiting the homes of more than 1,000 families to determine the effects of the German government's war food ration on the health of the people. In this population-based health and nutrition survey, they reported that

> the amount of sickness was striking. In three-fourths [of the homes] some member was sick. Scrofula and rickets [were] very common in children; pulmonary tuberculosis and influenza in adults.[49(p421)]

American medical personnel were also instrumental in providing aid to allied prisoners of war in German hands. Prior to repatriation, US preventive medicine personnel supervised German-run prisoner-of-war camps. These camps contained more than 45,000 men at the time that the Inter-Allied Commission took control. The original sanitary condition of all of these camps was "frightful." "Words can give only a slight idea of the filth and dirt in which these Russians lived."[50(p125)] From March to August 1919, there were 485 deaths from tuberculosis. Many of the Russian prisoners also suffered from trachoma. In response to these deplorable conditions, US Army medical officers employed Russian sanitary squads in a general cleanup campaign in all of the camps. Given the large number of men under these conditions, the occurrence of epidemic diseases in the camps was remarkably low. Only one case of smallpox was reported and six cases of diphtheria, but 45 deaths were attributed to influenza. At least 164 inmates had typhus; 17 of them died. German sanitary squads, under US supervision, deloused camp inmates. US Army Medical Corps officers even accompanied the Russians, Romanians, and Serbians on their repatriation trek back to their homelands.[50]

With the signing of the Treaty of Versailles on June 28, 1919, the American 3rd Army was inactivated and the majority of US forces sent home. About 8,000 US troops stayed behind for occupation duty as the American Forces Germany (later the American Department of the Inter-Allied Rhineland Commission).[16] Lieutenant Colonel Walter Bensel, MC, (and his successors: Major Morrison C. Stayer, MC, and Major Thomas J. Flynn, MC) organized and led the Department of Sanitation and Public Health for the American area of occupation. Continuing to exercise control of public health programs through German channels to the various *Kreisarzte*, these preventive medicine officers orchestrated the sanitation inspections of German prisons, hospitals, public bathing establishments, barber shops, cafes, hotels, theaters, cinemas, and slaughterhouses. In addition they established and enforced a civilian medical surveillance reporting system for contagious diseases, deaths, and births. Through their efforts in 1920 alone, they tracked and responded to epidemics of influenza (474 cases), paratyphoid (117 cases), and measles

(145 cases). Tuberculosis continued to be a problem for the pubic, given overcrowding and poor ventilation in many German homes. The prevalence of tuberculosis was estimated by survey at 2.2 per 1,000 (6.5 per 1,000 in Coblenz). With the revocation of antifraternization restrictions in September 1919, sexually transmitted disease rates among US soldiers saw a sharp increase to 422.65 per 1,000 annually (October 1919), necessitating the establishment of a court for vagrants (including prostitutes) with subsequent detention and treatment of those women found to be infected. American parentage was also alleged in over one-third of the illegitimate births in 1920 (411 of 1,134) occurring in the American area, especially in Kreis Mayen, where soldiers were billeted with private families instead of in barracks.[51] American forces formally ended their occupation of German soil on January 27, 1923.[15]

WORLD WAR II

With the fall of France to the German Army in June 1940, it became clear to the US military leadership that it was just a matter of time before the United States entered the war. By this date Lieutenant Colonel (later Brigadier General) James S. Simmons, chief of preventive medicine in the Army Surgeon General's Office, had already recruited professionals from civilian health positions to help him plan for the expected civil public health activities that would accompany and follow war in Europe. By late June, they had already submitted to the Army Surgeon General a plan for public health administration in occupied countries. The newly formed Medical Intelligence Division of the Preventive Medicine Service further provided essential medical and sanitary data on foreign countries for use in civil affairs training and planning.[10]

Even with this preparation, the vastness and complexity of Army civil public health activities throughout Europe and the Pacific at the close of World War II would prove to be a tremendous challenge. With the defeat and surrender of the Axis Powers in 1945, a relatively small cadre of US Army medical and sanitary officers had to help reestablish public health services for over 300 million people worldwide[7,52]:

> It is estimated that the number of our military government public health officers in World War II, including replacements, never exceeded about 700, of whom some 50 served in North Africa, Sicily and Italy, 175 in Germany and Austria, about 425... in the Philippines, Japan and Korea, and the re-

mainder in various other occupied and liberated areas from Norway to the Ryukyus. Added to this light brigade of 700 officers were about as many enlisted men of technician grade, some of whom performed highly responsible duties....about 1/3 of these 700 military government public health workers were medical officers...the remainder consisted of sanitary engineers and sanitarians, entomologists and parasitologists, bacteriologists and nutritionists, a few veterinarians and nurses, and other specialists...[52(p260)]

Although it would evolve and change names and organizational structure from 1943 to 1945, the Allied Military Government of Occupied Territory was activated by General Eisenhower in North Africa in May 1943. Its Public Health Division ultimately served only as an advisory, policy-making, information-providing agency with no direct control over public health operations in the field. These missions were instead handled by the medical and sanitary officers assigned to military government units by the Medical Regiment of the European Civil Affairs Division.[52,53] (Military government in the Pacific was organized and functioned somewhat differently and is described in the section on Japan.)

Italy

The military occupation was established in Italy while the war effort was still very active in Europe. This made it crucial to deal with the circumstances that were hindering the war effort. The unconditional surrender of Italy on September 8, 1943, placed the southern portion of the peninsula in Allied hands. Faulty intelligence reports had led military government planners to expect that the Italians would be self-sufficient, but the Allies soon found themselves in the midst of a major civilian relief effort, which greatly slowed the progress of military operations. Three immediate public health emergencies faced the people of southern Italy in the fall and winter months of 1943 into 1944: (1) poor harvests in Sicily and southern Italy, coupled with the retreating Nazis' scorched-earth policy, left the people near starvation, (2) the return of sick Italian soldiers from the Russian front a few months before the Allies arrived had "seeded" the lice-infested, overcrowded cities with typhus, and (3) at the encouragement of the retreating German Army, hundreds of thousands of displaced civilians streamed southward into the Allied-occupied area seeking food and shelter.[54,55]

A report from the city of Naples on the day after it was captured describes the situation:

> Medical supplies reported short. Number of doctors apparently adequate. Food situation serious. Reported that Germans took all stocks of food. Water situation acute. Viaduct and some of the reservoirs blown up, but 15 days supply of water on rationed basis available for present population....All transportation including electric trolley busses were taken by Germans. All industrial plants, warehouses and hotels reported destroyed. It was estimated 600,000 persons remained in city.[56(p240)]

The shortage of food, destruction of housing, overcrowding, loss of clean water and waste disposal, and social disruption all contributed to various infectious disease epidemics in the region. More than 12,000 people lived on a semipermanent basis in the deep tunnels and cellars (*ricoveros*) that had served as Naples' air raid shelters. Typhus proved to be a particular concern in the Naples area, jumping from 25 cases in October 1943 to more than 1,000 in January 1944.[55]

Unfortunately, a "multiplicity of commands"[55(p311)] and administrative confusion about who was responsible for the civilian crises resulted in a delayed Allied response. In December 1943, General Eisenhower provided the proper command emphasis to get adequate food relief flowing:

> It should be understood that our requisitions for food are not based on humanitarian or any other factor but that of military necessity. Conditions in

Southern Italy and Sicily are such that unless reasonable quantities of food are supplied very promptly, we will experience sabotage, unrest, and a complete cessation of all those activities considered necessary to our advance.[56(p315)]

Not waiting for a military response to the spreading typhus epidemic, Dr. Fred L. Soper and his colleagues from the International Health Division of the Rockefeller Foundation began a block-dusting effort in Naples with newly available DDT (dichloro-diphenyl-trichloroethane).[57] Having realized the potential threat to military personnel of such an outbreak, Brigadier General Leon A. Fox of the Typhus Commission, which had been established in 1942 to study typhus and devise methods to control it, took over the effort. He instituted a comprehensive, four-point campaign[56]:

1. Mass delousing of population of Naples,
2. Organization of a complete case-finding service with the cooperation of Italian-speaking physicians and priests,
3. Disinfection of contacts (at home and place of work), and
4. Immunization of key personnel (eg, hospital staffs, police, priests).

More than 1.5 million people were dusted with 5% DDT in talcum powder; special emphasis was given to those in air raid shelters and refugee camps. By February 1944, the epidemic was under control.[55] (American troops in Europe had already been immunized with the Cox-type typhus vaccine.[58]) In addition to the typhus situation, sexually transmitted diseases, smallpox, and malaria were also large problems that required aggressive control measures.[6,55]

An eruption of Mount Vesuvius (March 18–24, 1944) prompted the Allied Military Government and the American Red Cross to evacuate, feed, and shelter some 20,000 people from the towns in the vicinity of the volcano.[59] By the spring of 1944, the US 5th Army was daily feeding approximately 200,000 people. To the greatest extent possible, Italian Communal Public Assistance Boards (where they still existed) and Italian relief agencies were encouraged to take the lead in these areas, with the Allies providing supervision only.[56]

Germany

In the months immediately before the surrender of Germany, Allied leaders were given a glimpse of what to expect once the Third Reich finally collapsed:

> In recent months hundreds of thousands of displaced persons, refugees, and prisoners of war have been found, many in a pitiable state of nutrition and health, as a disorganized mass movement of huge proportions has taken place in eastern Germany.[58(p113)]

One report from the US 3rd Army in February 1945 stated:

> A great difficulty presents itself in that there are little or no medical facilities in some areas....There are no doctors, no hospitals, no medical supplies, no ambulances—a complete medical vacuum.[58(p113)]

When Germany did finally surrender on May 8, 1945, the nation was in chaos. Civil government, and with it the German public health system, had ceased to exist with the flight of Nazi officials. Thousands of Germans were homeless. Millions of foreign nationals who had been brought as slave labor to the industrial areas of the Third Reich were now displaced persons. Food stocks were almost totally exhausted in the cities. Little transportation existed.[60]

In the short term, US Military Government units were directed to "[assist] in the protection of our military forces and [prevent] unrest among Germans by the wise use of medical resources and the reestablishment of an adequate German public health service."[61(p943)] The ultimate objectives would be

> to insure that German health services and facilities were reestablished and maintained by the Germans, to prevent and control communicable diseases, and to eliminate health hazards that might interfere with the military administration of Germany, threaten occupation forces, or create hazards to other countries.[60(p496)]

Nutrition

Ascertaining the nutritional status of an entire population through scientific survey methods proved to be of enormous value to military public health planners of emergency feeding programs in Germany,[62] as well as Austria, Italy, and the Far East. The first US nutrition survey teams to reach the major cities of Holland (before the fall of Germany), for example, found a very thin and hungry people, who had suffered an average weight loss of 25 lbs. "Extreme emaciation and cachexia were common."[63(p138)] With the occupation of Germany, continuous appraisals and recommendations from the American nutrition survey teams were made

> in terms of minimal requirements for the prevention of disease, maintenance of reasonable standards of health, the maintenance of output of essential work, and the prevention of civil unrest which might be prejudicial to the occupying force.[64(p48)]

Readjustments in the international food commitment policy and a decrease in the amount of food available for distribution resulted in a ration cut in April 1946 and demonstrated just how precarious these "minimum requirements" were. The average body weights for adult men and women, which were already below the US standard, declined significantly within 30 days.

> In May 1946 serious malnutrition existed in Germany. Children could not grow properly, essential work could not be performed, and the aged and many other normal consumers were faced with starvation unless more food became available.[64(p51)]

Monthly street weighings of the civilian population showed that the low point in average adult body weight came in the second quarter of 1947. By January 1949, feeding programs had made such progress in restoring body weight that street weighings were discontinued.[65]

Infectious Diseases

German cities such as Cologne had been destroyed by extensive bombing and shelling. Water mains and sewer pipes 20 ft below the surface were ripped open in some of the strategic bombing.[66,67] During the harsh winter of 1945 to 1946, people found themselves severely crowded in the buildings that remained. In some cities, they had "as little as 28 square feet of floor space per person—just sufficient to permit a person to lie down."[68(p143)] Public health authorities were acutely aware of the transmission of respiratory diseases under these conditions. A lack of adequate housing still remained as a grave threat to the public's health as late as 1949.[61] War damage to the water and sewer systems resulted in epidemics of typhoid fever and dysentery through 1947, though the situation improved with the emergency use of chlorination.

Typhus, which was thought to have killed over 3 million people in the Balkans and Ukraine during and after World War I, had been introduced to Germany from the east by returning soldiers, forced laborers, and transports to concentration camps.[69] Heavily seeded with infection, the Rhineland was the site of explosive outbreaks in the spring of 1945. Many of the methods used in Italy worked in Germany: finding and isolating cases and mass delousing with DDT powder.[60] Over 15,800 cases of typhus from 518 locations were reported east of the Rhine river from March to June 1945. To protect Allied countries west of the Rhine, the Supreme Headquarters, Allied Expeditionary Force erected a *cordon sanitaire* for typhus control measures at all river crossings, entraining points, and airfields. (This tactic was also used successfully in Vienna to stop an epidemic of typhus there.[70]) All civilians and liberated prisoners of war travelling east to west were deloused at these points and given an endorsement on their identification papers. Individuals suspected of being sick with typhus were observed until diagnosed and given appropriate disposition. Personnel frequently exposed to typhus were immunized. By mid-July 1945, typhus was under control.[60]

Displaced Persons

As of October 1943, it was estimated that there were 21 million displaced persons (DPs) in Europe, mainly in Germany or in territory annexed by the Reich.[69] Ultimately, there would be 4.2 million DPs in the American occupation zone. Early in the occupation of Germany west of the Rhine, even before surrender, Military Government Public Health Officers supervised sanitation in the DP and refugee camps, while coordinating public health measures and communicable disease control activities (Figure 3-2). During the Allied period of rapid advance east of the Rhine, 50,000 combat and support troops of the 6th and 12th Army Groups became involved by necessity in the care, control, and repatriation of 4 million DPs.[60]

None of this prepared Allied personnel for the horror they would find in the numerous Nazi concentration camps. Among the atrocities found were human experimentation, forced labor, starvation, crowded unsanitary living conditions, and rampant disease. It is estimated that between 18 million and

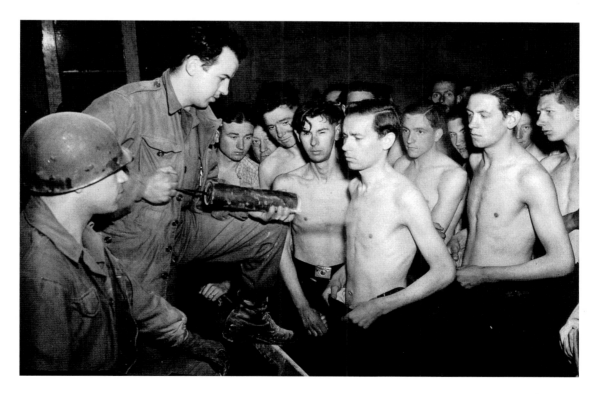

Fig. 3-2. In the aftermath of World War II, Europe held more than 21 million displaced persons, many of whom carried infectious diseases with them as they sought to return to their homes. Here Dutch refugees receive DDT dusting to kill the lice that transmit typhus. Photograph: Courtesy of the National Museum of Health and Medicine, Armed Forces Institute of Pathology, Catalog No. NCP 1965.

26 million people died in these camps from 1939 to 1945.[71] Public health and medical officers from the Military Government played a key role in trying to save and care for hundreds of thousands of inmates found still alive. In response to the extreme state of advanced starvation among the inmates, these officers mounted an emergency feeding program, which included intravenous feeding for those who were no longer able to take food by mouth.[60] More than half of the concentration camp inmates suffered from advanced tuberculosis. Typhoid fever and dysentery were widespread.[60,72] Typhus was rampant among the inmates, while louse infestation was universal; it was thought that the typhus epidemics in Austria were started by inmates. (It was at Bergen-Belsen that Anne Frank and her sister died of typhus, a matter of weeks before the camp was liberated.[73]) As in Italy, the American Typhus Commission took charge and brought the epidemic under control.[74] Since many inmates were too weak to move, the Allies found themselves operating the camps until the inmates were adequately restored to health.[60]

Local Involvement

From the start, Military Government policy made civil government (including public health) in Germany a civilian responsibility. This decision was made with the knowledge that German civil authorities would need a considerable amount of help. Military Government officials hoped to move as quickly as possible from operational control of civilian public health programs to a more advisory or supervisory role. Civil public health officers of the Military Government were expected to

> appraise a given situation, outline a few clear and practical objectives, organize and direct local health and medical personnel, and assist in obtaining medical supplies essential to the program. Except under unusual circumstances, for a public health officer to attempt to treat patients or to operate a clinic would be a misdirection of energy.[9(p132)]

Denazification of the German health care system was said to have

> removed nearly 95% of the experienced public health officers, nearly 85% of hospital staff personnel, and, in some areas, more than 50% of the doctors from private practice.[68(p143)]

Nonetheless, the German civilian public health system was gradually restored to reflect the same general objectives and procedures found in federal, state, municipal, and local public health departments in the United States. After 4 years of occupation and with a staff of 13 (down from the original 177 in 1945), Lieutenant Colonel Walter R. deForest, who was responsible for public health, wrote:

> Constantly until January 1948, it seemed as if we were just one step ahead of disaster. By that date the German State Public Health Departments were functioning satisfactorily in the United States Zone.[65(p32)]

Free elections in the combined French, British, and American zones in 1949 resulted in the recognition of the new nation, the Federal Republic of Germany, and the formal end of military government.

Okinawa, Japan, and Korea

Okinawa

In preparing for the invasion of Okinawa, US military government planners made the most of the lessons learned in Europe. The primary goal of Military Government during the combat phase would be to keep civilians out of the way of US fighting units. Priority would be given to preventing those diseases and conditions that might endanger the health of occupying troops. Unlike in Europe, civil affairs (CA) and Military Government would involve Navy as well as Army personnel. A full description of the CA units and Military Government on Okinawa can be found elsewhere.[75] The Allied attack on Okinawa commenced on April 1, 1945. By April 30th, 125,000 civilians were in refugee camps run by the Military Government. Compared with the Okinawans who had taken refuge in hillside caves and had a high incidence of impetigo, scabies, lice infestation, and pulmonary tuberculosis,[75] the health of the people in these camps was good. Strict preventive medicine measures in the camps and an educational program emphasizing personal hygiene and sanitation are credited with preventing serious epidemics.

The campaign for Okinawa officially ended July 2, 1945 after an enormous loss of life on both sides (12,000 Americans and more than 100,000 Japanese killed). Military Government officers made maximum use of Okinawan medical personnel and facilities to provide for the public health needs of the Okinawans. In 1952, Military Government was transformed into a civil administration with the creation of the Government of the Ryukyu Islands. For years thereafter, military preventive medicine and civilian public health activities were closely coordinated.[76,77] Okinawa was fully restored to Japan in 1972.

Japan

Japan's surrender on August 10, 1945, meant that US forces proceeded unopposed in their occupation of the main islands. A Public Health and Welfare Section, under the direction of Brigadier General Crawford F. Sams, MC, was established.[78] This section was organized "similar to that of any large modern state or territorial health department."[79(p634)] As Supreme Commander for the Allied Powers (SCAP), General MacArthur exercised his authority through the various ministries of the Japanese government and through the Emperor himself.[52,80] Within this framework, the Public Health and Welfare Section of General Headquarters, SCAP, directed government public health policy. For example, under the direction of Brigadier General Sams and under the authority of the SCAP, the Public Health and Welfare Section directed the Japanese Ministry of Health and Welfare to[80(pp669–670)]

- Initiate immediate surveys of disease prevalence, health care facilities, and medical supplies by prefecture,
- Initiate a communicable disease program that includes weekly reporting, disease control activities, and immunizations,
- Restore public sewer, water, and waste and garbage disposal systems,
- Reopen civilian hospitals, sanatoria, and leprosaria,
- Distribute Japanese military medical supplies and foodstuffs to the indigenous population,
- Inaugurate port quarantine control,
- Reopen or restore civilian public health laboratories,
- Expedite the collection, analysis, and reporting of vital statistics data, and
- Control venereal disease.

Even before the war, Japanese standards of sanitation had been far below those of Western societies. Water and sewer systems existed only in the larger cities and had been severely damaged by bombing.[79] According to the US Strategic Bombing Survey, 40% of the built-up areas of 66 Japanese cities was destroyed, and approximately 30% of the urban population was homeless.[81] A growing food shortage was clearly the greatest crisis facing the nation.[82]

The resources of [Japan during the war] had been used to support the activities of the Army, and the food of the civilian population had been officially restricted from the beginning of the war to approximately the basal metabolic level and had become so short that scientists were trying to determine how much farther the ration could be lowered without curtailing the ability of the people to support the [Japanese] Army.[83(p694)]

MacArthur ordered a report on the condition of the populace. This was accomplished through

(a) a review of autopsy reports of persons dying in public places, (b) obtaining reports from the Ministry of Welfare of deaths caused by malnutrition, and (c) institution of nutrition surveys (and physical exams).[83(p694)]

The incidence of smallpox increased throughout the war years in Japan. Despite 60 million people being immunized in the first 4 months of occupation, 17,800 cases of smallpox occurred in 1946. It was soon discovered that the technique of vaccination had been faulty—virus had been applied to the arm while it was still wet with alcohol. Seventy-five million people were revaccinated, bringing the epidemic to a halt. Only 29 cases were reported in 1948.[79] The US occupation troops did not escape unscathed. Of the 61 "previously vaccinated" servicemen who developed the disease, 21 died, prompting a rigorous revaccination program among the US forces also.[84] Noted military historian Albert Cowdrey stated it well:

American and Japanese health were interdependent, and the occupation authorities were obliged to improve the second in order to safeguard the first.[84(p47)]

As in postwar Europe, sexually transmitted disease (STD) loomed as an enormous problem for both the military and civilian communities. A campaign of health information for military personnel, placing red-light districts off limits, and outlawing prostitution (for the first time in Japan's history), did not seem to be sufficient to curb a STD rate that peaked at 150 cases per 1,000 troops per year in October 1946.[84] On the military side, STD control became a command responsibility, with coordination of program elements by the 8th Army's chief of preventive medicine. SCAP directed the Japanese government to require the reporting of venereal diseases; to establish STD control ordinances for each prefecture, including weekly examinations for prostitutes and bar girls; to treat those infected with

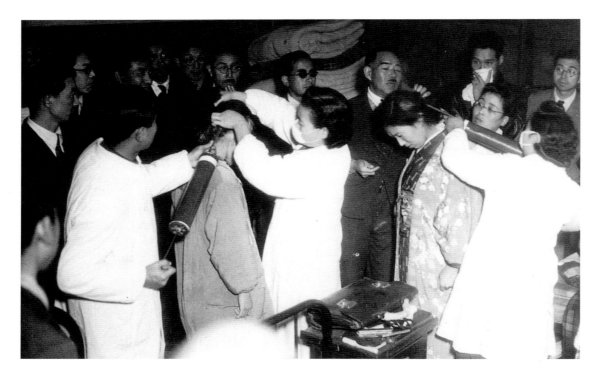

Fig. 3-3. Japanese health care workers are seen here dusting civilians with DDT in Tokyo's Komagoma Typhus Hospital in response to a widespread epidemic of typhus in December 1946. Photograph: Courtesy of the National Museum of Health and Medicine, Armed Forces Institute of Pathology, Catalog No. SC 287,308.

penicillin; and to set up training courses for laboratory and STD clinic staff. STD rates among personnel did moderate through the first half of 1947, yet the problem remained for the duration of the occupation.[84]

An epidemic of typhus in late 1945 led to the immunization of more than 8 million people and the dusting of 48 million with DDT powder (Figure 3-3). By 1948, the number of cases had fallen to less than 500, from over 31,000 in 1946. With the introduction of a new diphtheria vaccine and the vaccination of 18 million children, the morbidity rate for this disease dropped by 73% from 1945 to 1948. In similar fashion, a typhoid fever immunization program was started at this time. Cholera was kept in check largely by stringent quarantine measures focused on Japanese citizens returning from foreign countries. A nationwide BCG (bacille Calmette-Guerin) vaccination program started in 1946 is credited with reducing the tuberculosis mortality rate 36% by 1948. A country-wide effort to reduce the incidence of dysentery taught individuals about the importance of sanitation and personal hygiene. Particular efforts were made to discourage the centuries-old practice of using night soil (human excreta)

for fertilizer. In addition, in the spring of 1946, 9,000 trained and equipped six-man sanitation teams were assigned throughout the country so that every health district had its own team. The improvement in the safety of drinking water alone probably accounted for the 87% drop in the incidence of dysentery by 1948.[78,79]

After the adoption of a new constitution by the Japanese government and the signing of a peace treaty with the United States, which took effect April 28, 1952, Japan regained its full sovereignty and the military occupation formally ended.

Korea

The US troops who arrived in Korea after the surrender of Japan found no local indigenous government with which to work. The Japanese government had annexed the Korean peninsula in 1910 and had never allowed Koreans to occupy positions of leadership. The same was true of the nation's health care system. Virtually all key medical professional personnel had been Japanese, and they had all left. The public health infrastructure, in particular, was crippled. It was into this void that US Military Government stepped in 1945.[80]

The Headquarters, US Army Military Government, in Korea was formally established in January 1946. A Bureau of Public Health (later the Department of Public Health and Welfare) was quickly established. This department was staffed with 50 officers and 30 enlisted men from both the Army and the Navy. Provincial and community health departments were also established shortly thereafter. To fill the professional vacuum, the Military Government quickly instituted a 6-week training course in public health at Seoul University. Twenty-two students had completed this training by January 1946. In addition, the military worked with the Rockefeller Foundation to sponsor 10 Korean physicians in the study of public health.[80]

Although no fighting (and therefore no destruction of buildings) had occurred in Korea during World War II, the country shared many of the same sanitation and disease problems as postwar Japan. Water supplies were often polluted. Mosquitoes and flies were everywhere. As in Japan, night soil served as the chief fertilizer. Smallpox, cholera, typhus, typhoid fever, dysentery, and malaria were all endemic. Tuberculosis was common, killing 45,000 annually. Infant mortality stood at 300 per 1,000 live births, with half of all children dying before they reached the age of 5 years.[80]

So deep were the disease problems of Korea, so primitive was the people's lifestyle, and so few were the public health resources that the Military Government was able to conduct, at best, a holding operation during the occupation years. With few resources at their disposal, Army doctors primarily responded to epidemics "in the face of almost heartbreaking difficulties."[84(p57)] Recipients of the same "vaccination" program as pre-1945 Japan, Korea reeled from a smallpox epidemic in the winter of 1945 to 1946, which peaked at 19,809 cases in April. Typhus, also epidemic during these months, caused almost 6,000 cases and peaked with 1,064 cases in April. Despite the efforts of the American Typhus Commission to suppress the disease, typhus recurred the following winter (1946–1947), with 1,183 cases by May 1947. Koreans being repatriated from China were thought to have sparked a cholera epidemic in the summer of 1946 that resulted in 15,642 cases and 10,191 deaths. Nationwide efforts at immunization and sanitation followed all of these outbreaks. In addition to these outbreaks, two particular disease problems for occupation troops were malaria and venereal disease.[80]

The declaration of the Republic of Korea (South Korea) in August 1948 brought to an end 3 years of military government.

SUMMARY

This chapter has just scratched the surface in discussing the historic role of preventive medicine and public health in US armies of occupation and military government. In the aftermath of four major US wars, military preventive medicine personnel have distinguished themselves in protecting the health of US military occupation forces; providing organized, life-saving relief and epidemic disease control for suffering civilians in devastated, war-torn countries; and establishing or reestablishing sustainable civil government public health systems.

Public health is a vital and pressing function within military government, and it is most effectively delivered by well-trained and experienced military preventive medicine personnel and civilian public health officers assigned to work with the military. Within military government, the goals of preserving the health of the occupying personnel and improving the lot of a distressed civilian population are inextricably interdependent. Recognizing this, it is incumbent on medical professionals in the armed forces to ensure that preventive medicine personnel are well trained and ready to step forward when called on to serve with occupation forces and military government administrations in the future. The reputation of the United States as a humanitarian nation and its military heritage of professionalism demand the best.

REFERENCES

1. Gabriel RH. American experience with military government. *Am Political Sci Rev.* 1943;37:417.

2. Holborn H. *American Government: Its Organization and Policies.* Washington, DC: Infantry Journal Press; 1947.

3. Daugherty WE, Andrews M. *A Review of US Historical Experience With Civil Affairs, 1776-1954.* Bethesda, Md: Operations Research Office; 1961. Technical Paper ORO-TP-29.

4. Turner TB. Preface. In: Lada J, Hoff EC, eds. *Civil Affairs/Military Government Public Health Activities*. Vol 8. In: *Preventive Medicine in World War II*. Washington, DC: Office of the Surgeon General, Department of the Army; 1976.

5. US Army John F. Kennedy Special Warfare Center. *Public Health Functions, US Army Civil Affairs*. Fort Bragg, NC: USAJFKSWC; 1983. ST 41-10-7.

6. Simmons JS, Turner TB, Hiscock IV. Health programs under military government. *Am J Public Health*. 1945;35:35–41.

7. Bliss RW. Military responsibility for civilian health in war. *Mil Surgeon*. 1949;104:247–250.

8. Gordon JE. *A History of Preventive Medicine Division in the European Theater of Operations, US Army, 1941-1945*. Volume II, pt. XI, p 5. Mimeographed manuscript.

9. Turner TB. Civil public health in overseas theaters of operations. *Mil Surgeon*. 1945;96:131–134.

10. Turner TB, Hiscock IV. Problems of civilian health under war conditions—general concepts and origins. In: Lada J, Hoff EC, eds. *Civil Affairs/Military Government Public Health Activities*. Vol 8. In: *Preventive Medicine in World War II*. Washington, DC: Office of the Surgeon General, Department of the Army; 1976.

11. Scott W. *Memoirs of Lieut-General Scott, LLD*. Vol 2. New York: Sheldon and Co; 1864: 540–551.

12. Duncan LC. Medical history of General Scott's campaign to the City of Mexico in 1847. *Mil Surgeon*. 1920;47:436–470, 596–609.

13. Bowen TE. William Crawford Gorgas, physician to the world. *Mil Med*. 1983;148:917–920.

14. Newton R. Medical topography of the City of Mexico. *N Y J Med Collateral Sci*. 1848;1:298.

15. United States Army Institute for Military Assistance, Office of Nonresident Instruction. *Historical Development of Civil Affairs From the Romans to the Korean Conflict*. Fort Bragg, NC: USAIMA; 1972. IMA ST 41–170.

16. Bayne-Jones S. *The Evolution of Preventive Medicine in the United States Army, 1607-1939*. Washington, DC: Office of the Surgeon General, Department of the Army; 1968.

17. *The Report of the Surgeon General of the Army to the Secretary of War for the Fiscal Year Ending June 30, 1899*. Washington, DC: Government Printing Office.

18. Wood L. The military government of Cuba. *Ann Am Acad Political Soc Sci*. 1903;21:155.

19. Cosmas GA. Securing the fruits of victory: the US Army occupies Cuba, 1898–1899. *Mil Affairs*. 1974;38:85–91.

20. Gillett MC. *The Army Medical Department 1865–1917*. Washington, DC: Center of Military History, US Army; 1995.

21. *The Report of the Surgeon General of the Army to the Secretary of War for the Fiscal Year Ending June 30, 1900*. Washington, DC: Government Printing Office.

22. Gorgas MD, Hendrick BJ. *William Crawford Gorgas: His Life and Work*. Garden City, NY: Doubleday, Page & Co; 1924: 87–88.

23. *The Report of the Surgeon General of the Army to the Secretary of War for the Fiscal Year Ending June 30, 1901*. Washington, DC: Government Printing Office.

24. Reed W, Carroll J, Agramonte A. The etiology of yellow fever: An additional note. *JAMA*. 1901;36:431–440.

25. Hume EE. *Victories of Army Medicine: Scientific Accomplishments of the Medical Department of the United States Army*. Philadelphia: J.B. Lippincott Co; 1943.

26. *Yellow Fever, a Compilation of Various Publications: Results of the Work of Major Walter Reed, Medical Corps, and the Yellow Fever Commission.* Washington, DC: Government Printing Office; 1911.

27. *The Report of the Surgeon General of the Army to the Secretary of War for the Fiscal Year Ending June 30, 1907.* Washington, DC: Government Printing Office.

28. *The Report of the Surgeon General of the Army to the Secretary of War for the Fiscal Year Ending June 30, 1908.* Washington, DC: Government Printing Office.

29. *The Report of the Surgeon General of the Army to the Secretary of War for the Fiscal Year Ending June 30, 1909.* Washington, DC: Government Printing Office.

30. *The Report of the Surgeon General of the Army to the Secretary of War for the Fiscal Year Ending June 30, 1910.* Washington, DC: Government Printing Office.

31. Foster GM. *The Demands of Humanity: Army Medical Disaster Relief.* Washington, DC: Center of Military History, United States Army; 1983.

32. Hoff JVR. The share of the "white man's burden" that has fallen to the Medical Department of the Public Services of Puerto Rico. *Philadelphia Med J.* 1900;5:796–799.

33. Ashford BK, King WW. A study of uncinariasis in Porto Rico. *Am Med.* 1903;6:391–396.

34. Ashford BK. Notes on medical progress in Puerto Rico. *Mil Surgeon.* 1909;25:725–727.

35. Ashford BK. Where the treatment of all infected is the surest prophylactic measure: The problem of epidemic uncinariasis in Porto Rico. *Mil Surgeon.* 1907;20:40–55.

36. Bayne-Jones S, Hiscock IV, Stayer MC. The United States, its territories and possessions, and the Panama Canal Zone. In: Lada J, Hoff EC, eds. *Civil Affairs/Military Government Public Health Activities.* Vol 8. In: *Preventive Medicine in World War II.* Washington, DC: Office of the Surgeon General, Department of the Army; 1976: 120–125.

37. US Bureau of the Census. *Census of the Philippine Islands, Taken Under the Direction of the Philippine Commission in the Year 1903.* Vol 3. Washington, DC: Bureau of the Census; 17.

38. Beadnell CM. Reminiscences of the American–Filipino War, 1899. *Mil Surgeon.* 1927;61:129–152.

39. Lull GF. The development of the Philippine Health Service. *Mil Surgeon.* 1931;68:204–210.

40. *The Report of the Surgeon General of the Army to the Secretary of War for the Fiscal Year Ending June 30, 1902.* Washington, DC: Government Printing Office.

41. Vedder EB. *A Synopsis of the Work of the Army Medical Research Boards in the Philippines: Army Medical Bulletin.* Carlisle Barracks, Penn: Medical Field Service School; 1929.

42. Curry JJ. Report on parasitic disease in horses, mules and caribao in the Philippine Islands. *Am Med.* 1902;3:512–513.

43. Curry JJ. Surra or nagana. *Am Med.* 1902;4:95–99.

44. Woolley PG. Rinderpest. *Philippine J Sci.* 1906;1B:577–616.

45. Department of Sanitation and Public Health, German Occupied Territory: Administration. *American Expeditionary Forces.* Vol 2. In: *Medical Department of the United States Army in the World War.* Washington, DC: Government Printing Office; 1927: 821–827.

46. Marshall SLA. *The American Heritage History of World War I.* New York: American Heritage Publishing Company, Inc; 1964: 361–373.

47. Schule PA. A report on the intensive anti-typhoid campaign in southwestern Germany, including an analysis of data on seventy-one typhoid carriers under observation by the laboratory at Trier, Germany. *Mil Surgeon*. 1919;45:127–137,268–284.

48. Reasoner MA. German sanitation as observed during the American Occupation. *Mil Surgeon*. 1927;60:146–154.

49. Bruns EH. Report on the economic conditions of the poorer population of the city of Trier, as determined by house to house visits. *Mil Surgeon*. 1920;46:418–422.

50. Parsons AL. Extracts from the History, Medical Department, United States Military Mission, Berlin, Germany, August 10, 1919. *Mil Surgeon*. 1923;52:113–130.

51. Sanitation and public health. In: Assistant Chief of Staff, compiler. *American Representation in Occupied Germany, 1920-21*. Vol II. Germany: American Forces in Germany: chap 5.

52. Tobey JA. Military government and public health. *Mil Surgeon*. 1952;110:260–265.

53. News and comment: Medical Department officers in civil affairs. *Bull US Army Med Dept*. 1945;85:42–43.

54. Coles HL, Weinberg AK. Military necessity demands relief of civilian distress. *Civil Affairs: Soldiers Become Governors*. In: *US Army in World War II—Special Studies*. Washington, DC: Office of the Chief of Military History, Department of the Army; 1964: 306–339.

55. Turner TB. Sicily and Italy. In: Lada J, Hoff EC, eds. *Civil Affairs/Military Government Public Health Activities*. Vol 8. In: *Preventive Medicine in World War II*. Washington, DC: Office of the Surgeon General, Department of the Army; 1976: 293–342.

56. Coles HL, Weinberg AK. *Civil Affairs: Soldiers Become Governors*. In: *US Army in World War II—Special Studies*. Washington, DC: Office of the Chief of Military History, Department of the Army; 1964: 240.

57. Soper FL, Davis WA, Markham FS, Riehl LA. Typhus fever in Italy, 1943–45, and its control with louse powder. *Am J Hygiene*. 1947;45:305–334.

58. Civilian health problems in the European Theater. *Bull US Army Med Dept*. 1945;4:113–115.

59. Hume EE. The 1944 eruption of Vesuvius. *Mil Surgeon*. 1946;98:369–381.

60. Bayne-Jones S, Dehné EJ. The European Theater of Operations (1944-45). In: Lada J, Hoff EC, eds. *Civil Affairs/Military Government Public Health Activities*. Vol 8. In: *Preventive Medicine in World War II*. Washington, DC: Office of the Surgeon General, Department of the Army; 1976: 494.

61. Lundeberg KR. Public health survey of Germany. *Bull US Army Med Dept*. 1949;9:943–946.

62. Leone NC. Administrative aspects of an emergency nutrition program. *Bull US Army Med Dept*. 1949;9:198–206.

63. Civilian nutrition surveys in Western Europe. *Bull US Army Med Dept*. 1945;4:138.

64. Ashe WF Jr. The nutrition program in Germany: US Zone of Occupation in Germany May 1945–May 1946. *Bull US Army Med Dept*. 1948;8:47–58.

65. deForest WR. Public health in Germany under US occupation. *Med Bull US Army, Europe*. 1949;6:28–37.

66. United States Strategic Bombing Survey, Morale Division, Medical Branch Report. *The Effect of Bombing on Health and Medical Care in Germany*. Washington, DC: War Department; 30 Oct 1945.

67. Effects of strategic bombing on Germany's health. *Bull US Army Med Dept*. 1946;5:277–279.

68. Meeting on public health planning in German Occupied Zone. *Bull US Army Med Dept*. 1946;5:142–145.

69. Ziemke EF. *The US Army in the Occupation of Germany 1944–1946*. Washington, DC: Center of Military History, US Army; 1975: 53.

70. Farinacci CJ. Austria. In: Lada J, Hoff EC, eds. *Civil Affairs/Military Government Public Health Activities*. Vol 8. In: *Preventive Medicine in World War II*. Washington, DC: Office of the Surgeon General, Department of the Army; 1976: 512–513.

71. Concentration camp. *The New Encyclopaedia Britannica*. Vol 3. 15th ed. Chicago: Encyclopaedia Britannica, Inc; 1989: 513.

72. Howe PE, Sebrell WH Jr. Nutrition—Mauthausen and Gusen concentration camps. 3 July 1945. Memorandum. Quoted in: Bayne-Jones S, Dehné EJ. The European Theater of Operations (1944-45). In: Lada J, Hoff EC, eds. *Civil Affairs/Military Government Public Health Activities*. Vol 8. In: *Preventive Medicine in World War II*. Washington, DC: Office of the Surgeon General, Department of the Army; 1976: 484.

73. Anne Frank. *Encyclopaedia Britannica*. Volume 4. 15th ed. Chicago: Encyclopaedia Britannica, Inc; 1989: 1989: 936.

74. Davis WA. Typhus at Belsen, 1: Control of the typhus epidemic. *Am J Hygiene*. 1947;46:66–83.

75. Turner TB. The Philippines and Okinawa. In: Lada J, Hoff EC, eds. *Civil Affairs/Military Government Public Health Activities*. Vol 8. In: *Preventive Medicine in World War II*. Washington, DC: Office of the Surgeon General, Department of the Army; 1976: 621–623.

76. Daniels RG, Banta JE. The Public Health Council of Okinawa—a pathway to a coordinated, fruitful, tri-service preventive medicine program. *Mil Med*. 1958;123:265–273.

77. Vuturo AF, Jensen RT. Considerations for planning and implementing a Flying Health Service: experiences in the Ryukyu Islands. *Mil Med*. 1971;136:736–739.

78. Hume EE. Army medicine around the world. *Mil Surgeon*. 1949;105:110–116.

79. Bliss RW. The Army's interest in public health activities. *Bull US Army Med Dept*. 1949;9:633–639.

80. Turner TB. Japan and Korea. In: Lada J, Hoff EC, eds. *Civil Affairs/Military Government Public Health Activities*. Vol 8. In: *Preventive Medicine in World War II*. Washington, DC: Office of the Surgeon General, Department of the Army; 1976: 664.

81. World wars. *Encyclopaedia Britannica*. Vol 29. 15th ed. Chicago: Encyclopaedia Britannica, Inc; 1989: 1045.

82. News and comment: Health of Japanese civilians under assault. *Bull US Army Med Dept*. 1947;7:247–249.

83. Howe PE. Nutrition in public health in Japan. *US Armed Forces Med J*. 1950;1:694–702.

84. Cowdrey AE. *United States Army in the Korean War: The Medics' War*. Washington, DC: Center of Military History, US Army; 1987.

Chapter 4

PREVENTIVE MEDICINE IN MILITARY OPERATIONS OTHER THAN WAR

RALPH LOREN ERICKSON, MD, DrPH

INTRODUCTION

DOMESTIC ASSISTANCE AND RELIEF IN THE 19TH CENTURY

THE SAN FRANCISCO EARTHQUAKE: AN OPPORTUNITY FOR LOCAL INITIATIVE

DIGGING THE PANAMA CANAL

THE MEXICAN CRISIS

HUMANITARIANISM IN THE WAKE OF WORLD WAR I
Serbia
Armenia
Poland
Soviet Russia

HUMANITARIAN AND DISASTER RELIEF BETWEEN THE WORLD WARS

RELIEF EFFORTS IN THE EARLY COLD WAR

VIETNAM: NATION BUILDING, MEDICAL CIVIC ACTION, AND REFUGEE RELIEF

OPERATIONS OTHER THAN WAR IN LATIN AMERICA

THE MODERN ERA OF COMPLEX HUMANITARIAN EMERGENCIES
Iraq and the Kurds
Haitian Refugees

NATURAL DISASTER RELIEF IN RECENT TIMES

SUMMARY

R. L. Erickson; Lieutenant Colonel, Medical Corps, US Army; Chief, Preventive Medicine Service, Landstuhl Regional Medical Center, APO AE 09180

INTRODUCTION

At the direction of the National Command Authority and in support of US national interests, the men and women of the armed forces have served the United States throughout its history in a variety of missions that do not fit into the strict dichotomy of war versus peace. From the Jefferson administration onward, soldiers took the lead in the exploration of the North American continent and in protecting citizens on the frontier. They enhanced westward expansion by building roads, railroads, bridges, and canals. Following natural and man-made disasters (both in the US and abroad), entire operational units or task-appropriate, multidisciplinary teams provided assistance and relief to stricken populations. More recently, US military forces have found themselves engaged in peace operations in a variety of trouble spots around the globe.

With the ascendance of the United States as a world superpower in the latter half of the 20th century, such operations have quickened in their "pace, frequency and variety."[1chap13] These missions have been designated "stability and support operations" and military operations other than war (OOTW) and describe a wide range of military activities short of declared war.[1] These OOTW could call for the use of troops in actual combat, yet the focus is generally to resolve conflict and promote peace, nation building, disaster relief, and humanitarian assistance.[2] These OOTW may occur before or after war or during war in the same theater. In addition, it should be noted that many OOTW in the modern era are mixed in nature (eg, peace operations and humanitarian relief) and at times can be described as complex humanitarian emergencies (see Chapter 44, Complex Emergencies). These complex humanitarian emergencies are characterized by political turmoil, a lack of physical security, mass population movements, and high morbidity and mortality.

As in wartime, the priority mission for military preventive medicine professionals in OOTW remains the protection and maintenance of the health of the command (eg, through disease and injury prevention and control, health promotion, and surveillance). When so directed by the National Command Authority, these same preventive medicine skills have proven, however, to be of extraordinary worth in protecting of large civilian populations in need of help. In fact, as one moves along a continuum from high-intensity conflict (war) to the low-intensity activities of OOTW, the visibility and value of preventive medicine professionals increases dramatically. Where sustainability and long-term impact are the goals, missions involving humanitarian assistance, disaster relief, and nation building in particular should have a very strong public health and preventive medicine component. Exhibit 4-1 provides a list of the tra-

---

EXHIBIT 4-1

INVOLVEMENT OF PREVENTIVE MEDICINE PROFESSIONALS IN OPERATIONS OTHER THAN WAR

Preventive Medicine Professionals Providing Leadership

Humanitarian assistance (international and domestic)

Disaster relief (international and domestic)

Nation assistance, nation building and development

Preventive Medicine Professionals Providing Unique Support

Arms control

Counterterrorism operations

Support to domestic civil authorities

Security assistance

Support for insurgencies and counterinsurgencies

Preventive Medicine Professionals Providing Traditional Warfighter Support

Noncombatant evacuation operations

Counterdrug operations

Peace operations

Sanctions enforcement

Show of force

Attacks and raids

Support for preventive diplomacy

Sources: (1) Department of the Army. *Operations.* Washington, DC: DA; 1993. (2) US Army Field Manual 100-5. MHS 2020 Team. *Medical Health System 2020 OOTW Report.* Washington, DC: Department of Defense; 1998.

---

ditional missions and activities of OOTW subdivided by the degree of involvement of military preventive medicine personnel. This chapter, while not an exhaustive review of the subject, seeks to describe the critical and evolving role of preventive medicine in OOTW throughout the United States' history, through periods of domestic focus (isolationism) and international leadership.

DOMESTIC ASSISTANCE AND RELIEF IN THE 19TH CENTURY

Through the first half of the 19th century, the responsibility for providing domestic disaster and humanitarian relief rested on the local and state government within whose jurisdiction the calamity occurred. In the case of a major disaster, however, it did not seem reasonable that a devastated municipality should have to rescue itself. Nevertheless it remained a hot topic of constitutional debate.[3] One early exception to existing policy by the federal government came in 1832. With smallpox threatening the western Indian nations, Congress provided for a mass vaccination program to be carried out by both civilian and military physicians, especially those serving at frontier forts in Illinois and Michigan. Despite their efforts to immunize the nomadic tribes, it is estimated that half of the native Americans in this region died in an epidemic 5 years later.[4]

Thirty-three years later, at the conclusion of the Civil War and faced with over 4 million destitute former slaves, the federal government became much more involved in providing for the emergency needs of its citizens. In 1865, Congress established its first welfare agency (the Bureau of Refugees, Freedmen and Abandoned Lands[5]), appointing Major General Oliver Howard as its commissioner.

From this point on, the federal government became a more willing provider of humanitarian assistance, through a variety of agencies, when local governments were not capable of doing so. The US Army, in particular, participated in at least 17 such major relief efforts between 1868 and 1898, including the Chicago (1871) and Seattle (1889) fires, the Charleston earthquake (1886), the Johnstown (1889) and other major floods, and various yellow fever epidemics. More often than not, Army disaster relief was logistical in nature (as it frequently is today), taking the form of providing rations, clothing, bedding, and tentage.[3]

Armed with few effective disease control measures, military medical personnel did what they could to care for the sick and injured and to stem the spread of disease in these situations. In New Orleans (1853) and Key West (1877), military posts were made available (at the initiative of the local commanders) for the quarantine and treatment of yellow fever epidemic victims.[6] In 1869, under the threat of a smallpox epidemic in the town of Warsaw, Ky, one enterprising detachment commander quarantined an infected family and saw to it that his surgeon vaccinated most of the local civilian population.[7]

THE SAN FRANCISCO EARTHQUAKE: AN OPPORTUNITY FOR LOCAL INITIATIVE

Two violent tremors greeted the 450,000 inhabitants of San Francisco the morning of 18 April 1906. Within hours, more than 28,000 buildings had been destroyed by either the seismic events or the ensuing firestorm fed by broken gas mains. In the end, over a charred area of 4.7 square miles, 498 people had died, 415 were seriously injured, and nearly 300,000 people were left homeless.[8] Sensing the great need in the early hours after the earthquake, Lieutenant Colonel George H. Torney, the chief surgeon and commander at Letterman General Hospital, dispatched medical teams into the city and opened the doors of his facility to civilian casualties. By the end of the first day, the hospital had admitted 127 civilians. This number would increase dramatically the second day as more people learned of the services being offered at Letterman. With basic public services out of commission and the homeless huddled in makeshift camps in vacant lots across the city, the threat of epidemic disease loomed.[3]

The US Army's participation in the San Francisco relief effort was crucial in that they alone were local and still functioning. The organization that was intended to handle such a disaster, the Red Cross, was by its own admission not ready or able to respond.[9] The Army at the turn of the century possessed a complement of physicians and sanitarians trained and experienced in public health interventions for large populations. Military medical officers had been at the forefront of this era's medical-scientific advances in the etiology of infectious disease and the sanitation movement. In particular, many serving in uniform were veterans of the major sanitation cleanup campaigns in the occupied territories after the Spanish-American War (see Chapter 3, The Historic Role of Military Preventive

Medicine and Public Health in US Armies of Occupations and Military Government).

Brigadier General Frederick Funston, himself a veteran of the Philippine Insurrection and the acting commander of the Division of the Pacific, headquartered in San Francisco, ordered Lieutenant Colonel Torney to take charge of the sanitation of the city. Respecting this decision, the mayor and the president of the health commission of San Francisco quickly appointed Dr. Torney to serve as the head of a joint committee to control the sanitation of the city. In this capacity, Lieutenant Colonel Torney and his civilian and military medical staff supervised or ran more than 100 camps for more than 50,000 homeless citizens[10] (Figure 4-1). Retired Brigadier General Charles R. Greenleaf, a physician with firsthand experience from the sanitation cleanup of Cuba and Panama, also volunteered to help Lieutenant Colonel Torney in the effort. At his suggestion, the city was divided into six districts, each with an assigned health officer who would report back to Torney daily. Identified cases of contagious disease in the camps were transferred to a 200-bed hospital set up in Harbor View Park. Water in the camps was monitored closely for contamination. Smallpox vaccinations (3,500 doses per day) were given by Army personnel to all who were willing to receive them. A brief increase in typhoid fever

and smallpox cases was noted in the weeks following the earthquake, but these cases occurred outside of the Army-monitored camps and did not rise to epidemic levels.[9] In a resolution later unanimously adopted by the California Academy of Medicine, Lieutenant Colonel Torney was officially thanked for his efforts and those of the Army.[11] So efficient and effective was the relief effort mounted by the Army that military personnel had difficulty disengaging from the operation until July of that year, some 4 months later. The San Francisco earthquake marked the first time that military medical personnel played such a primary role in a major domestic disaster relief effort, but it also highlighted the danger to the military of being "stuck" with the mission beyond the emergency phase of the operation.

Over the next 10 years, the military would continue to participate in disaster relief efforts in the United States in a supporting or advisory role, with control remaining in the hands of local and state officials. An example of this came during the flooding of the Mississippi River in 1912, when the Surgeon General sent Major Reuben B. Miller and Captain Jacob M. Coffin to numerous refugee camps and centers. They distributed supplies and performed sanitary inspections, and the expert consultation (and accountability on follow-up visits) they provided was credited with preventing

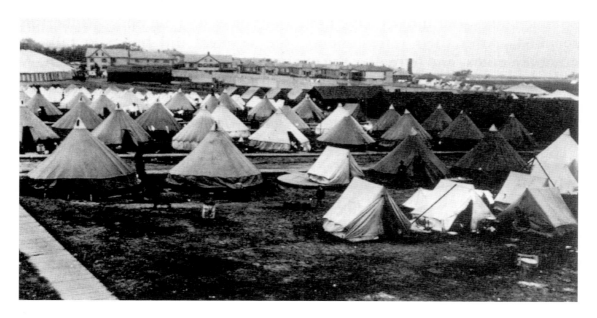

Fig. 4-1. US Army-run displaced person camp adjacent to Letterman General Hospital following the San Francisco earthquake, 1906. Army assets in San Francisco stepped in to help when civilian organizations were incapacitated. Source: Foster GM. *The Demands of Humanity: Army Medical Disaster Relief.* Washington, DC: Center of Military History, US Army; 1983: 59.

serious epidemics in the flooded areas.[12,13]

The flooding of the Miami and Ohio rivers the following year was equally devastating, requiring a significant commitment on the part of the US military. So hazardous were the health conditions within the city of Dayton itself that local officials in discussions with the visiting Secretary of War decided to appoint a federal officer to be in charge of the sanitation effort. Major Thomas L. Rhoads, who had been accompanying the Secretary of War (and was the President's personal physician), was placed in charge of a host of local and federal health care workers. These workers quickly set about making inspections of buildings and homes, treating and evacuating the sick and injured, isolating those with communicable disease, disseminating advice on preventing disease, and locating health and sanitation hazards. Once identified, various crews were tasked to eliminate these hazards, removing a huge amount of debris and filth while restoring potable water. Not only did these preventive medicine efforts successfully ease the burden on local hospitals, but no serious outbreaks of measles, scarlet fever or diphtheria occurred.[14,15]

During this same flood, Major Sanford H. Wadhams and Dr. M. S. Alexander worked side by side for 9 days to stem a meningitis epidemic, which had already claimed a number of lives in the predominantly black town of Deckerville, Ark. Though the state refused to help, these two individuals provided food, improved sanitation, successfully treated the sick with intrathecal serum and gave immunizations to more than 500 people, most of whom were trapped in railroad boxcars by the rising waters.[16]

In addition to these domestic disaster relief missions, military medical personnel were active on the American frontier in response to significant public health problems within native American populations. One such case was the comprehensive community needs assessment performed by Captain Paul C. Hutton among the Alaskan Indians in the Haines Jones Point and Hindustucky communities outside of fort william H. Seward in 1908. Identifying rampant poverty and squalor, endemic tuberculosis and trachoma, and an infant mortality rate of 275 per 1,000 births among the Alaskan Natives, Dr. Hutton established a hygiene and sanitation education program. In addition, he sent a detailed report of his findings to the Surgeon General of the Army with specific recommendations. A subsequent Grand Jury report on the diseases of Alaska, based on Captain Hutton's work, was forwarded to the US Congress, which took action that same year to develop a sanitation system for these communities.[17]

DIGGING THE PANAMA CANAL

A more exciting story of the victory of humans over communicable disease does not exist than that of the conquest of yellow fever, malaria, and plague that allowed for the building of the Panama Canal. The timely participation of military officers in the professional fields of medicine and engineering merits the inclusion of this event as an OOTW. The French had lost more than 22,000 men to tropical disease when, after 7 years of futility, the company constructing the canal went bankrupt. Ignorant that malaria and yellow fever are transmitted by the bites of mosquitoes (*Anopheles* and *Aedes* species respectively), French physicians in Panama did little to protect their workers. In fact, they were said to have placed the legs of hospital beds in water to keep crawling bugs from getting to their patients, thus increasing the available breeding sites for the vectors. After buying the rights to build the canal for 40 million dollars and compensating the Panamanians for their secession from Colombia, the US government took charge of this colossal project. Lieutenant Colonel George Washington Goethals was named engineer-in-chief of the project in 1907 after initial attempts at civilian leadership failed.[18]

Having earned an international reputation as a sanitarian in the cleanup of Havana, Cuba, Major William Crawford Gorgas was promoted to the rank of Colonel and appointed the Chief Sanitation Officer in charge of the isthmus. Applying the breakthrough work of Major Walter Reed and Sir Ronald Ross that linked the transmission of these diseases to mosquitoes, he established 25 sanitary districts within the Canal Zone, each with its own sanitary inspector. Within each of these districts, his teams drained every lake, pond, swamp, and ditch possible. Those that could not be drained were covered with a thin coating of oil to kill the mosquito larvae and eggs (Figure 4-2). Buildings were screened and fumigated. Tall grass was cut down, garbage burned, and rats destroyed.[19] So successful was this program that the last case of yellow fever among workers was recorded in December 1905. By 1913, the last year of canal construction, the incidence of malaria had fallen by

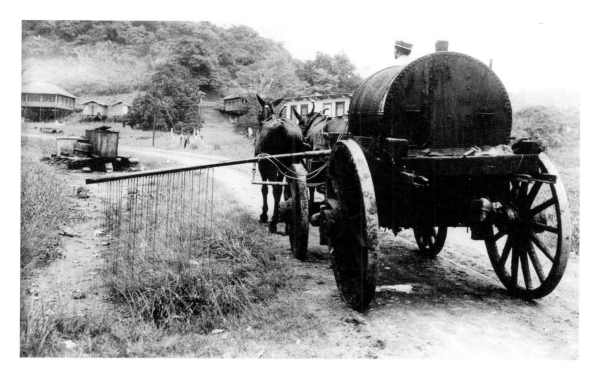

Fig. 4-2. Controlling mosquitoes and the diseases they carry was of vital interest to the builders of the Panama Canal. One method they used, shown here, was to deposit a thin film of oil onto standing water. Their success in disease control made possible the completion of the canal. Photograph: Courtesy of the National Museum of Health and Medicine, Armed Forces Institute of Pathology, Washington, DC. Catalog number: Reeve 62699.

90% from 1906 levels.[20] An estimated 78,000 lives were spared and 39 million work days from sickness saved as a result of these efforts.[21] Colonel Gorgas would be promoted to the rank of Major General and named the Surgeon General of the Army in 1914.

THE MEXICAN CRISIS

William Gorgas' tenure as Surgeon General was anything but boring as Mexico went through a period of revolutionary conflict, fledgling democracy, and a military coup d'etat that threatened vital US interests. An estimated 1 million Mexicans lost their lives during this period of instability between 1910 and 1920.[22] In addition to the immediate physical safety of US citizenry along the border and in Mexico were concerns for the spread of communicable disease from arriving refugees. By 1914, US Army medical personnel had already joined the Red Cross in detaining and providing relief to some 5,000 Mexican citizens who had crossed the border. The refugee camp at Fort Bliss, Tex, was in fact run by an Army medical officer and featured programs of mass immunization for typhoid fever and smallpox, malaria control, and strict sanitation. Despite these efforts, however, the death rate among those refugees was recorded at 21.8 per 1,000.[23,24]

HUMANITARIANISM IN THE WAKE OF WORLD WAR I

In the aftermath of World War I, Europe and parts of the Near East faced widespread famine, epidemics, and major migrations of displaced persons and refugees. A number of private organizations became involved in relief efforts soon after the cessation of hostilities, yet in many cases they were poorly resourced, understaffed, and without the required expertise to complete their intended missions. In response, President Wilson extended the wartime commitments of US military personnel who volunteered to work with these private US relief agencies being sent to Eastern Europe and the Near East. While still in the employ of the Department of War, these individuals engaged in situations where the presence of formal US military units would have been problematic. Historians have commented that the United States' intentions were both humanitarian and political.

> Herbert Hoover, who directed the American effort, and his boss, President Woodrow Wilson, sought through American relief measures to prevent civil disintegration, preserve a liberal world order, and thereby to check the spread of Bolshevism.[3(p80)]

Serbia

Major Edgar E. Hume (later Major General) was detailed with 25 other Army medical officers and 5 dental officers to work with the Red Cross Commission in postwar Serbia. From February 1919 to the summer of 1920, their priority was to control a typhus epidemic that had first entered the country in 1915. The US officers also helped establish a public health laboratory for the nation and supervised the cleanup of various prison camps.[25]

Armenia

Further to the east in the newly independent country of Armenia, Colonel William N. Haskell, US Army, led a military humanitarian relief mission from September 1919 to August 1920 under the auspices of the Near East Relief (NER), Caucasus Branch (a private philanthropic organization). The returning refugees were described as having survived

> five years of the havoc wrought by the destruction and devastation of war, with its accompanying famine, starvation and virulent epidemics. It is estimated that as a result of binding themselves unreservedly to the Allied cause, one million men in Turkish Armenia alone lost their lives by either massacre, starvation or deportation [sic]. Probably three-quarters of a million more perished as a result of disease and of epidemics of cholera, typhoid, dysentery, typhus, influenza, and relapsing fever.[26p140]

Many of those returning were women and children who had been rescued from Arabs, Kurds, and Turks who had taken them captive.

The NER team consisted of 20 US Army officers and 75 civilians (eg, relief workers, nurses, orphanage workers, chauffeurs). Major Walter P. Davenport served as the Director of Medical Relief. With

his US and Armenian staff, Dr. Davenport provided hospital care to about 4,000 individuals. In addition to distributing foodstuffs, the NER built pit latrines, native concrete latrines, baths, laundries, and delousing and disinfecting facilities. As a result of an NER campaign, 190,000 people received smallpox and tetra (cholera, typhoid, and paratyphoid A and B) vaccinations. It was estimated that 500,000 Armenians survived due to the feeding program alone. Sadly, the NER mission withdrew in advance of the Russian takeover of Armenia in the autumn of 1920.[26,27]

Poland

In 1919, the newly independent country of Poland faced two significant problems. The first was the ongoing war with Russia (the Bolsheviks) and the second was a raging epidemic of typhus, fed continually by the incessant flow of refugees and prisoners of war across its eastern frontier. Among the 2.4 million people crossing border checkpoints from the East for one 14-month period, at least 26,580 were found to have active typhus.[28] In the spring of 1919, some estimated that more than 10,000 died of typhus a day. Another estimate put the annual death toll from typhus to be some 200,000 by June 1920.[29] The mortality among health care providers was particularly heavy, with two hospitals losing seven-eighths and ten-twelfths of their doctors in the epidemic.[28]

To assist in the control of the epidemic, the first contingent of the American Red Cross Commission (headed by Lieutenant Colonel Walter C. Bailey) left Paris for Poland in February 1919.[29] By this point it was already clear that Poland represented the "rampart against the dangers of this disease"[28p623] for Europe and the world, but that the country itself lacked the resources to adequately respond. By April, the American Red Cross had established field units at Maciejow, Pruzana, Dolsk, and Bereza-Kartuska.[29]

Also working in Poland was Colonel Harry L. Gilchrist, US Army, who headed up the Polish Typhus Relief Mission, later redesignated the American Polish Relief Expedition. Dr. Gilchrist was hand-picked because of his public health experience with the military government in Manila and the San Francisco earthquake relief effort. More recently, Gilchrist had been in charge of the delousing programs in France to curb the spread of typhus there. Initially this mission was viewed as a direct extension of the Medical Department of the American Forces in Germany.[30]

Coordinating its actions with the Polish Ministry of Health, the American Polish Relief Expedition under Gilchrist had the goals of eliminating the typhus-carrying lice. This was attacked through the establishment of a strict sanitary cordon along the eastern border of Poland. All those crossing the border were required to undergo cleaning and delousing before being allowed through. In addition, bathing and delousing facilities were either constructed or brought in by mobile columns to local communities. US military personnel also helped run refugee camps, distribute food, and provide blizzard relief.[31] Three US servicemen died during this relief effort, one of typhus (Lieutenant Colonel Edward C. Register). In all, more than 40 commissioned officers and 500 enlisted personnel participated.[32] With over 2.5 million prisoners of war and civilian refugees flooding across the eastern border between 1 November 1918 and January 1920, the sanitary cordon was at times overwhelmed and bypassed. Likewise, the attempts to delouse local communities met with mixed success. By the summer of 1920, the Russian army overran the eastern border, effectively putting an end to the sanitary cordon supervised by the US military. With this, the United States focused its efforts on preparing for transport from Danzig to New York the 12,000 Polish-Americans (discharged soldiers of Haller's Army) who had fought for Poland before the US's entry into the war. Major Charles Halliday summarized the experience this way:

> the majority of physicians who went to Poland left feeling that, in so far as sanitation and preventive medicine were concerned, they had accomplished very little....many of the plans and recommendations made are now in force and are being extended as rapidly as means and circumstances will allow. Typhus, however, continues in epidemic form.[29p443]

Soviet Russia

Ironically, 1 year later (December 1921) the US government assigned Major F. H. Foucar MC, US Army, to work with the American Relief Administration, which was tasked to provide medical and sanitary relief to Russia. For 18 months, Dr. Foucar served as the district physician for the Samara region where severe famine and disease conditions prevailed. The American Relief Administration be-

gan an adult feeding program because many villages had exhausted their supplies of food. En route to Samara, Foucar described the misery of disease and death seen at the Kazan train station as "the most gruesome scene in [Dante's] Inferno."[33p692] Through the winter of 1921 to 1922, the incidence of louse-borne typhus rose to 19 new cases per 1,000 population per month. Major Foucar observed that "[s]oap was extremely dear and very bad and of ill reputation; public pay-baths were in operation, but charged more than the poor of the population, who most needed their facilities, could afford to pay."[33p692] The efforts of the ARA included rehabilitating hospital facilities, placing an ambulatory clinic in the train station, establishing feeding kitchens to feed the hungry, and establishing free bath houses (where more than 181,000 baths were given; also offered were haircuts, soap, and sterilization of clothing). By February 1923, the incidence of typhus had declined to 0.19 cases per 1,000 population per month—a 100-fold decrease.

More than 10,000 cases and 5,000 deaths from cholera also occurred in an epidemic in the Samara region in 1921. This was reduced to only 33 cases and 6 deaths in 1922 because of the institution of bacteriological testing of the city's water supply and the installation of two Wallace Tiernan, direct-feed chlorinating apparatuses at the city water-pumping station. More than 475,000 two-dose courses of a tetra vaccine were administered to the populace by the American Relief Administration in the summer of 1922, driving rates of cholera, typhoid fever, and paratyphoid fever to their lowest levels in 15 years. In addition, more than 10,000 smallpox vaccinations were given to adults and children who did not show evidence of previous protection. Programs were also initiated for the control and treatment of malaria, trachoma, and syphilis. The once-famous Roux laboratory, the maker of various vaccines and anti-toxins for the region, was not functioning when the American Relief Administration arrived at Samara. With the rehabilitation of its facilities and horse stables, purchase of equipment, and feeding of its personnel, the American Relief Administration returned this public health laboratory to full function within 2 years.[33,34]

HUMANITARIAN AND DISASTER RELIEF BETWEEN THE WORLD WARS

With the rise to prominence of the American Red Cross and the bolstering of state health boards, the role for the US military in domestic relief efforts diminished significantly after World War I. Army medical personnel continued to participate in a va-

riety of preventive medicine efforts as needed, though. In response to an outbreak of typhoid fever in 1921 in neighboring Jacobstown, NJ, soldiers and medical officers from Fort Dix established and administered an anti–typhoid fever program for the community.[35] In 1925, severe flooding hit southwestern Georgia, and Colonel Percy L. Jones led a team from Fort McPherson to the town of Newton, where they started an immunization program against typhoid and paratyphoid fevers for the townspeople. They also supervised mosquito control efforts and the distribution of Lyster bags for drinking water.[36] (Colonel Jones would later serve as a sanitation advisor to civilian health officials in West Palm Beach, Fla, following the hurricane of 1928.) Similar flooding in Arkansas in the spring of 1927 led to the mobilization of four Army physicians, who not only provided first aid, inoculations, and relief supplies but also conducted sanitation surveys and directed sanitation in camps.[37] With massive flooding of both the Mississippi and Ohio rivers in 1937, a hospital company (six medical officers and 93 enlisted personnel) was dispatched from Carlisle Barracks, Penn, to Louisville, Ky. Cooperating with the Red Cross, they established an emergency hospital in a local high school and took over the operation of an inoculation center from the City Board of Health. They provided 5,114 typhoid fever and 66 smallpox inoculations within the first 2 weeks of relief efforts.[38] Of note is the importance placed on immunization by the military during these disasters, with the provision safe drinking water being left to civilian relief agency workers.

With the exception of post–World War I Europe, US military relief operations overseas were few and far between during the 1920s and 1930s. The largest of these missions followed the Japanese earthquake of 1923, which initial estimates said left 2 million people homeless, 100,000 seriously injured, and 200,000 dead.[39] In light of the hostility of the Japanese government to the United States at the time, however, American involvement was limited to the restoration of St. Luke's hospital and the new construction of a 480-bed facility (the Bei-Hi hospital), which was turned over quickly to local control.[40]

A very different response was permitted following the Nicaraguan earthquake of 1931, which almost completely destroyed the capital city of Managua (by shock and fire) and left an estimated 5,000 people dead. US Navy physicians and corpsmen who were stationed locally went immediately to work caring for the injured. They would soon be joined by two Army surgeons (part of an engineering survey team) and personnel from the USS Lexington. All injured patients were automatically given prophylactic tetanus toxoid. In response to an early sanitary assessment that revealed a total cessation of public sanitation services and a lack of safe water, these professionals directed that water from the lake be boiled and chlorinated before consumption. Working with local officials and the Nicaraguan National Guard, relief camps holding 10,000 people apiece were established with strict sanitary regulations and vaccinations (ie, smallpox, typhoid fever). For fear of rabies, free-roaming dogs were ordered shot.[41]

RELIEF EFFORTS IN THE EARLY COLD WAR

In 1948, the United States assumed the responsibilities of world leadership with the passage by Congress of the Economic Cooperation Act, which established the European Recovery Program commonly known as the Marshall Plan. With Eastern Europe under the control of the Soviet Union, this plan offered more than just material assistance to 270 million Europeans in the west; it offered hope. When the Marshall Plan ended in 1951, Congress sought to link military and economic programs by creating the Mutual Security Agency. Leaders of the Army Medical Department, such as Major General Heaton, recognized early on that some of the United States' best diplomats in these endeavors would be her military medical personnel.[42]

An early example of this came in February of 1953 when more than 1,700 people died in the Netherlands due to flooding from unusually high tides and strong winds. At the request of the Dutch government, US military personnel assisted in the rescue and relief effort. Learning that the people were without safe water, the chief surgeon for US Army Europe, Major General Guy B. Denit, decided that the critical health care need was for emergency sanitation rather than casualty care. Military sanitary engineers took the lead in this effort, running water purification units in 19 areas. Those units ultimately furnished 75,000 gal of water a day for the populace.[43]

When the Brahmaputra River and its tributaries overflowed their banks in 1954, millions of Pakistanis were displaced from their homes. In response to their plight, a major relief effort was mounted by the US government that involved sending the chief of the Preventive Medicine Division of the Far East Command, along with the 37th Medical Company (Preventive Medicine) and 42 additional enlisted personnel, to Pakistan. With the region threatened by waterborne diseases, they formed 40 immunization teams with local military officials. In short order and at the same time that food and relief supplies were being distributed by others, these teams immunized more than 850,000 people against

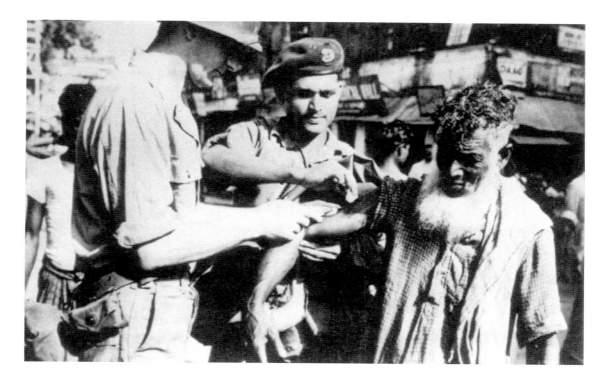

Fig. 4-3. The US military sponsored a typhoid fever and cholera immunization program in Pakistan after a devastating flood in 1954. This campaign immunized more than 850,000 people and provided high visibility for the US government. Photograph source: Armed Forces Institute of Pathology. As used in: Foster GM. *The Demands of Humanity: Army Medical Disaster Relief*. Washington, DC: Center of Military History, US Army; 1983: 150.

cholera and typhoid fever[44] (Figure 4-3). For the time and place, giving immunizations represented a high-tech, high-visibility intervention that the US military was uniquely prepared to deliver given its logistical muscle. No mention was made of efforts to secure safe drinking water for the masses or of the effectiveness of the immunization campaign.

In 1956, the US military deployed to Mexico to provide relief from Hurricane Janet in the Tampico area. As the Tamisi and Panuco river basins flooded, an estimated 800 people died, while some 5,000 were stranded on their roofs. Twelve US Navy medical officers and 24 corpsmen from Pensacola, Fla, and the USS Saipan worked with Mexican personnel to establish screened pit latrines and distributed hypochlorite compounds with which the people could treat their water. Together they vaccinated more than 54,000 people against typhoid fever, diphtheria, pertussis, and tetanus and sprayed much of the town with DDT and chlordane for vector control. Records indicate that no increase in typhoid fever or malaria was seen during this period.[45]

In response to a severe earthquake that rocked northwestern Iran in September 1962, killing more than 10,000 people, the US Army Europe sent the entire 8th Evacuation Hospital and the Preventive Medicine Surveillance Detachment from the 485th Medical Laboratory. Personnel from this detachment were instrumental in performing surveys, setting up delousing stations, supervising immunization teams, and providing sanitation instruction.[46,47]

Three months later, in January 1963, US Army Europe again responded to a major foreign disaster by sending an Army preventive medicine team to the flood-ravaged Moroccan province of Rabat to join US Navy and Air Force personnel already engaged in relief operations. Led by the US Army Europe Chief of Preventive Medicine (Lieutenant Colonel Joseph W. Cooch), this team of four physicians, three sanitary engineers, an entomologist, and eight preventive medicine technicians administered 41,000 doses of typhoid fever vaccine, deloused 9,000 people, and treated 75 wells.[48] These interventions were quite impressive in scope, yet no surveillance data were collected to assess their effectiveness.

Concurrent with these sporadic opportunities for US military involvement in goodwill missions overseas were institutional changes within the federal government as to which agency should orchestrate humanitarian assistance programs; they were felt to lack necessary focus and coordination. The issue itself was hotly debated during the 1960 presidential election. With his victory, John F. Kennedy made foreign assistance a top priority for his new administration. This prompted the US Congress to pass the 1961 Foreign Assistance Act, which called for the establishment of the US Agency for International Development (USAID) within the State Department. The first test for this new agency, the executor of all US foreign assistance programs, would be in the Republic of (South) Vietnam. In an effort to check the spread of Communism, USAID established a program based on counterinsurgency and democratic and economic development.

VIETNAM: NATION BUILDING, MEDICAL CIVIC ACTION, AND REFUGEE RELIEF

With the defeat of the French army at Dien Bien Phu by the Viet Minh and the resulting cease-fire agreement in Geneva, Vietnam was partitioned in 1954 at the 17th parallel into a procommunist north and an anticommunist south. As Ho Chi Minh's forces descended onto Haiphong and the rich Tonkin delta region to consolidate their gains, the US Navy mounted a 100-ship evacuation operation called "Passage to Freedom" that ultimately rescued 310,848 people fleeing the north. Key to this operation was Lieutenant (Junior Grade) Thomas A. Dooley who led the Navy's Preventive Medicine and Sanitation Unit at the refugee camps and embarkation sites in Haiphong. For his outstanding work with the fleeing refugees, Dr. Dooley was awarded the "Officier de l'Ordre National de Vietnam" by the President of South Vietnam in 1955.[49]

Within months of the political partition of Vietnam, the US government sent advisers to train the military of South Vietnam to deal with rebel forces known as the Viet Cong. The United States' first unconventional or guerilla war since the Philippine insurrection some 50 years before, the Vietnam War presented unique and serious challenges to the armed forces. Concurrent with the conduct of this war were OOTW known as medical civic action programs, which were complementary (in theory) to efforts in-country being managed by USAID. A mix of psychological operations and humanitarianism, these programs were intended to "win the hearts and minds" of the people while providing underutilized military medical personnel with an outlet for their skills.[50] The first of these programs, the Medical Civic Action Program (MEDCAP I), was begun in January 1963 to provide increased outpatient care for Vietnamese civilians living in rural areas. The strict intent was to enhance the "prestige" of the South Vietnamese government and army; US personnel were to have only a supporting role. US participation came primarily from advisory personnel assigned to Vietnamese Army units.[51,52]

In one example, MCA (Medical Civic Action) team #20 operated as a moving dispensary from April through December of 1963, visiting 121 villages and seeing some 20,000 civilian patients. With helminthiasis, conjunctivitis, and anemia among the most common diagnoses being made by his team, Captain James Anderson commented "it is obvious that a medical civic action program offers real opportunities for preventive medicine."[53p1056] In spite of this realization, no sustainable, long-term preventive medicine interventions were recorded by MCA team #20.[53]

By comparison, the US Special Forces (SF) working with the minority ethnic groups (eg, Montagnards, Nuongs, Cambodians) in the Vietnamese central highlands not only provided curative care but also sought to educate the people in basic sanitation and health measures. Captain Lowell Rubin, an SF physician who led much of this work, believed that the long-term objective of improving the health of these people could not be met any other way.[54] These tribes played a critical role in counterinsurgency efforts spearheaded by the SF. Referring to the Civilian Irregular Defense Group program of which these tribes were a part, Colonel Charles Webb (then the John F. Kennedy Special Warfare Center Surgeon and a preventive medicine physician) emphasized that comprehensive internal defense and development required that village health workers be trained appropriately. "A preventive medicine-oriented program, attacking the sources of disease, is necessary for any lasting contribution to local welfare... programs which provide safe water sources, sewage disposal, and the control of disease reservoirs and vectors."[55p392] According to Webb, veterinary officers also proved to be invaluable in these programs by assisting "in the prevention and eradication of zoonotic diseases, in slaughter and food preparation programs and in the treatment and care of domestic and pack animals."[55p394] The SF medical leadership (under Colonel Lewellyn Legters) was so serious about bringing state-of-the-art preventive medicine to unconventional warfare and medical civic action that they established the US Army Special Forces–Walter Reed Army Institute of Research Field Epidemiology Survey Team (Airborne).[56,57] Another demonstration of SF's commitment in this arena came in 1971, when the 1st SF Group in Okinawa helped quash typhoid fever epidemics in neighboring Malaysia and the Philippines by sending in immunization teams.[3]

Apparently these and other lessons were also being followed by the enemy. Captain Arthur Ahearn in his description of Viet Cong medicine states:

> The Viet Cong are quite conscious of public health, and they employ the principles of sanitation extensively in their civic action and propaganda efforts. During the recent flood in the Danang area, they launched an intensive campaign to educate the villagers about the dangers of water pollution and measures to be taken to protect water and food from contamination. Such slogans as "Prevention of Disease is Patriotism" and "Prevention of Disease is Fighting the Americans" have been observed.[58p221]

Declaring MEDCAP I a success because it had demonstrated that the government of South Vietnam cared about its citizens, the Military Assistance Command, Vietnam (MACV), phased the program out by 1965 (for all but SF) and replaced it with MEDCAP II. This new program had the same goals as MEDCAP I but would involve US and free-world military units of battalion size or larger in the direct provision of medical care to civilians. Each of these allied units had the option of conducting a MEDCAP II program in their area of operation if they had the approval of the local Vietnamese provincial authority, the US Overseas Mission, and the MACV sector advisor.[59] From 1 December 1967 to 31 March 1968, an average of 188,441 civilians received outpatient treatment and 17,686 were immunized through MEDCAP II activities each month. By 1970, the MEDCAP II program was seeing between 150,000 and 225,000 outpatients monthly. As part of these efforts, US Army veterinary personnel established training in swine husbandry for farmers and provided cattle vaccinations. As part of a rabies control program, 21,391 animals in civilian communities were immunized in 1967.[52]

In reviewing the conduct of MEDCAP programs, Lieutenant Colonel (later Major General) Floyd Baker, Surgeon of the 1st US Field Force, observed that

> the ultimate goal of medical assistance rendered to the Vietnamese is to have the Vietnamese themselves capable of maintaining a satisfactory level of preventive and therapeutic medicine. Although much has been contributed by US medical efforts, these efforts, at times, result in only temporary relief of a situation and contribute little to the long term improvement in the health status of the Vietnamese.[60p10]

In what would prove to be an instructive example of what MEDCAPs were intended to be, Dr. Baker described the appropriate disposition of an epidemic of plague in one hamlet. Thirty people were ill and three had already died. Although US military MEDCAP personnel were ready to handle the outbreak unilaterally, they instead coordinated with the provincial health director to have the Vietnamese authorities take charge, with US medical personnel in an advisory role only. The process took longer, but all cases of plague were identified and treated, and people in the surrounding area received appropriate immunization. Villagers learned the proper way to dust with 10% DDT (then in use) to control fleas. They also learned how to control the rat population.[60]

Jeffrey Greenhut in his excellent review of medical civic action programs in Vietnam perhaps sums up these efforts best in saying that

> The overall effectiveness of medical civilian assistance programs is difficult to measure. Medically they could make no real impact on the general health of the population ignorant of basic health measures....[It] must be kept in mind that the primary purpose of all the programs was to assist in winning the "hearts and minds" of the population and, in this, no reliable measure of effectiveness exists.[59p127]

Ironically, US involvement in OOTW in Vietnam ended much as it began some 20 years earlier. With the fall of South Vietnam in April 1975, the United States mounted Operation New Life to accommodate more than 120,000 refugees in camps in the Philippines, Guam, and the US mainland. Once again, preventive medicine personnel stepped forward in this humanitarian effort to provide camp sanitation, communicable disease control, health and hygiene education, and mass immunizations.[61,62]

OPERATIONS OTHER THAN WAR IN LATIN AMERICA

Since the establishment of the Monroe Doctrine, no part of the world has felt the dominant foreign intervention hand of the United States like the countries of the Western Hemisphere, particularly those of Latin America. While the US military buildup in Vietnam was just starting in April of 1965, there was increasing political turmoil in the Dominican Republic, a country the United States had occupied from 1916 to 1924. Fearing a Cuban-style communist takeover, President Johnson sent elements of the 18th Airborne Corps there. When the troops arrived and secured the capital city, they quickly learned that the civilian casualty rate had been greatly exaggerated. (In fact, it was several days before arriving hospital units could find any Dominican casualties to treat.) US battle casualties also proved to be relatively light, with 16 killed and 148 wounded, 68 of whom who required hospitalization. A common complaint was that the 22,000 servicemen participating in this operation (named Power Pack) found themselves with little to do.[63]

Preventive medicine personnel, however, found themselves to be in great demand. The threat of epidemic diarrhea spreading from the city to the troops spurred the 714th Preventive Medicine Detachment to quickly organize and train field sanitation teams (a total of 114 personnel) for the deployed force. The administration of immune globulin successfully curbed a nascent outbreak of hepatitis A in the troops. Vector control initiatives were credited with there being no reported cases of malaria or dengue among troops in the field.

In the civilian community, preventive medicine personnel worked closely with the Red Cross and the Ministry of Health to restore public services damaged in the fighting, such as the potable water system, and prevent the spread of disease by such activities as a typhoid fever immunization program. Through 1966, the emphasis for these public health cooperative efforts was placed on water testing, rodent control, restaurant inspection, field sanitation team training, venereal disease control, and garbage disposal.[63]

Although this intervention in the Dominican Republic to prevent anarchy proved to be a relative success with little loss of US service member life, the concurrent war in Southeast Asia proved to be otherwise. The Paris Peace Accords had allowed the United States to withdraw from South Vietnam in 1973, but the war itself left the United States with a severe reluctance to enter into another armed conflict. Instead, at the height of the Cold War, US military doctrine would focus for the next decade on the nuclear arms race and preparing to fight a conventional war with Warsaw Pact forces across the central plains of Germany. The military would engage in few humanitarian missions during this time. Peacekeeping missions, as we currently understand them, were not even a consideration.

A bloody coup by communist revolutionaries on the island of Grenada changed all of this. In October 1982, under the name Operation Urgent Fury, the US military and forces from six Caribbean nations flew to the island to restore order and to rescue approximately 1,000 US citizens being held captive. A myriad of preventive medicine issues confronted the preventive medicine officer (Colonel N. Joe Thompson) and the environmental science officer (Major John B. Czachowski) for the 18th Airborne Corps. (They would be joined by the 714/155 Preventive Medicine Detachment from Fort Bragg, NC.) After addressing preventive medicine issues involving US soldiers, these professionals moved on to the problem of caring for the basic sanitation and public health needs of some 800 detained Cuban and Grenadian personnel. With most of the senior leadership of the ministry of health killed in the coup, Colonel Thompson and Major Czachowski worked closely with representatives from USAID to restore the public health services of the island (eg, garbage disposal, sewage treatment, insect control, replacement of lost vaccines). Most notable were the efforts of an Army sanitary engineer from the US Army Environmental Hygiene Agency who established a system of "wash throughs" to clear a portion of the city water system of a toxin, paraquat, placed there by a saboteur.[64]

After the attempted communist takeover of Grenada, a significant concern arose that other countries in Latin America could slip into the Cuban and Soviet sphere of influence. A number of factors favored insurgency movements in these countries, such as the gross disparity in living conditions between rich and poor and an apparent lack of concern on the part of existing governments for the welfare of their own citizens. Following communist doctrine, Soviet surrogates would deploy civic action teams (eg, medical, engineering, teaching) to many rural areas to build support for their revolutionary cause while seeking to discredit the existing government. These rebels would further try to destabilize the government by disrupting its economy and ability to provide services to the people.

For struggling democracies to have their best chance to succeed against such a threat, they needed assistance from the outside. With health care matters and economic recovery being inexorably intertwined, the most appropriate role for military medicine in this low-intensity conflict (LIC) environment became that of nation building rather than the more traditional combat service support. While not usurping the State Department's job of development through the USAID, the Army Medical Department was nevertheless uniquely positioned to build on lessons learned from its MEDCAP programs in Vietnam.[65–67] It was important for the leaders and military of these countries to be seen as caring for their own people.

Throughout the 1980s, El Salvador was embroiled in a civil war between the Farabundo Marti Liberation Movement (Marxist-Leninist guerrillas supported by Cuba and Nicaragua) and the El Salvadoran democrats. Early in the insurgency, the guerrillas found it fairly easy to discredit the abusive military government and was known to have provided health care and other public services to the impoverished peasant farmers in the rural areas they controlled. Involvement of the US military in this conflict was severely limited by Congressional action. By the late 1980s, it became obvious to senior leaders of the El Salvadoran government that an end to hostilities could only be reached through significant government human rights reforms and free elections. Inherent in winning back the trust of the people was the need for significant civic action programs on the part of the El Salvadoran military. A team of officers and senior enlisted personnel from the Army Medical Department assisted in many of these efforts, which included the provision of prosthetic devices to those who had lost limbs to land mines, the establishment of an infectious disease reporting system, and the building of a human waste disposal system for the capital city of San Salvador.

The involvement of the Army Medical Department in Honduras largely began in 1983 with the military exercise Big Pine II (Ahuas Tara) through which US personnel of the Medical Element of Joint Task Force-Bravo (41st Combat Support Hospital) initiated a series of humanitarian civic action–type training activities termed Medical Readiness Training Exercises (MEDRETEs). In the first year, 135 villages were visited, 47,228 patients evaluated, 21,047 teeth extracted, and 37,067 animals treated. Medical personnel also participated with Honduran officials in providing 202,339 immunizations against polio, diphtheria, pertussis, tetanus, tuberculosis, and measles during the country's national immunization week.[68,69]

Over the next decade, MEDRETEs would be repeated frequently by many units deploying to Latin America and would provide training opportunities for health care professionals from all of the US armed services, including National Guard and Reserve units. Not unlike their MEDCAP forefathers in Vietnam, these MEDRETEs were planned with the best intentions yet too often proved to be ineffective and costly, providing but a transitory benefit to the rural populations served. In fact, many of these missions failed to even address the communities' public health requirements of potable water, human waste disposal, vector control, personal hygiene and sanitation, and basic health education.[70,71] Rarely, if ever, were medical outcomes followed in time to see if the interventions had a beneficial effect.

Because of the training benefit to the units involved, these missions continue to the present day, often involving National Guard units. Starting in the 1990s, these programs have come under greater scrutiny by the respective regional commander-in-chief and the Peacekeeping and Humanitarian Assistance Office of the Assistant Secretary of Defense to ensure that they are properly coordinated with the local ambassador and military attache and that their goals, methods, and content meet certain criteria. "Tailgate" medicine is no longer considered appropriate for these missions.

Distinct in funding and statutory authority from the humanitarian civic assistance–type projects mentioned above are humanitarian assistance programs, which enable the commanders-in-chief to finance projects customized to their regions' specific needs. Perhaps the best example of such a humanitarian assistance program funded by commander-in-chief initiative funds is the establishment of a sustainable computerized infectious disease surveillance system for a number of countries in the Caribbean region. This project, begun in 1997, has been a collaboration between preventive medicine professionals at the Walter Reed Army Institute of Research, the Pan American Health Organization, and the respective national ministries of health.

THE MODERN ERA OF COMPLEX HUMANITARIAN EMERGENCIES

Iraq and the Kurds

In March 1991, in the aftermath of the Gulf War, Saddam Hussein ruthlessly suppressed a popular uprising among ethnic Kurds in northern Iraq with the army divisions spared in the Persian Gulf War. Faced with certain retribution, 1.5 million people in this region attempted to flee the country in advance of Iraqi Army troops. More than 500,000 of these Kurds ended up massed along the austere mountainous border between Turkey and Iraq with no means to protect, feed, or shelter themselves. At the direction of President George Bush, the US military in Europe led a North Atlantic Treaty Organization relief effort (Operation Provide Comfort). This effort began with air drops of supplies in April 1991 (Figure 4-4) and culminated with the resettlement of the people into their towns by late summer (Figure 4-5). The 10th SF Group was the first and primary responder sent in to stabilize the situation in the mountains. First providing security for the people from hostile forces, these professionals quickly organized an efficient distribution system for food and relief supplies (Figures 4-6 and 4-7). Colonel Michael Benenson, an Army preventive medicine physician from the 7th Medical Command in Heidelberg, Germany, was named the Combined Task Force Surgeon for Operation Provide Comfort. Colonel Benenson and his staff supervised all of the medical aspects of the relief effort, assigning the placement of arriving military and civilian medical relief units where needed most. Two other preventive medicine physicians (Captain Ralph L. Erickson, US Army, from the US Army Special Operations Command, Fort Bragg, NC, and Lieutenant Commander Trueman Sharp, US Navy, from the 7th Preventive Medicine Unit, Sigonella, Italy) served with the Public Health Disaster Assistance Response Team (PH DART) from USAID's Office of Foreign Disaster Assistance in assessing the public health needs of the mountain "camps" on a daily basis. Working in both the camps and at the main staging base in Siloppi, Turkey, this team provided the coordinating link between the military (initially 10th SF Group, later numerous NATO allied units) and the follow-on civilian relief workers from private voluntary agencies. In this assessment and coordinating role, the team collected data concerning the incidence of in-

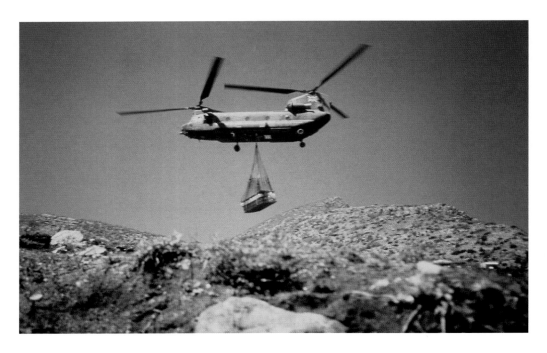

Fig. 4-4. Aerial food resupply of Kurdish refugee camp at Curcurcka, Iraq, during Operation Provide Comfort in 1991. The mountainous terrain of this border region made this form of resupply the only one practical. With significant rotary-wing airlift capability, the US military forged a productive collaboration with its civilian counterparts in the relief effort. Photograph: Courtesy of Lieutenant Colonel Ralph L. Erickson, Medical Corps, US Army.

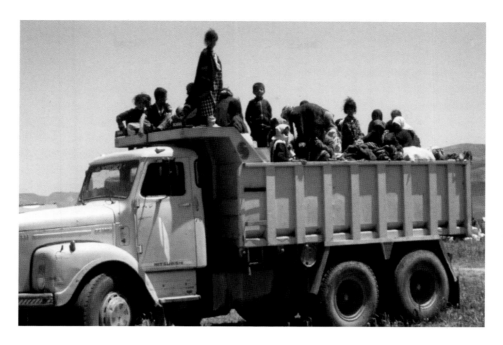

Fig. 4-5. Kurdish refugee families being transported from mountain camps back to their homes in northern Iraq during Operation Provide Comfort, 1991. Photograph: Courtesy of Lieutenant Colonel Ralph L. Erickson, Medical Corps, US Army.

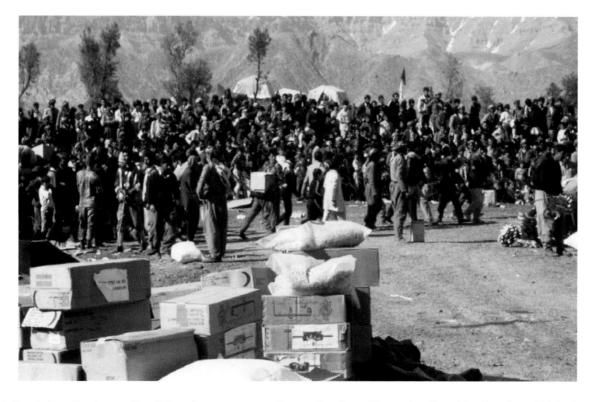

Fig. 4-6. Food distribution at Kurdish refugee camp at Curcurcka, Iraq (Operation Provide Comfort, 1991). In running this distribution network, the US military made use of the Kurd family-clan hierarchy. Mortality and health surveillance data were collected from the families at the time food was picked up. Photograph: Courtesy of Lieutenant Colonel Ralph L. Erickson, Medical Corps, US Army.

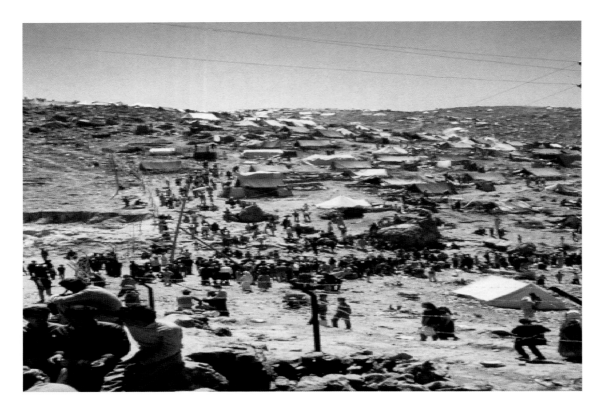

Fig. 4-7. At its peak, the Kurdish refugee camp at Curcurcka, Iraq, held 100,000 people (Operation Provide Comfort, 1991). With little protection from the elements and only a few intermittent streams from which to drink, hundreds of people, especially children, died from hypothermia or diarrhea. This excess mortality was greatly decreased with the provision of tents, food, and chlorinated water. Photograph: Courtesy of Lieutenant Colonel Ralph L. Erickson, Medical Corps, US Army.

fectious disease (eg, diarrhea) and mortality in the camps. It also helped prioritize necessary public health interventions, such as provision of safe water and sanitary facilities. Within this broad effort, a cholera epidemic was tracked and controlled. In response to an outbreak of measles, this team administered a program that led to more than 45,000 children under the age of 5 years being immunized (Figure 4-8). Members of the PH DART also conducted a cross-sectional health survey in this vulnerable age group, revealing significant acute malnutrition.[72,73]

Haitian Refugees

From 1991 to 1994, tens of thousands of Haitians fled their country because of a deteriorating economy and the violent repression of the ruling military junta. Many of those fleeing by small boats and rafts, hoping to travel to Florida, were interdicted by the US Coast Guard and brought to an established refugee camp at the US Naval Base at Guantanamo Bay, Cuba, where their immigration status could be further evaluated (Operation

GTMO). From October 1991 through May 1992, more than 34,000 Haitians were cared for at this camp, with 26,000 of them being eventually repatriated to their home country to apply for immigration through traditional channels. The infectious diseases carried by this predominantly male population included filariasis, malaria, tuberculosis, and human immunodeficiency virus infection. Though security was the number one public health priority at all times, the logistics of providing sanitation and safe food and water was an arduous task. These duties and others (eg, disease surveillance, vector control, immunizations) kept preventive medicine personnel from all of the uniformed services constantly busy.[74] Although the camp census fell considerably (to less than 1,000) following President George Bush's executive order to halt the bringing of migrating Haitians to Guantanamo (but rather to repatriate them directly to Haiti), conditions within Haiti continued to deteriorate through July 1994, prompting some to predict that more than 100,000 would attempt to flee within the coming months if something were not done.[75]

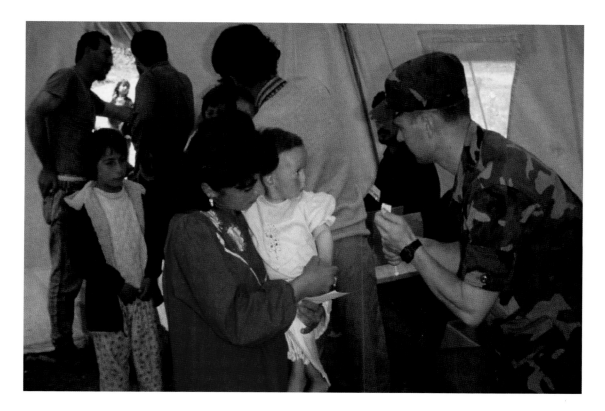

Fig. 4-8. A US preventive medicine officer provides measles immunizations to Kurdish refugee children during Operation Provide Comfort, 1991. Mortality from measles can be especially high in refugee settings where children are undernourished and stressed. In response to an outbreak of 26 cases of measles at the camp of Yekmal, more than 45,000 Kurdish children were immunized. Photograph: Courtesy of Lieutenant Colonel Ralph L. Erickson, Medical Corps, US Army.

In September 1994, US forces arrived in Haiti leading a multinational force to remove the military dictatorship and restore democracy (reseating President Aristide). Preventive medicine professionals deploying in support of Operation Uphold Democracy quickly established field sanitation, vector control, and safe water for the US (and later United Nations) camps.[76] An effective febrile disease surveillance system ultimately tracked incidence of dengue fever and hepatitis E among the peacekeepers, resulting in renewed emphasis on personal protective measures and sanitation.[77] The scope of preventive medicine services eventually expanded into the civilian community as personnel from the 61st Preventive Medicine Detachment conducted inspections of hotels, restaurants, and government institutions.[78] Personnel from the 94th Medical Detachment (Veterinary Medicine) also immunized nearly 50,000 dogs and cats for rabies as part of Operation Mad Dog.[79]

NATURAL DISASTER RELIEF IN RECENT TIMES

Following the deadly Alaskan earthquake of 1964, Army preventive medicine personnel assisted civilian public health officials in relief efforts in Anchorage, Valdez, and Seward. The Army personnel conducted sanitation surveys, provided a safe water supply, and provided immunizations where indicated. In the wake of three hurricanes hitting the United States (Betsy 1965, Beulah 1967, and Agnes 1972), Army units again participated as needed to ensure the public health safety of the populations affected through, respectively, the provision of typhoid immunizations, basic sanitation, and consultation.[3]

Responding to a December 1972 earthquake that leveled Managua, Nicaragua, leaving an estimated 5,000 people dead and another 20,000 injured, the US Southern Command deployed a Disaster Area Survey Team, commanded by Colonel Raymond L. Coultrip, to the city. In assessing the needs of the population and providing consultation to the US

Ambassador concerning US participation, this team performed two vital preventive medicine services. The first involved coordinating the repair of the city water system; the second was the turning back of an unnecessary typhoid fever immunization program even though political pressure was brought to bear to use some 900,000 doses of a vaccine contributed by another Latin American country.[80]

Hurricane Andrew swept ashore on 24 August 1992, destroying 25,000 homes and leaving 200,000 homeless or temporarily displaced in south Florida. In its eventual sweep through the Bahamas, Florida, and Louisiana, it would cause at least 48 deaths. Within hours, the 44th Medical Brigade under the command of Brigadier General (now LTG) James Peake formed a relief task force to aid civilian authorities in the devastated area, which happened to include Homestead Air Force Base. An early assessment revealed that the local public health system had collapsed and that tap water, though available, was not potable. Personnel from the 44th quickly established a series of 28 free clinics for both civilians and military members from the community. Efforts were also undertaken by the military to provide field sanitation facilities and water. Lieutenant Colonel Jose Sanchez and Captain Vincent Fonseca, representing the Epidemiologic Consultation Service of the Surgeon General (headquartered at the Walter Reed Army Institute of Research), established an outpatient surveillance system among the 28 clinics. With a complementary system established by the Dade County Public Health Unit, they demonstrated a sustained low prevalence of diarrhea and respiratory disease for the first month of relief operations. These data proved invaluable to senior leaders in the relief effort who were then able to prioritize interventions correctly (eg, avoiding an unnecessary typhoid fever immunization program, turning back an excess of health care volunteers), while reassuring the public that things were under control.[81]

Six years later, on 24 October 1998, Hurricane Mitch pummeled the Caribbean coast of Central America for more than 48 hours. The heavy, continuous rains and resulting landslides and flooding were estimated to have cost up to 25,000 lives in Honduras, Nicaragua, El Salvador, and Guatemala. In Honduras alone (the country most severely hit), more than 1.5 million people were affected, many without shelter.[82] In response to this immense human tragedy, the US Southern Command organized Operation Fuerto Apoyo (Strong Support), sending 5,400 servicemembers from all four armed services and 140,000 lbs of supplies to the region. Joint Task Force-Bravo spearheaded the effort in Honduras, while Task Force Aguila (Eagle) addressed the needs of El Salvador, Nicaragua, and Guatemala. Preventive medicine physicians and sanitarians from the US Army Center for Health Promotion and Preventive Medicine (Aberdeen Proving Ground, Md) played key roles through the initial assessment of the public health needs of these countries. The US military provided massive amounts of drinkable water (420,000 gal) at various locations and cleaned out contaminated wells. They also helped spray for vectors and provided consultation in the control of outbreaks of cholera, typhoid fever, leptospirosis, malaria, and conjunctivitis.[83]

SUMMARY

The participation of the US military in OOTW both within the United States and abroad, especially in the last 40 years, is perhaps best explained by necessity. Taking nothing away from the Federal Emergency Management Agency, the American Red Cross, the United Nations, and a host of nongovernmental organizations, the US military has unmatched capabilities and training that are useful in emergency situations. Transportation assets and logistical depth top the list. In addition, the Department of Defense's ability to provide credible physical security while maintaining command, control, communication, and intelligence in a highly unstable field environment is also unique. Though various groups are working to become self-sustaining under austere conditions, no other organization trains to the level of preparedness of the US armed forces.

The military's field medical capabilities, particularly the depth of preventive medicine equipment and expertise, allow for rapid employment without a prolonged period of acquisition or training.

With the dissolution of the Soviet Union and the end to the Cold War, the decades-long tensions between superpowers have eased considerably, but previously suppressed religious and ethnic rivalries have resurfaced with a vengeance. The collapse of the Soviet bloc has left a number of fragile, internally conflicted states, two of which in 2001 contain US military peacekeepers: Bosnia and Kosovo. Given decades of corruption, civil war, and rampant disease (eg, HIV), a number of profoundly weak nations, particularly in Africa, have nearly collapsed in recent years. Transitional nations—those trying to emerge from national conflict or political change)—are poised for either growth or chaos. The challenge for the US National Command Authority in this unstable, post–Cold War era is to be ready and to have established criteria for the employment of military forces in these OOTW.

The central role played by preventive medicine personnel in OOTW is best illustrated in the missions of humanitarian assistance, disaster relief, and nation building. From the earliest days on the American frontier to the aftermath of the San Francisco earthquake to the conquest of deadly disease in the building of the Panama Canal to complex humanitarian emergencies in places such as Poland or Northern Iraq to the devastated countries of Central America after a hurricane, these preventive medicine professionals have risen to the occasion. They have applied the latest science and practice of sanitation, water purification, immunization, and vector and disease control in service to those in desperate need. It remains a given that US military preventive medicine officers and enlisted personnel will continue to play THE leadership role for the military's medical departments in these and other similar missions of the future.

REFERENCES

1. Department of the Army. Operations other than war. *Operations*. Washington, DC: DA; 1993. Chap 13. US Army Field Manual 100-5.

2. Institute for National Strategic Studies. Strategic Assessment. Washington, DC: National Defense University: 1997.

3. Foster GM. *The Demands of Humanity: Army Medical Disaster Relief*. Washington, DC: Center of Military History, US Army; 1983: 6–22.

4. US Congress, House, Report of the Commissioner of Indian Affairs in Relation to the Act Extending the Benefit of Vaccination to the Indian Tribes, H. Doc. 82, 22d Cong., 2d sess., 1833; Ltrs, T. Hastley Crawford to Joel R. Poinsett, 11 Dec 1838 and 25 Nov 1838. Both in Report Books of the Office of Indian Affairs, 1838–85, M348 reel 1, National Archives. Cited in: Foster GM. *The Demands of Humanity: Army Medical Disaster Relief*. Washington, DC: Center of Military History, US Army; 1983.

5. Freedmen's bureau. *Encyclopedia Britannica*. Vol 4. 15th ed. Chicago: Encyclopedia Britannica, Inc; 1989: 965.

6. Duffy J. *Sword of Pestilence: The New Orleans Yellow Fever Epidemic of 1853*. Baton Rouge, La: Louisiana State University; 1966: 100–102.

7. Letter , C.A. Bell to R. Rinble, 25 Jun 1868, Letters Sent, Chief Medical Officer of Kentucky, entry 1091, Record Group 105, NA; Unlabeled newspaper clipping, in Medical Officers of the Civil War, p. 116, entry 86, Records of the Office of the Surgeon General, Record Group 112, National Archives. Cited in: Foster GM. *The Demands of Humanity: Army Medical Disaster Relief*. Washington, DC: Center of Military History, US Army; 1983: 20.

8. Russell Sage Foundation. *San Francisco: Relief Survey*. New York: Survey Associates; 1913: 4–5.

9. Greeley AW. *Earthquake in California, April 18, 1906: Special Report of Maj. Gen. Adolphus W. Greeley, Army, Commanding the Pacific Division, on the Relief Operations, Conducted by the Military Authorities of the United States at San Francisco and Other Points, With Accompanying Documents*. Washington, DC: US Government Printing Office; 1906.

10. *The Report of the Surgeon General of the Army to the Secretary of War for the Fiscal Year Ending June 30, 1906*. Washington, DC: Government Printing Office; 131–133.

11. News of the services. *Mil Surgeon*. 1907;20:513.

12. Normoyle JE. *Flood Sufferers in the Mississippi and Ohio Valleys: Report of James E. Normoyle in Charge of Relief Operations, April, May, June, July, 1912*. Washington, DC: US Government Printing Office; 1913: 122–34.

13. Bicknell EP. *Mississippi River Flood of 1912*. Washington, DC: American Red Cross; nd: 11.

14. Eckert AW. *A Time of Terror: The Great Dayton Flood*. Boston: Little, Brown & Co; 1965: 56–63.

15. Rhoads TL. Report of Chief Sanitary Officer on the Work of the Sanitation Department at Dayton, Ohio & Vicinity 29 March to 25 April. Records of the Office of the Chief of Engineers. National Archives. Record Group 77, file 88925. Cited in: Foster GM. *The Demands of Humanity: Army Medical Disaster Relief.* Washington, DC: Center of Military History, US Army; 1983: 75.

16. Wadhams. Letter to Fauntleroy. 24 April. National Archives. Record Group 94, file 2022074. As cited in: Foster GM. *The Demands of Humanity: Army Medical Disaster Relief.* Washington, DC: Center of Military History, US Army; 1983: 77.

17. Hutton PC. Diseases and sanitary conditions among Alaskan Indians. *Mil Surgeon.* 1908;22:449–454.

18. Panama Canal. *Compton's Encyclopedia.* Vol 18. Chicago: Encyclopedia Britannica, Inc: 1989: 95–104.

19. Breunle PC. William Crawford Gorgas: Military sanitarian of the Isthmian Canal. *Mil Med.* 1976;141:795–797.

20. Gorgas MD, Hendrick BJ. *William Crawford Gorgas: His Life and Work.* New York: Doubleday, Page and Co; 1924: 210.

21. Carmichael OC. *Endorsements, Resolutions and Other Data in Behalf of the Nomination of Dr. William Crawford Gorgas for Election to the New York University Hall of Fame for Great Americans.* Birmingham, Ala: np; 1950: 19.

22. United States of America: Imperialism, the Progressive Era, and the rise to world power. *Encyclopedia Britannica.* Vol 29. Chicago: Encyclopedia Britannica, Inc: 1989: 252.

23. *The Report of the Surgeon General of the Army to the Secretary of War for the Fiscal Year Ending June 30, 1914.* Washington, DC: Government Printing Office; 1914: 83, 164.

24. Johnson R. *My Life in the US Army 1899 to 1922.* p 174. Cited in: Gillette M. *The Army Medical Department 1865–1917.* Washington, DC: Center of Military History, US Army; 1995.

25. Hume EE. American relief work in Serbia. *Mil Surgeon.* 1921;49:188–201.

26. Davenport WP. General health conditions and medical relief work in Armenia. *Mil Surgeon.* 1921;48:139–158.

27. Lambert RA. Post-war medical conditions among Armenian refugees in southern Turkey and Syria. *Mil Surgeon.* 1921;49:314–332.

28. Gilchrist H. Typhus Fever in Poland. *Mil Surgeon.* 1920;46:622–629.

29. Halliday C. Conditions in Poland, 1919–1920. *Mil Surgeon.* 1922;51:418–443.

30. *The Report of the Surgeon General of the Army to the Secretary of War for the Fiscal Year Ending June 30, 1920.* Washington, DC: Government Printing Office; 378–379.

31. Bergman AN. Memorandum No. 20 Headquarters of American Typhus Fever Expedition, US Army. *Mil Surgeon.* 1920;47:485–486.

32. Headquarters, American Polish Relief Expedition Oct 1, 1920. *Mil Surgeon.* 1920;47:718–719.

33. Foucar FH. Resume of experiences and work accomplished in Russia with the American Relief Administration, 1921–1923: Part I. *Mil Surgeon.* 1924;54:680–698.

34. Foucar FH. Resume of experiences and work accomplished in Russia with the American Relief Administration, 1921–1923: Part II. *Mil Surgeon.* 1924;55:20–38.

35. Turnbull JS. Report on an outbreak of typhoid fever at Jacobstown, N.J. *Mil Surgeon.* 1922;50:306–309.

36. Rad, Commanding General 4th Corps Area to AG, 24 Jan 25; Letter, ET Conley to AG, 10 Mar 25; Letter William J. Harris, 4 Feb 25; Summary of Action Taken in Flooded Districts, by Thomas H. Darrel, 3 Feb 25; All in box 929, 400.38 Record Gp 407 National Archives. Cited in: Foster GM. *The Demands of Humanity: Army Medical Disaster Relief.* Washington, DC: Center of Military History, US Army; 1983: 108.

37. Memo for LTC R.L. Collins by T.J. Flynn, 25 Apr 27 and Financial Report of the Floods of 1927, both in box 2418, 400.38, Record Group 407, National Archives. As cited in: Foster GM. *The Demands of Humanity: Army Medical Disaster Relief.* Washington, DC: Center of Military History, US Army; 1983: 112.

38. Gorby AL. Army flood relief in the Ohio River flood area. *Army Med Bull.* 1937;39:45–50.

39. McNeal MJ. Destruction of Tokyo. *Catholic World.* 1924;118:315–316.

40. Munson EL. Report on the Medical and Hospital Service of the Japan Relief Mission. *Monthly Bull Philippine Health Serv.* 1924;4:57–60.

41. Hetfield WB. Medical activities in the Managua earthquake. *Mil Surgeon.* 1931;69:143–148.

42. Heaton LD, Tempel CW. The role of the Army Medical Service in America's People-to-People Program. *Mil Med.* 1961;126:256–58.

43. Ludwig HF. Sanitary engineering in "Operation Tulip." *Public Health Reports.* 1954;69:533–537.

44. Thisler, JO; On Mercy Wings; Army Information Digest 10 (Feb 55): 18–21; Office of the Surgeon General, Summary of Major Events and Problems, 1 July 1954 to 30 June 1955: 122–24, in Center for Military History files; Historical Summary, Office of the Chief Surgeon, US Army Forces, Far East and Eighth United States Army, 1954, in CMH files; *New York Times*, 17, 19, 27 Aug and 23 Sept 54. Cited in: Foster GM. *The Demands of Humanity: Army Medical Disaster Relief.* Washington, DC: Center of Military History, US Army; 1983: 149.

45. Gordon JJ, Luehrs RE. Medical aspects of a hurricane disaster in Mexico. *US Armed Forces Med J.* 1956;7:394–398.

46. Wergeland FL, Cooch JW. Operation Ida. *Mil Med.* 1963;128: 850–857.

47. Anon USAREUR Medics Aid in Iranian Earthquake. *Med Bull US Army Eur.* 1962;19(11):231–233.

48. Keating PJ. Moroccan flood relief: A personal report. *Med Bull US Army Eur.* 1963;20(4):96–99.

49. Medical officer honored. *US Armed Forces Med J.* 1955;6(1):1128.

50. Moncrief WH. The Provincial Health Assistance Program in the Republic of Vietnam. *USARV Med Bull.* 1967;2(1):39–43 (also called USARV Pam 40–1).

51. Eisner DG. Medical Civic Action Programs (MEDCAP). *USARV Med Bull.* 1966;1(7):27–29.

52. Neel S. Medical assistance to Vietnamese civilians. In: *Medical Support of the US Army in Vietnam 1965–70.* Washington, DC: Department of the Army; 1973. Chapter XIII; 162–168.

53. Anderson JE. The field Experience of a Medical Civic Action Team in South Vietnam. *Mil Med.* 1964;129:1052–1057.

54. Rubin LJ. MEDCAP with the Montagnards. *USARV Med Bull.* 1968;40(May-Jun):27–34.

55. Webb CR Jr. Medical considerations in internal defense and development. *Mil Med.* 1968;133:391–396.

56. Fuenfer MM. The United States Army Special Forces–Walter Reed Army Institute of Research Field Epidemiological Survey Team (Airborne), 1965–1968. *Mil Med.* 1991;156:96–99.

57. Driscoll RS. Medical surveillance in Vietnam: Meeting the challenge. *Army Med Dept J.* 1998;8(1/2):41–44.

58. Ahearn AM. Viet Cong medicine. *Mil Med.* 1966;131:219–221.

59. Greenhut J. Medical civic action in low intensity conflict: The Vietnam experience. Depauw JW, Luz GA, eds. *Winning the Peace: The Strategic Implications of Military Civic Action.* Carlisle Barracks, Penn: Strategic Studies Institute, US Army War College; 1990: Chap 9.

60. Baker FW. Medical assistance to the Vietnamese. *USARV Med Bull.* 1967;40(6):10–14.

61. Shaw R. Preventive medicine in the Vietnamese refugee camps on Guam. *Mil Med.* 1977;142:19–28.

62. Shaw R. Health services in a disaster: Lessons from the 1975 Vietnamese evacuation. *Mil Med.* 1979;144:307–311.

63. McPherson DG. *The Role of the Army Medical Service in the Dominican Republic Crisis of 1965.* Washington, DC: The Historical Unit, US Army Medical Service; Office of the Surgeon General, Department of the Army; 1970: 17–26, 50.

64. Thompson NJ. Czachowski JB. Preventive medicine in the Grenada intervention: Detained personnel and civilian populations. *J US Army Med Dept.* 1991;11/12(Nov-Dec):4–8.

65. Smith AM, Llewellyn C. Humanitarian medical assistance in US foreign policy: Is there a constructive role for military medical services? *DISAM J.* 1992;Summer:70–78.

66. Hood CH. The United States Army Medical Department in low-intensity conflict. *Mil Med.* 1991;156:64–67.

67. Taylor JA. Military medicine's expanding role in low-intensity conflict. *Mil Rev.* 1985;April:27–34.

68. Zajtchuk R. *Ahuas Tara II Honduras, Civil Affairs 41st Combat Support Hospital After Action Report 1983–1984.* Fort Sam Houston, Tex: 41st CSH; 1984.

69. Wittich AC. The medical system and medical readiness training exercises (MEDRETEs) in Honduras. *Mil Med.* 1989;154:19–23.

70. Hood CH. Humanitarian civic action in Honduras, 1988. *Mil Med.* 1991;156:292–296.

71. Weisser RJ Jr. The maturing of MEDRETEs. *Mil Med.* 1993;158:573–575.

72. Centers for Disease Control. Public health consequences of acute displacement of Iraqi citizens—March-May 1991. *MMWR.* 1991;40: 443–447.

73. Yip R, Sharp TW. Acute malnutrition and high childhood mortality related to diarrhea: Lessons from the 1991 Kurdish refugee crisis. *JAMA.* 1993;270:587–590.

74. Lillibridge SR, Conrad K, Stinson N, Noji EK. Haitian mass migrations: Uniformed service medical support, May 1992. *Mil Med.* 1994;159:149–153.

75. Gunby P. Military medicine undertakes peacetime mission, aiding in processing those fleeing from Haiti. *JAMA.* 1994;272:191–192.

76. Kolnick AA. Military physicians of 12 nations cooperate in Haiti. *JAMA.* 1995;274:1748–1750.

77. Centers for Disease Control and Prevention. Dengue fever among US Military Personnel—Haiti, September-November, 1994. *MMWR.* 1994;43:845–848.

78. Skolnick AA. Military physicians lend healing hands to Haiti. *JAMA.* 1995;274:1664–1666.

79. Carpenter L. Operation MAD DOG—A humanitarian civic action project in Haiti. *US Army Med Dept J.* 1996;7/8:17–20.

80. Coultrip RL. Medical aspects of US disaster relief operations in Nicaragua. *Mil Med.* 1974;139:879–884.

81. Lee LE, Fonseca V, Brett KM, Sanchez J, et al. Active morbidity surveillance after Hurricane Andrew—Florida, 1992. *JAMA.* 1993;270:591–594.

82. Anonymous. The devastating path of Hurricane Mitch in Central America. *Disasters: Preparedness and Mitigation in the Americas.* 1999;75(Suppl 1):S-1–S-3.

83. Silver FT. Mitch relief efforts winding down. *US Med.* 1999;February:1,9.

Chapter 5

CONSERVING THE FIGHTING STRENGTH: MILESTONES OF OPERATIONAL MILITARY PREVENTIVE MEDICINE RESEARCH

JOHN F. BRUNDAGE, MD, MPH

J.F. Brundage; Colonel, Medical Corps, US Army (Retired); Epidemiologist, Henry M. Jackson Foundation for the Advancement of Military Medicine, Army Medical Surveillance Activity, US Army Center for Health Promotion and Preventive Medicine, Aberdeen Proving Ground; formerly, Director, Epidemiology and Disease Surveillance, US Army Center for Health Promotion and Preventive Medicine, Aberdeen Proving Ground, MD 21010-5403

INTRODUCTION

Science, sanitation, technology, and medicine are entwined inextricably with the conduct of war, and, to a remarkable degree, the events and consequences of war have shaped human history.[1] Infectious diseases, for example, have consistently determined the rise and fall of armies, nations, and societies.[2,3] It is not surprising therefore that the benefits of military preventive medicine research extend far beyond the military exigencies that spawn that research. Given that fundamental understanding, this chapter limits its scope to military infectious diseases research conducted in direct support of military operations—either by investigators in the field or with materials collected there. The chapter does not reiterate the most often recounted military medical research achievements (eg, the Reed commission in Cuba; see Chapter 2, The Historical Impact of Preventive Medicine in War) nor provide an exhaustive account of research accomplishments with military operational relevance. Rather, it introduces readers to relatively unheralded efforts that established precedents, set standards, or elucidated principles of military operational preventive medicine research.

The latter half of the 19th century marked the beginning of the era of "scientific" military preventive medicine.[4] Pasteur developed the germ theory, which is the foundation of modern microbiology, immunology, public health, and preventive medicine. Koch devised methods of culturing and staining bacteria and developed tuberculin as immune therapy for tuberculosis.[5] Between 1870 and 1890, the bacterial etiologies of tuberculosis, leprosy, anthrax, gonorrhea, cerebrospinal meningitis, typhoid fever, pneumococcal pneumonia, diphtheria, tetanus, brucellosis, and relapsing fever were elucidated; Laveran described the link between plasmodium and malaria; Manson documented for the first time that insects transmit diseases; Finlay hypothesized that yellow fever was transmitted by a single species of mosquito; and Lister developed a system of "antiseptic" surgery that employed chemical and physical barriers to surgical wound contamination.[4]

In 1883, Baron Kanehiro Takaki of the Japanese Navy medical bureau suspected that beriberi resulted from "a wrong method of diet."[6] To test his hypothesis, he arranged for two ships to sail identical 9-month-long voyages during which one crew ate usual rations—raw fish and polished white rice—while the other ate a high-protein, low-carbohydrate diet. The former suffered high rates of beriberi, but the latter had few cases. By 1890, through nutritional intervention alone, beriberi was eliminated as a threat to the Japanese navy.[6] (Approximately 50 years later, vitamin B_1 [thiamin] was isolated from rice hulls, and its deficiency in diets was shown to cause beriberi.) Takaki's classic intervention trial foreshadowed an era of militarily focused, scientifically rigorous preventive medicine research conducted in the field.

ARMY SURGEON GENERAL STERNBERG

In 1893, George Miller Sternberg was appointed Army Surgeon General. For operational preventive medical research, there could not have been a more propitious time or man for this appointment. While serving as an Army physician, Sternberg became a pioneer in the emerging fields of bacteriology and immunology. He was the first in the world to recognize and describe the pneumococcus and the first in the United States to document plasmodium in a malaria patient. He did exhaustive research into methods and effects of disinfection.[7] He wrote the definitive bacteriology textbook of the time, and his investigations of yellow fever—in the laboratory and in the midst of multiple epidemics—disproved a succession of claims of bacteriologists around the world regarding the disease's etiology. Finally, Sternberg was the first to conduct virus neutralization assays, which remain a keystone of infectious disease research. Yet Sternberg was not one-dimensional. His scientific achievements were matched by remarkable and diverse military accomplishments. He was a skillful and courageous combat surgeon during the Civil War and the Indian wars, and he served in a variety of clinical and public health staff and leadership positions during peacetime.[8]

Thus at a time of exploding knowledge and expanding opportunities, the Army had a Surgeon General who was distinguished as a researcher, scientific innovator, and military officer. He understood the needs and concerns of commanders and soldiers, he knew the importance of basing military medical practices on sound scientific principles, and he perceived the long-term benefits of military medical research. Early in his tenure as Surgeon General, he equipped laboratories and encouraged medical staffs at Army hospitals to conduct research, and he developed an aggressive, multidisciplinary, and scientifically robust central research program. Of all of Sternberg's contributions, however, the following are seminal with regard to military research in operational preventive medicine.

Army Medical School

In 1893, Sternberg founded the Army Medical School, the first graduate school of preventive medicine and public health in the United States. Since its founding, the faculty and staff of the Army Medical School (later renamed the Army Medical Service Graduate School and now the Walter Reed Army Institute of Research [WRAIR]) have provided medical research support to the military services and many of the research efforts described in this chapter were conducted by officers from this institute.

Outbreak Investigation Teams

As Surgeon General, Sternberg pioneered the use of multidisciplinary specialist teams to investigate diseases that significantly threatened military operations. For example, in 1898 Sternberg commissioned the Reed-Vaughn-Shakespeare Board to determine the causes of the high rates of typhoid fever in Army training camps. Major Walter Reed of the Army Medical School led the team. Vaughn and Shakespeare were commissioned as majors in the US Volunteers for the specific purpose of serving on the board. The board's findings regarding asymptomatic carriage and modes of transmission of typhoid fever provided landmark insights into its epidemiology, pathophysiology, and methods of control.

Overseas Research Laboratories

Sternberg wanted to establish overseas laboratories so that military scientists on these research boards could work with local experts in the natural settings of tropical diseases of military operational concern. His first research board worked in the Philippines and established a laboratory there. Many officers who served on that board—including Simmons, Strong, Siler, Craig, and Vedder—became Army, national, and world leaders in the fields of tropical diseases, public health, and military preventive medicine.

Sternberg sent his second research board to Cuba,[9] where it also established a laboratory infrastructure. The board's primary mission was to determine the cause, modes of transmission, and means of prevention of yellow fever. The success of the Walter Reed Yellow Fever Commission is legendary. However, a major part of its success is attributable to collaborations with nonmilitary scientists such as Dr. Carlos Finlay, a renowned Cuban physician who developed the theory of yellow fever transmission by stegomyia mosquitoes. Dr. Finlay actively supported the definitive experiments of Reed in Cuba and thus enabled the preeminent military medical research achievement in US history.

Strong central and overseas laboratories staffed with world-class investigators do not ensure successful military preventive medicine research support. Research effort must be focused on operationally significant and militarily relevant problems. Thus, operational military preventive medicine research should begin and end in the field—where real-world problems occur and their effects are most keenly felt. In turn, individual care providers in field settings can play significant roles in military preventive medicine research programs.

HOOKWORM ANEMIA

In 1899, First Lieutenant Bailey K. Ashford commanded a small Army hospital in Ponce, Puerto Rico. While caring for hurricane victims, he was struck by the high prevalence of anemia with severe asthenia among the local, and particularly the poorest, civilians. He began systematically to examine the blood and stools of "tropical anemia" patients, and soon he noted that the most severely ill patients invariably had eosinophilia and hookworm. More importantly, however, patients whom he treated with thymol, an anthelminthic drug, rapidly increased their red blood cell counts and improved their states of general health. He concluded that hookworm caused tropical anemia and that both could be cured with anthelminthic therapy. In April 1900 in the *New York Medical Journal*, Ashford published his clinical, laboratory, and therapeutic observations and proposed his etiologic theory. The report and theory were largely ignored.

Although discouraged, Ashford asked to be reassigned to Puerto Rico so he could continue his studies and advocate for enhanced treatment and prevention of tropical anemia. In 1903, almost 4 years after publication of his initial observations, the Puerto Rico Anemia Commission was established (with a budget of $5,000). Under its auspices,

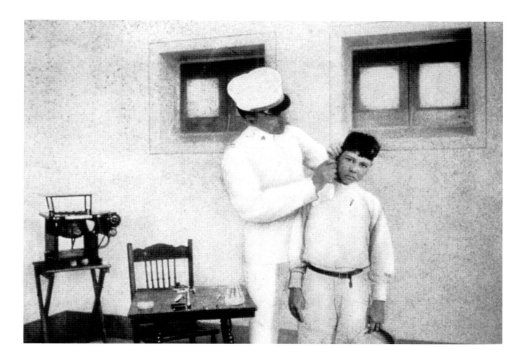

Fig. 5-1. As a young medical officer in Puerto Rico, Lieutenant Bailey K. Ashford, US Army, discovered that hookworm infestations caused a virulent anemia syndrome that was hyperendemic among local field workers. His subsequent clinical and public health activities inspired worldwide campaigns to diagnose, treat, and prevent hookworm anemia. Reproduced from Ashford. *A Soldier in Science*. New York: William Morrow (Harper Collins); 1934.

Ashford and colleagues established a model clinic in the town of Utuado. As the clinic's reputation grew, however, patients from throughout the island—as many as 1,200 in a day—sought care from Ashford and his staff. During the commission's 7-year existence, more than 300,000 patients were evaluated, treated, and counseled regarding prevention (Figure 5-1).[10]

The success of the Puerto Rico Anemia Commission motivated philanthropist John D. Rockefeller to form the Rockefeller Sanitary Commission to diagnose, treat, and prevent hookworm anemia in the southern United States. The Rockefeller Commission's success in the United States spawned the Rockefeller International Health Commission, which became the renowned Rockefeller Foundation.[10] Untold lives have been saved and countless more improved as a direct result of the dedication and persistence, as well as the skilled field research, of a junior Army medical officer.

WATER PURIFICATION

In 1909, the Secretary of War appointed a board of officers to investigate and make recommendations regarding water supplies for permanent military installations. In 1910, Major Carl Darnall, a physician assigned to the Chemistry Laboratory of the Army Medical School, began work on a system that used anhydrous chlorine gas to purify water in large quantities. By 1911, Darnall had constructed a prototype apparatus that was small, light (less than 200 lbs), effective, and reliable in laboratory tests. Before it could be accepted for military use, however, Darnall had to test the system's efficacy and reliability under field conditions. Darnall installed his apparatus next to the mechanical filter at the pump house at Fort Myer, Va. For 2 weeks, the systems worked side by side on the same "turbid, at times muddy"[11(p791)] Potomac River water. To explore its range of capabilities, the source water was at times deliberately contaminated with fresh horse manure or drawn downstream from a sewer drainpipe. The trials documented that Darnall's system was simple and inexpensive to install and operate—and was as efficient as other systems and more reliable. The board recommended that the system be used "at a military post with polluted water and no satisfactory purification system."[11(p796)]

Two years later, Major William Lyster, another Army physician, developed a field water system that used calcium hypochlorite for disinfection. To this day, chlorinated drinking water is stored in canvas bags, referred to as "lyster bags," that hang from tripods and tree limbs throughout military encampments.

Research and development of military water systems eventually became the responsibility of the Corps of Engineers.[12] But early in the 20th century, two Army physicians developed principles and systems for providing safe drinking water to soldiers and their families in the field and in garrison.

HEMOLYTIC STREPTOCOCCUS AND ACUTE RHEUMATIC FEVER

At the beginning of World War II, streptococcal infections and their acute and late sequelae were considered important childhood diseases but not significant military threats. In addition, there was remarkably little understanding of the natural history or pathophysiology of streptococcal infections, of the relationships between streptococcal infections and acute rheumatic fever, or of the capabilities of antibiotics such as sulfadiazine and penicillin to eradicate carriage, prevent clinical sequelae, or interrupt epidemics.

In 1943, there were rheumatic fever outbreaks at several military bases, particularly in the Rocky Mountain region. At the peak of epidemic activity at one installation, the rheumatic fever attack rate exceeded 10 per 100 persons per year.[13] The following year, prospective studies were conducted at Camp Carson, Colo. The investigators concluded that "if rheumatic fever is to be prevented, hemolytic streptococcal infections must be prevented.…The most urgent studies for the future should be directed toward…preventing hemolytic streptococcal infection and determining the manner in which hemolytic streptococci cause the rheumatic state."[14(p268)] For the next 6 years, though, fears of selecting for and disseminating resistant streptococcal strains precluded studies of penicillin prophylaxis in military populations.

In October 1948, representatives of the Armed Forces Epidemiological Board (AFEB) visited Camp Carson and Lowry Field in Colorado and Fort Francis E. Warren in Wyoming to select a site for long-term studies of streptococcal disease and rheumatic fever. The team chose Fort Warren because of the "high incidence of these diseases and the extreme [medical and command] interest.…"[14(p276)] A letter to the site visit team from Colonel John C.B. Elliott, the post's commanding officer, attested to his commitment: "I am determined to solve this problem if it is humanly possible.…I will throw every resource I can to the assistance of this unit if it will come in here and work with us."[14(p279)]

In January 1949, the Streptococcal Disease Laboratory began operations at Fort Warren, an Army (but soon to be an Air Force) technical training base. Dr. Charles Rammelkamp, the laboratory's director, and Army physicians First Lieutenant William Brink, First Lieutenant Floyd Denny, and First Lieutenant Lewis Wannamaker formed the initial professional staff. Army, Air Force, and local civilian personnel provided technical and administrative support. In a series of classic studies, the Laboratory demonstrated that penicillin G was the drug of choice for treating streptococcal pharyngitis, that rheumatic fever could be prevented by the treatment of acute streptococcal infections with penicillin,[15] that treatment lasting 10 days was more effective than shorter courses for eradicating the streptococcus, and that antibiotic therapy within 9 days of onset of acute pharyngitis was effective in preventing rheumatic fever.

The Laboratory also assessed the feasibility and determined the most efficient and effective regimens of mass penicillin prophylaxis to prevent or interrupt epidemics. In early studies, men were given oral, procaine, or benzathine penicillin in various dosages and schedules. The studies documented that complete eradication of streptococcal carriage depended on the penicillin dosage and the period of treatment. In other studies, airmen were given various doses of benzathine penicillin as prophylaxis against streptococcal infections. There was a strong correlation between the dose of benzathine penicillin and the duration of protection from subsequent streptococcal infections.

The elegantly designed and flawlessly executed studies of the Streptococcal Disease Laboratory produced much of the fundamental knowledge that underlies current treatment, prevention, and prophylaxis practices around the world. In recognition of its achievements, in 1954 the Laboratory received the Lasker Award from the American Public Health Association. The citation in part reads: "The success achieved is due in great measure to…keen awareness of the advantages afforded by military populations in epidemiological analyses. The collaboration of the medical departments of all three services in the work of the Laboratory, with minor exceptions, has been exemplary."[14(p303)]

The Laboratory formally closed in September 1955. Ironically, there was an outbreak of streptococcal pharyngitis among Air Force trainees at the renamed Warren Air Force Base the following spring. In the midst of the outbreak, Captain John Davis of the base hospital and Dr. Willard Schmidt of Western Reserve University—a veteran of the Streptococcal Disease Laboratory—gave a single injection of benzathine penicillin to each of 2,214 trainees at the start of their training. Trainees with histories of allergies (483) were exempted from penicillin treatment and served as controls. During the first 2 weeks of follow-up, there were no cases of streptococcal pharyngitis in the treated group and 19 in the controls. Three cases

"broke through" in the treated group during the third week, but there was still a significant protective effect. By the fourth week and thereafter, streptococcal pharyngitis rates in the two groups were comparable.[16] It was fitting that the real-world effectiveness of mass benzathine penicillin prophylaxis was demonstrated during an outbreak of streptococcal disease at Warren Air Force Base.

With the exception of Reed's Yellow Fever Commission, the legacy of the Streptococcal Disease Laboratory may be preeminent in the annals of operational military preventive medicine research. Today's military scientists and research managers would do well to study and emulate the methods and practices of the Streptococcal Disease Laboratory.

TROPICAL SKIN DISEASES

During the Vietnam War, skin diseases were the leading cause of clinic visits and the third leading cause of hospitalizations among soldiers, behind gastrointestinal and respiratory illnesses and ahead of malaria.[17]

In 1968, two US Navy physicians, Lieutenant Michael McMillan and Lieutenant Robert Hurwitz, were assigned to the hospital at Quang Tri Combat Base in the northernmost province of South Vietnam. Between October and December, they conducted a prospective study of 50 Marines who were evacuated from the field or otherwise hospitalized for disabling skin diseases ("jungle rot"). Patient histories indicated that most serious lesions developed at sites of minor scratches, mosquito bites, or leech attachments. Most cultures yielded group A beta hemolytic streptococci or *Staphylococcus aureus* or both. In every case, wound debridement and systemic penicillin therapy resulted in rapid healing and return to duty. The Navy physicians concluded that care and cleaning of minor wounds could prevent serious secondary infections, and they recommended the early use of systemic antibiotics to treat "tropical pyoderma."[18]

At about the same time at the southernmost end of Vietnam, infantrymen of the Army's 9th Infantry Division were exposed almost continuously, particularly during the rainy season, to rice paddy or swamp water during combat operations in the Mekong delta. In 1968, the WRAIR deployed a specially trained Field Dermatology Research Team led by Captain Alfred Allen.[17] The team was augmented by David Taplin, a civilian consultant from the University of Miami School of Medicine, who had conducted studies of skin diseases in the Florida Everglades (Figure 5-2).[19]

The team established its field laboratory in the Mekong delta, and between October 1968 and September 1969, it surveyed men of the 9th Division immediately on their return from combat operations (eg, patrols, reconnaissances in force). The investigators examined each soldier and recorded the location, size, and diagnosis of each skin lesion; suspicious lesions were cultured for bacteria and fungi. The team found that during the rainy season, skin diseases reduced the combat strength of rifle companies by as much as a third and that, even in the dry season, skin diseases accounted for nearly 80% of lost field-duty days in typical infantry battalions.[20] The surveys also revealed that bacterial and fungal infections were more prevalent and much more severe in combat troops than in support troops; that in combat troops, 20% of the fungal and most of the bacterial infections occurred in the area of the sock and boot; that the incidence of pyoderma was 2.5 times higher among white as compared to non-white infantrymen; and that group A beta hemolytic streptococci were responsible for as much as 90% of the most serious and disabling ulcerative pyodermas. The team also verified the effectiveness of early, systemic antibiotic treatment of bacterial pyodermas of infantrymen.[21] Based on these findings, the research team recommended the early and aggressive use of penicillin and griseofulvin, limitation of exposures to wet terrain during combat operations when possible, and mandatory removal of wet footwear during periods of "stand-down" from combat operations.

The presence of the research team in the Division area, combined with an aggressive education program, raised awareness among Division personnel regarding the nature and importance of skin infections. In turn, commanders became focused on

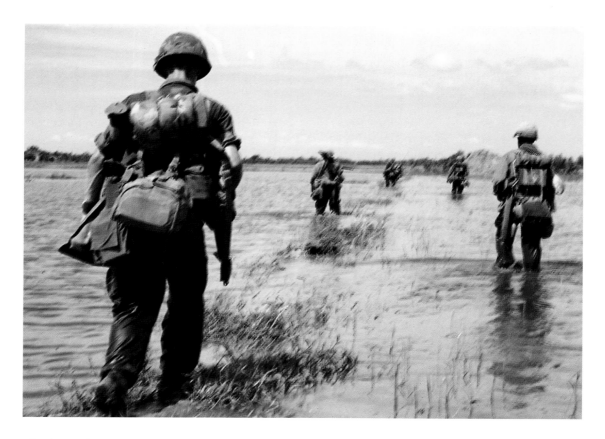

Fig. 5-2. In the Mekong delta region of South Vietnam and in other regions during rainy seasons, skin infections associated with continuous water immersion were leading causes of combat manpower losses. Studies conducted among front-line units in combat zones led to practical and effective treatments and preventive interventions. Photograph: Courtesy of the Walter Reed Army Institute of Research, Silver Spring, Maryland.

prevention, soldiers reported skin lesions earlier, and medics made more timely and accurate diagnoses. The result was more effective treatment. By the end of the tour of the research team, the 9th Division was losing fewer man-days each week than they had lost each day before the team's arrival.

In retrospect, the "jungle rot" of the Marines in the north was similar in etiology and pathogenesis to the "jungle sores" of infantrymen in the Mekong delta. In both settings, field studies led to preventive practices that decreased morbidity and conserved combat strength.

PLAGUE

Plague was known to be endemic in Vietnam since at least the start of the 20th century. Beginning in 1962, however, there was a countrywide epidemic that most significantly affected the large coastal cities. In the 5 years from 1962 through 1966, nearly 13,000 cases of plague were recorded among Vietnamese civilians.[22] As the United States expanded its presence in Vietnam in the mid-1960s, plague was considered a significant operational threat—particularly at logistical bases adjacent to foci of the civilian epidemic. To counter the threat, all US servicemembers before departing for Vietnam were immunized with a killed plague vaccine of unproven efficacy.

In 1964, WRAIR deployed a multidisciplinary team to study the plague epidemic and to document its effects on deployed US forces. In initial studies, the team trapped and examined more than 13,000 small mammals to document the distribution and concentration of the plague bacillus in its known natural hosts. Three species of rodents were identified as major plague reservoirs: *Rattus norvegicus*, *R exulans*, and *Suncus murinus*. Specimens of all three had antibodies to *Yersinia pestis*, plague's causative organism, as well as infestations with Oriental rat fleas (*Xenopsylla cheopis*), the classic vector of bubonic plague. Even though rats infected with *Y pestis* and fleas competent to transmit plague to humans infested Vietnamese cities and nearby US base camps, US servicemembers were spared. The research question was clear: Were environmental and personal protective measures preventing exposures of troops to infected rats and fleas or was the vaccine providing immunologic protection? Lieutenant Colonel Dan Cavanaugh and colleagues from WRAIR conducted studies to elucidate the answer.

The key turned out to be another disease: murine typhus. Like plague, murine typhus occurs when its etiologic agent (*Rickettsia mooseri*) is transmitted to humans by fleas living on infected rats. Their modes of transmission are similar, but murine typhus—unlike plague—was relatively common among US forces, particularly support personnel in rear areas.[23]

To assess the relative sizes of reservoirs of plague and murine typhus, the WRAIR team trapped 49 rats on US bases at Cam Ranh Bay, Cu Chi, and Ton Son Nhut. Eight (17%) rats had antibodies to *Y pestis* and ten (20%) to *R mooseri*.[24] Next, the team retrieved the stored serum samples of 58 soldiers who had been hospitalized with clinically diagnosed and serologically confirmed murine typhus. The titers

to *Y pestis* of 7 (12%) of the 58 confirmed murine typhus patients rose during their hospitalizations. The findings documented that typhus patients were frequently exposed to rat fleas infected with both *R mooseri* and *Y pestis*. Since no coinfected patients developed clinical manifestations of plague, the investigators concluded that the plague vaccine had conferred immunologic protection against flea-transmitted *Y pestis*.

The team's findings were consistent with the experience of US forces in Vietnam. During the entire war, there were only four cases of plague (three of whom had been immunized).[24] After the war, the team's findings helped inform plague vaccination policies in a variety of military and civilian settings.[25]

In retrospect, the legacy of the plague research team may lie more in its methods than its findings. It demonstrated that stored biological materials, particularly those linked to unique military or clinical circumstances, could yield significant, and unpredictable, military medical research benefits. Also, the team's ingenious use of specimens collected for studies of one disease to investigate an epidemiologically similar disease of greater military operational concern exemplified attributes essential to successful field research, especially in combat environments: focus on the military mission, ingenuity, resourcefulness, and technical excellence.

MENINGOCOCCAL MENINGITIS

In general, progress in military preventive medicine research has occurred over generations, with each advancing to the limits of the knowledge and technology of the day. The campaign against meningococcal disease, particularly in the setting of military training, exemplifies the value of patience, persistence, and focus across generations. For most of the 20th century, military researchers have led efforts to combat meningococcal meningitis in military trainee populations by developing and proving the efficacy of such interventions as acute respiratory disease wards, sulfa drugs for epidemic interdiction and chemoprophylaxis, and vaccines. This effort spanned 65 years and involved both Army and Navy researchers. The benefits have been felt by military recruits and the commanders who depend on them, but civilian populations have perhaps benefited the most.

In November 1917, during the mobilization for World War I, there was an outbreak of cerebrospinal meningitis among recruits at Camp Jackson, SC.[26] For 8 months, Major William Herrick, chief of the medical service at the camp hospital, system-

atically tracked the physical and laboratory results of 265 patients with meningitis. He documented fevers, malaise, and respiratory symptoms an average of 48 hours before the first signs of meningitis, and he recovered meningococci from the blood of patients before they had meningeal signs. He concluded that meningococcal disease was primarily a systemic infection, meningitis was a manifestation of secondary infection of the central nervous system, and the spread of meningococci from the nasopharynx to the meninges occurred by bloodborne rather than direct invasion. Special wards were established at Army basic training camps so that trainees with febrile respiratory illnesses could be removed from their units and systematically monitored to detect early signs of meningitis. For decades, the "ARD ward" (acute respiratory disease ward) was a cornerstone of recruit medicine.

In June 1941, Drs. John Dingle, Lewis Thomas, and Allan Morton reported that meningococci were eradicated from the nasopharynges of patients who were treated with sulfadiazine.[27] The findings suggested a potential use of sulfadiazine for epidemic control. In the midst of a meningitis outbreak at a naval training center in the winter of 1942 to 1943, Lieutenant Francis Cheever, Lieutenant Commander B.B. Breese, and their colleagues from the Naval Medical School, Bethesda, Md, studied the effects of sulfadiazine on meningococcal carriage. Men from a single barracks were divided into two groups: one group received sulfadiazine for 3 days and the other remained untreated. By the fourth day, carriage prevalence had increased among the controls, but all 161 carriers who were treated were negative.[28] The study demonstrated the potential value of mass sulfadiazine treatment to prevent or interrupt meningococcal outbreaks.

That same winter, Colonel Dwight Kuhns and colleagues tested the effects of mass sulfadiazine treatment during meningitis outbreaks at two Army training camps. More than 15,000 soldiers were given 2- or 3-day courses of sulfadiazine. Meningitis rates and carriage prevalences declined and remained low among those who were treated, in extreme contrast to the controls (2 cases among 15,000 given prophylaxis and 40 cases among 19,000 controls).

Kuhns and colleagues concluded that mass sulfadiazine chemoprophylaxis was safe and effective under the following conditions: first, all individuals in a closed group should be treated simultaneously; second, all personnel who later joined the group should be treated before they were incorporated; and third, once treated, the group should be protected from reinfection from outside sources.[29] These principles continue to guide the use of mass antibiotic chemoprophylaxis to control meningococcal and other militarily important communicable diseases.

In 1943, Dr. John Phair, Captain Emanuel Schoenbach, and Dr. Charlotte Root conducted meningococcal carriage studies among soldiers at Fort Meade, Md. While verifying sulfadiazine's effect on nasopharyngeal carriage, they warned that "care must be exercised in the prophylactic employment of the sulfonamides as its widespread and injudicious use might...lead to...infections with sulfonamide resistant meningococci."[30(p153)] The warning was prescient. Mass sulfadiazine chemoprophylaxis was a mainstay of military preventive medicine practice from its first widespread use in 1943 until the emergence of significant sulfa resistance 2 decades later.

In March 1963, there was an outbreak of meningococcal meningitis among recruits at the US Naval Training Center, San Diego. The epidemic continued despite sulfadiazine treatment of all trainees and cadre. An investigation was conducted by

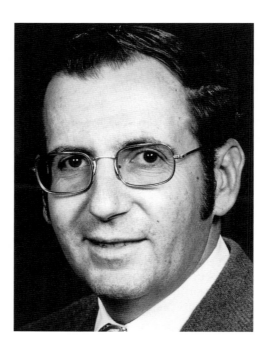

Fig. 5-3. In response to recruit camp meningitis outbreaks caused by antibiotic resistant strains of *Neisseria meningitidis*, Doctor Malcolm Artenstein led a team of military investigators in the development of vaccines against the most dangerous meningococcal serogroups. Photograph: Courtesy of the Walter Reed Army Institute of Research, Silver Spring, Maryland.

a Navy preventive medicine team that was augmented by Dr. Carl Silverman of the Public Health Service and Dr. Harry Feldman, chairman of the Committee on Meningococcal Infections of the Armed Forces Epidemiological Board. In a defining study, Commander Jack Millar supervised the administration of sulfadiazine to trainees of two companies with a combined carriage prevalence of 57%. When therapy was completed, carriage prevalence remained at 49%, and the predominant carriage strains were sulfonamide-resistant group B meningococci.[31]

The following year, 85 cases of meningitis occurred among military personnel at Fort Ord, Calif. When the fiancée of a trainee died of meningitis soon after they spent a day together, hysteria spread, the post was quarantined, and basic training was suspended.[32] In December 1964, Lieutenant Colonel Joseph Cataldo, deputy surgeon of the Special Warfare Center at Fort Bragg, NC, led a team that provided either sulfadiazine or sulfadiazine plus penicillin to 21,000 trainees, cadre, family members, and civilians who worked on post. Of 5,689 soldiers who gave samples for culture after completing the therapy, 207 (3.6%) were carriers of sulfa-resistant meningococci. Approximately 3 weeks later, sulfa-resistant strains were the predominant carriage strains in both the sulfadiazine and the sulfadiazine-plus-penicillin treatment groups.[33]

The Cataldo team's experience reinforced findings of Dr. Ross Gauld and colleagues from WRAIR earlier in the year. Gauld's team documented that sulfa-resistant group B meningococci consistently emerged as the predominant carriage strains in serial cohorts of Fort Ord trainees. They concluded that "control demands the development of ... a satisfactory immunizing agent."[34(p71)]

In response to the sulfa-resistance crisis, Dr. Malcolm Artenstein (Figure 5-3), a renowned virologist at WRAIR, with Captain Irving Goldschneider and Captain Emil Gottschlich, initiated studies of determinants of immunity against meningococci. They documented that immunity was serogroup-specific, so separate vaccines would have to be developed against each of the five epidemiologically significant serogroups: A, B, C, Y, and W-135. By 1968, they had produced a candidate vaccine against serogroup C meningococci, which caused the most cases at that time. In 1969 and 1970, they conducted large, controlled vaccine efficacy studies at Army basic training camps throughout the country. The results were compelling: only two cases of group C disease occurred among more than 28,000 recruit volunteers who received the experimental vaccine; 73 cases of group C disease occurred among nearly 115,000 unvaccinated controls. In these classic studies, the vaccine efficacy against group-homologous disease was 89.5%.[35] Since the fall of 1971, group C meningococcal vaccine has been given to all new Army and Navy trainees.[36,37]

Through the remainder of the 1970s, vaccines were developed against serogroups A, Y, and W135. Since the fall of 1982, recruits in all the services have received the tetravalent (serogroups A, C, Y, W135) meningococcal vaccine before the start of their basic training.[38] There have been few cases and no reported outbreaks of meningococcal disease by vaccine-homologous serogroups in immunized military populations.

Since their development, meningococcal vaccines have saved the lives of hundreds of military trainees. But the number of lives saved at recruit camps is small compared to the number of those—mainly children—who have been protected during epidemics around the world. It was recently estimated that 60 million to 80 million doses of meningococcal vaccine are required annually for worldwide epidemic control.[39]

LEPTOSPIROSIS ("FORT BRAGG FEVER")

In July 1942, soldiers at Fort Bragg, NC, began to seek medical care for an unknown but distinctive acute febrile illness. The syndrome included spiking fevers, chills, frontal headaches, and lumbar and periorbital pain. The defining feature, however, was a pretibial rash that appeared approximately 4 days after the initial onset of symptoms. Between late July and early September, 40 soldiers presented with the syndrome. Lieutenant Colonel Worth B. Daniels and Captain H. Arthur Grennan, physicians at the post hospital, led the investigation of what seemed a new disease. To assist the investigation, the Army Surgeon General appointed a special commission consisting of Dr. Paul Topping (National Microbiological Institute, National Institutes of Health), Dr. John Paul (Yale University School of Medicine), and Major Cornelius Philip.[32] Despite intensive epidemiologic, clinical, and laboratory investigations (including analyses of mosquitoes and flies and inoculations of patient fluids into humans, monkeys, chicken eggs, and rodents), the etiology could not be determined. The syndrome became known as "pretibial" or "Fort Bragg" fever.[40] Outbreaks of the illness recurred, and investigations into its etiology continued through the next 2 summers.

In 1943, First Lieutenant (later Captain) Hugh Tatlock was assigned to the Fort Bragg laboratory of the Commission on Acute Respiratory Diseases of the Armed Forces Epidemiological Board. In August 1944, Dr. Tatlock injected the fresh blood of a soldier with pretibial fever into laboratory animals. Eventually, the filtered plasma of a febrile guinea pig yielded a "virus" that was immunologically distinct from rickettsiae and viruses[41] that were known at the time to cause similar illnesses. Tatlock thought he had discovered the viral etiology of the new disease.

In 1951, Major William Gochenour and his colleagues at the Army Medical Service Graduate School in Washington, DC, decided to reexamine the sera of soldiers who had been diagnosed with Fort Bragg fever during the outbreak of 1944, including the patient from whom Tatlock had recovered the "new virus." Serum pairs were tested against antigens from a collection of strains of leptospirosis. Convalescent specimens had high titers of antibodies reactive with antigens of *Leptospira autumnalis*, a well-known cause of febrile illnesses in Japan. Additional studies confirmed that Fort

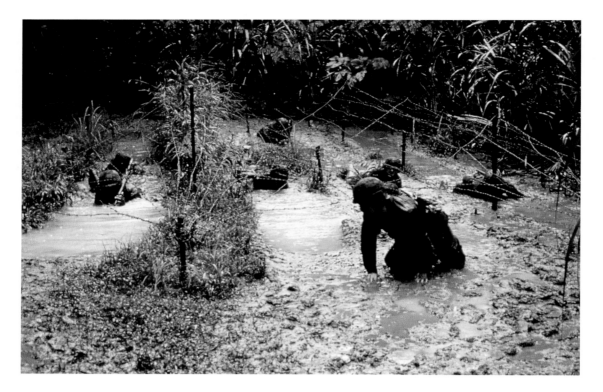

Fig. 5-4. Epidemiologic investigations documented that leptospirosis was a consistent threat to participants in jungle training during rainy seasons in Panama. Controlled studies among US-based units that deployed to jungle training during a rainy season demonstrated the clear effectiveness of doxycycline chemoprophylaxis. Photograph: Courtesy of Colonel Jerome J. Karwacki, Medical Corps, US Army.

Bragg fever was a leptospiral rather than a viral illness. The Fort Bragg strain of leptospirosis was eventually designated *L interogans,* serogroup *autumnalis,* serovar *fort-bragg.*[42] Thus, patient sera collected at Fort Bragg 8 years previously enabled military scientists in laboratories in Washington, DC, to link Fort Bragg fever to a strain of leptospirosis that was previously undocumented in the United States.[43]

But the book was not closed on leptospirosis. In 1981, epidemiologists from WRAIR investigated an outbreak of acute febrile illnesses among soldiers who had recently returned from jungle training in Panama (Figure 5-4). The team documented that leptospirosis caused the outbreak. Active surveillance of other units training in Panama revealed recurrent high attack rates of leptospirosis during the rainy season (September through December). In collaboration with the command surgeons of deploying airborne and ranger units, Lieutenant Colonels Ernest Takafuji and James Kirkpatrick and colleagues from WRAIR traveled to the Jungle Operations Training Center at Fort Sherman, Panama, to conduct a randomized, double-blinded, placebo-controlled field study of the effectiveness of doxycycline as prophylaxis against lep-

tospirosis. The results demonstrated an unequivocal preventive effect.[44] In March 1983, the AFEB recommended that all soldiers attending Panama jungle training during the rainy season receive doxycycline prophylaxis.[45] In August 1983, the AFEB's recommendation became Army policy.[46]

Dr. Daniels, who described Fort Bragg fever, commented that "the disease was described by Army clinicians, studied by Army medical personnel with the assistance of Army consigned consultants, transmitted to animals by an Army research worker, and finally proved as to etiology by an Army veterinarian and others."[32(p83)] He could have added that Army epidemiologists characterized its military importance, and Army physicians developed, tested, and fielded a safe, inexpensive, and highly efficacious preventive measure.

The success of military preventive medicine with regard to leptospirosis required transfers of information, insights, and precious clinical materials from field sites to central laboratories, among investigators of various specialties, and across generations. The overall experience stands as a model of effective operational military preventive medicine research.

JAPANESE B ENCEPHALITIS

Japanese encephalitis (JE), a mosquito-transmitted viral disease, is the predominant cause of outbreak-associated encephalitis in the world. Japanese B virus, the causative agent of JE, is enzootic in domestic animals throughout the southwest Pacific and southeast Asia. In endemic regions, there are seasonal increases in JE incidence and occasional large outbreaks.[47]

In July 1945, there were several cases of encephalitis among inhabitants of Heanza Shima, a small island close to Okinawa. A few days later, four cases were reported among residents of the main island. Naval Medical Research Unit 2 in Guam confirmed the diagnosis of Japanese B viral encephalitis and sent a team to assist medical officials from the US Military Government of Okinawa in an investigation.

Through July and August, cases of encephalitis continued to occur among the indigenous populations of Okinawa (91 cases) and two nearby islands (36 cases). Although more than 80% of cases were among children (nearly a third of all cases were fatal), the US occupation forces were not spared. Between July and September 1945, 38 Americans developed illnesses compatible with viral infections of the brain, 12 developed severe manifestations of encephalitis, and 2 died. Autopsy examinations of brain tissue and assays of convalescent sera implicated Japanese B virus as the cause. Lieutenant Colonel Albert Sabin of the Army Epidemiology Board joined the investigation.[48]

Sabin and colleagues observed that all cases of encephalitis among Americans occurred among the relatively few who were stationed in the northern part of the island. Factors that increased the risk for an outbreak included unsuccessful attempts to eradicate mosquito-breeding sites, particularly in the north because of its rough terrain, and the fact that for military reasons, most civilians and their domestic animals had been moved from the south to the north of the island before the outbreak. Also, serosurveys revealed that prevalences of virus-neutralizing antibodies increased with age among Okinawan residents (10 years or younger: 0%; 11 to 19 years: 55%; 20 years or older: 90%) and that indigenous domestic animals, including horses, goats, and cows, had serologic evidence of prior infections. Finally, there was a large outbreak of malaria in the island's northern provinces coincident with the encephalitis outbreak.

Sabin and local military public health officials concluded that there was an imminent and significant JE risk to American forces on Okinawa, particularly those deployed near foci of the civilian outbreak. The urgency of the public health situation, as well as the military operational circumstances, precluded a controlled study of the safety and efficacy of an inactivated mouse brain extract vaccine, the only product available for immediate use. Without delay, programs of aggressive mosquito control and mass vaccination were initiated. By the end of the summer, more than 60,000 personnel stationed in the north of the island had been immunized with remarkably few serious side effects.[48] The outbreak subsided coincident with the immunization campaign, but because there were no unimmunized controls, the independent effects of the vaccine could not reliably be determined.

Only a few years after World War II, US forces were again engaged in a JE-endemic theater. In 1946, Sabin and colleagues reported four cases of JE among American soldiers in southern Korea.[49] In 1949, Army physicians helped South Korean health officials investigate a large JE outbreak that included more than 5,500 cases, of which more than 40% were fatal. During the investigation, cattle, sheep, horses, and swine were found to have high prevalences of antibodies to Japanese B virus. Thus, by 1950, JE was known to be entrenched on the Korean peninsula,[50] and it soon showed that it could have an effect on military operations. During the summer of 1950, there was an outbreak among US forces that included an estimated 300 cases—of which at least 19 were fatal—among personnel who were defending the Pusan perimeter. At the peak of the outbreak, 10 cases per day—as many as 20 in a single night—were admitted to an Army evacuation hospital that was already overwhelmed with combat casualties.[51]

Approximately a decade later, Japanese B virus again attacked US forces but this time in southeast Asia. Between April and September 1969, Army physicians Captain W. Bruce Ketel and Lieutenant Colonel Andre J. Ognibene described the clinical courses of 57 patients with encephalitis who were evaluated at the 93d Evacuation Hospital in Long Binh, South Vietnam. Virus isolation and serologic studies implicated Japanese B virus as the principal cause. The authors estimated that during the outbreak as many as 10,000 US servicemembers may have been infected, most with mild or no symptoms. The authors asserted the need for a safe and effective vaccine.[52]

In 1984 and 1985, Lieutenant Colonel Charles Hoke and colleagues from the Armed Forces Research Institute of Medical Sciences in Bangkok,

Thailand, conducted a randomized, blinded, placebo-controlled trial of a highly purified, inactivated JE vaccine made from whole virus derived from mouse brain. Between November 1984 and March 1985, more than 60,000 children living in an endemic area of northern Thailand received either JE vaccine or placebo (tetanus toxoid). The vaccine's observed protective effect was 91%.[53] And in 1994, Major Jeffery Gambel and colleagues used sera routinely collected and stored in the Department of Defense Serum Repository to document persistence of antibodies to Japanese B virus up to 3 years after a primary immunizing series.[54]

Today, US forces are protected against JE, a persistent and widespread threat to military operations in the strategically critical Asia-Pacific region. Field studies during outbreaks in World War II, Korea, and Vietnam made clear the military importance of JE and the need for a safe and effective vaccine. Hoke's study among children in Thailand validated Sternberg's concept of 90 years earlier that military preventive medicine research, especially during peacetime, is often best conducted in *nonmilitary* settings of high disease risk. Finally, Gambel's study was the first to employ routinely archived serial serum specimens of active duty soldiers for the explicit purpose of military operational preventive medicine research.

MALARIA

Following World War I, Germany conducted intensive research to develop synthetic alternatives to quinine for preventing and treating malaria. In 1933, their efforts were rewarded with the discovery of quinacrine hydrochloride (Atabrine). When the United States and its allies lost access to natural sources of quinine at the beginning of World War II, quinacrine became, and remained throughout the war, the mainstay of Allied malaria prevention efforts.[55]

During World War II, there were more than 115,000 cases of malaria annually among US soldiers;[56] most were caused by South Pacific strains of *Plasmodium vivax* notorious for their propensity to relapse.[57] During the war, the malaria chemotherapy research program of the National Research Council supported the synthesis and testing of more than 14,000 candidate antimalarial compounds. Of approximately 80 that were tested against human malaria strains, the most promising was chloroquine, a member of the 4-aminoquinoline class.[58] In July 1945, the Board for Coordination of Malaria Studies of the National Research Council recommended a trial of the chemoprophylactic effects of chloroquine among troops in the Pacific. In August 1945, Major John Maier, on a leave of absence from the Rockefeller Foundation, began a study of weekly chloroquine (compared to daily quinacrine) among Army engineers operating on the Bataan Peninsula in the Philippines. Unfortunately from a medical research perspective, the war ended and units began demobilizing within weeks of the study's commencement.[59]

In the aftermath of World War II, Colonel John Elmendorf, commandant of the Army School of Malariology, Fort Clayton, Canal Zone, studied the long-term effects of various methods of malaria control in small towns in Panama.[60] Elmendorf and colleagues documented that weekly chloroquine was well tolerated and effective against *P falciparum* and erythrocytic forms of *P malariae* and *P vivax*. Elmendorf had to terminate his studies prematurely when the Army School of Malariology closed in December 1946.[61]

Following World War II, military malaria research flagged[62] as the threats to US forces waned. However, in 1950 when Korean forces from the north invaded the south, the United States again faced the challenge of deploying a large nonimmune force to a malaria-endemic theater. Through the summer of 1950, US servicemembers intermingled with multitudes of civilian refugees who poured into the collapsing beachhead at Pusan.[63] Conditions favored the rampant transmission of malaria, as housing, sanitation, and mosquito control failed. In July, the Army Surgeon General directed that troops in Korea receive weekly chloroquine prophylaxis. Because of limited supplies, however, the routine use of chloroquine ceased in October 1950, as the seasonal risk passed, and then resumed the following April. Still, in 1950 there were remarkably few cases of malaria among troops who complied with the prescribed prophylaxis regimen.[55]

With the start of routine troop rotations in the spring of 1951, however, the Korean malaria situation abruptly worsened. Vivax malaria emerged among thousands of servicemembers who had stopped their chemoprophylaxis[64] while en route to their homes or new duty assignments throughout the United States.[65] An answer was needed.

Of the thousands of compounds screened during World War II, only the 8-aminoquinolines displayed activity against exoerythrocytic ("tissue") forms of malaria. Primaquine, an 8-aminoquinoline synthesized at Columbia University, had the best margin between its minimal effective and maximal tolerated doses. In the 1940s, studies among inmate volunteers at federal penitentiaries documented that primaquine plus either chloroquine or quinine cured infections with prototypical strains of vivax malaria.[55] Unfortunately, when the Korean War began, primaquine was still experimental, and there had not been trials of its efficacy against strains of Korean origin. Clearly, in the summer of 1951, there was an urgent need for research and policy regarding the use of primaquine.

In August 1951, the Army Surgeon General established an expert mission to assess the feasibility of using mass primaquine therapy among returning Korean War veterans. The mission concluded that all troops leaving Korea should receive 15 mg of primaquine daily for 2 weeks—the maximum dose considered at the time to be safe without medical supervision. Before the policy could be promulgated, however, its feasibility and safety under real-world conditions had to be assessed.

In September 1951, Dr. Alf Alving of the University of Chicago, Major John Arnold, and Major Donald Robinson conducted studies of mass primaquine treatment without direct medical supervision aboard troop ships. On 18 September, in Sasebo, Japan, 1,493 servicemembers boarded the *USNS Sergeant Sylvester Antolak* destined for Seattle, Wash. The men were divided into two groups: one group received 15 mg of primaquine daily and the other received placebo. The voyage was rougher than usual for the season, but, remarkably, seasickness affected exactly the same number of men in each group. More importantly perhaps, there were no signs of toxicity associated with the primaquine, and, specifically, there was no evidence of hemolysis among black troops (approximately 17% of the total).[64] Shortly after the *Antolak* sailed, 2,060 servicemembers bound for the United States boarded the *USNS Marine Phoenix*. The men had taken daily primaquine for variable periods while awaiting embarkation, but once aboard, they were divided into two groups: one continued daily primaquine and the other took placebo. Again there were no significant differences in either seasickness or tolerance of the treatments between the groups.[64] The shipboard trials of Alving and colleagues documented the feasibility, tolerability, and safety of mass primaquine therapy even under the conditions of long and rough sea voyages. In short order, the Armed Forces Medical Policy Council advised the Services to begin routine primaquine therapy for all personnel leaving Korea.[66] The policy was instituted in December 1951.

As the malaria epidemic emerged among Korean War veterans, Alving and collaborators from the Army, Navy, Public Health Service, and civilian academic institutions conducted studies at Forts Breckenridge (Ky), Meade (Md), Dix (NJ), and Benning (Ga) and at Camp LeJeune (NC). Among hundreds of Korean War veterans with malaria, the investigators assessed the therapeutic and toxic effects of various regimens of primaquine plus chloroquine. Of numerous important findings, the studies revealed that 40% to 50% of vivax malaria of Korean origin relapsed after treatment with chloroquine alone;[63,67,68] that adding to chloroquine either 10 mg of primaquine daily for 14 days[67] or 15 mg of primaquine daily for 7 days[68] cured most cases; that 20 mg of primaquine daily for 7 days produced severe hemolysis in one black patient of 14 who were treated with the regimen;[67] and, finally, that 15 mg of primaquine daily for 14 days plus chloroquine was the treatment of choice for radical cure of Korean vivax malaria.[63] By the end of 1951, due in great part to the expeditious and incisive studies of Alving and his collaborators, the Services had safe and effective malaria control[66] and treatment[69] programs. In fact, much of current practice regarding the use of primaquine derives from studies conducted during the Korean War.

The military's experience in Korea helped foster unprecedented optimism regarding malaria's prevention, control, and even eradication. In 1960, however, the euphoria turned to apprehension with the first report of chloroquine-resistant *P falciparum*. Two American geophysicists working in Colombia, South America, were the first reported cases.[70] In short order, resistant falciparum strains were documented in other countries of South America and in southeast Asia. Years later, Brigadier General William Tigertt, commandant of WRAIR, recalled the "incredulity with which such reports were received by public health workers"[71(p605)] in southeast Asia. Major General Joe Blumberg, commanding general of the Army Medical Research and Development Command, recounted that "no organized effort to deal with resistant *P falciparum* was begun until, as has repeatedly happened in the past, it was fully recognized to be a problem of grave military importance."[62(p730)]

In August 1962, a US Marine captain stationed in Nha Trang, Vietnam, developed falciparum malaria despite weekly chloroquine prophylaxis. In November, he was transferred to the Navy Hospital at Great Lakes, Ill, after his infection had withstood three courses of escalating dosages of chloroquine. At Great Lakes, Captain Robin Powell and colleagues (including Dr. Alving) unequivocally documented the chloroquine resistance of the captain's Vietnam-acquired strain.[72] In 1964, Major Llewellyn Legters, Preventive Medicine Officer at the Army Special Warfare Center at Fort Bragg, NC, and colleagues reported three cases of chloroquine-resistant falciparum malaria among recent returnees from Vietnam.[73] The authors emphasized the urgent need for drugs that would "prevent infections with drug resistant strains of *P falciparum.*"[73(p175)]

Several years before significant US involvement in Vietnam, Lieutenant Colonel Stefan Vivona of WRAIR had conducted a study of more than 50,000 participants that demonstrated that weekly chloroquine plus primaquine (45 mg) formulated in a single tablet was a safe and feasible method of providing malaria chemoprophylaxis under field conditions.[74] In 1962, the weekly C-P tablet became the Army standard regimen for malaria chemoprophylaxis,[75] and it was the prescribed method of malaria control in the early years of US operations in Vietnam.

In late 1965, US force strength and cases of malaria (more than 98% *P falciparum*[76]) began to increase rapidly in Vietnam. Major Taras Nowosiwsky, Preventive Medicine Officer, Office of the Surgeon, US Army Vietnam, tracked malaria experience among US troops through a longitudinal system that "provided a continuous flow of information on the whereabouts of individual units each night by area of bivouac."[77(p462)] He documented few cases among troops who remained in base camps, but in five separate outbreaks during combat operations in endemic areas, he estimated that the average attack rate of *P falciparum* malaria was 10 per 1,000 men per day.[77]

In 1963, the Army launched the Antimalarial Drug Development Program to develop drugs to prevent or treat chloroquine-resistant *P falciparum* malaria. During the next 10 years, 27 of more than 200,000 compounds received Food and Drug Administration approval for advanced clinical testing in humans.[78] One drug tested early in the program was 4,4' diaminodiphenylsulfone (Dapsone), which was found to prevent patient infections with chloroquine-resistant strains of *P falciparum.*[79] In 1966, Major Robert J.T. Joy, chief of the Army Medical Research Team in Vietnam, conducted controlled studies of the chemoprophylactic effects of Dapsone (plus weekly C-P) among soldiers of the Army's 1st Cavalry Division and 25th Infantry Division during combat operations in Vietnam's Central Highlands, an area of known high malaria risk. All study participants continued weekly C-P chemoprophylaxis to which they added either daily Dapsone (25 mg) or placebo. Joy's studies documented significantly lower malaria attack rates in units that supplemented weekly C-P with Dapsone.[80,81] Despite uncontrollable differences among the units in the nature and intensities of their malaria exposures (eg, times, locations, and characteristics of combat operations) and in levels of compliance with prescribed chemoprophylactic regimens, Joy's findings were pivotal to the revision of Army malaria control policy. In July 1966, the Surgeon General directed that Dapsone be added to weekly C-P prophylaxis when troops in Vietnam were at high risk of exposure to drug-resistant *P falciparum* (as determined by the US Army Vietnam preventive medicine officer).[82]

Just as during the Korean War, malaria (mostly caused by *P vivax*) emerged in large numbers among returning Vietnam veterans in the late 1960s. In response, Army clinical investigators studied the responsiveness of *P vivax* of Vietnamese origin to the standard suppressive dose of chloroquine (300 mg) plus primaquine (45 mg). Of 42 patients with acute vivax malaria who were treated with a single C-P tablet, all had prompt clinical responses, and none had documented parasitic or clinical relapses.[83] To assess compliance with prescribed terminal prophylaxis regimens, Colonel O'Neill Barrett and colleagues surveyed 671 recent Vietnam returnees. Most respondents (70%) admitted failure to take terminal chemoprophylaxis as prescribed, and 25% reported taking no prophylaxis at all. Rank and personal experiences with malaria were not significant correlates of compliance.[76] Together, the studies documented that noncompliance, rather than drug refractoriness, accounted for most malaria cases among returning servicemembers.

The malaria experiences of the military services in World War II, Korea, and Vietnam have been replayed many times on smaller scales. For example, in December 1992, the United States deployed forces to Somalia to provide security and humanitarian assistance. Between December 1992 and May 1993, 48 cases of malaria occurred among deployed US servicemembers; most (85%) were caused by *P falciparum*. Risk factors were noncompliance with prescribed chemoprophylaxis and failure to use personal protective measures against arthropods.[84] Vivax malaria emerged in significant numbers after soldiers and Marines returned to the United States.[85] Beginning in May 1993, Lieutenant Colonel Bonnie Smoak and colleagues from WRAIR investigated an outbreak of malaria among recent Somalia returnees from the Army's 10th Mountain Division at Fort Drum, NY. Following initial clinical attacks, 60 soldiers received standard curative courses of primaquine: 15 mg daily for 14 days. Twenty-six (43%) of the sixty cases relapsed and required a second treatment course, and eight of them relapsed a second time. Higher doses of primaquine (30 mg daily for 14 days) were needed to achieve radical cures in these refractory cases. The experience suggested that primaquine-resistant *P vivax* strains were endemic at least focally in Somalia.[86]

At the turn of the century, Spanish-born American philosopher George Santayana wrote: "Progress, far from consisting in change, depends on retentiveness… when experience is not retained, as among savages, infancy is perpetual."[87(ch12)] Nearly 60 years later, Brigadier General William Tigertt reflected that "malaria can never be regarded with complacency and always must remain high on the military medical research priorities list. If we and those to follow us fail to recognize this, we and they deserve to be classified as savages in the sense the word was used by Santayana."[88(p82)]

SUMMARY

Nearly a century ago, Sternberg realized that there were medical threats unique to military service that were unlikely to be addressed by nonmilitary medical investigators. Thus, as Surgeon General, he established institutions (eg, central and overseas research laboratories) and procedures (eg, deployable multispecialty research teams, military-civilian collaboration mechanisms) to ensure that state-of-the-art research capabilities could be applied to and integrated with military operations worldwide. The field preventive medicine research successes recounted in this chapter attest to the value of the system and the procedures he established. Common characteristics of those successes include investigator selflessness, military operational relevance, medical command support, field command support, and collaboration with nonmilitary colleagues.

The preventive medicine researchers discussed in this chapter focused their studies on operationally critical aspects of militarily relevant questions. Their research agendas were not driven by their personal professional interests or the nonmilitary research priorities of others. Still, many military researchers gained professional prominence, acclaim, and respect for their studies that focused on military problems.

Military medical researchers require support (eg, administrative, logistical, monetary, technical) from parent institutions before, during, and after the field phase of studies. While the scope, level, and duration of necessary support are easily and often underestimated, the successful research programs described here were generally well supported. In addition, properly archived biological specimens often have provided the keys to success of military preventive medicine research programs. It is sobering, however, to note that gaps and inconsistencies in levels of support—generally due to shortsighted shifts in priorities, agendas, and budgets—frequently threatened the ultimately successful outcomes of even the most productive and widely acclaimed military research programs.

Operational preventive medicine research requires the sincere and dedicated support of the field (nonmedical) chain of command. Without exception, field commanders and their subordinate leaders provided access and support to the successful research programs discussed in this chapter.

The most successful military research programs consistently involved close collaborations with nonmilitary subject matter experts. Through the years, various mechanisms have been used to link military investigators with their civilian scientific and technical counterparts. For example, during war and other national emergencies, nonmilitary researchers have often been drafted into or volunteered for military medical service. Also, nonmilitary institutions (eg, academic centers, proprietary and nonprofit research and service organizations) have often collaborated with military research institutes on studies of mutual interest.

If necessity is the mother of invention, then military operations, particularly during combat, indeed provide fertile opportunities for military preventive medicine research. In turn, the military preventive medicine research successes of the past, such as those reviewed in this chapter, should challenge, motivate, and guide future military medical researchers and their leaders.

REFERENCES

1. Keegan J. *The History of Modern Warfare*. New York: Random House; 1993.

2. McLean WH. *Plagues and Peoples*. New York: Doubleday; 1976.

3. Zinnser H. *Rats, Lice, and Men: A Study in Biography*. Boston: Little, Brown, and Company; 1934.

4. Bayne-Jones S. *The Evolution of Preventive Medicine in the United States Army, 1607–1939*. Washington, DC: Office of the Surgeon General, Dept of the Army; 1968.

5. Edwards PQ, Edwards LB. Story of the tuberculin test from an epidemiologic viewpoint. *Am Rev Respir Dis*. 1960;8:1–47.

6. Takaki K. The preservation of health amongst the personnel of the Japanese navy and army, lecture II: the methods for investigating the cause of beri-beri. *Lancet*. 1906;May 26:1451–1454.

7. Kober GM. George Miller Sternberg, MD, LLD: an appreciation. *Am J Pub Health*. 1915;5:1233.

8. Gibson JM. *Soldier in White: The Life of General George Miller Sternberg*. Durham, NC: Duke University Press; 1958.

9. Writer J. Did the mosquito do it? *Am History*. 1997;February:45–51.

10. Ashford BK. *Soldier in Science: The Autobiography of Bailey K. Ashford*. New York: William Morrow and Company; 1934.

11. Darnall CR. The purification of water by anhydrous chlorine. *J Am Pub Health. Assoc*. 1915;1:183–197.

12. Black HH. Army field water developments. *Am J Pub Health*. 1944;34:697–710.

13. Holbrook WP. The Army Air Forces rheumatic fever control program. *JAMA*. 1944;126:84–87.

14. Denny FW, Houser HB. History of the commission on streptococcal and staphylococcal diseases. In: Woodward TE, ed. *The Armed Forces Epidemiological Board: The Histories of the Commissions*. Washington, DC: Office of The Surgeon General, The Borden Institute, US Dept of the Army; 1994.

15. Denny FW, Wannamaker LW, Brink WR, Rammelkamp CH, Custer EA. Prevention of rheumatic fever: treatment of the preceding streptococcic infection. *JAMA*. 1950;143:151–153.

16. Davis J, Schmidt WC. Benzathine penicillin G: its effectiveness in the prevention of streptococcal infections in a heavily exposed population. *N Engl J Med*. 1957;256:339–342.

17. Allen AM. *Skin Diseases in Vietnam, 1965–72*. Vol 1. In: *Internal Medicine in Vietnam*. Washington, DC: Office of the Surgeon General and Center of Military History; 1977: 30–32.

18. McMillan MR, Hurwitz RM. Tropical bacterial pyoderma in Vietnam: an improved therapeutic regimen. *JAMA*. 1969;210:1734–1736.

19. Taplin D, Zaias N, Blank H. The role of temperature in tropical immersion foot syndrome. *JAMA*. 1967;202:546–549.

20. Allen AM, Taplin D, Lowy JA, Twigg L. Skin infections in Vietnam. *Mil Med*. 1972;137:295–301.

21. Allen AM, Taplin D, Twigg L. Cutaneous streptococcal infections in Vietnam. *Arch Dermatol*. 1971;104:271–280.

22. Cavanaugh DC, Dangerfield HG, Hunter DH, et al. Some observations on the current plague outbreak in the Republic of Vietnam. *Am J Pub Health*. 1968;58:4:742–752.

23. Deaton JG. Febrile illnesses in the tropics (Vietnam). *Mil Med*. 1969;134:1403–1408.

24. Cavanaugh DC, Elisberg BL, Llewellyn CH, et al. Plague immunization, V: indirect evidence for the efficacy of plague vaccine. *J Infect Dis*. 1974;129(suppl):S37–S40.

25. Meyer KF, Cavanaugh DC, Bartelloni PJ, Marshall JD Jr. Plague immunization, I: past and present trends. *J Infect Dis*. 1974;129(suppl):S13–S18.

26. Herrick WW. Early diagnosis and intravenous serum treatment of epidemic cerebrospinal meningitis. *JAMA*. 1918;71:612–616.

27. Dingle JH, Thomas L, Morton AR. Treatment of meningococcal meningitis with sulfadiazine. *JAMA*. 1941;116:2666–2668.

28. Cheever FS, Breese BB, Upham HC. The treatment of meningococcus carriers with sulfadiazine. *Ann Intern Med*. 1943;19:602–608.

29. Kuhns DM, Nelson CT, Feldman HA, Kuhn LR. The prophylactic value of sulfadiazine in the control of meningococcic meningitis. *JAMA*. 1943;123:335–339.

30. Phair JJ, Schoenbach EB, Root CM. Meningococcal carrier studies. *Am J Public Health*. 1944;34:148–154.

31. Millar JW, Siess EE, Feldman HA, Silverman C, Frank P. In vivo and in vitro resistance to sulfadiazine in strains of *Neisseria meningitidis*. *JAMA*. 1963;186:139–141.

32. Jordan WS. History of the Commission on Acute Respiratory Diseases, Commission on Air-borne Infections, Commission on Meningococcal Meningitis, and Commission on Pneumonia. In: Woodward TE, ed. *The Armed Forces Epidemiological Board: The Histories of the Commissions*. Washington, DC: : Office of The Surgeon General, The Borden Institute, US Dept of the Army; 1994: 27.

33. Cataldo JR, Audet HH, Hesson DK, Mandel AD. Sulfadiazine and sulfadiazine-penicillin in mass prophylaxis of meningococcal carriers. *Mil Med*. 1968;133:453–457.

34. Gauld JR, Nitz RE, Hunter DH, Rust JH, Gauld RL. Epidemiology of meningococcal meningitis at Fort Ord. *Am J Epidemiol*. 1965;82:56–72.

35. Gold R, Artenstein MS. Meningococcal infections, II: field trial of group C meningococcal polysaccharide vaccine in 1969–70. *Bull World Health Organ*. 1971;45:279–282.

36. Artenstein MS. Control of meningococcal meningitis with meningococcal vaccines. *Yale J Biol Med*. 1975;48:197–200.

37. US Departments of the Air Force, Army, Navy, and Transportation. *Immunizations and Chemoprophylaxis*. Washington, DC: Department of Defense; 1 November 1995. Air Force Joint Instruction 48-110, Army Regulation 40-562, BUMEDINST 6230.15, CG COMDTINST M6230.4E.

38. Brundage JF, Zollinger WD. Evolution of meningococcal disease epidemiology in the US Army. In: Vedros NA, ed. *Evolution of Meningococcal Disease*. Vol 1. Boca Raton, Fla: CRC Press; 1987: 6–23.

39. Kreysler J. Personal Communication, 5 March 1997. E-mail.

40. Daniels WB, Grennan HA. Pretibial fever: an obscure disease. *JAMA*. 1943;122:361–365.

41. Tatlock H. Studies on a virus from a patient with Fort Bragg (pretibial) fever. *J Clin Invest*. 1947;26:287–297.

42. Memoranda: classification of leptospires and recent advances in leptospirosis. *Bull World Health Organ*. 1965;32:881–891.

43. Gochenour WS, Smadel JE, Jackson EB, Evans LB, Yager RH. Leptospiral etiology of Fort Bragg fever. *Public Health Rep*. 1952;67:811–813.

44. Takafuji ET, Kirkpatrick JW, Miller RN, et al. An efficacy trial of doxycycline chemoprophylaxis against leptospirosis. *N Engl J Med*. 1984;310:497–500.

45. Armed Forces Epidemiological Board. Doxycycline chemoprophylaxis against leptospirosis. Washington, DC: AFEB; 15 March 1983. Memorandum 83-2.

46. Headquarters, Dept of the Army. Administration of doxycycline to soldiers deployed to the Jungle Operations Training Center. 10 August 1983. Letter 40–83–12.

47. Vaughn DW, Hoke CH Jr. The epidemiology of Japanese encephalitis: prospects for prevention. *Epidemiol Rev.* 1992;14:197–221.

48. Sabin AB. Epidemic encephalitis in military personnel. *JAMA.* 1947;133:281–293.

49. Sabin AB, Schlesinger RW, Ginder DR, Matumoto M. Japanese B encephalitis in American soldiers in Korea. *Am J Hyg.* 1947;46:356–375.

50. Hullinghorst RL, Burns KF, Choi YT, Whatley LR. Japanese B encephalitis in Korea. *JAMA.* 1951;145:460–466.

51. Lincoln F, Silvertson SE. Acute phase of Japanese B encephalitis: two hundred and one cases in American soldiers, Korea. *JAMA.* 1952;150:268–273.

52. Ketel WB, Ognibene AJ. Japanese B encephalitis in Vietnam. *Am J Med Sci.* 1971;261:271–279.

53. Hoke CH Jr, Nisalak A, Sangawhipa N, et al. Protection against Japanese encephalitis by inactivated vaccines. *N Engl J Med.* 1988;319:608–614.

54. Gambel JM, DeFraites RF, Hoke CH Jr, et al. Japanese encephalitis vaccine: persistence of antibody up to 3 years after a three-dose primary series. *J Infect Dis.* 1995;171:1074.

55. Coggeshall LT. Treatment of malaria. *Am J Trop Med.* 1952;1:124–131.

56. Stone WS. Tropical medicine in the Armed Forces. *Am J Trop Med Hyg.* 1952;1(1):27–29.

57. Sapero JJ. New concepts in the treatment of relapsing malaria: the Charles Franklin Craig Lecture, 1946. *Am J Trop Med.* 1947;27:271–283.

58. Board for the Coordination of Malaria Studies. Wartime research in malaria. *Science.* 1946;103:8–9.

59. Maier J. A field trial of chloroquine (SN 7618) as a suppressive against malaria in the Philippines. *Am J Trop Med.* 1948;28:407–412.

60. Elmendorf JE, Barnhill KG, Takos M. Preliminary report on field experiments to demonstrate effectiveness of various methods of malaria control. *Am J Trop Med.* 1947;27:135–145.

61. Elmendorf JE, Barnhill KG, Hoekenga MT, Takos M. Second and supplementary report on field experiments to demonstrate effectiveness of various methods of malaria control. *Am J Trop Med.* 1948;28:425–435.

62. Blumberg JM. Welcoming remarks: workshop on biological research in malaria. *Mil Med.* 1969;September(special issue):729–730.

63. Alving AS, Hankey DD, Coatney GR, et al. Korean vivax malaria, II: curative treatment with pamaquine and primaquine. *Am J Trop Med Hyg.* 1953;2:970–976.

64. Alving AS, Arnold J, Robinson DH. Status of primaquine, I: mass therapy of subclinical vivax malaria with primaquine. *JAMA.* 1952;149:1558–1562.

65. Aquilina JT, Paparella JA. Malaria in returned veterans of the Korean war: clinical observations. *JAMA.* 1952;149:834–838.

66. Archambeault CP. Mass antimalarial therapy in veterans returning from Korea. *JAMA.* 1954;154:1411–1415.

67. Jones R, Jackson LS, DiLorenzo A, et al. Korean vivax malaria, III: curative effect and toxicity of primaquine in doses from 10 to 30 mg daily. *Am J Trop Med Hyg.* 1953;2:977–982.

68. DiLorenzo A, Marx RL, Alving AS, Jones R. Korean vivax malaria, IV: curative effect of 15 milligrams of primaquine daily for 7 days. *Am J Trop Med Hyg*.1953;2:983–984.

69. Hockwald RS, Arnold J, Clayman CB, Alving AS. Status of primaquine, IV: toxicity of primaquine in negroes. *JAMA*. 1952;149:1568–1570.

70. Moore DV, Lanier JE. Observations on two *Plasmodium falciparum* infections with an abnormal response to chloroquine. *Am J Trop Med Hyg*. 1961;10:5–9.

71. Tigertt WD. The malaria problem, past, present, and future. *Arch Intern Med*. 1972;129:604–606.

72. Powell RD, Brewer GJ, DeGowin RL, Alving AS. Studies on a strain of chloroquine-resistant *Plasmodium falciparum* from Viet-nam. *Bull World Health Organ*. 1964;31:379–392.

73. Legters LJ, Wallace DK, Powell RD, Pollack S. Apparent refractoriness to chloroquine, pyrimethamine, and quinine in strains of *Plasmodium falciparum* from Vietnam. *Mil Med*. 1965;130:168–176.

74. Vivona S, Brewer GJ, Conrad M, Alving AS. The concurrent weekly administration of chloroquine and primaquine for the prevention of Korean vivax malaria. *Bull World Health Organ*. 1961;25:267–269.

75. Ognibene AJ, Barrett O. Malaria: introduction and background. Ognibene AJ, Barrett O, eds. *General Medicine and Infectious Diseases*. Vol 2. In: *Internal Medicine in Vietnam*. Washington, DC: Office of the Surgeon General and Center of Military History, US Army; 1982: 271–277.

76. Barrett O, Skrzypek G, Datel W, Goldstein JD. Malaria imported to the United States from Vietnam: chemoprophylaxis evaluated in returning soldiers. *Am J Trop Med Hyg*. 1969:18:495–499.

77. Nowosiwsky T. The epidemic curve of *Plasmodium falciparum* malaria in a nonimmune population: American troops in Vietnam, 1965 and 1966. *Am J Epidemiol*. 1967;86:461–467.

78. Canfield CJ, Rozman RS. Clinical testing of new antimalarial compounds. *Bull World Health Organ*. 1974;50:203–212.

79. Degowin RL, Eppes RB, Carson PE, Powell RD. The effects of diaphenylsulfone (DDS) against chloroquine-resistant *Plasmodium falciparum*. *Bull World Health Organ*. 1966;34:671–681.

80. Joy RJ, McCarty JE, Tigertt WD. Malaria chemoprophylaxis with 4,4′ diaminodiphenylsulfone (DDS), I: field trial with comparison among companies of one division. *Mil Med*. 1969;134:493–496.

81. Joy RJ, Gardner WR, Tigertt WD. Malaria chemoprophylaxis with 4,4′ diaminodiphenylsulfone (DDS), II: field trial with comparison between two divisions. *Mil Med*. 1969;134:497–501.

82. Ognibene AJ, Conte NF. Malaria: chemotherapy. Ognibene AJ, Barrett O, ed. *General Medicine and Infectious Diseases*. Vol 2. In: *Internal Medicine in Vietnam*. Washington, DC: Office of the Surgeon General and Center of Military History, US Army; 1982: 320–321.

83. Hiser WH, MacDonald BS, Canfield CJ, Kane JJ. Plasmodium vivax from Vietnam: response to chloroquine-primaquine. *Am J Trop Med Hyg*. 1971;20:402–404.

84. Wallace MR, Sharp TW, Smoak B, et al. Malaria among US troops in Somalia. *Am J Med*. 1996;100:49–55.

85. Centers for Disease Control and Prevention. Malaria among US military personnel returning from Somalia, 1993. *MMWR*. 1993;42:524–526.

86. Smoak BL, DeFraites RF, Magill AJ, Kain KC, Wellde BT. *Plasmodium vivax* infections in US Army troops: failure of primaquine to prevent relapse in studies from Somalia. *Am J Trop Med Hyg*. 1997;56:231–234.

87. Santayana G. *The Life of Reason or The Phases of Human Progress*. New York: Charles Scribner's Sons; 1954.

88. Tigertt WD. Present and potential malaria problem. *Mil Med*. 1966;September(suppl):853–856.

MILITARY PREVENTIVE MEDICINE: MOBILIZATION AND DEPLOYMENT
Volume 1

Section 2: National Mobilization and Training

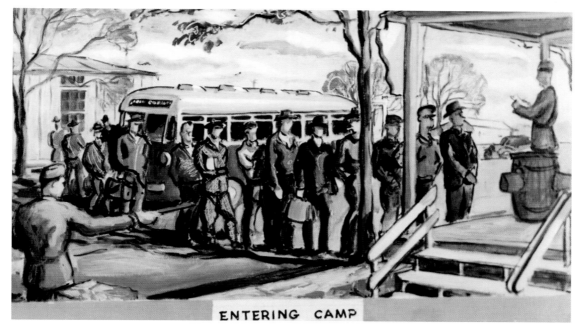

Louis H. Freund

Entering Camp

National mobilization requires turning large numbers of civilians into fit-to-fight military personnel and doing it quickly. The problems in disease control and injury prevention are immense, and their solutions are vital if trainees are to be kept on schedule.

Art: Courtesy of US Center of Military History, Washington, DC.

Chapter 6

THE RESERVE COMPONENTS: MEDICAL AND RELATED ISSUES OF MOBILIZATION

DALE A. CARROLL, MD, MPH; AND DAVID N. COWAN, PhD, MPH

D. A. Carroll; Colonel, Medical Corps, US Army (Retired); Senior Vice President–Medical Affairs and Performance Improvement, Rockingham Memorial Hospital, 235 Cantrell Ave., Harrisonburg, VA 22801; formerly, Chief, Consultants Division, US Army Medical Command and Preventive Medicine and Family Practice Consultant to The Surgeon General, US Army

D. N. Cowan; Lieutenant Colonel, Medical Service, USAR; Special Projects Officer, Division of Preventive Medicine, Walter Reed Army Institute of Research, Silver Spring, MD 20910-7500

INTRODUCTION

The tempo of deployments for the Armed Forces of the United States increased in the aftermath of the Cold War. By 1998 the US Army was involved in twice the annual deployments as it had undertaken in 1988, averaging 22,000 soldiers deployed overseas on any given day. Between 1991 and 1998, the number of US Air Force personnel deployed increased 4-fold. The US Navy reported an 8% increase in the number of ships at sea between 1993 and 1998. Before 1989, the US Marine Corps averaged one contingency or exercise every 15 weeks. By 1998 the average was one every 5 weeks.[1]

This marked increase in operational tempo (otempo) came at the same time as a drastic decrease in active duty personnel strength. The combined increase in otempo and the concurrent decrease in available strength has led to an increased role for the Reserve Component (RC) of the US Armed Forces. In addition to the large role played in the Persian Gulf War, the RC has contributed significantly to deployments ranging from disaster relief (eg, Hurricane Mitch in Central America) to peacekeeping (eg, Bosnia).

The role of RC forces has also increased in domestic operations. The support they provide has ranged from supporting law enforcement agencies to providing dental care to Native Americans and Eskimos.[2(p141)] The RC is also playing a critical role in the developing doctrine of homeland defense. The Army National Guard (ARNG) has been authorized to form Weapons of Mass Destruction Rapid Assessment and Initial Detection teams to provide rapid-response support to civilian authorities in the event of domestic use of such weapons.[3] The US Army Reserve (USAR) will field reconnaissance and decontamination teams and will enhance the capabilities of USAR medical units in the areas of combat stress control, triage, and patient decontamination.[4]

The RC has undergone significant force reductions—from 1.6 million reservists in 1989 to 1.3 million in 1998.[2(p133)] This trend of increasing reliance on the RC, even in the face of decreasing RC force structure, reaffirms that the RC is a crucial component in the successful implementation of US national security and military strategies, both internationally and domestically. This chapter will discuss the organization of the RC, the mobilization process, and medical issues associated with the RC. The RC plays a major role in the mobilization process and faces a set of medical issues somewhat different from those that affect the active component (AC). Knowledge of the RC structure and the mobilization process should facilitate the accession of the RC component upon mobilization. Sensitivity to the medical issues of mobilization should help improve the accession morbidity rates during and after deployment.

RESERVE COMPONENT ORGANIZATION AND FUNCTIONS

RC personnel in all the services belong to one of three major personnel classifications: the Ready Reserve, the Standby Reserve, or the Retired Reserve. Individual reservists may be assigned to units and drill with their units on a routine basis, while others may have no drill requirements and not be assigned to a unit.

The Ready Reserve

The Selected Reserve, the Individual Ready Reserve (IRR), and the Inactive National Guard make up the Ready Reserve. Selected Reservists are typically assigned to units that drill on a routine basis. These units may be operational units, which train and deploy as units, or augmentation units, which train together but when mobilized augment AC units. The Individual Mobilization Augmentee (IMA) is a reservist preassigned to a billet that must be filled on or shortly after mobilization in an AC organization, the Selective Service System, or the Federal Emergency Management Agency. IMAs train on a part-time basis with the organizations to prepare for mobilization.[2(p90)] Reservists on full-time active duty or full-time National Guard duty to support the RC (Active Guard/Reserve) are also considered part of the Selected Reserve.

IRR and Inactive National Guard personnel are typically individuals who have been previously trained by virtue of AC or RC service and have a remaining service obligation. IRR and Inactive National Guard personnel do not drill on a routine basis but may volunteer for annual training or military schooling.

The Standby Reserve

Members of the Standby Reserve are individuals who have completed their active duty or reserve service commitment and have requested assignment to the Standby Reserve. The Standby Reserve also includes individuals who have been released from the IRR or an RC unit because they have been elected to Congress, they hold a position as an essential government employee, they are pursuing graduate degrees in the health professions, or they have extreme temporary hardships. Members of the Standby Reserve are not required to attend drills and are not assigned to units.

The Retired Reserve

The Retired Reserve consists of individuals who are retired from the AC or who have served 20 or more years of qualifying service in the RC and are eligible for retired pay when they reach the age of 60. The Navy and Marine Corps, however, transfer enlisted members who retire after 20 or more years but fewer than 30 years of active duty to the Fleet Reserve or the Fleet Marine Corps Reserve until the individual reaches 30 years of service. Members of

the Fleet Reserve and the Fleet Marine Reserve can be involuntarily called back to active service. Retired personnel in the Army and Air Force are not subject to involuntary recall.[2(p94)]

Retired reservists are categorized based on the length of time since retirement and presence of a disability that would preclude mobilization. Category I includes those individuals who have no disability, are less than 60 years old, and have retired within the past 5 years. Category II comprises those individuals with no disability and who are under 60 years of age but who have been retired for longer than 5 years. Individuals of any age with a disability, regardless of time since retirement, make up Category III. Retirees in categories I and II are considered "mobilization assets"[2(p93)] and are included in the total DoD mobilization base. In contrast, retirees in Category III "with selected skills, primarily medical personnel, are considered mobilization assets on a case-by-case basis."[2(p93)]

RESERVE FORCES OF THE MILITARY SERVICES

Each of the four military services has a reserve force structure to augment and complement the AC. The Army and the Air Force have both reserve and National Guard forces within their respective reserve structures. National Guard personnel are considered part of the Ready Reserve. The US Coast Guard, although not usually considered a part of the Department of Defense (DoD), also has a reserve establishment. Exhibit 6-1 summarizes and contrasts the policies of each of the Services in regard to their RC mobilization and peacetime employment of RC assets.

US Army Reserve Components

US Army National Guard

In fiscal year 1998, the ARNG made up approximately 34% of the total Army personnel strength. It also contributed to the Total Army 54% of the combat arms units, 35% of the combat support units, and 35% of the combat service support units.[3]

The ARNG has a federal and a state mission. The federal mission is "to maintain properly trained and equipped units to be available for prompt mobilization for war, national emergencies or as otherwise needed....The state mission is to provide trained and disciplined forces for domestic emergencies or as otherwise directed by state law."[5(p26)] The ARNG of the separate states, territories, and District of Columbia are commanded while in state service by

the governor through the state adjutant general (or their equivalents). ARNG forces are permitted to engage in law enforcement activities only when in state service. Federalized ARNG units are prohibited, as are AC units, from engaging in law enforcement activities except in extremely limited circumstances.

US Army Reserve

The mission of the USAR is "to provide trained units and qualified individuals who are available for active duty in the United States Army in time of war or national emergency and at such other times as the national security requires."[5(p32)] USAR troop units are primarily combat support or combat service support. In fiscal year 1998, the USAR contained approximately half of the Total Army's combat service support force structure.[4]

US Naval Reserve Component

The mission of the US Naval Reserve (USNR) is analogous to that of the USAR. Approximately 30% of Selective USNR personnel serve in commissioned units. These are "completely operational entities that have their own equipment and hardware, including ships, aircraft squadrons, construction battalions, cargo handling battalions, mobile inshore undersea warfare units and special boat units. They are structured and equipped to come on active duty and function independently or alongside active

---

EXHIBIT 6-1

US SERVICE MOBILIZATION POLICIES

Army	• Heavy reliance on reserves for combat service support
	• Involuntary call-up to ensure access to units and to maintain unit integrity
Air Force	• Extensive peacetime use of reserves (especially strategic lift)
	• Volunteers used to fill missions
Marine Corps	• Volunteers used to augment
	• Reserves not required for initial operations
Navy	• Prefers involuntary call-up for unit integrity and visibility
	• Able to meet requirements with volunteers
Coast Guard	• Extensive use of peacetime reserves to augment active duty units
	• Some reserve units (Port Security Units) are required for initial operations

Source: US Department of Defense. *Joint Tactics, Techniques, and Procedures for Manpower Mobilization and Demobilization: Reserve Component (RC) Call-up*. Washington, DC: DoD; 1998. Joint Publication 4-05.1, III-4.

---

units."[2(p143)] The remainder of the Selective Reservists serve in augmentation units, which augment active units.

US Marine Corps Reserve Component

The mission of the US Marine Corps Reserve (USMCR) is consistent with the missions of the USAR and the USNR. The USMCR contributes a balanced force package of air, ground, combat, and combat support forces to the USMC total force. The USMCR, however, contributes 100% of the USMC civil affairs and adversary squadrons.[2(p148)]

US Air Force Reserve Components

US Air National Guard

The mission of the Air National Guard (ANG) is analogous to that of the ARNG, and, like the ARNG, the ANG is considered a state asset until it is federalized. The ANG is responsible for the air defense of the continental United States and is equipped with state-of-the-art aircraft. The ANG's capabilities span the spectrum of air operations. In fiscal year 1998, the ANG provided "one-third of the Air Force's tactical fighters, 43.2 percent of the KC-135 aerial refueling tankers, and 25.5 percent of the rescue and recovery capability…representing 34.4 percent of the total Air Force aircraft inventory."[2(p131)]

US Air Force Reserve

The mission of the US Air Force Reserve (USAFR) is to support the Air Force in its mission. The USAFR's contribution to the Air Force total force package includes tactical airlift, special operations, aerial refueling, rescue, heavy bombers, and tactical fighter aircraft. The USAFR also contributes a significant proportion of the Air Force's logistical, engineering, and medical support.[6] The USAFR and, to a lesser extent, the ANG frequently perform "real-world" missions as part of their training; they routinely conduct or participate in AC missions.

US Coast Guard Reserve Component

The US Coast Guard Reserve (USCGR) provides trained personnel to be activated in times of war and national emergency or when DoD requires additional personnel.[5] The Coast Guard is normally an agency of the Department of Transportation. Portions or all of the Coast Guard may be transferred to the Navy during wartime or at the direction of the President. The roles of the Coast Guard include maritime safety and law enforcement, marine environmental protection, and national defense. During wartime, these activities are expanded to include "preparing, coordinating and conducting operations in support of the coastal defense of both the United States and in-theater ports of debarkation."[5(p50)] USCGR forces are frequently tasked with drug and illegal immigrant interdiction missions, as well as domestic disaster assistance operations.

USCGR personnel and units are seamlessly integrated with the active component; most USCGR personnel are assigned to the active duty command that they would augment when they mobilize.[2] Certain capabilities are, however, concentrated in the USCGR. For example, the majority of the Coast Guard's deployable port security units are located in the USCGR. Reservists frequently perform "real-world" missions as part of their training and are often called on to fill AC shortfalls in day-to-day operations.[2(p158)]

MOBILIZATION

Mobilization is defined by the DoD as "the process of preparing for war or other emergencies..."[7(p1-1)] There are two components of mobilization: the military mobilization process and the national mobilization process.

Military Mobilization

Military mobilization refers to the process of bringing the military to an increased state of readiness. Mobilization connotes much more than just accession of personnel and units. Mobilized forces must be equipped, trained, and sustained. The mobilization process is designed to enable a flexible response to emergencies as part of a graduated response process. The graduated response process allows the National Command Authority (NCA) [the President and the Secretary of Defense] to respond to emergencies by choosing from a menu of mobilization options.

How the RC is Mobilized

Figure 6-1 depicts a notional scenario requiring a Presidential Selected Reserve call-up (PSRC). In the scenario, a Commander-in-Chief (CINC) of one of the geographical joint combatant commands is ordered to respond to a contingency. Geographical CINCs are responsible for planning for possible contingencies and unexpected events in their area of responsibility. The planning factors include an estimate of forces required, which typically include RC forces.

In the notional case shown in Figure 6-1, the CINC

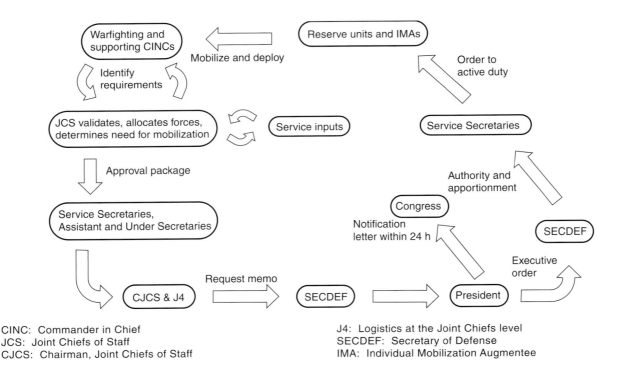

CINC: Commander in Chief
JCS: Joint Chiefs of Staff
CJCS: Chairman, Joint Chiefs of Staff

J4: Logistics at the Joint Chiefs level
SECDEF: Secretary of Defense
IMA: Individual Mobilization Augmentee

Fig. 6-1. Mobilization under a Presidential Selected Reserve Call-Up. Source: Goodbary RA. Reserve Forces of the United States Army. Presented at the United States Army War College; Dec 10, 1995; Carlisle, Pennsylvania.

identifies force requirements and submits the requirements to the Joint Chiefs of Staff for validation. The Joint Chiefs allocate forces and determine the need for mobilization. The Service Chiefs of the Army, Navy, Air Force, and Marine Corps join in the planning at an early stage. After the validated force package is approved by the various Service Secretaries and the necessary Under Secretaries and Assistant Secretaries of Defense, it is submitted to the Chairman of the Joint Chiefs of Staff, who requests that the Secretary of Defense inform the President of the need for RC mobilization. The President issues an executive order for the call-up and orders the Secretary of Defense to implement it. The President informs Congress within 24 hours of the executive order. In the meantime, the Secretary of Defense has ordered the Service Secretaries to mobilize the necessary forces. The identified RC units and personnel are mobilized and deploy to the crisis area in conjunction with AC units.

Levels of Military Mobilization

The NCA has a range of mobilization responses to apply to a crisis at any level of the continuum of military operations. The levels of mobilization are shown in Figure 6-2 and the legal authorities for mobilization are shown in Table 6-1. The range of responses available is shown in Figure 6-3. In addition to these options, other personnel management options are available to the services during a mobilization. Stop-loss actions enable the services to retain members beyond their terms of service. Stop-movement actions stabilize personnel by such methods as changing tour lengths or freezing all reassignments. Redistribution actions, such as cross leveling (ie, transferring) of personnel to high priority units, is another administrative action that may be used to respond to emergencies.

Mobilization of materiel and equipment is crucial if mobilized personnel are to carry out their assigned missions. The Persian Gulf War led to several logistics initiatives. These initiatives include the prime vendor concept whose aim is to realize cost savings by the selection of a single supplier for Class VIII (medical) supplies for medical treatment facilities in a specific geographic area. Another initiative is "just-in-time" delivery whose purpose is to ensure delivery of supplies when actually needed, thus enabling units to avoid accumulating large stockpiles of supplies and equipment. Finally "in-transit visibility" enables the logistician to pinpoint the exact location of an item anywhere in the logistical chain. A major

Fig. 6-2. Levels of Mobilization. Source: US Department of Defense. *Joint Tactics, Techniques, and Procedures for Manpower Mobilization and Demobilization: Reserve Component (RC) Call-up.* Washington, DC: DoD; 1998. Joint Publication 4-05.1, C-1.

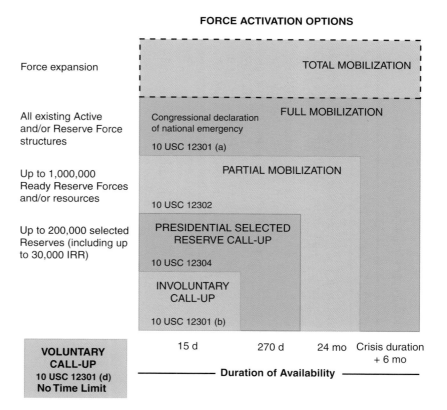

FORCE ACTIVATION OPTIONS

TABLE 6-1

LEGAL AUTHORITIES FOR MOBILIZATION

Level of Mobilization	Description	Action Required	Authority
Selective Mobilization (volunteer call-up and Service Secretary call-up)	Volunteers from National Guard and Reserves at any time under Title 10 USC 12301 (d). Units and individuals in an active status in an RC may be called without consent for not more than 15 days a year under 10 USC 12301 (b). Regular Retirees and Retired Reserve members with 20 years of active service may be ordered to active service involuntarily under 10 USC 688. Consent of state governors or the Commanding General of the District of Columbia National Guard is required for National Guard members serving under USC 12301 (b) or (d).	Publish order to active duty.	10 USC 331 10 USC 332 10 USC 333 10 USC 688 10 USC 12301 10 USC 12406
PSRC* (operational mission requiring augmentation of active force)	Units and individuals of Selected and Individual Ready Reserve; limited to 200,000 (including up to 30,000 IRR) at any one time (all Services) for up to 270 days without consent of the members. President must report to Congress within 24 hours of circumstances and anticipated use of forces. May not be used to perform any of the functions authorized by Chapter 15 or 10 USC 12406, or to provide assistance in time of serious natural or manmade disaster, accident, or catastrophe.	Presidential executive order to invoke authority. President delegates authority to the Secretary of Defense and the Secretary of the Department of Transportation. The Secretary of Defense may exercise stop loss authority IAW EO 12728.	10 USC 12304 10 USC 12305
Partial Mobilization (war or national emergency)	Ready Reserve units and individuals (NG and Reserve); limited to 1,000,000 (all Services) at any one time and not more than 24 consecutive months.	Presidential executive order declaring a national emergency. President delegates authority to the Secretary of Defense and the Secretary of the Department of Transportation. If not previously ordered, the President will usually invoke stop loss. The Secretary of Defense may exercise stop loss authority IAW EO 12728.	50 USC 1631 10 USC 12302 10 USC 12305 10 USC 671a 10 USC 671b
Full or Total Mobilization (war or national emergency)	National Guard and Reserve units, members of the Selected, Ready, and Standby Reserve, and Retired Reserve. The period of active service may be for the duration of the war or emergency plus 6 months.	Passage of a public law or joint resolution by the Congress declaring war or national emergency. The Secretary of Defense may exercise stop loss authority IAW EO 12728.	10 USC 671a 10 USC 671b 10 USC 12301 10 USC 12305 10 USC 12306 10 USC 12307

*PSRC: Presidential Selected Reserve call-up; IRR: Individual Ready Reserve; EO: executive order; NG: National Guard; IAW: in accordance with
Source: US Department of Defense. *Joint Tactics, Techniques, and Procedures for Manpower Mobilization and Demobilization: Reserve Component (RC) Call-up*. Washington, DC: DoD; 1998, B-2.

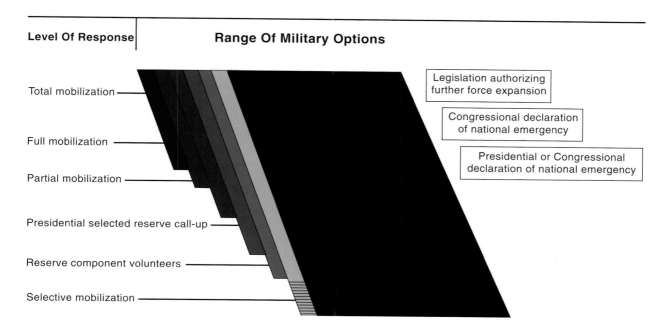

Fig. 6-3. Levels of Response. Source: US Department of Defense. *Joint Tactics, Techniques, and Procedures for Manpower Mobilization and Demobilization: Reserve Component (RC) Call-up.* Washington, DC: DoD; 1998. Joint Publication 4-05.1, III-5.

mobilization will severely test the validity of these concepts, especially in the area of medical logistics. The Persian Gulf War revealed problems with the availability of certain medical materiel items, such as immune serum globulin and anthrax vaccine. Shortages of other drugs and vaccines (eg, primaquine, adenovirus vaccine) have occurred when pharmaceutical and vaccine manufacturers have closed or mothballed facilities or production lines for items of military importance that either lack widespread civilian applicability or are no longer profitable.

Mobilization, especially full mobilization (the call-up of all reserve components) and total mobilization (full mobilization plus the addition of new force structure and personnel), requires coordination and action by numerous federal departments and agencies. The responsibilities of agencies such as the Federal Emergency Management Agency in domestic emergencies and the Office of Foreign Disaster Assistance in foreign emergencies are explained in chapters 45, The International Humanitarian Response System and the US Military and 46, Domestic Disaster Response: FEMA and Other Governmental Organizations.

RC forces are increasingly required to augment and complement AC forces in Security and Support Operations (SASO) such as foreign disaster assistance operations, complex humanitarian emergencies, and peacekeeping or peace enforcement operations. RC forces can be accessed for these op-

erations by any of the mobilization schemes shown in Table 6-1, dependent upon the decision of the NCA as determined by the scope of the operation.

The Military Health System and Mobilization

Demands on the System During Mobilization

Mobilization, at any level, involves the Military Health System (MHS) and will result in significant demands on that system. Increased rates of disease, for example, may become a concern. Massive numbers of mobilized personnel may be housed in overcrowded billets, with the consequent increased risk of respiratory diseases. A surge in the numbers of individuals undergoing initial entry training will result in the same risks. Increased demands on food service facilities may increase the risk of foodborne diseases. The social, family, and personal upheavals associated with mobilization may result in problems such as an increased rate of sexually transmitted diseases and increased rates of family violence and drug and alcohol use. Environmental and occupational concerns may arise due to reactivation of mothballed facilities and training areas. Increased production, transportation, storage, and use of chemicals, fuels, and munitions may result in increased risk of toxic material releases. All of these will need to be planned for by the MHS.

MHS assets will need to be allocated to perform medical and dental examinations and screening of RC personnel after mobilization begins. Preventive medicine personnel will play major roles in the screening of individuals before deployment. The difficulties encountered in evaluating individuals with symptoms associated with the Persian Gulf War and the lack of predeployment data have led to the development of joint predeployment screening protocols based on a DoD Directive[8] and a DoD Instruction.[9] Preventive medicine officers play key roles in the development of recommendations for predeployment immunizations and chemoprophylaxis. They prepare disease threat assessments and deliver disease threat briefings to deploying and deployed forces. Preventive medicine is also responsible for providing sustainment training of personnel and units in individual- and unit-level preventive medicine countermeasures.

Provisions for health care of non–active duty beneficiaries will be required. The number of non–active duty beneficiaries will be increased by the inclusion of family members of the newly accessed RC forces. One of the expected benefits of the military's TRICARE system will be the ability of the associated TRICARE networks to assume, during mobilization, a large portion of the health care workload for non–active duty beneficiaries. TRICARE is DoD's managed healthcare program designed to enhance the quality and accessibility of health care for beneficiaries while controlling costs. The plan consists of regional triservice medical coordination of health care in cooperation with private healthcare contractors. The contractors establish networks of nonmilitary healthcare providers to supplement DoD health care.

The preparation for receipt of casualties will result in the expansion of hospitals in the United States and the need for increased stocks of medical materiel. An increase in the requirement for blood and blood products will result in further strain on elements of the MHS. Preventive medicine activities can expect increased workload as they follow up on bloodborne infections (eg, hepatitis C) detected in donors.

Increased occupational health requirements from surging industrial activities can be expected. In addition, the Total Force Concept of full integration of DoD civilians will result in many DoD civilians with special skills being deployed to combat zones. The occupational health needs of these personnel must be met before and during deployment. Operations in the 1990s have reflected an increased role for DoD contractors and their personnel. The role of the MHS in health care for contracted personnel depends on the terms of the specific contract. In some operations, DoD has contracted for provision of certain preventive medicine functions after the area of operations has matured.

Demands on the System During Demobilization

Preventive medicine personnel will be active during redeployment and demobilization. The Persian Gulf War illness evaluation process has led to the development of more comprehensive postdeployment screenings.[9] Returning individuals will require information on diseases with long incubation periods to which they may have been exposed. In many cases, informational materials may need to be developed to assist primary care providers in providing health care to demobilized personnel. This is especially an issue with RC personnel. Individuals may return to the United States with latent diseases such as leishmaniasis or malaria. Tuberculosis screening will likely be required. Although political pressure tends to hasten demobilization, crowding of billets may still occur, leading to increased risk of airborne and foodborne infections.

Military Support to Civilian Authorities in the United States

Legal Authority

RC forces may be mobilized as part of a Joint Task Force established to provide military assistance to civilian authorities. DoD Directives 3025.1,[10] 3025.12,[11] and 3025.15[12] provide guidance for military support for civilian disasters, domestic civil disturbances, and domestic counterterrorism operations. Military assistance to civilian law enforcement officials is addressed in DoD Directive 5525.5.[13]

The level of mobilization and the actions required to mobilize forces for domestic operations are identical to those required for a wartime mobilization (Table 6-2). The NCA may order any level of mobilization to provide assistance dependent on the severity of the event. The following discussion focuses on the RC role in domestic disaster assistance or major terrorism incidents.

On declaration of a national emergency requiring DoD support, ARNG and ANG units are frequently already providing support as part of the state's emergency response plan. Guard medical units, along with Disaster Medical Assistance Teams (volunteers who can be called to federal service in times of emergency and so can provide care outside the states in which they are licensed or certified; see chapter 46, Domestic Disaster Response: FEMA and Other Governmental Organizations), are often the first health care support units to arrive in the emergency area. The ANG and the ARNG are not federalized in most emergencies.

TABLE 6-2

HEALTH SERVICE SUPPORT MOBILIZATION: SOURCES AND OPTIONS

Situation	Sources of Health Service Support	Mobilizing Health Service Support	Actions Required
Any level of emergency	RC health service support units and individuals	Mobilize volunteer individuals and units of the Selected Reserve	Military Departments order units and volunteer individuals to active duty within the limits of presidential authorities invoked
	Department of Veterans Affairs hospitals	Implement the Department of Veterans Affairs–DoD Contingency Plan	DoD and Department of Veterans Affairs act in accordance with the Department of Veterans Affairs and DoD Health Resources Sharing and Emergency Operations Act (38 USC 8111A) when DoD requirements exceed supply of continental US military hospital beds
	Host-nation health care systems	Activate host-nation support agreements	Geographic combatant commander requests support in accordance with agreements
National emergency or war	RC health service support units and individuals	Mobilize remaining RC health service support units and individuals	Military Departments order RC units and individuals to active duty
	Domestic civilian health care system	Transfer US Public Health Service commissioned members to DoD or US Coast Guard	US Public Health Service assigns members to DoD or US Coast Guard with request from Secretary of Defense or Transportation and presidential executive order
		Activate National Disaster Medical System	Secretary of Defense acts under provisions of Public Health Service Act when hospital bed requirements exceed capacity of DoD and Department of Veterans Affairs

Source: US Department of Defense. *Joint Doctrine for Mobilization Planning.* Washington, DC: DoD; 1995. Joint Publication 4-05, IV-20.

Maintaining state control of the Guard provides the governor with a more flexible force to respond to the emergency (as federalized Guard units lose their law enforcement authority).

The National Disaster Medical System

The National Disaster Medical System (NDMS) is a key component of the medical response to national mobilization and is also a key component in federal disaster and emergency assistance operations. NDMS and its functions in those situations are explained more fully in chapter 46, Domestic Disaster Response: FEMA and Other Governmental Organizations. The Assistant Secretary for

Health in the Office of Emergency Preparedness, Department of Health and Human Services, is responsible for the NDMS in peacetime. The DoD assumes control of the NDMS during wartime. The program is a partnership among the Departments of Health and Human Services, Veterans Affairs, and Defense. NDMS has two primary missions: "(1) to supplement State and local medical resources during major domestic natural and man made catastrophic disasters and emergencies; and (2) to provide backup medical support to the Department of Defense (DoD) and the Department of Veterans Affairs (VA) medical systems in providing care for U.S. Armed Forces personnel who become casualties during overseas conventional conflicts."[14(pII-1)]

MEDICAL CHALLENGES TO MOBILIZING THE RESERVE COMPONENT

The challenges of mobilizing RC units may not be widely appreciated by inexperienced AC or RC commanders or medical personnel. In addition to the medical concerns already mentioned and those

discussed below, there are myriad organizational hurdles to overcome, usually with limited time and support. A medical officer with an RC engineer battalion during the Persian Gulf War found that difficulties with medical clearance for deployment fell into three categories (administrative, logistic, and supply) and that careful planning would help overcome most of these problems.[15] Amato provides 12 specific recommendations related to administrative planning, use of chain of command, consistent medical qualification policies, use and maintenance of medical records, and appropriate use of medical personnel. He also reported that some medical personnel were overtly obstructive to the mobilization process because of their personal convictions regarding the propriety of the conflict. This article may be helpful to commanders and medical personnel who may be mobilized or assist with RC mobilization.

Medical and Fitness Issues

While the types of units found within each component vary even within branches of service, there are some commonalities about reservists among the various Reserve Components. RC members are generally older than active duty members of their parent services and usually have a civilian job, which may or may not be related to their military occupation. RC members have limited and intermittent contact with the active component, as they usually drill 1 weekend a month and perform 2 weeks of active duty each year. Physical training conducted during reserve duty sessions is insufficient in itself to ensure fitness. When physical training was conducted during drills, it was found not to be an effective or efficient method of improving the fitness of National Guard soldiers.[16] For several reasons, RC individuals can be a cause for preventive medicine concern during times of mobilization, deployment, and redeployment. While most reservists will perform their military tasks without becoming injured, ill, or otherwise a medical liability, the risk of such an event may be higher among reservists.

There have been several published reports regarding the physical and medical fitness of reservists. The physical fitness of these individuals has been found to be lower than that of active duty members in Canada[17] and in the United States.[18] Although there are limited data comparing the risk of injuries between RC and AC members during training exercises, reservists experience substantial levels of training-associated injuries. Korenyi-Both and colleagues[19] found that over a 4-year period, injuries accounted for over one third of sick call visits in a USAR mechanized infantry brigade, and that musculoskeletal injuries were the most common type. Foulkes[20] evaluated orthopedic injuries experienced by an ARNG brigade activated for Operation Desert Storm and found that 26%

were degenerative or due to overuse, two categories that may be difficult to differentiate and that may be related to fitness.[21]

There have been reports that substantial proportions of RC members were not medically fit for mobilization during the Persian Gulf War.[22] An earlier study[23] found that, on average, ANG members would need from 3 to 5 hours of dental treatment for necessary operative and rehabilitative dental care. One study[24] found that between 46% and 58% (depending on whether previous or current criteria were used) of Army RC soldiers examined in 1991 had a class 3 finding (ie, the existing condition is likely to result in a dental emergency within the next 12 months). During the mobilization for the Persian Gulf War, Rothberg and colleagues[25] studied 2,723 IRR soldiers called to active duty. Twenty-five percent were rejected for activation; the most common reasons were overweight (29% of rejections), sole parent of a minor child (25%), orthopedic problems (12%), and mental problems (10%).

In addition, based on the personal experience of one author (DNC) as the commander of a reserve unit, as well as anecdotal reports from senior RC medical officers, it is clear that falsification of weigh-in and physical fitness records occurs, and some reservists do not report medical conditions that would prevent their participation or deployment (eg, asthma, diabetes). On the other hand, some reservists intentionally do not complete specific predeployment tasks (eg, the family support plan) so they will be deferred from deployment. The limited contact RC members have with the AC military makes it easier than it would be if they were AC members for these deficiencies to go undetected. The impact this has on force readiness and medical assets has not been quantified.

Psychosocial Problems

RC members may face social and psychological challenges that differ from those of AC members. Active duty servicemembers generally deploy with members of the same unit they have been working with on a daily basis for months or years. Military units are frequently social units as well, with friendships existing between both the members and their families. Military families often live in government housing or at least in the general proximity of the military installation. When deployed, these families can constitute a social support network, giving mutual psychological and social assistance.

Although RC members also generally deploy with their units, many are individually assigned as fillers to other reserve or active units. In addition, the nature of reserve training (usually once a month and 2 weeks in the summer) is not conducive to developing close relationships. There is generally much less contact among the families, which often are scattered across a much wider area, and this provides fewer opportunities for developing effective social networks as compared to the situation with members of the active component.

Another important difference between an AC and an RC servicemember is the reservist's employment status. Active duty servicemembers continue in their usual occupation when deployed and have little change in their income level. While the jobs of mobilized RC members are secure by law, there can be very substantial changes in their incomes. Many RC enlisted members are highly educated professionals who maintain their military service both out of a sense of duty and to generate a small amount of additional income. However, their full-time military pay may be substantially lower than their full-time civilian pay. These differences may be even more dramatic when professionals such as physicians or attorneys are mobilized. A situation that can be even more financially devastating can occur when RC members are self-employed or own their businesses and employ others. There exists a potential for members in these situations to experience catastrophic financial setbacks, including the loss of businesses and subsequent unemployment for themselves and their employees. This has the potential to adversely affect morale and retention. Manglesdorff and Moses[26] compared the number of USAR medical department resignations for fiscal year 1990 (mostly before the Persian Gulf War) with fiscal year 1991 (during and mostly after the Persian Gulf War) and reported that Nurse Corps resignations rose from 82 to 429; Dental Corps from 28 to 115; Medical Corps from 99 to 435; and Medical Service Corps from 45 to 68. Many of these individuals reported suffering dramatic financial losses as a result of mobilization.

While there has been substantial research conducted evaluating psychological and social stressors on AC military personnel and their families, much less is known about RC personnel and their families. Black[27] reviewed stressors faced by active duty, National Guard, and Reserve servicemembers, based on data from the Defense Manpower Data Center, Monterey, California, collected in 1985 and 1986. He reported substantial differences in the spouses and families of RC members as compared to those of AC members. This included longer periods of marriage, older spouses, and a higher proportion of families with no children under 18 years of age. Compared to AC families, RC families were much more likely to have lived in their current location for more than 2 years. Black makes a number of reasonable recommendations regarding support groups but does not recommend how these can be oriented towards RC families. He does note that AC families are more likely to be distant from their extended families, while RC families may be socially isolated from other families in similar situations.

Since the end of the Persian Gulf War, there have been several studies evaluating concerns of RC members and their families. One study[28] evaluated indicators of stress among Air Force medical personnel shortly after the end of the war. Several areas of concern were found, including worries about families and financial concerns. A study of members of two USAR medical units was reported by Hammelman.[29] Soldiers reported being affected by the stressors more than their families. Several factors were associated with being affected more by the stressors, including being married, of higher rank, male, and a parent of preschool children. Unexpectedly, families of single parents were less affected than families with two parents. Apparently—but this was not explicitly stated—male reservists had greater concerns about financial difficulties than did female reservists.

A study[30] of mobilized Navy Reservists who responded to a questionnaire found that concerns of these personnel could be grouped into several categories, two of which were (1) financial and family hardship and (2) community and family support. Officers reported a higher level of financial difficulty than did enlisted members, which the authors attribute to the high proportion of physicians in the sample. Of the physicians, 63% reported a moderate-to-severe hardship on their civilian medical practice, and 42% reported a moderate-to-severe financial hardship. This article also reports on an unpublished Navy survey that found that more than 20% of the medical and dental officers reported a greater than 50% loss in income in the 6 months following their release from active duty. Less information was provided on community and family support, but the authors report a relatively high level of satisfaction with these issues among the study subjects.

Even less information is available regarding the reintegration of the RC member after release from active duty. Black[27] notes that a family's reunion may be more stressful than the separation and that readjustment may take up to 8 weeks but presents no RC-specific problems or solutions.

While psychological, social, and economic issues may not be routinely considered preventive medicine problems, these factors may directly affect preventive medicine personnel and programs. Malone and colleagues[31] evaluated a USNR Construction Battalion unit and speculated that increased morbidity reported by RC personnel may have been due to psychological, social, and economic stresses different in magnitude and type from those experienced by AC personnel. They hypothesize that rapid mobilization and demobilization does not allow adequate time for servicemembers to process adverse experiences or fears. They also discussed that the unexpected disruption of families and careers resulted in domestic and financial pressures that were magnified in the older age groups, which are overrepresented in the Reserve Components. Adverse health effects, generally self-reported and of a vague nature, have been observed years after mobilization and demobilization related to the Persian Gulf War.

Reservists are about twice as likely as active duty personnel to participate in the clinical evaluation programs operated by the DoD (ie, the Comprehensive Clinical Evaluation Program) and the Department of Veterans Affairs (ie, the Gulf War Health Registry), even though the actual types and degrees of morbidity among these personnel are not substantially different (Kang HK, 1997, unpublished data; DNC, 1997, unpublished data).[32,33] The reasons for the higher levels of participation are poorly understood, but the higher health care–seeking behavior and perceived health problems may present a military readiness issue and deserve further evaluation. It is largely the concern and activism by RC veterans that has driven the high degree of political and media interest in the health effects of serving in the Persian Gulf War.

SUMMARY

Mobilization, whether a military or a national mobilization, is a process that is vital to the national security of the United States. Access to the RC forces is a requirement for successful mobilization, and an understanding of the structure and function of the RC is crucial to understanding the mobilization process. RC personnel differ in a number of important characteristics from AC personnel, and there is substantial evidence that reservists have special physical, mental, and social concerns that affect both their ability to deploy and their health after they redeploy. All active duty and RC health care providers, and preventive medicine personnel in particular, need to understand these RC issues so they are prepared for the problems that may occur during a time of national emergency.

REFERENCES

1. Philpott T. Back on the edge. *The Retired Officer Magazine*. 1999;LIV:52–60.

2. Counts J, ed. *1999 Reserve Forces Almanac*. Falls Church, Va: Uniformed Services Almanac, Inc; 1999.

3. Schultz RC. The National Guard's secret to success. *Army Magazine*. 1998;48(10):95–100.

4. Plewes TJ. Army Reserve: A true partner in America's Army. *Army Magazine*. 1998;48(10):103–111.

5. Assistant Secretary of Defense for Reserve Affairs. *The Reserve Components of the United States Armed Forces*. Washington, DC: Department of Defense; 1996. DoD Pub 1215.15-H, 26.

6. Office of Public Affairs, Headquarters Air Force Reserve Command. Air Force Reserve Command briefing. January 1999. Available at: http://www.afres.af.mil.

7. US Department of Defense. *Joint Doctrine for Mobilization Planning*. Washington, DC: DoD; 1995. Joint Publication 4-05.

8. US Department of Defense. *Joint Medical Surveillance*. Washington, DC: DoD; 1997. DoD Directive 6490.2.

9. US Department of Defense. *Implementation and Application of Joint Medical Surveillance for Deployments*. Washington, DC: DoD; 1997. DoD Instruction 6490.3.

10. US Department of Defense. *Military Support to Civilian Authorities*. Washington, DC: DoD; 1993. DoD Directive 3025.1.

11. US Department of Defense. *Military Assistance for Civilian Disturbances*. Washington, DC: DoD; 1994. DoD Directive 3025.12.

12. US Department of Defense. *Military Assistance to Civilian Authorities.* Washington, DC: DoD; 1997. DoD Directive 3025.15.

13. US Department of Defense. *Department of Defense Cooperation with Civilian Law Enforcement Officials.* Washington, DC: DoD; 1986. DoD Directive 5525.5.

14. National Disaster Medical System. *National Disaster Medical System Strategic Vision.* Washington DC: NDMS; 1994.

15. Amato RS. Medical aspects of mobilization for war in an Army Reserve battalion. *Mil Med.* 1997;162:244–248.

16. Powell GD, Dumitru D, Kennedy JJ. The effect of command emphasis and monthly physical training on Army physical fitness scores in a National Guard Unit. *Mil Med.* 1993;158:294–297.

17. Song TM, Moore J. Physical fitness of militia forces. *Mil Med.* 1989:154:477–479.

18. Kokkinos PF, Holland JC, Newman R, Fiest-Fite B, Signorino CE. Physical activity, smoking, alcohol consumption, body mass index, and plasma lipid profiles of military reserve officers. *Mil Med.* 1989;154:600–603. Published erratum: *Mil Med.* 1990;155:51.

19. Korenyi-Both AL, Dellva WL, Juncer DJ. Prevalence of injuries and illnesses of a Reserve Separate Infantry Brigade (Mechanized) during annual training. *Mil Med.* 1991;156:280–282.

20. Foulkes GD. Orthopedic casualties in an activated National Guard Mechanized Infantry Brigade during Operation Desert Shield. *Mil Med.* 1995;160:128–131.

21. Jones BH, Cowan DN, Tomlinson JP, Robinson JR, Polly DW, Frykman PN. Epidemiology of injuries associated with physical training among young men in the Army. *Med Sci Sports Exerc.* 1993;25:197–203.

22. Loucks AB. Reserve readiness researcher studies NRRC Detroit. *Navy Med.* 1993;84(2):9.

23. Yacovone JA, Box JJ, Mumford RA. Dental survey of Air National Guard personnel. *Mil Med.* 1985;150:476–482.

24. Shulman JD, Williams TR, Tupa JE, Lalumandier JA, Richter NW, Olexa BJ. A comparison of dental fitness classification using different class 3 criteria. *Mil Med.* 1994;159:5–7.

25. Rothberg JM, Koshes RJ, Shanahan JE, Christman KW. Mobilization and rejection of Individual Ready Reserve personnel in Operations Desert Shield/Storm at a U.S. Army Quartermaster post. *Mil Med.* 1995;160:240–242.

26. Mangelsdorff AD, Moses GR. A survey of Army medical department reserve personnel mobilized in support of Operation Desert Storm. *Mil Med.* 1993;158:254–258.

27. Black WG Jr. Military-induced family separation: a stress reduction intervention. *Soc Work.* 1993;38:273–280.

28. Samler JD. Reserve unit mobilization trauma. *Mil Med.* 1994;159:631–635.

29. Hammelman TL. The Persian Gulf conflict: the impact of stressors as perceived by Army reservists. *Health Soc Work.* 1995;20:140–145.

30. Nice DS, Hilton S, Malone TA. Perceptions of US Navy medical reservists recalled for Operation Desert Storm. *Mil Med.* 1994;159:64–67.

31. Malone JD, Paige-Dobson B, Ohl C, DiGiovanni C, Cunnion S, Roy MJ. Possibilities for unexplained chronic illnesses among reserve units deployed in Operation Desert Shield/Desert Storm. *South Med J.* 1996;89:1147–1155.

32. Kang HK, Dalager NA, Watanabe KK. Persian Gulf Registry. Oral presentation at the National Institutes of Health Technology Workshop on the Persian Gulf Experience and Health; April 1994; Washington, DC.

33. Gray CG, Hawksworth AW, Smith TC, Kang HK, Knoke JD, Gackstetter GD. Gulf War veterans' health registries. Who is most likely to seek evaluation? *Am J Epidemiol.* 1998;148:343–349.

Chapter 7

EVOLUTION OF MILITARY RECRUIT ACCESSION STANDARDS

RAMY A. MAHMOUD, MD, MPH; KATHRYN L. CLARK, MD, MPH; AND LAUREL MAY, MD, MPH

R. A. Mahmoud; Lieutenant Colonel, Medical Corps, US Army Reserve; Group Director, Janssen Research Foundation, 1125 Trenton-Harbourton Road, PO Box 200, Room A11010, Titusville, NJ 08560-0200

K. L. Clark; Infectious Disease Analyst, Armed Forces Medical Intelligence Center, 1607 Porter Street, Fort Detrick, MD 21702-5004; Formerly, Major, Medical Corps, US Army; Division of Preventive Medicine, Walter Reed Army Institute of Research, Washington, DC; 20307-5100

L. May; Commander, Medical Corps, United States Navy, Lieutenant Commander; Epidemiologist, Navy Environmental Preventive Medicine Unit-6, 480 Central Avenue, Pearl Harbor, HI 96860-4908

INTRODUCTION

For as long as communities have raised armies, there has been a need to determine who is physically qualified to serve. One example shows that age and physical infirmity were considerations for military service millennia ago. In the Bible, it is written that God instructed Moses to "number the whole community of Israel by families in the father's line, recording the name of every male person aged twenty years and upwards fit for military service" (Numbers 1:2-3). The aged, infirm, and maimed were exempt from the Biblical census. Other armies throughout history have imposed a wide variety of physical standards.[1] It is also clear that these standards almost inevitably changed when the demand for soldiers increased, suggesting that what may be considered desirable soldierly characteristics in some situations may not be essential to effective war fighting.[2]

An accession standard is the application of a rule to determine fitness for military service following the screening of a group of people. From 1814 to 1986, accession medical standards for all of the US military services were set by the US Army, but today they are taken from Department of Defense Directive 6130.3.[3] This Department of Defense (DoD) directive provides physical standard goals

> to ensure that individuals under consideration for appointment, enlistment, and induction into the Armed Forces of the United States are:
> a. free of contagious diseases that would be likely to endanger the health of other personnel.
> b. free of medical conditions or physical defects that would require excessive time lost from duty for necessary treatment or hospitalization or would likely result in separation from the Service for medical unfitness.
> c. medically capable of satisfactorily completing required training.
> d. medically adaptable to the military environment without the necessity of geographical area limitations.
> e. medically capable of performing duties without aggravation of existing physical defects or medical conditions.[4(p1)]

Great difficulties lie in balancing standards so that the pressing needs of the community are fulfilled, that individuals who are less well suited to serve (or who might actually impair the effectiveness of a unit) are not permitted entry, and that when possible, each person is treated fairly. Controversy surrounded military medical standards even in antiquity. This was largely because of the difficulty of accurately predicting, based on information available at the time of accession, how a particular subgroup of people (much less a particular individual) will actually perform during a tour of military service. However, the importance of physical standards was recognized. Napoleon realized during his 100-days campaign that his last lot of troops (left over from previous campaigns' unsuitables) served "only to line the roadside and to fill the hospitals."[5]

A medical standard can pertain to a specific disease, injury, physical attribute, or symptom that is thought to be a indication of a more serious underlying condition. For example, in the past, height standards often served a health screening purpose entirely apart from any desire to select for men of a certain height. Short stature was sometimes felt to reflect underlying chronic disease or poor physical development. At times tall stature, especially in conjunction with low weight, was used as a marker of tuberculosis. "Lankiness" in Southern men was sometimes used as a sign of infection with malaria and hookworm.[2] Surrogate markers continue to be used today and will continue to be used as long as they remain a meaningful way of assessing an individual's health and as long as our knowledge of medicine and our ability to predict future performance remain imperfect.

Medical standards applied to screening programs are always intended to select individuals who are medically fit to fulfill necessary functions under the often rigorous conditions of military service and who are expected to remain so for a reasonable period of time.[6] Both common sense and real-world experience have taught the United States that it is too costly in terms of both dollars and readiness to allow persons to enter the military, train for a year or more, and be sent to new jobs, only then to discover that they cannot perform their assigned roles.

A variety of social, political, and doctrinal influences affect the various objectives of medical standards, whether those standards are applied during accession, retention, selection for special jobs (eg, aviator), or any other phase of military service. But there are two fundamental goals to medical standards. One goal is to improve military efficiency, and it has long been recognized that any enterprise employing men and women who are physically and mentally fit for their specialized occupations is more efficient.[7] Experience has also taught that the US government's liability for long-term medical care and disability care creates a huge financial burden that remains long after the service of any group of people. For this reason, and because it makes sense to protect the health of US citizens from needless harm, modern medical standards also have the goal of selecting those who are least likely to become disabled or injured in the normal performance of their duty.

Accession standards can be stiffened or relaxed as the manpower available for military service becomes either proportionately greater or less than the need for it. Changing medical standards are also used to meet objectives relating to force structure, (eg, target number of people in the service, median age of servicemembers, average number of tours of duty served). Other objectives of medical standards as previously applied or as conceivably applicable in the future to various parts of the armed forces may include offering special opportunities for certain subgroups of society, allowing the creation of a pool of individuals with a highly specialized civil-

ian expertise for call-up during wartime, permitting servicemembers with valuable experience to remain in a position to pass their experience on, and many others.

Clearly, many of these fundamental objectives are not achieved by using purely medical judgment, though fitness for combat duty naturally remains a critical criterion in selecting recruits. The philosophy and application of medical standards must necessarily incorporate both the changing needs of the military (eg, growing demands for special skills due to changing technology) and the social and political imperative to reflect the desires of the citizenry.[6] US military standards have evolved greatly and always with the goal of identifying from the pool of potential servicemembers those personnel capable of becoming the foundation upon which the armed forces' ability to meet the challenges of a complex world is built.

HISTORY OF MEDICAL STANDARDS IN THE UNITED STATES

Tracing the evolution of accession standards in the United States over time provides an excellent perspective from which to consider the current status of such standards.

The Early Years—A Blunt Tool

The second Continental Congress of the United States in July 1775 instructed that able-bodied men between 16 and 50 years of age be formed into loose organizations controlled by individual states and known as militias.[1] These were, in effect, the entire body of white male inhabitants who were felt able to preserve the peace. They fulfilled a role closer to that of police than to that of professional soldiery.

The first specific regulations governing the physical condition of recruits, issued in 1814, stated that all "free able-bodied men between the ages of 18 and 35 years who were active and free from disease were welcomed into the Army, but their healthiness had to be demonstrated."[1] Screening physical examinations ensured that each applicant "had perfect use of every joint and limb and that there were no tumors, diseased enlargement of bones or joints, sore legs, or rupture."[1]

The Civil War to World War I—Attempts to Be More Selective

Examination practices during the Civil War were lax and the induction physical something of a sham. One physician boasted that he examined 100 men

in an hour, and frequently applicants who were obviously too young, too old, or infirm were admitted. This was recognized even then to result in at least one problem still faced today when improperly qualified applicants are accepted: excessive discharges due to preexisting illnesses. According to a Sanitary Commission report of 1861, three quarters of the soldiers discharged from the Union Army were "diseased" at the time of enlistment and should never have been enlisted in the first place. The situation finally became so woeful that the Surgeon General demanded and got the physicians to perform physicals more conscientiously. Inspectors were sent to supervise examinations, and recruits entering camp were re-examined just to make sure.[8]

The massive manpower needs of this bloody war led to the passage of the Draft Act of 1863, which established the Enrollment Board to serve as the first independent federal agency charged with examining all prospective servicemembers for physical and mental fitness.[8] At about the same time, the Confederate States of America passed the similar Conscription Act, which called "all free Southern men between the ages of seventeen and fifty to the colors"[8(p108)] and also told recruiters "to accept anyone else who could pull a trigger or stop a minie [bullet]."[8(p108)] During times of exceptional need, "such matters as heart trouble and epilepsy are strictly academic."[8(p108)]

The military of the closing years of the 19th century and first part of the 20th century had a rich voluntary recruit applicant pool, and the armed forces became increasingly selective. Standards became more rigorous. From 1889 to 1915, 70.2% to 83.9% of all applicants could not meet standards and were rejected by the examination process as lacking in "...legal, mental, moral, or physical qualifications."[7]

World War I—The Need for Many Good Men

World War I brought many changes. The Selective Service Act provided for draft boards, in some ways precursors of today's military entrance processing stations. The draft boards screened the physical, mental, and moral fitness of prospective servicemembers. They were assisted by advisory boards, such as the medical advisory board and the legal advisory board, which were charged with establishing fitness standards and acting on complaints. The Provost Marshal General was placed in charge of the entire process.[9] Local boards were, as had historically been the case for entrance screening activities, very much overworked and undermanned in the face of a large flow of recruits.

Physical standards were revised several times during World War I. The first revision applied only to draftees, while the stringent standards described previously continued to apply to volunteers. It was not until the fourth revision, published in 1918, that the same, less-stringent standards were applied to both draftees and volunteers.[1] During the period from September 1917 through November 1918, records show that 2,801,635 men were inducted into the Army. Out of the approximately 10,000,000 registered men, roughly 2,510,000 were examined by local draft boards. During the first 4 months of mobilization, roughly one in three men were rejected on physical grounds, but the rejection rate dropped to one in four during the following 8 months.[9]

Reasons for Rejection

About 22% of rejections were for reasons of disease or defect that would interfere with so-called mechanical performance, such as problems with bones, joints, flat feet, and hernias. Fifteen percent were rejected because of imperfections of the sense organs and 13% for defects in the cardiovascular system. Roughly 12% were rejected for nervous and mental problems, in part due to "abnormal thyroid secretions." About 10% were rejected because of communicable diseases—in particular tuberculosis and venereal disease. Only slightly more than 1 out of 75 was rejected because he was judged to be men-

tally deficient or emotionally unstable.[10]

Recruiting officers were directed to exclude the mentally defective and those showing evidence of serious nervous disorders and to recognize and reject those exhibiting a "degenerate physique,"[7] that is, one marked by diminished stature and inferior vigor. Additional functional stigmata were defective mental qualities and moral delinquencies such as willfulness, deceitfulness, and indecency.[7]

Screening Problems

Pulmonary tuberculosis was screened for by history and physical and became an excellent example of problems resulting from unavailability of adequate screening tests. If not evident, tuberculosis was particularly suspected in tall persons, because tuberculous men were on average 1/2 inch taller and 12 pounds lighter compared to the average healthy World War I registrant.[2] Taking screening chest roentgenograms of every inductee at that time was neither possible nor practical, and radiography was used only as an adjunct in select cases. Unfortunately, these insensitive and non-specific screening methods allowed many men with tuberculosis to be inducted. This proved to be very costly to the government, which provided medical care and other benefits to many World War I veterans with tuberculosis.[11]

Between the Wars—Toward a More Scientific System

The years following World War I and into World War II saw publication of regulations intended to simplify and speed mobilization. Problems experienced during World War I, along with the increasingly technical demands of a modern military force, led to a need for greatly expanded training, which in turn led to the creation of military occupational specialties. Increasingly detailed classification of enrollees was performed, with attention to physical and intellectual proficiency and aptitude. The Army adopted the PULHES system of physical classification from the Canadian military.[12] PULHES is used to assess **p**hysical capacity, **u**pper extremities, **l**ower extremities, **h**earing(ears), **e**yes (vision), and overall **p**sychiatric impression. These areas are rated from 1 to 4, with 1 signifying no assignment limitations from a medical perspective, and as either temporary or permanent. Also, preinduction examining stations were opened to allow a more thorough evaluation of registrants. High school graduates and non-graduates, after orientation briefings, were given psychological tests separate from the medical examination. Skilled psychologists were employed to revise and improve classification procedures and testing, and the Army General Classification Test was implemented. Initially, those with high scores (over 100) on the test were routed largely into the Army Air Force; some went into the Special Services. Ultimately, the War Department sent 75% of those scoring over 100 to the Army Air Force. Ground commanders rebelled at this notion that intelligent men were not required in the ground forces and eventually prevailed, leading to a more equitable distribution of manpower.

The experience with tuberculosis in World War I sensitized the armed forces to the problem of nonspecific screening tools, but despite a decrease in cases of tuberculosis, it was still the primary disease-related cause of death among men of military age at the time of World War II. US Navy recruiters were especially interested in improving screening to prevent the spread of tuberculosis on crowded ships—a problem that continues to exist today. By early 1941, the US Navy had installed photofluorography units at seven training camps to examine recruits and personnel being reassigned to other units. By March 1942, the Army was also using radiography to screen all new recruits.[11] Ultimately, these military radiography screening programs demonstrated that 75% of early active tuberculosis could be discovered only by x-ray examination. Approximately 1% of apparently healthy young men and women were felt to have evidence of pulmonary tuberculosis extensive enough to warrant rejection.[11,13]

World War II—More Specific Screening

In September 1940, there were an estimated 1,024,789 men in the US Armed Forces, 519,805 of whom were in the Army. By the end of the war, more than 10 million men had served in the Army.[13] During the war, some men volunteered for military service, but for the most part, the armed services got their manpower through compulsion. Men were notified to appear for examination to determine their eligibility for service. In 1940, the armed services sought to avoid many potential difficulties by rejecting servicemen who they thought could not be readily converted into effective soldiers, sailors, airmen, or marines. The services had to assess whether a man's physical condition and stamina would enable him to keep the pace of the training schedule and withstand the stresses and strains of combat. The screening process became the anchor of military manpower policy and continued to be crucial throughout World War II.[10] Regulations actually allowed for up to 3 days of hospital observation and testing, if necessary, to clarify whether an individual was medically fit or not.[14] Some felt an even longer period to observe the individual reacting to military service should be allowed.[15]

The military believed that it also had to consider a potential servicemember's emotional stability. It was felt that in World War I sizable numbers of the American Expeditionary Force had "broken down" in battle. The services hoped to prevent a repetition of this experience. The advances made in psychological testing since the end of World War I encouraged many to believe that techniques had been developed that would distinguish the stable from the unstable, the bright from the dull, the well-motivated from the unmotivated.[10] After all, it is "[b]etter to enlist one man with normal intelligence than a dozen who are simply hewers of wood and drawers of water."[16(p302)]

The number of men disqualified for service exceeded all expectations while the need for manpower kept expanding.[13] For the period of November 1940 to August 1945, an estimated 17,954,500 men were examined for induction into military service, and 6,419,700 (35.8%) were rejected.[13] An army of 10 million men was possible only after changes were made to existing policies on physical and mental requirements, as happened in World War I. Although the US Army made changes in its physical and mental requirements throughout the war, it was during the first 2 years that the most telling changes had to be made to permit the induction of millions of men. Before changing standards and procedures, the Surgeon General's Office considered these three issues: (1) the contributions that could be made by persons with certain defects, (2) what the policy should be on the physical rehabilitation of men to make them capable of service, and (3) the legal and economic implications of inducting men with physical defects (thereby inviting future claims against the US government). The changes in physical standards that permitted the greatest addition of new men into the Army were those made for vision, venereal diseases, and teeth.[13]

Reasons for Rejection

Dental defects were the leading cause for rejection at local boards and accounted for 17.7% of all rejections. Providing treatment for dental defects resulted in the qualification of almost 1 million additional men for military service. During 1940 to 1941, eye defects caused 12.2% of all rejections and were the second leading cause for disqualification. After standards were lowered at the onset of the war, however, rejections for eye defects were exceeded consistently by those for mental disease, mental and educational deficiency, and musculo skeletal and cardiovascular defects. The change in standards for eye defects principally involved correcting vision by giving spectacles to those who could not meet the standards without them.[13]

Comparisons With World War I

The rejection rate during World War II was 80% above the rate during World War I. Differences between the two wars were least marked in rejections for physical defects, where the rate for World War II was only about one third higher. This increase must be evaluated in terms of the substantial improvement in the health of the nation since 1918. The higher rejection rate reflected a raising of the criteria, a more careful evaluation of selectees, or, as is most likely, a combination of both.[10]

Much more striking was the more than 4-fold increase in the overall rejection rate for mental and educational deficiencies in the face of a significant rise in the educational level of the population. In World War I, an estimated 29% of men of military age had no more than 6 years of schooling, while in 1941 only 14% had so little education. But perhaps the greatest contrast was in the proportions rejected for emotional disorders: World War II had a rate 11 times as great as that of World War I. Almost certainly, the marked increase in rejection rates reflects a significant raising of entry criteria as applied in practice. Of the 43,000 rejected in World War I, virtually all were truly mentally deficient (ie, unable to perform even unskilled work except under close supervision in a protective environment), but the majority of the 716,000 rejected during World War II were apparently rejected because they were uneducated.[10] In all, 1,992,950 men, or more than 30% of all rejections, were found by the Selective Service to be unfit for general duty because of mental and educational deficiency and neuropsychiatric conditions.[13] This prompted increased interest in psychiatric epidemiology and resulted in an expansion of and alterations in psychiatric nomenclature.[17] Prevalence of psychiatric disorders started to be established less from second-hand accounts and records and more from health care provider interviews. Many of these interviews used instruments based on the Psychosomatic Scale of the Neuropsychiatric Screening Adjunct, which was developed during World War II for Selective Service screening.[17]

Interestingly, despite stringent medical standards and a high initial rejection rate intended to prevent the entry of individuals with mental or educational deficits, 379,486 men were separated from the services for neuropsychiatric reasons from 1942 to 1945. These accounted for 45% of discharges for disability. An additional 356,000 were separated for ineptness, lack of required degree of adaptability, or enuresis.[13]

The 1960s—Weight Standards and Other Surrogate Measures of Fitness

In 1960, accession standards established minimum weights for heights and (in 5-year age increments) liberal maximum weights for height. Obesity, in its lesser forms, was considered treatable and not a reason for rejection or exemption. Until 1976, body weight was a screening tool that excluded only the extremes of underweight and obesity, while a separate regulation detailed physical fitness tests, which periodically assessed the physical performance of active duty military personnel. Then these standards changed from simple entry criteria to standards that must be maintained throughout a military career by appropriate nutrition and exercise.[2] Body weight and body fat standards are the only physical standards currently used by all the Services that actually exclude or eliminate individuals for unsuitability based on a surrogate measure of physical fitness and combat readiness.

Changes in enlistment criteria began early in the Vietnam War. With a shortage of people during the early war years, Secretary of Defense Robert McNamara came up with a plan to meet manpower needs and "salvage hundreds of thousands of young men from economic deprivation by bringing them into the armed services."[18(p15)] The plan significantly relaxed entry standards. During the 3-year span of Project 100,000 (as it was called), 240,000 persons entered active duty. These men were considered only marginally qualified mentally by many and were more likely to desert, not complete a full tour, and be court-martialed than other servicemembers.

Recent Changes

Accession standards have continued to change as new threats to military readiness have emerged. Screening for the human immunodeficiency virus (HIV) among applicants for all services of the military began in late 1985. From October to December of the first year of testing, the prevalence was 1.64 per 1,000 and was higher in males (1.77/1,000) than females (0.68/1,000).[19] The prevalence of recruit applicants infected with HIV has steadily declined since testing began. The prevalence fell to 0.82/1,000 in 1990 and then to 0.22/1,000 in 1994, and the differences in prevalences between the sexes disappeared.[19]

Increasing proportions of women in military accessions has made necessary more exploration of gender issues and medical accession standards. Conditions affecting women differently from men, such as genital chlamydia infections with their various sequelae, will need to be assessed for prevalence and importance relating to accession, attrition, medical costs, and military readiness. With continued scrutiny of the medical accessions process, it is likely that some entrance criteria will be deemed obsolete and new ones adopted as new disease entities arise and improved diagnostic tests are developed.

In the 1990s, the Army's approach to medical accession standards during war differed from that of prior wars. For the Persian Gulf War, retention standards were used instead of the more-lenient mobilization standards. The military services relied on the Reserve Component and National Guard for personnel instead of relaxing or modifying the standards for accession, as was done in World War I, World War II, and the Vietnam War.[3]

IMPLEMENTING ACCESSION MEDICAL STANDARDS IN THE 1990s AND BEYOND

Each individual service has the ultimate responsibility for determining which individuals will enter the service, be selected for a certain job, be retained in service, or otherwise pass a hurdle where medical evaluation plays a part. Beyond the guidance of DoD Directive 6130.3, individual service regulations address these issues, and authority for applying them resides with a variety of organizations. Much of the application of medical standards is a function of service medical facilities around the world, because that is where the examinations are done, whether retention and periodic screening examinations, special examinations for applicants to certain schools or special jobs, or other examinations to which standards apply. The exception to this is medical accession processing; it is not typically a function of service medical facilities and has been handled in the 1990s primarily by two organizations, the US Military Entrance Processing Command (MEPCOM) and the Department of Defense Medical Evaluation Review Board (DODMERB).

Military Entrance Processing Command

The MEPCOM is a joint service command operating under the executive agency of the US Army and is headquartered at the Great Lakes Naval Training Center in Great Lakes, Ill. It has the mission of helping determine if an applicant is qualified for enlistment into the armed forces based on standards set by each of the five individual services (ie, US Army, Navy, Air Force, Marine Corps, and Coast Guard).

The MEPCOM processes by far the largest number of potential servicemembers, mostly for enlistment rather than for the officer corps. In 1995, 340,530 medical examinations were performed by approximately 530 physicians, 474,820 people were tested with the Armed Services Vocational Aptitude Battery (ASVAB), and an additional 847,000 high school students were tested under the DoD student ASVAB testing program. The ASVAB attempts to improve the selection of applicants for enlisted service by measuring aptitude in multiple areas, such as general science, arithmetic reasoning, word knowledge, paragraph comprehension, numerical operations, coding speed, auto and shop information, mathematics knowledge, mechanical comprehension, and electronics information.[20] In the past, it had been a vehicle for examinees to avoid the draft by deliberately failing the battery. Computerized versions of the ASVAB can now detect deliberate failures. Ultimately 236,360 young men and women joined the armed forces from this pool of all who entered MEPCOM in 1995 (US Military Entrance Processing Command, North Chicago, Ill, 1996).

MEPCOM, initially called the Military Enlistment Processing Command, was created on 1 July 1976. It was formed under the jurisdiction of the Army Deputy Chief of Staff for Personnel at Ft. Sheridan, Ill, from elements of the US Army Recruiting Command and the Air Force Vocational Testing Group. Although it remains under the lead agency of the Army today and has a large number of Army personnel assigned to it, it is a tri-service command, is staffed by personnel from each service, and has had commanding officers from other services.

The first years of the command were devoted to standardization of testing and processing in reception and training centers. By September 1979, the command was made independent of the Recruiting Command by Department of the Army General Order 19. In 1980 the name was changed to the US Military Enlistment Processing Command. Replacing "enlistment" with "entrance" in 1983 created today's MEPCOM. The command moved in 1982 from Ft. Sheridan to the Naval Training Center at Great Lakes, Illinois. In that year the examination stations were named Military Entrance Processing Stations (MEPS). By 1985 the mission to process National Guard applicants was added, bringing virtually all applicants for enlistment in the US military under MEPCOM processing authority.

The early 1990s brought a downsizing and streamlining in the armed forces, and MEPCOM responded by instituting in 1992 "1-day" processing (a recruiter was given a "qualified" or "disqualified" decision in 1 day, pending only the results of HIV screening and drug testing), by moving toward a paperless testing system, and by playing a role in efforts to use evidence-based medical standards to best serve the changing manpower needs of US military services.

Service Prerogatives and Waivers

To process applicants efficiently, quickly, and accurately, MEPS use a single DoD standard; the exceptions are service-specific height and weight standards and visual standards for selected programs. It remains a service-specific prerogative, however, to either accept or reject individual applicants. This means that an individual who is determined to be disqualified by MEPCOM according to the DoD standard may still be accepted by a service if it grants the individual a waiver. After an individual is disqualified by the MEPS, his or her physical is then reviewed by the service-specific waiver authority. Some services have different waiver authorities for specific programs (eg, enlisted, Reserve Officer Training Corps, and academy appointments). The waiver authority then grants the waiver, denies the waiver, or requests more information. At certain times, each waiver authority follows temporary policies instituted by its Surgeon General for a specific condition. The DoD Directive also gives the secretaries of the military departments the authority to grant waivers.[4] While the decisions of some service waiver authorities are final, in the Navy and Marine Corps the final decision rests with the Chief of Naval Operations and the Commandant of the Marine Corps, respectively, with the recommendation from the Medical Department (Table 7-1).

DODMERB and the Service Academies

DODMERB is primarily responsible for evaluation of individuals applying for one of the service academies. As early as the mid-1960s, the superintendents of the US Military Academy, the US Air Force Academy, and the US Naval Academy would meet annually, and the surgeons of each academy would meet at the same time. These meetings provided for some coordination and a degree of consistency; however, by the late 1960s it was recognized that there would be great benefits from better coordination and standardization. Under the impetus of Colonel Kandel and others, largely at the Air Force Academy, an organization called the Service Academy Central Medical Review Board was established in January 1970. Later its name was changed to DODMERB. Its purpose, then as now, was to standardize and make more efficient the medical entrance processing for entry into the academies of the Army, Air Force, and Navy. Responsibility for Coast Guard academy examinations was moved from the Public Health Service to DODMERB in 1971 and responsibility for the Merchant Marines was added in 1972. This is an area of particular importance to the armed forces because every accepted applicant consumes a major investment of resources during academy training, and each is a potential career servicemember. Moreover, there have almost always been many more applicants than available positions in the academies. As a result, greater efforts and costs have always been incurred in screening such applicants with more complete examinations than might otherwise be employed, and high standards for entry have been imposed.

Because the Air Force examination was considered the most stringent, it was chosen as the initial unified examination. Academy entrance examinations had been performed at many locations, but it was found that many were not correctly performed. This was particularly a problem with the cycloplegic refractions. The Surgeons General of the services provided

TABLE 7-1

THE FIVE MOST COMMON MEDICAL REASONS FOR DISQUALIFICATION AT MILITARY ENTRANCE PROCESSING STATIONS IN 1995

Medical Reason	Disqualification Rate (%)	n
Hearing	1.42	5,145
Lower extremity	1.29	4,678
Lungs/chest	1.24	4,500
Feet	0.97	3,507
Psychiatric	0.97	3,506

Data Source: US Military Entrance Processing Command, 2834 Green Bay Road, North Chicago, IL 60064-3094.

DODMERB with a list of specific sites that were certified to perform the DODMERB examination. Use of other sites for entrance examinations was not permitted by DODMERB thereafter. DODMERB was responsible for the entire medical entrance processing of each applicant, regardless of service, and forwarded results directly to the director of admissions at each academy. DODMERB's pioneering use of computers and automated decision systems applying rule-based standards with over 1,500 decision rules led to recognized early success. In the 1970s, responsibility for most Reserve Officer Training Corps applicant examinations was added to DODMERB as a result. In the 1990s, DODMERB was responsible for processing 30,000 to 45,000 applicants per year, of whom approximately 12% are disqualified.[21]

MEPCOM and DODMERB examinations were not the same, and an examination performed at one did not satisfy the needs of the other. This was not a matter of minor additions or deletions: entirely different forms and procedures marked a total lack of coordination of the two systems for many years. In1994, a process was initiated that will lead to the compatibility of these examinations.

EVIDENCE-BASED ACCESSION MEDICAL STANDARDS

A movement is taking place, with the support of the General Accounting Office and both the military personnel and medical communities, toward developing and using more evidence-based, scientifically valid medical standards, not only for military accession but also for all the other situations in which the armed forces judge fitness for service based on medical screening. This movement is, at least in part, a response to an increasing awareness of the problem of attrition in the military.

The Drain of Attrition

It is recognized that approximately 30% to 35% of all enlistees entering the services are separated before the completion of their first term of service, and 10% to 15% are discharged in the first 6 months of duty.[22] These rates are similar in all the services. Many of the recruits that are separated in the first 6 months fail to meet minimum performance criteria or have medical problems. The most common reasons for medical separation in the first 6 months are asthma, psychiatric conditions, and orthopedic problems (Table 7-2). In fiscal year 1993, the cost of recruiting, screening, and training one individual was approximately $20,000. The General Accounting Office calculated that if the services could reduce this 6-month attrition by 4%, short-term savings as a result of transporting, feeding, clothing, and paying fewer recruits would be $4.8 million; $12 million would be saved after a reduction of 10%.[22] The savings would increase over time as infrastructure needed for recruiting and training could be reduced.

Objectives

This movement to develop and utilize evidence-based standards has multiple objectives. Recruiters want to ease the difficulty and reduce the cost of accessing high-quality volunteers by relaxing standards they hope will be found to have been needlessly strict. Recruiters also hope that by understanding predictors of successful completion of full tours of duty, premature losses can be reduced and the number of new recruits needed every month correspondingly reduced. Trainers hope to reduce injuries and improve the graduation rate from training by bringing in candidates who are more likely to succeed in training or by identifying physical or mental conditions for which better training can be devised. Line commanders ultimately may suffer less loss-of-duty time to medical problems, improved world-wide deployability, and a higher level of readiness among their personnel as individuals who are increasingly well suited for the job (and jobs increasingly well suited to individuals) are developed. The Department of Defense may reduce the risk young men and women face for disability

TABLE 7-2

DISCHARGES FOR CONDITIONS EXISTING PRIOR TO SERVICE IN 1995[*]

Condition	Discharge Rate (%)	n
Orthopedics (knee)	0.453	1,566
Chest and lungs (asthma)	0.453	1,502
Orthopedics (other)	0.426	1,471
Orthopedics (feet)	0.366	1,264
Orthopedics (back)	0.318	1,099
Psychiatric (other)	0.188	651

[*]Out of total number of people starting active duty in 1995.
Data sources: the Accession Medical Standards Analysis and Research Activity, Walter Reed Army Institute of Research, Silver Spring, Maryland 20910-7500; and the Defense Manpower Data Center, Monterey, California.

discharge or long-term medical problems, sparing our youth a degree of risk and saving the US Government some portion of the billions of dollars currently spent on long-term disability and medical liability payments.

Underlying these motivations is the clear benefit of setting policies and standards that are supported by the best available evidence and not solely by opinion or historical precedent. For example, flat feet had been accepted as a risk for injury and poor physical performance in recruits. However, a rigorously conducted study found that the data do not unconditionally support that assumption.[23] Asymptomatic individuals with low foot arches actually did not appear to be at increased risk of exercise-related injury. In another example, serologic testing for hepatitis C became available, and the routine screening of all recruit applicants was considered. Careful examination and analysis of the data and costs proved that universal serologic testing of recruit applicants for hepatitis C would not be a cost-effective policy (Tri-Service Accession Medical Standards Working Group, unpublished data, 1997). Evidence-based policy decisions are more easily defended and their impact can be more accurately predicted, monitored, and understood.

The Accession Medical Standards Analysis and Research Activity

The Accession Medical Standards Steering Committee, whose membership is drawn from the medical and personnel communities, was created to provide policy guidance and establish accession standards requirements. The Accession Medical Standards Working Group is subordinate to that committee and reviews accession policy issues and recommendations from the Accession Medical Standards Analysis and Research Activity. This activity was established in 1996 at the Walter Reed Army Institute of Research, Washington, DC, to support the development of evidence-based accession standards; it does this by guiding the improvement of medical and administrative databases, conducting epidemiologic analyses, and integrating into policy recommendations relevant operational, clinical, and economic considerations. Ideally, under the direction of the flag-level steering committee and with the efforts of the other bodies, medical standards will increasingly be based on rigorous studies, careful questioning of evidence, and methodologically appropriate analysis of data.

A variety of studies will be used to develop evidence-based policies and procedures and to validate current standards. This can be done by using survival analyses; for example, the group entering military service with asthma can be examined to determine whether the granting of waivers to certain people disqualified for asthma is appropriate (Figure 7-1). Certain diagnostic techniques and instruments need to be assessed. For example, understanding the sensitivity (the ability to detect those who truly have asthma) and specificity (the ability to accurately identify normals as normal) of the methacholine challenge test as a predictor of asthma is vital. Following over time indicators such as discharges for diagnoses that existed prior to service will allow for assessment of quality assurance measures at the waiver authorities and MEPS. Tools such as cost-benefit and cost-effectiveness analyses will be used to rigorously and quantitatively assess policy options, such as whether to continue screening for syphilis at the MEPS. Quality of experimental design, generalizability of findings from the medical literature to the target military population, and the presence of bias and confounding will be more widely and carefully considered by policymakers. After a change in policy is instituted, the impact on outcomes, such as attrition and hospitalization, must be monitored. In instances where expert opinion is all that can be relied on, standard methods with increased reliability, reproducibility, and validity (eg, the Delphi method) should yield more supportable results. This process will produce valuable new policies and procedures because of

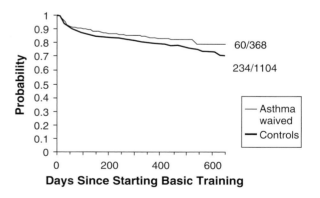

Fig. 7-1. Probability of remaining on active duty after accession. In a study of trainees from the Army, Navy, and Marine Corps in 1995, individuals given waivers for asthma appeared to have the same probability of remaining on active duty as their comparable non-waived counterparts. The waiver process as examined appeared adequate with respect to attrition. Graph: Courtesy of the Accession Medical Standards Analysis and Research Activity, Walter Reed Army Institute of Research, Silver Spring, Maryland 20910-7500.

its movement toward a scientific methodology in establishing and evaluating medical standards. However, a number of limitations and potential pitfalls exist.

Despite easier access to data and the shift toward more evidence-based decision making, the traditional method (in which subject experts based their judgments on personal assessments of available medical literature, on their own medical and operational experience, and on anecdote) will still be used when other options are not feasible. This may occur when resources or time do not permit rigorous analysis or when the potential value of a scientific approach is much less than the costs in time or money of such an approach. Using the "subject matter expert" approach is reasonable and desirable if its limitations, such as the propen-sity toward numerator bias, are explicitly recognized.

Numerator bias arises because clinical and administrative experience teaches a military physician a great deal about servicemembers who develop problems. Such experience also teaches the physicians about the relationship of a given problem to the prior conditions for which the servicemember could have been screened. However, the physician's experience may lack information about servicemembers who remain well (despite the same conditions) throughout their service. The result is an inappropriate emphasis when considering policy action on the performance of those who use the military medical system and underweighting of the performance of those who do not. Nevertheless, standards based on expert opinion will at times still be appropriate.

SUMMARY

There will always be a need to screen and select capable individuals for military service. Military medical accession standards have changed considerably throughout history and are likely to be altered further to adapt to the future needs of the military and the state of medical knowledge. Continuous improvements in accession and medical data collection are being made. Routine monitoring of the results of medical screening and the health of servicemembers is being done. Improved methods of assessing health are being developed. The capability to study this information epidemiologically allows potentially modifiable problem areas to be noted, trends to be monitored, and the impact of medical accession policy changes to be assessed. All this will improve the screening process, reduce medical attrition, and improve the capabilities of servicemembers in today's armed forces and so the forces themselves.

REFERENCES

1. Siegal DL. *An Evaluation of the Performance of the Medical Examination for Entrance into the Armed Forces*. Fort Leavenworth, Kan: US Army Command and General Staff College; 1971.

2. Committee on Military Nutrition Research, Body Composition and Physical Performance. Washington, DC: National Academy Press; 1992.

3. Wortzel CJ. *Medical Fitness Standards and Medical Examination Policies: Operation Desert Shield and Operation Desert Storm: An Individual Study Project*. Carlisle Barracks, Pa: US Army War College; 1993.

4. US Department of Defense. *Physical Standards for Appointment, Enlistment, and Induction*. Washington, DC: DoD; 1994. DoD Directive 6130.3.

5. Farenholt A. A plea for greater care in the performance of duty by medical officers at recruiting stations. *US Naval Med Bull*. 1917;11:318–325.

6. Karpinos BD. *Qualification of American Youth for Military Service*. Washington, DC: Office of The Surgeon General, Dept of the Army; 1962.

7. Hoffman FL. *Army Anthropometry and Medical Rejection Statistics*. Newark, NJ: Prudential Press; 1918.

8. Brook S. *Civil War Medicine*. Springfield, Ill: Charles C Thomas Publishers; 1966.

9. *Physical Examination of the First Million Draft Recruits*. Washington, DC: US Army Medical Department, Government Printing Office; 1919.

10. Ginzberg E, Anderson JK, Ginsburg SW, Herma JL. *The Lost Divisions*. New York, NY: Columbia University Press; 1959.

11. Haygood TM, Briggs JE. World War II military led the way in screening chest radiography. *Mil Med*. 1992;157: 113–116.

12. Department of the Army. *Medical Services Standards of Medical Fitness*. Washington, DC: Headquarters, DA; 1994. Army Regulation 40-501.

13. Foster WB, Hellman IL, Hesford D, McPherson DG; Wiltse CM, ed. *Physical Standards in World War II*. Washington, DC: Office of the Surgeon General, US Army Medical Dept; 1967.

14. Association Notes. *Mil Surg*. 1942;91:107.

15. Editorials. *Mil Surg*. 1941;88:425.

16. Bell RA. Recruit selection. *US Naval Med Bull*. 1940;38:301–306.

17. Dohrenwend BP, Dohrenwend BS. Perspectives on the past and future of psychiatric epidemiology. *Am J Public Health*. 1982;72:1271–1279.

18. Curry GD. *Sunshine Patriots*. Notre Dame, Ind: University of Notre Dame Press; 1985.

19. HIV-1 in the Army. *Medical Surveillance Monthly Report*. 1996;2(suppl):12–14.

20. *NLS [National Longitudinal Surveys] Users' Guide 1995*. Columbus, Ohio: Center for Human Resource Research, The Ohio State University; 1995: 52.

21. Mullen L. Personal communication, 1996.

22. General Accounting Office. *Military Attrition: DOD Could Save Millions by Better Screening Enlisted Personnel*. Washington, DC: GAO; 1997. GAO/NSAID-97-39.

23. Cowan DN, Jones BH, Robinson JR. Foot morphologic characteristics and risk of exercise-related injury. *Arch Fam Med*. 1993;2:773–777.

Chapter 8

THE BASIC TRAINING ENVIRONMENT

LAUREL BROADHURST, MD, MPH; K. MILLS McNEILL, MD, MPH, PhD; ROSE MARIE HENDRIX, MD, MPH; JAMES WRIGHT, MD; and LAUREL MAY, MD, MPH

L. Broadhurst; formerly, Major, Medical Corps, US Army; Epidemiology Consultant, 7th MEDCOM and 10th MEDLAB, APO AE 09180, Landstuhl, Germany; currently, Staff Physician, Weaverville Family Medicine Associates, 117 Hillcrest Dr, Weaverville, NC 28782

K. M. McNeill; Colonel, Medical Corps, US Army (Retired); formerly, Chief, Preventive Medicine Services, Dwight David Eisenhower Army Medical Center, Fort Gordon, GA 30905-5650; currently, Medical Director for Bioterrorism Preparedness, Office of Epidemiology, Mississippi State Department of Health, 570 E. Woodrow Wilson, PO Box 1700, Jackson, MS 39215-1700

R. M. Hendrix; Formerly, Lieutenant Colonel, Medical Corps, US Army; Chief, Preventive Medicine Service, US Army Medical Department Activity, Fort Jackson, SC 29207-5720, currently, Medical Director, Santa Cruz County Health Clinic, 1080 Emeline, Santa Cruz, CA 95060

J. Wright; Colonel, Medical Corps, US Air Force (Retired); formerly, AL/AOE, 2601 West Road, Suite 2, Brooks Air Force Base, Texas 78235-5241; currently, Occupational Medicine Physician, Concentra Medical Centers, 400 East Quincy, San Antonio, TX 78215

L. May; Commander, Medical Corps, US Navy; Epidemiologist, Naval Environmental and Preventive Medicine Unit 6, Naval Medical Clinic, 480 Central Avenue, Pearl Harbor HI 96860-4908

INTRODUCTION

Basic training is the process by which civilians enter one of the most honored of all careers, military service to one's country. This is a monumental process of transforming individual men and women into soldiers, sailors, airmen, and Marines prepared to defend their country. To understand military preventive medicine, one must understand the method of transition, which brings civilians into a military career, known as basic training.

Unlike college freshmen in dormitories across the country, military basic trainees, or recruits, eat, sleep, and breathe together in an intensely congested environment. There is little free time between classes, there is no choice of curriculum, and there is mandatory, daily physical training; recruits belong to the military 24 hours a day. Oftentimes, there is little change of pace even on weekends. Like a freshman year at college, this is a "coming of age" time for recruits. Many have never before been away from home, and even those who have may not have been outside their region of the country. The military promises opportunities to travel and often the first big trip is to a military basic training installation.

No civilian institution has as its goal to transform large numbers of individuals from all over the country into cohesive, combat-prepared units in a short time while maintaining consistently high training standards. This chapter will describe military basic training and the medical issues that characterize this environment. Each service has a specific term for its initial recruit training, but, for simplicity's sake, this experience will be referred to as "basic training" in this chapter. And, rather than referring to "basic trainees," "airmen basic," or "soldiers, sailors, airmen, and Marines," "recruits" will be used to describe new members of all four services.

GOALS OF BASIC TRAINING

The US Air Force, Army, Marine Corps, and Navy each have separate basic training facilities, but the services have the same goal for basic training. They attempt to transform civilian recruits into motivated, disciplined airmen, soldiers, sailors, and Marines who are trained and able to perform basic military skills in any assignment. This transformation results from the total immersion of recruits in the basic training environment. Basic training is an intensive, comprehensive process that transforms civilians into servicemembers by inculcating military values and teaching military skills.

Values

The atmosphere at basic training installations fosters patriotism, dignity, and pride in being part of the military. One of the most important tools for a successful basic training experience is the right attitude, for both drill instructors and recruits. The importance of the individual recruit to the military and to the nation is emphasized during the training. Training has been designed to bring about initial development and constant reinforcement of concepts that are important to the military. These concepts are integral parts of military tradition and include ethical standards, good order and discipline, teamwork, individual initiative, and commitment.

Skills

Training promotes a desire in recruits for self-improvement and achievement by providing knowledge and skills basic to all military personnel and rewarding performance in individual and unit tasks. Intensive training using military standards is an integral part of the environment, as are high standards in other study areas, positive military role models, and repeated opportunities to reinforce basic military skills. It is through challenging professional training that an individual gains the degree of confidence, self-discipline, commitment, and technical and physical competence required to make a contribution to the military mission. And it is through training that individuals develop the sense of team spirit necessary for success in a unit.

RECRUIT DEMOGRAPHICS AND ATTRITION

Despite the common goals of basic training in all the services, there are differences. To appreciate the differences in basic training environments for each service, it is useful to compare the demographics of each service's recruits (Table 8-1) and the number of individuals beginning and completing basic training programs annually. Rates of graduation from basic training in 1995 for the four services can

TABLE 8-1

RECRUIT DEMOGRAPHICS: HIGHEST EDUCATION STATUS AT THE TIME OF ACCESSION, 1995

Service	Mean Age (yrs)	Female (%)	HS* (%)	HS Diploma (%)	Some College (%)	Bachelor's Degree (%)	Graduate Degree (%)	Missing Data
Air Force	20.2	24.8	0.1	82.2	15.4	1.6	0.1	0.6
Army	20.6	18.6	0.3	87.0	6.1	3.3	0.2	3.1
Marine Corps	19.8	6.3	0.2	98.1	0.8	0.8	0.0	0.0
Navy	20.3	16.8	2.4	93.1	1.5	2.0	0.1	0.9

*without a high school diploma
Data source: Accession Medical Standards Analysis and Research Activity, Walter Reed Army Institute of Research, Silver Spring, Maryland.

be seen in Table 8-2. A total of 175,270 individuals completed military basic training in 1995. Since the draft ended in 1973, the US military has been an all-volunteer force. The number of individuals completing the initial physical examination and entering basic training is much smaller than during times of war. For example, draftees (not counting volunteers) in basic training in 1918 numbered 2,294,048. In 1943, during World War II, the number was 3,323,970. During the Korean War, 551,806 inductees were sent to basic training in 1951, and during the Vietnam War, the largest number of draftees entering basic training was over 382,000 in 1966.[1]

There was service-wide downsizing in the 1990s. In the Army, the number of recruits completing basic training went from a high of 89,539 in 1991 to 67,250 in 1995, and that downward trend will undoubtedly continue.[2] However, the percentage of female recruits has increased, as has the percentage of those having at least a high school diploma. As Table 8-1 shows, the service with the lowest av-

erage percentage of females is the Marine Corps at 6.3%. Nearly all recruits in all the services hold a high school diploma or general equivalency diploma, although the Air Force stands out with nearly 15.4% of its recruits having some college experience.[3] This is relevant because "[s]tudies of attrition have consistently shown that persons with high school diplomas and Armed Forces Qualification Test scores in the upper 50th percentile have lower first-term attrition rates."[4(p3)]

Table 8-2 details the attrition rates for each service. Rates of graduation from basic training of less than 100% are a problem not only for the recruits who fail to graduate but also for the military itself. It is expensive to recruit individuals, qualify them medically for basic training, transport them to basic training sites, pay them, clothe them, house them, feed them (all of this even while those who have failed await separation), and then transport them home. In 1994, there was an overall service attrition rate of 10.47% for recruits separated in the first 2 months

TABLE 8-2

RECRUIT ATTRITION IN THE FOUR SERVICES, 1995

Service	Males			Females		
	Entering	Graduating	Graduating (%)	Entering	Graduating	Graduating (%)
Air Force	27,300	24,570	90	7,700	6,930	90
Army	68,612	63,235	92	16,187	14,015	86
Marine Corps	30,535	26,367	86	1,952	1,523	78
Navy	36,784	31,744	86	9,246	6,886	74

Source: Preventive Medicine representatives in the four services

of service, with an average investment in each separated recruit estimated to be approximately $12,320. This cost the services over $230 million in 1994.[5] Many of these recruits are separated for preexisting medical conditions. In the era of voluntary enlistment, applicants who wish to join the service have an incentive to conceal medical conditions that may be disqualifying. Others are separated because they fail to meet minimum performance criteria (eg, failing physical training or weight standards), failing inspections, or failing to adapt otherwise to basic training. Recruits who are in good physical shape have a greater chance of meeting overall military performance standards. Those who struggle to meet physical standards often lose their motivation, both mental and physical, to meet other military requirements. Recruits are better prepared to succeed in basic training and are expected to have fewer injuries during training if recruiters have fully informed them of the physical fitness standards required and encouraged them to obtain those standards before reporting to basic training camps.

TRAINING ENVIRONMENT

Air Force

Air Force basic training occurs at one site: Lackland Air Force Base in San Antonio, Tex. Recruits complete a 30-day curriculum, which is spread over 6 weeks. Before training starts, recruits spend an average of 2 days on administrative inprocessing. They live in open-bay dormitories that routinely house 55 to 58 recruits (a maximum of 60) per bay. There are 20 separate bays per building, and each building regularly houses between 800 and 1,000 recruits. Recruits live, eat, and train together as a flight, which is about 55 recruits strong and is same-sex. Each large building has its own dining hall, academic classrooms, staff office complex, laundry room, small dispensary, and small post office. In addition to time spent in the classroom, a major portion of the training—notably, uniform and dormitory maintenance and inspections—occurs in the open-bay dormitories and adjacent dayrooms. Other activities, such as marksmanship, the Confidence Course, drill, physical conditioning, and ceremonies, are held outdoors year round.

In the Air Force, daily showers are mandatory, and antibacterial soap is provided. Dormitory cleanliness is strictly enforced, with laundry done at least twice a week and bed linens changed once a week. Recruits arrange their beds head-to-foot so that the transmission of airborne diseases while they sleep is reduced. Foot care is stressed, with special attention given to the prevention of blisters. Knowing that recruits prefer to sleep with their socks on (to save dressing time in the morning), there is a written policy that prohibits this practice, thus allowing feet to dry overnight. The recruits carry canteens at all times, and instructors encourage them to drink often and so reduce the cases of dehydration from training. Sports drink is available in the dining halls to add electrolytes to their diet and further aid in hydration. Every meal features low-fat, low-cholesterol menu items that recruits may choose. Using tobacco products and drinking alcohol is prohibited (24 hours a day, 7 days a week) during the program. Recruits undergo specific training designed to keep them from starting to smoke or from returning to this habit.[6,7]

Army

As of 1996, recruits are trained at six Army basic training centers (ie, Fort Benning, Ga; Fort Jackson, SC; Fort Knox, Ky; Fort Leonard Wood, Mo; Fort McClellan, Ala; Fort Sill, Ok) for 8 weeks. The traditional unit of housing is the barracks. The maximum number of recruits in a barracks area depends on the configuration of the building, but a minimum of 72 square feet is required per recruit to limit the spread of communicable diseases.[8,9] This space allocation does not include stairs, halls, latrines, utility rooms, recreation areas, storage rooms, or administrative areas. This square-footage rule also applies to temporary facilities and tents. Some post commanders, however, have obtained waivers that reduce the minimum to 62 square feet per recruit. In these cases, barracks are inspected every 6 months and the waiver renewed if the barracks passes the inspection.[10] Commanders must ensure that scheduling of common-use facilities, such as dining facilities, classrooms, theaters, and latrines, avoids overcrowding. Heating and ventilation in troop barracks is controlled for both health and comfort reasons.

Since 1994, the Army has emphasized sex integration. There is a 25% to 75% optimum ratio of females to males in each company of 60 recruits, and the companies are integrated down to and including the squad level, which consists of 8 recruits. Buddy teams are same-sex to facilitate the conduct of hand-to-hand and bayonet training. Both sexes must meet the same standards for order, discipline, health, welfare, and morale. Males and females are required to maintain high but different standards for physical training; road marches are integrated.

Marine Corps

Marine Corps recruits are trained for 11 weeks, with the first week consisting of induction time, at recruit depots in San Diego, Calif, and Parris Island, SC. The recruit depots attempt to maintain uniform training and administration except where differences in mission, geography, climate, or facilities require variations. All recruits are housed in open-squad bays in platoons (65 recruits per platoon). The length of the training day does not normally exceed 10 hours. This does not include routine time allotted for personal hygiene, barracks maintenance and cleaning, devotional services, and meals. Recruits are given at least 20 minutes to eat each meal. Recruits are permitted 8 hours of uninterrupted sleep, 1 hour of uninterrupted free time each day except when in the field, and 4 hours of free time on Sundays and holidays. Visits are allowed but only

during specified times established by the post commanders.[11,12] Males and females are trained separately.

Navy

US Navy recruits complete a 9.5-week training cycle at the Navy boot camp at Great Lakes Naval Training Center, Great Lakes, Ill. Recruits live in open-bay barracks with a maximum capacity of 88 recruits. Only one sex occupies a bay. Bathroom facilities are also open-bay style. Bed linens are changed weekly. Showers are required once daily. Shoes or shower flip-flops are required to be worn at all times except when in bunks. The recruits do everything as a large group: they eat together, shower at the same time, and sit in class together. They can march up to 25 miles a week traveling across the base to go to classes and meals. Field training for the Navy consists of fire fighting, weapons firing, and line handling training, all of which are conducted indoors. During the warmer weather months, physical training is held outdoors.[13]

INSTRUCTORS

Key leadership personnel in military basic training camps are the drill instructors. Besides the military recruiter, these are often the first military role models that the recruits have. Drill instructors hold at least at the rank of E-5, have usually been recommended by their commanders for training as drill instructors, and must have no disciplinary actions against them. The length of drill instructor training is roughly equivalent to the length of basic training for each service and consists of topics the drill instructors will be teaching the recruits plus effective teaching techniques. Their training includes such topics as leadership, stress management, counseling, fitness training, weapons training, drill and ceremony, wearing of the uniform, administrative issues, safety issues, equal opportunity issues, and integration of men and women. Drill instructors face a rigorous work schedule; days can last from 3:30 AM to 8:00 PM. The usual length of an assignment as a drill instructor is 2 to 3 years.[14]

All leaders who are associated with recruit training must ensure that training is conducted in a professional manner. Hazing, maltreatment, abuse of authority, or other illegal alternatives to leadership are counterproductive practices and are expressly forbidden. Instructors are strictly charged to treat all recruits firmly, fairly, and with dignity and are

held accountable for their actions. Instructors are trained to be constantly alert for recruits who have physical or other difficulties and are taught to question recruits demonstrating injury, illness, or other maladies regarding the nature of the problem. Safety is of the utmost importance in basic training and the priority of all instructors. Instructors who are not in the military attend training courses on how to train recruits in a military fashion and are certified annually. The selection, training, and supervision of drill instructors and civilian instructors have been improved; among other innovations, instructors now attend detailed training on sexual harassment issues and how to train recruits to respond if sexual harassment occurs.

With the integration of women into military units, the issues of sexual harassment and sex bias have needed to be addressed. As an organization, the military has several risk factors for sexual harassment. The traditional masculine identity and horizontal and vertical cohesion in military units may foster counterproductive attitudes toward women. In addition, several highly publicized allegations of sexual harassment (such as the Navy's "Tailhook" scandal in 1991 and the rape and sexual assault trials at Aberdeen Proving Ground, Md, and several other Army posts in late 1996 and early 1997) have focused the public's attention on this issue.

The Department of Defense has defined sexual harassment as "a form of sex discrimination that involves unwelcome sexual advances, requests for sexual favors, and other verbal or physical conduct of a sexual nature when (1) submission to such conduct is made either explicitly or implicitly a term or condition of a person's job, pay or career, or (2) submission to or rejection of such conduct by a person is used as a basis for career or employment decisions affecting that person, or (3) such conduct has the purpose or effect of unreasonably interfering with an individual's work performance or creates an intimidating, hostile or offensive working environment."[15] Program guidelines have been provided that

- outline training requirements for each unit and how these training methods will be evaluated to make sure they are working,
- explain how individuals who feel they have been subjected to sexual harassment may seek redress,
- prohibit reprisals against individuals because of their complaints,
- establish procedures to investigate these complaints,
- establish toll-free advice and counseling hotlines to provide information on sexual harassment, and
- inform military and civilian personnel that failure to comply with established policies may be reflected in negative annual performance ratings and could result in adverse administrative, disciplinary, or legal action.[15]

Air Force

Air Force military training instructors' demographics generally parallel that of their students; in 1998, out of a total of 307 training instructors, 15.6% were female. The training instructors represent virtually every Air Force specialty. All enlisted staff complete a 5-week instructor course, plus on-the-job training that spans an additional 14 weeks at Lackland Air Force Base.

Army

In 1995, US Army drill instructors numbered approximately 2,200, or 1 drill instructor for every 40 recruits, with 10% being female. Drill instructor training takes 8 weeks and is conducted at Fort Jackson, Fort Leonard Wood, and Fort Benning.

Navy

US Navy instructors are all petty officers (E-5 and above) and 16% are female. Six hundred seventy instructors were needed in 1998, and they were all trained for 8 weeks at the Navy Instructor Training and Recruit Division Commander "C" School at Great Lakes Naval Training Center.

Marine Corps

Each year, there are approximately 270 Marine Corps male and female drill instructors at either Parris Island (males and females) or San Diego (males). Drill instructor school is 8 weeks long, and approximately 20% of instructors are female. Drill instructors are selected from throughout the Marine Corps and encompass a cross-section of military occupational specialties.

ENTRANCE PROCESSING

Basic training begins at the reception battalion, where the recruit is brought under military control, completes entry processing, and begins the basic training process. This initial indoctrination from civilian to military life includes a "moment of truth." For example, in the Air Force's version of the "moment of truth," all recruits receive a "shakedown inspection" in their dormitories within 24 hours of arrival. The staff removes all nonprescription drugs, weapons, valuable items, pornography, tobacco, and other contraband from the recruits for the duration of basic training. Any illegal items are disposed of and the rest is returned to the recruit upon departure. All services have similar procedures. During the rest of entrance processing, hair is cut if needed, and military uniforms are issued along with name plates and identification tags ("dog tags"). Recruits are fitted for gas masks and helmets. Eyeglasses are issued if needed and hearing protection provided. Identification cards are provided, and all the paperwork needed to bring the recruit and his or her family into the military system is begun.

Screening

Medical screening is a significant part of entrance processing in basic training camps, although past medical records are not required. Recruits have already undergone and passed physical examinations for induction at military entrance processing stations, but when they arrive at the training site, they must be in good health and meet the required height and weight standards. To be eligible for military service, individuals are screened to ensure they have no acute diseases or physical impairments to training (see Chapter 7, Evolution of Military Recruit Accession Standards).[16] Recruits are not subjected to any form of physical conditioning, swimming, running, or unnecessary stress before receiving a medical examination. Blood group and type are determined.[17] This information is recorded in the medical records, on the military identification card, and on the dog tags the recruits are given, but the prevalence of errors in one or all of these has been estimated to be more than 10%.[18] Immunizations are given and tuberculosis skin tests are placed.[19] Female trainees are tested for pregnancy with urine tests at the entrance processing stations and again with serological tests at basic training; some installations also screen for rubella. Human immunodeficiency virus (HIV) screening is repeated for recruits whose preaccession test is more than 6 months old.[20] Medical records from the Military Entrance Processing Stations are screened for

incomplete physical examinations and deficiencies. Recruits with possibly disqualifying medical conditions discovered at this point will be evaluated and a decision made about granting them a waiver. Recruits with hearing or vision deficiencies are re-evaluated. Dental panographic x-rays for identification are performed.[16,21]

Immunizations

All accessions receive immunizations early during their processing for basic training (Table 8-3).[19] These immunization policies are coordinated by all the services, which often rely on counsel from the Armed Forces Epidemiological Board. Female recruits are tested for pregnancy before being shipped to basic training and are again tested after arrival and before receiving live virus vaccines. If the woman is not pregnant, all immunizations are given, along with precautions not to become pregnant for 3 months after the live-virus vaccines are administered. These include influenza, polio (inactivated), measles, tetanus-diphtheria, and rubella vaccinations. Recruits also have at times received immunizations against adenovirus types 4 and 7 and meningococcal meningitis. Additionally, Navy and Marine Corps recruits receive the mumps immunization year round.[19] As of January

TABLE 8-3

VACCINATIONS GIVEN TO MILITARY RECRUITS

Immunizing Agent	Air Force	Army	Marine Corps	Navy
Adenovirus (types 4, 7)*	—	x	x	x
Anthrax	†	†	†	†
Hepatitis A	x	†	x	x
Influenza	x	x	x	x
Measles‡	x	x	x	x
Meningococcal meningitis (A, C, Y, W135)	x	x	x	x
Mumps	—	—	x	x
Polio (inactivated polio vaccine, eIPV)	x	x	x	x
Rubella‡	x	x	x	x
Tetanus-diphtheria	x	x	x	x
Varicella	§	§	§	§

x: to be given
*Due to an interruption in the manufacture of this vaccine, no service is administering adenovirus vaccine at publication time.
†First priority is servicemembers deployed to high-risk areas, then other active servicemembers, then recruits
‡Services have the option of immunizing only seronegative recruits (based on testing)
§First recruits are screened, then susceptibles are vaccinated

1999, hepatitis A vaccine is given to Air Force, Marine Corps, and Navy recruits only. Varicella immunization policy differs among the services, and the Army is considering changing its policy of not administering this vaccine to any recruits. Anthrax vaccine has been instituted by all services for universal immunization but in phases based on priority; it will eventually be given to recruits.

The adenovirus vaccine has only been used by the military, specifically the Army, the Navy, and the Marines; the Air Force trains in a mild climate where adenovirus outbreaks may be less likely. Air Force recruits receive adenovirus vaccination only when there is evidence of active disease transmission. (At the time of publication, adenovirus vaccine production has been terminated by the manufacturer; a new source of vaccine remains to be found.) Adenovirus vaccine is ideally given year round. In years when the vaccine has been in short supply, however, stocks have been stretched by administering it only during the cold-weather months, when the virus is most prevalent. Any adenovirus outbreak must be investigated to ensure

that it is caused by adenovirus and not a more serious agent, such as group A streptococci.[22] In installations where high rates of respiratory virus infections have been identified, prophylaxis may be initiated against such streptococcal outbreaks with bicillin or erythromycin.

A device developed and used by the military since the 1950s to facilitate mass immunization is the jet injector gun. It uses compressed air to aerosolize vaccines and imbed the vaccine particles in the subcutaneous tissue or muscle. Personnel can be vaccinated at a rate of nearly 1,000 an hour. It is simpler, faster, and more economical than the classic method using a needle and syringe. Even though in 1988 the Armed Forces Epidemiological Board found that there was only a very small risk of transmitting hepatitis B or HIV from one vaccinee to the next if the guns were used and maintained correctly by trained technicians,[23] the issue of jet gun safety and maintenance was reconsidered by the Board in 1997. They concurred with the Department of Defense's decision to discontinue use of the jet gun except during public health emergencies.

CURRICULUM

Each service has unique training requirements, but all have classroom, field, and physical fitness components. The information taught during basic training is extensive because it must prepare civilians for their career as military servicemembers. Each service has specific curriculum requirements prescribed to the half hour for each academic topic to be covered. A general overview of each curriculum follows, and Table 8-4 holds a breakdown of broad topic areas.

Air Force

During the 6-week basic training course in the Air Force, topics such as uniform wear, weapons training, the history and mission of the Air Force, military codes of conduct, and health topics (eg, sexually transmitted disease prevention, substance abuse control, stress management) are taught. In addition to classroom training, drill takes place on

TABLE 8-4

HOURS (AND PERCENTAGE OF TOTAL TIME) SPENT BY RECRUITS IN VARIOUS SUBJECTS[*]

Topics	Army	Navy	Air Force	Marines
Military Subjects[†]	80 (26)	95 (66)	66 (30)	137 (31)
First Aid	18 (6)	NA	6 (3)	12 (3)
Military Training[‡]	81 (27)	38 (27)	113 (51)	98 (21)
Physical Training	47 (16)	NA	26 (12)	65 (14)
Weapons Training	78 (26)	11 (8)	10 (5)	145 (32)
Duration	8 wk	9.5 wk	6 wk	11 wk

NA: not applicable
[*]Based on the author's grouping of subjects into general categories
[†] Military subjects include service-specific missions, history, customs and courtesy, and code of conduct
[‡] Military training includes subjects such as base and barracks maintenance, drills, and service-specific missions

large asphalt pads adjacent to the dormitories. Recruits are detailed to perform groundskeeping tasks and basic maintenance of common areas within and around dormitories, plus familiar activities like "kitchen patrol," litter patrol, painting, and messenger service. Recruits wear necessary protective gear for these details, such as gloves, goggles, steel-tipped boots, ear protection, and coveralls.

Additionally, there are 4 hours of academic classes that teach recruits about principles of fitness and exercise. Recruits must complete a 2-mile run by the end of training in less than 18 minutes for males and 20 minutes 30 seconds for females. To prepare for this, recruits run in fitness ability groups on base roads for an average of 3 days per week and 25 minutes per session. Recruits also receive conditioning for the upper body, doing a series of strengthening exercises after each run. Recruits participate in a 21-obstacle "confidence" course. They do not run the course for time. The goal is to overcome each obstacle, meet the challenges, and gain confidence. Key commanders and staff meet monthly with the Preventive Medicine Group, an assemblage of health care professionals who advise the training cadre. The group's areas of expertise include preventive medicine, occupational medicine, orthopedics, public health, health promotion, nutrition, podiatry, sports medicine, and psychology. Together, the group members identify problems, identify opportunities for intervention, and work with the training staff to implement the most promising interventions.

Army

In addition to training in such subjects as use and care of weapons, military history, and military codes of conduct, recruits receive significant training in health and medical topics. As soldiers spend significant amounts of time in the field, recruits are trained to understand their increased susceptibility to disease and infection under field conditions. Individuals perform field sanitation duties, and foot and body hygiene practices are stressed. Recruits are trained in first aid so they can appreciate the significance of and provide prompt, effective first aid in the field. Each recruit is taught the skills needed to evaluate a casualty, basic cardiopulmonary resuscitation, how to treat burns, how to prevent bleeding and shock, and how to splint fractures. Training in how to transport a casualty is also stressed, as this is critical to the Army's mission in the field. An introduction is given to nuclear, biological, and chemical weapons, all military occupational hazards. Because recruits are exposed to the elements during field training exercises, preventive medicine topics, such as prevention and first aid for heat and cold injuries, are stressed. Personal protection measures against biting insects are emphasized and practiced.

Among the fitness topics taught are weight control, diet and nutrition, smoking cessation, control of substance abuse, and stress management. Personal health training includes the understanding of how to use the Army system of health care and preventive medicine and the importance of immunizations, self-examination for cancer, and hearing conservation. Infection with HIV is medically disqualifying for entry into military service, and HIV testing is done at regular intervals for soldiers. Therefore, a great deal of time is spent in basic training educating servicemembers about HIV. The difference between HIV infection and acquired immune deficiency syndrome is explained, methods of transmission of the virus and risk factors for HIV infection are discussed, and protective mechanisms that will reduce the risk of HIV transmission are emphasized. Recruits are well trained in what to expect if they acquire HIV, which includes counseling, medical care provided, changes in their status in the Army, and assignment restrictions.

Physical fitness has a direct impact on combat readiness, and physically fit recruits are assets to the Army. The Army emphasizes that exercise must be performed regularly to provide a training effect, and the intensity of exercise must gradually increase to improve the components of fitness. The physical fitness training program in basic training helps recruits make the transition from what can be a sedentary civilian life to a physically demanding military life. Recruits arrive at various levels of physical fitness and physical skill levels. While women are able to participate in the same program as males, often they must work harder to perform at the same level. Using ability groups for running, for example, alleviates this situation.

Special training is considered for recruits who fail to progress at the same rate as the unit or group.[24] Commanders are responsible for monitoring physical training to ensure training injuries are kept to an acceptable level and to monitor for overtraining, which can result in rhabdomyolysis. Recruits are encouraged to report excessively dark urine and excessive muscle pain, both symptoms of this condition.[10]

Installation commanders ensure that close working relationships develop among the training battalions, the supporting medical treatment facility, and their community mental health, preventive medicine, and occupational medicine activities. These activities can be especially helpful to unit commanders in establishing an effective heat and cold injury prevention program and health promotion program in basic training.

Marine Corps

The first week of recruit training is the induction into the Marine Corps, during which recruits receive medical and dental examinations, take aptitude confirmation tests, receive their initial issue of clothing and equipment, and are assembled into companies, series, and platoons. For the next 3 weeks of training, recruits concentrate on physical conditioning, academics, and close-order drill. Physical training (PT) is varied and progressive, with 64.5 hours spent in PT. Males are trained in close combat and bayonet fighting, as well as unarmed combat through hitting skills instruction and boxing matches. Female recruits do not receive training in these areas but focus on self-defense skills against armed and unarmed opponents. Additionally, combat water survival training is provided for both sexes, along with day and night navigation, hand and arm signals, camouflage, escape and evasion, and enemy vehicle recognition. Classroom instruction includes Marine Corps history, general military subjects, and first aid.

The next 2 weeks of recruit training concentrates on basic marksmanship with the M-16A2 service rifle. Recruits spend 1 week learning marksmanship fundamentals in the classroom and dry firing (grass drills). The following week is spent on live fire and culminates with initial rifle qualification.

After rifle qualification, the recruits spend a week performing either mess or maintenance duty. This supports the functioning of the basic training camp and gives the recruits a chance to work under the supervision of higher ranking recruits and not their drill instructors. This week also provides the opportunity to retrain recruits who experienced difficulty with either water survival or rifle qualification. They receive extra training and are given additional opportunities to qualify.

Recruits demonstrate mastery by successfully negotiating the obstacle and confidence course, completing a 10-mile march, and passing the PT test. Females run a slightly shorter distance and face different obstacles on the confidence course, which is designed to accommodate the height and upper body strength of women. To graduate, all recruits must pass the PT test and the combat water survival test, qualify with the rifle, pass the battalion

commander's inspection, and achieve mastery of the individual military subjects and combat basic tasks. If the recruit fails a graduation requirement, he or she will be recycled through training and given another opportunity to pass. The Crucible, a 48-hour field training exercise emphasizing teamwork and core values, is the climax of Marine Corps training.

Navy

Navy basic training addresses hazards unique to shipboard service. Training covers areas such as fundamental principles of amphibious operations, recognition of naval vessels, military seamanship, shipboard weapons, and damage control aboard ship. In addition, recruits receive classroom education in the medical areas of first aid, heat and cold injuries, health, pregnancy and parenting, and sexually transmitted disease. Instructors teach recruits to develop lifestyle habits that ensure health and to recognize the impact of health on quality of life and unit readiness.

All recruits are required to pass the Navy's physical fitness test before graduating. When recruits arrive, they are allowed 1 week to adjust to the new environment before starting their physical fitness training. They will take two physical fitness tests while at basic training. The first is a slower paced test to allow for assessment of individual abilities and weaknesses; the second test is for the record. Recruits who fail the second test are held at basic training for further physical training. Recruits are also required to pass the swim test. In the swim test, a recruit wearing the fatigue uniform without boots jumps from an 8- to 15-foot platform into deep water and treads water for 2 minutes. This is followed by 2 minutes of drown proofing, in which the recruit must perform blouse flotation (ie, filling the fatigue shirt with air so it can be used as a life preserver), before finishing with a 25-meter swim. By the end of basic training, the recruit must also become at least a third class swimmer, which consists of entering the water from a height of at least 5 feet, swimming 50 yards using any stroke, and using the water survival prone float for at least 5 minutes.[25] All recruits must meet the same standards with regard to academics, military drill, inspections, and the swim test. Physical fitness testing standards differ, however, for female and male recruits.

Since the Navy trains all recruits at one training site, they have a very well-prescribed PT program that is followed year round by all recruits. This consists of three modules: aerobic conditioning, muscle strength and endurance training, and low-intensity training and exercise (LITE); this is in addition to the 20 to 25 miles per week a typical recruit will walk in routine movements between training sites. Each module contains exercise routines that are time-efficient, are easy to perform, require no special equipment, and are modifiable to indoor, outdoor, and shipboard environments. General guidelines for the frequency and sequence of the modules throughout the Navy's basic training cycle include (*a*) two to three sessions per week of aerobic training on nonconsecutive days, (*b*) two to three sessions per week of muscle strength and endurance training on non-consecutive days, (*c*) LITE training during the 1 to 2 days preceding the physical readiness tests, and (*d*) a maximum of five scheduled exercise sessions per week with warm-up and cool-down periods for each session.[26]

PSYCHOLOGICAL ASPECTS OF BASIC TRAINING

Stress management is an essential aspect of basic training. Some stress is necessary to prepare recruits to operate effectively in the high-anxiety conditions of combat. Leaders must ensure, however, that the only stress placed on recruits is that which results from the recruit's performance of tasks. The stress created within a recruit by performance of a new or dangerous task is essential for motivation and learning. Stress should be positive and oriented toward attainable goals. Anxiety created by physical or verbal abuse is nonproductive and prohibited; stress should exist between the recruit and the task to be accomplished, not between the recruit and the instructors. Unwanted or unnecessary stress is harmful because it impairs performance and interferes with training. Stress management training for recruits identifies causes and effects of stress, teaches recruits to cope with stress, and provides information on ways to seek treatment for stress if needed.

For minor cases of anxiety and depression, recruits generally rely on the chaplains for counseling and guidance. Chaplains are especially crucial in counseling and responding to a recruit's experiences of sexual harassment, as they are often the only safety net a recruit will have. When a recruit becomes unable to handle stress, there are usually manifestations in his or her performance that clearly indicate that something is wrong. At this point, the recruit is referred to the installation mental health clinic, where diagnostic tests may be administered to ascertain the scope and degree of the underlying problem before deciding on a course of action. In many cases, short-term treatment will teach the recruit sufficient coping skills to deal with the specific stressor, allowing the recruit to graduate on time. In other cases, further training will only exacerbate the stress reaction, so the recruit is recommended for discharge and removed from training until the administrative action is complete.

On occasion, the anxiety of basic training becomes too intense for certain recruits and suicide may become an issue. Commanders and instructors teach their recruits suicide prevention techniques. Recruits are told to notify their chain of command if they become aware of someone who is contemplating suicide. Instructors watch for signs from recruits who may be depressed, lonely, despondent, or excessively stressed. Commanders counsel recruits who are reported to have discussed or alluded to suicide. The commander must refer any recruits suspected of contemplating suicide to mental health personnel for evaluation and counseling. Since recruits are supervised 24 hours a day, actual suicide attempts are rare, and successful suicides are exceedingly rare. If a recruit is genuinely suicidal, psychological care will begin immediately. Once the recruit is safely beyond the crisis, he or she will be discharged from the service and referred to a Department of Veterans Affairs hospital for follow-up treatment.

GRADUATION CRITERIA

All services have similar graduation criteria. All require recruits to pass the physical fitness tests, albeit with slightly different criteria and testing methods for each service. All recruits must pass basic field training skills, which are unique to each service. All must qualify with the service rifle, and all must pass inspections of different scope for each service. If a recruit fails to master any graduation requirement, he or she must be recycled through a phase of training or undergo additional instruction to correct the deficiency. Every attempt is made to allow recruits to master the required skill and graduate. When attempts to bring deficient recruits to satisfactory levels of knowledge, conditioning, behavior, discipline, or skill have failed, separation of the recruit from the service may be necessary. Usually the services will allow no more than 3 weeks of remedial training to pass the required training modules. On the other end of the recruit spectrum, commanders are encouraged to meritoriously promote recruits who have consistently demonstrated superior performance in the areas of

physical fitness, marksmanship, leadership, motivation, and academics.

SUMMARY

Basic training builds the essential foundation for military servicemembers in their new careers. The skills and indoctrination to military service obtained during basic training can be crucial to the servicemember's ability to defend his or her country. Essential aspects of basic training include teaching good health habits and avoidance of injury in an environment that is conducive to disease transmission and injury. Illness or injury distract a servicemember from the mission and reduce work

performance. To minimize this source of potential mission failure, recruits need to be trained to regard their health as being of equal importance to that of a properly functioning weapon. Recruits must be taught to value protective health measures, devices, and services. Failure to comply with health regulations results in casualties, which the commander cannot afford. There is no time in a recruit's career when sound health habits can be more successfully instilled than during basic training.

REFERENCES

1. Induction Statistics, Selective Services System, 1997. (www.sss.gov/induct.htm)

2. Pappa M. Personal Communication, 1996.

3. AMSARA, Accession Medical Standards Analysis and Research Activity, Walter Reed Army Institute of Research, Silver Spring, MD.

4. General Accounting Office. *Military Attrition: DoD Needs to Better Understand Reasons for Separation and Improve Recruiting Systems*. Washington, DC: GAO; 1998. GAO/T-NSIAD-90-109.

5. General Accounting Office. *Military Attrition: DoD Could Save Millions by Better Screening Enlisted Personnel*. Washington, DC: GAO; 1997. GAO/NSAID-97-39.

6. US Department of the Air Force. *Basic Military Training. Manual I (Military Training)*. Lackland Air Force Base, Tex: 37th Training Wing, 737th Training Group, DAF; May 1995.

7. US Department of the Air Force. *Basic Military Training. Manual I (Military Studies)*. Lackland Air Force Base, Tex: 37th Training Wing, 737th Training Group, DAF; June 1995.

8. US Department of the Army. *Preventive Medicine*. Washington, DC: DA; October 1990. Army Regulation 40-5.

9. Brodkey C, Gaydos JC. United States Army guidelines for troop living space: a historical review. *Mil Med*. 1980;145:418–421.

10. Yackovich A. Personal Communication, 1997.

11. Headquarters, United States Marine Corps. *Recruit Training*. Washington, DC: US Marine Corps; 25 March 1991. Marine Corps Order 1510.32B.

12. Marine Corps Combat Development Command. *Marine Corps Recruit Training*. Quantico, Va: United States Marine Corps; 4 November 1994. Point Paper C462 G.

13. US Navy Recruit Training Command. *1995 Command History*. Great Lakes, Ill: Dept of the Navy; 1996.

14. Mellendez MSG. Personal Communication, 1997.

15. The Office of the Secretary of Defense. *Prohibition of Sexual Harassment in the Department of Defense*. Washington, DC: The Chairman of the Joint Chiefs of Staff, the Inspector General of the Department of Defense, the Director of Administration and Management, the Directors of the Defense Agencies; 22 August 1994. Memorandum to the Secretaries of the Military Departments.

16. US Department of Defense. *Physical Standards for Enlistment, Appointment, and Induction.* Washington, DC: DoD; 31 March 1986. DoD Directive 6130.3.

17. US Department of the Army. *Medical, Dental and Veterinary Care.* Washington, DC: DA; 15 February 1985. Army Regulation 40-3.

18. Gaydos JC, Cowan DN, Polk AJ, et al. Blood typing errors on US Army identification cards and tags. *Mil Med.* 1988;153:618–620.

19. Headquarters, Departments of the Army, the Navy, the Air Force, and Transportation. *Immunizations and Chemoprophylaxis.* Washington, DC: DA, DN, DAF, DT; 1 November 1995. Air Force Joint Instruction 48-110, Army Regulation 40-562, BUMEDINST 6230.15, CG COMDTINST M6230.4E.

20. US Department of the Army. *Identification, Surveillance and Administrative of Personnel Infected with HIV.* Washington, DC: DA; 11 March 1988. Army Regulation 600-110.

21. US Department of the Army. *Process, Control and Distribution of Personnel at US Army Reception Battalion and Training Centers.* Washington, DC: DA; 24 April 1987. Army Regulation 612-201.

22. Shortage of adenovirus vaccine could precipitate outbreaks among trainees. *US Med.* 1997;33(February):1,19.

23. Armed Forces Epidemiological Board. *Recommendation on the Utilization of Hypodermic Jet Injector Guns for the Immunization of Military Personnel.* Washington, DC: AFEB; 7 March 1988. Memorandum to the Assistant Secretary of Defense (Health Affairs).

24. Headquarters, US Department of the Army. *Physical Fitness Training.* Washington, DC: DA: August 1985. Army Field Manual 21-20.

25. Schaffer R. Personal Communication, 1997.

26. US Naval Training Center, Great Lakes. *Physical Training Program 1996.* Great Lakes, Ill: US Naval Training Center; 1996.

Chapter 9

COMMUNICABLE DISEASE CONTROL IN BASIC TRAINING: PROGRAMMATIC ASPECTS

JEFFREY D. GUNZENHAUSER, MD, MPH

J. D. Gunzenhauser; Colonel, Medical Corps, US Army; Preventive Medicine Staff Officer, Office of the Surgeon General, 5109 Leesburg Pike, Suite 684, Falls Church, VA 22041

INTRODUCTION

The control of communicable disease in basic training or boot camp represents one of the greatest achievements of military medicine. The magnitude of this accomplishment is difficult to comprehend without first-hand experience of camp-based epidemics or extensive study of the lessons of medical history. This chapter provides a brief outline of the fascinating story of how this achievement has been accomplished. The technological tools and administrative controls that exist at basic training centers today combine to form an efficient, elegant approach to safeguarding the health of military recruits. An appropriate regard for time-worn lessons is the proper starting point for future efforts to raise health status. This chapter will highlight those lessons so that future efforts to minimize the threat of communicable disease to basic training populations can be successful.

Outbreaks of communicable disease at basic training installations have riveted the nation's attention. Not simply another national news item, these incidents have brought terror into the hearts of Americans. Typhoid fever during the Spanish-American War, influenza during World War I, scarlet and rheumatic fever during World War II, and meningococcal disease during the Vietnam War—these are a few notorious examples. The absence of significant outbreaks during the past 15 years is evidence of the success of control programs.

The control of communicable diseases in basic training is important for many reasons. Among these is the value of health maintenance to the individual recruit and the benefit of his or her optimal health to the initial training effort. [Note: rather than referring to "basic trainees," "airmen basic," or "soldiers, sailors, airmen, and marines," "recruit"

will be used to describe a new members of any of the four services.] The value of sustained health to the individual trainee is paralleled by the tremendous savings accrued by the military services through avoidance of retraining and additional recruitment. Another important reason for disease control is to minimize the potential of communicable disease spread to civilian populations. This is a major public health issue, as well as an item of political interest. Such concern resulted in the suspension of basic training at Fort Ord, Calif, in 1964.[1] Likewise, concern about community spread of measles and rubella was an important factor that led to routine recruit immunization against these infections.[2] On a grander scale, the National Immunization Program of 1976, which aimed to vaccinate all Americans against swine influenza, was initiated following an outbreak in Army basic trainees at Fort Dix, NJ.[3] Communicable disease control also enables military personnel to progress rapidly to more advanced training and immediate deployment, if necessary. Influenza outbreaks during World War I ravaged the health of large cohorts of soldiers who were scheduled to deploy to the front lines; this resulted in a need to reorganize and reconstitute units.[4] An ability to train and rapidly deploy large numbers of military personnel may be critical in future military campaigns. A final reason to minimize disease among training populations is to enable the service medical departments to be as efficient as possible in providing health service support to deployed forces: healthy trainees need fewer medical resources, resources that can be used by those on the front lines. These reasons underscore the importance of communicable disease control in recruit populations.

A PERSPECTIVE ON THE CONTROL OF COMMUNICABLE DISEASE

Programmatic aspects of communicable disease control are best viewed in terms of modes of transmission.[5,6] This viewpoint contrasts with the traditional medical curriculum, which normally assumes the perspective of agent taxonomy or organ system involvement. The major modes of disease transmission are the airborne, direct-contact, waterborne, foodborne, vector-borne, blood-borne, and sexual contact routes. Since the last two categories do not pose a substantial risk to today's basic trainee populations, they will not be discussed here. Exhibit 9-1 lists the major modes of transmission and their associated agents of communicable disease. All these

modes of transmission have played a major role in epidemics at basic training installations. A few examples will highlight the breadth of this spectrum.

In 1898, typhoid fever epidemics at numerous camps in the United States severely disrupted the operational ability of many commands during the Spanish–American War. Nearly 100 regiments were affected, with an average of more than 200 cases per regiment and a case-fatality rate of 7.6%. The Reed-Vaughan-Shakespeare Typhoid Board determined that person-to-person transmission through direct contact, as well as fly-borne transmission, played a more important role in the outbreaks than

---

EXHIBIT 9-1

ROUTES OF TRANSMISSION AND THEIR ASSOCIATED AGENTS OF COMMUNICABLE DISEASES

Airborne

Mycobacterium tuberculosis

Neisseria meningiditis

Influenza viruses

Measles virus

Varicella-zoster virus

Other viruses

Direct Contact

Influenza virus

Adenovirus

Streptococcus pyogenes

Neisseria meningitidis

Cold viruses

Streptococcus pneumoniae

Mycoplasma pneumoniae

Chlamydia pneumoniae

Foodborne or Waterborne

Salmonella typhi

Hepatitis A virus

Salmonella species (non-*typhi*)

Agents of food poisoning

Shigella dysenteriae and other *Shigella* species

Vibrio cholerae

Campylobacter jejuni

Vector-borne

Yellow fever virus

Dengue viruses

Plasmodium species

Borrelia burgdorferi

Rickettsia rickettsii

Ehrlichia chafeensis

---

improvements in camp sanitation dramatically reduced its occurrence in subsequent mobilizations.[7]

Tuberculosis was a major health problem for the military during World War I. Thousands of soldiers were hospitalized and more than 2,000 died. Although a substantial effort was made to bar from enlistment all individuals with evidence of pre-existing infection, approximately 5,000 with unrecognized active disease and up to 15,000 with radiologically detectable tuberculous infection were accepted into service. The crowding of basic training afforded prime conditions for transmitting infection from active cases to other recruits and also contributed to the total morbidity and mortality of that period.[8] Roentgen examination instituted during World War II resulted in reduced tubercular disease rates during that war.[9]

Disease caused by *Streptococcus pyogenes* exacted a terrible toll on military forces during World War II. Coburn and Young estimated that 21,209 naval personnel developed rheumatic fever during the war;[10] 83% of cases occurred within the continental United States (ie, were associated with initial training). The comparable figures for the Army were 18,339 and 77%, respectively.[11] The highest rates of streptococcal disease incidence occurred at the naval training center at Farragut, Idaho, where 2.2% (2,084 cases) and 10.4% (9,589 cases) of military personnel, recruits and cadre were hospitalized with rheumatic fever and scarlet fever, respectively, from 1943 through 1945.[10] In the Army, the highest rates of rheumatic fever were reported at Fort Warren, Wyo, where approximately 5% of soldiers were hospitalized with rheumatic fever during 1943.[11] Shortly after the end of the war, studies in military populations demonstrated the effectiveness of penicillin in controlling these types of outbreaks.

These three examples demonstrate subtle, important aspects of the interrelatedness of disease control efforts. The threat of typhoid fever, which was so devastating during the Spanish-American War, was eventually eliminated by development of an effective vaccination program and by general improvements in sanitation. While the vaccination strategy was unique to the military population, the sanitary improvements were largely the by-product of improving sanitary conditions across the United States. The eventual reduction in tuberculosis incidence may also be attributed to general improvements in the health of the nation as a whole. Yet, while these general improvements in the larger society undoubtedly contributed to the reduced incidence of typhoid fever, they appear to have had no or little impact on the occurrence of tuberculosis during World War I, which was then still a universal in-

the waterborne route. The outbreaks were so severe that the US Congress responded after the war by appointing a commission to investigate. The Dodge Commission severely criticized both the Medical Department and the War Department, eventually leading to a reorganization of the Army. Compulsory vaccination against typhoid fever beginning in 1911 and

fection by the age of 20 and remained the nation's leading cause of death. Hence, the military relied on screening procedures to minimize the number of enlistees with active disease. Unfortunately, this approach was ineffective. In addition to the substantial improvements in the quality and completeness of tuberculosis screening procedures between the two world wars, improvements in nutrition and the standard of living in the United States also favorably affected the threat of this disease. But the same improvements in sanitary conditions that eliminated the threat of direct-contact transmission of typhoid fever during the Spanish-American War and helped minimize the tuberculosis problem did not prevent the transmission of *S pyogenes* during World War II. To this day, environmental control measures (ie, interventions that reduce exposure to the agent) have had little impact on communicable infections that are spread primarily through direct-contact or airborne modes of transmission. These few illustrations demonstrate the interrelationships of communicable disease control efforts in the military and the United States as a whole.

These examples also show several general but critical aspects of disease control. First, communicable disease outbreaks occur with greatest frequency and impact during periods of mobilization. Second, the highest attack rates occur in unseasoned personnel, especially those in the earliest weeks of initial training (ie, basic training, boot camp). Third, during the period of mobilization for a particular campaign (even one of several years' duration), there is not sufficient time to develop means to control large outbreaks of previously unrecognized communicable disease threats. And fourth, current capacities to prevent disease outbreaks involve many components and are based on lessons from earlier periods and benefits accrued from general improvements in the larger community. These aspects will be discussed in the sections that follow.

PREVENTIVE INTERVENTIONS RELATED TO MODE OF TRANSMISSION

Preventive interventions for communicable diseases may target environmental reservoirs, transmission of agents from reservoir to host, or aspects of the agent-host interaction. Interventions may be classified as agent-specific if they target a single microorganism or as agent-generic if they affect multiple organisms. Agent-generic interventions make up much of what has come to be known as the "sanitary revolution" of the late 19th and early 20th centuries and have had a tremendous impact on the health status of all Americans, including trainees. In addition, numerous agent-specific interventions constitute a major portion of current communicable disease control programs in basic training centers.

Exhibit 9-2 lists some of the interventions in use today. For each agent and for each mode of transmission, elimination of the reservoir and immunization of the host—the trainee—are possible approaches. Thus, eradication of smallpox and vaccination against typhoid fever largely eliminate the need to consider how those organisms are transmitted, at least within the basic training environment. Between reservoir elimination and host immunization, however, exists a range of strategies linked to the mode of transmission. Most of these intermediary strategies can be classified as either environmental sanitation, "vector" reduction, or barrier approaches.

In developing and reviewing control programs, depth must be emphasized. The goal in disease control is not merely to identify and implement one effective strategy; rather, it is to implement sufficient layers of prevention so an adequate safety net exists in case one approach fails. Multiple preventive layers should exist for each agent and for each mode of transmission.

Airborne

Airborne contagion is distinguished from direct-contact transmission in that the former involves infective organisms suspended in air while the latter involves either immediate contamination of susceptible hosts or secondary transmission by "vectors" (ie, fomites). Of course, infections transmissible through airborne contagion may also be transmitted by direct contact, but environmental or host factors normally dictate a predominant mode. The suspended, infective vehicle of airborne contagion is the "droplet nuclei." Particles with a diameter between 0.1 μm and 50 μm are capable of suspension in air; the lower limit on the size of droplet nuclei is limited by the size of the organism itself.[12] Larger nuclei (10 μm to 50 μm in diameter) will fall to the ground relatively quickly. A 10 μm nuclei, for example, will fall the height of a room in 17 minutes.[13]

When inhaled, most nuclei larger than 5 μm in diameter deposit in the upper respiratory tract, while smaller nuclei deposit primarily in the lower respiratory tract. The ability of infectious organisms to be transmitted via this route is a function of the organism's accessibility to sites in the infectious host where droplet formation occurs, the stability and size of suspended particles, and the ability of suspended

EXHIBIT 9-2

PRIMARY APPROACHES TO DISEASE CONTROL BY ROUTE OF TRANSMISSION

Universal Approaches
Reservoir elimination
Environmental sanitation
  Continuous
  Intermittent
Vector reduction*
Barriers
  Reservoir-proximate
  Host-proximate
Host immunization

Airborne
Quarantine
Agent removal
Agent inactivation
Agent dilution
Barriers
Host immunization

Direct Contact
Reservoir removal (quarantine)
Environmental sanitation
Personal hygiene
Personnel dispersion
Bunk spacing and orientation
Masks
Host immunization

Foodborne
Reservoir elimination
Agent removal (filtration)
Agent inactivation
Restriction of sources
Proper waste disposal
Host immunization

Waterborne
Reservoir elimination
Agent removal (filtration)
Agent inactivation
Restriction of sources
Proper waste disposal
Host immunization

Vector-borne
Reservoir elimination
Vector elimination
Barrier protections against the vector
Host immunization

* Including such "vectors" as fomites

organisms to remain viable over time. Bacteria, fungi, and human by-products that contain viruses (eg, products of coughing or sneezing, fibers, or fragments of desquamated skin) when expelled into the air form droplet nuclei. Slight drafts or other air disturbances help such nuclei remain suspended for indefinite periods of time.

Airborne infections are a significant threat to the health of basic trainees. Influenza, multidrug-resistant tuberculosis, and varicella are notable concerns. In spite of considerable efforts to develop interventions against all airborne infections, virtually all preventive efforts in place today are agent-specific. There has been, for example, considerable effort to assess the contribution of crowding to the incidence of airborne infections.[14,15] John Shaw Billings, a distinguished Army physician of the 19th century, felt so strongly about the relationship of crowding to airborne infections that he disseminated a circular, stating "every man should have his sixty feet of floor space as much as his ration."[14p419] Designing epidemiological studies to assess the impact of crowding on respiratory disease rates is challenging, though, because "crowding" is a time-variant variable that is difficult to measure and interacts with agent endemicity (ie, if the influenza virus is not present, no one will get the flu, no matter how crowded it is). Despite considerable investigative effort, only scant evidence exists that crowding contributes to respiratory disease rates. Nonetheless, in 1943 the US Army adopted a standard requiring 50 square feet of space for each recruit in reception centers.[14]

The role of ventilation on incident infections has also been the subject of considerable study. While evidence exists that shows that ventilation pathways are associated with observed patterns of disease,[16–18] it is less clear to what extent variations in ventilation flow or in the amount of outside air introduced into a closed environment affect the magnitude of incidence rates. Brundage and colleagues[19] measured an association of modern, energy-efficient barracks with increased rates of respiratory disease. Before the institution of year-round adenovirus and influenza vaccination programs, trainees housed in energy-efficient barracks had a 50% greater risk of respiratory infection compared to trainees living in older, less tightly sealed barracks. Because other potentially confounding variables (eg, crowding) were not measured in the study, the authors were reluctant to endorse a causal relationship.

A variety of techniques have been attempted in the past to interrupt the airborne route of transmission. Quarantine procedures, such as the removal of affected individuals through mandatory hospitalization policies, have been used at basic training installations for many years. The effectiveness of these isolation procedures depends on a variety of factors, including the agent-specific duration of asymptomatic shedding, the willingness of affected trainees to report for medical evaluation, the logistical ease of reporting for evaluation, and the degree to which medical authorities adhere to hospitalization policies.

Studies have also been conducted to assess the effectiveness of procedures to inactivate or remove infectious agents from the environment. Wells[20] demonstrated that indoor ultraviolet irradiation has a modest effect in reducing infection rates in various populations. The recent emergence of multidrug-resistant *Mycobacterium tuberculosis* has prompted the Occupational Safety and Health Administration to recommend the use of ultraviolet irradiation as an adjunct in controlling the transmission of respiratory pathogens in health care facilities. Others[21] have reduced the frequency of nosocomial infections through the use of laminar airflow systems that incorporate filters capable of removing most microorganisms. Some advocates[22] recommend the development of techniques using small air ions to reduce the viability of suspended microorganisms. None of these approaches, however, has been applied or studied in military trainee populations.

During World War II, the Commissions on Acute Respiratory Disease and Air-borne Infections investigated the effect of oiling floors and bedding on acute respiratory infections.[23] These experiments were based on the concern that bedding or floor dust might serve as a "reservoir" for hemolytic streptococci that, when disturbed, could become airborne. Floors were treated using a petroleum-distillate floor oil, distributed through buckets with perforated bottoms, and spread with hair brooms.[24] Oiling of bedding (ie, blankets, sheets, pillowcases, and mattress covers) consisted of adding an oil-emulsion base during the rinse phase of machine laundering and resulted in an oil loading of 2% to 4% in the fabric.[25,26] General enthusiasm for these procedures was reported from participants due to the absence of dust and the reduced amount of work to maintain barracks cleanliness. In fact, the intervention was so popular that requests for the procedures were received from others not included in the study. Except for occasional staining of feet or clothes with oil, no complaints were received. During periods of endemic disease, this program reduced infection rates by 30% to 40%, but during epidemic periods rates were only reduced 6% to 12%.[1] For reasons that are not clear, the commission did not advocate this method as a means to control disease

rates. Because the commission presumed that *S pyogenes* was transmitted through the airborne route, it is possible that these studies underestimated the effect that oiling procedures may have on true airborne infections. This or other similar modes of intervention may warrant further evaluation.

Concerns over indoor air pollution and the effect that "tight" buildings may have on respiratory disease have resulted in several proposals and actions. Dilution of "polluted" indoor air may be accomplished by mixing with outside air. The American Society of Heating, Refrigerating, and Air-Conditioning Engineers (ASHRAE) publishes ventilation standards for indoor air quality. The standards address microorganisms as well as various gases, vapors, smokes, and other particulate contaminants. Most recently revised in 1989, the ASHRAE standard now requires 15 cubic feet of outside air per minute per person for "dormitory sleeping areas."[27] Before this revision, the requirement was only for 5 cubic feet per minute. The extent to which existing recruit barracks conform with the revised ASHRAE standard has not been comprehensively evaluated, and current military policy continues to emphasize minimal square footage requirements.

Control of airborne infections in basic training populations relies almost exclusively on agent-specific interventions. While none can deny the tremendous effect that these interventions have had, the health of trainees is vulnerable to a breakdown in any single strategy or to the emergence of new airborne agents of disease. The vulnerability of this posture was demonstrated in 1989 when a measles outbreak at Fort Leonard Wood, Mo, followed a delay in normal vaccination procedures until several weeks into the training cycle. The simple delay in vaccinations provided a sufficient "window" for a limited outbreak to occur among non-immune recruits. The agent-generic strategies the military has in place to control airborne infections (eg, requirements for segregation of sick trainees, minimal square footage of living space) can be expected to have at most a modest effect on limiting disease.

Direct Contact

Infectious organisms that can be transmitted through direct contact include many that have caused large epidemics in trainee populations in the past: adenovirus, influenza viruses, *S pyogenes,* and *Neisseria meningitidis.* Others in this group that cause respiratory infections include the common cold viruses, *S pneumoniae, Mycoplasma pneumoniae,* and *Chlamydia pneumoniae.* Other agents of disease, such as those that cause airborne or gastrointestinal infections, may also be transmitted through the direct contact route.

Direct-contact transmission may occur through several mechanisms. Sneezing, coughing, spitting, talking, and even normal breathing project microorganisms into the air[23] in the form of infectious droplets. These droplets are usually much larger in size than the droplet nuclei of airborne contagion, fall quickly, and come to rest on objects in the immediate environment. Susceptible persons become infected if the organisms enter directly into the body through portals such as the eye, nose, or mouth. Alternatively, viable organisms on the surface of environmental objects (fomites) may serve as a source of secondary, hand-inoculated infection. Direct-contact transmission may also result from physical contact between persons in either a primary (eg, kissing) or a secondary (eg, hand-shaking) mode.

The basic training environment (see Chapter 8) provides countless opportunities for direct-contact transmission. In fact, it is difficult to imagine conditions more conducive to contagion: crowding, groups containing individuals from diverse geographic locations, mandatory and continuous concentration of personnel, and vigorous activities involving physical contact both with other persons and with objects in the environment.

Control of infections transmitted through direct contact is similar in many aspects to the control of airborne infections. Reliance on vaccination is the primary mode of intervention for most organisms in this class. Year-round influenza immunizations appear to be very effective at preventing large outbreaks, such as those that have occurred in the past. Vaccines were developed to protect trainees from the tremendous morbidity of adenovirus infections and the risk of mortality from meningococcal disease. In contrast, outbreaks of *S pyogenes* infections have been controlled through the broad use of penicillin. Other agents of disease in this category have contributed to trainee morbidity in the past but have not caused repeated outbreaks over time or been associated with substantial mortality.

Quarantine of affected individuals with conditions transmissible by direct contact is normally routine and frequently mandatory. US Army policy, for example, has required the hospitalization of any trainee with an influenza-like illness, a temperature of 38°C or higher, and one or more respiratory symptoms. The degree to which these procedures are implemented determines the overall effectiveness of the policy. In addition, adherence to minimal square footage requirements in barracks areas probably decreases

case reproduction rates. Any measure that increases the distance between trainees could theoretically reduce the likelihood that infectious droplets expelled during a sneeze or cough would fall on and infect a susceptible person. Head-to-foot arrangements of bunks in sleeping quarters, for example, could have such an effect. One study[28] of the effect of double-bunking (ie, using bunkbeds) on the incidence of respiratory disease noted a 50% reduction in cases of acute respiratory disease (ARD) (excluding influenza, atypical pneumonia, and hemolytic streptococcal infections) in the intervention group in comparison to a control population.

Other measures of prevention are theoretically possible. Direct transmission of infectious droplets from one individual to another could be minimized, for example, through the use of masks, by dispersion of personnel, or by separation of symptomatic personnel from others. During the influenza epidemics of 1918 and 1919, several communities in the United States adopted programs of mask-wearing. There is some evidence that these programs had a modest effect.[4] Secondary transmission through fomite contact could be minimized through intermittent sterilization of environmental surfaces. Ultraviolet irradiation of air spaces or environmental surfaces, especially when personnel are absent, could be an efficient strategy in certain situations. Alternatively, surfaces might be developed that have inherent anti-microbiological properties. Finally, disease transmission rates could be reduced through changes in behavior. Mandatory, frequent handwashing and training to reduce contact between hands and facial portals of entry could have some effect.

In contrast to these potentially beneficial practices, one common practice probably has no effect. Often, as rates of respiratory disease increase, local personnel will open barracks windows and doors to increase ventilation. Because the most commonly encountered pathogens are transmitted through direct contact rather than airborne transmission, increased ventilation has no effect on this mode. It is conceivable that "fresh" air sterilizes the environment through an unspecified mechanism or that "fresh" air somehow enhances natural host immune defenses. However, these conceivable benefits have not been substantiated by trials.

Foodborne and Waterborne

Little information will be provided here on the threat of foodborne and waterborne infections to trainee populations. Other chapters in this volume address these diseases in detail (see Chapter 37, Diseases Spread by Food, Water, and Soil). Nonetheless, these conditions are of historical importance in the trainee environment. Intestinal infections were a horrendous problem in training camps before the sanitary revolution. Typhoid fever outbreaks during the Spanish-American War are the most notable example. Diarrheal diseases were also a common affliction that had a severe impact on training.

With the exception of typhoid fever, virtually all conditions in this foodborne and waterborne illness category are prevented through intermediary, agent-generic measures. These include policies to guarantee the procurement of safe water and food; routine inspection of food service facilities to ensure proper handling, preparation, and storage of food items; sanitary procedures for disposal of all forms of waste; and emphasis on handwashing and other personal hygiene measures. The success of these sanitary procedures to affect foodborne and waterborne disease transmission stands in stark contrast to the failure of all these approaches to affect transmission of airborne and direct-contact diseases.

Of course, sporadic outbreaks of foodborne or waterborne infections may occur in trainee populations whenever lapses occur in preventive strategies. The universal susceptibility of trainees to most agents of foodborne and waterborne disease and an inherent potential for diseases transmitted by this mode to affect many persons underscore the significance of these conditions. Thus, while the threat of foodborne and waterborne outbreaks may be small in comparison to the threat of diseases transmitted via other modes of transmission, it is imperative that the disease control officer emphasize procedures to prevent their occurrence.

Vector-borne

Other chapters in this volume have detailed discussions of the issues related to conditions in this category. While serious vector-borne infections, such as malaria, dengue fever, and yellow fever, were major problems in years past, their threat to current military trainee populations is not considered serious. These infectious agents were eliminated from the continental United States through vector control programs. Current trainee populations benefit from this situation, but re-establishment of viable vectors has occurred and warrants ongoing surveillance. Other vector-borne conditions, such as Lyme disease, Rocky Mountain spotted fever, and ehrlichiosis, are endemic in certain training locations. Successful control of vector-borne disease will, therefore, depend on avoiding re-introduction of previously eliminated organisms, as well as using personal protective measures.

SURVEILLANCE FOR COMMUNICABLE DISEASE

Control of communicable disease does not rely solely on the continuous implementation of proven strategies. It also requires a vigilant watchfulness for breakdowns in control practices and the emergence of previously unrecognized threats through the implementation of a comprehensive surveillance program.

A surveillance program for communicable diseases will have several goals. The first is, of course, to verify that prevention strategies are effective. While assuring the health of individual trainees, this goal also maintains accountability of the medical department to the public interest. A corollary of this goal is to identify outbreaks as soon as possible so that immediate corrective actions may be taken. Disease control programs should be designed in layers, with a pre-planned capability to add layers of prevention in response to an increased threat of disease. Another goal of surveillance is to trigger investigations that may identify risk factors, causes, and possible control strategies. While formal investigations are usually initiated only after one or more control strategies have failed, such investigations often identify shortcomings in these attempts or identify other alternatives for control that have not been considered. Another purpose of surveillance is to define disease trends so that resources may be efficiently distributed. Changes in the distribution of resources may be required both to meet the clinical health care needs of affected personnel and to assure disease prevention programs. A fourth goal of surveillance is to monitor the relative morbidity of various conditions so that prevention research can target those that cause the greatest problem. The ability of research and development agencies to revise and focus their efforts on conditions of greatest significance to the military community depends on their having current information concerning the health threat. All of these goals must be borne in mind when designing and evaluating surveillance systems.

Potentially, communicable disease surveillance programs may monitor any or all of the following elements: hazardous agents in the environment, exposures to those agents, and adverse health outcomes resulting from those exposures.[29] In addition, surveillance programs should collect and archive detailed information on potentially affected populations. Military basic training installations currently conduct only rudimentary surveillance programs. The Air Force conducts limited influenza surveillance in basic training, with collection of throat washings for viral cultures. Neither the Navy nor the Army performs routine environmental monitoring to identify circulating agents of respiratory disease. In the absence of information about which agents are present, it is impossible to monitor potential exposures of individual trainees to those agents.

All military services require medical personnel to report selected infectious conditions, including many that are of concern during basic training. In addition, personnel at Navy and Marine Corps training centers monitor total counts of positive cultures for *S pyogenes*. Personnel at Army basic training installations monitor trainee segregations for infectious respiratory conditions and laboratory-confirmed infections with *S pyogenes* among hospitalized trainees. Information on potentially exposed trainee populations is usually collected in aggregate form and does not normally provide more detail than the number and sex of trainees assigned to each company-sized training unit.

The current Army ARD surveillance program is an offspring of the now defunct adenovirus surveillance program.[30] In the early 1980s, the program was modified to collect specific information on streptococcal infections. A key component of the altered program has been the requirement to segregate trainees with an influenza-like illness, fever in excess of 38°C, and any respiratory symptom. Before the 1990s, this was usually on ARD wards, but with the arrival of managed care, cases are now often segregated in less-formal housing arrangements. Each week, surveillance personnel collect the following information for each training company: the number of recruits in training by sex, the number of trainees segregated with acute respiratory infections, the number of segregated trainees with at least one culture obtained for *S pyogenes*, and the number of positive throat cultures. These numbers are the building blocks for three indices, which are calculated each week (Table 9-1).

The ARD rate is a general measure of respiratory disease activity in trainee populations. The term "acute respiratory disease" as applied here is distinct from the term "acute respiratory disease of recruits," which from the 1940s to the 1970s applied to adenovirus infections.[30,31] ARD now means any acute, febrile condition primarily involving the respiratory system. As recently as 1986, the nominal epidemic threshold for the ARD rate was 2 hospitalizations per 100 trainees per week. When persistently low hospitalization rates were observed at all installations, the threshold was lowered to 1.5.

TABLE 9-1

MEASURES OF ACUTE RESPIRATORY DISEASE ACTIVITY AT US ARMY BASIC TRAINING INSTALLATIONS

Rate or Index	How Calculated	Threshold
ARD rate	100 x HOSP / POP	1.5
Streptococcal recovery rate	100 x GABHS / CULT	None[*]
Streptococcal-ARD surveillance index	ARD rate x streptococcal recovery rate	25

ARD: Acute respiratory disease
POP: The total number of individuals in the basic training population
HOSP: The number of trainees segregated with acute febrile respiratory conditions[†]
CULT: The number of throat cultures performed on hospitalized trainees
GABHS: The number of throat cultures positive for group A beta-hemolytic streptococci
[*]During outbreaks of virulent streptococcal disease, this rate often exceeds 50%. However, such high recovery rates may also be observed during periods of infrequent hospitalizations or during periods of hyperendemic infections with nonvirulent organisms. Therefore, this "rate" should never be used alone as a measure of streptococcal disease.
[†]Hospitalizations with any of the following diagnoses at the time of admission: acute respiratory disease, streptococcal pharyngitis, influenza-like illness, tonsillitis, upper respiratory infection, bronchitis, acute pharyngitis, pneumonia, peritonsillar abscess, retropharyngeal abscess, bacterial meningitis, mononucleosis, sinusitis, mycoplasma, otitis media, chickenpox (or varicella), or acute viral syndrome or illness.

Interpretation of ARD rates for groups of trainees smaller than the entire installation is problematic. Although the origins of large outbreaks can usually be traced to individual units, most elevations of ARD rates in less-than-installation-sized groups usually resolve spontaneously. For this reason, interpretation of the ARD rate for small-sized units is not recommended. Before the use of adenovirus vaccines, weekly ARD rates approached 10 per 100 during peak epidemic periods.[30] Following the initiation of year-round adenovirus 4 and 7 vaccination, ARD rates normally did not exceed 1 and only rarely approached or exceeded 2.[32]

Although the ARD rate is sensitive to outbreaks of adenovirus and influenza, it is a poor indicator of virulent streptococcal disease activity. This was demonstrated during an outbreak of acute rheumatic fever (14 cases) at Fort Leonard Wood in 1987 during a period when ARD rates remained well below the epidemic threshold.[33] Similar observations were made during subsequent outbreaks at other Army installations.[34]

In 1959, the Armed Forces Epidemiological Board suggested that weekly streptococcal pharyngitis rates in excess of 10 cases per 1,000 trainees may serve as an indicator of an increased risk for acute rheumatic fever.[35] The Navy applied this criterion in determining the need to reinstitute benzathine penicillin G prophylaxis at the Naval Training Center in San Diego, Calif, in 1987.[36] In contrast, the Army monitors the streptococcal-ARD surveillance index (see Table 9-1). This index includes a criterion for morbidity (defined as hospitalization) and, as such, is theoretically less susceptible to false alarms resulting from hyperendemic infections with nonvirulent strains and variations in screening behaviors of health care providers. In practice, either measure of streptococcal disease activity is sufficient as a tool for initiating penicillin prophylactic programs, especially when elevated rates are accompanied by independent evidence of virulent strain circulation in the trainee population (ie, cases of rheumatic fever or invasive sequelae). In some situations, penicillin prophylaxis may be indicated simply to prevent morbidity associated with streptococcal pharyngitis.

The ARD rate and either of these measures of *S pyogenes* activity are efficient indicators of outbreaks. In particular, because both adenovirus and streptococcal disease outbreaks require several weeks to reach peak activity and may extend over several months, sufficient time is normally available to interrupt an epidemic once the threshold is passed. In contrast, influenza epidemics start, reach their peak, and begin to subside within a 1- to 2-week period. The rapidity with which influenza can pass through a large population is not generally recognized. This contrast is demonstrated in Figure 9-1. For the purposes of influenza control, the currently implemented surveillance systems are only useful in that they may serve as sentinel indicators for unaffected installations.

CONTROL OF SPECIFIC DISEASES

This section builds on concepts already presented by discussing a handful of diseases that are of greatest concern today or for which unique control programs have been developed in the past. Fortunately, preventive strategies that affect the pathway along a particular mode of transmission are likely to affect more than one disease. Current environmental sanitation and personal hygiene practices have minimized waterborne, foodborne, and vector-borne infections to a level where they are not considered a substantial threat to the health of trainees. In contrast, virtually no effective agent-generic strategies have been developed for airborne and direct-contact contagion. All of the conditions discussed below fall into one of these two categories. Because this discussion highlights programmatic aspects of disease control, the reader is referred to Chapter 38, Diseases Spread by Close Personal Contact, for more information on the diseases themselves.

Influenza

The impact of influenza on US military operations during World War I was devastating. During 1918, over 43,000 members of the military died from influenza or pneumonia: 38,000 in the Army and over 5,000 in the Navy. These totals do not include deaths in 1919 for which statistics are somewhat less reliable. Of course, the tragedy wrought by influenza in US military forces was just a small part of the worldwide epidemic, in which up to 25 million died. In the United States, over 650,000 died during the two years 1918 and 1919.[4]

The rapidity with which influenza strains spread across the globe not only is a defining characteristic but also may be an important determinant of virulence enhancement. The rapid changes in the global distribution of influenza viruses were evident in the military population during World War

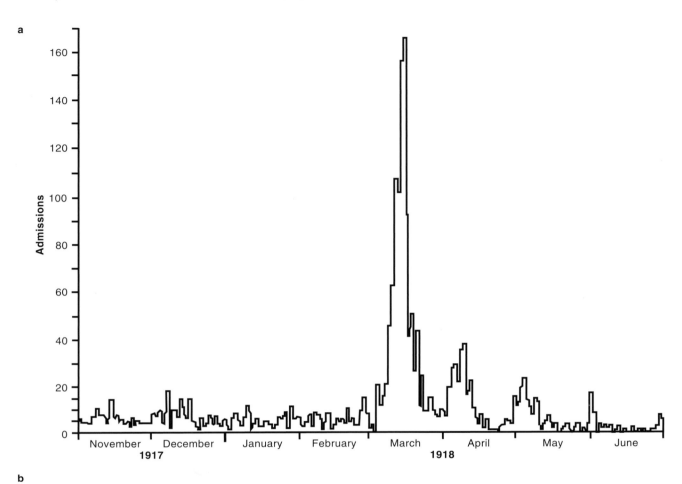

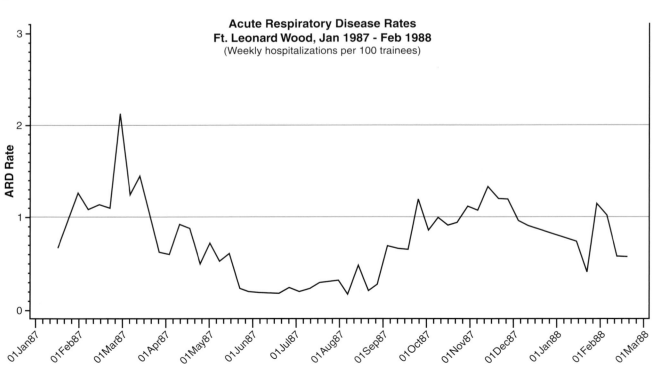

Fig. 9-1. These two graphs demonstrate the condensed epidemic curve of influenza virus outbreaks when compared with streptococcal-associated respiratory disease outbreaks. Graph **a** shows that an outbreak of influenza occurring at Camp Funston, Ks, in 1918 occurred during a 3-week period in March. In contrast, Graph **b** shows a rheumatic fever–associated outbreak of streptococcal disease among trainees at Fort Leonard Wood, Mo, during 1987 to 1988 that extended over a multimonth period (September 1997 to February 1988). Because of the extended duration of streptococcal-associated outbreaks, control programs can rely on surveillance and prompt intervention as an effective strategy, whereas the short duration of influenza outbreaks requires an emphasis on primary prevention (eg, vaccination) or prior preparation (eg, prepositioned medications).
Sources: (**a**) Opie EL, Freeman AW, Blake FG, Small JC, Rivers TM. Pneumonia at Camp Funston. *JAMA*. 1919;72:114. (**b**) Centers for Disease Control. Acute rheumatic fever among Army trainees—Fort Leonard Wood, Missouri, 1987-1988. *MMWR*. 1988;37:519–522.

I. An epidemic of non-lethal influenza affected military units in the continental United States during the spring of 1918. This original, less-virulent strain of virus subsequently spread around the world before being reintroduced into the United States in a more virulent form in the late summer. Almost instantaneously, the most-lethal form of influenza erupted at several sites around the world in September 1918. It exacted a horrible toll in human lives and misery for several months before beginning a prolonged, dwindling spiral that lasted into the second half of 1919. The fact that this form of influenza affected persons in the prime of life and that US forces in the continental United States were affected to a greater extent than those overseas ensured that trainee populations were among those most greatly affected. At Fort Devens, Mass, for example, up to 60 trainees died each day during the peak of the epidemic.

While many important questions concerning the epidemic of 1918–1919 remain unanswered, the effectiveness of current disease control practices can be interpreted in light of recent observations. Universal immunization of all military personnel with influenza vaccine is a Department of Defense policy. While seasoned personnel normally are vaccinated annually during the fall months, recruits receive the immunization in their first week of training, no matter what time of year. "Mass" prophylaxis of the entire force each year and continuous "tandem" prophylaxis of accessions results in a population that probably experiences the lowest age-adjusted attack rates in the world. The effectiveness of this approach, though, depends on the degree to which influenza vaccine components protect against circulating strains. The near complete absence of outbreaks of influenza in US armed services personnel during recent years[37] indicates that this strategy has been very effective. This success is probably attributable to a variety of factors. World Health Organization procedures for selecting strains for inclusion

in vaccine products have been remarkably accurate. Studies by Meiklejohn and colleagues[38,39] at Lowry Air Force Base, Colo, have documented that vaccines produced in industrial quantities for use in the elderly and other high-risk populations are highly immunogenic in military trainee populations. And notwithstanding the great number of deaths influenza continues to cause in susceptible populations, no recent strain of influenza has had a level of virulence comparable to that which ravaged the military force during World War I.

If a pandemic of influenza caused by a strain similar to the one that circulated in 1918 recurs, it is doubtful that current disease control strategies could provide much protection for military trainees. As previously discussed, no preventive strategies are currently in place that can interrupt the airborne or direct-contact modes of transmission, both of which are important routes for influenza.[39] Currently produced vaccines have low overall vaccine efficacy rates (70%–80%) and would not provide a substantial herd immunity barrier[40] against the spread of a virulent, highly transmissible strain. Even if strategies such as mask-wearing and environmental sanitation (eg, ultraviolet radiation) could provide protection, the absence of current materiel, training, and policy to direct these activities assures they will have a minimal role during early phases of a large-scale outbreak. One currently circulating proposal suggests stockpiling amantidine or rimantidine for use at basic training installations in the event of a large outbreak. Improvements in vaccine efficacy rates and reduced vaccine production times may be feasible in the near future. Such improvements in plans and technology could reduce the impact of a pandemic.

The National Influenza Immunization Program of 1976 highlights many of the difficulties that an effort to prevent a "killer flu" epidemic would entail. The origins of that effort[41–45] and the events that followed[46] (including cases of Guillain-Barré syndrome[47,48]) have caused many to reconsider how such national decisions are made.[49] The potential political liability of making an incorrect decision may make future efforts to respond to such a national threat extremely difficult. Nonetheless, efforts are in progress to outline such a strategy for the nation.[50]

Adenovirus

Adenovirus infections in military populations are of tremendous significance. Illness caused by adenovirus is characterized by high attack rates of a short-term, febrile, debilitating illness. Studies have shown that adenovirus types 3, 4, and 7 (and less commonly types 14 and 21) are the primary cause of febrile, acute respiratory disease in military trainees.[30,31,51,52] This organism was a nearly ubiquitous cause of outbreaks during the fall and winter seasons at basic training installations before the development of effective vaccines.[53] Typically, 50% or more of the entire trainee population would acquire this infection during the first few weeks of training, and most would be hospitalized. Thus, adenovirus infections took a heavy toll on the health of most trainees and cost the military many dollars in health care requirements, lost time from training, and the need to recycle trainees.

Isolation of the virus in the late 1950s and demonstration that enteric infections could induce protective immunity were milestones in the development of the live, enteric-coated vaccines. While some studies have demonstrated that live virus can be secondarily transmitted from the bowel of the vaccinated to the oropharynx of the susceptible,[1] such transmissions are relatively infrequent and have not been reported as a significant consequence of vaccination. Clinical trials conducted at Army basic training installations in the 1960s[54,55] demonstrated that vaccines against adenovirus types 4 and 7 were safe and efficacious, and they eliminated most acute respiratory disease in trainees. The tremendous savings afforded by these vaccines was summarized in a cost-benefit analysis performed by Collis and colleagues in 1973.[56] They showed that use of the type 4 and 7 vaccines at eight Army installations during just a few months in 1970 and 1971 prevented nearly 27,000 hospitalizations.

By the 1990s, all services except the Air Force required vaccination of male trainees within the first few days of accession to military service. Some installations have vaccinated female recruits, but installations that provide vaccine to males alone have not experienced outbreaks of adenovirus among non-immunized females. In 1984 (after observation

of summertime cases), the US Army instituted a program of year-round vaccination. Surveillance for emerging strains of adenovirus into the late 1980s demonstrated that the two vaccines were causally sufficient to prevent nearly all adenovirus infections (JDG, unpublished data, 1990). When production of the vaccines by their sole supplier lapsed in 1996, a policy of seasonal administration of vaccines was resumed and continued until supplies ran out in 1999.

The greatest current threat to the continued prevention of adenovirus-associated illness in military trainee populations is the lack of a commercial market for the vaccine outside of the armed services. In contrast to influenza, military problems with adenovirus infections have had little relevance for civilian populations. The sole US producer of adenovirus vaccines has disassembled its production facility and current lots of vaccine expired in the spring of 1997. In 1997 and 1998, the Food and Drug Administration extended the expiration date of existing vaccine lots, allowing vaccination through the 1998-1999 winter season. Despite current concerted efforts to re-establish a production capacity, it is inevitable that vaccines will not be available to protect trainees for a period of at least 2 years and that epidemics will recur.

While the commercial aspects of adenovirus vaccine production are unique among the conditions discussed in this section, the current crisis vividly demonstrates the vulnerability inherent in a communicable disease control program that is agent-specific and one layer thick. The absence of other preventive strategies, in particular the absence of mode-specific interventions for airborne and direct-contact transmission, is a continuing source of vulnerability.

Meningococcal Disease

Disease caused by *N meningitidis* has a long-standing relationship with the US military.[57] Notwithstanding recent policies to vaccinate military personnel deployed to parts of the world where meningococcal disease is endemic,[58] nearly 200 years of observations have demonstrated that meningococcal infections occur predominantly in recruits. In general, the prime determinant of large military epidemics has been mobilization for war, although smaller outbreaks may have been fueled by contemporaneous epidemics in civilian communities. During World War I and World War II, 2,279 and 559 deaths were attributable to meningococcal disease, respectively. The case-fatality rate during World War I was 39%.[57] Although disease caused by *N meningitidis* was the second leading cause of infectious disease death during World War II,[59] the overall case-fatality rate was substantially reduced through the use of sulfonamide prophylaxis.[60]

While many strains of meningococcus circulate freely among trainee populations, most "carriage" is asymptomatic. In fact, carriage rates among unaffected populations are similar to those observed during epidemics (20% to 80%).[57] Early suggestions that carriage rates in excess of 20% indicate a high risk of subsequent morbid disease have not been substantiated.[60] Transmission occurs presumably via respiratory droplets (airborne and direct contact) originating primarily from individuals with asymptomatic carriage. Fomites play a negligible role in disease spread.[61] Transmission among asymptomatic populations is very efficient and rapid, as documented by a 92% culture-positive rate in one study of 99 men over a 68-day period.[60]

The ability of meningococcal strains to circulate widely but cause disease only rarely may cause substantial psychological stress in affected populations. From the community viewpoint, the organism appears to strike randomly at helpless victims, a large proportion of whom succumb quickly. As a result, many community members may wait in fear to see who will be struck down next. This viewpoint infers both that the organism is extremely virulent and that susceptibility to life-threatening disease is high. In fact, both inferences are false. By the time cases occur, a large proportion of the population has probably already been exposed, but only those with the rare (and largely unknown) host susceptibility factors manifest disease. Agent-associated virulence factors undoubtedly exist, but these remain largely undescribed.

Antibiotic prophylaxis and vaccination have been the only two strategies in the prevention of meningococcal disease. From World War II through the early 1960s, strains of *N meningitidis* remained sensitive to sulfonamides. Complete reliance on this intervention and the eventual development of widespread resistance led to an 8-year period (1963–1971) during the Vietnam War era when no effective preventive strategies were available.[57] One of the initial outbreaks in this period—which occurred at Fort Ord—resulted in much local hysteria, considerable political pressure, and the eventual suspension of basic training at that installation. In the late 1960s, military investigators demonstrated that rifampin could effectively eliminate carriage, but the widespread development of resistance to this antibiotic limited its usefulness as a tool in outbreak interruption.[1]

Efforts in vaccine development intensified and eventually were fruitful. In October 1971, vaccination against serotype C was begun for all trainees;

vaccines against serogroups A, Y, and W-135 were subsequently developed and fielded during the late 1970s and early 1980s. Since the development and routine use of the tetravalent vaccine (A/C/Y/W-135), the occurrence of meningococcal disease has become extremely rare among recruits and due exclusively to serogroup B strains.[57] Several group B vaccines have been developed, but none demonstrates more than partial (approximately 50%) efficacy and all have only investigational new drug status.

As with other airborne infections, no effective prevention strategies have been developed that control meningococcal infections along its route of transmission. Although studies have shown associations of disease incidence with crowding, ventilation, and microclimate, few trials have been attempted to evaluate the effectiveness of modifying these factors.[62] Efforts attempted during World War I included quarantine, isolation of carriers, reduction of crowding, and increased ventilation.[60] The practical requirements of mobilizing a million soldiers during a very short period of time limited these attempts. Subsequent investigations focused almost entirely on chemoprophylaxis and immunoprophylaxis.

Nonavailability of a vaccine against serogroup B meningococcus remains a major threat to the health of trainees. The potential for this serogroup to cause substantial outbreaks was demonstrated in the early 1960s. The recent occurrence of large outbreaks of group B disease in other parts of the world highlights this potential threat. There is no logical reason to believe that these strains will not reappear. Furthermore, the causal connection between the fielding of vaccines and the disappearance of meningococcal disease in military recruits has been questioned by at least one prominent authority.[57] These shortcomings suggest that further inquiry into strategies to interrupt the transmission of meningococcal organisms within trainee populations may be warranted.

Group A Streptococcal Disease

The reemergence of rheumatic fever[63] and the identification of a previously unidentified syndrome (toxic streptococcal syndrome)[64] during the 1980s sparked substantial, renewed interest in *S pyogenes* infections. Increases in the occurrence of many of the known suppurative complications of streptococcal infections were reported from many locations. During this period, outbreaks of group A streptococcal infections occurred within the trainee populations of all military services.[33,35,37,65] Both the Army and Navy reported clusters of rheumatic fever cases. These outbreaks resulted in increased hospitalizations, substantial morbidity, and even death. Penicillin prophylaxis programs, which had been discontinued years before, were reinstituted to control disease.

Strategies to control streptococcal disease outbreaks in the military derive from the large outbreaks during World War II. As a result of those outbreaks, the armed services conducted numerous investigations to identify methods of disease control.[66] An early, remarkable victory was the demonstration that treatment of streptococcal pharyngitis with benzathine penicillin G (BPG) within 9 days of the onset of symptoms could prevent the development of rheumatic fever.[67] This intervention provided dramatic relief for installations where rheumatic fever attack rates after streptococcal pharyngitis approached 5%. However, because *S pyogenes* strains circulated widely among trainee populations and because many persons with rheumatic fever reported no antecedent episode of pharyngitis, treatment of symptomatic trainees was not effective in controlling outbreaks. Subsequent investigations at the Streptococcal Disease Laboratory at Fort Warren, Wyo,[67,68] and elsewhere[69–72] demonstrated that combined mass and tandem prophylaxis could control outbreaks in trainee populations.

Combinations of mass and tandem prophylaxis programs with BPG have been the mainstay of streptococcal disease control programs for the military ever since. Mass prophylaxis in this context consists of administering antibiotics to all trainees on an installation or in an affected group over a relatively short period of time. Tandem prophylaxis consists of routinely administering antibiotics to new cohorts of trainees shortly after arrival. An attempt to contain a broad-based disease outbreak with tandem prophylaxis alone[34] demonstrated the non-effectiveness of this approach. Current Army policies direct the administration of the tandem prophylactic dose (when used) within the first few days of arrival at reception stations, while at Marine Corps and naval training centers, this dose is administered on the 17th day. Hyperendemic infections among a Marine Corps trainee population receiving repeated courses of penicillin prophylaxis (on days 17 and 55) led Gray and colleagues to recommend erythromycin prophylaxis for individuals with penicillin allergy.[73]

The role of surveillance in the early identification of streptococcal disease outbreaks has already been discussed. Both the streptococcal-ARD index (Army) and the proportion of all throat cultures positive for *S pyogenes* (Navy and Marine Corps) serve as sensitive indicators of evolving outbreaks. A continuing difficulty, particularly at Army installations, is the lack of a reliable indicator to signal when prophylaxis programs may be terminated. A recurrent outbreak at Fort Leonard Wood in 1989 following 19 months of BPG prophylaxis demonstrated that absence of streptococcal disease in the local community was not a reliable indicator that prophylaxis could be safely discontinued.[34]

Although BPG may have benefits that extend beyond the prevention of streptococcal disease,[74] use of penicillin prophylaxis for disease control is not an optimal strategy. The potential for allergic reactions, the threat of developing resistant organisms, and the logistical burden of providing deep intramuscular inoculations warrant development of alternative control strategies. Although *S pyogenes* organisms have not yet demonstrated true resistance to penicillin, that is no guarantee that such resistance will not develop in the future. Selection of an alternative chemoprophylactic regimen may be problematic. While some suggest that development of a multi-M-type vaccine is a real possibility,[75,76] other experts believe that will not happen soon.

Efforts to contain the organism within the environment were attempted by investigators in the years immediately following World War II. Unfortunately, blanket- and floor-oiling experiments were predicated on the assumption that streptococci are transmitted through the airborne route. Subsequent investigations showed that direct contact transmission was, in fact, the principal mode. Environmental factors clearly play an important role in ongoing outbreaks of *S pyogenes*. For example, of 6,710 admissions for rheumatic fever reported in the Army during 1943, 43% occurred in the five states of Colorado, Utah, Idaho, Montana, and Wyoming.[11] This region of the country is recognized as an area of increased risk for streptococcal infections, but the reasons for this remain unknown.

Current approaches to the control of streptococcal infections suffer from the same limitations of all diseases discussed in this section. Reliance on chemoprophylaxis is agent-specific and at some point is liable to fail. Ongoing problems with streptococcal infections among Marine Corps trainees (eg, pharyngitis and less commonly suppurative sequelae) demonstrate that approaches that implement a single, final barrier within the susceptible host may not succeed.

Other Agents of Communicable Disease

Influenza viruses, adenovirus, *N meningitidis*, and *S pyogenes* are only four of numerous infectious agents that are a current threat to the health of military trainees. These organisms have had special significance in the past and remain among the most dangerous threats in the near future, but other organisms deserve at least brief mention.

Pneumococcal disease has been a major problem for military populations in the past, particularly in the 1940s.[77] Moreover, pneumonia caused by *S pneumoniae* is a significant threat to trainee health. Although these organisms were susceptible to penicillin in the past and an effective, multivalent vaccine[78] is available for long-term immunoprophylaxis, recent difficulties at the Naval Training Center indicate that prevention strategies are not likely to be simple. Reports of increasing resistance to multiple antimicrobials[79] and continuing outbreaks in closed populations[80–83] are a cause for concern.

Varicella infections continue as an unmanageable problem in recruit populations. Trainees arriving from tropical locations (eg, Puerto Rico) have low rates of childhood infection and therefore remain susceptible. Since the licensure of a varicella-zoster vaccine in 1995, its use in recruit populations has been endorsed by several services and may soon become a universal requirement for nonimmunes.

Chlamydia pneumoniae is a widely recognized cause of acute respiratory disease.[84] This organism has been identified as a significant cause of respiratory disease in recruit populations in other countries.[85] Retrospective analysis of one outbreak of pneumonia in Army recruits suggests that this organism has caused disease in this country as well. Chlamydial organisms are unique in their mechanisms of pathogenesis and could potentially cause unique problems in future trainee populations.

Streptococcal species other than group A could emerge as significant causes of respiratory disease in the future. Multiple serogroups have been incriminated as causes of disease outbreaks in other closed populations in the 1980s and 1990s.[86–90]

SUMMARY

Rates of communicable disease among military trainee populations have been brought to historical lows. Ongoing programs of environmental sanitation prevent the threat of vector-borne, foodborne, and waterborne diseases that plagued Army camps during the 19th century. Vaccinations against influenza, adenovirus, and the meningococcus have minimized the occurrence of these diseases. Nonetheless, the threat of virulent influenza, the lapse in adenovirus vaccine coverage, and the B serogroup "gap" in the tetravalent meningococcal armamentarium remain substantial threats to future trainee health. Similarly, the resurgence of *S pyogenes* infections during the 1990s and the sputtering patchwork approach of administering penicillin to massive populations of trainees suggests that a less-than-optimal strategy of disease prevention is being pursued. Other agents of communicable disease, which have not quite become leading players, loom in the background and are within an arm's reach of trainee wellness.

A currently prevailing attitude of complacency toward the prospect of trainee outbreaks probably has multiple causes. First, there are other aspects of military medicine and modern medicine, in general, that more easily attract and sustain attention and resources. These more-flashy areas compete with the ever-present and rather mundane need to sustain and enhance the health and readiness of that valuable asset: the newly enlisted sailor, soldier, airman, and marine. A second reason for the current lack of initiatives in the control of trainee communicable disease may derive from the belief that methods of immunoprophylaxis and chemoprophylaxis can inevitably be found to control all emerging threats. Yet it is this very belief that has perpetuated the emphasis on agent-specific strategies as the solution for disease control. These strategies have produced remarkable results, but they provide only limited solutions for what are essentially larger issues relating to modes of transmission. The need for renewing, revising, and recreating vaccines and antibiotic prophylactics will be as endless as the ability of organisms to emerge, adapt, and mutate. The continuing struggle to control agents transmitted by the airborne and direct-contact routes contrasts so clearly with the successes attained in the control of agents associated with other modes of transmission that the biomedical community should pause to consider redirecting at least some of its research efforts.

Environmental solutions that eliminate the threat of airborne and direct-contact contagion will not be easily obtained. Others who have investigated environmental factors related to the transmission of cold viruses eventually closed their laboratory with little to offer the world against its most common affliction.[91] The agenda of research that was left unfinished by the Commission on Airborne Infections when Sampson Air Force Base, NY, closed in June 1956 is a reasonable starting point for resuming work that is largely unfinished.[1] As one consultant familiar with these issues stated, "The field is wide open and merely awaits the arrival of some genius."[92(p768)]

REFERENCES

1. Jordan WS. History of the Commission on Acute Respiratory Diseases, Commission on Air-Borne Infections, Commission on Meningococcal Meningitis, and Commission on Pneumonia. In: Woodward TE, ed. *The Armed Forces Epidemiological Board, The Histories of the Commissions.* Washington, DC: Office of The Surgeon General, Dept of the Army: 1994; 5–137.

2. The Centers for Disease Control. Measles Surveillance Report No. 11, 1977–1981. Atlanta: Public Health Service; September 1982.

3. Boffey PM. Anatomy of a decision: how the nation declared war on swine flu. *Science.* 1976;192:636–641.

4. Crosby AW. *America's Forgotten Pandemic: the Influenza of 1918.* New York: Cambridge University Press; 1989.

5. Dunham GC. Basic principles of military epidemiology. *Military Preventive Medicine.* 3rd ed. Harrisburg, Penn: Military Service Publishing; 1940.

6. Chapin CV. *The Sources and Modes of Infection.* New York: John Wiley & Sons; 1910.

7. Bayne-Jones S. *The Evolution of Preventive Medicine in the United States Army, 1607–1939.* Washington, DC: Office of the Surgeon General, Dept of the Army; 1968.

8. Bushnell GE. Tuberculosis. Siler JF, ed. *Communicable and Other Diseases.* Vol 9. In: *The Medical Department of the United States Army in the World War.* Washington, DC: US Government Printing Office; 1928: 171–202.

9. Long ER. Tuberculosis. Coates JB, Hoff EC, Hoff PM, eds. *Communicable Diseases Transmitted Chiefly through Respiratory and Alimentary Tracts.* Vol 4. In: *Preventive Medicine in World War II.* Washington, DC: Office of The Surgeon General, Dept of the Army; 1958.

10. Coburn AF, Young DC. *The Epidemiology of Hemolytic Streptococcus during World War II in the United States Navy.* Baltimore: Williams and Wilkins; 1949.

11. Rantz LA. Hemolytic streptococcal infections. Coates JB, Hoff EC, Hoff PM, eds. *Communicable Diseases Transmitted Chiefly through Respiratory and Alimentary Tracts.* Vol 4. In: *Preventive Medicine in World War II.* Washington, DC: Office of The Surgeon General, Dept of the Army; 1958.

12. Morrow PE. Physics of airborne particles and their deposition in the lung. *Ann NY Acad Sci.* 1980;353:71–80.

13. Knight V. Viruses as agents of airborne contagion. *Ann NY Acad Sci.* 1980;353:147–156.

14. Brodkey C, Gaydos JC. United States Army guidelines for troop living space: a historical review. *Mil Med.* 1980;145:418–421.

15. The Personnel of Naval Laboratory Research Unit No. 1. Air-borne infections—a review. *War Med.* 1943;4:1–30.

16. Riley EC. The role of ventilation in the spread of measles in an elementary school. *Ann NY Acad Sci.* 1980;353:25–34.

17. Gundermann KO. Spread of microorganisms by air-conditioning systems. *Ann NY Acad Sci.* 1980;353:209–217.

18. Houk VN. Spread of tuberculosis via recirculated air in a naval vessel: the *Byrd* study. *Ann NY Acad Sci.* 1980;353:10–24.

19. Brundage JF, Scott RM, Lednar WM, Smith DW, Miller RN. Building-associated risk of febrile acute respiratory diseases in Army trainees. *JAMA.* 1988;259:2108–2112.

20. Riley RL. Airborne contagion: historical background. *Ann NY Acad Sci.* 1980;353:3–9.

21. Demling RH, Maly J. The treatment of burn patients in a laminar airflow environment. *Ann NY Acad Sci.* 1980;353:294–299.

22. Krueger AP, Reed EJ. Biological impact of small air ions: despite a history of contention, there is evidence that small air ions can affect life processes. *Science*. 1976;193:1209–1213.

23. Robertson OH, Hamburger M Jr., Loosli CG, Puck TT, Lemon HM, Wise H. A study of the nature and control of air-borne infection in Army camps. *JAMA*. 1944;126:993–1000.

24. Commission on Acute Respiratory Disease and The Commission on Air-Borne Infections. A study of the effect of oiled floors and bedding on the incidence of respiratory disease in new recruits. *Am J Hyg*. 1946;43:120–144.

25. Puck TT, Robertson OH, Wise H, Loosli CG. The oil treatment of bedclothes for the control of dust-borne infection, I: principles underlying the development and use of a satisfactory oil-in-water emulsion. *Am J Hyg*. 1946;43:91–104.

26. Loosli CG, Wise H, Lemon HM, Puck TT. The oil treatment of bedclothes for the control of dust-borne infection, II: the use of triton oil emulsion (T-13) as a routine laundry procedure *Am J Hyg*. 1946;43:120–144.

27. American Society of Heating, Refrigerating and Air-Conditioning Engineers, Inc. (ASHRAE). Ventilation for acceptable indoor air quality. ASHRAE, Atlanta, Ga, 1989.

28. Commission on Acute Respiratory Disease and The Commission on Air-Borne Infections. The effect of double-bunking in barracks on the incidence of respiratory disease. *Am J Hyg*. 1946;43:65–81.

29. Centers for Disease Control and Prevention. National surveillance for infectious diseases, 1995. *MMWR*. 1995;44:737–739.

30. Dudding BA, Top FH Jr, Winter PE, Buescher EL, Lamson TH, Leibovitz A. Acute respiratory disease in military trainees: the adenovirus surveillance program, 1966–1971. *Am J Epidemiol*. 1973;97:187–198.

31. Dingle JH, Langmuir AD. Epidemiology of acute, respiratory disease in military recruits. *Am Rev Respir Dis*. 1968;97(suppl):1–65.

32. Brundage JF, Gunzenhauser JD, Longfield JN, et al. Epidemiology and control of acute respiratory diseases with emphasis on group A beta-hemolytic streptococcus: A decade of U.S. Army experience. *Pediatrics*. 1996;97:964–970.

33. Centers for Disease Control. Acute rheumatic fever among Army trainees—Fort Leonard Wood, Missouri, 1987-1988. *MMWR*. 1988;37:519–522.

34. Gunzenhauser JD, Longfield JN, Brundage JF, Kaplan EL, Miller RN, Brandt CA. Epidemic streptococcal disease among Army trainees, July 1989 through June 1991. *J Infect Dis*. 1995;172:124–131.

35. Armed Forces Epidemiological Board. Recommendations of the ad hoc committee on prophylaxis of streptococcal infections of the commission on streptococcal disease. Washington, DC: Armed Forces Epidemiological Board, 1959.

36. Centers for Disease Control. Acute rheumatic fever at a Navy training center—San Diego, California. *MMWR*. 1988;37:101–104.

37. Meiklejohn G, Zajac RA, Evans ME. Influenza at Lowry Air Force Base in Denver, 1982-1986. *J Infect Dis*. 1987;156:649–651.

38. Meiklejohn G. Viral respiratory disease at Lowry Air Force Base in Denver, 1952–1982. *J Infect Dis*. 1983;148:775–784.

39. Cliff AD, Haggett P, Ord JK. *Spatial Aspects of Influenza Epidemics*. London: Pion Ltd; 1986.

40. Fine PE. Herd immunity: history, theory, practice. *Epidemiol Rev*. 1993;15:265–302.

41. Goldfield M, Bartley JD, Pizzuti W, Black HC, Altman R, Halperin WE. Influenza in New Jersey in 1976: isolations of influenza A/New Jersey/76 virus at Fort Dix. *J Infect Dis*. 1977;136(suppl):S347–S355.

42. Gaydos JC, Hodder RA, Top FH Jr, et al. Swine influenza A at Fort Dix, New Jersey (January-February 1976), I: case finding and clinical study of cases. *J Infect Dis.* 1977;136(suppl):S356–S362.

43. Gaydos JC, Hodder RA, Top FH Jr, et al. Swine influenza A at Fort Dix, New Jersey (January-February 1976), II: transmission and morbidity in units with cases. *J Infect Dis.* 1977;136(suppl):S363–S368.

44. Hodder RA, Gaydos JC, Allen RG, Top FH Jr, Nowosiwsky T, Russell PK. Swine influenza A at Fort Dix, New Jersey (January-February 1976), III: extent of spread and duration of the outbreak. *J Infect Dis.* 1977;136(suppl):S369–S375.

45. Top FH Jr, Russell PK. Swine influenza A at Fort Dix, New Jersey (January-February 1976), IV: summary and speculation. *J Infect Dis.* 1977;136(suppl):S376–S380.

46. Neustadt RE, Fineberg H. *The Swine Flu Affair: Decision Making in a Slippery Case.* Washington, DC: US Dept of Health, Education, and Welfare; 1978.

47. Roscelli JD, Bass JW, Pang L. Guillain-Barré syndrome and influenza vaccination in the US Army, 1980-1988. *Am J Epidemiol.* 1991;133:952–955.

48. Safranek TJ, Lawrence DN, Kurland LT, et al. Reassessment of the association between Guillain-Barré syndrome and receipt of swine influenza vaccine in 1976–1977: results of a two-state study. *Am J Epidemiol.* 1991;133:940–951.

49. Schoenbaum SC, McNeil BJ, Kavet J. The swine-influenza decision. *N Engl J Med.* 1976;295:759–765.

50. Hoke C, Division of Communicable Diseases and Immunology, Walter Reed Army Institute of Research. Personal Communication, 1995.

51. Buescher EL. Respiratory disease and the adenoviruses. *Med Clin North Am.* 1967;51:769–779.

52. Commission on Acute Respiratory Diseases. Acute respiratory disease among new recruits. *Am J Public Health Nation's Health.* 1946;36:439–450.

53. Bloom HH, Forsyth BR, Johnson KM, et al. Patterns of adenovirus infections in Marine Corps personnel. *Am J Hyg.* 1964;80:328–342.

54. Top FH Jr, Grossman RA, Bartelloni PJ, et al. Immunization with live types 7 and 4 adenovirus vaccines, I: safety, infectivity, antigenicity, and potency of adenovirus type 7 vaccine in humans. *J Infect Dis.* 1971;124:148–154.

55. Dudding BA, Top FH Jr. Scott RM, Russell PK, Buescher EL. An analysis of hospitalizations for acute respiratory disease in recruits immunized with adenovirus type 4 and type 7 vaccines. *Am J Epidemiol.* 1972;95:140–147.

56. Collis PB, Dudding BA, Winter PE, Russell PK, Buescher EL. Adenovirus vaccines in military recruit populations: a cost-benefit analysis. *J Infect Dis.* 1973;128:745–752.

57. Brundage JF, Zollinger WD. The epidemiology of meningococcal disease in the US Army. In: Vedros NA, ed. *Evolution of Meningococcal Disease.* Vol 1. Boca Raton, Fla: CRC Press; 1987: 5–25.

58. Moore PS, Harrison LH, Telzak EE, Ajello GW, Broome CV. Group A meningococcal carriage in travelers returning from Saudi Arabia. *JAMA.* 1988;260:2686–2689.

59. Gordon JE. General consideration of modes of transmission. In: Coates JB, Hoff EC, Hoff PM, eds. *Communicable Diseases Transmitted Chiefly through Respiratory and Alimentary Tracts.* Vol 4. In: *Preventive Medicine in World War II.* Washington, DC: Office of The Surgeon General, Dept of the Army; 1958: 3–52.

60. Phair JJ. Meningococcal meningitis. In: Coates JB, Hoff EC, Hoff PM, eds. *Communicable Diseases Transmitted Chiefly through Respiratory and Alimentary Tracts.* Vol 4. In: *Preventive Medicine in World War II.* Washington, DC: Office of The Surgeon General, Dept of the Army; 1958: 191–209.

61. Benenson AS, ed. *Control of Communicable Diseases in Man.* Washington, DC: Dept of the Army; 1995: 280–284. Army Field Manual 8–33.

62. Cvjetanovic B. Strategy for control. In: Vedros NA, ed. *Evolution of Meningococcal Disease.* Vol 1. Boca Raton, Fla: CRC Press; 1987: 135–143.

63. Veasy LG, Wiedmeier SE, Orsmond GS, et al. Resurgence of acute rheumatic fever in the intermountain area of the United States. *N Engl J Med.* 1987;316:421–427.

64. The Working Group on Severe Streptococcal Infections. Defining the group A streptococcal toxic shock syndrome: rationale and consensus definition. *JAMA.* 1993;269:390–391.

65. Centers for Disease Control. Group A beta-hemolytic streptococcal pharyngitis among U.S. Air Force trainees—Texas, 1988–89. *MMWR.* 1990;39:11–13.

66. Denny FW Jr, Houser HB. Commission on Streptococcal and Staphylococcal Diseases. In: Woodward TE, ed. *The Armed Forces Epidemiological Board: The Histories of the Commissions.* Washington, DC: Office of The Surgeon General, Borden Institute; 1994.

67. Davis J, Schmidt WC. Benzathine penicillin G: on effectiveness in the prevention of streptococcal infections in a heavily exposed population. *N Engl J Med.* 1957;256:339–342.

68. Morris AJ, Rammelkamp CH. Benzathine penicillin G in the prevention of streptococcic infections. *JAMA.* 1957;165:664–667.

69. Frank PF. Streptococcal prophylaxis in Navy recruits with oral and benzathine penicillin. *US Armed Forces Med J.* 1958;9:543–560.

70. Schreier AJ, Hockett VE, Seal JR. Mass prophylaxis of epidemic streptococcal infections with benzathine penicillin G, I: experience at a naval training center during the winter of 1955–56. *N Engl J Med.* 1958;258:1231–1238.

71. McFarland, Colvin VG, Seal JR. Mass prophylaxis of epidemic streptococcal infections with benzathine penicillin G, I: experience at a naval training center during the winter of 1956–57. *N Engl J Med.* 1958;258:1277–1284.

72. Frank PF, Stollerman GH, Miller LF. Protection of a military population from rheumatic fever: routine administration of benzathine penicillin G to healthy individuals. *JAMA.* 1965;193(10):119–127.

73. Gray GC, Escamilla J, Hyams KC, Struewing JP, Kaplan EL, Tupponce AK. Hyperendemic *Streptococcus pyogenes* infection despite prophylaxis with penicillin G benzathine. *N Engl J Med.* 1991;325:92–97.

74. Gunzenhauser JD, Brundage JF, McNeil JG, Miller RN. Broad and persistent effects of benzathine penicillin G in the prevention of febrile, acute respiratory disease. *J Infect Dis.* 1992;166:365–373.

75. Dale JB. Vaccine for strep A closer to reality. *US Med.* 1990;August:47–48.

76. Fischetti VA, Hodges WM, Hruby DE. Protection against streptococcal pharyngeal colonization with a vaccinia: M protein recombinant. *Science.* 1989;244:1487–1490.

77. Hodges RG, MacLeod CM. Epidemic pneumococcal pneumonia, I: description of the epidemic. *Am J Hyg.* 1946;44:183–192.

78. Shapiro ED, Berg AT, Austrian R, et al. The protective efficacy of polyvalent pneumococcal polysaccharide vaccine. *N Engl J Med.* 1991;325:1453–1460.

79. Breiman RF, Butler JC, Tenover FC, Elliott JA, Facklam RR. Emergence of drug-resistant pneumococcal infections in the United States. *JAMA.* 1994;271:1831–1835.

80. Hoge CW, Reichler MR, Dominguez EA, et al. An epidemic of pneumococcal disease in an overcrowded, inadequately ventilated jail. *N Engl J Med.* 1994;331:643–648.

81. Eskola J, Takala AK, Kela E, Pekkanen E, Kalliokoski R, Leinonen M. Epidemiology of invasive pneumococcal infections in children in Finland. *JAMA.* 1992;268:3323–3327.

82. Cherian T, Steinhoff MC, Harrison LH, Rohn D, McDougal LK, Dick J. A cluster of invasive pneumococcal disease in young children in child care. *JAMA.* 1994;271:695–697.

83. Centers for Disease Control. Outbreak of invasive pneumococcal disease in a jail—Texas, 1989. *MMWR.* 1989;38:733–734.

84. Grayston JT, Wang SP, Kuo CC, Campbell LA. Current knowledge on *Chlamydia pneumoniae,* strain TWAR, and important cause of pneumonia and other acute respiratory diseases. *Eur J Clin Microbiol Infect Dis.* 1989;8:191–202.

85. Kleemola M, Saikku P, Visakorpi R, Wang SP, Grayston JT. Epidemics of pneumonia caused by TWAR, a new *Chlamydia* organism, in military trainees in Finland. *J Infect Dis.* 1988;157:230–236.

86. Turner JC, Hayden GF, Kiselica D, Lohr J, Fishburne CF, Murren D. Association of group C beta-hemolytic streptococci with endemic pharyngitis among college students. *JAMA.* 1990;264:2644–2647.

87. Benjamin JT, Perriello VA Jr. Pharyngitis due to group C hemolytic streptococci in children. *J Pediatr.* 1976;89:254–256.

88. McCue JD. Group G streptococcal pharyngitis: analysis of an outbreak at a college. *JAMA.* 1982;248:1333–1336.

89. Meier FA, Centor RM, Graham L Jr, Dalton HP. Clinical and microbiological evidence for endemic pharyngitis among adults due to group C streptococci. *Arch Intern Med.* 1990;150:825–829.

90. Hill HR, Caldwell GG, Wilson E, Hager D, Zimmerman RA. Epidemic of pharyngitis due to streptococci of Lancefield group G. *Lancet.* 1969;2:371–374.

91. Andrewes CH. Adventures among viruses, III: the puzzle of the common cold. *Rev Infect Dis.* 1989;11:1022–1028.

92. Andrewes CH. The common cold: prospects for its control. *Med Clin North Am.* 1967;51:765–768.

Chapter 10

MUSCULOSKELETAL INJURIES IN THE MILITARY TRAINING ENVIRONMENT

DAVID N. COWAN, PhD, MPH; BRUCE H. JONES, MD, MPH; and RICHARD A. SHAFFER, PhD, MPH

D. N. Cowan; Lieutenant Colonel, Medical Service, US Army Reserve; Special Projects Officer, Division of Preventive Medicine, Walter Reed Army Institute of Research, Silver Spring, MD 20910-7500

B. H. Jones; Formerly, Colonel, Medical Corps, US Army (ret), Director, Epidemiology and Disease Surveillance, US Army Center for Health Promotion and Preventive Medicine, Aberdeen Proving Ground, Maryland 21010-5422; currently, Division of Unintentional Injury Prevention/National Center for Injury Prevention and Control, Centers for Disease Control and Prevention, 4770 Buford Highway, NE, Mailstop K-63, Atlanta GA 30341-3724

R. A. Shaffer; Commander, Medical Service Corps, US Navy; Head, Operational Readiness Research Program, Naval Health Research Center, PO Box 85122, San Diego CA 92186-5122

INTRODUCTION

Injuries in general have a greater impact on the health and readiness of the US military than any other category of medical complaint, and training injuries treated on an outpatient basis may have the biggest single impact on readiness. Physical training and physical fitness are required to accomplish military missions, and many military occupations routinely require a higher level of physical exertion and fitness than most civilian occupations, a fact recognized and enforced by regulation (eg, AR 350-41, *Training in Units*, Chapter 9, Physical fitness). During military training, all military personnel must attain and then afterward maintain a level of fitness much higher than usually found among civilians of the same age. In the military, physical training takes place in schools and in operational units. Generally, the training in schools is oriented toward rapidly increasing the physical strength and endurance of personnel, while training in units is oriented toward maintaining the level of fitness appropriate for the type of unit.

Physical training in basic training units accelerates healthy, young soldiers, sailors, airmen, and marines with varying levels of fitness to a fairly high level of fitness over a period of 8 to 13 weeks (Figure 10-1). After finishing basic training, individuals are either assigned to an operational unit or go on to further training. The fitness needed to function in an operational unit varies by the type of unit but, in general, will be higher in combat arms units (especially infantry) than in combat support or combat service support units. The level of fitness required in the schools that follow basic training varies by the type of school, with substantially more rigorous training required in special schools (eg, Airborne, Air Assault, Ranger, Special Forces, SEAL [Sea, Air, and Land] training) than in combat support or combat service support training programs. Indeed, physical training in special schools will often take servicemembers already in good physical condition and train them at levels similar to those of elite athletes.

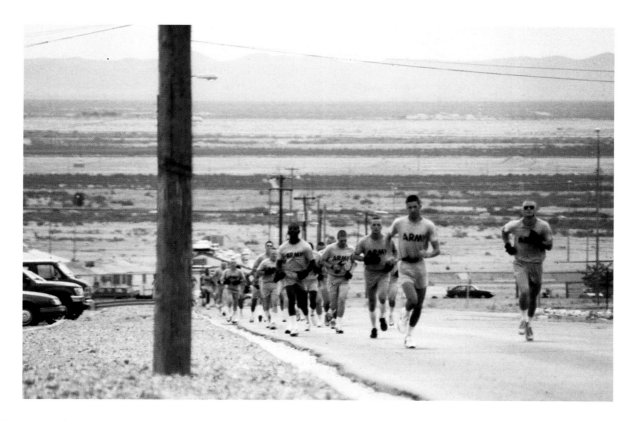

Fig. 10-1. Military training usually involves substantial amounts of running and marching. Some aspects of training, particularly running, are associated with increased risks of overuse injury. Photograph: Courtesy of Colonel Bruce Jones, US Army (Retired).

In addition to differences between types of units, there are often substantial differences in the personnel within the units. While most military personnel are young and fit, senior non-commissioned officers and officers are generally older, more sedentary, less fit, and may be less healthy. Many studies in civilian and military populations have demonstrated that being physically fit and active is protective against many health hazards, including injury.[1–5] However, obtaining desired levels of fitness through physical training is accompanied by substantial risk of injury. High risks of injury have been documented in many training situations, and the association between low levels of preexisting physical fitness and activity and the risk of injury in this environment has been established by numerous epidemiologic studies.

The need for fitness and the requisite physical training to maintain mission-readiness, the burden and impact of training injuries, and the protective effects of fitness in preventing subsequent injuries result in a complex and dynamic matrix of competing requirements. Understanding this matrix and optimizing the competing requirements is a difficult challenge for military policymakers, planners, commanders, and medical personnel. Nonetheless, only coordinated, well-planned, and multifaceted approaches based on an understanding of the many factors involved will have a positive impact on reducing the levels of injuries. Because of their importance, training-related injuries will be the primary focus of this chapter.

THE MAGNITUDE OF THE PROBLEM

The frequency of injuries and their effects on the military are not widely appreciated. Among US military personnel, injuries cause more deaths (about 50% more) than any other cause.[6] Injuries are implicated in a substantial proportion of disability discharges: nearly 50% of Army Medical Examination Board reviews of personnel assigned to an Army infantry division in 1994 were directly related to injury. Evaluation of Physical Examination Board data indicates that many chronic conditions leading to disability may result from service-related injuries. Acute and chronic effects of injuries are a major cause of hospitalization, causing about 30% of Army hospitalizations among active duty personnel in 1992. Injuries, particularly training injuries, create an enormous load on outpatient facilities. Among Army and Marine Corps trainees, rates of outpatient visits due to injuries of 20% to 40% per month have been observed, and rates of 20% per month have been reported among trained infantry soldiers. Furthermore, these problems are not unique to the US military; many other countries recognize the impact of injuries on their armed forces.[7]

For each death due to injuries among active duty Army personnel there are many more disabilities, hospitalizations, and outpatient visits (Figure 10-2). While deaths and disabilities due to injury cause concern because of their catastrophic and tragic impact on individuals, injuries resulting in less severe outcomes, such as loss to training, outpatient clinic visits, and hospitalizations, are of concern because of their frequency. In particular, it is noteworthy that the base of the Army injury pyramid is very broad, with more than 1,100 outpatient visits occurring for every death. Most of the injuries seen in military outpatient clinics are lower-extremity training-related injuries.[3,5,7] Injuries at all levels of severity cause a huge drain on military manpower and health care services and inflict enormous direct and indirect costs.[8]

Injury Incidence

As a consequence of their intense physical training, both basic training and combat unit populations have a high incidence of exercise-related injury. The volume of injured servicemembers seeking care in outpatient clinics creates long waiting times, reduces the time available per patient, and generally clogs the health care delivery system. In a study of Army infantry soldiers, the incidence of injuries was slightly higher than the incidence of illness (risk ratio = 1.3), but the number of lost duty days was 11 times higher for injury than for illness.[9] In another study,[10] training injuries among women trainees resulted in nearly 22 times as many lost training days compared to days lost due to illness. Numerous studies of military trainees[2,3,11–13] have documented the high risk of exercise-related injuries, ranging from 14% to 42% among men and from 27% to 61.7% among women. Most injuries are to the lower extremities, and most of these are overuse injuries.

Injury Types and Locations

The types of injuries experienced by military populations have been examined in several studies. Jones and colleagues[3] found that pain due to overuse was diagnosed in 24% of male trainees, muscle strains in 9%, ankle sprains in 6%, overuse

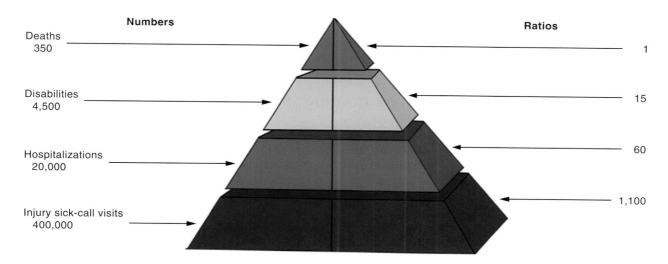

Numbers

Deaths
350

Disabilities
4,500

Hospitalizations
20,000

Injury sick-call visits
400,000

Ratios

1

15

60

1,100

Fig. 10-2. The Army Injury Pyramid. Army population figures and data from calendar year 1994 are the basis for this graphic. Reprinted from Jones BH. Conclusions and recommendations. In: The Injury Prevention and Control Work Group of the Armed Forces Epidemiological Board. *Injuries in the Military: A Hidden Epidemic.* Washington, DC: Armed Forces Epidemiological Board; 1996.

knee injuries in 6%, and stress fractures in 3%. Among 298 infantry soldiers, Knapik and colleagues[5] reported that musculoskeletal pain was most common, followed by strains, sprains, and cold-related injuries. Among male Marine Corps trainees, iliotibial band syndrome occurred most frequently, followed by blisters, stress fractures, ankle sprains, patellar tendinitis, shin splints, and patellofemoral syndrome.[14] The types of injuries diagnosed in male Navy trainees are also due mainly to overuse, with overuse knee injuries being the most common, followed by back pain, shin splints, ankle sprains, arm and shoulder pain, and stress fractures. Naval Special Warfare trainees were also evaluated and their most common injuries were found to be iliotibial band syndrome, stress fractures, patellofemoral syndrome, contusions, ankle sprains, low back injuries, periostitis, and Achilles tendinitis.[15]

In addition to experiencing higher risks of injury, the patterns of injury types found among female trainees differ somewhat from those found among men in the same program,[2] as shown in Table 10-1. Low back pain and tendinitis are the most common injuries among men, while muscle strains and stress fractures are the most common among women.

Impact of Injuries: Lost Time and Financial Costs

Most training injuries are not catastrophic or life threatening—most result only in limited duty for several days. The high incidence of injuries, how-ever, places a substantial burden on the medical care delivery system and leads to many lost training days and, frequently, to recruits having to repeat the training program (recycling). The costs are impressive. It has been estimated that stress fractures alone among 22,000 Marine Corps trainees in 1 year resulted in 53,000 lost training days and cost more than $16.5 million.[15] Extrapolation from the Marine Corps to all military trainees provides a reasonable estimate of costs related to all training injuries on the order of $100 million annually. Although stress fractures and stress reactions of bone occur fairly infrequently in basic training (risks reported include

TABLE 10-1

THE MOST COMMON INJURIES AMONG MEN AND WOMEN IN THE SAME ARMY BASIC COMBAT TRAINING PROGRAM

Injury Rank	Among Men	Among Women
1	Low back pain	Muscle strain
2	Tendinitis	Stress fracture
3	Sprain	Sprain
4	Muscle strain	Tendinitis
5	Stress fracture	Overuse knee injury

Data Source: Jones BH, Bovee MW, Harris JM 3d, Cowan DN. Intrinsic risk factors for exercise-related injuries among male and female army trainees. *Am J Sports Med.* 1993;21:705–710.

199

3.0%,[3] 2.4%,[2] 3.9%,[4] and 9.8%[15]), they are very debilitating and lead to more lost days of training and recycling than most other training-related injuries. The mean number of days lost per injury among Army infantry soldiers for stress fractures was 103, compared to 17 for sprains, 8 for other traumatic injuries, 7 for tendinitis, and 3 each for strains and musculoskeletal pain.[5]

RISK FACTORS FOR TRAINING-RELATED INJURIES

Identifying and understanding risk is key to developing effective prevention and treatment strategies for overuse injuries. Successful prevention depends on identification of *modifiable* risk factors. Since the early 1980s, much has been learned regarding risk factors for training- or exercise-related injuries in military populations (Exhibit 10-1), offering clues for effective interventions. These factors can usually be categorized as intrinsic (an attribute of the individual) or extrinsic (an attribute from some other source).

Intrinsic Risk Factors

A number of intrinsic risk factors have been identified among military populations. They include age, sex, anatomy, fitness, flexibility, and smoking.

EXHIBIT 10-1

RISK FACTORS FOR PHYSICAL TRAINING INJURIES IN MILITARY POPULATIONS

Intrinsic Factors

Age (risk generally increases with age)

Sex (risk is usually higher for women)

Anatomy (risk is associated with both leg and foot morphology)

Physical activity and fitness (risk is generally lower for more-fit individuals)

Flexibility (risk appears to be higher for those at the extremes of flexibility)

Smoking (risk is higher for cigarette smokers)

Extrinsic Factors

Absolute amount of training (risk is higher for more total distance covered)

Type of training (risk is higher for running versus walking or marching)

Acceleration of training (risk is higher after rapid increases in level of training)

Shoes and orthotics (inconsistent findings)

Training surface (inconsistent findings)

Age

Age has been evaluated as a risk factor for injury in a number of settings, but the findings have not been consistent. A number of studies have found that risks increase for older persons[3,5,16] even starting as early as age 25.[17] Others,[9,18–20] however, have found no association with age or an inverse association,[21] with the youngest at highest risk. The effect of age on risk has not been resolved and may prove to be a complex issue involving sex, previous history of exercise, existing level of fitness, nutritional and hormonal status, smoking, and the training environment, as well as the specific type of injury in question. If other risk factors are the same, older individuals are probably at greater risk of injury.

Sex

Most military studies have found women to be at increased risk of injury compared to men in the same training program.[1–3,22–24] Women entering military service are generally less fit than men, and this may account for some of the increase in risk among women. For example, Jones and colleagues[25] found that while female recruits were at an overall increased risk of injury, if the level of fitness was controlled for, there was no significant difference in risk of injury between the men and women. In addition, women have different lower extremity anatomy than men, including larger quadriceps angles (Q-angles) and greater degree of genu valgum (knock-knee).[26] Cowan and colleagues[27] found that among male trainees, these factors are associated with increased risk of overuse training injuries. The degree that these morphologic differences may account for differences in risk of injury has not yet been investigated. In contrast to women in training, women in operational units have been found not to be at increased risk of injury.[16] Lower rates of injury among women in operational units are probably due to lower levels of exposure to injury-causing activities relative to that found in training units.

Anatomic Factors

The effect of anatomic variations on the risk of

injury has been discussed for decades, but there has been remarkably little epidemiologic research conducted on this topic. Based on clinical impressions and case series, many characteristics have been proposed as risk factors, including flat feet and high arches (Figure 10-3), genu varum and valgum (Figure 10-4), excessive Q-angle, hyperextension of the knee (genu recurvatum), and leg length differences. However, a review of the literature conducted by Powell and colleagues[28] in 1986 concluded that the actual effect of lower limb anatomical variation on the risk of injuries in active populations has not been studied adequately in well-designed epidemiologic studies. He went on to state that "[n]one of the epidemiologic studies evaluated the role of anatomic factors in running injuries," that "case studies are unable to establish causality," and that "[c]areful, abnormality-specific studies should be a top priority for future research."[28(p100–101)]

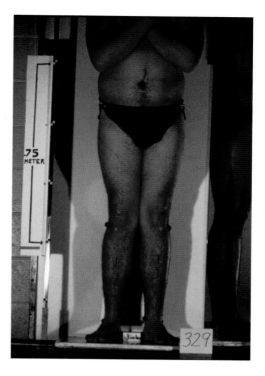

Fig. 10-4. Army infantry trainees with genu valgum, or knock-knees, were found to be more likely to experience an overuse injury. Photograph: Courtesy of Peter Frykman, MS, Research Physiologist/Biomechanist, US Army Research Institute of Environmental Medicine, Natick, Massachusetts.

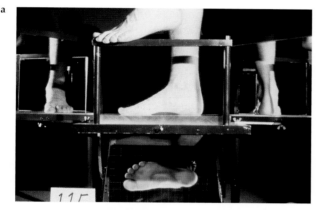

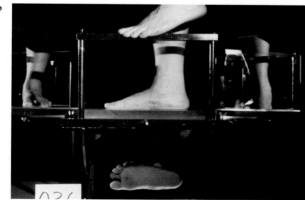

Fig. 10-3. Persons with high arches (**a**) are at increased risk of training injuries, while those with flat feet (**b**) may have a reduced risk, compared to those with "normal" arches. Photograph: Courtesy of John Robinson, Nike Sports Research, Nike, Inc., One Bowerman Drive, Beaverton, OR 97005-6453.

In the decade since that review, a few studies (mostly conducted by military scientists) evaluated prospectively the association between anatomic variables and risk of injury. The Israeli military studied anatomic risk factors for stress fractures and identified several factors that may be involved, including shorter tibial length, genu valgum, and excessive external rotation of the hip.[29,30] In US Marine Corps trainees, males diagnosed with stress fractures were shorter, lighter, and smaller in most bone structural girth dimensions than were uninjured trainees. In addition, bone structural geometric properties, such as cross-sectional areas, moments of inertia, section moduli, and width, were significantly smaller in those with stress fracture.[31]

The impact of foot[32] and leg[27] morphology on the risk of overuse training injuries was evaluated in the population studied by Jones and colleagues.[3] As shown in Table 10-2, infantry trainees with flat feet were at lowest risk, and those with high arches were at significantly increased risk. These findings are consistent with the findings of Giladi and colleagues,[33] who reported that low-arched Israeli sol-

TABLE 10-2

LOWER-EXTREMITY ANATOMY AND RISK OF INJURY AMONG ARMY TRAINEES

Characteristic	Injury Risk (%)	Source
Foot Morphology		1
Flattest 20% of arch heights	22	
Mid-60% of arch heights	39	
Highest 20% of arch heights	53	
Leg Morphology		2
Quintile 1 (most knock-kneed)	41	
Quintile 2	34	
Quintile 3	22	
Quintile 4	27	
Quintile 5 (most bowlegged)	28	
Quadriceps angle		2
≤ 10°	27	
> 10° to ≤ 15°	31	
> 15°	40	

Data Sources: (1) Cowan DN, Jones BH, Frykman PN, et al. Lower limb morphology and risk of overuse injury among male infantry trainees. *Med Sci Sports Exerc.* 1996;28:945–952. (2) Cowan DN, Jones BH, Robinson JR. Foot morphologic characteristics and risk of exercise-related injury. *Arch Fam Med.* 1993;2:773–777.

diers were at lowest risk of stress fractures. The findings of Kaufman and colleagues,[34] however, did not support those of Cowan.[32] Using different methods of measuring foot morphology among their population of SEAL candidates, they found that the flattest—and highest—arched tertiles had higher (but not significantly higher) risk of stress fracture, Achilles tendinitis, and iliotibial band syndrome. Army infantry trainees with genu valgum, shown in Table 10-2, had significantly increased risk of injury, as did those with excessive Q-angle. Genu recurvatum and leg length differences were not associated with increased risk of injury. This research provides some of the first quantitative descriptions of anatomic variances and estimates of risks for certain characteristics that should be further evaluated. As mentioned above, the anatomic differences between men and women may explain some portion of the differences in risk of training injuries, and this could best be evaluated in training units that contain both sexes.

Physical Activity and Fitness

Past physical activity and preexisting physical fitness are both important predictors of risk of training injury, and this is reflected in repeated findings that persons who enter military service with a history of high levels of activity and fitness are at significantly lower risk of injury.[1–5,9,35] There are several health-related parameters of fitness, including cardiorespiratory endurance, muscle endurance, strength, flexibility, and body composition. Not all of these factors are equally or consistently associated with risk of injury.

In a study of 303 infantry trainees,[3] there were significant univariate associations between risk of training injuries and several self-reported indicators of physical activity before entry into the Army. Compared to those reporting higher levels of activity, those reporting a more average activity level had a relative risk (RR) of injury of 1.8, while those who reported being inactive had an RR of 1.6. Compared to those running 4 or more days per week, those reporting running 1 to 3 days per week had an RR of 1.9, and those running less than 1 day per week had an RR of 2.2. Exercise frequency less than 1 day per week (RR = 1.5) was a significant predictor, but investigator-estimated energy expended per week in exercise (based on the reported intensity of exercise) was not associated with risk of injury. When fitness was assessed by several different methods, some measures of fitness were more strongly associated with injury than others. Body fat percentage was not a consistent predictor of injury, while those with both low and high levels of flexibility were at substantially increased risk (RR = 2.5 and 2.2, respectively) when compared to those of average flexibility. Dynamic lifting strength was not related to injury, but the number of pushups done (in 2 minutes) and 2-mile run time were somewhat associated with injury risk.

One- and two-mile run times have been found to be one of the most consistent predictors of injury risk in a number of studies, although there have been slight differences found in patterns and relative risks. Jones and colleagues[25] found that both men and women who ran faster had lower injury risks during basic training than those who ran slower, as is shown in Table 10-3. Faster women had a reduced risk of stress fracture.[2] Similar findings among trainees[20,36] and among trained infantry soldiers[5,9] have been reported by others. Based on the available evidence, it appears that endurance (as measured by run times) is the best fitness predictor of injury, with risks substantially higher among the worst performers.

TABLE 10-3

RUN-TIME PERFORMANCE AND RISK OF INJURY AMONG US ARMY PERSONNEL

Population	Sex	Distance (mile)	Grouping	Risk (%)	Source
Trainees	Male	1	Quartiles		1
			Q1 (Fastest)	14.3	
			Q2	10.0	
			Q3	26.3	
			Q4 (Slowest)	42.1	
Trainees	Female	1	Quartiles		1
			Q1 (Fastest)	36.1	
			Q2	33.3	
			Q3	57.1	
			Q4 (Slowest)	60.6	
Trainees	Female	2	Quintiles		2
			Q1 (Fastest)	50.0	
			Q2–Q4	67.3	
			Q5 (Slowest)	77.4	
Trainees	Male	2	Quintiles		3
			Q1 (Fastest)	25.9	
			Q2	34.6	
			Q3	42.9	
			Q4	55.5	
			Q5 (Slowest)	40.7	
Trainees	Male	2	Quartiles		4
			Q1 (Fastest)	25	
			Q2	24	
			Q3	39	
			Q4 (Slowest)	49	
Infantry Soldiers	Male	2	Quintiles		5
			Q1 (Fastest)	37.5	
			Q2	20.6	
			Q3	35.3	
			Q4	45.9	
			Q5 (Slowest)	61.1	
Infantry Soldiers	Male	2	Quartiles		6
			Q1 (Fastest)	33[*]	
			Q2	40[*]	
			Q3	48[*]	
			Q4 (Slowest)	52[*]	

[*]All data estimated from graph in Figure 3 in: Directorate of Information and Operations, Department of Defense. *Worldwide U.S. Active Duty Military Personnel Casualties Report, October 1979 through 1994.* Washington, DC: DoD; 1994.
Data sources: (1) Jones BH, Manikowski R, Harris J, et al. *Incidence and Risk Factors for Injury and Illness among Male and Female Army Basic Trainees.* Natick, Mass: US Army Research Institute of Environmental Medicine; 1988. Technical Report T-19-88. (2) Westphal KA, Driedl KE, Sharp MA, et al. *Health, Performance, and Nutritional Status of U.S. Army Women during Basic Combat Training.* Natick, Mass: US Army Research Institute of Environmental Medicine; 1996. Technical Report No. T96-2. (3) Jones BH, Cowan DN, Tomlinson JP, Robinson JR, Polly DW, Frykman PN. Epidemiology of injuries associated with physical training among young men in the Army. *Med Sci Sports Exerc.* 1993;25:197–203. (4) Canham ML, McFerren MA, Jones BH. The association of injury with physical fitness among men and women in gender integrated basic combat training units. *Medical Surveillance Monthly Report.* 1996;2(4):8–12. (5) Reynolds KL, Heckel HA, Witt CE, et al. Cigarette smoking, physical fitness, and injuries in infantry soldiers. *Am J Prev Med.* 1994;10:145–150. (6) Knapik J, Ang P, Reynolds K, Jones B. Physical fitness, age, and injury incidence in infantry soldiers. *J Occup Med.* 1993;35:598–603.

Lack of flexibility has been cited as a risk factor for injuries,[37,38] but this issue has not been adequately resolved. Jones and colleagues[3] found that infantry trainees at both extremes of flexibility were at increased risk of overuse injury, as did Reynolds and colleagues (Table 10-4).[9] Knapik and colleagues[5] reported a similar bimodal pattern in a study of female college athletes. While some have called for specific efforts to increase flexibility and range of motion,[39,40] there is no epidemiologic evidence that greater flexibility or stretching reduces injury risk. Military studies[3,5,9] suggest that maintenance of average or normal flexibility may be important.

Smoking

Cigarette smoking remains quite prevalent among military personnel, particularly among enlisted members. Currently, smoking is not permitted during basic training, but after completion of training, many individuals who were smokers before entry into service resume smoking, and some proportion of previous non-smokers begin smoking. Cigarette smoking has been found to be associated with lower levels of fitness among trainees,

even when other factors such as the level of exercise were controlled for.[41] Smoking has also been identified as a possible risk factor for overuse injury among military personnel. Jones and colleagues[3] found that infantry trainees smoking 10 or more cigarettes per day were approximately 50% more likely ($p < .05$) to experience a training injury than nonsmokers, as is shown in Table 10-5. Among trained infantry soldiers, smokers in one study[9] experienced a greater-than-65% increase in risk of injury ($p < .05$), and a survey[17] of 2,312 active duty female soldiers found that smokers had about a 50% increase in risk ($p < .001$) of stress fracture. Shaffer,[4] however, found no significant association between smoking and risk of stress fracture among male Marine Corps trainees. Ross and Woodward[19] found that among Australian Air Force trainees, smokers had increased risk of all training-related and overuse injuries, but that these increases in risk were not statistically significant.

Extrinsic Risk Factors

Several extrinsic factors have also been identified, and these may be even more appropriate ar-

TABLE 10-4

FLEXIBILITY AND RISK OF INJURY AMONG ARMY PERSONNEL

Grouping	Risk (%)	Source
Quintiles		1
Q1 (least flexible)	49.2	
Q2	38.3	
Q3	20.0	
Q4	33.3	
Q5 (most flexible)	43.6	
Quintiles		2
Q1 (least flexible)	48.5	
Q2	41.0	
Q3	33.3	
Q4	44.4	
Q5 (most flexible)	47.1	

Data Sources: (1) Jones BH, Cowan DN, Tomlinson JP, Robinson JR, Polly DW, Frykman PN. Epidemiology of injuries associated with physical training among young men in the Army. *Med Sci Sports Exerc.* 1993;25:197–203. (2) Reynolds KL, Heckel HA, Witt CE, et al. Cigarette smoking, physical fitness, and injuries in infantry soldiers. *Am J Prev Med.* 1994;10:145–150.

TABLE 10-5

SMOKING AND RISK OF INJURY AMONG ARMY PERSONNEL

Cigarettes Smoked	Risk (%)	Source
None in last year	28.7	1
None in last month	36.7	
1–9/day	34.5	
10–19/day	52.8	
≥ 20/day	49.2	
None	37.0	2
1–10/day	59.2	
> 10/day	64.0	
Nonsmokers	61.8	3
Smokers	77.4	

Data Sources: (1) Jones BH, Cowan DN, Tomlinson JP, Robinson JR, Polly DW, Frykman PN. Epidemiology of injuries associated with physical training among young men in the Army. *Med Sci Sports Exerc.* 1993;25:197–203. (2) Reynolds KL, Heckel HA, Witt CE, et al. Cigarette smoking, physical fitness, and injuries in infantry soldiers. *Am J Prev Med.* 1994;10:145–150. (3) Westphal KA, Driedl KE, Sharp MA, et al. *Health, Performance, and Nutritional Status of U.S. Army Women during Basic Combat Training.* Natick, Mass: US Army Research Institute of Environmental Medicine; 1996. Technical Report No. T96-2.

eas for intervention efforts than are intrinsic factors. The training itself (the total amount of activity and the scheduling of it), footwear, and running surface have all been postulated as being contributors to training injuries. Running more miles and a rapid increase in the level of activity have both been shown to be associated with a higher risk of injury. This is in contrast to running surface (which has not been tied to higher risk of injury) and various insoles (which have not been shown conclusively to protect military personnel from injury).

Training

Training itself has been identified as a risk factor for injuries. Rapid increases in the amount and intensity of training are postulated to be associated with increased levels of injury. Studies of civilian runners have found that those running high mileage have more frequent injuries.[42,43] An elegant experiment conducted in the mid-1970s demonstrated the association between the amount of training and risk of injury.[43] The researchers found that men who did not run had no injuries; those who ran 15 minutes (3 days per week) had an incidence of 22%; those who ran 30 minutes experienced 24% injuries; and those who ran 45 minutes had an injury rate of 54%.

The pattern of training among military recruits may also affect the risk of injury. As with any physical training program, the frequency, intensity, duration, and type of activity must take into account the physical condition of the trainees entering the program to prevent "training error," which increases the risk of injury. Military trainees who enter service with a history of being physically active are at reduced risk of injury, while those who have been more sedentary, and thus experience a rapid acceleration in activity when they enter the military, are at significantly higher risk of injury.[3] These populations must have gradual and appropriate "ramp-up" of physical activity with adequate rest included. Training patterns throughout basic training must also include the physical activity involved in personnel movement throughout the training schedule. For example, in 1996, Navy recruits marched in formation 25 miles in the first 5 days of training.[44] But Jones and colleagues[45] found that running mileage, rather than walking or marching, was most strongly associated with rates of injury. When they compared two companies of infantry trainees, they found that although both groups covered approximately the same total distance of running and marching, the company that did more running had significantly higher rates of injury but did not score

any higher on the final physical fitness test. A safe and effective exercise program will count all weight-bearing, and especially running, mileage and will ensure that all trainees develop an aerobic fitness base that balances running, marching, and other physical activities to avoid training levels above which injury rates increase but fitness does not.

Footwear

Footwear and orthotic devices have been proposed as risk (or protective) factors, but there is little evidence based on solid scientific investigation. US military personnel do not usually run in combat boots, but they routinely march, negotiate obstacle courses, conduct land navigation, train, and fight in boots. The combat boot has been evaluated and considered as an injury hazard.[12,46] Static and dynamic testing of existing combat boots in the laboratory suggests that properties theoretically associated with overuse injury, such as shock attenuation and stability, can be significantly improved with existing technology.

The use of inserts in military footwear as a method of reducing injuries has been evaluated in different settings with inconsistent findings. Smith and colleagues[47] conducted a controlled experiment among Coast Guard trainees in which randomly selected subjects received one of two inserts or no insert. At the end of training, the authors reported dramatic (greater than 50% for both types of insert) reductions in risk of injury, but the relevance of this study is questionable because over half of the injuries were calluses or blisters and no tests of statistical significance were given. Gardner and colleagues[36] conducted a similar randomized trial among Marine Corps recruits in which viscoelastic polymer insoles were provided to some while others used the standard non–shock-absorbing insoles. No significant reduction in the risk of musculoskeletal injury was demonstrated. (A planned, large-scale introduction of these insoles was canceled.) Another study[48] found that insoles made of this viscoelastic polymer did not reduce loading on the legs and feet. The material used in the inserts may be an important factor in determining the efficiency of inserts in reducing injuries. A study of South African military trainees[49] reported a significant and substantial reduction in the incidence of overuse injuries when neoprene (a different material) insoles were used during 9 weeks of training. The contradictory results of these studies indicate that using insoles as an injury reduction effort needs to be further studied before it is either rejected or accepted.

Running Surface

Some have speculated that a hard running surface is a risk factor in exercise-related injuries,[50] while others have found no association.[42] An interesting but not well-explained finding by Shwayhat and colleagues[20] indicated that men who ran on hard surfaces in preparation for entrance into an elite military school were at reduced risk of injury when compared to those who ran on soft surfaces. At present, there is inadequate evidence available for recommending any particular running surface for military training.

INJURY PREVENTION AND CONTROL

An appreciation of the magnitude and impact of training- and exercise-related injuries on military budgets, medical delivery systems, and mission readiness leads to an understanding of the importance of developing effective preventive methods and programs. However, the process of moving from identifying to resolving this problem is complex.

The problem—training injuries—is caused by certain intrinsic and extrinsic factors, including the training itself. There are no "magic bullets" that will eliminate the problem, but each promising intervention should be investigated and considered for implementation. Commanders and military policymakers need to be educated about all aspects of training injuries so they can make broad changes to effect improvements. Finally, research and evaluation of training injuries and intervention programs must be ongoing to identify the most effective and efficient preventive activities.

From a narrower, more scientific perspective, it is known that musculoskeletal injuries in military training populations result from multiple causes and are associated with a variety of risk factors acting together. Prevention of these injuries involves a combination of efforts and should have four main thrusts: (1) identification of intrinsic and extrinsic risk factors for injury, (2) pretraining modification of intrinsic risk factors, (3) modification of extrinsic risk factors, and (4) education of military training and medical personnel on the proper prevention and management of musculoskeletal injuries. There is no one plan or program that alone will be effective.

Once the problem in a military training program is identified, the next step in any effective prevention program is the sound scientific identification of the risk factors for injury. The nature of military training programs provides a controlled environment for valid assessment of injury incidence, physical activity, and lifestyle factors. Sound epidemiologic studies can be performed prospectively or retrospectively, generally in large sample situations. The largest logistical challenge in conducting these studies is integrating the research protocol into the daily activities of the training program and eliciting the support of the training cadre. The scientific challenge is understanding the relative contributions of the constellation of risk factors that make up the injury susceptibility profile.

Once the risk factors for injury have been identified for a given training population, targeted and successful modifications can begin to reduce the operational, fiscal, and health impact of these problems. The modification of any one factor will not eliminate the problem; because of the arduous nature of these training programs and the necessarily abrupt change to the trainee's lifestyle, some level of injury incidence will always be a cost of training. However, the potential for the reduction of injury incidence through modification of one or more factors can be great. For example, among 1,137 Marine Corps recruits in 1994, individuals who exercised less than 3 times per week at low intensity in the 2 months before training and ranked their level of fitness as fair to poor had a 40% excess risk of stress fracture during training.[14] By improving their level of fitness before beginning Marine Corps training, it may be possible to substantially lower their risk of injury. The general challenge of intrinsic risk factor modification is that it usually must be started before training, and in the case of basic training that involves dealing with individuals before enlistment or commission in the military. Regardless of when the modification of intrinsic risk factors begins, it must continue throughout the individual's military career. Screening of individuals with known risk factors for injury can also be employed, but these restrictions are usually only applicable to specific occupational specialties. For example, it may be possible to identify persons with specific risk factors or constellations of factors for injury and assign them to military occupations that require less marching and running than does the infantry.

Extrinsic factors such as operational training activities, physical fitness training activities, and training equipment should be evaluated for safety and effectiveness. Two of the goals of military training are instilling in a recruit an active military lifestyle and improving his or her physical fitness, so it is important to employ sound principles of physical conditioning in all aspects of the training schedule to minimize the effects of overuse injuries. A safe and effective physical conditioning program must consider all daily activities throughout training, such as military-specific training, movement mileage, and structured exercise. Modification of training activities to prevent injuries and improve fitness will have a goal of total body fitness that includes cardiovascular endurance, anaerobic capacity, muscular strength and endurance, high lean-body mass relative to body fat, and joint flexibility for optimal range of motion. The balanced training program for total body fitness is gradual and progressive (weekly training load increases not to exceed 10% to 15%). It stresses the cardiovascular and musculoskeletal systems, includes adequate rest, and is targeted to improve those activities that are important to the military goals of the program. These activities must be continued on a regular basis throughout training. An intervention to reduce injuries that followed these principles was implemented for males in Marine Corps basic training in 1995. An evaluation of this program compared to the existing training schedule demonstrated a significant reduction in overuse injuries, including a 50% reduction in stress fractures, with equal improvement in the physical fitness of recruits at the end of the program (Brodine SK, Shaffer RA, Naval Health Research Center, unpublished data, 1996).

The final and most important aspect of musculoskeletal injury prevention is the education of the military training and medical personnel in safe and effective methods for training and proper management of musculoskeletal problems. The military training cadre must understand and practice the principles of general conditioning and injury prevention with every trainee. The medical personnel supporting these programs need training in the prevention, early identification, and management of overuse injuries. Both of these groups must work closely in each training population to produce the optimum reduction of training injuries.

SUMMARY

Injuries in general, and training related injuries in particular, are a major cause of morbidity, lost duty time, and financial costs to the military. They are also a primary source of crowding in the military outpatient care system. Several modifiable risk factors have been identified, including physical fitness, cigarette smoking, and fitness training. It is known that training programs can be modified to prevent injuries yet still produce physically fit soldiers, sailors, airmen, and marines. Additional study is needed to evaluate the efficiency and effectiveness of modifying other factors, such as footwear. When intervention programs are implemented, rigorous evaluation is required to determine their benefits.

REFERENCES

1. Kowal DM. Nature and causes of injuries in women resulting from an endurance training program. *Am J Sports Med*. 1980;8:265–269.

2. Jones BH, Bovee MW, Harris JM 3d, Cowan DN. Intrinsic risk factors for exercise-related injuries among male and female army trainees. *Am J Sports Med*. 1993;21:705–710.

3. Jones BH, Cowan DN, Tomlinson JP, Robinson JR, Polly DW, Frykman PN. Epidemiology of injuries associated with physical training among young men in the Army. *Med Sci Sports Exerc*. 1993;25:197–203.

4. Shaffer RA, Brodine SK, Ronaghy S, et al. Predicting stress fractures during rigorous physical training simple measures of physical fitness and activity. *Med Sci Sports Exercise*. 1995;27:S78. Abstract.

5. Knapik J, Ang P, Reynolds K, Jones B. Physical fitness, age, and injury incidence in infantry soldiers. *J Occup Med*. 1993;35:598–603.

6. Directorate of Information and Operations, Dept of Defense. *Worldwide U.S. Active Duty Military Personnel Casualties Report, October 1979 through 1994*. Washington, DC: DoD; 1994.

7. Vogel JA, Vanggaard L, Hentze-Eriksen T. Injuries related to physical training. *Annales Medicinae Militaris Belgicae*. 1994;8:49–56.

8. The Injury Prevention and Control Work Group of the Armed Forces Epidemiological Board. *Injuries in the Military: A Hidden Epidemic*. Washington, DC: Armed Forces Epidemiological Board; 1996.

9. Reynolds KL, Heckel HA, Witt CE, et al. Cigarette smoking, physical fitness, and injuries in infantry soldiers. *Am J Prev Med*. 1994;10:145–150.

10. Jones BH, Manikowski R, Harris J, et al. *Incidence and Risk Factors for Injury and Illness among Male and Female Army Basic Trainees*. Natick, Mass: US Army Research Institute of Environmental Medicine; 1988. Technical Report T-19–88.

11. Shaffer RA, Brodine SK, Ito SI, Le AT. Epidemiology of illness and injury among US Navy and Marine Corps female training populations. *Mil Med*. 1999;164:17–21.

12. Bensel CK, Kish RN. *Lower Extremity Disorders among Men and Women in Army Basic Training and Effects of Two Types of Boots*. Natick, Mass: US Army Research and Development Laboratories; 1983. Technical Report NATICK/TR-83/026.

13. Jones BH. Overuse injuries of the lower extremities associated with marching, jogging, and running: a review. *Mil Med*. 1983;148:783–787.

14. Shaffer RA, Brodine SK, Corwin C, et al. Impact of musculoskeletal injury due to rigorous physical activity during U.S. Marine Corps basic training. *Med Sci Sports Exercise*. 1994;26:S141. Abstract.

15. Kaufman K, Brodine SK, Shaffer RA. *Musculoskeletal Injuries in the Military: Literature Review, Summary, and Recommendations*. San Diego, Calif: Naval Health Research Center; 1995. Technical Report 95–33.

16. Tomlinson JP, Lednar WM, Jackson JD. Risk of injury in soldiers. *Mil Med*. 1987;152:60–64.

17. Friedl KE, Nuovo JA, Patience TH, Dettori JR. Factors associated with stress fracture in young army women: indications for further research. *Mil Med*. 1992;157:334–338.

18. Linenger JM, Shwayhat AF. Epidemiology of podiatric injuries in US Marine recruits undergoing basic training. *J Am Podiatr Med Assoc*. 1992;82:269–271.

19. Ross J, Woodward A. Risk factors for injury during basic military training: is there a social element to injury pathogenesis? *J Occup Med*. 1994;36:1120–1126.

20. Shwayhat AF, Linenger JM, Hofherr LK, Slymen DJ, Johnson CW. Profiles of exercise history and overuse injuries among United States Navy Sea, Air, and Land (SEAL) recruits. *Am J Sports Med*. 1994;22:835–840.

21. Milgrom C, Finestone A, Shlamkovitch N, et al. Youth is a risk factor for stress fracture: a study of 783 infantry recruits. *J Bone Joint Surg Br*. 1994;76:20–22.

22. Protzman RR, Griffis CC. Comparative stress fracture incidence in males and females in an equal training environment. *Athletic Training*. 1977;12:126–130.

23. Brudvig TJ, Gudger TD, Obermeyer L. Stress fractures in 295 trainees: a one-year study of incidence related to age, sex, and race. *Mil Med*. 1983;148:666–667.

24. Pester S, Smith PC. Stress fractures in the lower extremities of soldiers in basic training. *Orthop Rev*. 1992;21:297–303.

25. Jones BH, Bovee MH, Knapik JJ. Associations among body composition, physical fitness, and injury in men and women Army trainees. In: Marriott BM, Grumstrup-Scott J, eds. *Body Composition and Physical Performance*. Washington, DC: National Academy Press; 1992: 141–173.

26. Hsu RW, Himeno S, Coventry B, Chao EY. Normal axial alignment of the lower extremity and load-bearing distribution at the knee. *Clin Orthop*. 1990;255:215–227.

27. Cowan DN, Jones BH, Frykman PN, et al. Lower limb morphology and risk of overuse injury among male infantry trainees. *Med Sci Sports Exerc.* 1996;28:945–952.

28. Powell KE, Kohl HW, Caspersen CJ, Blair SN. An epidemiological perspective on the causes of running injuries. *Phys Sports Med.* 1986;14:100–114.

29. Finestone A, Shlamkovitch N, Eldad A, et al. Risk factors for stress fractures among Israeli infantry recruits. *Mil Med.* 1991;156:528–530.

30. Giladi M, Milgrom C, Simkin A, Danon Y. Stress fractures: identifiable risk factors. *Am J Sports Med.* 1991;19:647–652.

31. Beck TJ, Ruff CB, Mourtada FA. Dual-energy X-ray absorptiometry derived structural geometry for stress fracture prediction in male U.S. Marine Corps recruits. *J Bone Miner Res.* 1996;11:645–653.

32. Cowan DN, Jones BH, Robinson JR. Foot morphologic characteristics and risk of exercise-related injury. *Arch Fam Med.* 1993;2:773–777.

33. Giladi M, Milgrom C, Stein M, et al. Exernal rotation of the hip: a predictor of risk for stress fracture. *Clin Orthop.* 1987;216:131–134.

34. Kaufman K, Brodine SK, Shaffer RA, Johnson CW, Cullison TR. The effect of foot structure and range of motion on musculoskeletal overuse injuries. *Am J Sports Med.* 1999;27:585–593.

35. Shaffer RA, Brodine SK, Almeida SA, Williams KM, Ronaghy S. Use of simple measures of physical activity to predict stress fractures in young men undergoing a rigorous physical training program. *Am J Epidemiol.* 1999;149:236–242.

36. Gardner LI Jr, Dziados JE, Jones BH, et al. Prevention of lower extremity stress fractures: a controlled trial of a shock absorbent insole. *Am J Public Health.* 1988;78:1563–1567.

37. Brody DM. Running injuries. *Clin Symp.* 1980;32:1–36.

38. Hoerner EF. Injuries of the lower extremities. In: Vinger PF, Hoerner EF, eds. *Sports Injuries: the Unthwarted Epidemic.* Littleton, Mass: PSG Publishing Company, Inc; 1986: 235–249.

39. James SL, Bates BT, Osternig LR. Injuries to runners. *Am J Sports Med.* 1978;6:40–50.

40. Micheli LJ. Lower extremity overuse injuries. *Acta Med Scand Suppl.* 1986;711:171–177.

41. Conway TL, Cronan TA. Smoking, exercise, and physical fitness. *Prev Med.* 1992;21:723–734.

42. Marti B, Vader JP, Minder CE, Abelin T. On the epidemiology of running injuries: the 1984 Bern Grand-Prix study. *Am J Sports Med.* 1988;16:285–294.

43. Pollock ML, Gettman LR, Milesis CA, Bah MD, Durstine L, Johnson RB. Effects of frequency and duration of training on attrition and incidence of injury. *Med Sci Sports Exerc.* 1977;9:31–36.

44. Almeida SA, Williams KM, Minagawa RY, Benas DM, Shaffer RA. *Guidelines for Developing a Physical Training Program for U.S. Navy Recruits.* San Diego, Calif: Naval Health Research Center; 1996. Technical Report 96-11K.

45. Jones BH, Cowan DN, Knapik JJ. Exercise, training and injuries. *Sports Med.* 1994;18:202–214.

46. deMoya RG. A biomechanical comparison of the running shoe and the combat boot. *Mil Med.* 1982;147:380–383.

47. Smith W, Walter J Jr, Bailey M. Effects of insoles in Coast Guard basic training footwear. *J Am Podiatr Med Assoc.* 1985;75:644–647.

48.   Nigg BM, Herzog W, Read LJ. Effect of viscoelastic insoles on vertical impact forces in heel-toe running. *Am J Sports Med*. 1988;16:70–76.

49.   Schwellnus MP, Jordaan G, Noakes TD. Prevention of common overuse injuries by the use of shock absorbing insoles: a prospective study. *Am J Sports Med*. 1990;18:636–641.

50.   Clement DB, Taunton JE, Smart GE, McNicol KL. A survey of overuse running injuries. *Physician Sportsmed*. 1981;9:47–58.

MILITARY PREVENTIVE MEDICINE: MOBILIZATION AND DEPLOYMENT
Volume 1

Section 3: Preparing for Deployment

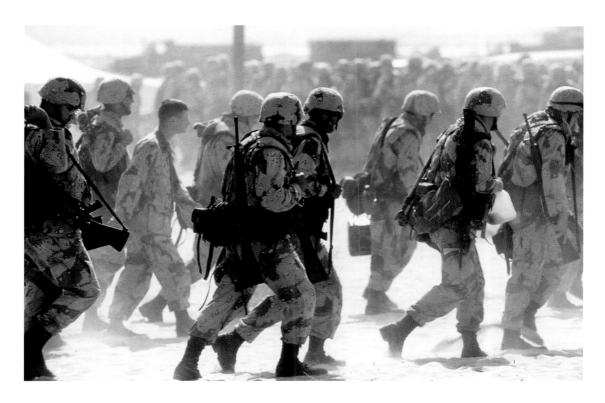

Before these Marines arrived in Southwest Asia for the Persian Gulf War, an impressive amount of planning and coordination had been done by preventive medicine professionals on their behalf. The health threats facing these Marines had been assessed, plans had been made to counteract those threats, and systems had been put into place to monitor their health status during and after the deployment. These efforts were focused on keeping disease and nonbattle injuries to a minimum—and they worked.

Photograph: Courtesy of the Defense Visual Information Center, March Air Reserve Base, California. Image 47 on the CD-ROM "U.S. Forces in Desert Storm."

Chapter 11

MEDICAL THREAT ASSESSMENT

BRUNO P. PETRUCCELLI, MD, MPH; AND BONNIE L. SMOAK, MD, PhD, MPH

B. P. Petruccelli, Lieutenant Colonel, Medical Corps, US Army; Director, Epidemiology & Disease Surveillance, US Army Center for Health Promotion and Preventive Medicine, 5158 Blackhawk Road, Aberdeen Proving Ground, MD 21010-5403

B. L. Smoak, Colonel, Medical Corps, US Army; Director, Division of Tropical Public Health, Department of Preventive Medicine and Biometrics, Uniformed Services University of the Health Sciences, 4301 Jones Bridge Road, Bethesda, MD 20814-4799

INTRODUCTION

Medical threat has been defined as "the composite of all ongoing or potential enemy actions and environmental conditions that will reduce combat effectiveness through wounding, injuring, causing disease or performance degradation."[1(p2)] During preparation for deployment, it is critical that commanders at strategic and operational levels acquire an estimate of the medical threat for the mission. Chapter 1 reviews the concepts of medical threat assessment, medical threat estimate, and the impact of the medical threat on commanders' operational plans. This chapter will describe the generic elements of a medical threat assessment in the predeployment phase, but as it is within a textbook emphasizing the preventive medicine aspects of military operations, it will not address estimating enemy force projection and weapons capabilities or planning the countermeasures to these intentional, hostile sources of harm. Instead, the following discussion focuses on the disease and nonbattle injury (DNBI) component of the medical threat.

Commanders must know what measures to take to protect their personnel from DNBI. A good assessment will identify medical threats that can decrease the fighting force by lowering fighting effectiveness and causing morbidity and mortality. Specific countermeasures can then be identified to reduce or eliminate these threats. The threat assessment is a dynamic process. After the initial information is obtained and countermeasures instituted, the assessment must be continually evaluated during and after the operation to ensure that the preventive measures are working and to identify new threats before significant casualties can occur. Typically, a threat assessment is developed when military personnel are sent to a foreign country, but this step is just as important when those servicemembers train in the United States. Medical casualties can occur from infectious agents and environmental elements, such as heat and cold, in the United States as well as abroad. Although it is not possible to fully predict disease and injury rates before a deployment, the assessment is used to guide medical policy.

FRAMEWORK FOR ASSESSMENT

Accurately identifying threats depends on knowing basic information that answers four essential questions: Who? What? When? and Where? Figure 11-1 illustrates how these questions correspond to the traditional epidemiologic triads of host-agent-environment and person-place-time. "What" refers to the nature of the operation itself and the related activities that are predicted to occur. Table 11-1 lists more specific questions to be considered in a threat assessment. The variable "who" (ie, the population) merits brief elaboration here.

The Population at Risk

Clearly defining the "who"—the group or population at risk—is the first step in developing a medical threat assessment. Generally, assessments are performed at the operational level, and the entire deployed force is treated as a single group. All threats in the area of operation are considered, but not all subgroups of personnel have the same risk of exposure to each of the threats. For example, soldiers having close contact with the indigenous population, such as military police or Special Forces teams, have a much different risk for particular diseases (eg, tuberculosis) than soldiers lacking that exposure. Sometimes, US medical officers may be asked to consider the indigenous population as the group at risk. For example, during Operation Uphold Democracy in 1994, there was initial concern that United Nations peacekeeping forces could bring chloroquine-resistant *Plasmodium falciparum* to the island of Hispaniola. Clearly, identifying the population to be protected is a prerequisite to developing a medical threat assessment.

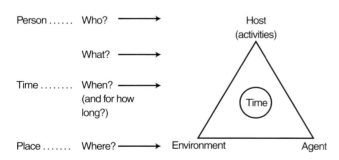

Fig. 11-1. This conceptual drawing shows the interdependent relationships among principal factors inducing a disease or injury. A host population and its activities encounter injurious agents in a given environment, during a specific time (eg, of day, of year) and for a specific duration. The synchronization or convergence of these factors determines the probability of injury and its magnitude in individuals or across groups.

TABLE 11-1

SPECIFIC FACTORS TO CONSIDER WHEN ASSESSING THE RISK OF DISEASE AND INJURY

Factors	Examples
Person Factors	
Number	Total population in the area of operations
Demography	Age, sex, culture
Health status	Medical history, current condition, immunity (eg, vaccinations, prior exposures)
Psychosocial	Psychological stress, sleep deprivation, desynchronosis, morale
Training	Combat, survival, physical, military occupational, hygiene
Equipment	Personal protection (eg, clothing, footwear, repellent)
Activity	Operation (eg, movement, work-rest cycles), occupation (eg, chemical, biological, physical, ergonomic), recreation (especially sports injuries, contact with water), behaviors (especially hygiene, sexuality, risk-taking)
Place Factors	
Global position	Latitude: arctic, temperate, tropical; longitude: Americas, Africa-Mediterranean, Asia, East Asia-Pacific
Development and stability	Sanitation, industrialization, waste management, vector control, stability food and water supplies, medical facilities
Terrain	Desert (eg, sand and dust, navigation), mountain (eg, altitude, energy expenditure), rain forest (eg, vectors, immersion), urban vs. rural setting
Climate	Temperature (hot vs. cold), relative humidity (wet vs. dry), wind
Biomass	Flora (eg, natural food supply, toxic plants, movement inhibition), fauna (eg, disease vectors and reservoirs, venomous animals)
Enclosures	Tentage, buildings, aircraft, ships, small vessels, vehicles, ventilation
Agent Factors	
Pathogens	Prevalence, infectivity, virulence, resistance (to immunity, drugs)
Vectors	Vector control measures applied by deploying force
Equipment	Passive safety devices in vehicles and equipment
Time Factors	
Year	Long-cycle variables (eg, pandemics)
Season	Seasonal or climate-dependent variables (eg, dry season and meningococcal disease, rainy season and malaria)
Time of day	Diurnally variable vectors, night safety, temperatures
Duration	Increased cumulative risk from longer stays

Once this is established, the other basic information of what, when, and where should be obtained. Information needed includes the planned activities of the group, the expected time and duration of the operation, and a more precise geographic location of the area of operation (see Table 11-1).

Information Sources

The next step in developing a threat assessment is to identify the potential threats themselves. Table 11-2 lists the principal military and civilian sources of pertinent information. An example of the depth of infor-

TABLE 11-2

SOURCES OF HEALTH RISK INFORMATION

Organization or Agency	Product Example
Military	
Armed Forces Medical Intelligence Center, Fort Detrick, Md	Medical Environmental Disease Intelligence and Counter measures (MEDIC) CD-ROM
Defense Pest Management Information Analysis Center, Silver Spriing, Md	Disease Vector Ecology Profiles (DVEP)
US Army Center for Health Promotion and Preventive Medicine, Aberdeen Proving Ground, Md, and subordinate units in Japan and Europe	Surveillance data
US Navy Environmental Health Center, Norfolk, Va, and Navy Environmental Preventive Medicine Units in Pearl Harbor, San Diego, Norfolk, and Sicily Profiles	Disease Risk Assessment Profiles (DISRAP), surveillance data
US Army Medical Research and Materiel Command, Fort Detrick, Md, and overseas laboratories in Thailand and Kenya	Research reports
US Navy Medical Research Command, Bethesda, Md, and overseas laboratories in Indonesia, Peru, and Egypt	Research reports
Civilian	
World Health Organization, Geneva, Switzerland, and Washington, DC Pan American Health Organization and Caribbean Epidemiology Centre	Weekly Epidemiologic Record
US Centers for Disease Control and Prevention, Atlanta, Ga	*Health Information for International Travel*
National Library of Medicine, Bethesda, Md	MEDLINE and other literature retrieval systems
US Department of State, Washington, DC	Travelers' Advisories, Background Notes
Ministries of Health of nations in region of interest	Ad hoc reports
Universities with overseas activities	Ad hoc reports
Medical publishers, electronic conferences	Textbooks, handbooks, travel web sites, consultants medicine software programs, ProMED Mail (NY State Dept of Health)

mation available from these sources is the extensive database on country-specific flora and fauna, including the arthropod vectors of militarily important diseases, maintained by the Defense Pest Management Information Analysis Center (Silver Spring, Md). The Armed Forces Medical Intelligence Center (Fort Detrick, Md) produces timely, detailed reports of country-specific environmental, infectious disease, and other health risks of military operational importance. It draws its information from multiple sources, including official, international reports of health, morbidity, and mortality; published scientific studies; and validated reports from the lay press.

The Internet, both through the World Wide Web and electronic mail services, offers countless possible sources of international health and safety information. A useful example is the Program for Monitoring Emerging Diseases (ProMED), a free electronic mail conference through SatelLife and HealthNet, which reaches participants throughout the world. Through this medium, epidemiologists and medical scientists can immediately report emerging or reemerging problems in specific geographic areas.

Not listed in Table 11-2 but also important are institutions that house military history resources; recent, peacetime data are best extrapolated in the context of past military operations in a comparable environment. Valuable collections may be accessed at the Center for Military History (Fort McNair, Washington, DC), the Uniformed Services University of the Health Sciences (Bethesda, Md), the National Library of Medicine (Bethesda, Md), and the individual services medical doctrinal centers (Army Medical Department Center and School, San Antonio, Tex; Naval School of Health Sciences, Bethesda, Md; Air Force School of Aerospace Medicine, San Antonio, Tex). Information is sometimes available from past deployments and from special assessment teams, such as those that might be part of the advanced party for a particular deployment. Other governmental agencies can also provide useful information. For example, the National Institutes of Health have active research projects in several foreign countries. Nongovernmental sources, such as missionaries or nongovernmental humanitarian organizations, can often provide current information about health threats in the countries in which they serve. A review of the scientific literature is extremely helpful. Note that disease and injury occurrence in native populations differs from that which might be expected among expatriates. Infectious disease rates in the indigenous pediatric population of an underdeveloped country may be the best model of expected disease risk in military personnel arriving from a developed country. Those servicemembers, unlike the indigenous adults, lack immunity to diseases that are usually acquired early in life in underdeveloped areas.

Regardless of its source, information should be carefully assessed for quality and completeness. It is rare, however, for any dataset or statement about health risks to accurately reflect the actual risks to be faced by deploying personnel. Typically, for example, reported rates of infectious diseases account for 10% or less of the actual number of cases that can be identified in a given geographic area through intensive surveys. Even in industrialized countries, where compliance with public health notification requirements tends to be better than in less-developed countries, published communicable disease rates should be at least doubled to reflect actual occurrence.[2] Exhibit 11-1 lists some of the main factors contributing to the nonreliability of risk information.

As a rule, published reports are more reliable quantitatively when they are describing significant epidemics or when the disease in question is distinct in its rarity, severity, or the reliability and relative simplicity with which a laboratory test can detect its presence. Reporting also tends to be more complete from regions where modern medical facilities are available and where there are no barriers to either medical care or disease reporting[2]. It should be remembered that many of the geographic areas to which the US military deploys have had years of civil strife and lack an adequate infrastructure to obtain current, accurate medical information. Thus an absence of information does not necessarily mean there is an absence of threat.

EXHIBIT 11-1

FACTORS COMPROMISING THE RELIABILITY OF PUBLISHED DISEASE REPORTS

Reporting Factors
  Nonreportable diseases
  Variable reporting criteria
  Underreporting
  Lack of communications
  Reporting biases
Data Collection Factors
  Biased studies
  Variable denominator
  Variable diagnostic capability
Social, Geographic Factors
  Borders that are political or economic, not ecological
  Cultural adaptation to endemic disease
Disease Factors
  Inapparent infections
  Long latencies
  Importations
  Variable immunization
  Disease periodicity
  Secular trends
  Variable persistence of agents, vectors, reservoirs
  Agent adaptation

THREAT CATEGORIES

Potential threats to health can be divided into cause-effect categories as follows: (a) battle injuries, (b) nonbattle injuries, (c) environmental injuries, (d) psychological stress, and (e) infectious diseases. Table 11-3 presents a summary of these.

Battle Injuries

Producing an estimate of combat casualties, while extremely important to medical planning, is not primarily a task of medical personnel. Likewise, the prevention of combat wounds is in the purview of military tactics and not preventive medicine. It should be noted, however, that these injuries have accounted for an increasing proportion of total mortality during wars as the sophistication and lethality of weapon systems has rapidly increased. At the same time, the sophistication of countermeasures to DNBI has also increased, accounting for fewer dramatic disease outbreaks and fewer transportation catastrophes during military operations. Nevertheless, DNBI remains the most likely cause of morbidity among deployed military personnel and has the potential to cause a large number of casualties, particularly during prolonged missions. However, medical readiness should not focus solely on the category or source of a particular threat. For example, an early medical response to mass casualties takes precedence over determining hostile versus nonhostile cause. Likewise the potential for enemy use of chemical or biological agents cannot be ignored when planning for medical countermeasures (eg, vaccinations) to toxic or infectious threats.

Nonbattle Injuries

Nonbattle injuries include those that result from aircraft, watercraft, or motor vehicle crashes, unintended fires or explosions, unsafe operation of heavy equipment, improper lifting of excessive weight, slips, trips, falls, and collisions during activities such as construction, bivouacking, and sports. Human risk factors include alcohol use, prescribed or self-administered drug ingestion, inadequate sleep, and time zone shift.

Environmental Injuries

Environmental hazards exist in every theater and can be divided into living and non-living threats. Living environmental hazards include venomous snakes and arthropods, poisonous plants and fishes,

and ectoparasites. Nonliving hazards include conditions such as heat, cold, dust, altitude, and pollution. The buildup of industrial waste, whether chemical or radioactive, in many countries has been uncontrolled and is difficult to quantitate as a health risk. The potential effects on personnel of inadvertent exposure to environmental and industrial hazards range from the chronic and subclinical to the acute and lethal. As is true with infectious diseases, there are intoxications that are "battle-stoppers" when acute effects predominate (eg, respiratory irritants in severe air pollution) and those that have little or no impact on operational effectiveness but may affect individuals over time (eg, adverse reproductive effects of a potent mutagen).

Psychological Stress

The importance of mental health in deployments is easily underestimated, partly because the real stresses of war can be neither reproduced nor simulated during even the most realistic training exercises. Ignoring the probability of psychological trauma, though, will almost surely have a major adverse impact on the health of the command. Such stresses as the absence of family and friends, uncertainties of personal safety, loss of privacy, new job requirements, and unresolved personal problems are to be expected during major deployments, even if there are no hostilities. These stresses significantly increase the risk of inappropriate behavior, anxiety disorders, depression, suicidal ideation, suicide, and homicide among deployed personnel. During hostilities, these behavioral shifts are further aggravated by the acute and delayed effects of combat stress, loss of companions, and friendly fire incidents.

Infectious Disease

Throughout human history, infectious diseases have caused the largest number of nonbattle casualties. Critical to the thoroughness and accuracy of medical threat assessments is an understanding of the basic epidemiology of significant human infections, including their modes of transmission and incubation periods, and the global distribution of geographically specific agents. In addition to the relevant, disease-specific sections of this textbook, there are numerous excellent textbooks and manuals available that permit a rapid review of all of these facts for any of the important human pathogens.

TABLE 11-3

CATEGORIES OF MEDICAL THREAT

Mode of Transmission or Etiological Group	Effects of Agents
Battle-related Injuries	
Small arms	Trauma from low and high velocity bullets, bayonets
Fragmentation ordnance	Trauma from artillery, mortars, bombs, rockets, grenades, mines
Blast effect munitions	Injuries from fuel-air explosives, blasts
Flame and incendiary munitions	Burns from napalm, white phosphorus
Directed-energy devices	Injuries from lasers, charged-particle beams, radio frequency
Chemical warfare agents	Toxicosis or tissue injury by cyanides, nerve agents, lung toxicants, vesicants, incapacitating agents, lacrimators, sternutators, vomiting agents
Biological warfare agents	Bacterial or viral disease; intoxication by bacterial, marine, fungal, plant, or venom toxins
Nonbattle Injuries	
Unintentional	Injuries from transportation, machinery, noise, fires, explosions, falls, sports, drowning, poisoning
Intentional	Homicide, suicide
Environmental Injuries	
Temperature	Heat stroke, immersion foot, frostbite, hypothermia
Solar radiation	Sunburn, photokeratitis
Altitude	Mountain sickness, pulmonary edema, cerebral edema
Plants	Dermatitis, toxic ingestion
Animals	Envenomation, bite wounds
Natural disasters and storms	Trauma, asphyxia, lightning strike
Psychological Stress	
Battle (Combat Stress Casualty)	Battle fatigue, combat and post-traumatic stress disorders
Nonbattle (Operational Stress Casualty)	Desynchronosis, depression, anxiety disorders, violence
Infectious	
Respiratory	Meningitis, pneumonia, influenza
Disease	
Fecal-oral	Diarrhea, typhoid fever, hepatitis
Arthropod-borne	Malaria, leishmaniasis, dengue
Soilborne, waterborne	Hookworm, schistosomiasis
Human contact	Sexually transmitted diseases
Animal contact	Q fever, brucellosis, rabies

Arthropod-borne diseases, such as malaria, arboviral fevers, leishmaniasis, and rickettsioses, have the potential to infect a large number of personnel and cause severe morbidity and mortality. Diseases that are transmitted by the fecal-oral route have also caused significant casualties in military forces[3–5]. Included in this category are the secretory and inflammatory enteritides that can manifest as severe diarrhea; the etiologic agents of these may be protozoal (eg, Giardia, Entamoeba), bacterial (eg, Escherichia coli, shigellae, salmonellae, vibrios), or viral (eg, caliciviruses, rotaviruses). Other enterically transmitted agents produce syndromes in which diarrhea is not a primary manifestation. Among these, typhoid fever and hepatitis A have the greatest potential for battle-stopping casualties if servicemembers are not appropriately immunized. A variety of helminthiases are also transmissible by ingestion but would rarely be expected to cause significant epidemics in the military setting.

Diseases that are transmitted by the respiratory route, either through secretions or as airborne particles, have historically been of greatest significance during basic training and not in the deployed setting. Even today, streptococcal and viral respiratory infections are mainly training camp hazards. However, the impact of respiratory pathogens on combat effectiveness may be underestimated because large, etiologically specific outbreaks have not often been identified while US forces are overseas. Medical surveillance data during large exercises and recent operations reveal that acute upper respiratory infections are a common reason for seeking medical care among deployed troops. Rates have been higher among personnel housed in fixed facilities (versus tents)[4] and among those afloat in smaller vessels (versus aircraft carriers)[6]. Universal use of meningococcal and influenza vaccines among basic trainees has nearly eliminated the diseases of greatest severity during basic training, although the potential remains for reemergence of group B meningo-coccus as a dominant organism since there is currently no licensed vaccine for it. The benefit of these vaccines very likely extends to overseas missions as well.

Sexually transmissible and bloodborne pathogens (eg, gonococci, treponemes, hepatitis B virus) and pathogens transmitted by contact with soil (eg, hookworm, strongyloides), water (eg, schistosoma, leptospira), and animals (eg, brucella, coxiella, rabies virus) have a wide range of virulence and of latency between infection and disease. Soil-transmitted helminths often cause subclinical infection, while rabies is universally fatal to the unimmunized. Leptospirosis, an acute systemic illness, can make personnel noneffective but full recovery without sequelae is typical, while syphilis is rarely disabling during its acute phase but can be severely disabling over the lifetime of individual patients. An epidemiologic characteristic that most of these agents share is that their potential for causing operationally significant epidemics involving large numbers of servicemembers is generally quite low. Still, the cumulative effect on clusters of individuals or relatively small, high-risk groups (eg, Special Forces units) could have a significant impact if enough persons are symptomatic during the critical phase of a mission.

A country's public health infrastructure and the availability of basic medical care to its population have an immeasurable impact on the level of disease and injury risks among nonindigenous personnel that occupy or reside in the country. Risks must be assessed from the standpoint of outcomes (eg, disease and injury rates, antibody seroprevalences) and existing controls (eg, quality and distribution of water supply, waste management, safety standards, disease case finding and treatment). Furthermore, whatever the available outcome data documented for a specific area, it can be assumed that war or natural disaster will have disrupted both the ecology and any industrial base.

PRIORITIZATION OF RISKS

Creating a list of all possible injuries and diseases that can affect personnel during the deployment is rarely helpful. A comprehensive list of possible risks for any given deployment is typically too long to be of practical value and can impede the medical staff officer's effort to focus the commander's attention on the most important countermeasures. Thus prioritization of the threat is one of the most critical steps in the entire assessment process.

Reducing the complexity of risk analysis to the two-dimensional categorization illustrated in Figure 11-2 can be helpful. Forming the axes of a four-quadrant table are (a) the likelihood that particular types of injury or disease will occur among personnel in the area of operations and (b) the potential for epidemic or mass-casualty presentation of the problem, which may be viewed as the population-level equivalent of acuteness. Events for which both of these are high (quad-

Probability of Occurrence

		High	Low
	High	I	II
Potential for Epidemics or Mass Casualties			
	Low	III	IV

Fig. 11-2. The projected impact of diseases, nonbattle injuries, and combat stress casualties on military operations is determined by two principal likelihoods: that of occurrence in the first place and that of causing multiple casualties within a relatively narrow time window. This categorical illustration simplifies the continuous distribution that these two probabilities, when multiplied, might produce for any given type of casualty. During operations planning, assignment of important, predicted casualties to two or more of these four quadrants is one way to prioritize countermeasures and limit the detail of command briefings, annexes, and rapid educational material.

rant I) must be reflected in the operational plan (OPLAN) and briefed as the significant threat (see chapter 13, Preventive Medicine and the Operational Plan). Less likely events deserve consideration in medical planning if they have the potential for affecting large numbers of personnel simultaneously within operational units (quadrant II). Events striking individuals in a sporadic fashion will generally not require special consideration by medical planners and logisticians, even though they may be quite likely to occur (quadrant III). Nevertheless, treatment and evacuation capabilities in the theater should be prepared for these expected events.

Within each quadrant, it is useful to prioritize predicted events further, giving greatest weight to events that are most likely to occur and to adversely affect military operations. For example, if a battalion based in the continental United States is deploying to a tropical area in February, heat casualties and arboviral fevers would probably be considered first quadrant events. Further prioritization might then depend on the timing of planned operations. For units expected to engage in battle soon after arrival, heat casualty prevention and treatment would be given top priority. Those expected to undergo a gradual build-up or remain in a defensive posture for a period of weeks will acclimatize, and any heat injuries that do occur will have little impact on the mis-

sion. For these units, arboviral fever prevention and treatment may be given the highest priority.

One of the most important determinants of epidemic or mass-casualty potential is the rapidity with which a particular event is expected to occur once a unit is in a position of risk for that event once they are exposed. In the context of infectious risks, this translates into the incubation period or latency. Short-latency conditions (2 weeks or less) are significantly more likely to disrupt operations. The incubation period in these cases varies little among exposed individuals, so events tend to occur nearly simultaneously among large numbers of servicemembers (for common-source exposures) or propagate over a relatively short period (for conditions spread from person to person). Thus diarrhea, while rarely serious in any individual, is likely to have a greater impact on the maneuver phase of an operation than schistosomiasis, even though it is likely to be a serious infection in those affected. This contrast holds true even if both of these conditions derived from a single, simultaneous exposure among hundreds of personnel. Many events may be assigned a low priority because nearly all servicemembers are resistant to them. For example, some infectious diseases are unlikely to manifest because of widespread immunity acquired through immunization (eg, typhoid, yellow fever) or natural disease (eg, varicella).

The prioritization of medical threats also depends on how successful countermeasures are likely to be during the deployment. In turn, the success of preventive measures in lowering DNBI rates depends on the degree to which personnel have been trained in these measures, on command emphasis and directives, and on the tactical situation. During the early stages of a deployment or in combat, personnel must often rely solely on individual prophylactic and preventive measures. This will work only if they have been adequately trained and that training is enforced routinely by the leaders of small units. In a more stable tactical situation, environmental controls can be instituted, such as area spraying with insecticides for vector control. Developing a medical threat assessment for a given operation is actually an art that balances the likelihood of any given disease or injury against the probability that countermeasures will prevent the disease or injury and against the expected impact of this casualty type on the operation.

QUANTITATION OF RISK

To understand the challenges and limitations presented by any attempt to estimate the anticipated

number of DNBI casualties in a particular operation, it is useful to consider a theoretical, idealized model. The chance that a soldier, sailor, Marine, or airman will suffer DNBI during a mission is the function of a baseline probability (b_0), unrelated to the deployment, plus the sum of numerous factors (x_i), each multiplied by its own probability coefficient (b_i):

$$PR(DNBI) = b_0 + b_1x_1 + b_2x_2 + b_3x_3 + \dots b_ix_i$$

Multiplying the probability of DNBI by the total number of military personnel taking part in the mission will deliver the total number of casualties not directly resulting from combat. The factors may vary by time and place. For example, if x_2 represents ambient temperatur—which directly affects the likelihood of heat injuries, cold injuries, and other adverse health events—it will have different values for different locations, seasons, and times of day. Each of the other factors is represented by another x_i. If enough data were available from a variety of previously completed missions, solving for all of the coefficients would construct a predictive model.

Multifactorial, mathematical models to predict disease, NBI, or combat stress casualties have not been applied in practice. Models to predict outcomes from specific physiologic stresses, such as heat,[7,8] have been described, but these have not been

correlated with actual casualty data. Models have been developed for predicting battle casualties, but estimates derived from applying those models to actual operations have often failed to approximate observed outcomes. Some experts have advocated the application of historical data to specific scenarios while adjusting for expected battle intensities and other variables in a very general way, without detailed formulae. Given the complexity of human, environmental, and other factors influencing force health, this same argument can certainly be made for prediction of DNBI.

In 1996, the Army Medical Department Center and School convened a subject-matter expert panel to develop estimates of DNBI hospitalization rates for the major contingency areas—namely, for a major regional conflict (MRC) in the East (ie, Southwest Asia scenario) and for an MRC in the West (ie, Korea scenario). A similar panel had been convened in 1992, and more consensus meetings are planned to continue refining the estimates. The 1996 panel members considered historical data from World War II, the Korean War, the Vietnam War, Operations Desert Shield and Desert Storm, and deployment experiences over the previous 5 years. They were assisted by decision support software. Projected rates were determined as medians of members' es-

TABLE 11-4

EXPECTED DISEASE AND NONBATTLE INJURY IN MAJOR CONTINGENCY AREAS, BY INTENSITY OF COMBAT AND POSITION IN THE AREA OF OPERATIONS[*]

Area of Operations	Intensity of Conflict				
	Expected Disease Rates, MRC[†] East (Southwest Asia)				
	None	**Light**	**Moderate**	**Heavy**	**Intense**
Division	0.60	1.62	2.13	2.51	2.89
Corps	0.59	1.32	1.69	1.96	2.15
COMMZ[†]	0.45	0.50	0.53	0.56	0.59
	Expected Disease Rates, MRC[†] West (Korea)				
Division	0.73	1.68	2.16	2.59	3.02
Corps	0.68	1.35	1.69	2.04	2.38
COMMZ[‡]	0.45	0.49	0.51	0.53	0.55
	Expected Nonbattle Injury Rates, MRC[†] East and West (Combined)				
Division	0.15	0.32	0.65	0.80	1.00
Corps	0.15	0.25	0.50	0.60	0.70
COMMZ[‡]	0.13	0.13	0.14	0.15	0.16

[*]The rates are per 1,000 personnel per day.
[†]Major Regional Conflict
[‡]Communications zone
Source: An expert panel convened at the US Army Medical Department Center and School, Fort Sam Houston, Tex: 1996.

EXHIBIT 11-2

EXPECTED RATIOS OF COMBAT STRESS CASUALTIES IN MAJOR CONTINGENCY AREAS

CS rapid return to duty:[*]
  Troop strength   1 : 1,000
CSC : Troop strength   0.025 : 1,000
CSC : Wounded in action   1 : 8
CSC : Disease   3 : 1,000

---

[*]Initial combat stress presentations that return to duty within 3 days; no diagnosis
Source: An expert panel convened at the US Army Medical Department Center and School, Fort Sam Houston, Tex: 1996.

---

timates. Their results are summarized in Table 11-4. A separate panel was convened to consider combat stress casualties (CSC) (Exhibit 11-2). Overall there was consensus on several assumptions and conclusions regarding prediction of DNBI and CSC:

- Rates depend on where troops are deployed, troops' linear position within the MRC (including distance from communications zone), and operational tempo.
- NBI rates vary little but disease rates differ between different MRCs.
- Rates vary by intensity of combat. (The difference in rates between moderate and light combat equals one-third of the difference in rates between moderate combat and no combat. Rates for heavy combat equal approximately the mean between moderate and intense combat.)
- Limited mobility, and thus greater concentration of troops within circumscribed areas, is correlated with higher disease rates (as reflected in data from the Korean War[9]).
- Combat, anticipated combat, and operational stress are likely to degrade emphasis on prophylactic measures and can have an adverse effect on immunity.
- Incidents such as inadvertent provision of contaminated food from host-nation or allied sources are unpredictable but can occur in any operation.
- The baseline medical condition of Reserve personnel may not be as good as that of Active Duty personnel.
- Many NBIs are due to sports and other recreational activities.
- At least 60% of CSC cases held for treatment at Level 2 (medical companies or clearing stations) will be returned to duty at that level within 3 days.
- One CSC may be expected for every eight wounded in action. (See Exhibit 11-2.)

Comparison of current estimates and ratios to historical statistics reveals moderate to marked decreases in predicted rates of disease, NBI, and CSC since previous major operations. A common conclusion of both the DNBI and the CSC panels was that improvements in training, leader development, and prevention capabilities account for these drops.

THREAT COMMUNICATION

The threat needs to be communicated to (a) commanders, to assist them in prioritizing the movement of specialized personnel and equipment and factor expected casualties into operational planning (eg, to consider time of day, season, acclimatization period), (b) medical personnel, to allow them to prepare mentally and logistically for the conditions they can expect to be treating, particularly those that are considered exotic in the United States, and (c) servicemembers, to raise their awareness, help them separate facts from myths, and induce them to use protective measures.

The format of the information, of course, will have to be suited to the recipient. For the commander, the highest priority threats should be clearly identified in a briefing or memorandum before the medical portion of the OPLAN is written. An example of this might be: "The major DNBI threats are the extreme heat, mosquito-borne fever illnesses, contaminated local food sources, and unreliable bottled water. The highest priority should be given to advanced deployment to allow for acclimatization, pretreatment of the BDU with permethrin and early shipment of deet insect repellent, rations, and water purification equipment." Threat and countermeasure information is normally placed in Annex Q of the OPLAN, but it may be appropriate to insert the most important elements of the threat into other parts of the plan, including the main body, where it will be more visible to commanders.

For the task force and unit surgeons, technical literature should be provided for transmittal to clinics and hospitals (eg, review articles or field manuals on the prevention and treatment of malaria). For the servicemembers, mass-produced educational cards or booklets should be written in clear and easily understood language and should emphasize the most important personal measures (eg, "Using your insect repellent can save your life from deadly diseases spread by mosquitoes.").

COUNTERMEASURES

Threat countermeasures that are instituted during the predeployment and sustainment phases are discussed elsewhere in this textbook. Assuming the best available engineering controls are in place, command emphasis on the enforcement of safety standards is the most important countermeasure to nonbattle injuries, and training should be as realistic as possible without compromising injury prevention. One important concept that applies equally to injury avoidance and disease control is that of preventive maintenance for the human. Unit cohesiveness, the buddy system, strong morale, fair discipline, personal hygiene, and adequate sleep are among the many elements that, though difficult to measure objectively, have a positive impact on every function of the human machine.

Psychological stresses can be reduced by simple actions, such as keeping personnel informed, ensuring mail deliveries, and scheduling recreation time and meals.

Excellent vaccines have been developed against diseases that several decades ago stopped military campaigns. Chemoprophylactic drugs are also available for diseases such as malaria and leptospirosis. When safe food and water are consumed and proper sanitation and hygiene are maintained, the incidence of diseases transmitted through the fecal-oral route will be very low. Similarly, the use of personal protection measures, such as repellent and proper wearing of the uniform, will decrease the likelihood of arthropod-borne diseases.

CONTINUAL REASSESSMENT

A medical threat assessment is an evolving process. It serves different functions at different times during the deployment. Prior to the operation, it is used to obtain command approval for the necessary preventive measures and to initiate appropriate immunizations. It can also be used to educate the deploying personnel about potential medical risks in the theater, as well as risks that could occur before deployment. For example, sexually transmitted diseases and unintentional injuries may increase just prior to deployment, so preventive measures should be instituted. The medical threat assessment must be continued during the deployment. Medical information must be continually gathered and analyzed. Disease and injury surveillance is critical in assessing the health of the force and the success of the preventive measures taken. Disease vectors and reservoirs should also be assessed once personnel are in-theater. Outbreaks and unusual clinical syndromes should be investigated in-theater to help identify those agents affecting personnel. During the initial weeks of Operation Restore Democracy (Haiti, 1994–1995), rates of febrile illness among the US forces increased unexpectedly. Dengue was suspected, and dengue virus was isolated later from the blood of several febrile soldiers.[10] Although dengue was known to be present in the Caribbean islands, the intensity of transmission was not appreciated until 20,000 nonimmune US servicemembers were sent to Haiti.

Medical assessments must continue even after the force has left the theater. Diseases with long incubation periods may become apparent only after the servicemembers return home. It was after the first soldiers and Marines returned to the United States from Operation Restore Hope (Somalia, 1992) and were diagnosed with malaria that medical officers became aware of the exposure of hundreds of personnel to *Plasmodium vivax* that may have occurred along the Jubba River in Somalia. Military physicians should seek continuing education experiences that reinforce their knowledge of geographic medicine so that serious illnesses acquired by servicemembers during deployments are not misdiagnosed.

Finally, assessments should not be made in a vacuum. Many elements of an OPLAN not directly related to preventive medicine are necessary variables in the medical threat equation. Examples of these include the number of personnel deploying, the number and types of medical facilities to be established, and the laboratory diagnostic capabilities that will be available. Accounting for as many of these variables as possible allows the preventive medicine officer to predict the rapidity with which small outbreaks can be interrupted before they become larger.

SUMMARY

Providing an assessment of the medical threat is among the important strategic and operational planning steps to be taken in adequately preparing commanders for a mission. From such an assessment should logically follow recommendations for effective countermeasures. Assessment begins with a thorough consideration of who is at risk, what operation is planned, when and for how long it will occur, and where it will take place. Multiple data sources may be consulted to characterize anticipated risks. Threats are categorized in a way that aids the prioritization of countermeasures, quantified to the extent possible, and communicated to appropriate levels of command. Specific countermeasure instructions are best disseminated to small unit leaders, who can then emphasize them to individual servicemembers. The threat is continually reassessed during the operation, based on medical surveillance, and commanders are updated as necessary.

REFERENCES

1. US Army Medical Department Center and School, Threat Support Office, Directorate of Combat and Doctrine Development. *The Medical Threat Facing a Force Protection Army*. Fort Sam Houston, Tex: USAMDCS: Feb 1994.

2. Wilson M. *A World Guide to Infections: Diseases, Distribution, Diagnosis*. New York: Oxford University Press; 1991.

3. Sanchez JF, Gelnett J, Petruccelli BP, DeFraites RF, Taylor DN. Diarrheal disease incidence and morbidity among US military personnel during short-term missions overseas. *Am J Trop Med Hyg*. 1998;58:299–304.

4. Hyams KC, Hanson K, Wignall FS, Escamilla J, Oldfield EC III. The impact of infectious diseases on the health of U.S. troops deployed to the Persian Gulf during operations Desert Shield and Desert Storm. *Clin Infect Dis*. 1995;20:1497–1504.

5. Harberberger RL, Scott DA, Thornton SA, Hyams KC. Diarrheal disease aboard a US Navy ship after a brief port visit to a high risk area. *Mil Med*. 1994;159:445–448.

6. Blood CG, Pugh WM, Gauker ED, Pearsall DM. Comparisons of wartime and peacetime disease and non-battle injury rates aboard ships of the British Royal Navy. *Mil Med*. 1992;157:641–644.

7. Reardon MJ, Gonzalez RR, Pandolf KB. Applications of predictive environmental strain models. *Mil Med*. 1997;162:136–140.

8. Gardner JW, Kark JA, Karnei K, et al. Risk factors predicting exertional threat illness in male Marine Corps recruits. *Med Sci Sports Exerc*. 1996;28:939–944.

9. Reister FA, ed. *Battle Casualties and Medical Statistics: US Army Experience in the Korean War*. Washington, DC: Office of the Surgeon General, Dept of the Army; 1973.

10. Trofa AF, DeFraites RF, Smoak BL, et al. Dengue fever in US military personnel in Haiti. *JAMA*. 1997;277:1546–1548.

RECOMMENDED READING

Blood CG, Gauker ED. The relationship between battle intensity and disease rates among Marine Corps infantry units. *Mil Med*. 1993;158:340–344.

Blood CG, Gauker ED, Jolly R, Pugh WM. Comparisons of casualty presentation and admission rates during various combat operations. *Mil Med*. 1994:159:457–461.

Blood CG, Jolly R. Comparisons of disease and nonbattle injury incidence across various military operations. *Mil Med*. 1995;160:258–263.

Carey ME. Learning from traditional combat mortality and morbidity data used in the evaluation of combat medical care. *Mil Med*. 1987;152:6–13.

Chin J, ed. *Control of Communicable Diseases Manual*. 17th ed. Washington, DC: American Public Health Association; 2000. Army Field Manual 8-33.

Hoeffler DF, Melton LJ 3rd. Changes in the distribution of Navy and Marine Corps casualties from World War I through the Vietnam conflict. *Mil Med*. 1981;146:776–779.

Legters LJ, Llewellyn CH. Military medicine. In: Wallace RB, ed. *Maxcy-Rosenau-Last Preventive Medicine and Public Health*. 14th ed. Stamford, Conn: Appleton & Lange; 1998.

Miser WF, Doukas WC, Lillegard WA. Injuries and illnesses incurred by an Army Ranger unit during Operation Just Cause. *Mil Med*. 1995;160:373–380.

Reister FA, ed. *Medical Statistics in World War II*. Washington, DC: Office of the Surgeon General, Dept of the Army; 1975.

Sanftleben KA. *The Unofficial Joint Medical Officers Handbook*. Bethesda, Md: Dept of Military and Emergency Medicine, Uniformed Services University of the Health Sciences; 1995.

Smoak BL, DeFraites RF, Magill AJ, Kain KC, Wellde BT. Plasmodium vivax infections in U.S. Army troops: failure of primaquine to prevent relapse in studies from Somalia. *Am J Trop Med Hyg*. 1997;56:231–234.

Stong GC, Kalenian MH, Hope JW. Medical evacuation experience of two 7th Corps medical companies supporting Desert Shield/Desert Storm. *Mil Med*. 1993;158:108–113.

US Dept of the Army. *Planning for Health Service Support*. Washington, DC: DA; 1994. Field Manual 8-55.

US Department of Defense. *Doctrine for Health Service Support in Joint Operations*. Washington, DC: DoD; 1995. Joint Publication 4-02. (Available at www.dtic.mil/doctrine/jel/logistics.htm).

Chapter 12

PREVENTIVE MEDICINE CONSIDERATIONS IN PLANNING MULTISERVICE AND MULTINATIONAL OPERATIONS

LAUREL BROADHURST, MD, MPH
DAVID ARDAY, MD, MPH
KENT BRADLEY, MD, MPH
RICHARD S. BROADHURST, MD, MPH
HOPPERUS BUMA, MD
BRIAN J. COMMONS, MSPH, MS
DAVID COWAN, PhD, MPH
STEPHEN CRAIG, DO, MTM&H

ROBERT LANDRY, MS
RELFORD E. PATTERSON, MD, MPH
RICHARD W. SMERZ, MD, MPH
HENRY P. STIKES, MD, MPH
RICHARD THOMAS, MD, MPH
RICHARD WILLIAMS, MD
JAMES WRIGHT, MD

L. Broadhurst, Staff Physician, Weaverville Family Medicine Associates, Weaverville, NC; Medical Advisor, North Carolina Department of Motor Vehicles, Raleigh, NC; formerly, Major, Medical Corps, US Army; Epidemiology Consultant, 7th MEDCOM and 10th MEDLAB, APO AE 09180

D. Arday, Medical Epidemiologist, Office of Clinical Standards and Quality, Health Care Financing Administration, 7500 Security Blvd., Baltimore, MD 21244; formerly, Assistant to Chief, Clinical Medicine and Wellness Programs Division, Health and Safety Directorate (G-WKH); US Coast Guard, Washington, DC 20593

K. Bradley, Lieutenant Colonel, Medical Corps, US Army; 7th Infantry Division Surgeon, Fort Carson, CO 80913

R. S. Broadhurst, Colonel, Medical Corps, North Carolina Army Guard, Commander, Company C, 161st Area Support Medical Battalion; formerly, Lieutenant Colonel, Medical Corps, US Army; Chief, Preventive Medicine and Medical Intelligence, US Army Special Operations Command, Fort Bragg, NC 28307

APCCH. Buma, Commander, Medical Branch, Royal Netherlands Army; Head of Naval Medical Training; P.O. Box 1010 (MCP 24D), 1201 DA Hilversum, The Netherlands

B. J. Commons, Colonel, Medical Service, US Army; US Army Center for Health Promotion and Prevention Medicine, Europe; CMR 402; APO AP 09180

D. N. Cowan; PhD, MPH, Lieutenant Colonel, Medical Service, USAR; Special Projects Officer, Division of Preventive Medicine, Walter Reed Army Institute of Research, Silver Spring, MD 20910-7500

S. Craig, Colonel, Medical Corps, US Army; Chief, Preventive Medicine, Keller Army Community Hospital, West Point, NY 10996; formerly, Surgeon, 96th Civil Affairs Battalion, Fort Bragg, North Carolina

R. Landry, Colonel, Medical Service, US Army; HHC, 18th MEDCOM, Unit 15281, APO AP 96205-0054

R. E. Patterson, Colonel, Medical Corps, US Air Force (Retired); formerly, Director, Military Public Health, Clinical Services, Office for the Assistant Secretary of Defense (Health Affairs); currently, Medical Director, General Motors Corporation Truck Group Assembly Plant, 2122 Broenig Highway, Baltimore, MD 21224

R. W. Smerz, Colonel, US Army (Retired); formerly, Surgeon, USSOCOM, 7701 Tampa Point Boulevard, MacDill Air Force Base, FL 33608-6001

H. P. Stikes, Colonel, Medical Corps, US Army; Commander, Lawrence Joel US Army Health Clinic, 1701 Hardee Avenue, SW; Ft. McPherson, GA 30330-1062; formerly, US Preventive Medicine Staff Officer, US Forces Command

R. Thomas, Captain, Medical Corps, US Navy; Naval Environmental Health Center, 2510 Walmer Ave., Norfolk, VA 23513-2617

R. Williams, Captain, Medical Corps, US Navy; Chief Clinical Consultant, Armed Forces Medical Intelligence Center, Fort Detrick, Bldg. 1607, Frederick, MD 21702-7581

J. Wright; Colonel, Medical Corps, US Air Force (Retired); formerly, AL/AOE, 2601 West Road, Suite 2, Brooks Air Force Base, Texas 78235-5241; currently, Occupational Medicine Physician, Concentra Medical Centers, 400 East Quincy, San Antonio, TX 78215

INTRODUCTION

In the US military of the 1990s, large unit operations have most often been joint operations, that is, operations composed of personnel from two or more of the services. This is not a new concept—many operations during World War II were joint, such as the amphibious invasions in the Pacific theater. Overall, military campaigns are won by occupying territory, which requires land forces of the Army or Marine Corps. But the Army and the Marine Corps cannot reach the area of operations without the Air Force, and the Navy and Marine Corps emphasis on mobility and flexibility means that they may require extensive Army logistics support once they have depleted their own combat service support. The services of the US military are interdependent for mission success.

Today's military units with significant preventive medicine (PM) assets, which generally reside at the division level and above, must interact with personnel from other services while sharing PM and other support assets. Additionally, Preventive Medicine Officers (PMOs) are placed in advisory positions to the Surgeons of joint forces, unified commands, and combined commands and so must be familiar with joint PM considerations. (Joint forces contain elements of at least two US military services; unified commands contain significant components of more than one US military service; and combined commands contain forces from more than one nation.) US military operations are conducted with such shared resources as a Joint Task Force (JTF) Surgeon, a Joint Blood Program Office, and a Joint Medical Regulating Office. In addition, increased US involvement in United Nations operations has meant that the operational force is likely to be a combined task force, which is sometimes called a multinational force. The PM planner in combined operations faces the difficult challenge of developing a comprehensive plan to keep the combined force healthy.

Major General Jonathan Letterman, Medical Director of the Army of the Potomac during the American Civil War, underscored the essential role of PM in military operations when he said:

> The leading idea, which should be constantly kept in view, is to strengthen the hands of the Commanding General by keeping his army in the most vigorous health, thus rendering it, in the highest degree, efficient for enduring fatigue and privation, and for fighting.[1(p100)]

That timeless wisdom calls on the medical leadership to employ PM to strengthen the warfighting capability of the commanding general of any task force, whether individual service, joint, combined, or unified. The essentials for planning and executing PM operations in joint, unified, and combined operations include knowledge of the policy-making process in the Office of the Assistant Secretary of Defense (Health Affairs) and the organization of PM in the Army, Navy, Marine Corps, Air Force, Coast Guard, and Reserve components. The PM mission in Civil Affairs and Special Operations is also relevant because these two organizations are often deployed as parts of joint, unified, or combined operations. Understanding the differences in structure and capabilities of these organizations is necessary to coordinate their efforts and provide effective PM services to all personnel.

OFFICE OF THE ASSISTANT SECRETARY OF DEFENSE HEALTH AFFAIRS

Preventive Medicine and Military Public Health Policy

The Assistant Secretary of Defense (Health Affairs)—the ASD (HA)—is the principal staff assistant and advisor to the Secretary of Defense and Under Secretary of Defense for Personnel and Readiness for all Department of Defense (DoD) health policies, programs, and activities. Preventive medicine is a principal component of the DoD's medical mission to maintain readiness, provide medical services and support to the armed forces during military operations, and provide continuing medical services and support to members of the armed forces, their dependents, and others entitled to DoD medical care. Current Joint Health Service Support Strategy demands delivering a healthy force and preventing and minimizing disease and nonbattle injury (DNBI).

Organizational Structure

Reporting to the ASD (HA) through the Principal Deputy Assistant Secretary are five Deputy Assistant Secretaries (DASDs); they are responsible for these functional activities: Clinical Services (CS), Health Budgets and Programs, Health Services Financing, Health Services Operations and Readiness (HSO&R), and Policy and Planning. The DASD (CS) establishes policies, procedures, and standards that govern DoD medical programs, such as quality management programs, human immunodeficiency virus programs, women's health issues, graduate medical education, health-related research, PM and public health, and all matters involving clinical policy. While the responsibility for formulation of PM and public health policy resides primarily with the DASD (CS), policy is routinely coordinated with two other offices. The first is the office of the DASD (HSO&R), which is responsible for assuring the adequacy of medical resources to meet the needs of national emergencies and armed conflict and for dedicating resources and personnel to implement policies affecting military public health. The other office with which the DASD (CS) coordinates is that of the Joint Staff's Deputy Director for Medical Readiness (J-4 MED) in the office of the J-4 (logistics). The Joint Staff performs military staff functions, which are discussed later in this chapter, for the Joint Chiefs of Staff (JCS). The J-4 MED provides the vital mechanism to implement PM policies affecting deployed forces and to incorporate them into JCS operations plans and joint doctrine.

The J-4 MED develops the joint force medical protection policy and PM strategies for diseases of operational importance, biological warfare, and the effects of exposure to environmental hazards. The mission of the J-4 MED Office is to plan for comprehensive medical readiness to support the national military strategy, while staying synchronized with the requirements of the Commander in Chief and the capabilities of the services; it also influences resource allocation and priority. The Office must coordinate with the services and defense agencies to determine PM requirements and capabilities. The officer filling this position at the J-4 MED also represents the Joint Staff on the Joint Preventive Medicine Policy Group, the Armed Forces Epidemiological Board, and the DoD's Global Surveillance and Response Committee.

Policy Formulation

It is DoD policy to enhance mission readiness, unit performance, and the health and fitness of individual military servicemembers (including Reserve and National Guard personnel), beneficiaries, and civilian employees through comprehensive health promotion and disease prevention programs and to provide healthy environments for workers and visitors. PM policy issues may emerge from the office of the ASD (HA), from the services, from legislative mandate, or from operational requirements. The process can be complex, involving interaction among multiple agencies within the DoD, including Health Affairs, General Counsel, Legislative Affairs, Comptroller, and

Public Affairs. For example, the policy determining the use of tick-borne encephalitis vaccine by US forces during Operation Joint Endeavor in Bosnia involved extensive review and coordination among the aforementioned DoD offices, the Centers for Disease Control and Prevention, and the Armed Forces Epidemiological Board.

The office of the ASD (HA) relies on internal analysts to formulate policy; however, it routinely solicits external review and consultation from the Surgeons General, the Armed Forces Epidemiological Board, the Armed Forces Medical Intelligence Center (AFMIC), and civilian public health institutions. PM expertise is provided through the Surgeons General from the Center for Health Promotion and Preventive Medicine, Aberdeen Proving Ground, Md; the Naval Environmental Health Center, Norfolk, Va; and the Air Force's Institute of Environmental Risk Analysis, San Antonio, Tex. On occasion, as in the situation involving the health concerns of Persian Gulf War veterans, external institutions such as the National Academy of Sciences may be commissioned to provide consultation and recommendations. As policies are formulated, they are coordinated by the Surgeons General of the various services.

Priority Programs

As the office of the ASD (HA) prepares for the challenges of the 21st century, several PM issues will likely predominate. Experiences in the aftermath of the Persian Gulf War have increased the emphasis being placed on comprehensive medical surveillance. This medical surveillance will integrate and fully coordinate the efforts of the Surgeons General, JCS, and subordinate units before, during, and after deployment. As the nature of modern warfare evolves, participation in low-intensity conflict and humanitarian assistance operations will become increasingly important. Prevention and control of DNBI will continue to be of paramount importance, but surveillance systems must also be capable of detecting chronic morbidity that might be associated with participation in deployments.

The DoD, which administers the largest managed care organization in the United States, has begun to recognize the potential benefit of PM approaches to the assessment of health services. Quality management review will become increasingly important to study the performance and outcomes of key clinical preventive services, such as screening tests, routine counseling, and immunizations, and has been incorporated into health care benefit plans for active duty and other DoD enrollees.

US ARMY FIELD PREVENTIVE MEDICINE

Army field PM is organized and staffed to provide soldiers and commanders with the same PM services in the field environment as they have in garrison. These services are critical to soldiers, whether they are engaged in training exercises or deployed in combat operations. The prevention of disease and injury reduces manpower losses, patient loads, and evacuation requirements. The timely and effective implementation of appropriate PM measures to counter the medical threat serves as a combat multiplier, enhancing unit effectiveness and reducing the individual soldier's exposure to disease and environmental threats. Command interest and commitment to the PM program are essential to its success, since the military public health program is a command program and not actually a medical program.[2]

The scope of field PM services available in a theater of operations includes providing assistance to the commander in preparing staff estimates by identifying the medical threat and recommending appropriate PM countermeasures. PM assets provide oversight for the health-related aspects of water and ice production, distribution, and consumption; entomological control measures; environmental conditions; and waste disposal practices. Another key responsibility is the training and assessment of field sanitation teams.[3]

Unit-Level Preventive Medicine Assets

PM functions are performed at the soldier and unit level across the theater, from the forward line of troops to the rear areas. Specialized PM personnel are organic to the divisions and armored cavalry regiments, as well as to medical functional units at echelons above the division level. These personnel are trained and ready to provide flexible PM assistance within their areas of concern. But PM support for both training and combat operations begins with the individual soldier and continues up through the unit and higher echelons. Individual- and unit-level PM measures are a command responsibility. The individual soldier must perform basic PM measures, such as maintaining physical and mental fitness and guarding against heat and cold injury, other physical injury, biting insects, and diarrhea. Organic medical personnel and the unit field sanitation team provide assistance.[2–4]

The field sanitation team advises the unit commander on issues essential to reducing DNBI. It also ensures that appropriate field sanitation facilities are established and maintained, effective sanitary and control measures are applied, and effective PM mea-

sures are practiced. The team instructs, supervises, assists with, inspects, and reports on field sanitation activities. Field sanitation teams are required for units that are company- or battery-sized or larger.[3,5]

The field sanitation team normally consists of company medics, trained medically as military occupational specialty designation 91As. If these specialists are not available, at least two soldiers in the unit will be picked and trained; at least one must be a noncommissioned officer (NCO). They are trained in the use, maintenance, and care of the field sanitation team equipment, such as water purification kits, food service disinfectant, personal protective equipment, tools needed for spraying insecticide, mouse and rat traps, and rodenticide. The team members provide unit training in personal protective measures for disease control. They also inspect the unit's food service operations, ensure that the unit leaders are supervising the disinfection of the unit's water supply, and instruct the troops in methods of individual water purification. The team members monitor the construction of garbage and soakage pits and inspect the arrangements for waste disposal. The field sanitation team also monitors the construction of field latrines and urinals and inspects them regularly. They use arthropod and rodent control, and sometimes this includes pesticide spraying.[5]

Divisional Preventive Medicine Assets

The PM sections of the divisions and armored cavalry regiments are responsible for assessing the medical threat and determining PM countermeasures; advising commanders and staffs of PM requirements; training, monitoring, and providing technical assistance to unit field sanitation teams; monitoring the training of all soldiers in PM measures; and conducting surveys, inspections, and control activities. Divisional PM assets include a PM physician, an environmental science officer or sanitary engineer, and PM NCOs and enlisted specialists. Division PM sections are typically located in the medical company of the main support battalion. Within the armored cavalry regiment, a single PM NCO is assigned to the medical troop of the regimental support squadron.[2]

Preventive Medicine Assets at Echelons Above the Division Level

Above the division level, direct PM support is typically provided by the PM section of the area support medical battalion (ASMB) or by specialized PM detachments attached to the battalion. The ASMB includes a PM section identical to that found in the divisions. The staffing of this section permits it to have an extensive capability for epidemiologic (eg, infectious disease) investigations and sanitary engineering support. PM personnel conduct evaluations to identify actual and potential health hazards, recommend corrective measures, and assist in training personnel in disease prevention programs. Support is coordinated with PM detachments and other units within the ASMB. As PM detachments are normally attached to an ASMB, the PM section within the ASMB assumes technical supervision of the attached detachments to coordinate assignment of specific missions. ASMBs and PM support are normally allocated based on the anticipated medical threat and the mission.[6]

PM general support at echelons above the division level is provided by functional teams on an area basis. On occasion, these teams can be attached to specific units in a direct support role and may be used as far down the organization chain as the division level. These functional PM teams provide support within a theater of operations in the specialties of epidemiology, entomology, environmental science, and environmental engineering. Teams are allocated based on the number of troops supported and the medical threat. These teams depend on other units for logistical support. The two types of teams presently available are (1) the Medical Detachment, Preventive Medicine (Entomology) and (2) the Medical Detachment, Preventive Medicine (Sanitation). The teams are similar in structure and function but differ in their primary emphasis. They both have an entomologist, an environmental science officer or sanitary engineer, and enlisted technicians. Both types of team are capable of monitoring vector control activities, field sanitation, water treatment and storage, waste disposal, and DNBI control practices within their assigned area and of making appropriate recommendations. Other functions they perform include medical data collection, investigations, and environmental sampling. Capabilities unique to the entomology team include area and aerial spraying.[2]

PM consultative capabilities are organic to the medical command and control elements at the corps level and above. The medical group's capabilities include consultation services and technical advice in PM, environmental health, and sanitary engineering. The medical brigade provides similar consultation and technical services, plus medical entomology and radiological health. At the theater level, the medical command is also staffed to provide PM consultation and technical services. PM consultative services at all these levels include assessment of the medical threat, evaluation of the PM program, technical advice on medical aspects of nuclear, biological, chemical, and directed-energy weapons, and staff coordination of PM services.[2]

An additional theater asset currently available is the Theater Army Medical Laboratory. This Laboratory provides a broader range of laboratory functions than those normally found in theater hospitals, to include microbiological identification and characterization, biochemical and toxicological analyses, and serological testing for disease diagnosis and prevention. Other functions it provides include food contamination analyses, detection and diagnosis of zoonotic diseases, entomological laboratory support, epidemiologic analyses, and environmental health assessments (Exhibit 12-1). Army PM assets are also found in Civil Affairs and other Special Operations units and are discussed later in this chapter.

EXHIBIT 12-1
THE CAPABILITIES OF THE THEATER AREA MEDICAL LABORATORY

- Provides analytical, investigative, and consultative capabilities to identify nuclear, biological, and chemical threat agents and other samples from the area of operations
- Provides analytical, investigative, and consultative capabilities to assist in the identification of occupational health, environmental health hazards, and endemic diseases
- Provides special environmental control and containment to evaluate biomedical specimens for the presence of highly infectious or hazardous agents of operational concern
- Provides data and data analysis to support medical analyses and operational decisions
- Provides medical laboratory analysis to support the diagnosis of zoonotic and significant animal diseases that impact on military operations
- Provides tailorable force projections to support war and operations other than war

Source: Chambers WR. Command Briefing, 520th Theater Army Medical Laboratory, 1997.

Future Directions

As part of the Medical Reengineering Initiative process, several changes to this PM organization are planned. The current entomology and sanitation detachments are to be replaced with consolidated detachments that retain the capabilities of the two detachments while removing the duplication. A disease surveillance system that is effective, timely, and responsive to the line commander's needs is key to the future PM mission and is being developed. The Theater Area Medical Laboratory is to be reorganized to create a corps-level area medical laboratory, with its focus on endemic disease and environmental and occupational health threats. It is anticipated that these changes, among others, will make the PM support in the field even more effective.

NAVY AND MARINE CORPS FIELD PREVENTIVE MEDICINE

The US Navy and Marine Corps are two separate yet interdependent services within a single military department. The organization of PM services in the Navy and Marine Corps reflects this dichotomy within the Department of the Navy. Medical support is provided to both services by the Navy Medical Department in three ways: (1) direct support from Navy medical personnel assigned to Navy ships, squadrons, and units, (2) direct medical support from Navy medical personnel assigned to Marine Corps units, and (3) medical support to Navy and Marine Corps units from Bureau of Medicine and Surgery (BUMED) activities such as hospital, clinics, and PM units.

Preventive Medicine Services in Peacetime

Key PM support to operational units during routine operations is provided by Preventive Medicine Technicians (PMTs) assigned to medium- and larger-sized ships (ie, aircraft carriers and most amphibious ships) and by Independent Duty Corpsmen providing some PM services to smaller ships such as destroyers. Approximately 50% of ships with sailors and Marines are at sea at any one time. Programs in the prevention of foodborne and waterborne illnesses, heat injuries, communicable diseases, and occupational injuries and illnesses are active on all ships. Operational staffs may have PM personnel, such as Aerospace Medicine residency–trained flight surgeons, Environmental Health Officers, Industrial Hygiene Officers, and PMTs, filling staff positions.

PM support to Marine units consists of PMTs distributed to battalions and squadrons; a larger PM section is located within the medical battalion and consists of Environmental Health Officers, Entomologists, and PMTs. Marine staffs may have PM personnel involved with contingency and exercise planning. Examples include a physician PMO and a PMT assigned to the Marine Expeditionary Force (Command Element) staff, a residency-trained flight surgeon and PMT on the Marine Air Wing Staff, and an Environmental Health Officer and a PMT assigned to the Marine Division staff.

PM support from BUMED activities includes personnel from hospitals and clinics. They provide an entire spectrum of occupational health and PM services to Navy and Marine Corps units and commands both afloat and ashore. A major focus of PM programs has been at recruit commands, which have had recurrent communicable disease problems.[7] Navy– and Marine Corps–wide programs in all areas of PM, occupational health, and environmental programs are developed and managed by the Navy Environmental Health Center, Norfolk, Va, and its subordinate units: four Navy Environmental and Preventive Medicine Units and two Disease Vector Ecology and Control Centers, which specialize in entomological threat reduction.

At any time, PM personnel are forward deployed in Aircraft Carrier Battle Groups, in Amphibious Ready Groups, and at overseas bases throughout the world providing "routine" public health services and participating in combined and joint military exercises. PM plays a major role in complex humanitarian relief operations, such as those in Rwanda, Guantánamo Bay, and Haiti[8]; in civic action programs associated with annual military exercises, such as Operation Cobra Gold in Thailand; and in public health training operations deployed with engineering and dental units in the Caribbean region.

Preventive Medicine During Mobilization

During a major mobilization, additional PM personnel are assigned from BUMED activities and the Naval Reserve to operational units. Two major advancements occurred in field PM during the Persian Gulf War: (1) the development of methodologies to collect disease rates faster and provide commanders a real-time assessment of DNBI rates that had previously been available months to years after a conflict, and (2) the formation of Navy Forward Deployable Laboratories, through the efforts of personnel from the Navy Medical Research and Development Command, the Environmental and

Preventive Medicine Units, and the Disease Vector Ecology and Control Centers, to provide public health services beyond the capabilities of operational units.[9] These units have been so successful that those laboratories are now part of Navy medical doctrine.[10]

The Navy Forward Deployable Laboratory is an advanced infectious disease diagnostic laboratory that can aid in the recognition and treatment of clinical infectious disease cases, as well as the detection of biological warfare agents. The Laboratory is designed to function anywhere, from the cramped quarters of Navy ships to tents in remote Third World locations. Its diagnostic capabilities are extensive, including the classic bacteriological culture methods but also providing antibiotic susceptibility testing, enzyme-immunoassay, fluorescent microscopy, diagnostic DNA probes, and polymerase chain reaction. It is designed to function as a state-of-the-art, comprehensive, onsite diagnostic laboratory when large numbers of sailors and Marines are deployed to regions with a high risk of infectious disease transmission.[9]

In a major regional conflict, an entire PM unit of approximately 40 personnel, who provide environmental health, entomology, industrial hygiene, and epidemiologic specialty services, can be deployed as part of the Navy Advanced Base Functional Component system. This is a major-theater asset, but it is limited by the extensive airlift capability it requires and by the engineering, transportation, and logistical support it needs when deployed.

PM in the Fleet Marine Force reflects the task organization philosophy behind the differing sizes of Marine Air Ground Task Forces formed to meet the potential threat.[11] The smallest of the task forces is a Marine Expeditionary Unit, which is routinely deployed in both the Pacific and the Atlantic and Mediterranean regions; it consists of 2,000 Marines and sailors deployed on three to five amphibious ships. Its PM support consists of PMTs assigned to the Ground and Air Combat Elements, with a larger PM section in the Combat Service Support Element. The task forces increase in size in increments until they become a Marine Expeditionary Force (MEF) of 50,000 Marines and sailors fully equipped for 60 days of sustained combat. All the PM assets assigned to a MEF in garrison would deploy, as well as active duty and reserve billets that are only filled at mobilization. The majority of PM services reside in the medical battalion, the unit that is responsible for providing additional support (from the Combat Service Support Element) above what organic unit personnel can provide. Specific additional capabilities can be added from the Navy deployable laboratories and the Advanced Base Functional Components, if needed. Each MEF can also be tasked to perform such operations as humanitarian relief or the evacuation of US or allied nation noncombatants from a combat or disaster situation.

AIR FORCE FIELD PREVENTIVE MEDICINE

Air Force PM manpower assets differ markedly from those of the other services. General PM physicians are few in number and assigned primarily to the Force Health Protection and Surveillance Branch and the Office for Prevention and Health Services Assessment, both at Brooks Air Force Base in San Antonio, Tex. PM and public health duties at Air Force bases are performed by flight surgeons, public health officers, and bioenvironmental engineers.

Flight surgeons are physicians who complete a 7-week course in Aerospace Medicine. This training includes some public health and environmental medicine. Larger bases or bases with more complex missions or disease risks have flight surgeons assigned who are graduates of the residency in Aerospace Medicine.

Air Force public health officers may be veterinarians, nurses, or biomedical specialists. Many have a Master of Public Health degree, and all attend a 10-week course in public health and environmental health. They receive extensive training in all aspects of public health, including epidemiology, environmental sanitation, food safety, occupational health, and medical entomology. They are trained to conduct health threat assessments before deployments and disease surveillance during deployments.

Most medical facilities have several flight surgeons, two public health officers, and two bioenvironmental engineers. These officers, along with public health and environmental technicians, compose the PM team that manages all aspects of public health, occupational health, and environmental surveillance. Bioenvironmental engineers must possess a degree in engineering and attend a 3-month course at the School of Aerospace Medicine, with extensive training in water sanitation, pollution control, industrial hygiene, and occupational and environmental surveillance.

Deployed PM assets vary, depending on the size and type of the operation. Air Force squadrons on routine deployments are accompanied by a Squadron Medical Element, which provides basic medical and public health support. A typical Squadron Medical Element comprises a flight surgeon, an aeromedical technician (trained in basic medical care and administration), and a public health technician. It will be supplemented with an additional flight surgeon for prolonged deployments. These elements are not normally deployed for operations other than war. In those types of deployments (which include humanitarian crises, natural disasters, and peacekeeping operations), additional physicians, such as family practitioners, could be assigned. An Air Transportable Clinic (ATC) or an Air Transportable Hospital (ATH) are normally deployed for these operations. As training for these types of operations is limited, experienced flight surgeons and public health officers are deployed.

When wing-size organizations are deployed, an ATC is usually deployed. The ATC has basic medical care capability similar to a clinic and has PM assets. Flight surgeons, family practice physicians, and surgeons provide basic medical care, while flight surgeons and public health officers and technicians provide PM and public health expertise. Bioenvironmental engineers and technicians are responsible for water testing and sanitation, pollution control, and surveillance for and decontamination of nuclear, biological, and chemical contamination.

In organization- or theater-size deployments, an ATH is deployed. An ATH provides medical and surgical capability with minimal laboratory and radiological services. PM assets are similar to those of an ATC and include flight surgeons, public health officers, bioenvironmental engineers, and technicians. The flight surgeon is normally residency trained in Aerospace Medicine and has public health experience. Additional PM assets may be requested by the theater commander or theater surgeon.

Specialized PM assets exist at the Epidemiologic Research Division at Brooks Air Force Base. Normally these officers provide epidemiologic, public health, and travel medicine consultation to all Air Force medical treatment facilities and conduct disease surveillance for the Air Force. The Laboratory Services Branch of the Epidemiologic Research Division provides extensive reference laboratory services to Air Force facilities worldwide and extensive microbiology laboratory services to physicians during disease outbreak investigations.

The Epidemiologic Research Division can field two theater epidemiology teams to provide deployed Air Force units with health threat assessments, public health consultations, disease surveillance capability, and on-site disease outbreak investigations. Each team has one PM physician, one public health officer, and one public health technician. The team can be supplemented with an entomologist, a laboratory officer, or an infectious disease physician as needed.

PREVENTIVE MEDICINE IN THE US COAST GUARD AND OTHER FEDERAL AGENCIES

US Coast Guard

Although it is one of the five armed forces of the United States, during peacetime the US Coast Guard is an agency within the Department of Transportation. Coast Guard medical assets are limited and focus on primary care and support of operational requirements. Units deployed outside the United States during contingency operations generally rely on collocated DoD units for care beyond that which can be provided by an independent duty medical corpsman. Although PM is emphasized throughout the Coast Guard medical program, there is no formal PM structure. The Director of Health and Safety is responsible for the medical and safety programs and is the primary point of contact for any medical issues involving coordination with outside agencies.[12]

The Coast Guard endeavors to be the world's leading maritime humanitarian and safety service.[13] It is the smallest of the military services, consisting of approximately 37,000 active duty, 8,000 reserve, 6,000 civilian, and 36,000 auxiliary personnel in 1995.[14] The Coast Guard Reserve is organized into 51 groups and 311 units, which are controlled directly by the Commandant, US Coast Guard, through the headquarters operations and personnel directorates. In addition, there are nondrilling ready reservists who, as in the DoD, may be mobilized for domestic emergencies or military support operations, as well as national emergencies and war. The Coast Guard's four main missions are maritime law enforcement, maritime safety, environmental protection, and national security.

Most Coast Guard units are organized, trained, and equipped to perform more than one of those four main missions and cannot be neatly typed by function. While most units are armed, they are usually equipped with only small arms and defensive weapons and are not designed to operate independently in a high-threat environment. Because of its historic relationship with the Navy, the Coast Guard frequently trains and operates with naval units and can be most easily integrated into the Navy's structure during contingencies.[15] Specific duties usually assigned to Coast Guard units participating in contingency operations are port safety and security, search and rescue, law enforcement (eg, interdiction of merchant vessels for contraband), and ensuring the safety and security of maritime commerce and transportation.

Forces most likely to work closely with DoD units during contingency operations include port security units (Figure 12-1) and visit and search teams, in addition to forces on cutters, patrol boats, and aircraft. Elements may be assigned individually to contingency operations or, more likely, they may be part of organized, larger joint harbor defense commands or composite naval coastal warfare units.

There are four methods under three legal authorities that may be used to place Coast Guard forces under DoD operational control: declaration of war [14 USC 3], presidential action [14 USC 3], assistance to other federal agencies [14 USC 141], and training and education [14 USC 144-145]. The President may direct by executive order that either the entire Coast Guard or part of it become a service in the Department of the Navy. The exact status of support for those forces would be negotiated at the time of the transfer. Under the statute allowing transfer for assistance to other federal agencies, the Secretary of Transportation may allow Coast Guard forces to work for the DoD when the Secretary of Defense so requests. Assignments are made for specific purposes and can be of unlimited duration. Return of forces is automatic when the purpose is ended, the DoD releases the forces, or the Department of Transportation revokes its consent.[15] Currently, there are two major field command, control, and support elements—Atlantic and Pacific Areas—each of which is subdivided into several districts. Operational units, such as cutters, small boat stations, air stations, and marine safety offices, report to their respective districts for tactical command and control.

The Coast Guard is extensively involved in stopping illegal immigration into the United States through alien migrant interdiction operations. During the summer of 1994, Coast Guard units involved in Operations Able Manner and Able Vigil intercepted 56,000 Haitian and Cuban boat people in the Caribbean Sea.[16] Boats containing alien migrants are often unseaworthy, overcrowded, and unsanitary (Figure 12-2). These operations may expose US personnel to foreign nationals and environments harboring communicable diseases. The Coast Guard has taken an active approach to controlling the health risks associated with alien migrant interdiction operations by such methods as education in sanitation practices, selective immunization and chemoprophylaxis, appropriate use of personal protective equipment, and operational policies.[17]

Federal Emergency Management Agency

The Federal Emergency Management Agency (FEMA) is responsible for coordinating disaster assistance to states and territories; this assistance saves lives and protects public health, safety, and property. FEMA prepares the Federal Response Plan (FRP)[18] in compliance with the provisions of the Stafford Act.[19] The FRP is designed to address the consequences of any disaster or emergency situation in which there is a need for federal assistance. The FRP applies to natural disasters, technological emergencies (eg, hazardous material spills), and certain other incidents. During the period immediately following a disaster requiring a federal response, FEMA directs other federal agencies to identify requirements and mobilize and deploy resources to the affected area in accordance with the FRP.

The FRP outlines the organization and contains the responsibilities of the various federal agencies tasked to provide assistance in any of twelve emergency support functions: transportation, communications, public works and engineering, firefighting, information and planning, mass casualty care, resource support, health and medical services, urban search and rescue, hazardous materials, food, and energy. Under the current FRP, the DoD has primary responsibility in two areas, public works and engineering and urban search and rescue, but has supporting roles in all other areas.[20]

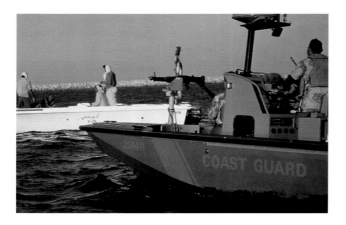

Fig. 12-1. US Coast Guard members of a Port Security Unit are operating under the command and control of the US Navy in the Persian Gulf during the Persian Gulf War. Photograph: US Coast Guard.

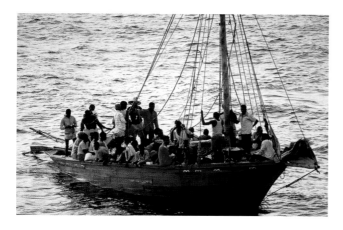

Fig. 12-2. This boat overcrowded with alien migrants is about to be boarded by Coast Guard personnel as part of its alien interdiction mission. Photograph: US Coast Guard.

US Public Health Service

The US Public Health Service is an agency within the Department of Health and Human Services that has the lead federal role in coordinating and ensuring public health and medical services during any federal disaster response.[21] The Public Health Service sponsors a number of Disaster Medical Assistance Teams across the country, as part of the National Disaster Medical System. Most of these are locally sponsored, community-based teams of approximately 35 civilian volunteers with skills and experience in both hospital and field emergency service. These teams can be rapidly mobilized, at which time the members temporarily become federal employees.[21] In addition to the local teams, the Public Health Service maintains a larger team (the PHS-1 DMAT), based in Washington, DC, which is mostly made up of officers of the Public Health Service Commissioned Corps. This team can rapidly deploy to disaster sites to provide both acute medical care and PM services, including basic field sanitation, water potability testing, and entomological assessments. The PHS-1 DMAT is generally the first medical disaster team to be sent to a federally declared disaster area when local resources have been overwhelmed.[22]

The Public Health Service Commissioned Corps is a uniformed, nonmilitary corps of more than 6,000 officers, including medical, dental, nursing, engineering, and sanitarian professionals. With the exception of the DoD and the Department of Veterans Affairs, federal agencies rely on the Public Health Service Commissioned Corps as a source of professional medical personnel and expertise. By law, this Commissioned Corps is a source of personnel to augment DoD health care activities in the United States and, on a limited basis, other activities during national emergencies.[23] The Corps is the only uniformed backup to the armed services that can be rapidly mobilized and ordered into areas of danger for indefinite periods of time. Since 1988, there has been a memorandum of understanding between the Public Health Service and the DoD outlining procedures for the mobilization and deployment of Public Health Service commissioned officers to the DoD, including emergency mobilization services.[24]

The Centers for Disease Control and Prevention (CDC) is another Public Health Service agency that has major responsibilities for preparing for and responding to public health emergencies, such as disasters, and for conducting investigations into the health effects and medical consequences of disasters.[25] It is also a source of epidemiologic and scientific support services and information, and it publishes numerous materials that can be useful for operational planning.[26,27]

THE RESERVE COMPONENTS

There are Reserve branches in all the military services: the Army Reserve (USAR), the Naval Reserve (USNR), the Marine Corps Reserve (USMCR), and the Air Force Reserve (USAFR). The Reserves are elements of and are directly controlled by the individual services, and their primary function is to augment and support the service in periods of war or other national emergency.

The Reserve components consist of the above elements and the two National Guards: the Army National Guard (ARNG) and the Air National Guard (ANG). Both are normally controlled by the states, with the governor of each state serving as the commander-in-chief of guardsmen in his or her state during peacetime. All 50 states, the District of Columbia, Guam, Puerto Rico, and the US Virgin Islands have National Guard units. The primary role of the Guard during peacetime, operating as a state agency, is to assist in natural or other disasters and to aid in the control of uprisings or civil disturbances. During wartime, the Guard can be federalized, becoming assets of the Army and Air Force. The National Guard can also be federalized during national emergencies and may come under the control of FEMA.

In any future military action, the medical assets, including PM units, of the various Reserve components will be mobilized and integrated into the active military forces. There are no PM units in the ARNG, but there are two types of units in the USAR: sanitation detachments and entomology detachments, with about 10 of each currently in existence. Each detachment or team includes two officers and nine enlisted technicians and has its own transportation assets. These teams have the same primary missions as their active component counterparts.[28]

The Reserve force structure, including PM and other medical assets, is currently under review, and the structure and mission may change substantially in the future. It is anticipated that by 2001, the entomology and sanitation teams will be reconfigured as PM detachments, with one environmental science officer and one entomologist per team. Two enlisted technicians will be added, bringing team strength to 13. These new teams will have both environmental sanitation and entomology functions, as well as other general PM missions. New equipment will improve the mobility and communications capability of the detachments and will allow for real-time transmission of health and disease data. Approximately 16 teams will be assigned to the USAR.[29]

The Air Force, including its Reserve component, is also changing its PM structure. PM teams have been developed to be deployable at the wing level. These teams will likely be composed of a flight surgeon, a bioenvironmental engineer, a public health officer, and enlisted personnel (including public health, bioenvironmental, and emergency medical technicians). The role of this team will be to advise the wing commander on the health of the airmen, identify health threats and environmental and occupational hazards, evaluate general sanitation, approve food and water sources, direct the control of disease vectors, control communicable diseases, and perform disease surveillance and epidemiologic investigations of disease outbreaks. The force structure will be similar in active duty, USAFR, and ANG units, but the ANG may have additional PM and epidemiologic assets at the theater, base, and wing level.[30]

THE PREVENTIVE MEDICINE MISSION IN SPECIAL OPERATIONS

While Special Operations Forces (SOF) have played a role in US military operations throughout our nation's history, it was only during World War II that the concept and organization of SOF became more formally developed. The Office of Strategic Services was created to provide unconventional and psychological warfare capabilities at the strategic and tactical levels. The 1st Ranger Battalion, Alamo Scouts, 1st Marine Raider Regiment, Navy Combat Demolition Units and Underwater Demolition Teams, and the 885th Bomb Squadron are a few of the units in the services that provided specialized tactical support to conventional forces.

Until the 1980s, these forces were considered unconventional, outside of mainstream military operations. During the 1980s, SOF assets and capabilities became integrated into strategic and tactical planning and then established in individual service and joint doctrine. The US Special Operations Command (USSOCOM) was created on 16 April 1986, consisting of the Air Force Special Operations Command, the Naval Special Warfare Command, the US Army Special Operations Command (USASOC), and the Joint Special Operations Command[31] (Figure 12-3).

Missions

Primary SOF missions include Special Reconnaissance, Foreign Internal Defense, Direct Action, Unconventional Warfare, Combating Terrorism, Counterproliferation, Civil Affairs, Psychological Operations, and Information Warfare/Command and Control Warfare.[31] These missions frequently place the special operations servicemember under physical, mental, and environmental stresses not generally encountered by conventional forces. These stresses are compounded by isolation from conventional military support elements.

PM is involved in the success of SOF from selection and training through mission completion. Special medical fitness requirements ensure the SOF candidate is physically and mentally equipped to meet physical challenges and perform specialized duties, such as parachuting, flying, and scuba diving.[32] Environmental education and training ensures that SOF personnel understand the importance of field sanitation and hygiene and can operate in the extremes of heat, cold, and altitude. Missions frequently place SOF personnel in isolated areas in close contact with indigenous populations where diseases not seen in the United States are common. Under such conditions, susceptibility to endemic and epidemic disease is increased. SOF personnel are also often isolated from upper echelon medical care provided by conventional support units. PM issues that are critical to mission success include detailed disease and vector threat information, recommendations for special immunizations, chemoprophylaxis, special equipment (eg, individual water filters), and postmission disease surveillance.

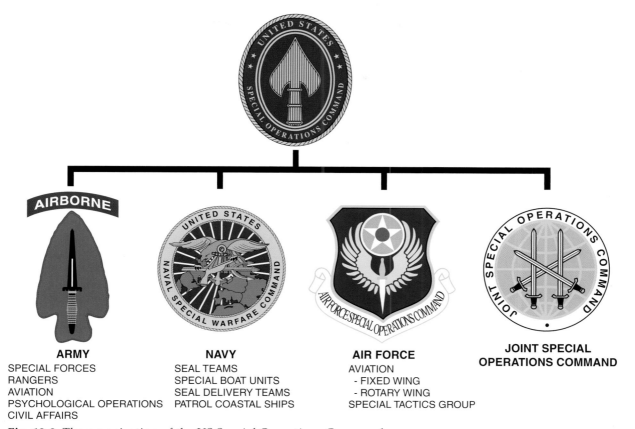

ARMY
SPECIAL FORCES
RANGERS
AVIATION
PSYCHOLOGICAL OPERATIONS
CIVIL AFFAIRS

NAVY
SEAL TEAMS
SPECIAL BOAT UNITS
SEAL DELIVERY TEAMS
PATROL COASTAL SHIPS

AIR FORCE
AVIATION
- FIXED WING
- ROTARY WING
SPECIAL TACTICS GROUP

**JOINT SPECIAL
OPERATIONS COMMAND**

Fig. 12-3. The organization of the US Special Operations Command.
Source: US Special Operations Command. Special Operations in Peace and War. SOC: 1996.

Preventive Medicine Assets in Special Operations Forces

PM assets are found at all levels of command in SOF. At USSOCOM, a PM sciences officer coordinates PM planning and execution for the command surgeon. The Joint Special Operations Command Surgeon has a full-time PMO on staff. Due to its mission requirements for extensive operations in developing countries with tremendous disease threats, the Army's SOF command has more PM personnel than the other SOF commands. PMOs and NCOs are assigned to USASOC and the US Army Civil Affairs and Psychological Operations Command. Each Special Forces Group has an environmental science officer; Special Forces medics, highly trained in PM techniques, are organic to each group, battalion, company, and operational detachment. PM NCOs are assigned to the Special Forces battalions, the Special Operations Support Command, the Special Operations Medical Training Center, and the civil affairs units.

The Navy Special Warfare Command and the Air Force Special Operations Command have no dedicated PM specialists on staff. Navy Independent Duty Medical Technicians and Corpsmen (on duty with SEAL [Sea Air Land] teams and Special Boat Squadrons) and Air Force Pararescuemen are trained in basic PM techniques to support their missions.[33] Physicians and physician assistants serving as unit flight surgeons, diving medical officers, general medical officers, and in other similar positions provide limited PM expertise to support these NCOs.

Deployment Considerations

SOF mission planning and preparation must have a different focus than that of conventional forces. Since SOF have very limited organic medical assets, units place greater emphasis on preventing health problems and quickly addressing those that do develop. Intelligence preparation must be detailed and extensive, including the locations and capabilities of host-nation hospitals. Evacuation routes must be coordinated, to include possible military transport from isolated countries. Unusual or investigational immunizations, along with an emphasis on personal protective measures and education, allow SOF to maintain a high posture of prevention against environmental and infectious disease threats.

Even with meticulous execution, preventive strategies can fail. SOF use post-deployment PM briefings to remind servicemembers about disease exposures, the need for continuing chemoprophylaxis, and actions to be taken should symptoms arise and to establish appropriate postdeployment surveillance systems in garrison. Illnesses can thus be diagnosed and treated in a timely fashion, with a high index of suspicion for exotic diseases.

THE PREVENTIVE MEDICINE MISSION IN CIVIL AFFAIRS

The need to deal effectively with a civilian populace in military operations has long been understood. According to US Army doctrine, the mission of Civil Affairs (CA) is to support the commander's relationship with civil authorities and the civilian populace, promote mission legitimacy, and enhance military effectiveness.[34] The first CA division was activated on March 1, 1943, in response to the anticipated demands of dealing with the civilian population of Europe during World War II. CA personnel had previously been under the purview of the Provost Marshal.[35] The end of the Cold War did not end conflict, though. CA has an important role to play during conflict and immediately after a conflict. However, CA has become actively involved in operations during peacetime to support national strategic objectives.

Mission and Role

The role of PM in CA is to alleviate human suffering among civilians in accordance with Article 56 of the Geneva Convention, prevent and control communicable disease that may impede military operations, and institute necessary health measures in the reconstruction of a country's public health program.[36] This role can be expanded based on the nature of the environment in which CA forces may be deployed. In a Foreign Internal Defense (FID) mission, the role of public health teams may be to provide individual or team advisors or provide assistance in the conduct of civic action projects. In peacetime, public health teams may be required to provide support operations and render humanitarian assistance. Public health specialists or teams in CA are often the coordinators and planners of action to accomplish the mission. CA units have a regional focus; they are often trained in languages specific to their region, and they understand the cultural complexities of their area of concern.[37]

The public health team has various responsibilities based on its mission. Generally, direct involvement in the provision of health services is not its mission except for the Foreign Internal Defense CA battalion. The team is best suited to provide guidance, assessments, and oversight. The actual rendering of recommended services or interventions requires effective coordination with medical assets from other US military units, the host nation, or donor agencies. Humanitarian assistance missions often involve other agencies outside of the DoD, such as the State Department, and they may be designated lead agent for a particular operation. CA personnel often find themselves working with personnel from the State Department and various United Nations organizations. In their delivery of public health services to a community, the CA units coordinate closely with agencies in country (eg, UN High Commissioner for Refugees, UN Development Program, US Agency for International Development, various non-governmental organizations) regarding any ongoing projects. Public health teams must ensure their activities are in support of national strategic objectives and in accordance with embassy guidance.

Capabilities and Structure

Only the Army and Marine Corps have CA units, and the vast majority (approximately 96%) are in the Reserves. Many of the personnel in the CA units perform jobs in their civilian life that directly enhance their ability to perform their CA mission. For example, a public health physician may work in their state health department as a civilian and then be the public health team leader in his or her CA unit. Although medical skills can be transferred to the civilian arena, this may not be the case in all of the 20 functional areas of CA expertise (Exhibit 12-2).[34] There are five CA commands or brigades in the Army, each of which is aligned with one of the five regionally oriented unified commands. Embedded within the CA structure are significant public health assets. The only physicians in the structure by doctrine are public health or preventive medicine specialists. In the RC, physicians trained in various specialties perform the role of a PM physician (Exhibit 12-3).

EXHIBIT 12-2

FUNCTIONAL SPECIALTIES IN CIVIL AFFAIRS

Government Section
Civil defense
Labor
Legal
Public administration
Public education
Public health
Public safety
Public welfare

Public Facilities Section
Public communications
Transportation
Public works and utilities

Special Functions Section
Arts, monuments, and archives
Civil information
Cultural affairs
Dislocated civilians

Economic Section
Civilian supply
Economics and commerce
Food and agriculture
Property control

EXHIBIT 12-3

MEDICAL PERSONNEL IN CIVIL AFFAIRS (CA) UNITS

Medical Personnel at the CA Brigade Level

Government Team
Public Health Physician (Team leader)
Veterinarian
Community Health Nurse
Health Service Material Officer
Environmental Science Officer
Sanitary Engineer Officer

Public Health Team
Public Health Physician (Team leader)
Veterinarian
Environmental Science Officer
Sanitary Engineer Officer
Medical NCO
Professional Service NCO

Medical Personnel at the CA Battalion Level (Foreign Internal Defense/Unconventional Warfare)

Public Health Team
Public Health Physician (Team leader)
Veterinarian
Field Medical Assistant
Sanitary Engineer Officer
Dental Officer
Entomologist
Medical Supply NCO
Chief Dental NCO

Civic Action Team
Veterinarian (Team leader)
Environmental Science Officer
Physician Assistant
Emergency Treatment NCO
Preventive Medicine NCO
Animal Care NCO

Direct Support Team
Medical NCO

Medical Personnel at the 96th CA Battalion Level (only CA unit on active duty)
Public Health Physician (Team leader)
Veterinarian
Special Forces Medic (one per Tactical Support Team)

Deployment Considerations

Before deployment, PM personnel will need to perform a thorough mission analysis. CA units are expected to develop extensive country studies, which include the epidemiology of diseases in the area of operations and the health of the indigenous population. Other information of concern includes the medical capabilities of the country; the number, type, and location of non-government organizations in the area; and any unique cultural considerations in dealing with the indigenous population.

MANAGING PREVENTIVE MEDICINE ASSETS IN THE FIELD

To the casual observer, US military operations conducted in recent years may not appear to meet the common definition of *war*. In fact, each of these missions falls somewhere on the spectrum of operations between war at one end and peace at the other and are termed operations other than war. Humanitarian assistance and peacekeeping operations in Somalia and Haiti are examples, as are non-combatant evacuations, hostage rescues, raids, shows of force, and other operations short of war. The rules of engagement and the logistics required to support these operations change with the type of mission. The mission may change its focus and move from one category to another (eg, peacekeeping to raids). These types of operations tend to be multi-service or multinational, requiring coordination among supporting services and countries and thus increasing the logistical challenges. There are three core PM missions that support any of these operations: identification of all medical threats, development of countermeasures to those threats, and surveillance for diseases and injuries. To achieve success, each PMO must effectively manage the assets available, then provide the resulting PM information to the unit surgeon and elicit support from unit commanders.

Variables Influencing Management Structure

A number of factors must be considered when establishing an organizational structure for the effective utilization of PM assets. The size and geography of the area of operations will influence the distribution of PM personnel and equipment. The presence of a Theatre Army Medical Laboratory (TAML) or Forward Deployed Laboratory (FDL) and the specific PM specialties represented, such as entomology, influence the services that can be offered. These can be augmented by host-nation and contractor service agreements. The health status and demographic profile of the indigenous population, as well as that of coalition forces, may become important if the PMO is called on to use PM resources to support them. Finally, the facilities for eating, living, and sanitation for all populations supported may demand undue attention if they are not properly maintained. Often the PMO will have very limited authority over PM assets in theater but retain responsibility for the overall success of the PM mission in the eyes of the command. Consequently,

negotiation skills, networking skills, and determination are invaluable. On arrival in theater, the PMO must rapidly assess the PM capabilities and materiel available and review the medical surveillance plan with personnel at each medical treatment facility.

Mission Planning Process

Regardless of the type of mission, the military follows a deliberate decision-making procedure to plan and direct the operation. Medical officers, and PM personnel in particular, must understand this system to have an impact when they address public health and general medical issues. Typically when a warning order or mission is received, the unit staff refers to the standing operational plan (OPLAN) for that particular situation and begins mission analysis, which is covered in some detail below. The staff then develops a specific mission and briefs this restated mission to the unit commander. After it is approved, the mission is used as the basis for the staff to develop several courses of action (COAs) to achieve the mission. During COA development, the staff analyzes, compares, and "wargames" each COA, finally deciding on one to recommend to the commander. When the commander approves the COA, the staff modifies the OPLAN, complete with specified, implied, and essential tasks for subordinate units to complete. This slow process is inadequate when staffs are responding to an emergency situation. Crisis action planning was developed to address this problem and is less complex and faster. Because of the imminent deadline for the OPLAN, the commander may work more closely with the staff, since they cannot afford the time to digress or consider many COAs. Consequently, the commander will probably forgo formal briefings and approve the results from the working sessions.[38]

Mission Analysis

During mission analysis, unit surgeons and PMOs must seize the opportunity to provide medical input into the OPLAN and its medical annex. To provide intelligent and cogent comments, medical personnel must assemble information from various sources, including the TAML and FDL staff sections at the unit headquarters. Copies of both the warning order from the higher command and the commander's guidance should be kept in the Operations Section: S-3 at battalion and brigade, G-3 at division and corps, and J-3 at joint staffs. The Intelligence Section (S-2, G-2, or J-2 at the respective levels) develops the Intelligence Preparation of the Battlefield. This document analyzes the enemy's capabilities, weaknesses, and strengths, as well as the terrain, the weather, and other relevant factors, and it may include information from the Defense Intelligence Agency and the Central Intelligence Agency. The Operations Section will also develop the Concept of the Operation, based on the information from the intelligence staff and the commander's guidance. Medical personnel must be familiar with this document since it describes what the unit will do and what the medical assets will have to support. In a similar fashion, the Logistics Section (S-4, G-4, or J-4) will develop the Logistics Estimate, which describes what support, including medical, will be provided.[38,39]

To provide optimum service to the unit and commander, the PMO must work closely with the command surgeon and interact with the other staff elements. With the surgeon and the Personnel Section (S-1, G-1, or J-1), the PMO should help develop casualty estimates and reports with a DNBI emphasis, because rates of DNBI always exceed rates of combat injuries. Additionally, the PMO should review the plan for handling enemy prisoners of war and refugees from a disease control and public health perspective. The S-2, G-2, or J-2 is the source to answer questions from or research any intelligence requirements needed by medical and nonmedical planners about such issues as enemy medical care facilities and equipment, nuclear, biological, and chemical weapons types and capabilities, and weather projections to support aeromedical evacuation. Medical personnel must work very closely with unit support components to develop a good Service Support Annex to the OPLAN. The PMO in particular should review this document and can have a tremendous public health impact. The PMO can ensure the appropriate provision of field services, including such issues as food (ie, its selection, procurement, storage, preparation, and disposal), water (adequate amounts and safe), laundry, graves registration, and hazardous waste disposal.[2,39]

As a part of the Service Support Annex, the Surgeon's Office should write Annex Q, Health Service Support. This document should have several sections, including one on PM (an example of which can be seen in Chapter 13, Preventive Medicine and the Operation Plan). The PM portion should emphasize DNBI and public health by including recommended countermeasures to the threat, estimates of the im-

pact of DNBI on combat power, information on educating servicemembers and commanders, immunization and chemoprophylaxis recommendations, outbreak investigation guidance, and occupational and environmental health requirements. The Logistics portion of Annex Q should address whether the Army will be the Class VIII (medical supply) source for the DoD, as is usually the case; the support relationships between medical units and their associated line units; the use, source, safety, and transport of blood; and whether or not coalition partners will use combined logistics, in which the US bears a disproportionately large burden of support, or national logistics, in which each country supports itself. Annex Q should also discuss veterinary services such as food supply inspection and zoonoses, which are also of interest to the PMO.

PMOs may interact with clinicians when reviewing casualty reports and conducting epidemiological investigations of disease outbreaks. Of particular interest must be the reports of nuclear, biological, or chemical weapons casualties, since the PMO may be the local "expert" for medical issues regarding weapons of mass destruction. Clinicians and PM personnel in subordinate units will need to know the level of medical support available, so the location and diagnostic capability of supporting laboratories must be included in Annex Q, as well as the locations and support relationships of combat stress control teams. Finally, subordinate PM units must know the identity and location of their next higher echelon of medical support for additional PM expertise, medical supply, and similar issues.[3]

Preventive Medicine Assets in Joint Operations

The JTF commander does not have ultimate authority over joint operations. That responsibility rests with the Commander-in-Chief (CINC) for that geographical portion of the worldwide system of unified commands, such as the Southern Command (Figure 12-4). The CINC, in turn, answers to the National Command Authority in the person of the Secretary of Defense or the President. For a specific or limited purpose, the CINC, as combatant commander, will relinquish operational control of various forces of any service under his control to the JTF commander, who is often from a different service[38] (Figure 12-5). With operational control, the JTF commander can control the events in the entire area of operations.

The PMO in the JTF functions just as he or she would in a single service force, except that requirements and resources of all services must be considered and coordinated (Figure 12-6). For example, the

Marines Corps, unlike the Army, has no dedicated medical evacuation helicopters and must request this support from other services. And Air Force involvement in an operation can make it easier to obtain a Mobile Aeromedical Staging Facility to hold and process casualties for fixed-wing evacuation.[2]

Preventive Medicine Assets in Unified Commands

The role of the PMO at the unified command is broad in scope and deep in responsibility; it is also extremely vital to the unified commander and the surgeon in both peace and war. Each geographic CINC is a combatant commander with a broad, continuing mission and significant components from two or more services. The CINC also has the responsibility for coordinating and integrating health service support within the theater of operation and exercising this responsibility directly through the unified command surgeon. The surgeon's joint staff must coordinate medical initiatives, solutions to regional medical issues, standardized approaches to national issues, and interoperability, and the health service support plans

and operations of subordinate units. The surgeon's office must be able to assess the health service support requirements and capabilities of component commands and provide guidance to enhance their effectiveness. Each unified command surgeon should have a PMO on staff whose primary function is to address the medical threats in the entire theater of operations. Similar to PMOs at other levels of command, he or she then promulgates recommended policies and countermeasures to obviate or mitigate those threats, monitors the health of deployed forces through an established surveillance mechanism, and modifies and updates policies and countermeasures based on ever-changing intelligence and surveillance data. An asset that must be employed early in operations is the TAML, which is designed to operate directly for the theater surgeon. This asset provides the theater surgeon a rapid diagnostic capability to monitor the health of the force and identify biological or chemical threats early. At the unified command level, the impact of medical threats as contributing factors to social, political, and economic stability in both peace and other operational environments

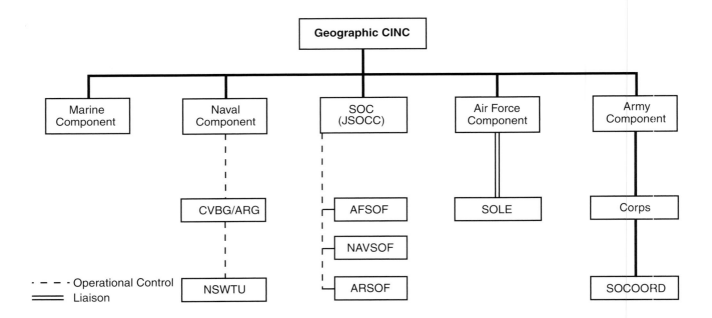

SOC: Special Operations Command
JSOCC: Joint Special Operations Component Commander
CVBG/ARG: Carrier Battle Group/Amphibious Ready Group
AFSOF: Air Force Special Operations Command

NAVSOF: Navy Special Operations Command
ARSOF: Army Special Operations Command
SOCOORD: Special Operations Coordination Element
SOLE: Special Operations Liaison Element
NSWTU: Naval Special Warfare Task Unit

Fig. 12-4. The Geographic Commanders in Chief Special Operating Forces with Integrating Elements.
Source: US Special Operations Command. *Special Operations in Peace and War.* SOC: 1996.

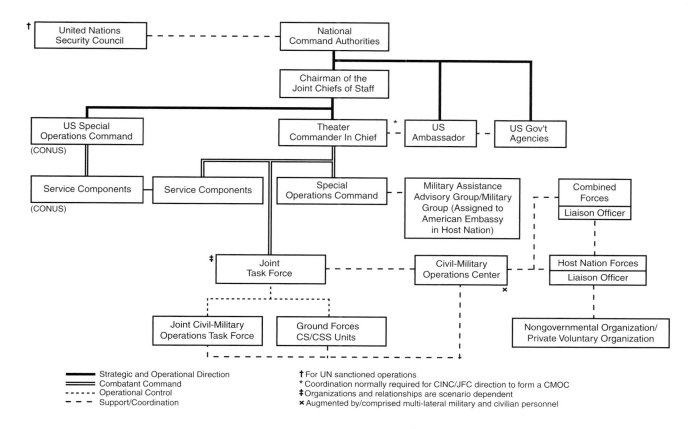

Fig. 12-5. The Organization of a Joint Task Force.
Source: US Special Operations Command. *Special Operations in Peace and War*. SOC: 1996.

must be considered. In addition to the traditional threat assessment, then, the PMO must attempt to determine the adequacy of the health infrastructure in the various countries in the theater and, in collaboration with civil affairs teams and the respective ministries of health, may be called on to make appropriate recommendations for ameliorating these deficiencies under unstable conditions.

Preventive Medicine Assets in Combined Operations

A combined task force, frequently referred to as a multinational force, consists of the forces of two or more nations acting together for the accomplishment of a single mission, and it may be organized from an alliance or coalition of nations. An alliance is the product of a longstanding, formalized agreement among political, diplomatic, and military officials. It offers the advantage of time for planners to adopt uniform warfighting (including PM) doctrine and standards among participating nations. Member nations of the North Atlantic Treaty Orga-

nization have worked for decades on developing many of the standarization agreements (known as STANAGS) now in effect. Implementing PM countermeasures and conducting medical surveillance in a combined task force derived from a coalition presents the most difficult challenge in military PM. Coalitions are less formal, ad hoc agreements among nations organized to meet short-term objectives.[38] In 1990, President Bush spearheaded a coalition that contributed to the combined force that removed the Iraqi Army from Kuwait. Before arriving in the theater of operations, contingents had no time to agree on standard procedures.

In US operations in the 1990s, including the Persian Gulf War and missions in Haiti and Bosnia, the United States participated in combined operations with forces from allies and other friendly countries. This added many layers of complexity to an already massive PM undertaking. Additional countries bring additional cultures and languages and different military training, doctrine, equipment, and objectives. Participating nations may have very limited health services support doctrine or capability, particularly in PM issues. Attitudes about staying healthy and patient care may differ markedly among the national components of a combined force. In other cases, force elements may share doctrine and cultural attitudes but lack essential resources. Health services support planning also may be influenced by the nationality of the combined force commander or the combined force medical authority. For these and other reasons, provision of health services support typically remains a national, not a combined, responsibility.

Most military forces of the world depend on domestic civilian resources for all aspects of their health care. These forces typically are not strategic and rarely deploy beyond their borders unless assisted. Therefore, military personnel from these countries are unlikely to encounter exotic health threats with any

greater frequency than the civilian population they come from. Consequently, the military organizations of most countries lack an organized PM capability. Only those countries, such as the United States, Canada, and France, that routinely deploy strategic ground forces beyond their borders are likely to have developed military PM doctrine. In combined operations, the obvious implication of this situation is that the responsibility for military PM operations falls to the country fielding the capability. If any part of the force lacks the capability to employ PM countermeasures or rejects employing them for cultural reasons, the public health threat to the entire force increases. The keys to success of combined operations are trust and teamwork.

Compared to joint operations, assessing the

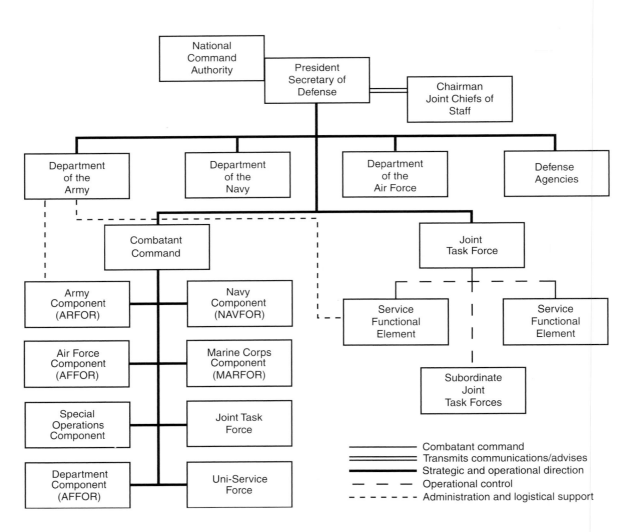

Fig. 12-6. Joint Task Force Relationships.
Source: US Department of the Army. *Operations*. Washington, DC: DA; 1993. Field Manual 100-5.

health threat in combined operations is more complicated because the health status among the combined force lacks homogeneity. However, each participating contingent joins the combined force healthy by its own set of deployability standards and shares a unique disease exposure and immunization history. Servicemembers may join a combined force harboring active infections endemic to their country of origin but exotic to other contingents of the force. For example, the exposure experience to hepatitis or Japanese encephalitis among Thai soldiers is greater than that of their US or Canadian counterparts.

In combined operations, medical surveillance techniques and procedures are limited to North Atlantic Treaty Organization alliance forces. Agreement among contingent forces on conducting medical surveillance is unlikely until the operation is weeks old. Consequently, useful medical surveillance of the combined force during the most critical early phase of an operation is unlikely. Except in those contingents with the most sophisticated PM capability, environmental survey and lab support capability will not be available.

SUMMARY

For the PMO or other health services planner to understand how to properly plan and execute PM services on deployments, it is essential to appreciate the big picture of military preventive medicine. This chapter has reviewed the process of PM policy development from the strategic JCS level to the operational JTF level to the tactical field unit. Although there are unique aspects to PM among the different US military services and these must be anticipated in the planning of any joint operation, there are additional considerations in providing PM support to government agencies or to operations with units from the Reserve Component, combined forces, Civil Affairs, or Special Operations Forces. With an understanding of these differences and an appreciation of the intricacies and complexities of military planning and operations, PM personnel can provide great benefit in conserving the fighting strength for their unit or command.

REFERENCES

1. Clements BA. *Medical Recollections of the Army of the Potomac by Jonathan Letterman, MD, and Memoir of Jonathan Letterman, MD*. Knoxville, Tenn: Bohemian Brigade Publishers; 1994: 100.

2. US Department of the Army. *Health Service Support in a Theater of Operations*. Washington, DC: DA; 1991. Field Manual 8-10.

3. US Department of the Army. *Unit Field Sanitation Team*. Washington, DC: DA; 1989. Field Manual 21-10-1.

4. US Department of the Army. *First Aid for Soldiers*. Washington, DC: DA; 1991. Field Manual 21-11.

5. US Department of the Army. *Preventive Medicine*. Washington, DC: DA; 1990. Army Regulation 40-5.

6. US Department of the Army. *Area Support Medical Battalion: Tactics, Techniques and Procedures*. Washington, DC: DA; 1993. Field Manual 8-10-24.

7. Thomas RJ, Conwill DE, Morton DE, Brooks TJ, Holmes CK, Mahaffey WB. Penicillin prophylaxis for streptococcal infections in US Navy and Marine Corps recruit camps (1951–1985). *Rev Inf Dis*. 1988;10:125–130.

8. Massart EL. USNS Comfort supports Operation Sea Signal. *Navy Med*. 1995;86(1):3–5.

9. Hyams KC, Hanson K, Wignall FS, Escamilla J, Oldfield EC. The impact of infectious diseases on the health of US troops deployed to the Persian Gulf during Operations Desert Shield and Desert Storm. *Clin Infect Dis*. 1995;20:1497–1504.

10. US Department of the Navy. *Navy Forward Deployable Laboratory*. Washington, DC: DN; 1995. Naval Warfare Publication 4-02.4, Part C.

11. US Marine Corps. *Health Services Support Manual*. Washington, DC: USMC; 1990. Fleet Marine Field Manual 4-50.

12. US Department of Transportation. *US Coast Guard Medical Manual*. Washington, DC: USCG; 1990. Commandant Instruction M6000.1(series).

13. Kramek RE. Commandant's direction. *Commandant's Bulletin*. 1995;2:insert. Commandant Publication P5720.2.

14. US Coast Guard data, 1995.

15. US Department of Transportation, US Coast Guard. *Coast Guard Manpower Mobilization and Support Plan*. Washington, DC: USCG; 1996. Commandant Instruction M3061.1.

16. Peña F. Citation for the Department of Transportation Gold Medal for Outstanding Achievement. *Commandant's Bulletin*. Commandant Publication.1995; P5720.2.;1:2.

17. US Department of Transportation, US Coast Guard. *Public Health and Communicable Disease Concerns Related to Alien Migrant Interdiction Operations (AMIO)*. Washington, DC: USCG; 1994. Commandant Instruction M6220.9.

18. Federal Emergency Management Agency. *Federal Response Plan (for Public Law 93–288, as amended)*. Washington, DC: FEMA; 1992.

19. Robert T. Stafford Disaster Relief and Emergency Assistance Act, Pub L No. 93-288, amended by 49 USC § 5121 et seq (1988).

20. US Department of the Army. *Domestic Support Operations*. Washington, DC: DA; 1993. Field Manual 100-19.

21. Ginzburg HM, Jevec RJ, Reutershan T. The Public Health Service's response to Hurricane Andrew. *Public Health Rep*. 1993;108(2):241–244.

22. Hess WA, Administrative Officer, Public Health Service-1 DMAT. Personal communication, 1996.

23. Public Health Service Act, Pub L No. 78–410, amended by 42 USC § 204, 212, 216, 217 et seq (1990).

24. Department of Health and Human Services, US Public Health Service. Response of the Department of Health and Human Services to the GAO Draft Report Relating to the Commissioned Corps of the Public Health Service. Rockville, Md: PHS Office of the Surgeon General; 1995. Memorandum.

25. Noji EK. Centers for Disease Control: Disaster preparedness and response activities. *Disasters*. 1992:177–178.

26. Gregg MB, ed. *The Public Health Consequences of Disasters 1989*. Atlanta: US Department of Health and Human Services, Public Health Service, Centers for Disease Control and Prevention; 1989.

27. Centers for Disease Control and Prevention. Famine-affected, refugee, and displaced populations: Recommendations for public health issues. *MMWR*. 1992;41(No.RR-13):1-76.

28. US Department of the Army. *TOE, Medical Detachment, Sanitation and Entomology*. Washington DC: DA; 1987.

29. Lynch L, Environmental Health Consultant, USAMEDCOM. Personal communication, 1996.

30. Savory B, Chief, Bioenvironmental Engineering Management Branch, HQ, AFRES Health Services Directorate; Nizoloski P, Superintendant of Public Health, Air National Guard, ANCRC/SGB; personal communication, 1996.

31. US Department of the Army. *Special Operations in Peace and War*. McDill AFB, Fla: US Southern Command; 1996. US Special Operations Publication 1.

32. US Department of the Army. *Standards of Medical Fitness*. Washington, DC: DA; 1991. Army Regulation 40-501.

33. Magnum M, Scott B, Joint Special Operations Command. Personal communication, 1996.

34. Department of the Army. *Civil Affairs Operations*. Washington DC: DA; 1993. Field Manual 41-10.

35. Sandler S. Seal the victory: A history of US Army Civil Affairs. *Special Warfare.* 1991;4(1)39.

36. US Department of the Army. *Public Health Functions.* Fort Bragg, NC: US Army John F. Kennedy Special Warfare Center; 1983. ST 41-10-7.

37. Carnes L, Brinderhoff J, Carlton P, Muller K, Quinn D. *Civil Affairs: Perspectives and Prospects.* Institute for National Strategic Studies, National Defense University; 1993: 3.

38. US Department of the Army. *Operations.* Washington, DC: DA; 1993. Field Manual 100-5.

39. US Army Medical Department Center and School. *AMEDD Staff Officer's Handbook.* Fort Sam Houston, Tex: AMEDDC&S; 1993. General Reference SISC-68.

Chapter 13

PREVENTIVE MEDICINE AND THE OPERATION PLAN

STEVEN YEVICH, MD, MPH

S. J. Yevich, Colonel, US Army (Retired); Director, VA National Center for Health Promotion and Disease Prevention, 3000 Croasdaile Drive, Durham, NC 27707; formerly, Colonel, Medical Corps, US Army, Command Surgeon, US Special Operations Command,7701 Tampa Point Blvd., MacDill Air Force Base, FL 33608-6001

INTRODUCTION

Operation plans (OPLANS) are large-scale deliberative processes, accomplished by unified commands during the calm of peacetime to minimize the negative effects on rational tactical and strategic planning caused by the emotions and confusion of rapid deployments. The plans provide a basic framework for a military operation to combat specific potential threats, defining such things as the chain of command, initial employment of forces, logistical support, medical support, and any other details that would help direct the conduct of operations against that specific threat.

There are nine unified commands in the US military forces, each with different responsibilities: Atlantic Command, European Command, Southern Command, Pacific Command, Central Command, Special Operations Command, Transportation Command, Space Command, and Strategic Command. These are commonly abbreviated as "CINCs" (colloquially named for the title of the Commanding General: Commander-in-Chief). Of the nine CINCs named above, the first five are unified combatant commands, responsible for specific geographic regions (AORs or Areas of Responsibility) of the world. Each CINC, in conjunction with the Joint Chiefs of Staff, identifies the major threats to the United States from within his AOR and deliberately develops OPLANS to address each of those threats if a contingency situation should arise. Examples of regional threats that could be anticipated, and for which OPLANS could be developed, include the invasion of South Korea by North Korea, the invasion of Kuwait and Saudi Arabia by Iraq, or a missile attack on the United States from Cuba. The OPLANS for each regional threat are given and referenced by specific numbers.

Guided by the OPLANS of the CINCs, each component service of a unified command devises a plan to support the master, or basic, CINC OPLAN, defining in increased detail its methods and means of implementing the plan. Component units configure their personnel, equipment, and training to support these plans. To test the plans, the component services and the CINCs engage in exercises patterned on the threat scenarios. They use the force structure designated by the OPLANS for actual implementation of the OPLAN. These exercises provide a way to assess the effectiveness and feasibility of implementing the OPLAN—they serve as a reality check. The OPLANS are living documents, subject to continual revision to reflect new concepts, lessons learned, better intelligence (such as increased or decreased enemy capability), new technology, and better ideas.

THE PREVENTIVE MEDICINE OFFICER'S ROLE IN OPLAN DEVELOPMENT

The Preventive Medicine Officer (PMO) should become familiar with all the major OPLANS for his or her unit or AOR and evaluate the adequacy of the planning preparation. There is no rigid format for an OPLAN; traditionally, though, Annex Q is the Medical Services section of the OPLAN, and Appendix 7 is the Preventive Medicine section. Within each of these sections, the format is not rigidly structured; guidance is offered in the Joint Chiefs of Staff publication.(See Reference f below.) In addition to Annex Q and Appendix 7, the PMO may be best informed and equipped to provide input into several other sections, such as the Medical Intelligence section (Appendix 11) and the Veterinary section (Appendix 12). Information addressing the following issues may also best come from the PMO: biological and chemical warfare, enemy prisoners of war, care of refugees, public health aspects of the reconstruction of friendly and enemy states, and other humanitarian assistance projects. Major OPLANS should be updated and verified annually.

THE PREVENTIVE MEDICINE OFFICER'S CONTRIBUTIONS TO THE OPLAN

In this chapter, Appendixes 7, 11, and 12 from a CENTCOM OPLAN, which were devised for an extensive operation, are used as a well-detailed example of the types of contributions preventive medicine can make to an OPLAN. This can serve as guidance and a checklist for a PMO required to develop an OPLAN de novo. All OPLANS may not require the amount of preventive medicine input shown here, but the preventive medicine contribution to Appendix 7 should be maximized. The regional command and its component services follow the specifications in an OPLAN very carefully, so it is exceedingly important to plan for and detail all possible issues that could arise during an operation, especially those that could be ignored during the confusion of an operation—from predeployment to redeployment. The example should be cut, elaborated, updated medically and scientifically, and otherwise tailored to the operation profile and the AOR threat. The importance of certain issues will vary by region or country of deployment, the intensity of combat, the geographic expanse, and other specific threats. Many

of the entries in this OPLAN example have generic applications to other regions. But do not use this example for its specific medical information or for its references, as these are constantly changing.

Note the following points: all paragraphs must have a classification (eg, Unclassified, Confidential, Secret, Top Secret—shown here by the placeholder (X), and italicized text represents the author's commentary.

APPENDIX 7 TO ANNEX Q TO USCINCCENT OPLAN ### (X)
PREVENTIVE MEDICINE SERVICES (X)

(X) REFERENCES: *Listing all references can save time for both the writer and the users of the OPLAN. These references are for illustration purposes only—they are not necessarily current, nor is the list necessarily thorough.*

a. (X) *Control of Communicable Diseases Manual.* 17th ed; Chin J, ed.; American Public Health Association, 2000. (NAVMED P-5038; USA FM 8-33)

b. (X) *Contingency Pest Management Pocket Guide;* Armed Forces Pest Management Board, 1998. Technical Information Memorandum No. 24.

c. (X) *Immunizations and Chemoprophylaxis.* AR 40-562, NAVMEDCOMINST 6230.3, AFR 161-13, CG COMDTINST M6320.4D; *1 Nov 1995.*

d. (X) *Health Information for International Travel, (1996–97).* HSS Publication No. (CDC) 93-8280, Centers for Disease Control and Prevention, Atlanta, Ga: *1997.*

e. (X) *General Recommendations on Immunization.* US Department of Health and Human Services, Centers for Disease Control and Prevention; *MMWR;* Vol. 43(RR-1); *1994.*

f. (X) *Doctrine for Health Service Support in Joint Operations.* Preliminary coordination 11 Aug 2000. Joint Publication 4-02.

g. (X) *Core Curriculum on Tuberculosis.* US Department of Health and Human Services, Centers for Disease Control.

h. (X) *Disease Vector Ecology Profile* (by country). Defense Pest Management Information Analysis Center, Forest Glen Section, Walter Reed Army Medical Center, Washington, DC.

i. (X) *Medical Reference Guide.* Travel Health Information Service, Shoreland Medical Marketing, Inc., Milwaukee, Wis; *Updated regularly.*

j. (X) *Venomous Snakes of the Middle East.* Defense Intelligence Agency, Armed Forces Medical Intelligence Center, Ft. Detrick, Md; DST-1810S-469-91.

k. (X) *The Risk of Disease and Non-Battle Injury to US Forces in Southwest Asia.* Division of Preventive Medicine, WRAIR, Washington, DC; 1994.

l. (X) *Staying Healthy in Southwest Asia.* Division of Preventive Medicine, WRAIR, Washington, DC; 1994.

m. (X) *Heat Illness: A Handbook for Medical Officers.* US Army Research Institute of Environmental Medicine, Natick, Mass; USARIEM Technical Note 91-3; Jun 1991.

n. (X) *Sustaining Health and Performance in the Desert: A Pocket Guide to Environmental Medicine for Operations in Southwest Asia.* US Army Research Institute of Environmental Medicine, Natick, Mass; USARIEM Technical Note 91-2; Dec 1990.

o. (X) *Travel and Routine Immunizations.* Thompson RF, Shoreland Medical Marketing, Inc., Milwaukee, Wis.

p. (X) *Health Hints for the Tropics.* 12th Edition, 1998. Published and distributed by The American Committee on Tropical Medicine and Traveler's Health of the American Society of Tropical Medicine and Hygiene.

q. (X) Immunization for Biological Warfare Defense. (*Nov 1993*) DOD Directive 6025.3.

r. (X) Medical Environmental Disease Intelligence and Countermeasures (MEDIC), Defense Intelligence Agency, Armed Forces Medical Intelligence Center, Ft. Detrick, MD. Updated every 6 months.

1. (X) <u>Purpose</u>. To provide a comprehensive concept of operations, define the threat, and assign tasks for preventive medicine support of the Basic Plan.

2. (X) <u>Abbreviations, Definitions, and Assumptions</u>. *Note: This list is for demonstration purposes only; it may not be complete, accurate, or current.*

a. (X) <u>Abbreviations</u>. *Make sure all abbreviations used in the Annex are listed here.*
  (1) AFMIC—Armed Forces Medical Intelligence Center
  (2) AOR—area of responsibility
  (3) ARCENT—US Army component, US Central Command
  (4) ASD(HA)—Assistant Secretary of Defense (Health Affairs)
  (5) BW—biological warfare
  (6) CENTAF—US Air Force component, US Central Command
  (7) CENTCOM—USCENTCOM; the joint regional command,
US Central Command
  (8) CHPPM—Center for Health Promotion and Preventive Medicine
  (9) CINC—Commander-in-Chief; also can refer to the regional command
(eg, CENTCOM)
  (10) CINCCENT—Commander in Chief, US Central Command
  (11) CONPLAN—Concept plan
  (12) CW—chemical warfare
  (13) DEET—N,N-diethylmeta-toluamide insect repellent
  (14) DIA—Defense Intelligence Agency
  (15) DNBI—Disease, nonbattle injury
  (16) DPMIAC—Defense Pest Management Information Analysis Center
  (17) EPW—enemy prisoner of war
  (18) ER—emergency room
  (19) FRAGORD—fragmentary order
  (20) HCA—humanitarian civic assistance
  (21) HIV—human immunodeficiency virus
  (22) ICU/CCU—intensive care unit/cardiac care unit
  (23) JCS—Joint Chiefs of Staff
  (24) MEDIC—Medical Environmental Disease Intelligence and Countermeasures
  (25) MOPP—mission-oriented protective posture
  (26) NAMRU—Naval Medical Research Unit
  (27) NAVCENT—US Navy component, US Central Command
  (28) NBC—nuclear, biological, and chemical
  (29) NCO—Noncommissioned Officer
  (30) NEPMU—US Navy Environmental and Preventive Medicine Unit
  (31) OCONUS—outside the continental United States
  (32) OPLAN—operation plan
  (33) OPORD—operation order
  (34) PM—preventive medicine
  (35) PMO—Preventive Medicine Officer
  (36) PPM—personal protection measures
  (38) STD—sexually transmitted disease
  (39) TAML—Theater Area Medical Lab
  (40) TB—tuberculosis
  (41) WRAIR—Walter Reed Army Institute of Research
b. (X) <u>Definitions</u>.
  (1) (X) Component Surgeon—The ARCENT, CENTAF, or NAVCENT Surgeon in theater or their designated in-theater representatives.
  (2) (X) Theater Surgeon—The CENTCOM Surgeon, when deployed to the theater; otherwise, this is the Command Surgeon designated by the CENTCOM Surgeon in his or her place. This may be the Component Surgeon from the component with the largest in-theater representation.
  (3) (X) Theater Medical Surveillance Team—A team of medical and scientific experts with its own inherent rapid diagnostic laboratory capability that is assigned directly to the Theater Surgeon. The team's major purpose is to minimize casualties, in part by establishing a theater network of disease surveillance, investigating disease outbreaks, identifying health hazards, and providing a high level of preventive medicine technical expertise not normally found in

one location in a combat zone. The Theater Area Medical Lab is the Army unit currently fielding this function.

    c. (X) <u>Assumptions</u>.

       (1) (X) That US forces must be entirely self-sufficient in their PM support and that host-nation or allied coalition PM services cannot be expected to be adequate or even present.

       (2) (X) That the target region will harbor a plethora of infectious diseases to which US military forces will be immunologically naïve and therefore be more susceptible to increased morbidity and mortality than the indigenous people.

       (3) (X) That current and specific disease prevalence information reflecting actual "field conditions" may not be available from US military medical intelligence sources or international health organizations before deployment.

       (4) (X) That the specific types and prevalence of health threats will change throughout the deployment.

3. (X) <u>Concept of Operations.</u> A PM program that (1) is included in initial operation planning, (2) is deployed and installed with the earliest forces, and (3) is fully supported by the command will result in effective implementation of measures required to minimize disease and injury. Institution of a thorough disease surveillance network, employment of a forward diagnostic laboratory, continual education of commanders and service members, and utilization of immunizations and the highest possible standards of sanitation and hygiene are the simple keys to maintaining combat effectiveness and overcoming what have been historically the greatest medical threats to the mission. Continual reevaluation of effectiveness, anticipation of problems, and flexibility in theater PM policies are required to accommodate newly discovered or developing health threats.

    a. (X) <u>Theater Preventive Medicine Priorities</u>.

       (1) (X) <u>Disease Surveillance</u>. Obtaining immediate disease surveillance data is the key to filling the gap in current, country-specific disease intelligence and the key for early identification of disease and injury trends during the operation. A theater medical surveillance team must deploy early with the initial forces to the theater, must possess a rapid diagnostic laboratory capability, and must fall under the direct control of the Theater Surgeon. A tri-service network of all medical treatment facilities will report centrally to the Theater Surgeon using the weekly JCS Disease Reporting format (see Tab A to Appendix 7). In this manner, timely disease outbreak information will be obtained for trend analysis and for disease investigation.

       (2) (X) <u>Disease Outbreak Investigation</u>. PM assets will investigate disease outbreaks locally. To ensure accurate disease surveillance during the initial stages of deployment, outbreaks must be thoroughly investigated with laboratory assistance. The theater medical surveillance team, with its diagnostic laboratory capability, can aid unit PM assets during large-scale outbreaks or those of cryptic etiology. All outbreak results must be reported to the Theater Surgeon for trend analysis and theater disease awareness.

       (3) (X) <u>Predeployment and Initial Deployment Preparation</u>. Medical, specifically PM, personnel must alert and caution commanders and service members about preventable medical problems likely to arise as a result of geo-environmental changes and the high tempo of activity during the initial phases of deployment. Factors that should be addressed include injuries due to lifting or dropping objects and other accidents, proper nutrition, time zone acclimatization (jet lag), climatic acclimatization, water intake, and psychological stressors.

       (4) (X) <u>Climatic Injury Prevention</u>. Medical assets within each respective unit must make commanders and service members aware of the dangers, prevention, and treatment of heat and cold injuries. During the early phase of deployment, commanders and senior NCOs must be aware of physical activity precautions and acclimatization measures.

       (5) (X) <u>Potable Water</u>. PM assets must ensure proper source selection for all water (including ice) sources. They must continually verify water quality and perform periodic inspections of all utilized water facilities (eg, bottled water, bulk chlorinated supplies, well water, local tap water).

       (6) (X) <u>Food Safety</u>. No bulk food sources for service members will be used unless inspected and sanitarily approved by US military PM or veterinary personnel. Periodic inspection of products while in storage is required (see also Appendix 12 Veterinary Services).

       (7) (X) <u>Personal Hygiene Measures</u>. Unit-level medical assets must provide education and

training for all service members to ensure awareness of basic personal hygiene measures.

(8) (X) <u>Dental Hygiene</u>. Dental problems are a potential cause of high morbidity among personnel living under stress and in field conditions. Dental hygiene must be continually emphasized and dental statistics closely monitored for adverse trends.

(9) (X) <u>Theater Arthropod Vector Control</u>. Education of service members in use of PPMs and provision of area control measures are the responsibility of unit PM assets. All aerial spraying will be coordinated through the Theater Surgeon. The use of herbicides is prohibited except as coordinated with the JCS through the Theater Surgeon.

(10) (X) <u>Other Environmental Threats</u>. When other environmental hazards are identified or anticipated, PM assets must bring these to the attention of commanders so that service member education and protection against the threats are provided. Examples of environmental hazards include altitude, dusts, and intense sunlight.

(11) (X) <u>Combat Stress</u>. All medical assets must be continually alert for subtle manifestations of combat stress. Diagnoses should be communicated per the JCS reporting format to the Theater Surgeon. The Theater Surgeon is responsible for identifying the extent of this problem, informing the Command, and recommending activation or supplementation of Combat Stress teams. Education of commanders, senior NCOs, and service members in identifying common presentations must also emphasize the need to treat combat stress as an illness and not a mental weakness. Early recognition results in effective treatment and early return to duty. Periodic service member and commander meetings should be organized by medical assets or commanders or both to elicit and discuss individual concerns that could give rise to stress reactions.

(12) (X) <u>Redeployment Considerations</u>. Because service members will constantly be exiting the AOR, redeployment medical considerations must be contemplated and addressed early in the operation; they must also be updated continually to reflect the most current medical problems arising within the AOR. While the redeployment program is a Command program, the medical assets are key to providing timely and appropriate advice concerning its extent. At a minimum, individual medical records should contain a notice of the service member's deployment to the AOR, diseases prevalent within that area, and clinical precautions to be taken when medical problems arise. Redeployment medical briefings should be conducted before service members leave the AOR to address topics such as STDs, signs and symptoms of endemic diseases, education on terminal drug prophylaxes (when needed), and awareness of possible psychological readjustment problems. Appropriate medical screening (eg, blood tests, tuberculin skin tests) should be conducted at this time. Terminal prophylaxes, if indicated (eg, the AOR is in a malarious region), should be emphasized and the full drug regimens should be given to the service member as he or she leaves the AOR.

b. (X) <u>Immunizations and Chemoprophylaxes</u>. Comprehensive and precise information will be promulgated in a CENTCOM FRAGORD to the CONPLAN OPORD.

(1) (X) <u>General</u>. The CENTCOM Surgeon Preventive Medicine Office has prepared and published guidance on immunizations and chemoprophylaxes. This information is an essential part of this Appendix and has been provided to Components and Service Headquarters under separate cover to obtain quad-service consensus and compliance on this vital aspect of service members' preparation for deployment. The objective is to deploy personnel with the right immunological profile quickly and effectively in time of crisis.

(2) (X) <u>Specific Immunizations</u>. *(Note: Currency and applicability of these immunizations to the region of deployment may change.)* Precise guidance in the FRAGORD will cover these issues: routine immunizations for diseases such as hepatitis A (vaccine or immune globulin alternative), influenza, measles, rubella, meningococcal meningitis (quadrivalent vaccine), polio (oral vaccine), tetanus-diphtheria, typhoid fever, varicella, yellow fever, and plague; special immunizations for diseases such as hepatitis B, rabies, Rift Valley fever, pneumococcal infection, Japanese encephalitis, and cholera; and chemoprophylaxes for malaria and other diseases. *Determining the status of a predeployment tuberculin skin test may be indicated.*

(3) (X) <u>Vaccination Against Biological Agents</u>. (Dependent on DoD Decision Process in Execution Planning)

(a) (X) <u>General</u>. Reference P provides guidance concerning immunization for BW defense. When appropriate and subject to exceptions approved by the Chairman of the JCS, the following personnel will be immunized against validated BW threat agents for which suitable vaccines are available in sufficient time to develop immunity before deployment to high-threat areas:

<u>1</u> (X) Personnel assigned to high-threat areas.

<u>2</u> (X) Personnel predesignated for immediate contingency deployment (eg, crisis response).

<u>3</u> (X) Personnel identified and scheduled for deployment on an imminent or ongoing contingency operation to a high-threat area.

(b) (X) <u>Approval Sequence for Nonlicensed Vaccines</u>. HQ CINCCENT submits a BW threat analysis to the Chairman of the JCS. The Chairman, in consultation with the CINC, the Service Chiefs, and the Director of DIA, will validate and prioritize the BW threat. This prioritized list is then forwarded through the ASD(HA) to the Executive Agent (US Army). The Executive Agent consults with the Service Secretaries and the Chair of the Armed Forces Epidemiological Board. The Board makes recommendations on the safety and effectiveness of the vaccines, and the coordinated recommendations go forward to the ASD(HA). The ASD(HA) then coordinates with the Chairman, JCS, before issuing vaccinations guidance.

(c) (X) *Specific Vaccines. Discuss various vaccines for BW agents that may be encountered. Include a statement about the safety and effectiveness of the vaccine, its Food and Drug Administration licensure, its vaccination schedule, the lag period before attaining protective immunity, the booster schedule, any contraindications or potential adverse side effects, the availability of vaccine, and any alternative or additional countermeasures to address the threat (eg, antibiotics, disinfectant procedures).*

<u>1</u> *(X) Address population to be vaccinated (eg, everyone, front-line troops only, pilots, medical personnel).*

<u>2</u> *(X) Address indications for proceeding with BW agent vaccinations (eg, on unambiguous threat of BW attack), whether to inoculate before deployment, whether to complete vaccine series before deployment, or whether to delay deployment until immunity is gained.*

(d) (X) <u>Differential Diagnosis for Certain BW or CW Agents</u>. *Similar information to that included in Table 13-1 may be helpful to deploying or deployed medical personnel as a handy synopsis of material that may be difficult to research before deployment.*

(4) (X) <u>Chemoprophylaxes Against Biological and Chemical Agents</u>. Because of the possible BW and CW threats, nerve agent and BW agent prophylaxes may be required. All service members should be knowledgeable in the use of these chemoprophylaxes.

(a) (X) <u>BW Prophylaxis</u>.

<u>1</u> (X) <u>Specific BW Agent</u>. *Present the medical defenses against each specific agent (eg, vaccine, antibiotic, combination).*

<u>a</u> *(X) If a chemoprophylactic agent (eg, antibiotic) is used as a countermeasure after exposure to the agent, delineate how it would be distributed (eg, given to each service member, kept with medical personnel), when and how often it would be administered, and how long it would be continued.*

<u>2</u> (X) <u>Specific BW Agent</u>. *See above.*

(b) (X) <u>CW Prophylaxis</u>. *Present each of the chemoprophylaxes that may be used by the service member in the event of CW attack.*

<u>1</u> (X) <u>Chemoprophylaxis #1</u>. *Describe the reason for usage, when the medication or injection should be administered, how often it should be given, and for how long it should be continued.*

<u>a</u> *(X) Address how units should distribute the chemoprophylaxis. Also stress the need for service member education on instructions for usage and usual side effects.*

<u>2</u> (X) <u>Chemoprophylaxis #2</u>. *See above.*

(c) (X) <u>Training and Education</u>.

<u>1</u> (X) <u>Service Members</u>. Commanders will ensure that, in addition to the standard personal and unit training in BW and CW, all service members receive training and demonstrate knowledge in the use of the BW and CW chemoprophylaxes.

<u>2</u> (X) <u>Health Care Workers</u>. All service members who are involved in the direct health care of

TABLE 13-1

DIFFERENTIAL DIAGNOSIS OF CHEMICAL NERVE AGENT, BOTULINUM TOXIN, AND STAPHYLOCOCCAL ENTEROTOXIN B INTOXICATION FOLLOWING INHALATION EXPOSURE

	Chemical Nerve Agent	Botulinum Toxin	Staphylococcal Enterotoxin B
Time to Symptoms	Minutes	Hours (12–48)	Hours (1–6)
Nervous System	Convulsions, twitching	Progressive paralysis	Headache, muscle ache
Cardiovascular System	Slow heart rate	Normal rate	Normal or rapid rate
Respiratory System	Difficulty breathing, airway constriction	Normal, then progressive paralysis	Nonproductive cough; in severe cases: chest pain, difficulty breathing
Gastrointestinal System	Increased motility, pain, diarrhea	Decreased motility	Nausea, vomiting, diarrhea
Ocular	Small pupils	Droopy eyelids (conjunctival injection)	May have "red eyes"
Salivary	Profuse, watery saliva	Normal, but swallowing difficult	May be slightly increased salivation
Death	Minutes	2–3 days	Unlikely
Response to Atropine and 2 PAM-Cl*	Yes	No	Atropine may reduce gastrointestinal symptoms

*pralidoxime chloride
Source: US Army Medical Research Institute of Infectious Diseases. *Medical Management of Biological Casualties Handbook.* 2nd ed. Fort Detrick, Md: USAMRIID; 1996.

patients should be familiar with protocols to administer special vaccines, identify BW and CW agent exposure, and handle and treat BW and CW casualties, according to their level of expertise.

   c. (X) Medical Intelligence Sources. See Appendix 11.

   d. (X) Command Responsibilities.

      (1) (X) Component Commands. Through their Command Surgeons, the component commands ensure implementation of PM countermeasures to health threats and compliance by service members with these countermeasures.

        (a) (X) Component commands should recognize that PM assets provide disease surveillance, investigate health hazards (including disease outbreaks), provide specific advice concerning implementation of PM countermeasures, and provide feedback to commanders on the effectiveness of PM countermeasures.

        (b) (X) Component commands ensure that PM personnel are fully integrated into mission planning, logistics, and operations for early implementation of PM guidance and to avoid poorly planned contingency measures in the future.

          1 (X) PM assets must be included in advance-party activities and site surveys and should be deployed in the earliest phase of operations.

          2 (X) Command emphasis should include high priority for PM logistical needs to fulfill the PM mission, to include communications, computer, and vehicular support.

      (2) (X) Subordinate Unit Commands. Subordinate commands are responsible for unit compliance with theater PM countermeasures. Important specific measures are as follows but are not limited to these listed.

        (a) (X) Field Sanitation Teams. Ensure that units have designated, equipped, and trained field sanitation teams and that these teams deploy with equipment to the theater.

(b) (X) <u>Disease Surveillance</u>. Ensure compliance by unit medical assets with weekly disease surveillance reports per JCS format.

(c) (X) <u>Environmental Threats</u>. Ensure that environmental threats are identified and addressed and that proper precautions are implemented.

(d) (X) <u>Water Safety</u>. Ensure that all water for service member use is potable.

(e) (X) <u>Food Safety</u>. Ensure that all foods, food production facilities, and food handlers are sanitarily approved.

(f) (X) <u>Pregnancy</u>. Ensure that no pregnant service member deploys to the AOR.

(g) (X) <u>STDs</u>. Ensure compliance with theater policy discouraging sexual intercourse.

(h) (X) <u>Pets</u>. Ensure enforcement of "no pets, no mascots" policy.

(i) (X) <u>Combat Stress</u>. (See Section 3.a.11). Provide command support for a combat stress program and for treatment.

(j) (X) <u>Redeployment</u>. Anticipate redeployment and ensure all service members receive medical outprocessing before redeployment as prescribed by the Theater Surgeon.

e. (X) <u>Theater Laboratory Support</u>.

(1) (X) A laboratory with rapid diagnostic capability will accompany the early initial deployment as part of the theater medical surveillance team. The laboratory maintains diagnostic capabilities to support disease surveillance activities, investigate environmental health threats, and provide rapid identification of BW agents.

(2) (X) As the theater develops, the theater medical support system will fully complement, support, and integrate PM efforts in the theater of operations, to include providing laboratory support.

f. (X) <u>Veterinary Support</u>. See Appendix 12.

g. (optional) (X) <u>Enemy Prisoners of War</u>. PM and veterinary assets must assist in site location decisions, design, and maintenance of EPW camps. Specific responsibilities include ensuring proper environmental and sanitary location of the EPW site; proper number, type, and maintenance of sanitation and hygiene facilities; hygienic handling of food and water supplies; insect control; administration of immunizations, if necessary; EPW education in PM measures; disease surveillance of the camp; and disease outbreak investigation.

i. (optional) (X) <u>Humanitarian Civic Assistance</u>. When US military forces oversee HCA programs, as with refugee populations and disaster management, PM and veterinary assets must be included in the initial planning stages to determine short- and long-term goals, attainability and impact of relief measures, and breadth of impact of those measures on the target population. During the conduct of the HCA, PM assets continually assess the general health of the target population, conduct disease surveillance, investigate and address health threats, and reevaluate the direction of the HCA operation. When medical relief operations are conducted in conjunction with civilian nongovernmental organizations, PM assets must work directly with the leadership of those organizations in establishing goals and priorities to produce broad-based improvements in the health of the population, in the organization of the operation, and in the allocation of labor in these projects.

4. (X) <u>Health Threat</u>. *Research and annually (or more frequently) update the information in this section. The information offered below may not be current or accurate for the particular region of deployment. Many units will rely on this guidance alone as the sole direction for planning.* The priority of health risks will vary among the targeted countries, vary according to season, and change during the deployment. The risks of disease in several categories can be predicted and should be anticipated in medical planning. However, current medical intelligence must be gathered (Section 3.a.3, 3c, and Appendix 11) before deployment and must be continually updated during the deployment.

a. (X) <u>Diseases of Operational Importance</u>. The following are ubiquitous and are not AOR-specific. However, they may become even more significant under conditions of high stress and poor hygiene.

(1) (X) <u>Acute Respiratory Infections</u>. Climatic changes, fatigue, fine airborne dusts, and service member crowding can all contribute to high levels of acute respiratory infections. Countermeasures aimed at decreasing the risk factors should be implemented.

(2) (X) <u>Dermatological Conditions</u>. Hot and dry, hot and wet, and cold and wet climates are all encountered within the CENTCOM AOR. Service member education should include foot and skin care appropriate to the environment.

(3) (X) <u>Heat- and Cold-related Problems</u>. Heat-related injuries can be a significant category of illness if command attention is not paid to adequate hydration, proper work-rest cycles, and acclimatization. In addition, cold temperatures (even freezing temperatures) can be encountered in the desert, as well as in the mountainous areas. Commanders and senior NCOs must be aware of nighttime drops in temperature and ensure that preventive measures are implemented.

b. (X) <u>Diseases with Short Incubation Periods</u> (usually less than 15 days).

(1) (X) <u>Acute Diarrheal Disease</u>. Acute diarrheal disease constitutes the greatest immediate disease threat to the health of the force. Emphasis must be placed on the principles of field sanitation and hygiene if DNBI rates are to be kept to a minimum. Prophylaxis is not generally indicated but may be required in special circumstances, as determined by the Theater Surgeon.

(2) (X) <u>Enteric Protozoal Diseases</u>. Proper food preparation and water treatment will minimize acquisition of these diseases.

(3) (X) <u>Malaria</u>. Malaria is a serious threat in certain areas (see Section 3.b.2). For service members entering these areas, compliance with chemoprophylaxis and other preventive measures must be ensured through education and command influence.

(4) (X) <u>Typhoid and Paratyphoid Fevers</u>. Again, proper food and water treatment and handling will minimize risk of contracting these. Fly control by screening, proper garbage disposal, and other sanitary practices are needed. Typhoid fever immunization may be indicated.

(5) (X) <u>Arboviral Fevers</u>. There is a plethora of arthropod-borne viral diseases within the general AOR (eg, sandfly fever, West Nile fever, Crimean-Congo hemorrhagic fever, Sindbis fever, dengue). A high degree of suspicion, with keen disease surveillance and a forward rapid diagnostic laboratory, can provide early identification of these diseases. Commanders must enforce the use of PPMs, with judicious use of area and regional insect control measures.

(6) (X) <u>Sexually Transmitted Diseases</u>. Incubation periods may vary from days to years. All known STDs exist within the AOR. The restrictions and anxieties accompanying military operations make sexual relations a potential outlet for these tensions. As a result, "common source" infections from contacts with the limited female population, as well as with indigenous people, could make STDs a major risk. Penicillin-resistance can be assumed. HIV screening for OCONUS travel should be done in accordance with service regulations. Avoiding exposure is the key to prevention.

(7) (X) <u>Meningococcal Meningitis</u>. Crowded conditions exacerbate the spread of meningitis. Immunization and adequate physical spacing of individual personnel are measures commanders and PMOs should enforce.

(8) (X) <u>Cholera</u>. Proper food preparation and water treatment will minimize acquisition of cholera.

c. (X) <u>Diseases with Long Incubation Periods</u> (usually greater than 15 days).

(1) (X) <u>Enterically Transmitted Acute Viral Hepatitides (A and E)</u>. Immunization (in the case of hepatitis A) and proper food and water sanitation will minimize these threats.

(2) (X) <u>Schistosomiasis</u>. Acquisition is by exposing skin to fresh water sources (eg, by wading or swimming). These activities should be avoided.

(3) (X) <u>Parenterally Transmitted Acute Viral Hepatitides (B, C, and D)</u>. Exposure via blood transfusions, contaminated needles, and contaminated wounds may occur in the field setting or possibly through substandard medical treatment (eg, when rendered by allied or coalition forces). Drug abuse may occur even in well-controlled combat zones. Sexual transmission can also be an avenue for these infections.

(4) (X) <u>Leishmaniasis</u>. Adequate use of PPMs to prevent sandfly bites must be emphasized.

(5) (X) <u>Tuberculosis</u>. The endemicity of TB in the AOR, as well as its high prevalence in some allied and coalition forces, could account for a high rate of exposure of US service members. Multidrug resistance should be presumed. Early identification of active TB cases in indigenous or other non-US camp workers (eg, food handlers) can minimize personnel exposure. Redeployment PPD testing is required.

(6) (X) <u>Sexually Transmitted Diseases</u>. See Section 4.b.6.

d. (X) <u>Insect and Arthropod Vectors</u>. Diseases transmitted by arthropod vectors (eg, mosquitoes, sand flies, ticks, lice, fleas) are numerous and will have a significant effect on the health of the force unless PPMs are enforced. Examples of disease these vectors carry include plague, flea-borne typhus fever, tick-borne relapsing fever, louse-borne typhus fever, and louse-borne relapsing fever. The use of the following are required of all personnel: (1) clothing treatment (permethrin), (2) "buddy checks," (3) personal insect repellents, (4) insect bar (mosquito netting with suspension system) sprayed with permethrin, and (5) proper wearing of the uniform (sleeves down). All personnel should sleep under insect bars.

e. (X) <u>Pets</u>. Domestic animals (eg, dogs, cats, sheep, goats) or wild animals (eg, monkeys, rodents, reptiles) are not to be kept as pets or mascots. These animals are infected with a variety of zoonotic diseases that can be transmitted to humans. They can also harbor vectors capable of transmitting diseases that have a high potential for adversely affecting the health of the command, including rabies, African tick typhus fever, Q fever, Crimean-Congo hemorrhagic fever, and leishmaniasis.

5. (X) <u>Tasks</u>. *This is the section where tasks are apportioned to various levels of the Command and down to the Component Services. Central Command is used here as an example. By delineating specific tasks in the OPLAN, emphasis and verification of the importance of the task is established and specification of distinct responsibilities can be assigned. Note that heavy emphasis is placed on Theater Medical Surveillance because this has been a chronically weak area in PM theater support.*

a. (X) <u>US Central Command</u>. Through the CENTCOM Surgeon, USCINCCENT provides command support for PM initiatives and issues. The CENTCOM Surgeon will ensure that health-related issues in the theater are brought to the attention of USCINCCENT as well as the Component Surgeons, project and identify DNBI casualty trends before they become significant, and ensure that PM issues are addressed and preventive measures are instituted. Important specific corollary responsibilities include the following.

(1) (X) Establish a theater disease surveillance network. A theater medical surveillance team (see 3.e), under direction of the CENTCOM Surgeon, will deploy to the theater with the advance party to accomplish the following:

(a) (X) Initiate the theater disease surveillance network.

(b) (X) Analyze disease surveillance data.

(c) (X) Investigate disease outbreaks and other health hazards.

(d) (X) Provide an on-site, technologically advanced diagnostic capability, to include BW agent identification.

(e) (X) Provide education and guidance in special health-related issues to health care providers, commanders, and service members.

(2) (X) Ensure that Component Surgeons comply with periodic disease surveillance reporting according to the JCS reporting format.

(3) (X) Ensure that Component Surgeons receive disease surveillance findings and proper guidance in addressing health issues.

(4) (X) Ensure PM education and training of appropriate personnel (eg, health care providers, commanders, service members).

(5) (X) Before deployment, and as other indications arise, identify immunization and chemoprophylaxis requirements for the theater.

(6) (X) Ensure that redeployment issues are addressed in a timely fashion.

b. (X) <u>Components</u>. *(The services: US Army, Navy, Air Force, and Marine Corps.)*

(1) (X) Will institute effective PM countermeasures; comply with the DNBI Surveillance Program; provide for and effectively employ PM resources to meet their own or joint missions; and ensure commanders are kept informed of the health of their commands.

(2) (X) Will submit the Weekly Medical Surveillance Report. DNBI data will be logged and reported by all deployed units using the JCS Weekly Medical Surveillance Report format (see Tab A, Appendix 7). These weekly reports will be forwarded from all medical facilities, beginning from Aid Station level to each subsequent higher level until reaching the office of the Theater Surgeon. The theater medical surveillance team (or the theater PMO) will collect these reports and analyze the data. If the CENTCOM Surgeon is not the Theater Surgeon, the theater Surgeon will forward these reports to CENTCOM Surgeon's Office weekly.

(3) (X) ARCENT, as executive agent, will provide veterinary coverage within the theater of operations.

(4) (X) Will ensure all deploying personnel are briefed by PM or other medical personnel on the following issues.

(a) (X) Endemic diseases, specifically the infectious disease risk as outlined in MEDIC.

(b) (X) Water and food consumption. No food or water is to be consumed unless first approved by US military medical authorities. Personnel must know proper water treatment procedures and recognize unsafe food and water situations.

(c) (X) Proper field sanitation techniques.

(d) (X) Use of permethrin clothing treatment and DEET lotion.

(e) (X) Personal hygiene.

(f) (X) Prevention of environmental (heat and cold) injuries.

(g) (X) Inappropriateness of maintaining pets or mascots in theater, including the diseases carried by these animals and the dangers of handling snakes, spiders, scorpions, and centipedes.

(h) (X) Sexually transmitted diseases.

(i) (X) Malaria (and other) chemoprophylaxis, if indicated.

(5) (X) The Theater Area Medical Laboratory deploys with its own diagnostic laboratory capability. Other laboratory support can be provided by ... *(list all higher-level laboratory capabilities within or near the AOR, whether fixed facility, afloat, or mobile).*

(6) (X) CENTAF will provide fixed-wing aerial spraying capability.

c. (X) <u>Commanders' Responsibilities</u>. Commanders at all levels are responsible to maintain the health of their personnel.

(1) (X) Commanders should recognize that medical and PM assets provide disease surveillance, investigate health hazards (including disease outbreaks), provide specific advice concerning implementation of PM countermeasures to health threats, and provide feedback to commanders on the effectiveness of those countermeasures.

(2) (X) Commanders should fully integrate PM personnel into mission planning, logistics, and operations for early implementation of PM guidance.

(a) (X) PM assets must be included in advance-party activities and site surveys and should be deployed in the earliest phase of operations.

(b) (X) Command emphasis should include high priority for PM logistical needs to fulfill the PM mission, to include communications, computer, and vehicular support.

(3) (X) Commanders are responsible for the following specific PM measures, which will affect the health of the service members.

(a) (X) <u>Field Sanitation Teams</u>. Ensure that units have designated, equipped, and trained field sanitation teams and that these teams deploy with equipment into the theater. Note: This unit responsibility is often overlooked or intentionally avoided, resulting in serious PM problems upon deployment.

(b) (X) <u>Disease Surveillance</u>. Ensure that medical assets comply with weekly disease surveillance reports per the JCS format. Provide command support for the theater medical surveillance team in acquiring data.

(c) (X) <u>Disease Outbreak Investigations</u>. Provide command support for all disease outbreak investigations by medical assets and the theater medical surveillance team.

(d) (X) <u>Preventive Medicine Advisories</u>. Ensure PM precautions are implemented and enforced.

(e) (X) <u>Environmental Threats</u>. Ensure that environmental threats are identified and addressed and that proper precautions are implemented. Ensure that time is allowed for time-zone, altitude, and climatic acclimatization by newly arrived personnel. Enforce water discipline (especially if MOPP gear is worn). Provide equipment for service members to be protected from other environmental threats (eg, dust, sun).

(f) (X) <u>Use of Personal Protection Measures</u>. Ensure all service members are educated in measures to protect themselves from arthropod vectors. Ensure service members are provided with equipment and means for protection from these vectors.

(g) (X) <u>Personal Hygiene</u>. Ensure all service members receive education and training in personal hygiene; ensure this guidance is practiced.

(h) (X) <u>Water Safety</u>. Ensure all water sources are inspected, treated, and sanitarily approved before being used. Ensure periodic inspections of these sources.

(i) (X) <u>Food Safety</u>. Ensure that all food stuffs, food handlers, and mess facilities are periodically inspected and sanitarily approved. Ensure that all food stuffs are procured from US military–approved production facilities.

(j) (X) <u>Pregnancy</u>. Ensure that no pregnant service member deploys to the AOR; all service members identified in theater as being pregnant will be reassigned out of the AOR as soon as possible.

(k) (X) <u>HIV Screening</u>. Ensure compliance with HIV screening in accordance with service regulations.

(l) (X) <u>Sexually Transmitted Diseases</u>. Ensure that sexual intercourse is discouraged in accordance with theater policy. Ensure that service members receive training in awareness and prevention of STDs.

(m) (X) <u>Pets</u>. Ensure that no pets or mascots are kept by service members in the theater.

(n) (X) <u>Combat Stress</u>. (See Section 3.a.11.) Provide command support for a combat stress program and for treatment. Ensure that personnel have free access to these programs without subsequent discrimination.

(o) (X) <u>Redeployment</u>. Ensure that all service members receive medical briefings and medical outprocessing as prescribed by the Theater Surgeon before redeployment. When applicable, ensure that all service members are aware of terminal chemoprophylaxis and have received all necessary medication before redeployment.

6. (X) <u>Coordinating Instructions</u>.

a. (X) <u>Unit Surgeons</u>. Unit Surgeons must maintain close, continual contact with PMOs, PM detachments, and the theater medical surveillance team to obtain current information on the status of health risks and threats and to identify their concerns about health issues that may arise within their units. The Unit Surgeons coordinate the delivery of disease surveillance reports to their Component Surgeon and for PM support when required from veterinary units, PM units, and the theater medical surveillance team.

b. (X) <u>Preventive Medicine Units</u>. PM units must keep commanders and medical personnel informed of health concerns as they arise. They must convey all information on potential health threats, outbreak investigations, and health hazards to Unit and Component Surgeons, as well as to the theater medical surveillance team. PM units coordinate with veterinary assets and the theater disease surveillance team for additional support when required.

c. (X) <u>Veterinary Assets</u>. Veterinary assets must provide the Component Surgeon, theater disease surveillance team, and Theater Surgeon with timely activity reports, as well as report health hazards and potential disease threats within their areas of responsibility.

d. (X) <u>Component Surgeons</u>. Component Surgeons must keep the Theater Surgeon apprised of disease surveillance data from their respective components. They must coordinate through their subordinate units to provide timely disease reporting, institution of PM measures, and compliance with theater PM guidance.

e. (X) <u>Theater Area Medical Lab</u>. As the theater medical surveillance team, the TAML coordinates through the Component Surgeons for the establishment of a theater disease reporting network, the investigation of disease outbreaks and health hazards, and the implementation of other special PM measures to address casualty prevention issues. The team advises components through the Theater Surgeon on precautions and preventive measures to be instituted when adverse health trends are recognized in the surveillance data.

f. (X) <u>Theater Surgeon</u>. The Theater Surgeon coordinates through the Component Surgeons for overall theater casualty prevention and minimization. The Theater Surgeon keeps the Component Surgeons informed of the results of the analyzed data from the disease surveillance network so precautions and countermeasures can be instituted.

Although the Joint Disease Surveillance report is a JCS requirement for all deployments, awareness of this requirement or understanding of the report format and mechanism for reporting is often limited. For this reason, it should be included as a Tab to Appendix 7 for convenient reference. Remember that the report can be tailored to identify special diseases and problems (see paragraph 4 of the form) that may be sentinel issues for the AOR (eg, malaria, tick-borne encephalitis, "rashes," asthma). Also note that references and specific scientific details are subject to change based on region of deployment and current medical thinking.

TAB A TO APPENDIX 7 TO ANNEX Q TO USCINCCENT OPLAN *NUMBER* (X)

JOINT DISEASE SURVEILLANCE REPORT (X)

Ref: USCENTCOM Reg 525-1 Annex P Weekly Medical Surveillance Report *(USCENTCOM Reg 525-1 is a CINC-specific Regulation, published by the CINC, which stipulates duties and requirements of all components on deployment to the CINC's AOR.)*

1. (X) Instructions. This report applies to Service components participating in all joint exercises and operations, including those commanded by Joint Task Force and Sub-Unified Command organizations.

    a. (X) Frequency. A timely, comprehensive medical surveillance program can inform commanders of the health of their commands and identify trends that can be attacked before significant casualties occur. Component Surgeons will report disease and injury incidence in the enclosed format. Reports will be sent weekly to the responsible Unified Command Surgeon, and are due within 5 days after the end of the reporting week. Within components, data should be collected from the levels where initial diagnosis is made to ensure that reports include cases involving loss of duty time without hospitalization. The basis for this report is INITIAL DIAGNOSIS OF NEW CASES, not initial complaint, hospital admission, or follow-up visits.

    b. (X) Application. For Army and debarked Marine and Navy components, the primary level for data collection should be the Battalion Aid Station or equivalent; for the Air Force component, the primary level should be in the Air Transportable Clinic if present or the Squadron Medical Element if not. For the shipboard Navy and embarked Marines, the primary level should be Sick Bay. Components are encouraged to implement this reporting format at the levels where data are collected and to automate the format within existing data processing systems.

    c. (X) Other Details.

        (1) (X) This is not a hospital admission/disposition report. At medical treatment facilities with inpatients and holding capabilities, only two types of cases should appear in this report: those INITIALLY DIAGNOSED at "sick call" or equivalent held for the facility staff, collocated units, and walk-ins and those emergency cases that bypassed lower reporting levels during evacuation.

        (2) (X) In facilities where patients from other services are seen for initial diagnosis, report cases by service in separate reports or in a single consolidated report, per the component Command Surgeon's guidance. Where applicable, list other service average strength as "unknown" and briefly explain in paragraph 5.

        (3) (X) To simplify reporting, battle and nonbattle injuries should be reported in appropriate general diagnostic categories but listed by type in paragraph 5. "Battle injuries" are those caused during hostile actions directly by munitions or other weapons (eg, bullet or shrapnel wounds) or by their proximal effects (eg, burns from battlefield explosions, lacerations from flying debris). All others are reported as nonbattle injuries, including those occurring on the battlefield but not associated with munitions, weapons, or direct hostile action (eg, injuries from vehicles accident not caused by enemy action).

        (4) (X) It is important from a PM standpoint to identify in paragraph 5 any unusual or recurring causes of medical visits. The surveillance report content will be used to achieve a unified understanding of and response to the theater PM challenges. The actual format of the surveillance report will be provided on execution of the OPLAN (Exhibit 13-1).

APPENDIX 11 TO ANNEX Q TO USCINCCENT OPLAN #### (X)

MEDICAL INTELLIGENCE SUPPORT TO MILITARY OPERATIONS (X)

Input to the Medical Intelligence section of an OPLAN often is best provided by the PMO. All possible sources for medical intelligence should be listed. During the scramble of a deployment, this allows subordinate units to obtain current information directly from the sources.

The following Appendix from CENTCOM is an example. Note that the information is fairly generic and can apply to all regional commands. Exact sources and telephone numbers and information in this example may not be accurate or current.

EXHIBIT 13-1

USCENTCOM WEEKLY MEDICAL SURVEILLANCE REPORT

(CLASSIFICATION)

WEEKLY MEDICAL SURVEILLANCE REPORT[*]

1. TO: _____ DTG SUBMITTED: _____

OPERATION/EXERCISE: _____

2. FROM (COMPONENT/UNIT/SECTION): _____

   a. REPORTING PERIOD (DTG to DTG): _____

   b. AVERAGE TROOP STRENGTH DURING REPORTING PERIOD: _____

3. **GENERAL DIAGNOSTIC CATEGORIES**

NEW CASES

_____ a. HEAT/COLD INJURIES (H/C). Heat stroke, heat cramps, heat exhaustion, dehydration, sunburn, frostbite, chilblain, hypothermia

_____ b. GASTROINTESTINAL ILLNESSES (G-I). Diarrhea, gastroenteritis, dysentery, gastritis, food poisoning, constipation, intestinal parasites

_____ c. RESPIRATORY ILLNESSES (RES). Upper respiratory infections, colds, bronchitis, asthma, pneumonia, pharyngitis, otitis, sinusitis

_____ d. DERMATOLOGICAL ILLNESSES (DER). Viral rashes or lesions, cellulitis, fungal or bacterial infections, contact dermatitis, dermatitis caused by insect bites, skin ulcers, eschars

_____ e. OPHTHALMIC ILLNESSES/INJURIES (EYE). Conjunctivitis, eye infections or irritations, corneal abrasions, foreign bodies, solar injury, laser injury, trauma not associated with trauma reported under Orthopedic/Surgical Injuries, para 3g

_____ f. PSYCHIATRIC ILLNESSES (PSY). Depression, situational reactions, anxiety, neuroses, psychotic reactions, suicide attempts, behavioral reaction to medication or substance abuse

_____ g. ORTHOPEDIC/SURGICAL INJURIES (INJ). Fractures, sprains, lacerations, abrasions, internal injuries, burns and thermal injuries (not sunburn), nonenvenomating animal bites (usually mammal or reptile), other trauma; includes battle, nonbattle, occupations, and recreation incidents

_____ h. MEDICAL ILLNESSES (MED). Cardiac-related problems such as chest pain and hypertension; neurological problems such as headaches, convulsions, and syncopal episode; allergic reactions including systemic reactions to venomous bites and stings; hepatitis; urogenital illnesses not associated with sexually transmitted disease; internal conditions not related to trauma (eg, appendicitis)

_____ i. SUBSTANCE ABUSE (ABU). Abuse of alcohol, illegal drugs (including marijuana), pharmaceuticals (prescribed or unprescribed), or other substances

_____ j. DENTAL (DEN). Dental injury, disease, or conditions requiring care by a dentist

_____ k. FEVERS OF UNDETERMINED ORIGIN (FUO). Fevers not apparently associated with diagnosed illness or injury

_____ l. SEXUALLY TRANSMITTED DISEASES (STD). Gonorrhea, syphilis, chlamydia, genital herpes, pelvic inflammatory disease, venereal warts/chancres

4. **SPECIAL DIAGNOSTIC CATEGORIES**

NEW CASES

   Diseases, injuries or medical conditions of special interest within the command or as directed by higher authority (eg, malaria, barotrauma), including cases already reported under a General Diagnostic Category (eg, the number of Orthopedic/Surgical Injuries that were sports-related).

     a. _____

     b. _____

(Continue as necessary)

5. **COMMENTS/REMARKS:** Clarify or explain specific entries in paragraph 3 and 4, as needed. Reference applicable paragraph and subparagraph.

[*]This format is provided for illustrative purposes only. Categories and specific diseases will vary by regions.

1. (X) <u>Situation.</u>
   a. (X) <u>Enemy.</u> Refer to Annex B.
   b. (X) <u>Friendly.</u> Refer to Basic Plan.
   c. (X) <u>Assumptions.</u> See Preventive Medicine Appendix 7 to Annex Q.
2. (X) <u>Mission.</u> Support the mission outlined in Basic Annex Q.
3. (X) <u>Execution.</u> All deployed medical assets will provide the Theater Surgeon with appropriate medical intelligence feedback when appropriate or as required. Medical assets upon redeployment will also provide the Component Command Surgeons' Offices and the USCENTCOM Surgeon's Office with a debriefing in the general format of the AFMIC "Medical Information Report," but all items may not apply to the mission. Information should be as complete as possible. (The briefing may be handwritten.)
   a. (X) <u>Intelligence Sources.</u> The following medical intelligence sources may be helpful for mission planning purposes and for obtaining current information.
      (1) (X) <u>Armed Forces Medical Intelligence Center.</u> Can provide specific summaries of current medical intelligence, by country. Can provide a Quick Response report to high priority medical intelligence requests that require less than 40 person-hours of research. They also publish MEDIC, which includes suggested PM countermeasures and Medical Capabilities Studies for most countries within the CENTCOM AOR. Specific medical threats are also published on a weekly basis, disseminated by weekly electronic message traffic. AFMIC Operations telephone: DSN 343-7574; Commercial (301) 619-7574; Fax -2649 (Secure), -2409 (Unclassified). All lines are STU-III compatible.
      (2) (X) <u>Defense Pest Management Information Analysis Center.</u> Publishes Disease Vector Ecology Profiles for many countries within the CENTCOM AOR. Provides current and extensive information on medical zoological threats (eg, arthropods [spiders, ticks, mosquitoes, etc.], leeches, snakes, some parasites, some poisonous plants), by specific country or by geographic distributions of specific threats. Telephone: DSN 295-7479; Commercial (301) 295-7479.
      (3) (X) <u>US Navy Environmental and Preventive Medicine Unit #7 (NEPMU-7).</u> Located in Sigonella, Italy, NEPMU-7 publishes Annual Disease Risk Assessment Profiles for countries within the AOR. It constitutes a major source for medical threat estimation and general PM recommendations; specific consultation and updates by NEPMU-7are also available. Telephone: DSN 314-XXX-XXXX, Commercial 011-XX-XX-XXX-XXXX, Secure 011-39-XX-XXX-XXXX.
      (4) (X) <u>Center for Health Promotion and Preventive Medicine.</u> The Center houses experts in all PM specialties who can address broad PM issues, as well as highly technical and arcane topics. These issues include epidemiology, entomology, communicable diseases, bioenvironmental engineering, occupational medicine, water and air quality, and medical readiness. Telephone: 1-800-222-9698 (24 hours); DSN 584-7374, Commercial (410) 436-7374; Fax -7301 (secure).
      (5) (X) <u>Walter Reed Army Institute of Research.</u> The Preventive Medicine Division is a collection point for PM information, technical experts, and points of contact for many PM and disease aspects of most countries within the AOR. They have extensive in-house experience with theater disease surveillance, investigation, and research on numerous PM issues pertinent to the AOR. Telephones: DSN 285-9600; Commercial (301) 319-9600; Fax -9104.
      (6) (X) <u>US Army Medical Research Institute of Infectious Diseases.</u> This institute is a source of information on infectious diseases, including the latest medical research, BW agents, vaccine developments, and therapeutic regimens. Telephone: DSN 343-2772/2833; Commercial (301) 619-2772/2833; Fax -4625.
      (7) (X) <u>Naval Medical Research Unit #3 (NAMRU-3).</u> This regional research center, located in Cairo, Egypt, conducts medical research on diseases within the CENTCOM AOR. NAMRU-3 is the source of specific disease information and scientific developments and can be contacted directly for practical medical experience within the AOR. Commercial telephone 011-202-284-1375, Fax -1382.
      (8) (X) <u>US Air Force Institute for Environment, Safety, and Occupational Health Risk Analysis, Force Health Protection and Surveillance Branch.</u> This branch has expertise in epidemiology, health promotion, biostatistics, and database development. Telephone: DSN XXX-XXXX; Commercial (XXX) XXX-XXXX; Fax -XXXX.
      (9) (X) <u>USAF School of Aerospace Medicine.</u> The School has consultants in epidemiology, ento-

mology, communicable diseases, bioenvironmental engineering, occupational medicine, food sanitation, and medical readiness. Telephone: DSN 240-3500; Commercial (210) 536-3500; Fax -3419.

(10) (X) Armstrong Labs. Formerly a part of the Air Force, this is now a private organization that works on a fee/contract basis. DSN 240-2002, comm (210) 536-2002, fax –2025.

b. (X) <u>Medical Intelligence Estimates</u>. See Preventive Medicine Appendix 7. *This is also the section in which to emphasize disease threats within the local population that may affect combat service support and civil affairs efforts by US military personnel.*

c. (X) <u>Environmental Health.</u> See Preventive Medicine Appendix 7. *Identify key features in the area that could affect the health of military personnel, to include the status of public infrastructure (eg, water, sewage), industrial pollutants and other industrial hygiene threats, and zoonotic disease threats.*

d. (X) <u>Non–US Military Health Care Infrastructure</u>. *List all host-nation military medical facilities that can be used within the AOR. List their capabilities, to include location (state miles or time from airports or known US military compounds or ports), beds, specialties available, operating capabilities, diagnostic equipment, reputation of facility and doctors, and any other specific information that may become important when choosing a facility for US casualties.*

(1) (X) <u>Host-Nation Military Hospital #1</u>. #1 Hospital is the military hospital on the ZZZ Air Base. It is a 300-bed multi-specialty hospital. It is about 30 minutes away from Yippee Kiyay Apartments. It is expandable to 1,000 beds in a contingency. It also is the referral hospital for decompression sickness. It has a 20-bed, level II ER and an ICU/CCU with 10 beds.

(2) (X) <u>Host-Nation Facility #2</u>. #2 military hospital is available, but mass casualty cases or trauma should not be taken here. Instead, refer to the nearby University Hospital.

e. (X) <u>Civilian Facilities</u>. *As with the host-nation military medical facilities (see above), list all the host-nation civilian hospitals that can be used within the AOR, as well as their capabilities and reputation, if known.*

(1) (X) <u>Host-Nation Civilian Hospital #1</u>. #1 Hospital is comparable to some of the best hospitals in the United States. It is an ultramodern, complete, multi-specialty hospital. It is located approximately 10 minutes from the Marriott Hotel in the capital city. It is available for use by all US forces through a previously arranged agreement.

f. (X) <u>Tasks</u>. See Preventive Medicine Appendix 7 for surveillance and reporting.

APPENDIX 12 TO ANNEX Q TO USCINCCENT OPLAN NUMBER (X)

VETERINARY SERVICES (X)

The Veterinary appendix to Annex Q of the OPLAN may become the responsibility of the Command PMO for review (if not for generation of the entire document). The following covers generic topics important for the CENTCOM AOR. When adapting this appendix for another AOR, it should, of course, be tailored to the region, operation, and availability and safety of food sources within that AOR. As in the other OPLAN appendixes, each paragraph must have a security classification.

1. (X) <u>Purpose</u>. To provide the concept of operations and assign tasks for veterinary support of the Basic Plan. The threat is outlined in Appendix 7, Preventive Medicine.

2. (X) <u>Assumptions</u>. See Appendix 7, Preventive Medicine.

3. (X) <u>Concept of Operations</u>. Within the theater, US military veterinary assets must inspect and approve all bulk food sources in the theater, including both non–US sources and US government prepackaged, acquired, or produced foods. Food production facilities not located within the United States must be inspected periodically and sanitarily approved by military veterinary authorities for continued usage. The theater veterinary officer maintains a list of approved host-nation food sources.

a. (X) Preventive medicine assets within the theater are responsible for periodic inspection and sanitary approval of food preparation and handling techniques in food production facilities.

b. (X) When non–US military personnel are involved in food preparation and handling, the Theater Surgeon is responsible for setting health standards for the hiring of these employees, as well as standards of health to be maintained for continued employment. Medical and preventive medicine assets must ensure implementation of these standards, verify the continued state of good health of these employees, and ensure that proper food handling standards are being taught to these employees. Food handler certificates, issued by military preventive medicine assets, must be obtained by all food handlers.

c. (X) Contaminated rations or rations suspected of contamination by NBC agents must be inspected and tested by veterinary personnel before issue or consumption.

d. (X) Captured rations must be first certified for use by veterinary food inspectors before distribution or consumption.

e. (X) Veterinary assets must be informed of suspected or confirmed endemic animal and zoonotic disease occurrences. They are responsible for advising the Theater Surgeon on appropriate treatment and prevention protocols and monitoring the implementation of these programs.

4. (X) <u>Health Threat</u>. See Appendix 7.

5. (X) <u>Tasks</u>. Veterinary support will be provided by _____ (*usually the Army*). The Veterinary Services, under the direction of the Theater Surgeon, have the following theater responsibilities. The Xth Unit located in _____(*location*) will maintain all veterinary files within the CENTCOM AOR.

a. (X) <u>Weekly Activity Reports</u>. Submit a Veterinary Service Weekly Activity Report to the theater disease surveillance team and the Theater Surgeon. This report will cover activities concerned with animal medicine, food inspection, zoonotic diseases, and other significant events.

b. (X) <u>Food Safety</u>. Inspect and approve all foodstuff sources used by US military personnel within the theater. Military veterinary services will also conduct periodic sanitary inspections of bulk food supplies and the facilities from which these originate. Locally acquired foodstuff must be inspected and approved before purchase, before entry into the theater supply system or issue, and periodically while in storage.

    (1) (X) <u>Contaminated Rations</u>. Contaminated rations or rations suspected of contamination by NBC agents must be inspected and tested by veterinary personnel before issue or consumption. Decontamination of rations contaminated by these agents is a unit responsibility.

    (2) (X) <u>Captured Rations</u>. Captured rations must be first certified for use by veterinary food inspectors before consumption or distribution.

c. (X) <u>Zoonotic Diseases</u>. Provide theater consultation, as needed, for zoonotic diseases and their vectors.

d. (X) <u>Rabies Program</u>. Draft the theater rabies and animal bite protocol for the Theater Surgeon. Address the quarantine, handling, diagnosis, and disposition of animals suspected to be rabid.

e. (X) <u>Antivenins</u>. Locate and coordinate procurement of appropriate antivenins against venomous threats within the AOR.

f. (X) <u>Military Working Dogs</u>. Ensure the safety of the food supply and the health care of military working dogs.

6. (X) <u>Coordinating Instructions</u>. The Theater Surgeon will ensure there is a senior veterinary officer on the medical staff and maintain close contact with ancillary veterinary medical staffs.

SUMMARY

Appendixes 7, 11, and 12 of the Annex Q of each of a CINC's operation plans should be thorough and detailed, written well in advance, and constantly updated. These appendixes provide the preventive medicine–related guidance by which the components can make their own preparations for their missions. In the chaos accompanying mission preparation, robust CINC OPLANS assist the subordinate component commands by reducing the chances of accidental omission of critical information and decreasing the likelihood of ill-conceived planning by serving as a checklist. They also provide a ready source of mission and regionally oriented information for each specific OPLAN, thereby decreasing the need for multiple-source research. Premission planning is excellent preventive medicine.

Chapter 14

MEDICAL PREPARATION FOR DEPLOYMENT

MARGOT R. KRAUSS, MD, MPH; AND STEPHANIE BRODINE, MD

M. R. Krauss, Colonel, Medical Corps, US Army; Deputy Director, Division of Preventive Medicine, Walter Reed Army Institute of Research, Silver Spring, MD 20910-7500

S. Brodine, Captain, US Navy (Retired); formerly, Head, Clinical Epidemiology Division, Naval Health Research Center, San Diego, CA 92186-5122, currently, Professor and Head, Division of Epidemiology and Biostatistics, Graduate School of Public Health, San Diego State University, San Diego, CA 92184

INTRODUCTION

The concept of medical and dental preparation for deployment came from lessons learned during the two world wars, when overwhelming numbers of individuals were inducted into or volunteered for military service. In 2 months (September and October) of 1917 alone, 482,000 US men were called to serve their country. Recruits were often quickly screened, trained, and sent directly to battle. But medical personnel were not prepared to handle the mass examinations; they had themselves reported only shortly before the draft contingents arrived at base camps.[1]

Principles of personal health maintenance were established and practiced long before World War II, but the concept was first clearly validated during World War II, when "sanitary teams" were created in the Army and the Navy to control disease. Outbreaks of shigella dysentery were successfully aborted with the initiation of strict personal hygiene measures for food handlers and shipboard personnel.[2] Since World War II, the importance of preventive measures has been demonstrated repeatedly in successive conflicts, such as the Korean War and the Vietnam War, and education continues to play a central role in integrating preventive measures into military operations. More recently, the power of health education was demonstrated during Operations Desert Shield and Desert Storm by the near total absence of heat casualties in an extremely high-risk environment.[3]

Lessons learned during these conflicts led to the concept of preparing for deployment or "readiness" in the 1990s. Readiness means that military personnel are medically fit and protected from known disease threats so that they can deploy worldwide with little or no notice.

READINESS

Service-Specific Considerations

"Soldier readiness" in the Army, "operational readiness" in the Navy, and "readiness" in the Air Force all refer to service-specific programs to ensure that soldiers, sailors, Marines, and airmen are administratively ready for deployment at all times. Organizational differences between the services dictate various methods for ensuring readiness. Readiness encompasses a broad range of issues, including the relevant skill requirements specific to the particular unit, platform, or wing involved. This chapter addresses only the medical and dental aspects of predeployment preparation and education.

The medical officer assigned to the unit, platform, or wing may be the sole medical planner for a specific deployment. As a staff officer and medical planner, he or she must be familiar with occupational medicine, preventive medicine, environmental medicine, general medicine, medical planning, medical logistics, and field sanitation, among other necessary areas.[4] The medical officer plays a key role in all aspects of readiness, overseeing all medical preparation for deployment and providing appropriate preventive medicine education and advice to the commanders.[5]

In the Army, manpower staffing requirements include "checking the status of individual soldier readiness during in-processing; once annually as a unit or an individual; during out-processing; and within 30 days of an actual deployment."[6(p20)] A soldier readiness processing team from the installation accomplishes the annual checks for units and individuals and the predeployment checks under the general leadership of the chief of the Military Personnel Division (G1/AG). The team consists of representatives from such offices as personnel, medical, dental, provost marshal, finance, security, legal, logistics, and operations. One goal is to eliminate the nondeployment status of individuals with correctable medical and dental conditions.[6]

In the Navy, the Chief, BUMED (Bureau of Medicine and Surgery), is responsible for ensuring the readiness of the medical personnel assigned to various platforms (eg, Fleet Hospital, Casualty Receiving and Treatment Ships, Fleet Marine Force).[7] Operational readiness for sailors and Marines is the responsibility of the commanding officers of shore-based medical treatment facilities.[8]

For the Air Force, predeployment health assessment is routinely conducted to ensure dental and medical records are in order and immunizations are up to date. Once an airman is placed on mobility status, a mobility processing unit provides health education, immunizations, and a last check to ensure the airman is ready to deploy.[9]

Each service ensures the active duty member has received appropriate immunizations, human immunodeficiency virus (HIV) testing, DNA testing, hearing testing, eyeglasses and gas mask inserts, identification (eg, dog tags, Geneva convention status card, medical warning bracelet), and dental screening. In addition, predeployment processing verifies that the service member has a complete medical record, a current physical exam, and a deployable physical profile.

Special Considerations

There are four programs that affect readiness and so require elaboration: the Exceptional Family Member Program (EFMP), DNA testing, physical profiling, and the HIV policy.

The EFMP is a personnel requirement that identifies service members whose family members have chronic medical problems.[10] This identification assists the personnel commands in making appropriate assignments, ensuring that the necessary medical capabilities are available to the family within 40 miles of an assignment within the United States or country-wide for an assignment outside the United States. Although EFMP referral is an aspect of readiness, it does not affect deployability status. A service member in the EFMP is fully deployable.

As of March 1994, the Assistant Secretary of Defense (Health Affairs) directed that no service member, civilian employee, or civilian contractor shall be deployed into an imminent danger zone without first leaving a specimen in the DNA Registry and Depository.[11] This policy has resulted in steps to acquire DNA specimens from all active duty service members. On November 13, 1996, the eventual adoption of the DNA Registry as the standard for positive casualty identification was approved, so the requirement to store duplicate dental panographs was rescinded.[12]

The Army physical profile system used to classify general aspects of overall health is referred to by the acronym PULHES (P—general physical stamina and strength, U—upper extremities, L—lower extremities, H—hearing, E—eyes, S—psychiatric evaluation). Each letter has four potential grades; grades 3 and 4 require a medical review board to determine medical fitness and deployability. Medical conditions that make service members of any service nondeployable require a physical evaluation board to determine whether they may remain on active duty.[13] Temporary profiles are issued for conditions that usually resolve with time. For example, a pregnant service member is considered non-deployable for up to 179 days after delivery. Although not explicitly stated in any regulation, it makes medical sense not to deploy the pregnant service member because of the relative contraindication of giving live vaccinations during pregnancy and the concern of complications arising in a developing country or during hostile actions.

Service members who have tested positive for HIV may remain on active duty but are considered nondeployable. This policy reflects the current knowledge of the natural progression of HIV infection, to include the relative contraindication of giving live vaccinations to infected individuals[14–16] and their increased susceptibility to diseases that are endemic where personnel may deploy. Most HIV-positive service members remain on active duty until their immune systems are compromised, when they are medically retired.

RESERVE COMPONENT

A major shift from a large standing force to an increasing reliance on the reserves has led to an even greater challenge in ensuring readiness. Reservists tend to be older than active duty service members and have little contact with the military other than weekend drills and 2 weeks of active duty time per year. There is little physical training conducted during reserve duty sessions. When physical training has been conducted, it was not been found to be an effective or an efficient method of improving the fitness of the National Guard.[17]

The impact of the Reserve Component on readiness was apparent during the Persian Gulf War, where reservists made up approximately 17% of the deployed force.[18] There have been reports that substantial proportions of Reserve Component service members were not medically fit for mobilization for Operation Desert Shield.[19] Of 2,723 persons from the Individual Ready Reserve called to active duty, 25% were rejected for activation. The most common reasons for rejection were being overweight (29%), being the sole parent of a minor child (25%), having orthopedic problems (12%), and having mental problems (10%).[20] In one reserve battalion, 7% were not able to deploy due to medical reasons, the two most common being psychiatric problems and back problems.[21]

The Persian Gulf War also demonstrated that Reserve Component personnel were not dentally prepared.[22] One hundred percent of those in the reserves (ie, Individual Mobilization Augmentee and Individual Ready Reserve) required a dental examination, while only 8.6% of those on active duty required one. Dental treatment was required by 17% and 27% of the reservists and National Guardsmen, respectively; only 8% of those on active duty required treatment.

DENTAL PREPAREDNESS

Oral health is a readiness issue because of the chronic disease that is endemic in American service members. A 1994 survey of the oral health status of 2,711 recruits and 13,050 active duty personnel from the Army, Navy, Marine Corps, and Air Force indicated that 99.3% of all recruits and 92.4% of active duty service members had oral conditions that required some form of treatment. Almost half (49.1%) of recruits and 14.5% of active duty service members had oral problems severe enough that they were considered to be at high risk for dental emergencies that would interfere with operational effectiveness.[23]

The chronic nature of dental diseases implies that the oral health of personnel who have deployed will deteriorate during periods of fatigue, nutritional deficiencies, and psychological stress. This will be compounded by their use of tobacco, especially when field hygiene is not practiced and if dental care is not provided. The magnitude of the potential problem for today's military can be appreciated by looking at the dental emergency rate in Vietnam: 142 per 1,000 soldiers per year and 182 per 1,000 Marines per year.[24] These numbers were considered underestimates because of the difficulty in collecting data in an operational environment.

Considering the need to minimize emergency and routine dental care in the area of operations, the preferred intervention is being prepared for deployment. All three military services use the Department of Defense Dental Classification System[25] to identify an individual's level of risk for needing an unplanned dental visit, to target higher risk personnel for care, and to profile the status of the unit's dental health for the commander. This requires that all service members be examined and classified at least annually.

All three services target Class 3 personnel (those with at least one dental condition that predisposes them to a dental emergency within a year) for treatment as a readiness issue, but dental emergencies do occur among Class 2 (minor dental needs) and Class 1 (no dental needs) individuals. In one study, the Class 3 emergency rate was 530 per 1,000 troops per year, the Class 2 rate was 145 per 1,000 per year, and the Class 1 rate was 67 per 1,000 per year.[26] The reason for the lack of sensitivity of this predeployment screening index is that some emergencies, like trauma, are unpredictable. The effect of predeployment screening has been estimated to reduce dental emergency rates by 478 per 1,000 soldiers annually.[27]

In addition to the secondary prevention described above, all three services provide or assist in providing primary preventive dental care to promote oral health and prevent oral disease and injury. These include systemic fluorides, topical application of fluorides, plaque control education, dietary counseling, oral prophylaxis, protective mouthguards, pit and fissure sealants, tobacco risk education, and preventive orthodontics.[28] Oral disease and injury are inevitable during military operations, but many oral emergencies can be prevented by predeployment preparation.[26,29] It remains clear, however, that it is the command's responsibility to ensure that service members are available for dental examinations and care.

PREDEPLOYMENT IMMUNIZATIONS AND CHEMOPROPHYLAXIS

Immunizations are a well-known and accepted means of protecting individuals and military forces against disease. Knowing which vaccinations are needed or required depends on knowing who is the controlling authority for the deployment. The Commander in Chief of a unified command, in coordination with the appropriate Surgeons General or Commandant of the Coast Guard, establishes specific immunization requirements based on special disease threat assessments for each deployment area. Current health threat assessments based on disease prevalence in specific geographic regions are maintained by each service preventive medicine authority using federal, Department of Defense, and other relevant sources of information (see chapter 11, Health Threat Assessment). Medical leadership ensure that the appropriate vaccinations for area-specific threats are given to active duty personnel.

A tri-service regulation[30] documents generally required immunizations for the uniformed departments of the Army, Navy, Marine Corps, Air Force, and Coast Guard (Active and Reserve), nonmilitary persons under military jurisdiction, selected federal employees, and family members eligible for care within the military health care system.

The services require all active duty members to receive influenza vaccination annually and tetanus vaccination every 10 years. In addition, the present tri-service regulation covers vaccines against hepatitis B, Japanese encephalitis, meningococcal meningitis, plague, rabies, yellow fever, and typhoid fever. Although there appears to be some uniformity between services on immunization requirements, the interpretation of "high-risk" deployment and "high-risk" occupational group varies between services.

Immune globulin, once the mainstay of prevention against hepatitis A, was often a source of confusion because of the issue of timing its injection with that of live-virus vaccines. This is no longer a problem because immune globulin has been replaced by the more-efficacious hepatitis A vaccine. The timing of giving other vaccines may still be raised. All of the routinely given militarily relevant vaccines may be given simultaneously without reduced effectiveness or increased reactogenicity. Live-virus vaccines may be given at the same time as immune globulin without inhibiting the immune response. If live-virus vaccines are not given at the same time, 4 weeks should be allowed to elapse between sequential vaccinations. There are no current data on possible interference between the yellow fever vaccine and the vaccines for typhoid fever, plague, rabies, typhus, paratyphoid fever, or Japanese encephalitis.[31]

A major challenge in the military is ensuring all active duty personnel are up to date on their immunizations. The rapid turnover of personnel and frequent deployments, plus the mandate to vaccinate the entire force against anthrax, makes using a standardized method of tracking immunizations a priority. In a decentralized troop medical clinic setting, confusion about regulations and deployment requirements can result in individuals being over-vaccinated. According to one Army study[32] conducted in 1994 and 1995, 30% of soldiers were "inappropriately" vaccinated. Those inappropriately vaccinated included soldiers who received vaccinations for deployment when they did not deploy or received booster vaccinations 6 months or more earlier than recommended. A standardized method of tracking immunizations should reduce the percentage of inappropriately vaccinated individuals and ensure that service members do not go unvaccinated.

Any major adverse reaction resulting from vaccination should be noted in the individual's medical record. Information to be included consists of identification of the vaccine used, lot number and manufacturer, date of administration, name and location of the medical facility, and type and severity of the reaction. Health care providers are required by the National Vaccine Injury Compensation Program to report reactions via the Vaccine Adverse Events Reporting System (VAERS) of the Department of Health and Human Services using form VAERS-1.[30,33] Only reactions requiring hospitalization or lost time from duty of over 24 hours are reported. Low-grade fevers, local soreness, and redness for less than 24 hours are not reported unless contamination of the lot is suspected. Military medical authorities are required to report to both VAERS and their own service.[30]

Investigational New Drugs and Vaccines

New drugs and vaccines designed to treat or prevent diseases that threaten the fighting strength of the military have strategic importance and so are critically important to the military. These new drugs and vaccines usually have little application within the civilian community (eg, botulinum vaccine). Often the military develops these unique products and then provides the technology to civilian companies who produce the drug or vaccine and conduct the clinical trials necessary to gain Federal Drug Administration (FDA) approval. New drugs and vaccines undergo years of testing for safety and efficacy before acquiring investigational new drug (IND) status, but that is only one step in the long process of winning FDA approval. Having the ability to use effective new drugs and vaccines under IND application has been key to providing the active duty military with needed vaccinations before they have received FDA approval.

The use of investigational new drugs and vaccines in the military is evaluated and approved by a human subjects review board under the authority of the Army Surgeon General. According to regulation,[34] even vaccines that have been approved for use by foreign countries may only be used in the United States under IND protocols until FDA approval is obtained. As an example, the Japanese encephalitis vaccine had been successfully used in Japan for more than 20 years; it took more than 10 years of use in the United States under IND status before sufficient data were gathered for FDA approval. Military members must give informed consent to take drugs or biologics under IND status.

An exception was made during the Persian Gulf War when a waiver of the requirement for informed consent for use of investigational drugs and vaccines was sought by the military. The justification was military expediency due to the perceived threat of chemical and biological warfare. The FDA granted the request and issued a new general regulation, rule 23(d), that permits waivers on a case-by-case basis when consent is "not feasible in a specific military operation involving combat or the immediate threat of combat."[35] This ruling allowed the use without consent of an IND vaccine (ie, pentavalent botulinum-toxoid vaccine) and of an approved drug being used for an unapproved reason (ie, pyridostigmine bromide as a pretreatment for nerve-gas attacks).[36] These particular products had been extensively tested and found to be safe, yet lacked the two well-controlled studies demonstrating safety and efficacy in humans required by the FDA for approval. This criterion will never be meet as it would be unethical to expose subjects to botulinum or nerve agents.[37] As new vaccinations and drugs become available, the ability to use them under the IND protocol will remain a vital means to the goal of preventing disease and disability in deploying service members.

Chemoprophylaxis and Personal Protective Supplies

Of the diseases that are amenable to chemoprophylaxis and personal protection measures, the most commonly encountered by service members is malaria. Disease manifestations and treatment of all diseases that can be prevented by chemoprophylaxis or personal protection measures or both are dealt with in other sections of this book. The major issue for predeployment is how to start large units on effective chemoprophylaxis and how to acquire the necessary protective equipment and supplies (eg, bednets, permethrin, deet repellant).

The Commander in Chief and his or her medical staff, using the medical threat assessment will choose the medication needed and write the guidance for personal protection measures. The OPLAN (operational plan) will outline the medications to be given and protective measures. The commanders of the assigned units, platforms, and wings are expected to ensure compliance with the OPLAN. Medication is provided by the local medical treatment facility, but it is unlikely to stockpile adequate amounts for large deployments. Likewise, units may not be able to afford stockpiling supplies for routine preventive measures. Therefore, rapidly deploying units may not be able to acquire the required medications or supplies before departure. This recurring problem highlights the need for the medical officer to be involved early in the medical planning for deployment and to work closely with logistics personnel.

Distributing the medication and ensuring compliance is a commander's responsibility, but the implementation can be expected to vary. Distribution of medication at a routine unit formation is the preferred method but may not be feasible throughout the deployment. Education and good information dissemination are other key elements to a successful program; this has been learned in every operation, from World War II to Somalia, when malaria chemoprophylaxis and personal protective measures were needed.[38] The same issues are faced, whether the instruction is about malaria chemoprophylaxis, leptospirosis chemoprophylaxis, or pretreatment for potential nerve gas exposure.

HEALTH EDUCATION

Once military members have been administratively prepared, medically screened, and vaccinated against endemic medical threats, health education prepares the active duty service member and the commander for disease threats that may be encountered during the deployment. For a predeployment education program to be effective, military personnel must integrate the recommended preventive measures into operational units' deployment procedures. Preventive measures that rely solely on the activities of a small group of specialized personnel, such as in a deployed Air Force fixed base, are usually the easiest to implement.[39] Adherence to recommendations aimed at the individual is more difficult to achieve.[40] Success has been most clearly linked to support and strong emphasis by the commanding officer, expressed through the chain of command to the noncommissioned officer level. An example includes the malaria and dengue experience in Operation Restore Hope in Somalia; outbreaks of these vector-borne diseases occurred primarily in those units whose leadership did not enforce the prescribed countermeasures.[41] This emphasizes the importance of targeting the commanders and the entire chain of command, including the noncommissioned officers and company commanders, to inform them of the anticipated medical threats and convince them of the requirement to enforce appropriate countermeasures.

A lack of compliance with preventive measures, which can result in disease and nonbattle injuries and reduced combat efficiency, can signify a lack of unit discipline. This helps to explain the trend to hold the senior leadership accountable for breakdowns in preventive measures as a readiness issue. Convincing the leadership may be particularly challenging when the disease threat is unfamiliar and thus somewhat theoretical to the leadership and line personnel. The experience of Army troops in the Middle East during World War II is an example; strong recommendations to avoid skin contact with fresh water in the Middle

East were not heeded until a large number of personnel were incapacitated by schistosomiasis.[42] In contrast, preventive measures for heat injury, which are very familiar to most service members, have been successfully built into the routine logistics of training, tactical maneuvers, and handling water in both the Army and the Marine Corps.

The type of health education possible depends on the type of deployment. Deployments can be planned (scheduled in advance), crisis (a rapid response to political events), or combination (the itinerary of a planned deployment changes in response to current events). In crisis or combination deployments, the procedures and depth of predeployment education depends on the imminence of deployment and the availability of resources. In the case of planned deployments, the process and materials for predeployment education are usually incorporated into the standard preparation procedures. In the Marine Corps, for example, Navy Preventive Medicine Technicians, Environmental Health Officers, Preventive Medicine Officers (PMOs), and Aeromedical Safety Officers are intimately involved with the complete predeployment process of logistically preparing deploying battalions. Classes are given for the senior enlisted personnel, company commanders, and junior enlisted personnel. PMOs, Environmental Health Officers, or Battalion Surgeons brief the deploying commander and the senior officers and enlisted leaders. If possible, the more-senior PMOs give a final predeployment briefing to the operational leadership, emphasizing the anticipated threats and the leadership's accountability for service member compliance. Others can help in this process. For example, the Naval Environmental Preventive Medicine Units have participated, primarily through providing the deploying personnel the most up-to-date medical intelligence.

The methods used for predeployment education vary from an informal discussion to a lecture with or without visual aids (Figure 14-1). Briefing packets of printed materials are also often prepared for service members' future reference. More recently the US Army has developed pamphlets, prepared for particular areas of operations, delineating the personal protection measures required for that region. This represents a significant advance in getting key information to the individual service member. These pamphlets served as a major means of educating line personnel in such large-scale "crisis" deployments as those to the Persian Gulf and to Bosnia-Herzegovina.[43]

The topics selected for predeployment education

depend on the deployment platform and the scenario—the who, what, when, how, and where of the deployment. For instance, predeployment education for shipboard personnel usually centers on port visits, with an emphasis on motor vehicle accidents and urban diseases such as dysentery and sexually transmitted diseases. Accurate, up-to-date information on the endemic disease rates in the local populations should be provided, when possible, to reinforce the importance of preventive measures (eg, the prevalence rate of HIV infection in commercial sex workers). For the Special Forces, Army, and Marine Corps infantry, the threat potential can be greater due to their more extensive contact with an uncontrolled environment and indigenous populations. The operation scenario becomes critical to planning an effective predeployment education program. Components of the operation necessary for planning an education package include information regarding the food and water supply, waste storage and disposal, climate, terrain, diseases endemic to the area, health of local populations, plant and animal threats, and vectors. Specific topics are prioritized based on the operation scenario and the amount of time allotted for predeployment briefings. General categories include environmental injury, sanitation, vector-borne diseases, foodborne and waterborne diseases, and other infectious diseases.

Sources of information for predeployment education are myriad. A recent tri-service innovation is the Armed Forces Preventive Medicine Recommendations, produced by the Armed Forces Medical Intelligence Center. Called the MEDIC, it is a short country-by-country summary (one to two pages per country) of preventive medicine recommendations appropriate for a joint land-based exercise or contingency operation and is distributed on a CD-ROM disk. Nonmilitary agencies such as the State Department and World Health Organization can also be sources of medical information. A recent addition to information resources are the internet infectious disease discussion groups, such as PROMED, and various World Wide Web sites. Any information gleaned from non–US government sources (especially Internet sources) requires confirmation before being used in briefings to commanders and service members.

There is increasing interest in evaluating the quality and efficacy of education programs with measurable outcomes, with the goal being continued improvement and refinement. This is a very difficult process to incorporate into predeployment

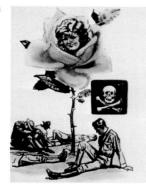

a

A syphilitic woman
may be as fair as
a rose to the
glance—

—but more dangerous
than a leper.

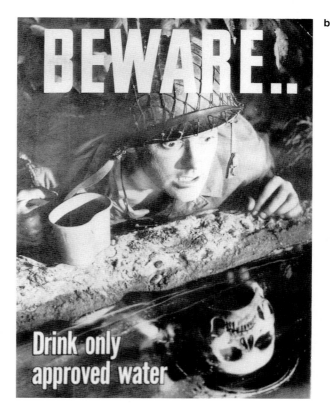

b

BEWARE...

Drink only
approved water

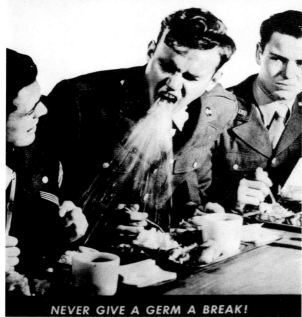

c

COVER COUGHS
COVER SNEEZES

NEVER GIVE A GERM A BREAK!

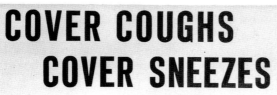

d

44	JANUARY					44
SUN	MON	TUE	WED	THU	FRI	SAT
						1
2	3	4	5	6	7	8
9	10	11	12	13	14	15
16	17	18	19	20	21	22
23 30	24 31	25	26	27	28	29

SKEETER'S DINNER TIME,
SUNDOWN TO SUNUP.

DON'T BE MOSQUITO BAIT.
KEEP YOUR SHIRT ON.

MALARIA & EPIDEMIC DISEASE CONTROL · SOUTH PACIFIC

Fig. 14-1. Efforts to educate service members about the dangers of infectious diseases have taken many forms, and the flier or poster is one of the cheapest and most easily distributed. The World War I flier shown in (**a**) decorously warns doughboys against syphilis, while posters (**b**) and (**c**), both from World War II, warn against diseases transmitted by water and airborne droplets. Calendars were also used to teach or remind personnel about preventive measures. The example in (**d**) reminds service members to wear their shirts from sundown to sunup to keep mosquito bites, and mosquito-borne disease, to a minimum. Photographs: Courtesy of National Museum of Health and Medicine, Armed Forces Institute of Pathology: Catalogue numbers: (a) WWI lantern slides, (b) REEVE 35086, (c) REEVE 35036, (d) REEVE 88266.

education programs. Certain elements of the process can more-easily be assessed. For instance, education materials can be piloted to examine such issues as readability and comprehension for the target population.[43] One of the most effective ways to evaluate the efficacy of a predeployment education program is to measure disease incidence, the ultimate outcome measure for a prevention program. Real-time disease surveillance during deployment can rapidly identify outbreaks in sentinel disease categories, which may signify a breakdown in preventive measures. Outbreak investigations expeditiously conducted can pinpoint the appropriate military units and identify areas of noncompliance.

It has been well documented that information alone is not enough to induce changes in established behaviors. One of the newer trends in education is to incorporate skill building into educational programs—a concept that is relevant to predeployment education in which military personnel are being trained in certain behaviors as countermeasures for disease threats. This methodology has been successfully applied to STD prevention. An intensive, multi-session, military-specific prevention program

was designed based on research done in target groups with Marine Corps infantry personnel and Navy preventive medicine personnel, and it was associated with a decrease in risky sexual behavior in a Western Pacific deployment.[44] Central themes were port-liberty behaviors, peer influences, transmission of asymptomatic STDs, and perceived invulnerability. Skill building centered on communication, appropriate use of alcohol, and safe sexual practices. As these types of educational programs are very labor-intensive, it is likely that implementation will be best accomplished in targeted, high-risk groups.

Over the past few decades, the assets and the process of health education for deploying forces have become more formalized. Each of the armed services has its own mechanism through the chain of command to accomplish this goal. Efforts to standardize preventive medicine recommendations where possible across the three services are desirable. As joint operations among US forces are becoming more common, it is becoming crucial that each service component of a joint command both understand and support the need for a common preventive medicine strategy.

SUMMARY

Medical and dental predeployment preparation must not be perceived as a last-minute activity but be a concerted effort throughout the military training year, with close monitoring by unit commanders. Last-minute activity must only be used to identify the few who have slipped through the cracks. Immunizations remain a major component of military force protection and need to be addressed on a continual basis. Deployments to particular geographic areas may require additional vaccines, to include IND products. Health education needs to be an integral part of the deployment process and with

strong command support and emphasis can result in adherence to preventive recommendations and decreased morbidity and mortality. Investment in predeployment medical and dental preparation will avoid or decrease degradation of mission effectiveness caused by medical or dental emergencies. Although medical and dental personnel are intimately involved in the process of predeployment readiness, commanders have the authority and ultimate responsibility to ensure their most valued weapon system, the soldier, sailor, Marine, or airman, is in an excellent state of readiness.

REFERENCES

1. Bowen AS. *Activities Concerning Mobilization Camps and Ports of Embarkation*. Vol 4. In: *The Medical Department of the United States Army in the World War*. Washington, DC: US Government Printing Office; 1928, 21.

2. Thompson CM, While BV. Clinical observations on dysentery caused by *Shigella flexneri*. *Naval Med Bull*. 1946;6.

3. Wasserman GM, Martin BL, Hyams KC, Merrill BR, Oaks HG, McAdoo HA. A survey of outpatient visits in a United States Army forward unit during Operation Desert Shield. *Mil Med*. 1997;162:374–379.

4. Seay WJ. Deployment medicine: Emporiatrics military style. *Army Med Dept J*. 1995;July–August:2–9.

5. Withers BG, Erickson RL, Petruccelli BP, Hanson RK, Kadlec RP. Preventing disease and non-battle injury in deployed units. *Mil Med*. 1994;159:39–43.

6.   Department of the Army. *Personnel Processing (In- and Out- and Mobilization Processing)*. Washington, DC: DA; 1989. Army Regulation 600-8-101.

7.   Department of the Navy, Bureau of Medicine and Surgery. *Medical Augmentation Program*. Washington, DC: DN; 1994. BUMED Instruction 6440.5A.

8.   Department of the Navy, Bureau of Medicine and Surgery. *Mobile Medical Augmentation Readiness Team Manual*. Washington, DC: DN; 1993. BUMED Instruction 6440.6.

9.   Department of the Air Force. *Aerospace Medical Operations*. Washington, DC: DAF; 1994. AF Instruction 48-101.

10. Department of the Army. *Exceptional Family Member Program*. Washington, DC: DA; 1996. Army Regulation 608-75.

11. DAPE-HR-PR. Subject: Deoxyribonucleic Acid (DNA) Specimen Collection. 27 Jun 94. Memorandum.

12. DAPE-MPE. Subject: Deployment Criteria, Duplicate Panographs. 10 Dec 96. Memorandum.

13. Department of the Army. *Standards of Medical Fitness*. Washington, DC: DA; 1995. Army Regulation 40-501.

14. Department of the Army. *Identification, Surveillance, and Administration of Personnel Infected with Human Immunodeficiency Virus (HIV)*. Washington, DC: DA; 1994. Army Regulation 600–110.

15. Department of the Air Force. *Human Immunodeficiency Program*. Washington, DC: DAF; 1994. AF Instructions 48–135.

16. Department of the Navy. *Management of Human Immunodeficiency Virus-1 (HIV-1) Infection in the Navy and Marine Corps*. Washington, DC: DN; 1990. SECNAV Instruction 5300.30C.

17. Powell GD, Dumitru D, Kennedy JJ. The effect of command emphasis and monthly physical training on Army physical fitness scores in a National Guard Unit. *Mil Med*. 1993;158:294–297.

18. Defense Manpower Data Center. *Desert Shield/Desert Storm Participation Report*. Vol 2. Monterey, Calif: DMDC; 1994: 1.

19. Loucks AB. Reserve readiness researcher studies. *Navy Med*. 1993;84:9.

20. Rothberg JM, Koshes RJ, Shanahan JE, Christman KW. Mobilization and rejection of Individual Ready Reserve personnel in Operations Desert Shield/Storm at a U.S. Army Quartermaster post. *Mil Med*. 1995;160:240–242.

21. Amato RS. Medical aspects of mobilization for war in an Army Reserve battalion. *Mil Med*. 1997;162:244–248.

22. King JE. US Army dental support for Operation Desert Shield/Storm. *Dental Corps Intl*. 1992;3(1):4–6.

23. York AK, Poindexter FR, Chisick MC. *1994 Tri-service Comprehensive Oral Health Survey*. 1995. Available from Defense Technical Information Center in two volumes: ADA299414 and ADA299418.

24. Ludwick WE, Gendron EG, Pogas JA, Weldon AL. Dental emergencies occurring among Navy-Marine personnel serving in Vietnam. *Mil Med*. 1974;139:121–123.

25. Department of Defense. *Standardization of Dental Classification*. Washington, DC: DoD; 8 November 1990. DoD Instruction 6410.1.

26. Teweles RB, King JE. Impact of troop dental health on combat readiness. *Mil Med*. 1987;152:233–235.

27. King JE. Dental status impact on unit readiness. *Med Bull US Army, Europe*. 1986;43(5/6):18–21.

28. Assistant Secretary of Defense (Health Affairs). *Glossary of Healthcare Terminology*. Washington, DC: Department of Defense; 1996.

29. Payne TF, Posey WR. Analysis of dental casualties in prolonged field training exercises. *Mil Med.* 1981;146:265,269–271.

30. Departments of the Air Force, Army, Navy, and Transportation. *Immunizations and Chemoprophylaxis.* Washington, DC: DoD; 1995. Air Force Joint Instruction 48-110, Army Regulation 40-562, BUMEDINST 6230.15, CG COMDTINST M6230.4E.

31. Centers for Disease Control and Prevention. *Health Information for International Travel, 1996–1997.* Atlanta: Department of Health and Human Services, CDC; 1997. HHS publication CDC 97-8280.

32. Klamerus S, Chief, Preventive Medicine Service, Fort Polk, La. Personal communication, 1995.

33. Chen RT, Rastogi SC, Mullen JR, et al. The Vaccine Adverse Event Reporting System (VAERS). *Vaccine.* 1994;12:542–550.

34. Department of the Army. *Use of Investigational Drugs and Devices in Humans and the Use of Schedule 1 Controlled Drug Substances.* Washington, DC: DA; 1991. Army Regulation 40-7.

35. Informed consent for human drugs and biologics; determination that informed consent is not feasible. *Fed Reg.* 1990;55:52, 814–817. As cited in: Annas GJ. Changing the consent rule for Desert Storm. *N Engl J Med.* 1992;326:770–773.

36. Annas GJ. Changing the consent rule for Desert Storm. *N Engl J Med.* 1992;326:770–773.

37. Berezuk GP, McCarty GE. Investigational drugs and vaccines fielded in support of Operation Desert Storm. *Mil Med.* 1992;157:404–406.

38. Weina PJ. From atabrine in World War II to mefloquine in Somalia: the role of education in preventive medicine. *Mil Med.* 1998;163:635–639.

39. Legters LJ, Llewellyn CH. Military medicine. In: Last JM, Wallace RB, eds. *Maxcy-Rosenau-Last Public Health & Preventive Medicine.* 13th ed. Norwalk, Conn: Appleton & Lange; 1992: Chap 71.

40. Gambel JM, Brundage JF, Burge RJ, DeFraites RF, Smoak BL, Wirtz RA. Survey of U.S. Army soldiers' knowledge, attitudes, and practices regarding personal protection measures to prevent arthropod-related disease and nuisance bites. *Mil Med.* 1998;163:695–701.

41. Hanson K, Preventive Medicine Residency Director, Uniformed Services University of the Health Sciences. Personal communication, 1996.

42. Larimore GW, Rubin LD. Health education. In: Anderson RS, Hoff EC, Hoff PM, eds. *Special Fields.* Vol 9. In: *Preventive Medicine in World War II.* Washington, DC: Office of the Surgeon General, Dept of the Army; 1969.

43. Huycke KA, Gambel JM, Petruccelli BP, Wasserman GM. Lessons learned from producing health information booklets for deploying U.S. military personnel. *Mil Med.* 1997;162:209–214.

44. Boyer CB, Shafer MA, Brodine SK, Shaffer RA. Evaluation of an STD/HIV intervention for deployed military men. Presented at the Eleventh Meeting of the International Society for STD Research; August 28, 1995; New Orleans, La.

MILITARY PREVENTIVE MEDICINE: MOBILIZATION AND DEPLOYMENT
Volume 1

Section 4: Occupational and Environmental Issues During Sustainment

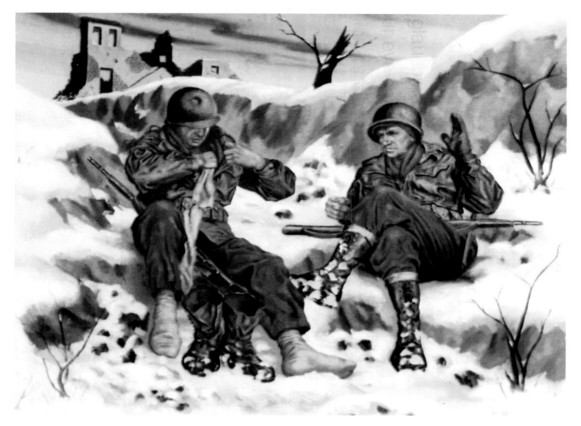

Frederick W. Toelbe   *Control of Trench Foot*

Frederick W. Toelbe, an Army artist in the European theater during World War II, captures one of the less glorious moments of warfare. A soldier is about to replace his wet socks with the dry pair he has been carrying inside his shirt. Trench foot, a debilitating condition caused by immersion in water and made worse by tightly laced boots, can take a soldier out of action just as completely as a gunshot wound. Benjamin Franklin's advice in the 1733 edition of *Poor Richard's Almanac* still applies to today's military: "Keep your mouth wet, your feet dry."

Art: Courtesy of US Center of Military History, Washington, DC.

Chapter 15

JET LAG AND SLEEP DEPRIVATION

NANCY JO WESENSTEN, PhD; CARLOS A. COMPERATORE, PhD; THOMAS J. BALKIN, PhD; AND GREGORY BELENKY, MD

N. J. Wesensten, Research Psychologist; Department of Neurobiology and Behavior, Division of Neuropsychiatry, Walter Reed Army Institute of Research, Silver Spring, MD 20910-7500

C. A. Comperatore, Research Psychologist; US Coast Guard Research and Development Center, Niantic, CT 06357

T. J. Balkin, Research Psychologist, Chief, Department of Neurobiology and Behavior, Division of Neuropsychiatry, Walter Reed Army Institute of Research, Silver Spring, MD 20910-7500

G. Belenky, Colonel, Medical Corps, US Army; Director, Division of Neuropsychiatry, Walter Reed Army Institute of Research, Silver Spring, MD 20910-7500

INTRODUCTION

Current and projected US military strategies call for rapid deployment of forces based in the continental United States to any part of the globe. These rapidly deployed forces will travel by air across multiple time zones and will need to be operationally effective immediately on arrival. These forces will conduct operations 24 hours a day, with the bulk of fighting occurring at night. Such rapid transmeridian travel will lead to desynchrony between external time cues at the new time zone and the service member's internal timing (circadian) system. Desynchronosis refers generally to situations in which external time cues are out of synchrony with the body's internal rhythms, the body's internal rhythms are out of synchrony with each other, or both. Jet lag is a specific instance of desynchronosis caused by crossing time zones. The symptoms of jet lag include cognitive performance impairment, sleep difficulties, gastrointestinal problems, fatigue, and mild depression.[1] Many of the body's physiological processes (eg, body temperature, hormonal rhythms) are cyclic; peaks and troughs recur at predictable times relative to external time (eg, body temperature reaches a nadir between 4 and 6 AM and begins rising again toward the end of the sleep period) and to each other. These cyclic processes readjust slowly to changes in external cues. In the case of deployment across multiple time zones, it takes 5 to 8 days for these cyclic processes to synchronize with the new local time. During this 5-to-8-day readjustment period, the individual suffers from jet lag. Shift work causes many of the same symptoms as jet lag because individuals are attempting to remain awake at times when bodily rhythms are synchronized for sleep.

During deployment, military personnel who rapidly cross time zones and work in shifts will suffer desynchronosis from both. Deployments increase the risk of jet lag, and they also increase demands on the service member's alertness and cognitive performance because of the advanced technology used by today's US military services and increases in operational tempo. For purposes of managing sleep to sustain alertness and performance before and during deployments, the researchers at the Walter Reed Army Institute of Research (WRAIR) are developing a Sleep Management System (SMS). The SMS will consist of six elements:

1. means to measure sleep under operational conditions,
2. a computer-based algorithm to predict performance on the basis of prior sleep,
3. recommendations for safe, effective stimulant drug use when no sleep is possible,
4. recommendations for safe, effective sleep-inducing drugs to promote good sleep under non–sleep-conducive conditions,
5. systems for on-line, real-time monitoring of alertness and performance, and
6. guidelines and doctrine for managing sleep to sustain alertness and performance during deployments.

Efforts toward managing sleep and alertness are also under way by other branches of the military and at the National Aeronautics and Space Administration. Each of these efforts focuses on one or more individual components of the WRAIR SMS. A comprehensive listing of fatigue-related resources is maintained by the Department of Transportation and can be found at the website http://olias.arc.nasa.gov/zteam.

This chapter is divided into two sections. The first section describes jet lag and factors influencing its duration and severity, effects of jet lag on sleep and of consequent sleep deprivation on performance, and a review of general approaches aimed at alleviating jet lag effects. The second section describes the Army Aviation Fighter Management System (AAFMS). The AAFMS is a practical guide for maximizing crew endurance by minimizing fatigue and performance degradation throughout a mission. The AAFMS describes practical applications of certain components of the WRAIR SMS but, in addition, provides specific guidance for coordinating scheduled unit activities such as aircraft maintenance cycles, refueling, briefing, and meals. The AAFMS can be used as a guide for scheduling activities to reverse desynchronosis occurring after transmeridian flights or during shift work. In a more general sense, however, the AAFMS is a guide that can be applied to any military scenario in which the goal is to improve crew endurance through sleep management.

JET LAG

Flight Factors

Several factors have been identified that affect the severity and duration of jet lag. These include the direction of travel, number of time zones crossed, and flight duration. In the case of the first factor, direction of travel, an eastbound flight crossing six time zones is perceived as more stressful than a westbound flight crossing the same or even a greater number of time zones.[2,3] Fragmented sleep (sleep with frequent awakenings) is a common problem following eastbound travel particularly, because sleep is being initiated during the individual's physiological day. On the other hand, after westbound travel, sleep is generally initiated at some point within the individual's physiological night.

The second factor affecting jet lag is the number of time zones crossed; jet lag duration is a direct function of number of time zones crossed.[2,3] As a general rule, one day of recovery is required for each time zone crossed. Whether a flight is homebound or outbound appears to have no effect on either severity or duration of jet lag. A homebound flight in an easterly direction will be perceived to be as stressful as an outbound flight in the same direction.

Flight duration, the third factor, affects jet lag severity but has no effect on its duration. Longer flights across the same number of time zones cause more severe jet lag. Flight duration probably causes general fatigue; some malaise is reported[4] after long north-south flights in which no time zones are crossed. In addition, long flights often involve some degree of sleep deprivation. It is likely that longer flights increase jet lag by increasing sleep loss.

Individual Differences

Individual differences are thought to affect severity and duration of jet lag, and they include chronotype (whether an individual is a morning person or an evening person), age, and personality (whether an individual is an introvert or an extrovert).[5] Only age, however, has a demonstrated objective effect on jet lag. When crossing the same number of time zones, individuals as young as 37 to 52 years of age suffer more severe and longer-lasting jet lag as measured by objective criteria (eg, performance, sleep quality) than younger (18–25 years old) individuals.[6] It is unclear whether this discrepancy is due to age-related declines in circadian system flexibility, in overall health, or in sleep pattern consistency in general (regardless of time zone transition). Individuals reaching early middle age, therefore, may require jet lag interventions for a longer period than young adults.

Rate of Adaptation to Time Zone Change

Over time, individuals become adapted to the new local time. One factor affecting rate of adaptation is exposure to social cues. Individuals allowed social contacts adapt up to two times more quickly to new time zones than individuals who remain isolated from social contact by, for example, remaining inside hotel rooms or barracks.[7] Similarly, regular exercise and regularly scheduled meal times may hasten subjective adaptation to new time zones.[5] The success of those two activities may reflect a more general effect of engagement in regular activity, no matter what the source. Factors such as social cues, exercise, and meals may act as general "zeitgebers" (time cue providers). Any activity occurring regularly may act as a zeitgeber and thus hasten adaptation to new time zones.

JET LAG AND SLEEP

Although jet lag is a consequence of desynchronosis, a growing consensus suggests that the most important component of jet lag is desynchronosis-induced sleep deprivation.[8] Indeed, many of the symptoms of jet lag (eg, degradation in performance, alertness, and mood) mimic those of sleep deprivation, suggesting that sleep loss is one of the main factors contributing to jet lag symptomology, such as sleep difficulties and fatigue.

The effects of transmeridian travel on sleep are well described.[9] Following eastbound travel, both the ability to fall asleep (sleep initiation) and to stay asleep (sleep maintenance) are adversely affected. These effects can last up to 8 days following a 7-hour time zone shift. Following westbound travel, the ability to fall asleep is unaffected, but the ability to stay asleep in the second half of the sleep period is impaired[10] because this portion of the sleep period occurs during the individual's physiological morning. Both eastbound and westbound flights also affect the balance of the various sleep stages.[9] The consequences for performance and well-being are probably marginal, however, because there is no evidence that any one sleep stage is more important than any other, as long as duration of sleep is preserved. Because the recuperative value of sleep, in terms of next-day performance and ability to maintain alertness, is dependent on duration,[11] eastbound travel in particular diminishes sleep's recuperative value by decreasing sleep duration through increased time spent either awake or in very light, nonrecuperative sleep. A repeating pattern of a night of poor sleep followed by a night of good sleep is often experienced by jet-lagged individuals, particularly after eastbound flights. This zigzag pattern of alternating good and poor sleep reflects the combined effects of desynchronosis, which leads to a poor night's sleep, and subsequent sleep deprivation, which drives "good" sleep on the following night.

Flight scheduling also affects the amount of sleep deprivation incurred with transmeridian travel. Eastbound flights are generally scheduled as night flights, with passengers arriving in the morning of the new local day; this requires them to miss more than 24 hours of sleep if they did not sleep during the flight. Westbound flights are usually day flights arriving in the afternoon of the new local day, therefore resulting in only several hours of sleep deprivation (equal to the number of time zones crossed) before nocturnal sleep.

The most important consequences of transmeridian travel on sleep are the inability to fall asleep and, once asleep, frequent awakenings throughout the night. Both these effects lead to decreased quantity and impaired quality of sleep and result in diminished performance and alertness.

SLEEP DEPRIVATION AND PERFORMANCE

Partial sleep deprivation, total sleep deprivation, and fragmented sleep (even if the normal total hours of sleep are accumulated) have deleterious effects on alertness, cognitive performance, and mood. A variety of studies suggest that higher-order mental operations (ie, those involving the prefrontal cortex) are particularly sensitive to sleep deprivation. Complex cognitive performance, including the ability to understand, adapt, and plan in rapidly changing circumstances, is affected.[12] In a detailed and realistic simulation of artillery fire operations,[13] five-person teams were evaluated for their ability to conduct simulated continuous combat operations lasting 36 hours. Each team's task was to plot target locations; derive range, bearing, and angle of gun elevation; and charge immediately on receipt of the target and update situation maps. Across 36 hours of sleep deprivation, each team's ability to derive range, bearing, and elevation accurately and to charge was unimpaired. After approximately 24 hours without sleep (about the same amount of sleep deprivation incurred following nighttime eastbound flights of more than 6 hours), however, team members stopped updating their situation maps and stopped computing preplanned targets immediately on receipt of new information. As a consequence, the teams disrupted their smooth, accurate flow of work, fired on prohibited targets, and generally lost control of the operation. This is exemplary of the types of performance deficits seen in real-world situations involving partially or totally sleep-deprived individuals.

In laboratory simulations, sleep fragmentation and sleep deprivation result in a decline in overall performance (primarily because of reduction in speed), but accuracy is relatively preserved. Performance degradation in the laboratory across time, when no sleep is allowed, is characterized by a gradual, systematic decline (Figure 15-1). In actual operations, this systematic decline in performance may be of no great consequence if the task is simple and familiar and if accurate (albeit slower) performance is sufficient. However, if the task is complex, unfamiliar, intrinsically time-limited, or any combination of these, sudden failure may occur when the time needed to reach an accurate decision exceeds the time available. When time runs out, the individual is forced to guess, and performance drops to chance levels. In actual operations, a gradual decline in performance may still maintain the appearance of adequacy until performance drops below some critical threshold, at which point sudden failure occurs. If the individual is a critical element in a complex system, the sudden performance failure may result in catastrophic consequences.

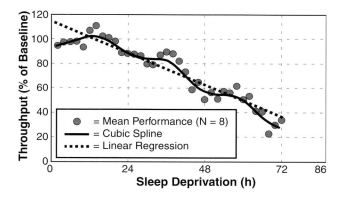

Fig. 15-1. This graph illustrates performance on a computerized, serial, addition-subtraction task across 72 hours of total sleep deprivation within the laboratory. Data are from eight healthy young males undergoing 72 hours of total sleep deprivation in the laboratory. In this task, subjects mentally added or subtracted two numbers appearing sequentially on the screen (followed by an arithmetic operation sign), and entered the answer on a numeric keypad. The spheres represent mean performance on the serial addition or subtraction task. Data points represent the product of speed and accuracy, and as a percent of baseline (presleep deprivation) performance. The speed * accuracy product is noted as "throughput." Throughput is the same as productivity, the amount of useful work performed per unit of time. Superimposed on this linear decline is the normal circadian rhythm shown here as the cubic spline fit to the data.

JET LAG INTERVENTIONS

The most important consequence of transmeridian travel is impaired sleep. Impaired sleep leads to performance degradation, so most interventions are aimed at either improving sleep or, when sleep is not possible, improving alertness. Approaches aimed at overcoming poor sleep, as well as boosting performance under sleep-deprived conditions, have been successful and are well documented.[14–16] Interventions aimed at speeding the rate of reentrainment (ie, overcoming the desynchronosis component of jet lag) have had less success,[5] with the exception of carefully timed bright light.[17]

Speeding Reentrainment

Chronobiotics

The search for a chronobiotic agent, an agent that speeds reentrainment of the body's clock to new local time, has met with only limited success. Dietary interventions receiving some attention include combination carbohydrate-protein diets and tryptophan. None of these approaches has been shown to speed reentrainment or to prevent or alleviate jet lag as measured objectively by performance, body temperature, or sleep-wake cycles. Positive effects on subjective ratings of performance and mood, however, have been noted. Pharmacological approaches to speeding reentrainment have included using caffeine, benzodiazepines, and melatonin.[5] Although these compounds have not yet been shown definitively to speed adaptation to time zone changes, they have demonstrated objective effectiveness for improving either alertness or sleep.

Bright Light

There is substantial evidence[17] that properly timed exposure to bright light can speed rates of reentrainment (as measured by body temperature) to new time zones. Timed bright light, however, requires scheduled, controlled exposures and therefore is impractical for most military operational settings. Conversely, improperly timed light exposure can slow reentrainment. Ambient daylight is bright light. Appropriate timing of exposure to ambient daylight is important for adjustment to new time zones and to shift work. Thus, management of ambient light exposure is an important element in adaptation to new time zones and is being incorporated into the WRAIR SMS.

Prophylaxis

Prophylactic measures attempt to minimize desynchronosis on arrival at the new time zone. The most straightforward approach consists of gradually shifting bedtime to match the destination's local time before embarking. This proactive approach is impractical, however, because it requires the individual to overcome powerful environmental cues and social demands, such as going to bed several hours before the norm. It is unreasonable to expect an individual planning to take a trip crossing eight time zones to go to bed at 4 PM for 1 week before he or she leaves.

Interventions for Improving Sleep and Alertness

Interventions aimed at improving sleep quality and alertness have been used successfully to combat sleep loss caused by transmeridian travel and sleep loss during continuous or sustained operations. These interventions are being incorporated into the WRAIR SMS.

Naps

Naps aimed particularly at alleviating sleep deprivation may be a useful strategy because in continuous operations naps can significantly improve performance.[18] As with the main sleep period, naps must be of sufficient duration and continuity to be effective. For example, a 1-hour nap that is fragmented with awakenings and shifts to light, nonrecuperative sleep may not be as effective as a 30-minute nap that is unfragmented. Prophylactic naps taken during transmeridian flights offer some benefit, particularly on eastbound flights when individuals arrive in the morning of new local time and must begin work immediately. Even though there may be opportunity to sleep on transmeridian flights, conditions are rarely conducive: sleep is interrupted by meals and other in-flight services, the cabin is well-lit and noisy, and the seats are uncomfortable for sleep. Nap quality can be improved by the use of nonpharmacological sleep aids (eg, ear plugs, sleep masks) and pharmacological ones.

Caffeine

Stimulants may be useful in the short-term management of alertness following a night of reduced sleep. Caffeine in doses from 300 to 600 mg (a cup of coffee contains approximately 100 mg of caffeine) is effective in reversing the cognitive performance deficits of 48 hours of sleep deprivation, with effects lasting up to 12 hours.[19] In situations where an opportunity to sleep becomes available after caffeine administration, however, the ability to fall asleep, even in the face of sleep deprivation, may be impaired.[14] In addition, caffeine cannot replace sleep itself. Thus, caffeine may be used as a short-term solution to sleep deprivation, but it has no effect on speed of reentrainment and may adversely affect subsequent sleep.

Pharmacological Sleep Aids

Orally administered benzodiazepines represent the most widely prescribed class of sleep-inducing agents. Their effects on improving duration and continuity, and hence recuperative value, of sleep are well documented.[20–22] Drugs such as triazolam (Halcion), temazepam (Restoril), and zolpidem (Ambien—a nonbenzodiazepine that has effects similar to benzodiazepines) improve sleep by reducing the time taken to fall asleep and the number of awakenings, thus improving sleep duration by reducing fragmentation.

To be useful in a military setting, sleep-inducing agents should act quickly and should not impair postsleep performance. In laboratory studies[23] of sleep during and following a simulated eastbound flight, the short-acting agents triazolam and zolpidem substantially improved sleep by putting people to sleep quickly and keeping them asleep in spite of a bright, noisy environment in which the subjects were sitting upright. However, at sleep-inducing doses (0.5 mg of triazolam, 20 mg of zolpidem—twice the currently recommended dose of both drugs), triazolam and zolpidem produce cognitive performance impairments (primarily impairing the ability to learn new material) if individuals are forced to awaken and perform mental work when the drug is having its peak effect. Thus, the benefits of drug-induced sleep under operational conditions may be offset by potentially hazardous performance impairments if personnel are required to awaken and perform before the drug effects have dissipated. Performance impairments due to sleep-inducing drugs may not be immediately apparent because individuals are able to perform tasks and recall information that was learned before taking the drug. However, if military personnel are given a new task or instructions while

still under the effects of the drug, their subsequent memory for this new information is likely to be impaired. In a field study[24] involving long-range deployment by air, 0.5 mg of triazolam (the only dose found to be sleep-inducing under non–sleep-conducive conditions) had equivocal effects on sleep during the 8-hour eastbound flight. More important, triazolam produced operationally significant impairments in new learning on arrival in Germany, 8 hours after drug administration. In fact, other studies[16,23] have shown that the more effective triazolam and zolpidem are for inducing sleep, the greater the performance decrement at estimated peak drug plasma concentrations, approximately 1.5 hours after oral ingestion for both drugs. Because high doses of triazolam and zolpidem (as well as other sleep-inducing agents) appear to be necessary to substantially improve sleep in healthy, young adults in non–sleep-conducive conditions, up to 8 hours of downtime is required following administration of 20 mg of zolpidem and up to 12 hours may be necessary following administration of 0.5 mg of triazolam.[15,16] Lowering the dosage (eg, 0.25 mg of triazolam or 10 mg of zolpidem, the maximum doses currently recommended) would reduce the risk of postsleep performance impairments. It might also reduce the amount of recuperative sleep obtained, particularly in non–sleep-conducive environments or in relatively well-rested individuals. Pharmacological sleep aids can improve the recuperative value of sleep, but they carry the risk of impaired postsleep performance if the duration of downtime following drug administration is inadequate. Given with adequate downtime in the schedule, both drugs are considered safe and effective for improving sleep.

An alternative to extended downtime following administration of pharmacological sleep aids is the administration of an "antidote" drug that reverses within minutes the effects of the sleep-inducing agent. The combination of triazolam followed by caffeine has been investigated, but caffeine has little effect on reversing triazolam-induced performance deficits.[25] Flumazenil (Romazicon), a nonstimulant drug used to reverse benzodiazepine anesthesia and overdose, has been tested in simulated deployment situations.[15] Flumazenil fully reversed the performance-impairing effects of sleep-inducing doses of triazolam and zolpidem. A two-drug system, consisting of a combination sleep-inducing agent (triazolam or zolpidem) followed by a rapid-reawakening agent (flumazenil), is currently under development for the WRAIR SMS.

Melatonin

Melatonin may be useful for improving sleep, speeding adaptation after transmeridian travel, and speeding adaptation to shift work. The potential benefits of a low pharmacological dose of melatonin (10 mg or less) are its lack of toxicity,[26] short duration of action,[27] minimal side effects, and putative resynchronization[28] and sleep-inducing properties.[29] Melatonin (5 mg) decreases sleep latency, improves sleep quality, and increases next-day alertness,[30] although to a lesser degree than triazolam or zolpidem. Similarly, melatonin increases subjective sleepiness following administration of 2 mg and 5 mg.[2,31] A study[32] of efficacy in the prevention of sleep loss and cognitive degradation in volunteers traveling eastward across eight time zones and working nighttime duty hours showed that a 7-day melatonin regimen (10 mg administered twice, once at 7 PM and again at 8 PM) resulted in longer sleep duration and improved postsleep performance.

Following eastbound flights, melatonin administration during the late afternoon and early evening of the new local time may hasten sleep onset. Following westbound travel, administration during the second half of the night may reduce sleep maintenance problems. For the latter, a time-release formula taken before bedtime would avoid disrupting sleep to take medication. It is unclear what dosage of melatonin is optimal for chronobiotic effects, because recent findings indicate that larger doses (eg, 5 mg) are more effective than smaller doses for inducing phase shifts.[28] As with the benzodiazepines, however, melatonin doses of greater than 1 mg may impair postsleep performance. In particular, the time required for the return of full alertness following a given dose of melatonin has yet to be determined, and currently there is no available "antidote." Research is under way to determine melatonin's effectiveness during multiple rapid deployments, its effects on flight performance, grounding time for aviators, possible interactions with the menstrual cycle, and appropriateness for incorporation into the WRAIR SMS.

The most deleterious consequence of desynchronosis due to jet lag or shift work is its effects on sleep quality. Impaired sleep quality, in turn, adversely affects performance and mood. Interventions aimed at either improving sleep or bolstering alertness when sleep is not possible have been successful. Conversely, with the exception of bright light and possibly melatonin, attempts to speed reentrainment have been unsuccessful. Impaired sleep and sleep deprivation have thus been identified as causing impaired performance and mood following transmeridan travel or shiftwork. The above interventions aimed at improving sleep and alertness, however, are general in nature. Guidelines for identifying specific activities that could potentially interfere with crew sleep and improving coordination of these activities are also required. The US Army Aviation Fighter Management System was developed in response to these needs.

THE US ARMY AVIATION FIGHTER MANAGEMENT SYSTEM: A SYSTEMS APPROACH TO CREW ENDURANCE

Because the most deleterious, and avoidable, consequence of desynchronosis is sleep deprivation, the Army Aviation Fighter Management System (AAFMS) focuses on controlling sleep and factors that affect it. The implementation of a desynchronosis prevention plan requires an integrated system that encompasses a crew endurance plan and a sleep and daylight exposure plan. To be successful, this effort must include everyone from the individual service member through the upper management strata. The AAFMS is a guide to creating this integrated system. Although the AAFMS describes activities relevant to Army aviation missions, activities specific to any branch of the military could be substituted.

The crew endurance plan is a set of activities that must be coordinated for any mission. These activities, or elements, are best arranged by order of flexibility (Figure 15-2). Mission objectives are the least flexible of these elements so cannot be changed by the crew, while materiel activities (eg, maintaining and operating aircraft) are the most flexible and usually can be scheduled by the crew. The most flexible elements or activities are scheduled around the least flexible.

Mission Requirements

At the center of the crew endurance management system are mission requirements, the activities over which the unit has no control. Mission requirements determine how the crew rest plan evolves and determine the unit's work-rest cycles, mission flight schedules, operational tempo, and flight environment. Elements of a crew rest plan for a particular mission are determined by the unique requirements of that mission.

Individual-Level Activities

The individual level is composed of strategies that, although developed by unit planners based on the mission requirements, must be adjusted by the

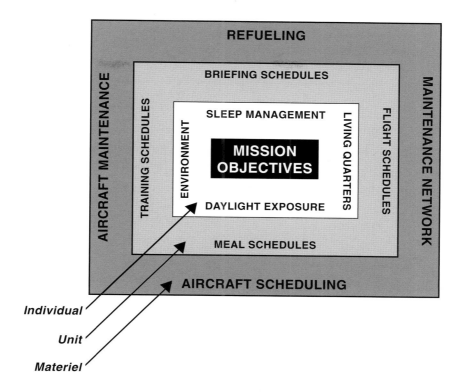

Fig. 15-2. Schematic of the Crew Endurance Management System. At the core of the system-and driving the other elements-are mission objectives. Individual-, unit, and materiel-level elements for improving crew sleep and alertness are coordinated around mission objectives.

individual service member to meet his or her needs. These controls are nonpharmacological. The use of pharmacological means of improving sleep and alertness should be restricted to special instances in which the outlined controls are inadequate or impractical. The potential risks of using pharmacological sleep inducers or alertness enhancers or both must be weighed against the potential benefits to accomplishing mission objectives. These individual-level critical strategies help prevent sleep deprivation following transmeridian deployment or shift work. They include a sleep management plan, a daylight exposure management plan, and an environmental management plan (Table 15-1).

Sleep Management Plan

Sleep management requires the identification of bedtimes and awakening times that are likely to provide sufficient rest and return military personnel to duty at their maximum alertness. A knowledge of mission requirements, such as deployment timing and tactics, must precede the design of the sleep management plan. Bedtimes and awakening times are scheduled around the deployment schedule or flight mission. Other schedule elements at the unit and materiel levels (eg, meals, briefings, aircraft maintenance) are then adapted to the sleep management plan.

After the sleep management plan is approved, it should be reviewed by the chain of command. Each person in the chain should be trained regarding the plan's implementation. This ensures that each service member understands his or her individual strategies. Although the sleep management plan is tailored to the individual, its controls generally are applied to small groups. For example, sound masking (a technique to help individuals sleep in a noisy environment) benefits all personnel trying to sleep in the immediate area. Both individual and small-unit responsibilities are involved in implementing a sleep management plan.

Light Management Plan

The daylight exposure management plan provides a schedule of daylight exposure or avoidance that will synchronize the body clock to the mission-driven work-rest cycle. The plan is based on how the body's circadian rhythm responds to light, depending on time of day. In general, most people's circadian rhythms respond to light exposure at a given time of day by shifting in the same direction.[33] The light exposure

TABLE 15-1

PRACTICAL CONTROLS FOR SLEEP, AMBIENT LIGHT, AND ENVIRONMENTAL MANAGEMENT AT THE INDIVIDUAL LEVEL

Goal	Practical Control
Ensure adequate duration and continuity of sleep	Schedule one continuous sleep period lasting 6–8 h
Ensure that sleep takes place in darkness	Black out windows if sleep is taken during the day
	Use sleep masks if sleep is taken during the day
Improve sleep-conducive quality of noisy environments	Provide ear plugs to dampen noises
	Mask sounds using rushing sounds but a constant rate and volume
Improve sleep-conducive quality of hot environments	Improve evaporative cooling by providing fans
Improve sleep-conducive quality of cold environments	Warm tents before the sleeping period to avoid disruptive effects of fire inspections required when heaters are used during sleep
Hasten adaptation from day work to night work	Avoid varying initial daylight exposure after awakening
	Avoid daylight immediately before or during sleep period
	Wear dark sunglasses at other times to reduce the amount of light reaching the eyes
	Retire as soon as possible after night operations
Hasten adaptation from night work to day work	Seek as much daylight exposure as possible within the hours dictated by the light management plan

Source: Comperatore CA. The crew rest system. In: Comperatore CA, Caldwell J, Caldwell L, eds. *Leader's Guide for Crew Endurance.* Fort Rucker, Ala: US Army Safety Center; 1996.

plan is designed to enhance speedy adaptation to a new work schedule or time zone or both, without the need for timed exposure to artificial bright light. Individuals traveling eastward who have daytime duty hours should avoid daylight from sunrise to approximately 10:30 AM, particularly when they have crossed more than five time zones. They should seek daylight exposure after 10:30 AM because the exposure will stimulate the advance of the sleep-wake cycle and promote adaptation to the new time zone. This approach should be implemented during the first 2 days after arrival. Thereafter, daylight exposure may begin at sunrise.

When nighttime operations are combined with travel across more than five time zones, military personnel need only advance sleep onset by 2 to 3 hours relative to their bedtime at the home time zone. In this case, if night operations extend into the early morning hours (eg, 4:00 or 5:00 AM), service members should retire before sunrise; if the duty period extends past sunrise, they should avoid exposure to daylight by, for example, wearing dark sunglasses that prevent light intrusion into the eyes. In-

dividuals should seek daylight exposure after 10:30 AM. This process will eventually result in the advance of the sleep-wake cycle by approximately 2 to 3 hours in the first week after arrival.

Environmental Management Plan

Noise and daylight intrusions into sleeping quarters degrade sleep and hence its recuperative value for sustaining subsequent alertness and performance. This is particularly problematic when personnel are sleeping in the field. Similarly, extreme temperatures in sleeping quarters will degrade sleep.

Unit-Level Activities

The unit level includes coordination of scheduled activities within groups of service members. These elements must be scheduled after considering the individual-level schedule of activities. For example, unit and aircrew mission briefings should be scheduled to occur before or after the designated sleep

TABLE 15-2

PRACTICAL CONTROLS FOR SLEEP, AMBIENT LIGHT, AND ENVIRONMENTAL MANAGEMENT AT THE UNIT LEVEL

Unit-Level Activity	Practical Control
Briefings	Schedule briefings to occur outside the designated sleep period
Training for night operations personnel	Modify training schedule to accommodate designated sleep periods
	Segregate day crews from night crews to reduce ambient noise levels during scheduled sleep periods
Meals	Schedule breakfast as first meal after awakening for both night and day workers
	Schedule all meals outside of designated sleep period

Source: Comperatore CA. The crew rest system. In: Comperatore CA, Caldwell J, Caldwell L, eds. *Leader's Guide for Crew Endurance.* Fort Rucker, Ala: US Army Safety Center; 1996.

period. Most elements at this level can be customized by the unit. Common unit activities that must be considered within the crew rest plan are summarized in Table 15-2.

Materiel-Level Activities

The materiel level involves work schedules and activities associated with equipment used to accomplish mission objectives. For example, in an aviation unit, elements in the materiel level are primarily concerned with maintaining and operating aircraft. This level is the most flexible and can often be tailored to schedules at the individual level. The unit's management of aircraft involves scheduling maintenance, refueling, air crews, and aircraft flight times. Each of these activities may potentially disrupt the crew rest plan if coordination is neglected. Materiel-level elements and practical controls for their coordination within the crew rest plan are found in Table 15-3.

TABLE 15-3

PRACTICAL CONTROLS FOR SLEEP, AMBIENT LIGHT, AND ENVIRONMENTAL MANAGEMENT AT THE MATERIEL LEVEL

Materiel-level Activity	Practical Control
Aircraft maintenance	Submit maintenance requests immediately after arrival from night missions to prevent disruption of crew rest
Refueling	If near designated sleep areas, schedule refueling to occur before or after sleep period
Aircraft scheduling and operations	Keep aircraft keys and log books in a tent separate from where crew are sleeping to prevent disrupting crew rest to get access to keys and log books
	Plan approach routes into field landing zones and bivouac areas so that aircraft do not fly over designated sleep areas
	Direct visiting aircraft to landing areas that are not adjacent to sleeping personnel

Source: Comperatore CA. The crew rest system. In: Comperatore CA, Caldwell J, Caldwell L, eds. *Leader's Guide for Crew Endurance.* Fort Rucker, Ala: US Army Safety Center; 1996.

Further Information

Detailed descriptions of crew endurance management plans for specific missions, such as night operations and rapid deployment, are contained in the Army's *Crew Endurance Leader's Guide*[34] published by the Army Safety Center, Fort Rucker, Ala. For more information on crew endurance and light management plans, contact Dr. Lynn Caldwell, US Army Aeromedical Research Laboratory, Aeromedical Fac-tors Branch, ATTN: MCMR-UAS-AF, PO Box 620577, Fort Rucker, AL 36362-0577, DSN: 558-6858, (334) 255-6858. For more information on sleep and performance in general, and the WRAIR SMS, see the WRAIR Division of Neuropsychiatry's home page on the World Wide Web at *http://wrair-www.army.mil* or contact COL Gregory Belenky, Director, Division of Neuropsychiatry, Walter Reed Army Institute of Research, 503 Robert Grant, Silver Spring, MD 20910-7500; e-mail: gregory.belenky@na.amedd.army.mil.

SUMMARY

Optimum mental performance is critical to successful combat operations at all levels of command and control today, and all visions of future combat demand even-more-sophisticated cognitive operations of military personnel at all levels. Adequate sleep is central to sustaining cognitive performance. The disruptive effects of rapid deployment across time zones on sleep and subsequent performance imperil the military's capability to perform its mission, but there are techniques and pharmacological agents that can ameliorate these effects. The evolving US Army SMS and AAFMS will provide software, hardware, and doctrine that will unobtrusively measure and effectively manage sleep to sustain performance in combat situations.

REFERENCES

1. Graeber RC. Alterations in performance following rapid transmeridian flight. In: Brown FM, Graeber RC, eds. *Rhythmic Aspects of Behavior*. NJ: Laurence Earlbaum Associates; 1982:173–212.

2. Hauty GT, Adams T. Phase shifts of the human circadian system and performance deficit during the periods of transition, I: East-west flight. *Aerospace Med*. 1966;37:668–674.

3. Hauty GT, Adams T. Phase shifts of the human circadian system and performance deficit during the periods of transition, II: West-east flight. *Aerospace Med*. 1966;37:1027–1033.

4. Hauty GT, Adams T. Phase shifts of the human circadian system and performance deficit during the periods of transition, III: North-south flight. *Aerospace Med*. 1966;37:1257–1262.

5. Redfern PH. "Jet-lag": Strategies for prevention and cure. *Hum Psychopharmacol*. 1989;4:159–168.

6. Moline ML, Pollak CP, Monk TH, et al. Age-related differences in recovery from simulated jet lag. *Sleep*. 1992;15(1):28–40.

7. Honma K, Honma S, Nakamura K, Sasaki M, Endo T, Takahashi T. Differential effects of bright light and social cues on reentrainment of human circadian rhythms. *Am J Physiol*. 1995;268(Suppl 2):R528–R535.

8. Dement WC, Seidel WF, Cohen SA, Bliwise NG, Carskadon MA. Sleep and wakefulness in aircrew before and after transoceanic flights. *Aviat Space Environ Med*. 1986;57(Suppl 12):B14–B28.

9. Endo S, Yamamoto T, Sasaki M. Effects of time zone changes on sleep—west-east flight and east-west flight. *Jikeikai Med J*. 1978;25:249–268.

10. Nicholson AN, Pascoe PA, Spencer MB, Stone BM, Green RL. Nocturnal sleep and daytime alertness of aircrew after transmeridian flights. *Aviat Space Environ Med*. 1986;57(Suppl 12):B43–B52.

11. Wesensten NJ, Balkin TJ, Belenky G. Does sleep fragmentation impact recuperation? A review and reanalysis. *J Sleep Res*. 1999;8:237–254.

12. Horne JA. *Why We Sleep: The Functions of Sleep in Humans and Other Mammals.* Oxford: Oxford University Press; 1988.

13. Banderet LE, Stokes JW, Francesconi R, Kowal DM, Naitoh P. Artillery teams in simulated sustained combat: performance and other measures. In: Johnson LC, Tepas DI, Colquhon WP, Colligan MJ, eds. *The Twenty-Four Hour Workday: Proceedings of a Symposium on Variation in Work-Sleep Schedules.* Washington, DC: Government Printing Office; 1981: 581–604. DHHS, NIOSH Report 81-127.

14. Moline ML, Zendell SM, Pollak CP, Wagner DR. Acute effects of caffeine on sleep in simulated jet-lag. *Sleep Res.* 1995;24:529.

15. Wesensten NJ, Balkin TJ, Davis HQ, Belenky GL. Reversal of triazolam- and zolpidem-induced memory impairment by flumazenil. *Psychopharmacology (Berl).* 1995;121:242–249.

16. Wesensten NJ, Balkin TJ, Belenky GL. Effects of daytime administration of zolpidem and triazolam on memory. *Eur J Clin Pharmacol.* 1995;48:115–122.

17. Czeisler CA, Allan JS. Acute circadian phase reversal in man via bright light exposure: Application to jet-lag. *Sleep Res.* 1987;16:605.

18. Rosekind MR, Smith RM, Miller DL, et al. Alertness management: Strategic naps in operational settings. *J Sleep Res.* 1995;4(S2):62–66.

19. Penetar D, McCann U, Thorne D, et al. Caffeine reversal of sleep deprivation effects on alertness and mood. *Psychopharmacology (Berl).* 1993;112:359–365.

20. Donaldson E, Kennaway DJ. Effects of temazepam on sleep, performance, and rhythmic 6-sulphatoxymelatonin and cortisol excretion after transmeridian travel. *Aviat Space Environ Med.* 1991;62:654–660.

21. Seidel WF, Roth T, Roehrs T, Zorick F, Dement WC. Treatment of a 12-hour shift of sleep schedule with benzodiazepines. *Science.* 1984;224:1262–1264.

22. Walsh JK, Schweitzer PK, Sugerman JL, Muelbach MJ. Transient insomnia associated with a 3-hour phase advance of sleep time and treatment with zolpidem. *J Clin Psychopharmacol.* 1990;10(3):184–189.

23. Balkin TJ, O'Donnell VM, Wesensten N, McCann U, Belenky G. Comparison of the daytime sleep and performance effects of zolpidem versus triazolam. *Psychopharmacology(Berl).* 1992;107:83–88.

24. Penetar DM, Belenky G, Garrigan JJ, Redmond DP. Triazolam impairs learning and fails to improve sleep in a long-range aerial deployment. *Aviat Space Environ Med.* 1989;60:594–598.

25. Roehrs T, Zwyghuizen-Doorenbos A, Smith D, Zorick F, Roth T. Reversal of caffeine by triazolam-induced impairment of waking function. *Psychopharmacol Ser.* 1988;6:194–202.

26. Sugden D. Psychopharmacological effects of melatonin in mouse and rat. *J Pharmacol Exp Ther.* 1983;227:587–591.

27. Aldhous M, Franey C, Wright J, Arendt J. Plasma concentrations of melatonin in man following oral absorption of different preparations. *Br J Pharmacol.* 1985;19:517–521.

28. Deacon S, Arendt J. Melatonin-induced temperature suppression and its acute phase-shifting effects correlate in a dose-dependent manner in humans. *Brain Res.* 1995;688:77–85.

29. Zhdanova IV, Wurtman RJ, Lynch HJ, et al. Sleep-inducing effects of low doses of melatonin ingested in the evening. *Clin Pharmacol Ther.* 1995;57:552–558.

30. Arendt J, Borbely AA, Franey C, Wright J. The effects of chronic, small doses of melatonin given in the late afternoon on fatigue in man: A preliminary study. *Neurosci Lett.* 1984;45:317–321.

31. Dollins AB, Lynch HJ, Wurtman RJ, et al. Effect of pharmacological daytime doses of melatonin on human mood and performance. *Psychopharmacology (Berl).* 1993;112:490–496.

32. Comperatore CA, Lieberman HR, Kirby AW, Adams B, Crowley JS. Melatonin efficacy in aviation missions requiring rapid deployment and night operations. *Aviat Space Environ Med.* 1996;67:520–524.

33. Daan S, Lewy AJ. Scheduled exposure to daylight: A potential strategy to reduce "jet lag" following transmeridian flight. *Psychopharmacol Bull.* 1984;20:566–568.

34. Comperatore CA. The crew rest system. In: Comperatore CA, Caldwell J, Caldwell L, eds. *Leader's Guide for Crew Endurance.* Fort Rucker, Ala: US Army Safety Center; 1996.

Chapter 16

COMBAT STRESS CONTROL AND FORCE HEALTH PROTECTION

JAMES W. STOKES, MD; HARRY GREER, MD; AND PAUL S. HAMMER, MD

J.W. Stokes; Colonel, Medical Corps, US Army; Combat Stress Control Program Officer, Behavioral Health Division (MCHO-CL-H), Health Policy and Services, US Army Medical Command, 2050 Worth Road, Fort Sam Houston, TX 78234-6010

H. Greer; Captain, Medical Corps, US Navy; Instructor, Defense Medical Readiness Training Institute, Fort Sam Houston, TX

P.S. Hammer; Commander, Medical Corps, US Navy; Staff Psychiatrist, Mental Health Department, Naval Medical Center, San Diego, CA 92136

INTRODUCTION

Preventive Medicine and Combat Stress Control (CSC) are recognized as important, autonomous military medical functional areas by the US Army and by the Department of Defense. They are now combined under the umbrella concept, or battlefield operating system, of "Force Health Protection." Both are ultimately the responsibility of the commander and the noncommissioned officers (NCOs) at all echelons. The general medical personnel in units serve as monitors, advisers, educators, and action teams to correct identified problems. The unit chaplains provide important support because of their access to the service members and the confidential nature of their discourse. But those personnel have their own urgent primary duties demanding their attention in combat and other high-risk missions. Preventive medicine personnel and the mental health personnel assigned to CSC duties both have force health protection as their primary mission.

The CSC operational concept and published Army doctrine[1–3] define CSC as primary, secondary, and tertiary prevention to be conducted in support of command in the military unit context by members of the five mental health professional disciplines and their enlisted assistants. Department of Defense Directive 6490.5 directs the US military services to ensure

appropriate prevention and management of Combat Stress Reaction (CSR) casualties to preserve mission effectiveness and warfighting, and to minimize the short- and long-term adverse effects of combat on the physical, psychological, intellectual and social health of all Service members.[4(p1)]

The directive mandates training of all ranks in the CSC principles appropriate to their rank and responsibilities, including primary, secondary, and tertiary prevention.

In both the Marine Corps and the Army, preventive medicine and mental health are intrinsic parts of the force structure. Unfortunately, these two disciplines, in both the civilian world and in the military, often find it difficult to work as a team. Mental health workers need training in epidemiology and familiarization with sanitation, environmental hazard monitoring, and vector and infectious disease control. Preventive medicine workers need some training in community mental health. Both need training in risk communication. It is often the case that deployed senior preventive medicine assets are located at the corps or higher levels and the mental health personnel are at the subordinate division level. Preventive medicine officers, therefore, may have the responsibility to see that mental health programs are effective. This pattern is also consistent with that found in most civilian health departments. It is important, then, that preventive medicine physicians understand principles involved in mental or behavioral health promotion.

As with preventive medicine in general, preventive stress control must be applied across the full continuum of operations, from garrison and peacetime training to the battlefield. The best preventive interventions and training must be made before the units are involved in high-stress, high-risk action.

COMBAT STRESS CONTROL'S RELATIONSHIP TO PREVENTIVE MEDICINE IN THE OPERATIONAL SETTING

Good preventive medicine discipline usually means good stress control. Effective camp hygiene and preventive medicine measures imply strong, concerned, caring leadership, good buddyship, mentoring of new arrivals by veterans, and effective initial training. Strong preventive medicine discipline gives each unit member pride, a sense of professionalism and competence, and trust in leaders and comrades. (An exception may be when the good preventive medicine discipline is one positive effect caused by a martinet who is in other ways mistreating personnel.) Pride, professionalism, and trust in leaders and comrades are strong protections against becoming a stress casualty.

Conversely, poor preventive medicine discipline often implies poor stress control. Inadequate pre-

ventive medicine measures suggest inadequate unit training or ignorant, uncaring or preoccupied (perhaps overstressed) leaders, buddies, and veterans. Those factors are predictive of stress casualties, as well as of diseases and nonbattle injuries.[5] Low-grade illnesses and injuries further sap energy and self confidence, leading to stress, disease, and nonbattle injury casualties. The remaining unit members see their comrades evacuated and replaced by strangers who are at higher risk from stress, and demoralization can build on demoralization.

Physical threats identified in the medical threat assessment are also stress threats. Unfamiliar harsh climates or terrain, dangerous fauna or flora, and warnings of exotic diseases cause stress and anxiety unless service members are confident in their protective measures. The threats posed by nuclear, biological, and chemical warfare agents can produce current and long-term stress, as illustrated by the concerns about illnesses in veterans of the Persian Gulf War.[6] Rumors about the protective measures can arouse fears of side effects such as impotence, sterility, genetic damage, and autoimmune diseases, among other disabilities. Anthrax immunization and prophylactic and pretreatment medications, such as anti-malarials or pyridostigmine for nerve agent, are two examples of such fears from the Persian Gulf War. These fears can cause high-risk behaviors, such as noncompliance with the protective measures. Service members have even accepted court martial or resigned from the service rather than take required anthrax vaccinations.[7–9]

The stress threat can increase the preventive medicine threat. Mission tempo, arousal, and anxiety decrease sleep and cause fatigue. Sleep debt and fatigue disturb immune system function, so susceptibility to illnesses increases.[10] Distraction or fatigue causes decreased attention to safety, hygiene, and other self care, increasing the risk of disease and nonbattle injury. This process can result in an "evacuation syndrome," as overstressed service members unconsciously commit the same negligence that they saw got others "honorably evacuated" from greater danger.[11] The extreme version is deliberate, self-inflicted illness or injury, a form of malingering.

Combat stress or boredom stress can result in high-risk behaviors such as substance abuse, fighting, and unsafe sexual fraternization, which also contribute to preventable diseases and injuries.[1,11] Unless preventive actions are taken at the early signs, these behaviors can escalate quickly to misconduct stress behaviors that demand disciplinary action for breaches of military regulation or criminal acts. Post-traumatic and postdeployment stress can continue this negative interaction long after the operation is finished and contribute to medical as well as psychiatric symptoms and diagnoses.

THE PSYCHOLOGICAL RESPONSE TO THE COMBAT ENVIRONMENT

The combat environment is associated with a variety of psychological stresses. Some of the psychological stressors inherent in the physical and social aspects of the combat environment are listed in Exhibit 16-1.

Anxiety, anger, fear, guilt, envy, suspiciousness, and frustration are all normal emotional reactions. In the average environment, the higher-functioning individual is expected to cope with feelings without pathological responses. In the combat environment, however, even higher-functioning people may fail to cope and manifest adjustment disorders with exaggerated emotional responses, instability, rage outbursts, withdrawal, isolation, impulsive behavior, alcohol and substance abuse, or poor judgment. On the clinical level, service members may exhibit anxiety and depressive conversion reactions, dissociative reactions, acute stress reactions, subsequent post-traumatic stress disorders, and even brief reactive psychoses. The real task, then, of any stress control effort is to attempt to prepare individuals and commands to cope with the psychological environment without debilitating psychological responses.

EXHIBIT 16-1

PSYCHOLOGICAL STRESSORS INHERENT IN THE COMBAT ENVIRONMENT

Separation from familiar psychological support systems

Isolation from information

Mistrust of the information received from higher authority

Fear of physical hazards and enemy action

Fear of physical mutilation or death

Fear of the loss of emotionally close peers

Fear of failure and loss of self-esteem

Fear of social embarrassment and of loss of community status

Anger and envy toward those seen as better off

Anger toward those seen as failing to give needed support

Anger over physical discomfort or privation

Anger over perceptions that one is being used or manipulated

Anger toward the enemy and their real or seen atrocities

Anger over the death or injuries of peers

Anger over the "rules" and their seen unfairness

Guilt over leaving dependents without support

Guilt over the injuries or death of peers

Guilt over real or imagined failure to accomplish a mission

STRESS, ANXIETY, AND FEAR

Some of the earliest literature in psychology and psychiatry attempted to develop a scientific picture of anxiety. One theory of anxiety sees anxiety developing in stages and posits that as individuals grow and develop, they are able to perceive more complex threats to their emotional and physical well-being.[12] A closer look at the tenets of this theory may be helpful in understanding CSC.

The first anxiety is postulated to occur in infants and is one of being or not being. The second level of anxiety is separation anxiety. The feeling of being lost or completely alone can produce an intense and uncomfortable feeling of anxiety in most people. The theory describes children as learning to cope with separation anxiety by identifying and incorporating a psychological picture of the parent into their own makeup. Children also learn to take their security with them symbolically and to maintain contact at a distance. Knowledge of these mechanisms can be used in a program of prevention.

The next level of anxiety concerns being in control of self. This level is related to the anxiety we all experience over failure to control our own bodily functions, such as excretion. This anxiety, as we get older, evolves into anxiety over being able to control the immediate environment in terms of personal security. Mastery of this anxiety as a child is by achieving physical control of one's own body, by growing competence to provide for one's own basic needs, and by learning to communicate basic needs effectively to an immediate care giver. In later life, the need to master this anxiety may be expressed symbolically. The emphasis Marines place on never being without their rifles may be a symbolic way of their feeling safe and in control.

Anxiety about physical injury or mutilation and its social consequences is the next level. Mastery of this anxiety is by identification with individuals and institutions that are seen as powerful and invulnerable. The connection to the efforts of all services to promote identification with the institution, such as uniforms and flags, is obvious. Less obvious is the use of special unit identifiers and uniform items to promote a feeling of invulnerability to injury in the individual.

Higher levels of anxiety have been described,[13] such as fear of loss of personal competence in a higher skill or anxiety over social embarrassment or loss of status. Most institutions use these anxieties to maintain cooperation and productivity in the organization. These are the anxieties mastered by getting certifications or good grades or by earning special recognition, awards, or promotions. In real life, all of these psychological mechanisms operate simultaneously and may frequently reinforce each other.

Fear is anxiety with the threat of immediacy. Fear is accompanied by a psychological press to action. Fear is a healthy protective emotion when individuals possess the equipment, competence, and freedom of action that allows them to cope effectively with the immediate threat. When individuals lack or are deprived of the capacity or option to protect themselves, they usually exhibit desperate or destructive behavior or pathological withdrawal. It is important for the command to recognize that pathological reactions to fear are more of a failure of the organization to prepare the individual than a characteristic of the individual.

Shame is a fear of loss of love. This emotion is more complex than anxiety or fear and represents an incorporation psychologically of a parent figure who represents love and approval to the individual. Higher-functioning social organizations and individuals operate on this level most of the time. The resulting positive emotions are pride and self-esteem.

Guilt is a fear of punishment. Internalized, this may become a punitive, self-destructive emotion leading to self-destructive actions. Guilt can lead to evasive and deceptive behavior and is often expressed by anger. Organizations that use punishment as a means control are often faced with the constant acting-out of angry, aggressive behavior. The preoccupation of an individual or an organization with blame or punishment can bring paralysis as the organization becomes focused on the past and individuals become defensive, fearing being the scapegoat. An example of the destructive effects of an organizational system based on punishment is the "better weasel" principle: in organizations that use negative reinforcement, those individuals most adroit at avoiding punishment—the better weasels—will rise to the top of the hierarchy.

COPING WITH EMOTION

From an early age, individuals learn psychological mechanisms that help them cope with emotions.[12] Some of the earliest and most primitive are denial, projection, and incorporation. Higher-level coping involves identification, sublimation, rationalization, and intellectualization. The highest level of coping is adaptation. All of these mechanisms may be used simultaneously by an individual and, with some modification, may describe the coping of an organization. An understanding of these mechanisms underpins the techniques of preventing maladaption to stress.

Denial may be understood by thinking of infants turning away from food that they do not want to eat even though the food meets their nutritional needs. Psychologically, denial means turning away from perceptions and thoughts that are unpalatable, even if the individual needs to know the truth (eg, the alcoholic who denies that he or she has a problem). Projection may be understood as "the devil made me do it." This blaming of others is a very common defense. In organizations where projection is used by the majority of individuals, scapegoatism, with its associated paranoia and suspiciousness, is common. Identification is usually a healthy way to adapt, but it can be a problem when someone identifies with a negative role model. Incorporation is an uncritical identification with an individual or group—the individual swallows the "whole party line." Incorporation can be the basis for cults. Some of the worst atrocities of warfare have been committed by individuals who incorpo-

rated uncritically a group identity. Examples include the Japanese Army in the rape of Nanking (1937 to 1938), German SS and Wehrmacht units in the Soviet Union in World War II, and Serbs, Croats, and Muslims engaged in ethnic cleansing in the Balkans before World War II and in the 1990s.

The higher levels of coping include rationalization and intellectualization. Rationalization involves convincing oneself that the threat is exaggerated or manageable without real evidence or study. That is, we tell ourselves what we want to hear. Intellectualization is a bolstering of our rationalizations with internal and often philosophical arguments. In organizations, these types of defenses can produce a dream-world atmosphere at headquarters, with no one willing to accept or cope with an unpalatable reality.

PATHOLOGICAL REACTIONS TO STRESS

The essence of stress prevention from a military standpoint is to keep individuals as functional as possible in the face of stress. When the individual

fails to cope with psychological stress, a number of pathological reactions can occur. They have in common some loss of functional efficiency. In the most

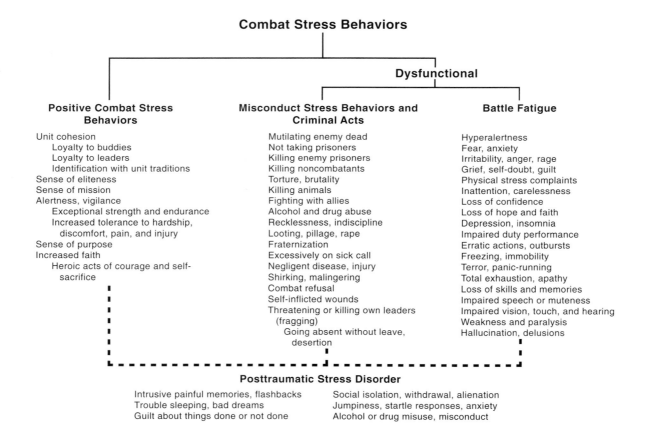

Fig. 16-1. Symptoms of combat stress behaviors.
Source: Department of the Army. *Leaders' Manual for Combat Stress Control.* Washington, DC: DA; 29 September 1994. Field Manual 22-51.

extreme cases, the individual is lost to duty entirely.

Figure 16-1 lists symptoms of battle or contingency fatigue, misconduct stress behaviors, and post-traumatic stress. The table also lists the positive combat stress behaviors that bring out heroic behavior and can protect service members (somewhat) against becoming stress casualties during battle. The positive stress behaviors do not protect against the misconduct stress behaviors unless leadership and unit identity make clear the standard and rigorously enforce it. No amount of combat stress can be allowed to justify or excuse criminal misconduct. The positive combat stress behaviors also do not in themselves confer immunity against post-traumatic stress. For example, death or mutilation of beloved comrades is an especially long-lasting and painful trauma. Immunization against stress requires special stress control actions, including debriefings, memorial services, justly awarding special recognition for valor, and long-term social validation of the value of the sacrifices.

Mild stress reactions include chronic feelings of anxiety with disturbances of sleep, impulsiveness, frequent startle reactions, and an increase in "neurotic" behavior, such as obsessiveness or compulsive rituals. Panic and freezing are severe reactions to anxiety. More complex reactions may occur with long-term stress. These reactions frequently result from mixtures of anxiety, anger, fear, guilt, and shame. They may include irritability, explosive rages, despondency, social isolation, excess drinking, and diverse psychophysiological reactions. Psychophysiological responses include appetite disturbances, headaches, upset stomach, irritable bowel, and insomnia or hypersomnia. Physical discomfort, fatigue, heat or cold, and physical loss of function (eg, overuse syndromes) exacerbate the stress and may be hard to distinguish from the effects of psychological stress. Prolonged and severe stress coupled with fatigue and the wear and tear of a harsh environment may produce in the individual the complex entity of acute combat/operational stress reaction.

PRIMARY PREVENTION

As with other aspects of preventive medicine, primary prevention is concerned with preventing the occurrence of disease or disability that may become evident either immediately or not until after weeks, months, or years. CSC primary prevention involves the effort to monitor, identify, modify, avoid, or reduce stressors before they cause dysfunction, just as preventive medicine seeks to do the same with pathogens before they cause disease, and build stress-coping skills within individuals.[3] Effective CSC starts with good mental health in garrison during peacetime.

One approach to primary prevention is to screen service members to identify those at high risk of becoming stress or psychiatric casualties, then either strengthen their resistance or remove them from danger. CSC personnel can provide advice regarding "immunizing" service members from the pathological dimensions of stress by progressive exposure to stressors in realistic training and measuring the effects of such efforts. They can also advise on how to promote unit cohesion and to provide education on stress management, stress control techniques, mental hygiene, and other protective issues. CSC personnel, especially the enlisted specialists, talk routinely with service members at squad and crew level, "taking the pulse of the unit" through informal or structured group interviews. Short questionnaire surveys can also be used. CSC personnel also facilitate or provide "preventive maintenance." This includes encouraging and mentoring small unit leaders to conduct their own

debriefings after any difficult or unsuccessful action. End-of-tour debriefings, which summarize, clarify, and give closure to the minor as well as major irritations and emotionally charged memories of the deployment, should be done at the team level before the redeployment home. Closure ceremonies, memorial services, and fair allocation of awards and decorations should be encouraged. Briefings and discussions that give realistic expectations of the common frictions of reunion with families and coworkers, and skills to cope with them, should also be encouraged and facilitated.

A mnemonic for primary prevention of stress reactions is "C4 times two," with the obvious reference to the primary combat casualty care course. This model is based on well-established principles but not on an empirical test—that remains for future research. The eight Cs are confidence and competence, communication and coordination, community and cooperation, and comfort and concern. The first word in these mnemonic phrases pertains to the individual and the second to the organization. The job of the preventive medicine officer or the mental health team is to teach these principles at both the individual and organizational level.

Confidence and Competence

First, individuals need to see their training as a means of developing their ability to survive and their confidence in themselves. Individuals should be instructed to take a personal interest in the training and be assertive about asking questions, as well as requesting clarification and demonstration. For this to be successful, the trainers need to be encouraged to develop a partnership with each student and to use consistent and skillful positive reinforcement. The trainer must demonstrate appropriate confidence and trust in the trainee and see the trainee's competence as a compliment to the trainer. The trainer becomes a role model and a nonpunitive parent figure, with whom the trainee identifies and from whom the trainee seeks approval. These are basic principles applied by flight instructors with great success. A challenge for preventive medicine and mental health is to apply these same principles in teaching medical and command personnel.

Communication and Coordination

Fundamental to building self-esteem and in bonding the individual to the goals of the group is feeling included and worth talking to. Communicating feelings and attitudes in an appropriate way is a skill that can be taught. People fail to communicate for many reasons, including lack of verbal facility, learned fear and anxiety, remembered embarrassment, and nonverbal or direct messages from an authority figure that suppress communication. While teaching communication may be perceived as effete sensitivity training, accident studies among air crews reveal that failure to communicate is a major "human factor" in aircraft accidents.[14] Commanders must realize that to get a group to act as a coordinated whole, two-way, effective communication is essential. For example, peers and commanders need to listen for clues that an individual is considering suicide. Studies have shown that up to 80% of individuals who kill themselves have given indications of their intent to peers or supervisors.[15]

Community and Cooperation

"Being in the same boat" and "misery loves company" are trite sayings, but they are also true. Each service member should be highly encouraged to be part of a group. Sports, religious services, and other opportunities to share interests foster community. Most military organizations do a good job of building community among service members, but the individual is frequently torn between loyalty to family and loyalty to the unit. The command should be encouraged to secure the cooperation and loyalty of the unit members' spouses. While intense family-like bonds in a unit can be troublesome, these same feelings can be the best protection against psychological deterioration in a stressful situation, whether in combat or in garrison.

Comfort and Concern

Comfort is not considered a major military virtue; however, taking care of oneself is very important in a combat environment. The length of time that an individual can remain effective partly depends on the level of comfort that can be achieved in the combat environment. Psychologically, a child learns early to trust the people who are concerned for his or her comfort. Lack of concern for comfort is frequently one of the most deeply felt resentments. Furthermore, learning to take care of oneself and learning to suffer as little as possible in objectively difficult circumstances is a source of pride and self-esteem. The commander who shows a genuine concern for the comfort of the service members and who shares the necessary discomforts will be able to ask for and receive a greater level of sacrifice in the face of danger.

Working With Units

Primary prevention involves incorporating the "C4 times two" principle into the everyday fabric and function of the unit. The essence of primary prevention is behavioral and attitudinal changes on the part of a large number of individuals. How to accomplish these changes is neither obvious nor easy. One strategy is to target specific groups. In a division, groups to be targeted ought be the general staff, senior staff NCOs, unit staff, unit commanders down to company level, and division medical personnel. The most difficult part is developing credibility with these groups. Prevention is often ignored or neglected because it is difficult to get busy people's attention when talking about problems that have not yet occurred. Leaders are often preoccupied with current problems and will practice denial if they cannot see that a problem is close at hand. Breaking through that denial is difficult enough with such preventive problems as food and water sanitation or infectious disease prevention, but it is even more difficult with prevention of stress casualties and psychiatric casualties. This is why the force health protection team that combines personnel from mental health and preventive medicine must invest a large amount of time laying the groundwork for their consultation. They must sell themselves and their function to the units they serve. This groundwork involves three steps. The team must first have a deep and thorough understanding of the unit they serve. In the second step, the team must develop a sense of membership and identity with that unit. The third and last step is doing the actual force health protection work. When the first two steps are completed, the team will be able to deliver their force health protection message in a way that the unit can hear, understand, and implement.

The First Step (Understanding the Unit)

The first task of clearly understanding the type of unit the team serves goes far beyond mere knowledge of the mission, table of organization, standard operating procedures, and operating functions of the unit. It involves knowledge and respect for the history, traditions, customs, and personality of the unit. The team must seek a depth of understanding of the unit that enables them to communicate and gain cooperation easily. It has been the experience of medical officers and NCOs involved in prevention that their credibility and hence effectiveness has depended on spending time in the field with the various units. Further, they had to be seen as competent in the field as far as military skills were concerned. Acquiring field competence involves more than going to a week-long school; it involves a dedication to pursue and practice these skills on a daily basis. It also involves a personal commitment to physical fitness, beyond that involved in merely passing the semiannual physical fitness test.

The Second Step (Identifying With the Unit)

An attitude of participation and membership in the unit is key for those providing mental health services. The force health protection team must become a part of the unit, and the unit should think of the team members as "one of us." If this does not happen, the force health protection team finds itself on the outside, resented by the command as yet another advisor telling them how they should do their job. The force health protection team must be seen as an ally, not as enemy or an irrelevant entity making demands from on high.

In developing this sense of understanding and membership, there is one vital consideration to be kept in mind. The underlying principle that allows a unit to function in combat is trust. Members of a unit must trust one another with their lives. If a force health protection team is to work effectively with a unit, then they too must earn the trust of that unit and the trust of the commander. Trust and credibility are established as the team works to develop and implement a comprehensive preventive mental health plan for the unit.

The Third Step (Doing the Work)

In actually providing force health protection services, the team must convince the various commanders to allot training time to mental health promotion in an already very crowded training schedule. To get this time, the force health protection personnel must prove their worth and the worth of the training to the various commanders. One way to do this is to make themselves available to commanders for consultation on specific problems. For the mental health members of the team, usually this will involve seeing suicidal individuals or helping with individuals who have mental health or family problems. These cases can provide opportunities to suggest training staff and subordinate commanders in prevention, as well as to increase rapport between team members and the unit. The team should develop information handouts that explain the concepts of prevention to unit leaders and presentations (ie, "road shows") complete with audiovisual aids and handouts that can be presented with little notice. Above all, the team must be alert for opportunities to reach out to help the unit.

There is a strategy to using educational opportunities as a way of gradually approaching a higher level of trust and influence in the unit. Giving a class is not merely an opportunity to present the preventive medicine and stress control information. It is an opportunity to become known, to be seen as a useful resource, and to foster the process of integration of the team into the unit. Giving stand-alone, unintegrated classes is not adequate. To be effective, the team must develop a specific and comprehensive preventive plan tailored to the needs of the unit they serve. The necessity for this can be seen in the frustration some military leaders have experienced in attempting to grapple with suicide prevention, alcohol abuse, and other problems—difficult mental health and social problems that have plagued US society for years. Commanders have attempted to solve these problems by attacking them with the same vigor they would attack an enemy on the battlefield, but they have been frustrated by the vague and ethereal nature of these issues, lack of measurable progress, and continued worsening of the problems despite their best efforts. The Marine Corps has developed programs to address these sorts of problems.[16] Exhibit 16-2 is a more detailed example of how one such primary prevention program developed and how it addressed mental health problems to encourage lifestyle changes and practice true primary prevention in the areas of nicotine addiction, nutrition, alcohol abuse, and suicide prevention.

EXHIBIT 16-2

AN EXAMPLE OF A MARINE CORPS PRIMARY PREVENTION PROGRAM

The development of a comprehensive preventive mental health program for the First Marine Division will be used as an example. The commanding general of the division was highly receptive to preventive mental health measures in general and having his division psychiatrist focused on prevention in particular because of the problem all Marine commands in southern California were having with suicides. The commander's support was crucial in establishing the program.

The program developed on two fronts: having the division psychiatrist become more fully integrated into the daily lives of the units and developing teams of chaplains and peer Marines led by the psychiatrist to provide stress management education and a network for support and referral.

The division psychiatrist became a "circuit rider," spending most of his time out at the units introducing himself to the commanders and offering to consult on individual cases and to provide lectures on appropriate topics at maintenance stand-down periods. He went out to the field with units and provided quick, convenient care for Marines. Being in the field also gave the psychiatrist the opportunity to educate the leaders. He became their unit psychiatrist, and they confided in him with their difficult issues.

One issue clearly surfaced as a major concern to many leaders—the problem of manipulative suicidal ideation. No other problem caused more consternation, frustration, and bad feeling between the commands, patients, and mental health professionals. After extensive study and trial and error, the division psychiatrist developed an education strategy for leaders. A presentation on personality development and personality disorders was developed for senior NCOs and officers. This lecture acknowledged the difficulties and frustrations leaders experienced in having Marines with personality disorders and offered specific, practical tips on how to handle their behavior. It became a very popular lecture and became a regular part of the 1st Sergeant's Course. Another presentation, this one targeted at NCOs, compared mental fitness with physical fitness and so correlated mental health with something comfortable and familiar to Marines.

Chaplains had been the de facto mental health representatives for each unit, but under this program chaplains became members of teams that included the division psychiatrist and peer Marines trained in critical event debriefing, peer counseling, and stress management. This trained peer is able to get past the "image armor" of Marines and get them to talk about a stressful incident or hear a presentation on stress management. A group of trained peers took on the task of educating the rank and file and was much more effective than those who had traditionally been assigned that task, the psychiatrist and the unit chaplain.

As this new approach was brought to bear on the problem of suicides, the concept of suicide prevention was changed from crisis intervention referral to stress management and stress prevention. Large-scale suicide prevention lectures were no longer given. Instead, trained peers gave presentations designed to improve coping skills in small unit classes with homogeneous groups. NCOs were targeted because they have the most influence over junior Marines. Marines who experienced this new approach felt that it was much more useful than the large classes. They felt free to discuss their concerns regarding mental health prevention issues in a more supportive and open atmosphere, thus decreasing the stigma associated with mental health issues. Psychiatric preventive mental health was made relevant and palatable to the Marines through the concept of comprehensive stress management. This approach also had the advantage of assuming and encouraging health rather than focusing on treating disease.

—Dr. Hammer

SECONDARY PREVENTION

To fulfill the second priority of CSC—secondary prevention—CSC personnel train leaders, chaplains, and medical personnel to make very early identification of dysfunctional stress reactions in individuals and organizations. Those front-line resources, supported by CSC personnel (when available), intervene at the duty site and treat the overstressed service member as close to the unit as feasible to maximize rapid return to duty. This far-forward intervention limits contagion of stress symptoms.

A very useful guide for preventive mental health surveillance of individuals presenting for primary care is contained in the report of the US Preventive Services Task Forces.[17] Teaching primary care health providers to diagnose and do basic early interventions is a major challenge for preventive medicine.

Surveillance

Preventive medicine, because of its roots in infectious disease, can provide credibility for the mental health providers when they interact with primary health care providers. Preventive medicine officers can also lend the mental health components support through surveillance and the presentation of epidemiologic data to commanders. One example would be seeing that the major commanders and health care providers are aware of the periodic DoD Survey of Health-Related Behaviors Among Military Personnel.[18] This regular report can dramatically show how preventable mental health problems and substance abuse saps manpower and efficiency from the force. Inclusion of alcohol screening data and behavioral incidents in the regular ongoing surveillance program can further support preventive mental health efforts by keeping primary care providers and commanders constantly aware of these losses.

Department of Defense Directive 6490.5, *Combat Stress Control Programs*, directs that the services shall collect combat (and operational) stress casualty rates separate from the neuropsychiatry and disease and nonbattle injury rates.[4] The two categories of Combat/Operation Stress Reactions and Psychiatric Mental Disorders are now included on the Joint Weekly DNBI Report.[19]

Specific Populations and Problems

The presence of women in an expanding range of military roles presents a new and challenging problem in the mental health area. Each service's medical department needs to be sensitive to women presenting with stress or post-traumatic stress disorder symptoms masked as somatic complaints. Many of these individuals may need specialized psychological treatment not available in a deployment environment. With sensitivity and support, though, they can complete a deployment successfully before receiving more definitive treatment.

Sexually transmitted diseases have been seen traditionally as preventive medicine problems, with emphasis on treatment and prevention. On deployment, the perception of what is acceptable behavior may be distorted. Further, alcohol and peer pressure may compromise individuals' expectations of themselves. Dangerous or injudicious sexual behavior involving commercial sex workers, pressure on female peers for sex, and even unusual or deviant sexual behavior may result. The medical departments should help the commands in dealing with these behavior problems to prevent the adverse consequences. This should involve a structured counseling program. Every individual should be educated regarding appropriate and safe sexual behavior. The occurrence of an STD should trigger a specific and documentable intervention modeled after the evaluation of an alcohol incident. (In many cases it will also be an alcohol incident.) Here again the attitude of commanders and the cooperation between mental health teams and preventive medicine assets is very important.

A few individuals will develop serious mental illness during the course of any deployment. These individuals should be identified and referred for psychiatric care. Many of these individuals can be treated as outpatients and can continue with their duties, depending on the operational situation. Some will, of course, be unfit and require evacuation, hospitalization, and administrative action to release them from service.

TERTIARY PREVENTION

The third priority of CSC is tertiary prevention or rehabilitation of manifest problems to prevent worsening and chronic disability. Established cases are provided with aggressive treatment to prevent chronic disability. This treatment is best provided at successive echelons of care in the combat zone (and communications zone, when present), before evacuation to the United States. This has the lowest priority of CSC activities, however, and may often be deferred until patients arrive at US facilities.

COORDINATING PREVENTIVE MEDICINE AND COMBAT STRESS CONTROL EFFORTS

Preventive medicine detachments and teams and CSC detachments and teams share similar territories and have common operational problems. Both CSC and preventive medicine personnel serve as advisers, consultants, and assistants to the chain of command. It is the commanders who have primary responsibility for controlling stress and for preventive medicine measures; many of preventive medicine's and CSC's recommendations are basic tenets of good leadership. Leaders under stress must focus on their primary operational mission, sometimes to the unintentional detriment of preventive medicine or CSC concerns, so the personnel from these areas serve as the system's institutional memory or "conscience."

Preventive medicine and CSC units share many characteristics. Both are small, dispersed, mobile teams that are dependent on their changing host units for logistical and administrative support. Both need to travel to visit units, inspect and survey, and give constructive feedback to commanders. They may both be put at risk by their movement and must provide their own security. Preventive medicine and CSC teams need operational intelligence about what is going to happen. Both need data about the occurrence of specific types of casualties, and both contribute input to statistical databases.

One lesson learned from operations in the Persian Gulf, Somalia, Haiti, and Bosnia is that preventive medicine and CSC should work closely with each other. (In Somalia, preventive medicine and CSC personnel were greeted with "Here comes the Bugs and Hugs team.") Personnel from the two disciplines can watch for each others' indicators and share observations of relevance. They should cross-train in each other's basic data collection techniques or temporarily cross-attach personnel between teams, so one team can serve both functions on a single site visit. They can cover for each other's interests at daily staff meetings when it is contrary to the mission for both small teams to have a representative present.

BRIEF REVIEW OF EACH SERVICE'S COMBAT STRESS CONTROL ORGANIZATION

Military organization is always a moving target, but it is useful to examine the CSC assets of each service, how they are deployed, and how they interact with their preventive medicine colleagues. The numbers and distributions of specialists related here were current as of 2000.

US Army

The US Army Medical Department's organizational and operational concept for CSC, like that for preventive medicine, requires basic coverage of all units that may be at risk, plus flexibility to concentrate additional resources to deal with shifting workloads and unpredictable eruptions. The first line of defense to assist commanders with basic force medical protection from combat and operational stress is the team of a behavioral science officer and an enlisted specialist, with a HMMWV (high mobility, multi-wheeled vehicle), in each combat maneuver brigade. The officer can be either a clinical psychologist or a social worker. This team should work out of the medical company, throughout the brigade support area, and forward to units in relatively safe locations; it interacts with all the unit leaders, chaplains, and medical teams. Unlike the preventive medicine sergeant at the brigade echelon, this Mental Health Section provides direct clinical evaluation and care to those soldiers who need it, preferably while they are still in their units. A similar two-person officer and enlisted team may be available at the area support medical companies in the corps and communications zone. At the division support medical company in the division rear (and in the area support medical battalion headquarters further to the rear), the officer in the Mental Health Section is a psychiatrist. The psychiatrist provides additional diagnostic and treatment capabilities and technical supervision for the brigade mental health teams and general medical personnel throughout the division.

The additional flexibility required by the CSC concept is provided by CSC teams from medical CSC detachments or a medical CSC company allocated to the corps or the echelon above corps. One CSC detachment is normally allocated per division. These units provide CSC Preventive Teams, which come forward as far as the maneuver brigades, preferably before combat commences, to augment the mental health sections. The preventive teams have a social worker and a psychiatrist (or psychologist), two enlisted specialists, and HMMWV. The CSC Restoration/Fitness Team has a psychiatric clinical nurse specialist, a psychologist (or psychiatrist), an occupational therapist, five behavioral science specialists and two occupational therapist NCOs, and two vehicles. They bring tents, cots, and equipment to hold up to 50 stress casualties. They normally reinforce the division support medical company or an area support medical company but can send personnel further forward, especially to support units undergoing reconstitution after heavy attrition. Task-organized elements of the company or detachment also can collocate with combat support hospitals to provide tertiary prevention treatment (called "reconditioning") for stress casualties who do not return to duty within 3 days. With an additional 1 to 2 weeks of treatment outside of hospitals, many of these soldiers may return to duty in the theater rather than be evacuated to the United States.

The Army's medical headquarters, which provides command control in the corps, has mental health staff officers and NCOs to monitor the daily reports of the CSC units, as well as the general medical and preventive medicine surveillance statistics. They coordinate the redistribution of the mobile CSC teams to cover the shifting workload. Operational Stress Assessment Teams deployed from the Walter Reed Army Institute of Research, Silver Spring, Md, also may deploy into the theater to conduct questionnaire and interview surveys to assess stressors and stress for the Department of Army and the local commander. It is part of the CSC concept to strengthen the linkage between the Operational Stress Assessment Teams, the corps medical commands, the organic Mental Health Sections, and mobile CSC unit teams. Further development of automated data processing and the Theater Medical Information Program will greatly enhance capabilities for getting trends in stressors and stress and providing commanders with useful and timely recommendations on how to correct the problems.

The concept of having behavioral health expertise organic to the maneuver brigades, to serve as sensors, mentors, first responders, and receptor sites for reinforcing mobile CSC teams, is being incorporated into Army doctrine. The future operational concept for force health protection may integrate combat stress control, preventive medicine, veterinary teams, an area medical laboratory, epidemiology, and operational stress assessment teams under a single Medical Force Protection headquarters in the corps, both in garrison and on deployment.

US Navy

The US Navy deploys Special Psychiatric Rapid Intervention teams (SPRINT) from shore hospitals to assist command, survivors, and families after shipboard accidents, air crashes, and other highly

traumatic events. Personnel are chosen for each specific mission from a roster of psychiatrists, psychiatric nurses, other mental health officers and technicians, and chaplains. They are not equipped to live and operate in the field environment. The neuropsychiatric service personnel aboard a hospital ship or in a Fleet Hospital ashore can function in the preventive mode; during the Persian Gulf War, one of the hospital ships sent a SPRINT to the amphibious assault ship *Iwo Jima* following a fatal boiler explosion. Recently, a clinical psychologist has been deployed on 6-month sea duty aboard the air craft carrier in some large task forces, to work primarily in preventive activities.[20]

US Marine Corps

Marine Corps medical support is provided by the Navy. Marine divisions have a division psychiatrist and psychiatric technician in the division surgeon section of the headquarters. The two surgical support companies of the medical battalion in the division's Force Service Support Group each have had a clinical psychologist assigned on mobilization. The Marine Corps has requested that the Navy provide a Combat Stress Platoon to the medical battalion. This could allocate one psychiatrist, two psychologists, and three psychiatric technicians to each "surgical company," which replaces the collection and clearing company in support of each brigade. However, these billets are not filled before deployment, and their future is uncertain.

US Air Force

The Air Force 50-bed Air Transportable Hospital included a Combat Stress Unit of up to two officers and two enlisted personnel. These teams deployed with their hospitals to Saudi airfields during the Persian Gulf War and to several humanitarian assistance missions. The Air Force is moving toward the concept of the Expeditionary Air Force, which will replace the fixed structure of the old hospitals with a modular design (often compared to Lego blocks). This will allow the assembly of a flexible medical support tailored to the specific situation. Two types of modular stress control teams have been organized and trained and are available from fixed Air Force hospitals for rapid deployment to augment any type of field medical facility, including a mobile air staging facility or an Army CSC element. The Mental Health Rapid Response Team consists of a clinical psychologist, a social work officer, and an enlisted technician; they have only light equipment and provide preventive interventions and outpatient counseling. The Mental Health Augmentation Team has a psychiatrist, three psychiatric nurses, and two technicians. It deploys with a pallet of tents, cots, and supplies to join a Mental Health Rapid Response Team and provide a holding treatment facility, as well as more preventive assets. In addition to these teams, which are designed for deployments of up to 90 days, Air Force medical facilities also maintain Critical Incident Stress Management Teams of mental health personnel and chaplains who are on call to provide preventive interventions following crashes or other disasters.

SUMMARY

The military operations of the United States over the next 20 years cannot be predicted with great precision, but it is safe to predict that they will usually be joint operations under the Combined Combatant Commands. They are likely to continue to include training exercises with our coalition allies, humanitarian assistance and disaster relief, peace support and peace enforcement, and other stability operations but may escalate to major theater wars that may involve weapons of mass destruction. There is also the mission of federal military support to US civilian authorities in the event or threat of disaster or terrorist attack with chemical, biological, or radiation agents. While some of these diverse military operations may allow ample planning time, and even become routine, others will be contingency operations requiring haste and perhaps secrecy in the planning. Most will be conducted under the scrutiny of the worldwide media and commented on over the Internet. American and world society will continue to hold the US military to a very high standards for protecting its own personnel and other innocent people involved in the operation against both immediate and long-term harm from toxic exposures, diseases and other injuries, and the consequences of harmful psychological stress. The consequences of stress will include acute performance breakdown and misconduct stress behaviors, as well as post-traumatic stress disorder and undiagnosed chronic physical syndromes. To meet the challenge across this broad continuum of operations and problems and to do so efficiently in a resource-constrained situation, preventive medicine and CSC must forge a close, working alliance.

REFERENCES

1. Department of the Army. *Leaders' Manual for Combat Stress Control*. Washington, DC: DA; 29 September 1994. Field Manual 22-51.

2. Department of the Army. *Combat Stress Control in a Theater of Operations: Tactics, Techniques, Procedures*. Washington, DC: DA; 29 September 1994. Field Manual 8-51.

3. Department of the Army. *Planning for Health Service Support*. Washington, DC: DA; 9 September 1994. Field Manual 8-55.

4. Department of the Army. *Combat Stress Control (CSC) Programs*. Washington, DC: DA; 23 February 1999. Department of Defense Directive 6490.5.

5. Manning FJ. Morale and cohesion in military psychiatry. *Military Psychiatry: Preparing in Peace for War*. In: *Textbook of Military Medicine*. Washington, DC: Office of the Surgeon General and the Borden Institute; 1994.

6. Stokes JW, Banderet LE. Psychological aspects of chemical defense and warfare. *Mil Psychiatry*. 1997;9:395–415.

7. Airman is ousted as rebellion against anthrax vaccine grows. *New York Times*. March 11, 1999. National Desk Section.

8. Marine convicted in anthrax-shot case. *New York Times*. June 20, 1999. National Desk Section.

9. Funk D. Some continue to balk at anthrax shot. *Army Times*. February 22, 1999.

10. Khansari DN, Murgo AJ, Faith RE. Effects of stress on the immune system. *Immunol Today*. 1990;11:170–175.

11. Jones FD, Sparacino LR, Wilcox VL, Rothberg JM, Stokes IW, eds. *War Psychiatry*. Part 1. In: *Textbook of Military Medicine*. Washington, DC: Office of The Surgeon General, US Dept of the Army, and Borden Institute; 1995.

12. Freud A. Baines C, trans. *The Ego and the Mechanisms of Defense*. London: Hogarth Press; 1968.

13. Erickson E. *Childhood and Society*. New York: Norton; 1950.

14. Ciavarelli A. *Human Factors*. Monterey, Calif: School of Aviation Safety, Naval Postgraduate School; 1995. Available at http://web.nps.navy.mil/~avsafety/courses/

15. Schneidman ES. A conspectus of the suicidal scenario. In: Maris RW, ed. *Assessment and Prediction of Suicide*. New York: Guilford Publications; 1992.

16. US Marine Corps. *US Marine Corps Semper Fit Program Manual*. USMC: 2000. MCO P1700.29.

17. US Preventive Services Task Force. *Guide to Clinical Preventive Services*. 2nd ed. Baltimore: Williams & Wilkins; 1996.

18. Bray RM, Froutil LA, Wheeles SC, et al. *Department of Defense Survey of Health Related Behaviors Among Military Personnel*. Research Triangle Park, NC: Research Triangle Institute; 1995.

19. Joint Chiefs of Staff. *Deployment Health Surveillance and Readiness*. Washington, DC: JCS; 4 Dec 1998. Memorandum.

20. Paige-Dobson B. Personal communication, 1997.

Chapter 17

NUTRITIONAL CONSIDERATIONS FOR MILITARY DEPLOYMENT

PATRICIA A. DEUSTER, PhD, MPH; and ANITA SINGH, PhD, RD

P.A. Deuster; Human Performance Laboratory, Department of Military and Emergency Medicine, Uniformed Services University of the Health Sciences, 4301 Jones Bridge Road, Bethesda, MD 20814

A. Singh; Food and Nutrition Service, US Department of Agriculture, 3101 Park Center Drive, Alexandria, VA 22302; formerly, Human Performance Laboratory, Department of Military and Emergency Medicine, Uniformed Services University of the Health Sciences, 4301 Jones Bridge Road, Bethesda, MD 20814

INTRODUCTION

Deployment of military personnel, either for armed conflict or humanitarian assistance operations, inevitably requires large numbers of people to be fed. Military operations, often in hostile environments, combine periods of strenuous physical activity with periods of minimal activity or isolation. Such alternations in rest and activity impose perturbations in the body's homeostasis, with particular strains on the circulatory, respiratory, metabolic, and hormonal systems.[1] Thus, nutritional considerations for service members during deployment are complex and require awareness of environmental issues, as well as knowledge of physical demands.[2] Nutritional issues of particular importance in extreme environments include energy balance, hydration status, substrate utilization, and micronutrient needs. If these nutritional issues are not considered, fatigue may ensue, and both physical and cognitive performance may become limiting.

Although the importance of nutrition and dietary patterns in sustaining physical and cognitive performance has been recognized for many centuries, only in recent years have investigators attempted to document the dietary interventions that are most effective. Initial investigations focused on dietary manipulations for sustaining physical activity under thermoneutral environments; more recently, interactions between nutrition and physical activity under various environmental extremes have been considered. This chapter will first provide a brief overview of the physiological adaptations to physical activity, followed by a discussion of nutritional considerations for military operations. Specific nutritional issues of military operations under various environmental conditions, including heat and cold, and during acute exposure to altitude will be presented. Finally, military rations and what types of rations are available for various military operations are discussed.

PHYSIOLOGICAL RESPONSES TO PHYSICAL ACTIVITY

When physical activity is of low intensity and short duration, the strain on various physiological systems may be minimal, but when physical activity is prolonged or sustained, the strains are more pronounced and adaptations become more apparent. With both extended submaximal and extended high-intensity resistive activities, strains on the circulatory, respiratory, and energy balance systems are paramount. During the early phase of submaximal, steady-state activity, transient strains on oxygen delivery stress oxygen balance. Until the circulatory system adapts and the flow of substrate increases, anaerobic glycolysis is the initial system that provides energy. As soon as fuel and oxygen delivery capabilities respond, however, the individual adapts to the strain, and metabolic substrates are delivered aerobically to the working muscle. In contrast, when the activity is anaerobic, such as during heavy lifting activities, strains on the circulatory, respiratory, and energy balance systems may be sig-

nificant. Such activities are of extremely short duration, and adaptations are limited.

In all environments, maintenance of blood glucose within a physiologic range, of adequate carbohydrate stores in the form of muscle and liver glycogen, and of plasma volume are essential. For example, if troops have been marching for 2 to 3 hours without a carbohydrate source, blood glucose levels will typically fall and fatigue will ensue.[3–5] Moreover, both prolonged marches and moving heavy gear for extended periods can result in significant decreases in muscle glycogen,[6] an indication of diminishing energy stores. Thus, dietary measures that strive to maximize glycogen stores in preparation for physically demanding tasks will reduce strains on energy metabolism. Similarly, drinking fluids at regular intervals during exercise will minimize strain on the circulatory system and help maintain plasma volume.

NUTRITIONAL CONSIDERATIONS FOR MILITARY OPERATIONS

The stress of deployment, in particular during prolonged marching, multiple shorter bouts of activity, and extreme thermal conditions, can impose significant demands on the fluid balance and energy stores of service members. Commencing any type of military operation in a compromised nutritional status, such as with inadequate glycogen stores or having failed to restore energy or replace

fluids lost during previous operations, can affect how the body adapts to strains on the system. Unless service members are adequately nourished, physiological sequelae (eg, hypoglycemia, hypovolemia, dehydration, glycogen depletion, hyponatremia) and performance decrements can ensue.[7–10] For sustained operations in which physical effort is low (< 50% of $\dot{V}O_2max$) to moderate (50% to 70% of $\dot{V}O_2max$), hypoglycemia, hypovolemia, and dehydration are of the greatest concern. The nutrients of greatest importance for maintaining hydration status and energy balance include water, electrolytes, and the energy-providing nutrients: carbohydrate (CHO), fatty acids, and protein.

Hydration Status

Water is considered the most essential nutrient, and when hydration status becomes compromised, decrements in cognitive and physical performance are inevitable (Figure 17-1). Fluid within cells and tissues maintains plasma volume and serves as the medium wherein metabolic reactions proceed; given that physical exertion and cold exposure can increase metabolic activity 5- to 20-fold, fluid requirements under such conditions can be substantial.

Hydration status should be a primary consideration during exercise of all types. Assessing hydration status is best accomplished by observing urine color and monitoring body weight, which should be 0.5 to 1.5 kg higher than usual. Clear to light urine suggests a well-hydrated state, while dark or odorous urine suggests a degree of dehydration unless vitamin B supplements are being taken.[11] Frequency of urination can also be used as an indicator of hydration status.

The major determinant of fluid loss during physically demanding tasks is sweat rate; the amount of sweat lost depends on ambient temperature, radiant load, air velocity, clothing, exercise intensity, and physical conditioning. Many studies demonstrate marked variability in sweat rates and emphasize the importance of exercise intensity in determining the volume of sweat lost.[12] Figure 17-2 provides an approximation of sweat rates in liters per hour; these estimates can serve as guidelines for amounts of fluid to drink during and after exercise. If sweat and urine losses are not replaced by drinking water and other beverages, dehydration will become a significant problem. Dehydration may occur at any temperature and even under conditions when physical activity levels are low. Mild dehydration can decrease appetite and cause lethargy, moderate dehydration decreases work capacity, and severe dehydration can be fatal.

Drinking fluids before and at regular intervals during exercise is essential for maintaining health and performance. Although the type of activity will dictate the specific characteristics of the fluid replacement beverage, the beverage should (*a*) be palatable to promote adequate intake, (*b*) cause no gastrointestinal discomfort, (*c*) be rapidly absorbed; and, preferably, (*d*) have an osmolality of less than

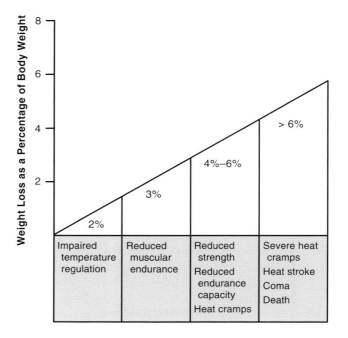

Fig. 17-1. Effects of Dehydration on Body Functions
Source: Original to authors

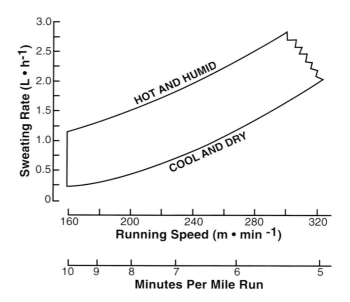

Fig. 17-2. Approximate hourly sweating rates and water requirements for runners based upon metabolic rate data. Reproduced with permission from Sawka MN, Pandolf KB. Effects of body water loss on physiological function and exercise performance. In: CV Gisolfi, DR Lamb, eds. *Fluid Homeostasis During Exercise*. Vol 3. *Perspectives in Exercise Science and Sports Medicine*. Indianapolis: Benchmark Press; 1990.

350 mOsm/L. If the exercise is to be continued for an extended period of time, the fluid replacement beverage should provide CHO and electrolytes, primarily sodium and potassium; extensive amounts of electrolytes can be lost when exercise is performed in the heat for a long time period or over extended days.[8–10] Water, CHO-containing beverages, and diluted fruit juices have all been recom-mended, but the CHO content should not exceed 12%; 6% to 8% solutions are optimal.[8,9] Carbonated beverages should be avoided during exercise as their consumption may cause gastrointestinal distress. In addition, the caffeine content of sodas may make them undesirable under some conditions. Table 17-1 compares the composition of selected fluid replacement beverages. The most commonly

TABLE 17-1

COMPARISON OF SELECTED FLUID REPLACEMENT BEVERAGES

Beverage (8 oz)	CHO Source* and Concentration	Sodium (mg)	Potassium (mg)	Other Nutrients	Osmolality (mOsm/L)
Gatorade	6% sucrose/glucose	110	25	Chloride, phosphorus	280–360
Exceed	7.2% glucose polymers/fructose	50	45	Chloride, calcium, magnesium, phosphorus	250
All Sport	8.0% high-fructose corn syrup	55	50	Thiamin, niacin, chloride, phosphorus, vitamins B_6 & B_{12}, pantothenic acid	525
10-K	6.3% sucrose/ glucose/fructose	52	26	Phosphorus, vitamin C, chloride	350
POWERade	7.9% high-fructose corn syrup/glucose polymers	55	30	Phosphorus	388
Coca Cola	11% high-fructose corn syrup/sucrose	9.2	Trace	Phosphorus	600–715
Sprite	10.2% high-fructose corn syrup/sucrose	28	Trace	——	695
Cranberry Juice Cocktail	15% high-fructose corn syrup/sucrose	10	61	Vitamin C, phosphorus	890
Orange Juice	11.8%fructose/ sucrose/glucose	2.7	510	Calcium, niacin, iron, vitamins A & C, thiamin, phosphorus, riboflavin	690
Water	——	Low	Low	——	10–20

*Sucrose = fructose and glucose
high-fructose corn syrup = a 54%:46% mixture of fructose and glucose derived from processed and converted corn starch
glucose polymers = long chains (> 3 molecules linked) of glucose

studied fluid replacement beverages contain electrolytes and either simple or complex CHO (maltodextrin or glucose polymers); these beverages usually taste good, promote rapid absorption of water, and provide substrate for the working muscles.[8–10] CHO-electrolyte (CHO-E) beverages have been studied in military populations and have shown positive results.[13–17] Importantly, CHO-E beverages can be ingested at any time—with meals, as a snack, or before, during, and after physical training sessions—to compensate for sweat losses and to maintain plasma volume.

Recommendations include drinking 0.30 to 0.50 L (0.25 to 0.5 qt) of cool, plain water 1 hour before starting a physical training exercise or any intense physical exertion[9,10] to minimize strain on the thermoregulatory system. However, excessive water intake during exercise may lead to electrolyte imbalances in hot weather.[18,19] Ideally, 0.25 to 0.75 L (0.26 to 0.8 qt) of a beverage supplemented with CHO-E (5% to 8% CHO) should be drunk every 30 minutes throughout strenuous exercises lasting more than 60 minutes, depending on the environmental conditions, to prevent hypoglycemia and extend performance[8–10] (Figure 17-3). In most studies that show benefits of CHO-E supplementation, subjects were provided 25 to 60 g of CHO per hour of exercise.[8,10] Providing CHOs 15 to 30 minutes before the anticipated onset of fatigue may extend performance for a short time.[20] If exhaustion has been reached before provision of the CHO-E,

though, work capacity will not be extended because the rate of glucose absorption is slower than the rate at which blood glucose can be taken up and used by exercising muscles. Evidence also indicates that ingesting CHO-E (1.0 g/kg body weight) immediately after prolonged exercise and again 2 hours later will enhance endurance capacity 4 hours later.[21]

Energy Balance

One of the biggest nutritional problems in the field is the failure to maintain energy balance. Monotony of the diet, decreased appetite, and lack of time to eat contribute to decreased energy intake, whereas sustained activity with heavy loads increases expenditure.[22] In combination, these factors contribute to weight loss. Weight loss in the field is common, regardless of the thermal strain,[23] and may compromise mental and physical performance. Service members should be made aware of the importance of consuming their daily field rations for maintaining readiness.

Depending on the type and duration of the maneuver, soldiers have been known to expend 3,000 to 6,000 kcal/d during cold weather operations.[23,24] The primary energy substrates used during military operations are CHO and fatty acids; less than 10% of the energy expended is derived from the oxidation of protein. An 80-kg man stores approximately 1,800 kcal of CHO as glycogen in liver and muscle and 75,000 to 150,000 kcal as fat. In spite of

Concentration of Beverage (%)	Carbohydrate (CHO) Delivered by Beverage of Given Concentration				
	25 g/h	30 g/h	40 g/h	50 g/h	60 g/h
	Approximate Volume (mL) of Beverage Required to Deliver Desired Amount of CHO per Hour				
3	825	1,000	1,325	1,675	2,000
5	500	600	800	1,000	1,200
6	425	500	675	825	1,000
7	350	425	575	725	850
8	300	375	500	625	750
10	250	300	400	500	600
12	200	250	325	425	500

Fig. 17-3. The volume of fluid required to provide varying amounts of carbohydrate (CHO) each hour for a given concentration of CHO in the beverage. Beverage concentrations are on the left (3% to 12%) and amount of CHO is across the top (25 to 60 g/h). The shaded section represents the volumes of beverage that are adequate for fluid replacement (500 to 1500 mL/h). The unshaded sections are volumes that are either too low (< 500 mL/hr) or too high (> 1500 mL/hr) to be beneficial.

Adapted with permission from Coyle EF, Montain SJ. Carbohydrate and fluid ingestion during exercise: Are there trade-offs? *Med Sci Sports Exerc.* 1992;24:671–678.3.

the large stores of fat, overall performance is most affected by CHO stores. Once glycogen stores are exhausted, physical and mental performance will deteriorate and exhaustion will ensue. Overall, the relative contribution of CHO and fatty acids is determined by the intensity and duration of the physical activity, prior nutritional status, conditioning level of the service member, and ambient environmental conditions.[25]

Regulation of energy balance depends on the balance of CHOs, proteins, and fats in the diet. However, evidence indicates that only CHO and protein balances are precisely regulated.[26] Because CHO (glycogen) stores are limited, CHO oxidation is adjusted to the intake of CHO over a period of 24 hours. It has been shown that depletion of glycogen will induce an increase in CHO intake.[27] Given that glycogen is an important energy substrate for the active muscle, liver and muscle glycogen stores should be replaced after an intense military operation to maintain CHO balance.

Similarly, protein balance is a function of energy intake and expenditure. When energy intake matches energy expenditure, protein intakes above requirements induce an increase in protein oxidation and only a transient increase in positive nitrogen balance. Furthermore, an increase in protein intake results in a marked postprandial thermic effect.[27] Unlike CHO, protein is a minor energy substrate for working muscle. Thus, protein balance is only minimally disturbed by physical exertion.

In contrast to CHO and protein, fat (fatty acids or lipids) balance does not appear to be intrinsically regulated: ingestion of fat does not promote oxidation of fatty acids but rather energy needs determine the degree of dependence on fatty acids as substrate.[27] Physical exertion is one physiological stress that induces an increase in fatty acid oxidation, an indication that exercise may be one mechanism to minimize a surplus of fat. Maintaining energy balance when the energy demands are high requires a basic knowledge of the appropriate amount of each of the three energy-providing nutrients.

Carbohydrate Requirements

It is generally acknowledged that a diet high in CHO is required to replenish glycogen stores between consecutive days of training; when CHO intake is low, rigorous training over several days will result in a gradual depletion of muscle glycogen stores.[7,28,29] Costill and colleagues[7] demonstrated that when subjects who trained 2 hours each day consumed a diet providing only 40% (as compared

to 70%) of the energy from CHO, glycogen depletion was evident after only 3 days. Others[30] observed a decline in muscle glycogen over a 7-day period in runners and cyclists who exercised for 1 hour daily and ate a diet that provided only 42% (5.0 g CHO/kg of body weight per day) of their energy from CHO. Despite the decline in muscle glycogen stores, daily training capacity remained similar over the 7-day period, so a short-term decrease in muscle glycogen stores may not impair performance. However, another study[31] reports that CHO intake during strenuous exercise can delay fatigue by decreasing the rate of muscle glycogen depletion.

A diet high in CHO for several days before a sustained training operation has the potential to increase liver and muscle glycogen stores and thereby extend the time to exhaustion. This may be accomplished by frequent snacking, or "grazing," on foods high in CHO to achieve an intake of 6 to 10 g of CHO per kilogram of body weight; approximately 60% to 70% of the total energy intake from CHO may be required each day to maintain glycogen stores.[32–34] A good premission meal can increase glycogen stores in muscles and liver and delay the onset of hypoglycemia. Goforth and colleagues[35] have shown glycogen supercompensation achieved by ingestion of a high-CHO diet (720 g/d) for 3 days was sustained for an additional 3 days when the subjects were inactive but maintained a moderate intake of CHO (332 g/d).

If a high-CHO diet cannot be eaten before an operation, ingestion of up to 4.5 g of CHO per kilogram of body weight 4 hours before a prolonged, physically demanding march or other field maneuver may maintain or extend performance by augmenting glycogen stores or maintaining blood glucose levels.[36,37] A premission meal should have limited amounts of fat and protein, since these nutrients take longer to digest and, if consumed less than 1 hour before a physical training or activity session, may cause gastrointestinal distress. A high-protein meal should be avoided because excessive protein can increase fluid requirements and may cause dehydration. CHO and CHO-E beverages are excellent choices in this situation. A smaller (400-500 kcal) high-CHO meal could be eaten 2 to 3 hours before the exercise.[36] Again, a CHO-E beverage 1 to 2 hours before a mission will leave the stomach faster than a solid meal.

Service members should know their individual tolerances for timings of meals and their ability to perform endurance activities. In general, they should allow more time for digestion before events that require intense physical activity. During extended field maneuvers, they should be encouraged to drink CHO-E beverages; however, some individuals may prefer to eat solid foods, primarily various energy bars or dried fruits. These foods will serve as a source of CHO to maintain blood glucose during prolonged events.[38] A study[13] that examined the effects of drinking a CHO-E beverage during several days of military training concludes that:

- CHO-E beverages can increase energy intake during field exercises,
- service members drinking CHO-E and eating their food were more likely to sustain physical performance than those eating only part of their food, and
- CHO-E beverages provide a readily accessible source of energy, which can be advantageous when inadequate food consumption is likely.

Food selections are personal choices, but dietary manipulations should always be tested in training sessions to ensure the foods selected will not cause gastrointestinal distress,[33] a common problem among endurance athletes.[38–40] Fasting, as an effort to reduce gastrointestinal distress and enhance fatty acid oxidation during physical exertion, is discouraged because it may impair physical performance by depleting liver glycogen stores and compromising blood glucose levels.[41]

Use of non-issue food items as substitutes for meals or rations should be limited since non-issued items may be lacking in several important nutrients, be high in fat, or be both. Such items, however, can be used as snacks to supplement total daily intakes. Also, high-CHO items, such as crackers, dried fruits, trail mixes, and sports bars, can be used. It is important to check the fat content of snack items, such as sports bars, because if it is greater than 3.0 g/100 kcal (27% or 27 kcal/100 kcal), absorption may be delayed and stomach cramping may occur. To maintain energy intake and blood glucose levels during sustained physical exercises, when possible service members should be encouraged to drink 25 to 50 g of CHO an hour.

Protein Needs

There is no consensus as to whether protein requirements are influenced by physical activity.[42] Amino acids can be oxidized during exercise, but the extent of oxidation depends on the exercise intensity, the availability of glucose and free fatty acids, and prior nutritional state. In particular, oxi-dation of the amino acid leucine appears to be enhanced when exercise is enforced in a fasted state as compared to a postabsorptive state. Moreover, increased nitrogen excretion in response to exercise has been demonstrated.[42] Interestingly, it has been shown that women exhibit a lower nitrogen excretion than men during exercise.[43] Whether this reflects their lower muscle mass or a decreased protein use during exercise has not been determined. Despite these exercise effects on amino acid and protein metabolism, the extent of the obligatory protein losses with exercise remains unresolved. As of 1999, protein's recommendations are still derived from a study by Tarnopolsky and colleagues[44] comparing the protein needs of body builders and endurance athletes. The highest values were found for the endurance athletes, and it was concluded that protein needs may depend on the intensity and volume of training.[32,33,44] A protein intake of 1.6 g/kg body weight was deemed adequate to maintain nitrogen balance in endurance athletes,[44] but strength athletes need less. In general, these protein needs can be met when 12% to 15% of daily energy intake is derived from protein and when energy balance is maintained.[32] When energy intakes approach 4,500 kcal/d, protein needs can be met when protein constitutes only 8% of the total energy intake.

Micronutrient Needs

Requirements for vitamins and minerals are typically met when service members eat a balanced diet. During deployment this may not be the case. In particular, when energy needs are not met through the diet, inadequate amounts of essential micronutrients will be consumed. A shortage of vitamins decreases the work capacity of personnel, and it has been shown that strenuous military missions are accompanied by an increased utilization of vitamins and minerals.[45] When military rations are the major source of energy, it is important for unit leaders to encourage consumption of those items that have been fortified to optimize nutrient intake.

In addition to inadequate energy intakes contributing to a potential deficit in vitamins and minerals, most deployment environments pose specific problems. By being outdoors and being physically active, service members are exposed to intense sunlight and high metabolic rates, and these exposures may result in significant oxidative stress.[2] Individuals may benefit from taking additional amounts of the antioxidant nutrients, such as vitamins E and C, but the amounts of particular nutrients that should be taken to offset environmental stressors are controversial. Recommendations to meet the increased micronutrient requirements at altitude can be found below in the section on altitude and may be used as a guide for both hot and cold environments in the absence of definitive data.

NUTRITIONAL CONSIDERATIONS BETWEEN MISSIONS

Recovery from prolonged operations may be critical, especially if only short rest periods are possible. Research has shown that if adequate nutritional strategies are implemented, additional physical work can in fact be achieved despite fatigue.[21] The three primary nutritional interventions that can influence recovery are glycogen restoration, rehydration, and electrolyte (particularly sodium) replacement.

Replacement of glycogen stores should start immediately or soon after completing a sustained effort. Providing 1.5 g of glucose per kilogram of body weight immediately after and again 2 hours after exercising for 2 hours significantly enhances replenishment of muscle glycogen stores.[46] Ingestion of CHO should continue even after the first 2 hours, though. Blom and colleagues[47] presented a schedule to maximize glycogen stores wherein subjects ingested 50 g of CHO every 2 hours after exercise for 6 hours. Glycogen resynthesis proceeded at a relatively constant rate as long as blood glucose remained elevated; ingestion of greater amounts of CHO does not further accelerate glycogen resynthesis.[46] Importantly, CHO foods with a low glycemic index (ability to raise blood glucose concentration) were not as effective as foods with a moderate-to-high glycemic index.[47,48] The importance of consuming foods with a high glycemic index has been confirmed.[49]

In addition to sustained, low-intensity aerobic exercise, high-intensity resistance exercise is associated with a rapid utilization of glycogen; only 30 minutes of intense exercise resulted in a 25% decline in muscle glycogen.[50] Ingestion of 1.5 g of CHO per kilogram of body weight immediately and again 1 hour after resistive exercise is effective in repleting glycogen stores.[6] It is reasonable to assume that foods with a high glycemic index would be restorative after heavy anaerobic activities as well. The glycemic index of selected foods is presented in Table 17-2.

For rehydration after strenuous exercise, forced fluid ingestion may be essential because the sensation of thirst can be blunted. Typically, voluntary consumption of fluids will restore only half of the fluid lost.[51] Body weight should be monitored to estimate fluid losses, so that over a period of several hours, a liter of fluid is ingested for every kilogram of body weight lost. Most commercially available fluid replacement beverages are appropriate for rehydration and appear to be as effective, if not more so, than water.[52]

TABLE 17-2

A SELECTION OF FOODS AND THEIR GLYCEMIC INDEXES*

Foods	Amount of Food That Provides 50 g of Carbohydrate
Highly Glycemic Foods (GI > 85)	
Bagel	1.3 bagel
Bread (white or whole wheat)	4.2 slices
Cornflakes	2.5 cups
Honey	2.9 tbsp
Maple syrup	3.1 tbsp
Potato, baked w/ skin	1 medium
Raisins	0.4 cup
Shredded wheat cereal	1.4 cups
Sweet corn, cooked	1.5 cups
Watermelon	4.5 cups
Moderately Glycemic Foods (GI between 60 and 85)	
Baked beans	1.0 cup
Banana	1.8 medium
Grapes	55 grapes
Oatmeal, cooked	2.0 cups
Orange juice	2.0 cups
Rice, cooked	1.0 cup
Sweet potato, boiled	0.8 cup
Low Glycemic Foods (GI < 60)	
Apple	2.5 medium
Peaches	5 medium
Pear	2 medium
Green peas, cooked	2.2 cups
Ice cream	1.6 cups
Spaghetti and other pasta, cooked	1.4 cups
Yogurt, nonfat plain	2.9 cups

*The glycemic indexes (GI) in this table are based on a relative GI of 100 for white bread.
Reproduced from Coyle. Timing and method of increased carbohydrate intake to cope with heavy training, competition and recovery. *Sport Sci.* 1991;9:2–51.

NUTRITIONAL CONSIDERATIONS FOR SPECIFIC ENVIRONMENTS

Exposure to extreme environments always poses unique nutritional problems that must be considered, before deployment if possible. The three environments most often encountered during military operations are heat, cold, and high altitude (see chapter 19, Environmental Medicine: Heat, Cold, and Altitude). Service members may be deployed to environments that are hot and humid, hot and dry, cold and wet, or cold and dry. The environments may be even more varied, depending on the geographical location and time of year. Acclimation is desirable for maintaining performance, but nutritional interventions may also be of benefit.

Hot Environments

Any type of activity in the heat presents a challenge to maintenance of temperature homeostasis and plasma volume. As the intensity of activity increases, the generation of metabolic heat increases, and this heat must be dissipated to achieve thermal balance. The effectiveness of heat loss mechanisms depends on the ambient temperature and the humidity. The circulatory system adapts to the strain by invoking two primary events: an increase in blood flow to the skin and the onset of sweating, both of which facilitate heat transfer to the skin surface, where it can be dissipated into the environment.[53] Major concerns in a warm or hot environment are fluid and electrolyte balance, since water and electrolytes are lost through sweating. Working at a high intensity in hot, humid surroundings can result in significant fluid and electrolyte losses. One to two liters can be lost each hour and even more when special protective clothing is worn. The highest sweating rate ever reported was approximately 4 L/h.[12] Therefore, maintaining fluid status is the primary nutritional consideration for adapting to a hot environment. Electrolyte balance and energy needs are other nutritional concerns in hot environments.

Fluid Requirements

The detrimental effects of dehydration on physical performance are well known and have been described earlier (see Figure 17-1). Failure to replace fluids lost through sweating will result in dehydration and eventually in heat injury.[8-10] Because thirst is not a sufficient stimulus for maintaining body water during physical exertion, forced drinking of fluids is often necessary in warm environments.[51,54]

The level of dehydration was 4% in men and women who drank approximately 10 mL of fluid per kilogram of body weight each hour (0.50 to 0.80 L/h) while running in a hot, humid environment.[55] Thus, 0.50 to 0.80 L of fluid each hour was not sufficient for strenuous activities under hot and humid conditions.

Approximately 0.5 to 0.75 L (0.5 to 0.8 qts) of fluid should be drunk every 30 minutes, depending on whether service members are working continuously or are using work-rest cycles. Regardless of the temperature and work conditions, service members cannot absorb more than 0.80 L (0.85 qt) every 30 minutes. The upper limits for fluid replacement in a warm environment are set by the maximal gastric emptying rates, which approximate 1.2 to 1.6 L/h for an average adult male.[54,56] In hot weather when the physical demands require efforts greater than 70% of $\dot{V}O_2$max, fluid losses can be as high as 2.0 L/h (2.1 qt).[51] Thus, fluid intakes of up to 1.6 L/h (1.7 qt) may be necessary when military personnel are required to perform in the heat for 3 or more hours;[9] ingestion of more than 1.6 L/h may cause gastric distress. US Army recommendations for 1999 have 1.5 qt/h and no more than 12 qt/d as the upper limit for water requirements during hard, continuous work in the heat. This volume of water is needed to replace fluid lost during heavy work, but service members should also drink this additional fluid (0.25 to 1.0 qt/h) during periods of rest when water requirements are lower.[57] Ideally, the fluid replacement beverage should contain electrolytes and a 5%- to 7%-concentration of CHO to promote fluid absorption and provide exogenous glucose, respectively, when the activities exceed 1 hour.[58]

Once the activity is over, weight loss can be used to estimate the degree of dehydration and amount of fluid to be replaced. The rehydration beverage should contain 2.32 g of sodium chloride or 40 mEq of sodium per liter of fluid to accelerate rehydration, maintain the osmotic drive for drinking, and minimize the water clearance associated with a reduction in serum electrolytes.[9,59] Conversely, unusual weight gains can and should be used as a sign of overhydration.

Electrolyte Concerns

Electrolytes are lost in the sweat, and excessive losses of electrolytes can lead to cramping of muscles or severe medical problems. Losses of sodium, in particular during prolonged physical exertion, can be significant, and these losses will initially result in a proportional contraction of the extracellular volume to maintain normal serum sodium levels. Further losses can lead to hyponatremia. Hyponatremia has been observed in athletes who exercise for extended periods of time in the heat. Although drinking too much water or fluid with a low sodium content during prolonged exercise may result in hyponatremia,[19] excessive sodium loss through sweating is also a likely cause.[19,60] Hyponatremia is rare [19] but can be life-threatening.[61]

The best way to maintain electrolyte balance over prolonged exposure to heat is to drink CHO-E replacement beverages. Gisolfi and colleagues[9] concluded that 20 to 30 mEq/L of sodium in a sports drink should be protective; most commercial fluid replacement beverages provide sufficient sodium so that hyponatremia should not be a significant concern. The beverage selected should provide no more ions than indicated in Table 17-3.[62,63] The National Academy of Sciences recommends that chloride be the only "anion" (negatively charged electrolytes) accompanying sodium and potassium; no other electrolytes are recommended.[63] Typically, magnesium and calcium are present in most sport beverages but in amounts well below the recommended upper limits. If a rehydration solution containing 40 mEq of sodium per liter is consumed during the first 2 hours after prolonged exercise, sodium replacement will help restore fluid volume. In addition, foods that are high in water and rich in potassium should be eaten.

Energy Balance and Carbohydrate Needs

Although minimal information on the metabolic cost of military maneuvers in hot environments is available, several studies indicate expenditure values of over 4,000 kcal per day in a hot, humid

TABLE 17-3

UPPER LIMITS FOR SODIUM AND POTASSIUM IN FLUID REPLACEMENT BEVERAGES DURING HEAT STRESS

Units	Sodium	Potassium
mg/8 oz	165	46
mg/L	690	195
mEq/8 oz	7.2	1.2

Source: Commentary and summary. In: Marriott GM, ed. *Nutritional Needs in Hot Environments: Applications for Military Personnel in Field Operations.* Washington, DC: National Academy Press; 1993.

jungle[64], hot-dry environments,[23] and hot-wet swamps.[65] In all cases, energy intakes were well below expenditures.[23,64,65] Others have reported an increased metabolic rate with acute heat exposure[66] and a 5% increase in oxygen uptake to perform a given task in the heat as compared with more comfortable conditions.[23] Thus, energy balance may be compromised when service members reside and work in a hot environment, and appetite may be suppressed in the hot weather, especially the first few days after arrival. This means that when living and working in temperatures ranging from 30°C to 40°C (86°F to 104°F), energy intakes should be increased somewhat, unless activity level decreases accordingly. One measure to offset any potential energy deficit is to enforce regular ingestion of CHO-E beverages, but the concentration of CHO should be lower under conditions of heat stress (5% to 7%) than in thermoneutral conditions so that the fluid is rapidly absorbed.

Cold Environments

Exposure to a cold environment, be it air or water, disrupts homeostasis and imposes a significant physiological strain. The consequences of cold stress are related to the severity of the cold stimulus. Performing daily activities and, ultimately, survival in such environments require that a new balance between heat production and heat loss be achieved. Under conditions of rest, the body's adaptive response to cold exposure is cutaneous vasoconstriction to minimize heat loss, followed by the onset of shivering, or cold-induced thermogenesis, to enhance heat production. When living or performing military training operations in the cold, the physiological strain may be mitigated by selected nutritional measures. These interventions strive to compensate for the adaptive responses to cold of increased urine output and energy expenditure. Therefore, the most important aspects of nutrition in a cold environment are hydration status, energy balance, and CHO intake.

Hydration Status

The initial physiological response to a cold environment is diuresis, which contributes to a reduction in plasma volume and ultimately dehydration. In addition, fluid losses in the cold are increased through respiration, reduction in fluid intake, and sweat lost from physical exertion. Urinary excretion of sodium, potassium, and other ions is also increased in the cold, but fluid losses are of greater concern. Plasma volume has been shown to decrease by as much as 17% during prolonged immersion in cold water.[67] Thus, maintenance of hydration status by drinking fluids is absolutely critical. Dann and colleagues[68] demonstrated that exertion in a cold environment is associated with a decrease in voluntary fluid intake, dehydration, and a reduction in glomerular filtration rate. They estimated that 0.15 L (0.16 qt) of fluid should be ingested each hour to avoid compromising kidney function. Given that the cold-induced diuresis results in a loss of sodium, potassium, and other cations in the urine, drinking fluids that provide electrolytes may be preferable,[67] but this intervention has not been carefully examined. In general, body weight and urine color should be monitored to ensure fluid needs are met. As in the heat, forced fluid ingestion of 0.25 to 0.75 L every 30 minutes may be required to achieve fluid balance. A CHO-E beverage, preferably a 5% to 7% solution, has been shown to improve physical performance in cold environments.[69]

Energy Balance

Studies of individuals and groups of civilians and military personnel indicate that exposure to cold environments can increase energy requirements 2- to 5-fold.[53,70] Expenditures as high as 7,500 kcal/d have been reported for Arctic expeditions.[71] Studies of military populations under conditions of moderate activity and extreme cold (–30°C to –15°C [–22°F to 5°F]) have noted energy expenditures of 4,200 to 4,750 kcal/d.[23,64,72] Coupled with these expenditures were intakes of fewer than 3,000 kcal/d. Thus, one of the major problems in the cold is maintaining energy balance.

Factors that may serve to increase energy needs include the added exertion due to wearing heavy clothing, shivering, the increased activity associated with traveling over snow and icy terrain, and the increased activity to keep warm. In general, energy requirements will increase in proportion to the intensity of shivering, the duration and relative intensity of the physical exertion, and the severity of the cold insult. Under resting conditions, a 3°C to 4°C decrease in core temperature invokes shivering and a significant increase in resting oxygen uptake.[73] Physical exertion is one way of promoting thermal balance by increasing metabolic heat production. However, physical exercise will increase energy requirements as well as heat loss due to increased blood flow to the skin and active muscles.[70] Metabolic heat production during exercise in cold air can override cold-induced heat losses when the exercise intensity is sufficiently high, but even intense exercise in cold water may not be adequate to compensate for heat losses.[74] Energy requirements should be unaltered in persons who are adequately clothed and protected from the environment.[70]

Carbohydrate Requirements

Both fats and CHOs are used as metabolic fuels, but CHO may contribute more to total energy metabolism in cold as compared with temperate environments.[70] Theoretically, dependence on CHO as the primary energy substrate might minimize heat loss by increasing metabolic heat production during exposure to cold. However, investigations have not supported the hypothesis that preferential metabolism of CHO will improve thermal balance. Vallerand and colleagues[75] demonstrated that feeding of high-CHO foods (100% and 68%), as compared with water, did not induce any detectable changes in either cold-induced thermogenesis, heat loss, or body temperature under resting conditions, despite a greater reliance on CHO as the energy substrate.

One of the adaptations to cold in the absence of adequate clothing and protection is shivering. As shivering increases, so does oxygen uptake, with the magnitude of increase being greater in cold water than cold air.[70] Because shivering requires a continuous supply of energy substrate to support the contractile process, significant research has focused on what substrate is preferentially used to maintain muscular contraction. Some investigators believe that CHOs are the primary source of energy for shivering thermogenesis, but this is controversial.[53,73,75,76] If CHOs were the only suitable energy substrate, glycogen stores would be rapidly depleted, and exposure time would be severely limited.

Numerous studies have been conducted to determine whether CHO or free fatty acids are preferentially utilized; protein oxidation is minimal. Vallerand and colleagues[73] demonstrated a 7-fold increase in CHO oxidation and a less than 2-fold increase in the oxidation of fatty acids during resting conditions. However, Martineau and Jacobs[77] were unable to demonstrate impaired thermal balance when intramuscular glycogen stores were low and the availability of plasma free fatty acids was reduced. Similarly, Young and colleagues[76] demonstrated that thermal balance was not compromised when initial muscle glycogen levels were low. Thus, it appears that when resting, the body compensates by using metabolic substrates other than muscle glycogen to maintain energy production.

It has been postulated that when exercise is performed in the cold, CHOs serve as the preferred substrate,[78] but utilization and mobilization of free fatty acids is accelerated during exercise in the cold.[79] Numerous studies have shown a relative decrease in the respiratory gas exchange ratio during low-to-moderate intensity exercise, whereas an increase or no change has been noted when the exercise is more vigorous.[78,79] The relative proportion of each substrate appears to depend on a variety of individual factors, such as percent of body fat, physical fitness, prior dietary patterns, and cold acclimation, as well as the type and intensity of the exertion and degree of cold stress.[78,80] When exercise and shivering occur in combination, the rate of muscle glycogen breakdown may be considerably accelerated as compared with an equivalent exercise bout in a warmer temperature.[78] Given that lipid stores are rarely limiting, a high-CHO diet would be preferable when exercising in the cold to ensure maintenance of glycogen stores necessary for maintaining metabolic heat production.[75] In addition, glycogen loading, or supercompensation, achieved by maintaining a diet high in CHO with minimal physical activity, may be effective in enhancing muscle and liver glycogen stores for exercise in the cold.

High-Altitude Environments

Ascent to altitude (> 3,050 m [10,000 ft]) imposes the stress of hypoxia in addition to stresses imposed by cold exposure. Hypoxia-induced adaptations of the oxygen delivery system include increased respiratory drive to increase oxygen delivery and enhanced extraction of oxygen by tissues; an increase in blood hemoglobin is a later adaptation. As with cold exposure, vasomotor adaptations strive to minimize heat loss and metabolic responses serve to generate heat, which is lost to the environment. Failure to invoke these multiple physiological adaptations can have serious consequences, even in the absence of physical activity.

With respect to physical training at altitude, emphasis has focused on substrate utilization, induction of energy pathways within the musculature, and respiratory fluid losses. One notable physiological response to exertion at altitude is an exaggerated blood lactate concentration for a given relative exercise workload;[81] this response may reflect an enhancement in glycolysis and preferential utilization of glycogen.[53] Interestingly, the exaggeration of blood lactate is diminished by acclimation,[81] which has been interpreted as a reduced reliance on glycolysis.[82] Nonetheless, several investigators have shown that there is a dependence on blood glucose for physical exercise at altitude; this reliance is further enhanced with acclimation.[82] These observations suggest that CHO is the preferred substrate and indicate the importance of nutritional interventions for maintaining performance and readiness. The major nutritional concerns at altitude include hydration status, energy balance, intake of CHO, and micronutrient needs.

Hydration Status and Electrolyte Needs

As in all environments where physical training is part of the daily activities, hydration status is a primary concern. At altitude, fluid balance becomes increasingly important because dehydration may be a factor in the development of acute mountain sickness. The rates and routes of fluid loss at altitude will depend on environmental conditions, including barometric pressure and consequent hypoxia, temperature, and humidity. These specific factors will determine the magnitude of the physiological adaptations affecting fluid balance. Adaptations include diuresis and natriuresis, which result in reduced volume of plasma and interstitial and intracellular fluid.[83] Moreover, respiratory fluid losses are increased because of the increased ventilatory drive in a dry and cold environment. Fluid losses are increased at altitude, and these losses must be compensated for to prevent dehydration and preserve personnel performance. Physical exertion may in part override the apparent reductions in total body water at altitude. Withey and colleagues[84] observed a small positive water balance in those who exercised over several days. This was attributed to an exercise-induced increase in plasma aldosterone. Despite a potential compensatory effect of exercise on overall body water, maintenance of hydration status remains essential. Forced fluid ingestion may be needed because a failure to drink enough water at altitude has been noted[85–88] and thirst does not always keep pace with fluid needs.

There are no recommendations for the exact amount of fluid required to maintain fluid balance at altitude. Reports[89] of water losses approximating 7.0 L/d have been challenged; these losses were based on the assumption that expired air is fully saturated with water vapor, and others have since shown this assumption to be incorrect.[90] Studies on Mount Everest and other locations have estimated fluid losses to be between 2.6 and 4.0 L/d; water balance has been achieved with intakes of 1.8 to 4.0 L/d.[85,87,88] Water losses of 2.5 to 5.1 L/d have been noted in subjects exposed to altitudes between 5,900 and 8,046 m over a 7-day period.[86] The losses were not met by water input, which ranged from 2.1 to 3.9 L/d. Worme and colleagues[91] demonstrated that fluid balance was maintained in men who ate a dehydrated ration and exercised vigorously for 31 days at moderate altitude (2,400 to 3,500 m) and drank approximately 5 L of fluid a day. They were, however, extremely conscientious about regular fluid ingestion. In general, the magnitude of sweat lost, CHO in the diet, activity level, range of daytime temperatures, absolute altitude reached, and duration of acclimation will determine the amount of water required to maintain hydration status. At a minimum, 1 L should be ingested for every 1,200 to 1,500 kcal consumed, and body weight should be monitored to ascertain needs. Future research should address this issue so that definitive recommendations can be provided.

Energy Balance

Virtually all persons who go to moderate or high altitudes experience some weight loss and loss of lean body mass. Many investigators have concluded that weight loss can be prevented by increasing energy intake at altitudes below 5,000 m, but a 5% to 10% weight loss may be inevitable at altitudes above 5,000 m due to decreased food intake.[86,92,93] Reasons for weight loss at high altitude include greater energy requirements, a reduction in food intake, loss of body water from increased ventilation and dry air, decreased fluid intake, malabsorption of nutrients, and acute mountain sickness, which can cause nausea, vomiting, headache, and decreased appetite.

Several studies have indicated a 6% to 50% increase in basal metabolic rate and the energy cost of physical exertion with altitude exposure[85,87,91,94]; these responses may be early adaptations to altitude. One report[94] noted increased oxygen uptake requirements of 3% to 35% at various exercise workloads at altitude as compared with sea-level requirements. Others[85] noted an initial 28% increase in basal metabolic rate when men were acutely exposed to altitudes of 4,300 m; after 10 days the increase was only 17%. Comparable increases have

previously been estimated for women at similar altitudes.[95] Doubly labeled water has been used to determine the energy expenditure of climbers during ascent of Mount Everest,[88,92] with reported values ranging from 3,000 to 5,000 kcal/d. The high-energy expenditures have been attributed to an enhanced sympathetic drive in response to the initial stress of exposure, but an understanding of the mechanisms will require further study.

Another issue to address is the purported decline in energy intake. Subjects maintained in a hypobaric chamber for 40 days and who reached a final altitude of 8,884 m decreased their energy intake 43% and lost an average of 7.4 kg.[96] These results reinforce the notion of a declining food intake with altitude exposure, but not all studies support this finding. Subjects who remained at 5,050 m for 1 month increased their daily energy intake 45% (from sea-level intakes of 2,100 kcal to 3,200 kcal); weight loss averaged approximately 2.6 kg, or 3.8% of preexposure weight.[97] Similarly, others[91] have reported a 45% increase in daily energy intake (from about 2,350 kcal to about 3,500 kcal) in subjects who spent 1-month at 3,000 m, with a 1.9 kg loss (2.5% of initial body weight). Another study[85] reported increased intakes from 3,000 to 3,400 kcal/d; the subjects lost only 1% to 2% of their initial body weight. In contrast, energy intake averaged only 2,200 kcal/d during the Mount Everest expedition of Westerterp and colleagues[88] and only 1,900 kcal/d for the Mount Everest expedition of Reynolds and colleagues.[92] Part of the differences may reflect the altitude attained, the amount of activity, and the overall conditioning level of the participants, but it is also reasonable to conclude that weight loss can be minimized when palatable foods are provided and leaders emphasize the importance of food intake to maintain weight for strength and performance.

Intake of Carbohydrate

Given that glycogen stores may be a limiting factor for physical exertion at altitude, high-CHO foods have been considered the preferred energy substrate. In addition to repleting glycogen stores depleted by strenuous physical activity and shivering, CHO may improve metabolic efficiency by requiring less oxygen than fatty acids for complete oxidation. Moreover, a preferential reliance on CHO may be advantageous for the pulmonary system because it effectively decreases the physiological altitude by 305 to 610 m.[83] The higher respiratory quotient with CHO results in an increased alveolar oxygen partial pressure for a given alveolar carbon dioxide pressure.[98] A high-CHO diet has also been shown to increase physical performance after a rapid ascent to altitude.[99] Other studies indicate that consumption of CHO can blunt or delay the progression or severity of symptoms of acute mountain sickness. It has been suggested that individuals develop a preference for CHO-rich foods after ascending to altitude,[97] but this is not always the case.[92,93,96]

Investigations that have monitored CHO intake at altitude reveal inconsistent outcomes. Worme and colleagues[91] provided subjects a high-CHO diet (65% or approximately 575 g/d) and were careful to ensure that weight loss was minimal, even if complaints of bloating, flatulence, and abdominal distress were frequent. Kayser and colleagues[97] provided subjects a wide variety of palatable foods and found that CHO increased from 62% of energy intake at sea level to 77.3% after three weeks at 5,050 m; this finding supports a preference for CHO foods. In contrast, when subjects had free access to palatable food in a hypobaric chamber for 40 days, the percent of CHO in the diet declined from 62% before the exposure to 53%. Rose and colleagues[96] concluded that prolonged altitude exposure was associated with a reduction in their selection of foods high in CHO. However, their findings in a hypobaric environment may reflect a response quite different from what might be encountered on a mountain, so a diet that derives a major proportion of energy from CHO is still recommended.

Energy expenditure estimates should be used to determine the absolute amount of CHO. In general, the breakdown of energy should be 60% to 65% from CHO, 10% to 15% from protein, and 20% to 30% from fat. When energy requirements are above 4,000 kcal, however, more fat may be required because it is difficult to obtain sufficient calories from CHO alone. Recommendations for the approximate gram amounts of CHO, protein, and fat for various energy levels are shown in Table 17-4. At a minimum, 400 g of CHO should be consumed; this can be accomplished by eating high-CHO snacks between meals and drinking warm CHO-E beverages during activity and recovery periods.

Micronutrient Needs

Increased intakes of selected vitamins and minerals may be needed for maintaining performance at altitude where hypoxia and thermal challenges prevail. For example, the classic response to hypoxia is blood volume expansion, increased erythropoiesis, and increased hemoglobin concentration 1 to 3 weeks after ascent. The primary nutrient required for hemoglobin synthesis is iron.[100] For this reason,

TABLE 17-4

APPROXIMATE NUMBER OF GRAMS OF CARBOHYDRATE, PROTEIN, AND FAT RECOMMENDED FOR VARIOUS ENERGY INTAKE LEVELS DURING SUSTAINED AND HIGH-TEMPO OPERATIONS

Energy Level (kcal)	Carbohydrate (g)	Protein (g)	Fat (g)
3,000	450	110	85
3,500	525	115	100
4,000	600	125	120
4,500	675	135	140
5,000	700	160	170

TABLE 17-5

SUGGESTED ADDITIONAL AMOUNTS OF VITAMINS AND MINERALS FOR SOJOURNS TO ALTITUDE

Nutrient	Suggested Amount	% of RDA
Vitamin E	400 IU	4,000
Vitamin B$_1$ (thiamin)	3 mg	200
Vitamin B$_2$ (riboflavin)	2 mg	118
Vitamin B$_3$ (niacin)	5 mg	26
Pantothenic acid	5 mg	100
Folic acid	200 μg	100
Vitamin B$_{12}$	1 μg	50
Iron	5 mg	33
Magnesium	200 mg	57
Zinc	5 mg	33

Sources: Reynolds R. Nutritional needs in cold and in high-altitude environments. In: Marriot BM, Carlson-Newberry SJ, Institute of Medicine Committee on Military Nutrition Research. *Nutritional Needs in Cold and in High-altitude Environments: Applications for Military Personnel in Field Operations.* Washington, DC: National Academy Press; 1996; Committee on Dietary Allowances, Food and Nutrition Board, National Research Council. *Recommended Dietary Allowances.* 10th ed. Washington, DC: National Academy Press; 1989.

many investigators have examined changes in iron stores, hematocrit, hemoglobin, and serum iron with altitude exposure.[91] Adequate iron stores are necessary for hematological adaptations to the hypoxia of altitude[101] but supplementation with iron is beneficial only when iron stores are inadequate.

Requirements of vitamins used for energy metabolism, including thiamin, riboflavin, and niacin, may also increase. When energy intake is sufficient to meet energy needs, the intake of these nutrients is also sufficient. Given that energy intake is typically compromised at altitude, however, supplemental intake of specific nutrients may be necessary to meet the increased requirements.[102] In addition, higher intakes of certain vitamins and minerals may be protective against some of the pathological changes that occur at altitude.[103] The increased metabolic rate and hypoxic conditions at altitude can increase the production of harmful free radicals, which may compromise the circulatory system and impair physical performance. Taking greater amounts of the antioxidant vitamin E may be protective against oxidative injury. Preliminary findings indicate that taking 400 mg of vitamin E daily at high altitude reduced free radical production and maintained anaerobic performance in men.[104] Vitamin E supplementation also appears to prevent some of the rheological disturbances induced by high altitude.[102] Vitamin and mineral recommendations were proposed in 1995 to account for possible increased requirements of specific nutrients at altitude.[105] The recommendations were derived from intake data from field studies, urinary excretion of nutrients, other measures of "nutrient status," and the well-documented reduction in food intake. Table 17-5 presents the suggested additional amounts of nutrients that may be necessary when working in the cold at altitude.

OPERATIONAL RATIONS

When the tactical situation and unit missions preclude the use of kitchen equipment for preparing warm meals for the group, individually packaged rations are the next line of field feeding. Individually packaged operational rations may be wet-pack (sealed in a pouch without any of the food's moisture being removed) or dehydrated and can be consumed hot or cold. The dehydrated rations can usually be reconstituted with hot or cold water or consumed dry. All of the individual field rations are specifically designed to supply adequate energy and nutrients for particular types of missions. Since the duration and environmental conditions of missions vary, different types of operational rations have been developed. These rations provide different amounts of energy, with varying proportions of CHO, protein, and fat, to meet the nutritional demands of various operational scenarios. Although many people think that military rations are suboptimal, they have been carefully designed and will sustain service members during deployment. A number of rations are available, and these rations are discontinued, improved, or modified based on an annual ration review. Some of the rations introduced after 1995 include the Unitized Group Ration and the Go-To-War Ration. The Unitized Group Ration is for sustaining groups of service members during deployments where organized food service facilities can be set up. In contrast, the Go-To-War ration is for sustaining an individual during the early states of mobilization when other options are not available. This ration augments other rations and does not replace them. In addition, Food Packet, Survival rations have been reformulated and have several types, such as General Purpose, Improved; Abandon Ship; and Aircraft, Life Raft. Detailed information about these operational rations can be obtained elsewhere.[106] Commonly used operational rations are described below.

Meal, Ready-to-Eat, Individual

The ration known as the MRE (Meal, Ready-to-Eat) is used to sustain the individual service member during operations when organized food service is unavailable. The MRE menus are revised periodically, and the number of menus doubled to 24 between 1995 and 1998, with the production of MRE XVIII. The ration for 1 day comprises three meals and provides about 3,900 kcal (51% CHO, 13% protein, and 36% fat; sodium content: 5.5 g). Each MRE contains an entree, crackers, a spread (cheese, peanut butter, or jelly), a dessert or snack, beverages, an accessory packet, a plastic spoon, and a flameless ration heater (Table 17-6). When included, the supplemental pouch bread will provide an additional 200 kcal (55% CHO, 12% protein, and 33% fat). About 23 oz of water is required to rehydrate the beverages.

MREs provide the essential nutrients and maintain readiness if they are consumed by the service members. Three MREs may need to be eaten each day when MREs are the sole source of nutrition. Some components of the MRE have been supple-

TABLE 17-6

12 MENUS FOR MEAL, READY-TO-EAT, INDIVIDUAL (MRE XVIII)

Menu 3	Menu 4	Menu 6	Menu 7	Menu 8	Menu 9
Chicken stew	Ham slice	Grilled chicken	Pork chow mein	Chicken w/ rice	Beef stew
Pretzels	Buttered	Mexican rice	Chow mein	Fudge brownie	Tavern nuts
Pound cake	noodles	Pound cake	noodles	Jalapeno cheese	Jalapeno cheese
Jelly	Pound cake	Jelly	Cookie,	spread	spread
Cocoa	Cheese spread	Cocoa	choc-covered	Beverage base	Cocoa
Packet C	Cocoa	Packet D	Peanut butter	Packet A	Packet B
	Packet C		Beverage base		
			Packet A		

Menu 10	Menu 12	Menu 15	Menu 16	Menu 18	Menu 20
Chili w/ mac	Cheese tortellini	Beef franks	Bean & rice	Turkey breast w/	Spaghetti w/
Fig bar	(vegetarian)	Potato sticks	burrito	potatoes	meat sauce
Peanut butter	Applesauce	Peanut butter	(vegetarian)	Pound cake	Cheese curls
Cocoa	Granola bar	Candy*	Fruit	Cheese spread	Peanut butter
Packet D	Peanut butter	Beverage base	Fruit-filled bar	Chewy choc bar	Candy*
	Candy*	Packet A	Peanut butter	Beverage Base	Cocoa
	Packet D		Peanut brittle	Packet D	Packet C
			Packet D		

Each menu contains crackers, hot sauce, flameless ration heater, and spoon.
Packet A: coffee, cream substitute, sugar, salt, chewing gum, matches, toilet tissue, towelette
Packet B: coffee, cream substitute, sugar, salt, chewing gum, matches, toilet tissue, towelette, candy (vanilla caramels or Tootsie Rolls)
Packet C: lemon tea w/sugar, salt, chewing gum, matches, toilet tissue, towelette
Packet D: lemon tea w/sugar, apple cider, salt, chewing gum, matches, toilet tissue, towelette
*Jolly Rancher candy, heat stable M&Ms, Peanut Munch bar, or Skittles.
Menus listed in this table are reviewed annually and may change over time.

mented with selected vitamins (ie, A, B_1, B_2, niacin, B_6, and C) and minerals (ie, calcium), and so these items must be eaten to meet nutrient requirements. Fortified items include cocoa beverage powder, cheese spread, peanut butter, crackers, and the coatings of the oatmeal cookies and brownies.

Ration, Cold Weather

The Ration, Cold Weather (RCW) was designed to sustain individuals during operations in cold conditions, and each menu provides 4,500 kcal (60% CHO, 8% protein, and 32% fat; sodium content: 5 g). The six menus, which come as two meal bags (Bag A and Bag B), should provide sufficient energy to meet requirements during strenuous activities in the extreme cold. The various menus are shown in Table 17-7. The RCW is high in CHO since this macronutrient is believed to generate more metabolic heat. Each menu should be sufficient for a 24-hour period, but more can be eaten when en-

ergy demands are higher. The RCW is also lower in salt and protein than the MREs to reduce daily water requirements and lessen the possibility of dehydration. A 1-day ration requires 90 oz (about 9 cups or 3 canteens) of water for rehydration.

Food Packet, Long Range Patrol II

The Food Packet, Long Range Patrol II (LRP II) ration was designed for initial assaults, special operations, and long-range reconnaissance missions. The LRP II is a restricted calorie ration, and one packet is issued to an individual per day for up to 10 days. Eight of the twelve menus, consisting of dehydrated entrees, cereal bars, cookies and candy, instant beverages, accessory packets, and plastic spoons, are shown in Table 17-8. Each menu provides 1,560 kcal (50% CHO, 15% protein, 35% fat; sodium content: 2.6 g) and requires approximately 28 oz of water to prepare, although some of the foods may be eaten dry. It is lightweight, has been

TABLE 17-7

12 MENUS FOR RATION, COLD WEATHER

BAG A					
Menu 1	**Menu 2**	**Menu 3**	**Menu 4**	**Menu 5**	**Menu 6**
Oatmeal, strawberry & cream	Oatmeal, apple & cinnamon	Oatmeal, apple & cinnamon	Oatmeal, maple & brown sugar	Oatmeal, apple & cinnamon	Oatmeal, apple & cinnamon
Nut raisin mix	Nut raisin mix	Nut raisin mix	Nut raisin mix	Nut raisin mix	Nut raisin mix
Cocoa beverage powder (2)	Cocoa beverage powder (2)	Cocoa beverage powder (2)	Cocoa beverage powder (2)	Cocoa beverage powder (2)	Cocoa beverage powder (2)
Apple cider mix	Apple cider mix	Apple cider mix	Apple cider mix	Apple cider mix	Apple cider mix
Chicken noodle soup	Chicken noodle soup	Chicken noodle soup	Chicken noodle soup	Chicken noodle soup	Chicken noodle soup
Fruit bars (fig or blueberry)	Fruit bars (fig or blueberry)	Fruit bars (fig or blueberry)	Fruit bars (fig or blueberry)	Fruit bars (fig or blueberry)	Fruit bars (fig or blueberry)
Crackers (2)	Crackers (2)	Crackers (2)	Crackers (2)	Crackers (2)	Crackers (2)
Spoon	Spoon	Spoon	Spoon	Spoon	Spoon
Accessory packet	Accessory packet	Accessory packet	Accessory packet	Accessory packet	Accessory packet

BAG B					
Menu 7	**Menu 8**	**Menu 9**	**Menu 10**	**Menu 11**	**Menu 12**
Chicken stew	Chicken stew	Chili con carne	Chicken a la king	Chicken & rice	Spaghetti w/ meat sauce
Granola bars (2)	Granola bars (2)	Granola bars (2)	Granola bars (2)	Granola bars (2)	Granola bars (2)
Oatmeal cookie bars (2)	Oatmeal cookie bars (2)	Oatmeal cookie bars (2)	Oatmeal cookie bars (2)	Oatmeal cookie bars (2)	Oatmeal cookie bars (2)
Chocolate-covered cookie or brownie	Chocolate-covered cookie or brownie	Chocolate-covered cookie or brownie	Chocolate-covered cookie or brownie	Chocolate-covered cookie or brownie	Chocolate-covered cookie or brownie
Orange beverage powder	Orange beverage powder	Orange beverage powder	Orange beverage powder	Orange beverage powder	Orange beverage powder
Tootsie Rolls	Tootsie Rolls	Tootsie Rolls	Tootsie Rolls	Tootsie Rolls	Tootsie Rolls
M&Ms	M&Ms	M&Ms	M&Ms	M&Ms	M&Ms
Lemon tea (2)	Lemon tea (2)	Lemon tea (2)	Lemon tea (2)	Lemon tea (2)	Lemon tea (2)
Spoon	Spoon	Spoon	Spoon	Spoon	Spoon

Accessory packet: coffee, cream, sugar, chewing gum, toilet paper (2), matches, closure device (2)

accepted by military personnel, and is relatively inexpensive. To obtain adequate CHO and calories during extended operations, at least two menus would need to be eaten; only 195 g of CHO are provided. Alternatively, the LRP II and the MRE can be combined to meet additional calorie requirements; the two rations are nutritionally compatible.

Other Information

The best way to select a ration is to estimate the anticipated energy expenditure during the deployment. The ration for any mission that involves strenuous physical activity should provide at least 400 g of CHO. One distinct advantage of the military ration is that the nutritional content is known; there is no need to count calories on labels to get the desired energy distribution. For example, if the mission is in a cold environment, the RCW is an excellent ration to choose because it provides 4,500 kcal/d with an appropriate distribution of CHO, protein, and fat. If the rations are prepared as instructed, freeze-dried rations will not increase the need for water unless greater amounts of sodium

TABLE 17-8

EIGHT OF THE TWELVE MENUS FOR THE FOOD PACKET, LONG RANGE PATROL II (LRP) FOR FISCAL YEAR 1996

Menu 1	Menu 2	Menu 3	Menu 4
Chicken Stew	Beef Stew	Sweet & sour pork w/rice	Turkey tetrazini
Fruit-filled cereal bar	Granola bar	Chocolate sports bar	Granola bar
Oatmeal cookie bar	Chocolate-covered cookie	Jelly	Chocolate-covered cookie
Peanut Munch bar	Tootsie Roll (4pk)	Crackers	Caramels
Apple cider drink	Cocoa beverage	Apple cider drink	Cocoa beverage
Accessory packet	Accessory Packet	Accessory packet	Accessory packet
Spoon	Spoon	Spoon	Spoon

Menu 5	Menu 6	Menu 7	Menu 8
Chicken & rice	Spaghetti w/meat sauce	Chili con carne	Beef w/rice
Apple cinnamon pastry	Chocolate sports bar	Fruit-filled bar	Cornflake bar
Peanut butter	Fig bar	Crackers	Fig bar
Crackers	Crackers	Starch jellies (Chuckles)	M&Ms
Lemon tea (2 pkts)	Cocoa beverage	Orange beverage	Beverage base (MRE)
Accessory packet	Accessory packet	Accessory packet	Accessory packet
Spoon	Spoon	Spoon	Spoon

Accessory packet: coffee, creamer, sugar, chewing gum, toilet paper (2), matches, salt

or protein are added to them.

As long as the package is left unopened, stored properly (low humidity and at less than 27°C [80°F]), and not handled excessively, most military rations will be usable for at least 3 years; the MRE and RCW have shelf lives of 3 years. The ration with the longest shelf life is the LRP II, which has an estimated life of 10 years at 27°C.

SUMMARY

During deployment, military personnel typically undergo sustained operations under a variety of environmental extremes. Exposure to these multiple physiological challenges can result in performance decrements, often due to dehydration and weight loss. Nutritional interventions that minimize such physical changes will mitigate physiological strain, facilitate adaptation, and promote readiness. The primary nutritional considerations for deployment are maintaining fluid, electrolyte, and energy balance and obtaining the right proportion of energy from CHO, protein, and fat.

REFERENCES

1. Farhi LE. Exposure to stressful environments. In: *Dejours' Comparative Physiology of Environmental Adaptations.* 2 vols. Basel, Switzerland: Karger; 1987: 1–14.

2. Askew EW. Environmental and physical stress and nutrient requirements. *Am J Clin Nutr.* 1995;61(suppl):631S-637S.

3. Coggan AR, Swanson SC. Nutritional manipulations before and during endurance exercise: Effects on performance. *Med Sci Sports Exerc.* 1992;24(9 Suppl):S331–S335.

4. Coggan AR, Coyle EF. Effect of carbohydrate feedings during high-intensity exercise. *J Appl Physiol.* 1988;65:1703–1709.

5. Mitchell JB, Costill DL, Houmard JA, Fink WJ, Pascoe DD, Pearson DR. Influence of carbohydrate dosage on exercise performance and glycogen metabolism. *J Appl Physiol.* 1989;67:1843–1849.

6. Pascoe DD, Costill DL, Fink WJ, Robergs RA, Zachwieja JJ. Glycogen resynthesis in skeletal muscle following resistive exercise. *Med Sci Sports Exerc.* 1993;25:349–354.

7. Costill DL, Miller JM. Nutrition for endurance sport: Carbohydrate and fluid balance. *Int J Sports Med.* 1980;1:2–14.

8. Coyle EF, Montain SJ. Carbohydrate and fluid ingestion during exercise: Are there trade-offs? *Med Sci Sports Exerc.* 1992;24:671–678.

9. Gisolfi CV, Duchman SM. Guidelines for optimal replacement beverages for different athletic events. *Med Sci Sports Exerc.* 1992;24:679–687.

10. Millard-Stafford ML, Sparling PB, Rosskopf LB, DiCarlo LJ. Carbohydrate-electrolyte replacement improves distance running performance in the heat. *Med Sci Sports Exerc.* 1992;24:943–940.

11. Singh A, Pelletier PA, Deuster PA. Dietary requirements for ultra-endurance athletes. *Sports Med.* 1994;18:301–308.

12. Sawka MN, Pandolf KB. Effects of body water loss on physiological function and exercise performance. In: CV Gisolfi, DR Lamb, eds. *Fluid Homeostasis During Exercise.* Vol 3. *Perspectives in Exercise Science and Sports Medicine.* Indianapolis: Benchmark Press; 1990.

13. Montain SJ, Shippee RL, Tharion WJ, Kramer TR. *Carbohydrate-electrolyte Solution During Military Training: Effects on Physical Performance, Mood State, and Immune Function.* Natick, Mass: US Army Research Institute of Environmental Medicine; 1995. T95–13, Technical Report AD A297258.

14. Mudambo KS, Leese GP, Rennie MJ. Dehydration in soldiers during walking/running exercise in the heat and the effects of fluid ingestion during and after exercise. *Eur J Appl Physiol.* 1997;76:517–524.

15. Mudambo KS, Scrimgeour CM, Rennie MJ. Adequacy of food rations in soldiers during exercise in hot, day-time conditions assessed by doubly labelled water and energy balance methods. *Eur J Appl Physiol.* 1997;76:346–351.

16. Tharion WJ, Cline AD, Hotson N, Johnson W, Niro P. *Nutritional Challenges for Field Feeding in a Desert Environment: Use of the Unitized Group Ration (UGR) and a Supplemental Carbohydrate Beverage.* Natick, Mass: US Army Research Institute of Environmental Medicine; 1997. T97–9, Technical Report ADA328882.

17. van Dokkum W, van Boxtel LBJ, van Dijk MJ, Boer LC, van der Beek EJ. Influence of a carbohydrate drink on performance of military personnel in NBC protective clothing. *Aviat Space Environ Med.* 1996;67:819–826.

18. Murray R. Nutrition for the marathon and other endurance sports: Environmental stress and dehydration. *Med Sci Sports Exerc.* 1992;24:S319–S323.

19. Noakes TD, Norman RJ, Buck RH, Godlonton J, Stevenson K, Pittaway D. The incidence of hyponatremia during prolonged ultraendurance exercise. *Med Sci Sports Exerc.* 1990;22:165–170.

20. Coggan AR, Coyle EF. Reversal of fatigue during prolonged exercise by carbohydrate infusion or ingestion. *J Appl Physiol.* 1987;63:2388–2395.

21. Fallowfield JL, Williams C, Singh R. The influence of ingesting a carbohydrate-electrolyte beverage during 4 hours of recovery on subsequent endurance capacity. *Int J Sports Nutr.* 1995;5:285–299.

22. Knapik J, Harman E, Reynolds K. Load carriage using packs: A review of physiological, biomechanical and medical aspects. *Appl Ergonomics.* 1996;27:207–216.

23. Burstein R, Coward AW, Askew WE, et al. Energy expenditure variations in soldiers performing military activities under cold and hot climate conditions. *Mil Med.* 1996;161:750–754.

24. King N, Roberts DE, Edwards JS, Morizen RD, Askew EW. Cold-weather field feeding: An overview. *Mil Med.* 1994;159:121–126.

25. Coyle EF. Carbohydrate feeding during exercise. *Int J Sports Med.* 1992;13(Suppl 1):S126–S128.

26. Flatt JP. Importance of nutrient balance in body weight regulation. *Diabetes Metab Rev*. 1988;4:571–581.

27. Jequier E. Body weight regulation in humans: The importance of nutrient balance. *News Physiolog Sci*. 1993;8:273–276.

28. Costill DL, Bowers R, Branam G, Sparks K. Muscle glycogen utilization during prolonged exercise on successive days. *J Appl Physiol*. 1971;31:834–838.

29. Sherman WM, Costill DL, Fink WS, Miller JM. Effect of exercise-diet manipulation on muscle glycogen and its subsequent utilization during performance. *Int J Sports Med*. 1981;2:114–118.

30. Sherman WM, Doyle JA, Lamb DR, Strauss RH. Dietary carbohydrate, muscle glycogen, and exercise performance during 7 d of training. *Am J Clin Nutr*. 1993;57:27–31.

31. Coyle EF, Coggan AR, Hemmert MK, Ivy JL. Muscle glycogen utilization during prolonged strenuous exercise when fed carbohydrate. *J Appl Physiol*. 1986;61:165–172.

32. Applegate EA. Nutritional considerations for ultraendurance performance. *Int J Sport Nutr*. 1991;1:118–126.

33. Houtkooper L. Food selection for endurance sport. *Med Sci Sports Exerc*. 1992;24:S349–S359.

34. O'Keeffe KA, Keith RE, Wilson GD, Blessing DL. Dietary carbohydrate intake and endurance exercise performance of trained female cyclists. *Nutr Res*. 1989;9:819–830.

35. Goforth HW Jr, Arnall DA, Bennett BL, Law PG. Persistence of supercompensated muscle glycogen in trained subjects after carbohydrate loading. *J Appl Physiol*. 1997;82:342–347.

36. Hargreaves M, Costill DL, Fink WJ, King DS, Fielding RA. Effect of pre-exercise carbohydrate feedings on endurance cycling performance. *Med Sci Sports Exerc*. 1987;19:33–36.

37. Sherman WM, Brodowicz G, Wright DA, Allen WK, Simonsen J, Dernback A. Effect of 4 hour preexercise feedings on cycling performance. *Med Sci Sports Exerc*. 1989;21:598–604.

38. Rehrer NJ, Brouns F, Beckers EJ, et al. Physiological changes and gastro-intestinal symptoms as a result of ultra-endurance running. *Eur J Appl Physiol*. 1992;64:1–8.

39. Baska RS, Moses FM, Deuster PA. Cimetidine reduces running-associated gastrointestinal bleeding: A prospective observation. *Dig Dis Sci*. 1990;35:956–960.

40. Rehrer NJ, Beckers EJ, Brouns F, Saris WH, Ten Hoor F. Effects of electrolytes in carbohydrate beverages on gastric emptying and secretion. *Med Sci Sports Exer*. 1993;25:42–51.

41. Dohm GL, Beeker RT, Israel RG, Tapscott EB. Metabolic responses to exercise after fasting. *J Appl Physiol*. 1986;61:1363–368.

42. Millward DJ, Bowtell JL, Pacy P, Rennie MJ. Physical activity, protein metabolism and protein requirements. *Proc Nutr Soc*. 1994;53:223–240.

43. Tarnopolsky LJ, MacDougall JD, Atkinson SA, Tarnopolsky MA, Sutton JR. Gender differences in substrate for endurance exercise. *J Appl Physiol*. 1990;68:302–308.

44. Tarnopolsky MA, MacDougall JD, Atkinson SA. Influence of protein intake and training status on nitrogen balance and lean body mass. *J Appl Physiol*. 1988;64:187–193.

45. D'iakonov MM. [The current nutritional problems of servicemen.] *Voen Med Zh (Russia)*. 1994;55–58.

46. Ivy JL, Lee MC, Brozinick JT, Reed MJ. Muscle glycogen storage after different amounts of carbohydrate ingestion. *J Appl Physiol*. 1988;65:2018–2023.

47. Blom PC, Hostmark AT, Vaage O, Kardel KR, Maehlum S. Effect of different post-exercise sugar diets on the rate of muscle glycogen synthesis. *Med Sci Sports Exerc*. 1987;19:491–496.

48. Coyle EF, Coyle E. Carbohydrates that speed recovery from training. *Phys Sports Med*. 1993;21:111–123.

49. Burke LM, Collier GR, Hargreaves M. Muscle glycogen storage after prolonged exercise: Effect of the glycemic index of carbohydrate feedings. *J Appl Physiol*. 1993;75:1019–1023.

50. Tesch PA, Colliander EB, Kaiser P. Muscle metabolism during intense, heavy-resistance exercise. *Eur J Appl Physiol*. 1986;55:362–366.

51. Greenleaf JE. Problem: Thirst, drinking behavior, and involuntary dehydration. *Med Sci Sports Exerc*. 1992;24:645–656.

52. Gonzalez-Alonso J, Heaps CL, Coyle EF. Rehydration after exercise with common beverages and water. *Int J Sports Med*. 1992;13:399–406.

53. Young AJ. Energy substrate utilization during exercise in extreme environments. *Exerc Sport Sci Rev*. 1990;18:65–117.

54. Sawka MN. Physiological consequences of hypohydration: Exercise performance and thermoregulation. *Med Sci Sports Exerc*. 1992;24:657–670.

55. Millard-Stafford ML, Sparling PB, Rosskopf LB, Snow TK, DiCarlo LJ, Hinson BT. Fluid intake in male and female runners during a 40-km field run in the heat. *J Sports Sci*. 1995;13:257–263.

56. Mitchell JB, Voss KW. The influence of volume on gastric emptying and fluid balance during prolonged exercise. *Med Sci Sports Exerc*. 1991;23:314–319.

57. Montain SJ, Latzka WA, Sawka MN. Fluid replacement recommendation for training in hot weather. *Mil Med*. 1999;164:502–508.

58. American College of Sports Medicine. Position stand: Exercise and fluid replacement. *Med Sci Sports Exerc*. 1996;28:i–vii.

59. Nose H, Mack GW, Shi XR, Nadel ER. Role of osmolality and plasma volume during rehydration in humans. *J Appl Physiol*. 1988;65:325–331.

60. Hiller WD. Dehydration and hyponatremia during triathlons. *Med Sci Sports Exerc*. 1989;21(5 Suppl):S19–S21.

61. Garigan TP, Ristedt DE. Death form hyponatremia as a result of acute water intoxication in an Army basic trainee. *Mil Med*. 1999;164:234–238.

62. Brouns F, Saris W, Schneider H. Rationale for upper limits of electrolyte replacement during exercise. *Int J Sport Nutr*. 1992;2:229–238.

63. Marriott GM, ed. *Nutritional Needs in Hot Environments: Applications for Military Personnel in Field Operations*. Washington, DC: National Academy Press; 1993.

64. Forbes-Ewan CH, Morrissey BL, Gregg GC, Waters DR. Use of doubly labeled water technique in soldiers training for jungle warfare. *J Appl Physiol*. 1989;67:14–18.

65. Moore RJ, Friedl KE, Kramer TR, et al. *Changes in Soldier Nutritional Status and Immune Function During the Ranger Training Course*. Natick, Mass: US Army Research Institute of Environmental Medicine; 1993. T43–93, Technical Report AD A257437.

66. Consolazio CF, Shapiro R, Masterson JE, McKinzie PSL. Energy requirements of men in extreme heat. *J Nutr*. 1961;73:126–134.

67. Deuster PA, Smith DJ, Smoak BL, Montgomery LC, Singh A, Doubt TJ. Prolonged whole-body cold water immersion: Fluid and ion shifts. *J Appl Physiol*. 1989;66:34–41.

68. Dann EJ, Gillis S, Burstein R. Effect of fluid intake on renal function during exercise in the cold. *Eur J Appl Physiol*. 1990;61:133–137.

69. Febbraio MA, Murton P, Selig SE, et al. Effect of CHO ingestion on exercise metabolism and performance in different ambient temperatures. *Med Sci Sports Exerc*. 1996;28:1380–1387.

70. Young AJ, Sawka MN, Pandolf KB. Physiology of cold exposure. In: Marriot BM, Carlson-Newberry SJ, Institute of Medicine Committee on Military Nutrition Research. *Nutritional Needs in Cold and in High-altitude Environments: Applications for Military Personnel in Field Operations*. Washington, DC: National Academy Press; 1996.

71. Stroud MA, Coward WA, Sawyer MB. Measurements of energy expenditure using isotope-labelled water (2H2(18)O) during an Arctic expedition. *Eur J Appl Physiol Occup Physiol*. 1993;67:375–379.

72. Jones PJ, Jacobs I, Morris A, Ducharme MB. Adequacy of food rations in soldiers during an arctic exercise measured by doubly labeled water. *J Appl Physiol*. 1993;75:1790–1797.

73. Vallerand AL, Jacobs I. Energy metabolism during cold exposure. *Int J Sports Med*. 1992;13(Suppl 1):S191–S193.

74. Toner MN, McArdle WD. Physiological adjustments of man in the cold. In: Pandolf KB, Sawka MN, Gonzalez RR, eds. *Human Performance, Physiology and Environmental Medicine at Terrestrial Extremes*. Indianapolis: Benchmark Press; 1988: 361–399.

75. Vallerand AL, Tikuisis P, Ducharme MB, Jacobs I. Is energy substrate mobilization a limiting factor for cold thermogenesis? *Eur J Appl Physiol*. 1993;67:239–244.

76. Young AJ, Sawka MN, Neufer PD, Muza SR, Askew EW, Pandolf KB. Thermoregulation during cold water immersion is unimpaired by low muscle glycogen levels. *J Appl Physiol*. 1989;66:1809–1816.

77. Martineau L, Jacobs I. Effects of muscle glycogen and plasma FFA availability on human metabolic responses in cold water. *J Appl Physiol*. 1991;71:1331–1339.

78. Shephard RJ. Metabolic adaptations to exercise in the cold: An update. *Sports Med*. 1993;16:266–289.

79. Doubt TJ, Hsieh SS. Additive effects of caffeine and cold water during submaximal leg exercise. *Med Sci Sports Exerc*. 1991;23:435–442.

80. Doubt TJ. Physiology of exercise in the cold. *Sports Med*. 1991;11:367–381.

81. Green HJ, Sutton JR, Wolfel EE, Reeves JT, Butterfield GE, Brooks GA. Altitude acclimatization and energy metabolic adaptation in skeletal muscle during exercise. *J Appl Physiol*. 1992;73:2701–2708.

82. Brooks GA, Butterfield GE, Wolfe RR, et al. Increased dependence on blood glucose after acclimatization to 4,300 m. *J Appl Physiol*. 1991;70:919–927.

83. Kayser B. Nutrition and energetics of exercise at altitude: Theory and possible practical implications. *Sports Med*. 1994;17:309–323.

84. Withey WR, Milledge JS, Williams ES, et al. Fluid and electrolyte homeostasis during prolonged exercise at altitude. *J Appl Physiol*. 1983;55:409–412.

85. Butterfield GE, Gates J, Fleming S, Brooks GA, Sutton JR, Reeves JT. Increased energy intake minimizes weight loss in men at high altitude. *J Appl Physiol*. 1992;72:1741–1748.

86. Pulfrey SM, Jones PJ. Energy expenditure and requirement while climbing above 6,000 m. *J Appl Physiol*. 1996;81:1306–1311.

87. Westerterp KR, Kayser B, Brouns F, Herry JP, Saris WH. Energy expenditure climbing Mt. Everest. *J Appl Physiol.* 1992;73:1815–1819.

88. Westerterp KR, Kayser B, Wouters L, Le Trong JL, Richalet JP. Energy balance at high altitude of 6,542 m. *J Appl Physiol.* 1994;77:862–866.

89. Pugh LGCE. Physiological and medical aspects of the Himalayan scientific and mountaineering expedition, 1960–61. *Br Med J.* 1962;5305:621–627.

90. Ferrus L, Commenges D, Gire J, Varene P. Respiratory water loss as a function of ventilatory or environmental factors. *Respir Physiol.* 1984;56:11–20.

91. Worme JD, Lickteig JA, Reynolds RD, Deuster PA. Consumption of a dehydrated ration for 31 days at moderate altitude: Energy balance and physical performance. *J Am Diet Assoc.* 1991;91:1543–1549.

92. Reynolds RD, Lickteig JA, Howard MP, Deuster PA. Intakes of high fat and high carbohydrate foods by humans increased with exposure to increasing altitude during an expedition to Mt. Everest. *J Nutr.* 1998;128:50–55.

93. Reynolds RD, Lickteig JA, Deuster PA, et al. Energy metabolism increases and regional body fat decreases while regional muscle mass is spared in humans climbing Mt. Everest. *J Nutr.* 1999;129:1307–1314.

94. Johnson HL, Consolazio CF, Daws TA, Krzywicki HJ. Increased energy requirements of man after abrupt altitude exposure. *Nutr Rep Intl.* 1971;4:77–82.

95. Hannon JP, Sudman DM. Basal metabolic rate and cardiovascular function of women during altitude acclimatization. *J Appl Physiol.* 1973;34:471–477.

96. Rose MS, Houston CS, Fulco CS, Coates G, Sutton JR, Cymerman A. Operation Everest II: Nutrition and body composition. *J Appl Physiol.* 1988;65:2545–2551.

97. Kayser B, Narici M, Milesi S, Grassi B, Cerretelli P. Body composition and maximum alactic anaerobic performance during a one month stay at high altitude. *Int J Sports Med.* 1993;14:244–247.

98. Hansen JE, Hartley LH, Hogan RP III. Arterial oxygen increase by high-carbohydrate diet at altitude. *J Appl Physiol.* 1972;33:441–445.

99. Consolazio CF, Matoush LO, Johnson HL, Krzywicki HJ, Daws TA, Isaac GJ. Effects of high-carbohydrate diets on performance and clinical symptomatology after rapid ascent to high altitude. *Fed Proc.* 1969;28:937–943.

100. Berglund B. High-altitude training: Aspects of haematological adaptation. *Sports Med.* 1992;14:289–303.

101. Worme JD, Moser-Veillon PB, Douglas LW, Deuster PA. Changes in iron status during exposure to moderate altitudes. *J Wilderness Med.* 1992;3:18–26.

102. Deuster PA, Gallagher KL, Singh, Reynolds RD. Consumption of a dehydrated ration for 31 days at moderate altitudes: Status of zinc, copper and vitamin B_6. *J Am Diet Assoc.* 1992;92:1372–1375.

103. Simon-Schnass IM. Nutrition at high altitude. *J Nutr.* 1992;122:778–781.

104. Simon-Schnass IM, Pabst H. Influence of vitamin E on physical performance. *Int J Vitam Nutr Res.* 1988;58:49–54.

105. Marriot BM, Carlson-Newberry SJ, Institute of Medicine Committee on Military Nutrition Research. *Nutritional Needs in Cold and in High-altitude Environments: Applications for Military Personnel in Field Operations.* Washington, DC: National Academy Press; 1996.

106. Natick Research, Development and Engineering Center. *Operational Rations of the Department of Defense.* 3rd ed. Natick, Mass: US Army Soldier Systems Command. Natick PAM 30–25.

Chapter 18

HEALTH CARE FOR WOMEN IN MOBILIZATION AND DEPLOYMENT

LISA KEEP, MD, MPH

L. Keep; Lieutenant Colonel, Medical Corps; Residency Director, General Preventive Medicine Residency, Walter Reed Army Institute of Research, Silver Spring, MD 20190-7500

INTRODUCTION

There is a long history of individual women or small numbers of women in the US military. It has not been until recently, though, that women have been present in larger proportions and fully integrated into the services, including in jobs with greater exposure to hardship and combat. From a medical standpoint, this change has meant that medical needs particular to women must be met in garrison, on deployment, and on redeployment. The new roles filled by women make the logistics of providing appropriate supplies and equipment and trained health care personnel wherever women may be in the theater more challenging than in the past. In addition, women as a population may have somewhat different risk factors than men for adverse outcomes such as injury or posttraumatic stress disorder. Knowledge of such differences could lead to changes in equipment or training to minimize the risk. Because the integration of large numbers of women has been such a recent phenomenon, little is known about many of the factors that may affect the health of deployed women. Most of the studies that have been done have focused on populations that were accessible to study, such as those in initial entry training, rather than deployed populations. This chapter attempts to summarize both what is known about factors influencing the health and health care of women in mobilization and deployment and what remains to be studied. If the reader wants more specific information, a CD-ROM containing lectures and videos on common problems in obstetrics and gynecology and references, including manuals, treatment protocols, and Department of Defense Instructions, is now available.[1] It includes information on treatment of refugees and prisoners of war and includes telephone numbers to military hospital obstetrics and gynecology clinics and labor and delivery decks to allow users to contact expert help at any time. Forms needed to document care can be printed, and a correspondence course covering the contents of the CD-ROM and which grants Continuing Medical Education credit is included.

Most of the issues regarding health on deployment concern both men and women. However, because women constitute an increasing proportion of the military and because the female's social circumstances, anatomy, and physiology may relate to the military environment differently than the male's, the Committee on Defense Women's Health Research was convened in 1995 under the auspices of the Institute of Medicine of the National Academy of Sciences. Its mission was to advise the US Army Medical Research and Materiel Command on gaps and strengths in current research relating to the health and performance of military women and to provide guidance on establishing research funding priorities. Factors affecting health care while deployed that were identified by the Committee included austere conditions, harsh geography and weather, primitive housing and sanitary facilities, potential for limited supplies and difficult access to health care personnel or facilities, and exposure to diseases and prophylactic medications and immunizations. Potential military health hazards identified by the Committee included fuels and lubricants, pesticides, dust, smoke, obscurants, electromagnetic radiation (eg, laser range finders and target designators; radio-frequency, microwave, and millimeter-wave communications; electronic warfare equipment) and chemical warfare defense using prophylaxis with drugs.[2] While the differences between men and women regarding these factors and potential military health hazards are fewer than are the similarities, there are issues for which differences are significant enough to warrant consideration or for which differences may exist but data are insufficient to either confirm or refute any hypothesis.

DEMOGRAPHICS

In 1997, the approximately 200,000 women on active duty constituted approximately 14% of the US force.[2,3] There were roughly 140,000 women in the Reserve Component in 1995, constituting 16% of the Reserve force.[2] Projections are that women may constitute 20% of the active duty force in the near future.[2,4] By contrast, women constituted 2% of the force in 1972.[4] In 1995, there were approximately the same proportion of female officers as enlisted in each service. Among officers, 61% were in either health care or administrative primary occupations. Among enlisted women, 49% held primary occupations in functional supply/administrative or health care fields.[2] The distribution of all women between services in 1995 is shown in Figure 18-1, their racial distribution is shown in Figure 18-2, and their age distribution is shown in Figure 18-3. In 1997, women were disproportionately single (44%) compared to men (37%) on active duty.[3] Women were also disproportionately single parents: 11% versus 2.6% for men.[5]

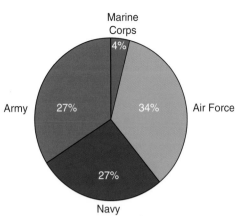

Fig. 18-1. Distribution of All Active Duty Females by Service, 1995.
Source: Committee on Defense Women's Health Research, Institute of Medicine. *Recommendations for Research on the Health of Military Women*. Washington, DC: National Academy Press; 1995: 8.

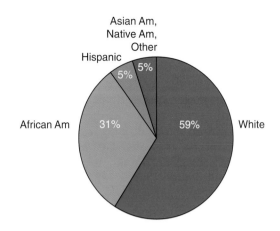

Fig. 18-2. Distribution of All Active Duty Females by Race and Ethnic Group, 1995.
Source: Committee on Defense Women's Health Research, Institute of Medicine. *Recommendations for Research on the Health of Military Women*. Washington, DC: National Academy Press; 1995: 8.

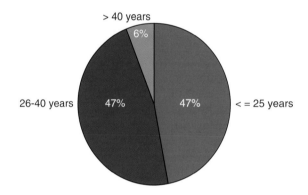

Fig. 18-3. Distribution of All Active Duty Females by Age, 1995.
Source: Committee on Defense Women's Health Research, Institute of Medicine. *Recommendations for Research on the Health of Military Women*. Washington, DC: National Academy Press; 1995: 9.

GENERAL HEALTH CARE NEEDS AND UTILIZATION

Few studies have been done on health care needs and utilization among women service members, but there are data to support that they use health care more often than their male counterparts and for different complaints. A large 1997 prospective outpatient morbidity study was done among US soldiers serving in South Korea and at Fort Lewis, Wash.[6] South Korea is considered by some to represent a "semideployed" environment. The study captured outpatient data for approximately 6,500 women and 28,000 men. Women were found to access clinics at rates approximately twice that of men even after standardization for age, race, rank, level of civilian education, and type of unit (weekly clinic visits per 1,000 population for females: South Korea 116.8,

Fort Lewis 103.4; for males: South Korea 59.7, Fort Lewis 60.4). This rate ratio did not change significantly even after excluding sex-specific diagnoses. Women in South Korea had clinic utilization rates 10% greater than that of their Fort Lewis counterparts, resulting in an additional 11 visits per 1,000 per week. The category with the highest proportion of visits was "injuries and other orthopedic conditions" for all but women at Fort Lewis, for whom "medical illness" conditions prevailed. Clinic visit rates for the injuries category for both sexes were roughly equal, unlike the results found in most other studies. Injuries accounted for more than 40% of all visits for men at either location but for women at either location, injury visits accounted for less than 25% of all visits.

GYNECOLOGIC CARE, SEXUALLY TRANSMITTED DISEASES, SEXUAL RISK BEHAVIORS, AND PREGNANCY

Gynecologic care, sexually transmitted diseases, sexual risk behaviors, and pregnancy are interrelated and constitute the area of greatest difference between deployed men and women since they are related to our most significant biological differences.

Gynecologic Care

The need for routine gynecologic care is an area of women's health during deployment that requires significant resources. A review of women's health needs during the Persian Gulf War by Murphy and colleagues[4] showed that, although men and women had similar complaints in general, 20% to 25% of women's outpatient visits were for gynecologic complaints. The most common reasons for gynecologic visits were requests for oral contraceptives, fungal vaginitis, and abnormal menses (thought to be primarily related to stress and discontinuation of oral contraceptives). Few women required hospitalization for gynecologic complaints. The most common reason for a woman to be evacuated out of theater was pregnancy. Another common reason was for evaluation of abnormal cervical cytology for Papanicolaou (Pap) smears for which results were not available before deployment. (There was no colposcope in-theater, so those needing evaluation were sent to Germany.)[7]

A 1998 Navy study of sailors on four ships stationed on the east coast of the United States surveyed 1,154 volunteers drawn from those who were present for duty on the day of the study.[8] Women reported attending sick call significantly more often than men (189 vs. 117 visits per week per 1,000 personnel). Non–sex-specific reasons for attending sick call were generally similar and were most often for a cold, sore throat, cough, headache, or accident or injury. The female-specific reasons reported for attending sick call were requests for oral contraceptives, vaginal discharge or yeast infection, menstrual cramps, menstrual irregularity, pregnancy check, and Pap smear. Eleven percent of these women reported having been unable to obtain their usual form of birth control during deployment.

Adequacy of Training and Supplies

A Navy study of health care providers' perceptions of shipboard women's health care showed that 56% of the 32 health care providers (all represent-

ing different ships) thought their clinics were understaffed, though 91% reported having an Authorized Medical Allowance List (AMAL) designed specifically for women at sea and 81% reported adequate pregnancy testing supplies.[9] Their primary recommendation for improvement was to increase the amount and types of birth control available. They also reported insufficient budgets (47%) and AMALs (44%). Suggestions for improvement of AMALs included increased supplies of injectable depo-medroxyprogesterone acetate (Depo-Provera), a greater variety of oral contraceptives, and more accurate pregnancy and sexually transmitted disease (STD) testing kits. Sufficient obstetrics and gynecologic training was reported by 81%, and 75% reported having ample female-specific diagnostic equipment. However, there was a statistically significant difference between medical officers and Independent Duty Corpsmen (IDC) or senior enlisted corpsmen regarding their evaluation of the sufficiency of their training in obstetrics and gynecology, with medical officers expressing greater confidence in their level of training.

Potential problems related to these issues can be anticipated and many of them prevented. Health care providers who deploy and who can be expected to care for women should be trained to provide a basic, minimum level of routine gynecologic care. Medications, supplies, and equipment should be on hand or ordered before deployment, and the literature can provide guidance on specific items and planning factors.

Medications

Deploying service members should carry a 6- to 12-month supply of personal medications, and this should reflect consideration of the potential need for contraception and nonsteroidal antiinflammatory drugs for treatment of menstrual cramps. Self-treatment packs issued to women before deployment for treatment of fungal vaginitis and urinary tract infection (UTI) may be considered. Some authorities suggest that supplies of Depo-Provera may be given to the service member to be carried, then administered by medical personnel.[10] Since spotting and intermenstrual bleeding are common, however, this method of birth control may not be tolerated if started just before deployment. Note should be taken that six 28-day oral contraceptive pill (OCP) cycles do not equal 6 calendar months; a minimum of 7 cycles of OCPs may be necessary to ensure a sufficient supply until the medical logistic system can be expected to supply refills of routine medications.[10] Even though a woman may not anticipate having sexual intercourse while deployed, she should be cautious about discontinuing her oral contraceptives, as the subsequent possible increase in menstrual flow and cramping may cause her to seek medical evaluation.

Birth Control

Methods of birth control other than the above-mentioned oral contraceptive pills and Depo-Provera may be particularly convenient for some deployed women. These include Norplant, a continuous-release levonorgestrel product contained in six matchstick-sized (34 mm x 2.4 mm) silicone rubber tubing capsules, which are implanted under the skin of the arm and which provide protection for 5 years; and the intrauterine device (IUD), which can last for up to 10 years. A common reason Norplant users request removal of the device is frequent and irregular menstrual spotting, so users should be informed of this possibility before implantation. If implantation is carried out shortly before deployment and the woman becomes dissatisfied with the method, access to a physician with experience in removal could be problematic while she is deployed. Placement of the rods under the skin of the upper arm may interfere with comfortable wear of the rolled Battle Dress Uniform sleeve. Not all service members will be appropriate candidates for an IUD, since it is associated with increased rates of pelvic inflammatory disease, especially in those who are not in permanent monogamous sexual relationships. Those in monogamous relationships that follow one after another are also at increased risk of pelvic inflammatory disease. It should be kept in mind that the social forces and stress of deployment may result in situations in which service members have unanticipated sexual relationships. None of the above-mentioned methods provide protection against sexually transmitted diseases. Barrier methods of birth control, which do provide such protection, can be used in addition to these methods, but the service member must carry all supplies and should be aware that extremes of temperature during storage can decrease the integrity of latex. Used alone for prevention of pregnancy, barrier methods have higher failure rates than do IUDs or hormonal methods.

Drug Interaction and Metabolism

As with any drug, there may be adverse events associated with drugs commonly used by women.

Incidence of candidal vaginitis increases after use of antibiotics such as doxycycline, which may be used as an antimalarial. Antimicrobials may also reduce the effectiveness of oral contraceptives in a small subset of women.[11] It may be advisable to recommend use of an additional method of birth control, such as a barrier method or abstinence, while the woman is taking antimicrobials.

There are incomplete data on the effects and interaction of sex, ethnicity, and menstrual cycle on drug metabolism. Drugs of interest include those more likely to be used by military personnel (eg, those for chemical or biological defense, antimalarials) or used frequently in military women (eg, OCPs, antifungals, analgesics). The Committee on Defense Women's Health Research recommended research in these areas,[2] but until such research is conducted health care practitioners should consider the possibility that there may be such effects in women that could change the bioavailability of medications.

Sexually Transmitted Diseases and Sexual Risk Behaviors

Because of their generally young age (and corresponding maturity level) and because of their often sudden popularity in a population that is 85% male, women service members, particularly those in the lower enlisted ranks, are at risk for STDs and unintended pregnancy. The results of the few studies that have been done to quantify sexual risk behaviors may help health care providers to plan interventions. A survey of 594 unmarried in-processing female US Army recruits showed that although 87% reported having had vaginal sex, 26% reported a previous pregnancy, and 14% reported a previous STD infection, almost 41% of respondents used condoms "never," "rarely," or "occasionally."[12] Recruits who reported using alcohol were significantly less likely to report using condoms and were more likely to report a higher total number of sexual partners. Twenty-nine percent of the respondents reported "rarely" or "never" receiving pelvic examinations, and 19% reported receiving "occasional" pelvic examinations. Forty-five percent of the respondents reported that they would feel embarrassed to ask a health care provider about STDs even though 88% of these reported being sexually active. "Friends" were reported as the most common source of sex education. Asked about STD prevention methods with casual sex partners, 42% were nonresponders, 16% reported "no method," and 36% reported using a condom or a condom with spermicide. Almost 47% of respondents did not consider themselves to be at risk for contracting an STD.

Among a convenience sample of 104 US Army recruits presenting to the gynecology clinic for an appointment[13], 29% reported using no method of birth control, 29% reported using a condom, and 43% reported using oral contraceptives. Thirty-four percent reported the combined set of risk factors of more than one lifetime sexual partner, a new sexual partner in the last 6 months, and not using a condom.

Among 165 ship- and shore-based Navy women surveyed[14], 41% did not use any method of protection against STDs and 48% used a condom. Fifty-eight percent reported not worrying about getting an STD, but 72% reported worrying about their ability to have their partner use a condom.

Actions

Periodic routine predeployment checks, such as Soldier Readiness Checks, could mandate periodic pelvic and breast exams to ensure that these are done and that results are known before deployment. Since the Persian Gulf War, newer methods of cervical screening (eg, automated cytologic testing, fluid-based monolayers, human papillomavirus DNA testing, cervicography, Polarprobe optoelectronics) have become available and are likely to change patient management. These changes may make it possible to obtain more definitive diagnoses more quickly so that the burden of following up indeterminate Pap smear results will be either reduced or eliminated.

As part of a program to reinforce health and safety measures to all service members in the predeployment period, information about and access to effective methods of birth control and STD prevention can be provided. Ideally, information about sexual decision-making could be offered on a routine basis, since time for such education might be too short in the predeployment period. Pregnancy testing should be offered just before deployment to those who think they could possibly be pregnant. Female service members should be informed that there are known and unknown risks to the fetus from a variety of sources during deployment. The only ways to absolutely protect a fetus from these risks are either to not become pregnant or to detect the pregnancy before deployment and so avoid deploying (Figure 18-4).

Mandatory predeployment pregnancy testing for all women may not be cost-effective. Some time limit would have to be set such that the mandatory test would be conducted "x" or fewer days before departure. Deployment dates often change more than once before actual departure, so multiple tests might be required to satisfy the time requirement. Some units, especially those not collocated with other elements of their larger unit, travel from their home stations to

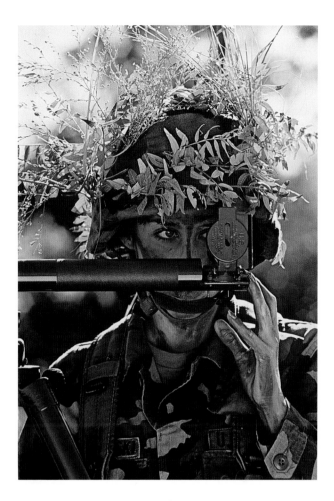

Fig. 18-4. There are known and unknown infectious, toxic, and environmental risks to the fetus during deployment. The possible risks for this soldier include heat injury and prophylaxis against malaria or chemical weapons. Photo source: Department of Defense photograph. Defense Visual Information Center. *Women in the U.S. Armed Forces*. CD-ROM. March Field, Calif: DVIC; 1998. Image 88-04612.

other locations before deploying, often spending a number of weeks at the new site. Testing might be required before departure from each station, increasing costs. Because of the duty positions women hold, some units have far more than the tri-service average of females, and repeated absence for testing by such a large percentage of the unit could adversely affect predeployment preparation. There are women who are not sexually active or who either use an effective method of birth control or have been sterilized; the likelihood of pregnancy in these women is low to nonexistent, but they could well be included in any such mandatory pregnancy testing program. Any testing program can miss those who become pregnant after the test but before deployment. In addition, some of those redeployed because of pregnancy become pregnant in-theater. Given the results of the above studies regarding sexual risk behaviors, the possibility must be conceded that not all of those who would be at risk of being pregnant would recognize their situation or take the initiative to obtain the pregnancy test. Formal studies of the cost-effectiveness of predeployment pregnancy testing would be welcome.

Pregnancy

Unplanned Pregnancy

One of the concerns identified by the Defense Advisory Committee on Women in the Services (DACOWITS) in 1994 was for the effects of unplanned pregnancy on the individual woman, on military women as a whole, and on the unit.[2] Unplanned pregnancy in an unmarried service member presents her with difficult decisions on such issues as termination of the pregnancy, adoption, single motherhood, and marriage. Each of these decisions affects the child as well as the mother. The emotional burden on the mother of aborting her child or giving it up for adoption may be significant. Military life can be challenging for single service members even without children; the responsibility of caring for children adds enormously to this challenge. For all of these reasons, unplanned pregnancy has significant effects on the individual involved. Because pregnancy is such a visible condition, because it may be regarded by unit members as voluntary or intentional, and because it impacts significantly on a woman's deployability and sometimes on her ability to fully perform in her primary occupation for most of a year, it can affect unit morale and readiness. Some may view women as less useful service members or resent the special treatment of pregnant women.

Clark and colleagues[15] studied pregnant soldiers presenting for prenatal care at Fort Lewis, Wash. The authors found that junior enlisted women had the highest percentage of unintended pregnancies in this population. Rank was strongly associated with other factors that themselves are associated with higher rates of unplanned pregnancy, such as age, marital status, and education level. They state that "…rank may be used…as an easily available surrogate marker…for identification of soldiers at greatest risk of unintended pregnancy."[15p447] Among those whose pregnancies were unintended, 62% did not use contraceptives and 38% experienced contraceptive failure. The most common reasons for not using contraception were adverse effects of contraceptives, not planning to have sex, and not believing they would become pregnant. Lack of access to care was not given

as a reason for not using contraceptives in this study, though this factor may vary by branch of service, duty location, or type of unit. The methods employed by those using contraceptives were not the most effective methods and required "motivation and consistency,"[15(p448)] in the words of the authors. The study recommends five strategies developed by the Institute of Medicine to reduce unintended pregnancy (Exhibit 18-1).

Classes to educate women, especially those in the lower enlisted ranks, and to discuss issues surrounding sexual decision making, methods of birth control, the consequences of unintended pregnancy, and STD prevention could be offered periodically or at the time of each transfer to a new duty station, perhaps with an additional class or classes offered when a unit is notified it may be deploying. In-processing procedures could include offering women the opportunity to be seen by a health care provider, which would allow them to obtain advice, contraceptives, or the Pap smear that can be required before prescription of hormonal contraceptives. Any such program to prevent unintended pregnancies and STDs should be designed to include its evaluation for effectiveness.

Vaccines and Pregnancy

Women and men in deployable status should have their immunization status screened routinely and immunizations updated accordingly. In most instances, therefore, a woman will have already been

---

EXHIBIT 18-1

FIVE STRATEGIES TO REDUCE UNINTENDED PREGNANCIES

1. Improve knowledge about contraception and reproductive health

2. Increase access to contraception

3. Address feelings, attitudes, and motivation associated with contraception and avoiding unintended pregnancies

4. Evaluate the results of any programs designed to prevent unintended pregnancies

5. Stimulate research

Reprinted with permission from *Military Medicine: International Journal of AMSUS*: Clark JB, Holt VL, Miser F. Unintended pregnancy among female soldiers presenting for prenatal care at Madigan Army Medical Center. *Mil Med.* 1998;163:444–448.

immunized before pregnancy occurs. At the time for immunizations to be updated, there is a small chance that a woman will be in the early stages of pregnancy and unaware that she is pregnant. Risk of serious adverse effects from vaccines, even live vaccines, are primarily theoretical. In some cases, a vaccine may even be recommended in pregnancy because the disease the vaccine prevents carries more risk to the fetus than does the vaccine. The military regulation governing immunizations and chemoprophylaxis says the following about immunizing females of childbearing age:

> A pregnancy screening test is not routinely required prior to administering vaccines or toxoids, including live virus vaccines, to females of childbearing age. Take the following precautions to avoid unintentional immunization during pregnancy:
>
> Ask if pregnant. If the answer is "yes" or "maybe" exclude from immunization or refer for evaluation. If the answer is "no," immunize. If a live virus vaccine is administered, counsel the individual to avoid becoming pregnant for three months and document in the health record.[16p3–4]

Drugs and Pregnancy

If a female service member is diagnosed as pregnant in a theater of operations, immediate consideration must be given to the potential effects of maternal medications on the fetus. The woman may be taking certain medications for operational reasons so consideration must also be given to the effect of stopping or prohibiting use of such medications. For example, if the service member is on flight status or is deployed to certain geographic areas, she may be taking doxycycline as an antimalarial, and this drug can adversely affect fetal bones and teeth. While this prophylactic medication should be discontinued immediately, the service member will have to be housed in such a way as to protect her from potential exposure to mosquitoes to ensure that she is not infected with malaria while awaiting evacuation. If there is a threat of biological or chemical weapon use in the theater, the service member must be counseled on whether to use any available prophylactic medication while awaiting evacuation. This topic is too broad for thorough coverage in this format, and the clinician should consult standard texts or seek expert consultation for such cases.

Infections and Pregnancy

Some infections, such as malaria, rubella, and toxoplasmosis, result in higher rates of morbidity and mortality in pregnancy (see chapters in Section 6: Infectious Diseases of Concern). The female service member may be at higher risk of exposure to agents causing such diseases in a deployed setting, and the clinician should keep this possibility in mind.

URINARY TRACT INFECTIONS

UTIs are more common among women than men and may be more common in the field. There may be no latrine facilities available and privacy may be minimal. In such conditions, some women will wait as long as possible before urinating. Maintaining a full bladder increases risk for UTI. Some women will intentionally dehydrate themselves to avoid urinating. Such dehydration puts them at risk for heat or cold injury. Educating women about UTIs and the risks associated with dehydration, providing latrines with privacy if possible, and educating women about field-expedient methods to avoid exposure of the body during urination are actions that can be taken to decrease the risk of UTI and dehydration. Simple measures such as using a urinary diversion device, donning a poncho to use as a privacy screen while squatting outdoors, or urinating while inside a tent or other field-expedient enclosure into a ziplock bag, coffee can, or other container for later disposal can be effective in affording some privacy to women while urinating. Urinary diversion devices are funnel-like devices that allow a woman to urinate through the trouser fly while standing.

PRIVACY

Although military women prefer privacy for elimination functions, they may also prefer to be housed with their unit in the field rather than in a separate women's area. One concern identified by DACOWITS was "avoidance of artificial separations for women, eg, overconcern for special female facilities."[2(p30)] Men's concerns for privacy or their desire not to be close to women in their living quarters should be given equal consideration.

PERSONAL HYGIENE

Information can be provided to women on personal hygiene in the field and may help reduce the number of cases of vaginitis and UTI. Army Community Health Nurses and their equivalent in the other services, family practitioners, nurse practitioners, obstetrician-gynecologists, and others can assist with such training. The information can include advice to

- use unscented products (eg, soaps, sanitary pads) because perfumes can cause chemical vaginitis
- use tampons and sanitary pads without deodorant or baking soda (these can alter vaginal pH),
- use tampons with cardboard applicators (plastic applicators can abrade vaginal mucosa; dirty hands can soil tampons without

applicators before insertion),
- change tampons and pads frequently,
- clean pubic area with unscented wet wipes if showers are not available, and
- wear loose-fitting trousers.[10]

There is no medical need for special shower facilities for women or for more frequent showers for women. If shower facilities are available, women may prefer to shower more frequently than men. Maintenance of good personal hygiene in both sexes reduces the incidence of skin disease caused by extended contact with filth. Since the dermatological diagnostic category typically has one of the highest rates of outpatient visits, provision of showers or other facilities that encourage personal hygiene may decrease such visits and improve service member health.

ERGONOMICS, INJURY, AND FITNESS

Ergonomics

Another of the concerns identified by DACOWITS regarded the fit of uniforms, boots, and masks. The Committee on Defense Women's Health Research found in 1995 that the risk of injury may be higher for women using clothing, equipment, tools, protective gear, and prescribed methods designed for

men (Figure 18-5). Data on this subject are incomplete, and the Committee recommended further research on anthropometric data for sizing and design to fit a variety of body shapes, differences in thermal balance when wearing body heating and cooling systems, and endurance when loads are mounted in different configurations on various body locations.[2]

a
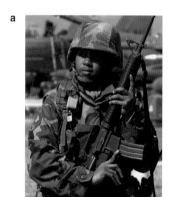
b
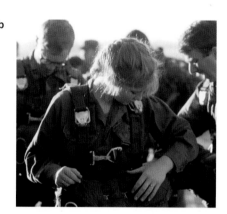
c
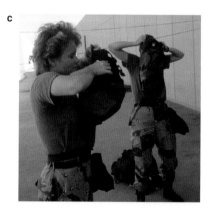

Fig. 18-5. Every day, female soldiers use gear designed for their male counterparts such as load-carrying equipment and weapons (**a**), parachute harnesses (**b**), and gas masks (**c**). It is unclear whether use of clothing and equipment by women that was designed for use by men leads to increased rates of injury or other adverse outcomes.
Photo sources: (a) Department of Defense photograph. Operational Medicine and Fleet Support Division, Bureau of Medicine and Surgery, Department of the Navy. *Operational Obstetrics and Gynecology: The Health Care of Women in Military Settings.* 2nd ed. CD-ROM. Washington, DC: DN; 2000. NAVMEDPUB 6300-2C. Image "Field Gear." (b) Department of Defense photograph. Defense Visual Information Center. *Women in the U.S. Armed Forces.* CD-ROM. March Field, Calif: DVIC; 1998. Image 87-02152. (c) Department of Defense photograph. Defense Visual Information Center. *Women in the U.S. Armed Forces.* CD-ROM. March Field, Calif: DVIC; 1998. Image 92-06818.

Factors in women that can adversely affect thermoregulation relative to men include generally higher surface-to-mass ratio, higher percentage of body fat, and lower maximal aerobic power. A 1992 review of temperature regulation in women[17] stated that "[t]here is little support for the theory that gender affects thermoregulatory ability if all factors that independently and/or collectively affect thermoregulation, such as maximal aerobic power, state of training, or heat acclimation, are controlled."[17p201] It also noted that "during light exercise in hot environments, little difference is seen in exercise core temperature during different menstrual cycle phases."[17p205] However, there is an upward shift in the temperature set-point of about one half of one degree (0.4°C, 0.7°F) during the luteal (post-ovulatory) phase of the menstrual cycle, and this shift seems to delay onset of sweating and cutaneous vasodilation. There are also changes in fluid volume control with menstrual phase, which can affect thermoregulation. These temperature and fluid shifts may be statistically significant, but whether they are clinically significant for the work performance of female service members remains unclear.

A small study compared oxygen uptake ($\dot{V}o_2$) and heart rate in men and women performing nine occupational tasks in both standard military uniform and chemical protective ensemble (CPE; ie, M-17 mask and chemical protective clothing).[18] It showed that tasks requiring mobility across a distance, such as load carriage or lift and carry, resulted in significant increases in both $\dot{V}o_2$ and heart rate among both men and women wearing the CPE. Stationary tasks (eg, lifting and lowering) resulted in no differences in $\dot{V}o_2$ or heart rate between the two clothing conditions in either men or women. The meager data available indicate that the similarities between men and women are greater than the differences regarding work effort while wearing the CPE. More studies must be done, however, before conclusions can be drawn.

Injuries

Most of the data on injuries in military women focus on the basic training or initial entry environment (Figure 18-6). A 1997 review[19] of the patterns and risk factors for exercise-related injuries in all military women found that level of aerobic fitness is a primary risk factor for exercise-related injury in both women and men, with higher levels of fitness associated with lower injury rates. The review also noted that basic training injury rates are generally 1.5 to 2 times higher in women than in men.

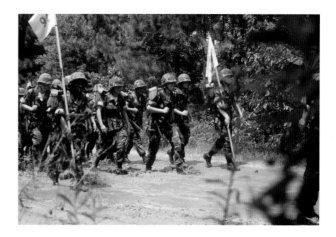

Fig. 18-6. Activities like running and marching can cause overuse injuries. Women, such as these Marine Corps recruits, are at higher risk of overuse injuries than are men. Photo source: Department of Defense photograph. Defense Visual Information Center. *Women in the U.S. Armed Forces.* CD-ROM. March Field, Calif: DVIC; 1998. Image 84-11808.

A study[20] among Army basic trainees showed that though women's relative risk for injury was 2.1 times that of men, multivariate analysis revealed that female sex was no longer predictive of injuries, but physical fitness, particularly aerobic fitness, remained significant. The authors concluded that women enter training less physically fit relative to both their own fitness potential and to men. Women, however, made much greater improvements in fitness than men, indicating that remedial training for those who enter training less fit could potentially reduce both total injuries and the difference in risk of injuries between men and women.

Overuse injuries, rather than acute injuries, are more common in women than in men and tobacco may be one risk factor. A study[21] found that recruits who reported smoking at least one cigarette in the month before beginning basic training had significantly higher rates of any injury during basic training than those who did not. Thirty-five percent of both women and men reported having smoked at least one cigarette in the month prior to basic training, but only women had significantly higher rates of overuse injury. A 1994 study[22] in an all-male infantry unit also found cigarette smoking to be an independent risk factor for injury.

A 1999 prospective study[23] of all female trainees at the Marine Corps Recruit Depot (MCRD), Parris Island, SC; the Navy Recruit Training Command (RTC), Great Lakes, Ill; and the Marine Corps Officer Candidate School (OCS), Quantico, Va, showed that most (32% to 45%) of the visits for a new health problem were for musculoskeletal disorders. Musculoskeletal injuries occured in 44% of female recruits at MCRD, 37% of female recruits at RTC, and 62% of female officer candidates at OCS. The most common category of musculoskeletal injury in all three populations was overuse injury. Stress fractures were diagnosed in about 6% of recruits at MCRD, 4% of recruits at RTC, and almost 10% of OCS candidates. Comparison data for males at the sites were not available.

The Institute of Medicine's Subcommittee on Body Composition, Nutrition, and Health of Military Women of the Committee on Military Nutrition Research recommended that female recruits either undergo a structured fitness program before entry into basic or initial entry training or a similar program within basic training.[24] The program would be designed to start at a lower level of activity and gradually increase so that stressed bones would have time to remodel before stress fractures occur. Fitness Training Units operate in Army basic training, and a 1998 study[25] showed that the Unit appeared to be effective in reducing injuries and increasing training success in women, but the authors recommended modifications for male participants to improve outcomes. The other services use similar units to improve fitness before releasing recruits to initial entry training.

A study[26] of injury among male and female Army parachutists found that though women jump under less hazardous conditions than men, they have a higher risk of serious injury. This result could be because women were more likely to be in a cadet or student status than men, but the study did not address this issue. Based on data reported to the US Army Safety Center during a 10-year period, women jumped more often than men in daylight and in static-line, nontactical environments and were more likely to have had their injury caused by an improper parachute landing fall, which are all consistent with cadet or student status. It is also possible that the design of the parachute and harness results in more injuries in females than in males. However, over the course of the 10-year period, women's injury rates dropped more than, and in fact began to approach, men's injury rates. It can be speculated that this was because women gained experience and proficiency, but no data are available on which to base a conclusion. Further research is needed to answer questions regarding the relationship of injury in military women to flexibility, body composition, tobacco and alcohol use, anatomic and biomechanical characteristics, and level of training and experience.

Hospitalizations for sports and physical training injuries were studied using the Total Army Injury and Health Outcomes Database (TAIHOD).[27] The rate (number of injuries per 10,000 person-years) of such injuries was approximately twice as high among men as among women, the opposite of the rate usually found in studies of the basic training environment. The study's authors note, however, that a major limitation of the study was the lack of data on level of exposure of the subjects to each activity; the denominator for rates was person-time on active duty. The body parts most commonly injured by both men and women were the knee and ankle. Among men, basketball and football were associated with the highest hospitalization injury rates. Among women, "other" sports—those not included in specific categories, such as running and volleyball—were associated with the highest hospitalization injury rates. In the specific sport categories, physical training and basketball posed the greatest risks. A study[28] using data accessed through the Defense Medical Surveillance System showed that females were 28% more likely to have injury-related outpatient visits but 35% less likely to be hospitalized for injury than males.

A study of musculoskeletal-related disability among Army personnel used data from the US Army Physical Disability Agency database and was restricted to cases from 1990 to 1994 in which the soldier was found unfit for duty and either separated from service or temporarily or permanently retired.[29] Musculoskeletal disability rates were reported by Military Occupational Specialty (MOS) (cases/1,000 in the MOS during the same time period). Among the 20 MOSs with the highest musculoskeletal disability rates for women, women's rates significantly exceeded men's in 15. The authors recommend prospective studies of job type and musculoskeletal disability.

Fitness and Job Performance

How the physical strength and fitness of military women affect job performance in the field is a controversial topic. The Committee on Defense Women's Health Research noted that the repeal of the Combat Exclusion Law opened up many new and dangerous jobs to women. Some of these jobs may have high requirements for strength and endurance, but the physical fitness testing programs in the Armed Forces relate to general health, physical fitness, or appearance, not to specific job performance.[30] Physical fitness has three components: muscular strength, muscular endurance, and cardiopulmonary fitness.[31]

Strength distribution curves for Army men and women overlap least when comparing absolute strength, with overlap increasing when adjusted for body mass and reaching near-parity when adjusted for fat-free body mass. The quantity of muscle mass differs between men and women, resulting in differences in absolute strength, though relative strength is approximately equal. On average, female soldiers weigh 20% less and have 10% more body fat and 30% less fat-free body mass than male soldiers.[31] Performance on tasks reflective of muscle strength that have relevance to military jobs, such as lifting, pulling, pushing, and carrying loads, is related to fat-free mass but is related little if at all to the proportion of body fat (Figure 18-7).[30,31]

Similarly, women and men have been shown to have essentially equal muscular endurance when exercising at a given percentage of maximal strength.[31] For any given absolute load, however, the average woman will use a greater percentage of her maximum strength than the average man and will therefore fatigue faster.

Cardiopulmonary fitness or aerobic power is measured by maximal oxygen uptake, $\dot{V}o_2$max. Women have a lower $\dot{V}o_2$max than equally trained men because of men's greater fat-free mass and women's greater body fat, lower hemoglobin levels, and lower cardiac output. Among Army basic trainees, the female-to-male $\dot{V}o_2$max ratio was 0.63 in absolute terms and 0.75 when adjusted for body weight. Among cadets at the US Military Academy, the ratios were 0.67 and 0.82, respectively.[31]

Overcoming Strength Limitations

Physical training may be able to overcome some of the differences in these three components of physical fitness between the average man and the average woman. Progressive resistance training can result in increases in muscular strength and aerobic exercise, and training can result in increases in $\dot{V}o_2$max. The lower the initial state of training or fitness, the more potential there is for improvement. Such improvements in muscular strength and endurance and in cardiopulmonary fitness may enable women to adequately perform many physically demanding jobs.[31,32]

Changes in aerobic power and muscle strength were measured in male and female cadets attending the US Military Academy between 1979 and 1982.[33] The authors conclude that even given a 2-year experience in similar training programs and with similar social, cultural, and environmental factors, the gap in aerobic power and muscle strength did not narrow significantly. On arrival, women scored at the high end of the "good" category of the American Heart Association's cardiorespiratory fitness classification, whereas men far exceeded the lower limit of the "high" category. Females, but not males, significantly increased their $\dot{V}o_2$max after the initial 6-week training program in which all cadets participate. Among men, change in $\dot{V}o_2$max seemed to be related to level of fitness and activity before arrival; those who were most fit lost $\dot{V}o_2$max over the 6-week period, while those who were least fit gained. Both males and females significantly reduced their maximum heart rate and percent body fat. Additional measurements were taken before and after the second summer training program and after the second academic year. Percent body fat had returned to initial values in both men and women. $\dot{V}o_2$max among females decreased over the course of the second academic year, possibly due to time lost from training because of injury. Lean body mass increased, but maximal isometric strength showed no change. Among males, $\dot{V}o_2$max and lean body mass increased significantly over the 2-year period, as did strength of the upper torso (arm and shoulder) and leg extensors. For all strength measures, women averaged 30% to 40% lower than males.

The influence of physical fitness training on the manual material-handling capability of female sol-

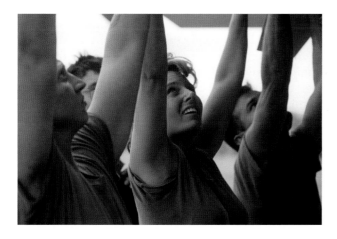

Figure 18-7. Airmen load a missile onto an F-15 Eagle aircraft. Differences in absolute strength between men and women are related to fat-free body mass; women's absolute strength is typically less than men's, but when adjusted for fat-free body mass, it is approximately equal. Photo source: Department of Defense photograph. Defense Visual Information Center. *Women in the U.S. Armed Forces.* CD-ROM. March Field, Calif: DVIC; 1998. Image 90-09800.

diers was evaluated in a small study published as a technical report in 1996[34] and in the peer-reviewed literature in 1997.[35] The women underwent a progressive resistance and aerobic training program over 14 weeks. The training program did not include any specific material-handling tasks. The time required was about 1 hour per day, 5 days a week. The program was effective in improving manual material handling such that those who completed the program met the lifting qualifications for 15 to 21 additional MOSs, depending on the assumptions used about lift height. However, carrying requirements were ignored. Road-march times were improved to a level of statistical significance, representing a decrease in time of about 1.5 minutes over 5 km of flat paved road.

Other methods that may allow women to perform physically demanding military tasks include self-pacing (if the task allows), redesigning the task to reduce the physical demands, modification of the task through use of performance aids (such as stretcher-carry harnesses), and use of teamwork (Figure 18-8). When allowed to self-pace while backpacking with equal loads, both men and women maintained the same relative exercise intensity of 45% of $\dot{V}O_2$max, though women were walking at a lower speed.[31]

A July 1993 General Accounting Office report titled "Women in the Military: Deployment in the Persian Gulf War" concluded that "[o]verall, the unit commanders and focus group participants gave primarily positive assessments of women's performance in the Persian Gulf War."[36(p2)] But it was also noted that "[s]ome people expressed concerns about women's physical strength capabilities; however teamwork was frequently cited as a way physical strength limitations were overcome for both women and men."[36(p3)] This concept was supported by a study of team lifting in military personnel.[37] As might be expected, individual males and all-male lifting teams could lift more than individual females or all-female lifting teams; mixed-sex teams could lift weights that were intermediate between the male and female maximums. The major limitation of team-lifting is the potential loss of a lifting partner, particularly in a combat environment, when such a situation might leave an average female ineffective in the lifting task until another partner is available.

If none of these methods proves satisfactory for a particular task, then a performance standard could be used as a screen to be sure that only those either already capable of a task or likely to be trainable to be so are permitted to do it.

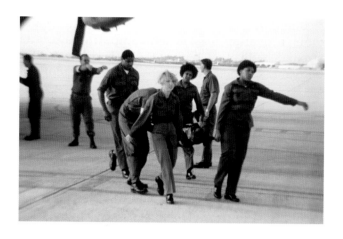

Fig. 18-8. As can be seen in this photograph of Air Force medical personnel assisting simulated casualties during a mass casualty evacuation drill, use of teamwork is one way to allow women to perform physically demanding military tasks.
Photo source: Department of Defense photograph. Defense Visual Information Center. *Women in the U.S. Armed Forces.* CD-ROM. March Field, Calif: DVIC; 1998. Image 84-05647.

Fitness Standards

In the late 1970s, a system was developed to establish occupationally-related, sex-neutral physical fitness standards.[38] A list of physically demanding tasks for each MOS was compiled, and MOSs were grouped into five clusters with similar physical demands for both muscular strength and aerobic capacity (rated as low, medium, or high for each category). From each cluster, the four to six most demanding tasks were selected. For each task, actual weights lifted and distances moved were verified and the actual energy or force required to perform these tasks to standard was measured. The 8-hour average energy cost rate was converted to the necessary aerobic capacity to perform the task, allowing for sufficient reserve to permit recovery and repetition. The standard was then established in liters per minute of oxygen consumption for aerobic demand and weight and distance for strength demand. This standard was then converted to two sets of physical fitness standards, one to be used as an entrance qualification and one for retention. This system was never used (Figure 18-9).

In 1981, the Women in the Army Policy Review Group repeated this task analysis and MOS grouping but based grouping primarily on lifting requirements.[39,40] A set of physical fitness tests, called the Military Enlistment Physical Strength Capacity Test (MEPSCAT), was developed by the US Army Research Institute of Environmental Medicine, Natick,

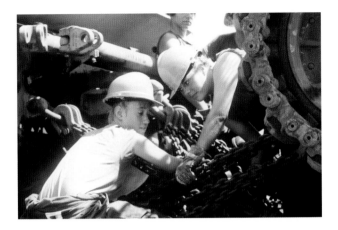

Fig. 18-9. Task-specific, sex-neutral standards for accession and retention in various military occupational specialties have been developed but never put into effect. If they were, potential resentment of females for not "carrying their load" in physically demanding jobs would be diminished or eliminated.
Photo source: Department of Defense photograph. Defense Visual Information Center. *Women in the U.S. Armed Forces.* CD-ROM. March Field, Calif: DVIC; 1998. Image 85-04882.

and described above.[38] Although the lifting test was given to all soldiers entering the Army for several years, the standard was not used to determine eligibility for any MOS, and the effectiveness of the test was never evaluated. It has since been eliminated.[31]

A Navy study[41] showed that Physical Readiness Test scores can be used to predict performance of carry-and-lift tasks representative of general shipboard work, though the authors recommend that critical carry-and-lift task parameters be defined before their method is used for job screening or selection. Studies have shown poor correlation between the Army Physical Fitness Test and lifting and load carriage.[42]

This topic remains politically charged. Among the recommendations of the Committee on Defense Women's Health Research regarding fitness was for research on scientific methods to assess fitness and then to use these assessments as a basis for fitness standards. (This topic is also addressed in the Nutrition section below.) The Subcommittee on Body Composition, Nutrition, and Health of Military Women recommended

> development of task-specific, gender-neutral strength and endurance tests and standards for use in the determination of placement in MOSs that require moderate and heavy lifting. Additional fitness programs should be created and enforced to develop and maintain the strength, endurance, and flexibility required by these MOSs.[43(p14)]

Mass, to use for screening new accessions for MOS classification. A study was done to validate the MEPSCAT using the Policy Review Group's MOS task analysis as a basis for the job-related tasks (eg, lift, carry, push, pull). A single measure of lifting capacity was the best predictor of job performance as defined by success on the job-related tasks, though the authors caution that their study has significant limitations and recommend a system that sounds similar to the one developed in the late 1970s

It remains unclear how further research would be helpful absent the political will to implement programs based on the results.

NUTRITION AND WEIGHT

In spite of abundant supplies of food and nutrients in the United States, the diets of many American women are lacking in some nutrients. Female athletes have additional dietary requirements that are not always met, and some may also have disordered eating. Military women are similar to the general population from which they volunteer, have activity levels that may approach or equal those of athletes, and are subject to weight and body fat standards, so they may also be subject to the nutritional deficiencies of their civilian counterparts. The stress and altered level and schedule of activity during deployment may create additional nutritional requirements. Unfortunately, data on the nutritional status and needs of women on deployment are lacking. Most data derive from studies of women in initial entry training, since this population is more easily studied, but recruits may have similar nutritional needs to deployed women.

Nutrients

One 1993 study[44] at Fort Jackson, SC, was designed specifically to evaluate the nutritional intake of female soldiers during US Army Basic Combat Training. This study showed that the women in the study had suboptimal mean intake of vitamin B_6, folic acid, calcium, magnesium, iron, and zinc. Almost half of the soldiers had mean intakes of less than 60% of the Military Recommended Daily Requirement (MRDA) of calcium and folic acid. Some women in the study also had suboptimal consumption of total calories, protein, vitamin C, thiamin, riboflavin, niacin, vitamin B_{12}, vitamin A, and phosphorous. The authors reviewed data obtained from previous Army nutritional surveys that included women and found that these women consumed fewer total calories in the field compared with garrison settings and that intake of both macronutrients and micronutrients was suboptimal in the field. They also compared these data with national data for women ages 20 to 29 years of age, including the second National Health and Nutrition Examination Survey and the Continuing Survey of Food Intakes by Individuals for 1985. They found that the nutrient intakes for women in field settings and in their study were similar to those of the civilian population—both are deficient in some nutrients. This situation may put military women at more risk for undernutrition and underperformance than their civilian counterparts because increased physical activity results in increased requirements for some nutrients and adequate nutrition is important in achieving peak physical performance. In addition, nutrition early in life can affect health status later in life; variation in calcium nutrition during adolescence accounts for 5% to 10% of the difference in adult bone mass, but this difference itself accounts for 50% or more of the risk for hip fracture in later adulthood.[45]

Military rations must feed both male and female service members, but because their requirements for some nutrients (eg, total calories, calcium, iron) differ, it is difficult to design rations to meet all of these needs. For example, if a female service member's energy requirement is 2,400 kcal ("calories") and she is eating Meals, Ready-to-Eat (MREs), she would have to consume approximately 131% of her energy requirement to meet the calcium MRDA of 1,200 mg or 166% of her energy requirements to meet the iron MRDA of 18 mg.[43] In the study by King and colleagues[44], subjects who discarded more than 50% of any food item they had selected were asked to give a reason. The two most common reasons were "not hungry" and being "full." This finding may support the idea that some women may not be able to eat enough of military rations to ensure adequate nutrition. To increase calcium content, ultra–high temperature treated milk has been added to Tray Pack (T) Rations and dehydrated filled-milk products are being developed and will be added to the B Ration and MRE. MRE Pouch Bread is fortified with calcium and iron.[46]

MREs are fortified with vitamins and minerals, but fortification varies by food item. To ensure intake of the broad range of vitamins and minerals, service members should consume part of each item in the MRE. There is an average of 1,200 calories in an MRE. If service members are consuming only MREs, women should be encouraged to eat half of the MRE at each meal to provide an intake of 1,800 calories per day (see Chapter 17, Nutritional Considerations for Military Deployment, and Chapter 19, Environmental Medicine: Heat, Cold, and Altitude).

The Committee on Defense Women's Health Research recommended that further research be conducted on the acceptability and consumption of field rations and fluids in the field and on factors that affect intake, such as environmental conditions, menstrual status, and level of physical activity. They also recommended research on nutrient and fluid requirements for optimal performance of specific categories of jobs or tasks under both normal and extreme environmental conditions.[2]

Weight and Body Fat

Some service members, both male and female, use deployment or a field training exercise (FTX) as an opportunity to lose unwanted excess weight. The soldiers in the study mentioned above[44] participated in a 4-day FTX during Basic Combat Training. Though nutrient intake data were not collected during the FTX, a questionnaire was administered to all soldiers, male and female, on their return. Of the 153 soldiers, 85.5% reported that they ate less than their usual dining hall intake while in the field. Of the reasons for consuming less, the most common were "the food did not look good" (62.7%) and "I was not hungry" (49.7%), but 16.3% of these soldiers not yet out of Basic Combat Training answered "I wanted to lose weight." In a survey study,[8] 46% of women (vs. 26% of men) reported having lost weight during deployment, and 22% of women (vs. 13% of men) reported having gained weight during deployment. Service members who lose weight while in the field, whether intentionally or not, are at risk for undernutrition, which is itself a risk factor for heat and cold injury in the short term and for less than optimum performance and health in the long term. Some service members may also develop eating disorders, either as a reaction to stress or as a result of their attempts to meet retention weight and body fat limits, and women may be at higher risk for eating disorders. An Air Force study showed that weight standards in Air Force Instruction 40-502 allowed most men a maximum allowable weight equivalent to a body mass index (BMI) of 28, whereas the cutoff point for women is only a BMI of 25.[47] (BMI is weight in kilograms divided by the square of height measured in meters.) Female service members may resort to disordered eating to maintain these more-stringent standards. Registered Dieticians can assist service members, their commanders, and their health care providers in developing a plan to achieve the service member's desirable weight while maintaining adequate nutrition in a variety of settings, including the field, and on all matters regarding diet and nutrition.

Fitness and Body Fat

Though body fat is related to cardiopulmonary fitness and performance on tasks such as unloaded walking or running, it is less important in tasks such as load carriage or backpacking and unrelated to tasks of moving external weights, such as pushing, pulling, lifting, and carrying.[30] The most common physically demanding tasks in the Army are lifting and carrying (including load carriage, such as backpacking). There is little evidence that unloaded running ability relates to military performance, and in fact a correlation of only 0.16 was found between the 2-mile run time and a 20-km load carriage time.[42] It may take different body types to carry loads well and to run fast. Higher lean (or fat-free) body mass is associated with faster load carriage and with better performance on lifting, pushing, carrying, and exerting torque, and the associations are stronger for lean body mass than for percent body fat.[42] Some have suggested that there be a requirement for minimum lean body mass rather than maximum body fat for entry and retention on active duty.[30,42]

The Army's initial body fat standards, established in 1982, were based on estimates of body fat percent that correlated with desired levels of physical fitness as measured by $\dot{V}o_2max$. Subsequently, these measures were also found to correlate well with the 2-mile run standard. However, the result was that the body fat standard was based on a measure of aerobic fitness, excluded any measurement of muscular strength or endurance, and was unrelated to job performance or other objectively based need.[30]

The Subcommittee on Body Composition, Nutrition, and Health of Military Women recommended revision of the current two-tiered body composition (weight for height, then body-fat measurement) and fitness screen. The new system would emphasize fitness as measured by ability to pass the physical training test. Specific criteria would determine whether the service member would be returned to duty, referred to a fitness program, referred to a weight management program, or referred to both programs. The Subcommittee further recommended development of

> a single service-wide equation derived from circumference measurements for assessment of women's body fat, to be validated against a four-compartment model using a population of active-duty women or a population that is identical in ethnic and age diversity to that of military women.[43(p14)]

The Subcommittee believed that such an equation could result in changing the BMI cut-off values.

The Subcommittee recommended that in the postpartum period, women should be allowed up to 1 year to attain body weight standards as long as satisfactory progress is being made, a potential increase of 6 months for all four services. The Subcommittee also recommended that fitness testing should not be required for 180 days after delivery, an increase only for the Army of 45 days. Finally, the Subcommittee recommended an increase in the length of exemption from deployment after childbirth to 6 months from the current 4 months for all four services.

PSYCHOLOGICAL STRESS

With the rapid changes in the demographic make-up of the military since the 1970s, concern has arisen over the success in integrating women into a primarily male organization and the prevalence and effect on women of sexual harassment and posttraumatic stress disorder (PTSD). Further discussion of these topics appears in chapter 49, Psychological Aspects of Deployment and Reunion.

Sources of Stress and Coping Behaviors

The 1995 Department of Defense Survey of Health Related Behaviors Among Military Personnel[48] included questions about mental health. The authors reported that about one in three military

women and almost one-half of women in the Marine Corps reported experiencing high stress as women in the military. They further reported that stress associated with being a woman in the military was higher among "other" racial or ethnic groups, those with a high school education or less, younger personnel, unmarried personnel, and enlisted personnel. Comparable conclusions for men are not provided. Personnel of both sexes and from all services reported higher levels of stress from their military duties than from their personal lives. Among men responding to the survey, the most frequently mentioned sources of stress were being away from family (23.7%), deployment (17.1%), increases in work load (16.6%), financial problems (15.0%), and conflicts between military and family responsibilities (13.0%). For women, these were being away from family (21.1%), major changes in family, such as birth or death of a loved one (17.0%), increases in work load (15.9%), problems in work relationships (15.7%), and problems with supervisors (13.1%). The sources of stress on which men and women differed the most in this survey were deployment (men 17.1%, women 6.9%), changes in family (men 12.3%, women 17.0%), and personal health problems (men 4.0%, women 8.6%). For both men and women, the most frequently mentioned coping behaviors were thinking of a plan to solve the problem, talking to a friend or family member, and exercising or playing sports. Men chose "talk to a friend or family member" significantly less frequently than did women (men 69.7%, women 87.6%). Men were more likely to cope by having a drink (men 24.4%, women 16.8%). Women were more likely to cope by getting something to eat (men 45.5%, women 57.2%). The authors conclude that stress among women in the military may be related to work and family roles and from being female in a predominantly male environment. They suggest broadly disseminating to military women stress management techniques that address issues of coping in a male environment. These data may help noncommissioned officers, commanders, and health care providers identify and ameliorate sources of stress in service members.

A study was carried out in 1991 of sex differences in stress among combat support and combat service support soldiers deployed to the Persian Gulf during the Persian Gulf War.[49] The study was done during the deployment but after the end of the war. None of the volunteers had been in combat. The males were significantly older and more likely to be noncommissioned officers than the females. Three stress categories were studied: operational, personal, and anticipation of combat. Personal stress was the most highly correlated with psychological symptoms for both sexes, with no significant difference between the sexes. Hardiness, a measure of resilience, was associated with having fewer psychological symptoms for both sexes, with no significant difference. Women reported significantly higher stress from anticipation of combat.

The authors of a study among National Guard and Reserve personnel comparing those who did and did not deploy conclude that "ethnic minorities but not necessarily women may be more vulnerable to psychological risk." [50(p415)] They found that those who deployed and those of nonwhite race scored higher on the Beck Depression Inventory scale; that those who deployed scored higher on the Depression and Anxiety scales of the Brief Symptom Inventory; and that those who deployed and women scored higher on the

Health Symptom Checklist.[50] Women's scores on the Health Symptom Checklist did not vary by deployment status, nor did women report greater symptoms of psychological distress than men or score higher on measures of PTSD symptomatology.

Sexual Harassment

Sexual harassment is an issue that has received increased attention as the proportion of women in the military has increased. A 1995 Army study[51] used self-report surveys on sexual harassment among combat support and combat service support soldiers at three Army posts. Subjects were administered the Sexual Experiences Questionnaire, which measures actual experiences rather than perceptions of harassment. Seventy-nine percent of females and 68% of males reported having experienced "gender harassment," such as sexist jokes or crude comments. Fifty-five percent of women and 38% of men reported experiencing unwanted sexual attention. Fifteen percent of women and 9% of men reported experiencing sexual coercion, imposition, or assault. After being given the Department of Defense definition of sexual harassment, "a form of sexual discrimination involving deliberate, repeated unwelcome sexual advances, requests for sexual favors, and other verbal or physical conduct of a sexual nature,"[51(p65)] 30% of women and 8% of men reported they had been sexually harassed. Reporting coercion was predictive of lower psychological well being for men. The only predictor of lower psychological well being for women was gender harassment.

Posttraumatic Stress Disorder

Some scientists have addressed the prevalence of PTSD symptoms in military populations and the relationship of sexual and nonsexual trauma to PTSD symptoms. One study of soldiers at six active duty Army posts used self-report questionnaire data and an algorithm to determine prevalence of PTSD symptoms. It showed that the current and lifetime prevalences of "potential PTSD" were higher in women.[52] Among all study participants, regardless of PTSD status, women reported a significantly higher number of PTSD symptoms than men. The overall prevalence of current symptoms was 6.7%, with 5% prevalence in men and 8.6% in women. Of those with "potential PTSD," women reported more sexual trauma and men reported more nonsexual trauma, but women's traumatic episodes were more likely to have occurred before their military service than men's. In the same study population, 22.6% of women reported experiencing a completed rape, with 81.2% of these occurring before entry to military service.[53] Thirty percent of the women reported experiencing attempted rape and assault other than attempted rape, and 29% reported experiencing completed rape. Seventy-five percent reported that the sexual assaults occurred before they entered the service, with approximately 12% each reporting sexual assaults occurring only on active duty and both before and during active duty. The authors suggest that a history of attempted and completed rape in childhood may be more common among female soldiers than among civilian women and that sexual assault history should be elicited to permit appropriate care for any lingering physical or psychological effects.

A similar self-report survey of premilitary adult sexual victimization and aggression among Navy recruits revealed that 45% of the women reported being the victim of either attempted or completed rape and that 15% of the men reported perpetrat-ing either attempted or completed rape.[54] The authors note that women who have been victimized and who are exposed to a variety of stressors, such as those that can occur during deployment, may have an increased need for certain medical and psychological services. They also note that a history of sexual aggression is predictive of future sexual aggression in nonmilitary populations and suggest that interventions among these men may be helpful.

The Committee on Defense Women's Health Research identified several avenues of research in the area of psychological stress during deployment.[2] These include possible sex differences in the nature, intensity, and optimal treatment of combat stress reaction or PTSD; phobias and other psychological effects related to the use of protective clothing and equipment; the impact of family issues such as separation from children and adequacy of child care; and methods of preparing women for the sex-specific aspects of captivity.

SUMMARY

Women make up an increasing proportion of active duty service members. More jobs with the potential for a variety of hazardous exposures are open to military women. Most of the issues regarding health during mobilization and deployment concern both men and women, and the similarities between men and women regarding potential military health hazards are greater than are the differences. However, there are differences significant enough to warrant consideration. It is important to understand the differences for many reasons. These dif-ferences must be taken into account to ensure that female service members receive the same quality of care as do males, even if the content of the care differs somewhat. A better understanding of all service members' capabilities and limitations will permit maximal use of those capabilities for the good of the service and the country while minimizing preventable harm to the individual. There remain many questions requiring additional research, and the current state of knowledge in this area will likely undergo significant change as data accumulate over time.

REFERENCES

1. Operational Medicine and Fleet Support Division, Bureau of Medicine and Surgery, Department of the Navy. *Operational Obstetrics and Gynecology: The Health Care of Women in Military Settings.* CD-ROM. 2nd ed. Washington, DC: DN; 2000. NAVMEDPUB 6300-2C. To receive a copy, call the Naval Operational Medical Institute, Pensacola, Fla, at (850) 452-2292/4487.

2. Committee on Defense Women's Health Research, Institute of Medicine. *Recommendations for Research on the Health of Military Women.* Washington, DC: National Academy Press; 1995: 8.

3. Army Medical Surveillance Activity. Defense Medical Epidemiologic Database. http//:amsa.army.mil. Accessed on October 23, 1999.

4. Murphy F, Browne D, Mather S, Scheele H, Hyams KC. Women in the Persian Gulf War: Health care implications for active duty troops and veterans. *Mil Med.* 1997;162:656–660.

5. Thomas MD, Thomas PJ. Surveying pregnancy and single parenthood. In: Rosenfeld P, Edwards JE, Thomas MD, eds. *Improving Organizational Surveys.* Newbury Park: Sage; 1993. Cited in: Committee on Defense Women's Health Research. *Recommendations for Research on the Health of Military Women.* Washington, DC: Institute of Medicine, National Academy Press; 1995: 9.

6. Gunzenhauser JD. *Comparative Morbidity Study of Active Duty Women Serving in Korea and Ft. Lewis*. Ft Belvoir, Va: Defense Technical Information Center; 1997. ADA 332962.

7. Hawley-Bowland C. Epidemiologic overview of common gynecologic disorders and first-trimester complications among active-duty women. *Womens Health Issues*. 1996;6:353–355.

8. Means-Markwell M, Hawkins R, Reichow K, et al. A survey of women's health care needs on U.S. Navy ships. *Mil Med*. 1998;163:439–443.

9. Schwerin MJ, Sack DM. Shipboard women's health care: Provider perceptions. *Mil Med*. 1997;162:666–670.

10. Hawley-Bowland C. Women's issues during deployment. Perez RP, ed. *Military Unique Curriculum Handbook for Physicians*. Tacoma, Wash: Madigan Army Medical Center; 100–101.

11. Weisberg E. Interactions between oral contraceptives and antifungals/antibacterials: Is contraceptive failure the result? *Clin Pharmacokinet*. 1999;36:309–313.

12. Eitzen JP, Sawyer RG. Sexually transmitted diseases: Risk behaviors of female active duty U.S. Army recruits. *Mil Med*. 1997;162:686–689.

13. Abel E, Adams E, Stevenson R. Sexual risk behavior among female Army recruits. *Mil Med*. 1996;161:491–494.

14. Abel E. Sexual risk behaviors among ship- and shore-based Navy women. *Mil Med*. 1998;163:250–256.

15. Clark JB, Holt VL, Miser F. Unintended pregnancy among female soldiers presenting for prenatal care at Madigan Army Medical Center. *Mil Med*. 1998;163:444–448.

16. Departments of the Air Force, Army, Navy, and Transportation. *Immunizations and Chemoprophylaxis*. Washington, DC: Department of Defense; 1995. Air Force Joint Instruction 48-110, Army Regulation 40-562, BUMEDINST 6230.15, CG COMDTINST M6230.4E.

17. Kolka MA. Temperature regulation in women. *Med Exerc Nutr Health*. 1992;1:201–207.

18. Murphy MM, Patton JF, Mello RP, Harp ME, Bidwell TE. Physiological impact of wearing a chemical protective ensemble (CPE) during occupational task performance of men and women. *Med Sci Sports Exerc*. 1993;25(Suppl):S138. Abstract 768.

19. Deuster PA, Jones BH, Moore J. Patterns and risk factors for exercise-related injuries in women: A military perspective. *Mil Med*. 1997;162:649–655.

20. Bell NS, Mangione TW, Hemenway D, Amoroso PJ, Jones BH. High injury rates among female Army trainees: A function of gender? *Am J Prev Med*. 2000;18(Suppl 3):141–146.

21. Altarac M, Gardner JW, Popovich RM, Potter R, Knapik JJ, Jones BH. Cigarette smoking and exercise-related injuries among young men and women. *Am J Prev Med*. 2000;18(Suppl 3):96–102.

22. Reynolds KL, Heckel HA, Witt CE, et al. Cigarette smoking, physical fitness, and injuries in infantry soldiers. *Am J Prev Med*. 1994;10:145–150.

23. Shaffer RA, Brodine SK, Ito SI, Le AT. Epidemiology of illness and injury among U.S. Navy and Marine Corps female training populations. *Mil Med*. 1999;164:17–21.

24. Subcommittee on Body Composition, Nutrition, and Health of Military Women. *Reducing Stress Fracture in Physically Active Military Women*. Washington, DC: Committee on Military Nutrition Research, Food and Nutrition Board, Institute of Medicine, National Academy Press; 1998: 10 (internet version). www.nap.edu/readingroom/books/stress. Accessed on April 7, 1999.

25. Knapik JJ, Sharp MA, Canham ML, et al. *Injury Incidence and Injury Risk Factors Among U.S. Army Basic Trainees*

at Ft. Jackson, SC, 1998 (Including Fitness Training Unit Personnel, Discharges, and New Starts). Aberdeen Proving Ground, Md: US Army Center for Health Promotion and Preventive Medicine; 1999. Report 29-HE-8370-99.

26. Amoroso PJ, Bell NS, Jones BH. Injury among female and male Army parachutists. *Aviat Space Environ Med*. 1997;68:1006–1011.

27. Lauder TD, Baker SP, Smith GS, Lincoln AE. Sports and physical training injury hospitalizations in the Army. *Am J Prev Med*. 2000;18(Suppl 3):118–128.

28. Washington SC. Injury-related morbidity in relation to military occupations, active duty U.S. Armed Forces, 1998–1999. *Med Surveillance Mon Rep*. 2000;6(2):10–14.

29. Feuerstein M, Berkowitz SM, Peck CA Jr. Musculoskeletal-related disability in US Army personnel: Prevalence, gender, and Military Occupational Specialties. *J Occup Environ Med*. 1997;39:68–78.

30. Vogel JA. Obesity and its relation to physical fitness in the U.S. military. *Armed Forces Society*. 1992;18(4):497–513.

31. Sharp MA. Physical fitness and occupational performance of women in the U.S. Army. *Work*. 1994;4(2):80–92.

32. Knapik JJ, Wright JE, Kowal DM, Vogel JA. The influence of U.S. Army Basic Initial Entry Training on the muscular strength of men and women. *Aviat Space Environ Med*. 1980;51:1086–1090.

33. Daniels WL, Wright JE, Sharp DS, Kowal DM, Mello RP, Stauffer RS. The effect of two years' training on aerobic power and muscles strength in male and female cadets. *Aviat Space Environ Med*. 1982;53:117–121.

34. Knapik JJ, Gerber J. *The Influence of Physical Fitness Training on the Manual Material-handling Capability and Road-marching Performance of Female Soldiers*. Aberdeen Proving Ground, Md: US Army Research Laboratory: 1996. Technical Report ARL-TR-1064.

35. Knapik JJ. The influence of physical fitness training on the manual material handling capability of women. *Appl Ergon*. 1997;28:339–345.

36. US General Accounting Office. *Women in the Military: Deployment in the Persian Gulf War*. Washington, DC: GAO; 1993.

37. Sharp MA, Rice VJ, Nindl BC, Williamson TL. Effects of team size on the maximum weight bar lifting strength of military personnel. *Hum Factors*. 1997;39:481–488.

38. Vogel JA, Wright JE, Patton JF, Dawson J, Eschenback MP. A *System for Establishing Occupationally-related Gender-free Physical Fitness Standards*. Natick, Mass: US Army Research Institute of Environmental Medicine; 1980. Report T-5/80.

39. Teves MA, Wright JE, Vogel JA. *Performance on Selected Candidate Screening Test Procedures Before and After Army Basic and Advanced Individual Training*. Natick, Mass: US Army Research Institute of Environmental Medicine; 1985: 4. Report T13/85.

40. Myers DC, Gebhardt DL, Crump CE, Fleishman EA. *Validation of the Military Entrance Physical Strength Capacity Test*. Alexandria, Va: US Army Research Institute for the Behavioral and Social Sciences; 1984: 6. Technical Report 610.

41. Beckett MB, Hodgdon JA. *Lifting and Carrying Capacities Relative to Physical Fitness Measures*. San Diego: Naval Health Research Center; 1987. Report 87-26.

42. Harman EA, Frykman PN. The relationship of body size and composition to the performance of physically demanding military tasks. In: Committee on Military Nutrition Research, Food and Nutrition Board. *Body Composition and Physical Performance: Applications for the Military Services*. Washington, DC: Institute of Medicine, National Academy Press; 1992: 115–117.

43. Subcommittee on Body Composition, Nutrition, and Health of Military Women. *Assessing Readiness in Military Women: The Relationship of Body Composition, Nutrition, and Health.* Washington, DC: Committee on Military Nutrition Research, Food and Nutrition Board, Institute of Medicine, National Academy Press; 1998: 14 (internet version). www.nap.edu/readingroom/books/mwomen. Accessed on April 7, 1999.

44. King N, Arsenault JE, Mutter SH, et al. *Nutritional Intake of Female Soldiers During the U.S. Army Basic Combat Training.* Natick, Mass: US Army Research Institute of Environmental Medicine; 1994. Report T94-17.

45. Marriott B. Nutrition and health in military women: A lifelong issue. *Womens Health Issues.* 1996;6:371–374.

46. King N, Fridlund KE, Askew EW. Nutrition issues of military women. *J Am Coll Nutr.* 1993;12:344–348.

47. Haddock CK, Poston WS, Klesges RC, Talcott GW, Lando H, Dill PL. An examination of body weight standards and the association between weight and health behaviors in the United States Air Force. *Mil Med.* 1999;164:51–54.

48. Bray RM, Kroutil LA, Wheeless SC, et al. *Highlights, 1995 Department of Defense Survey of Health Related Behaviors Among Military Personnel.* Research Triangle Park, NC: Research Triangle Institute; 1996: 67–73.

49. Rosen LN, Wright K, Marlowe D, Bartone P, Gifford RK. Gender differences in subjective distress attributable to anticipation of combat among U.S. Army soldiers deployed to the Persian Gulf during Operation Desert Storm. *Mil Med.* 1999;164:753–757.

50. Sutker PB, Davis JM, Uddo M, Ditta SR. Assessment of psychological distress in Persian Gulf troops: Ethnicity and gender comparisons. *J Pers Assessment.* 1995;64:415–427.

51. Rosen LN, Martin L. Psychological effects of sexual harassment, appraisal of harassment, and organizational climate among U.S. Army soldiers. *Mil Med.* 1998;163:63–67.

52. Stretch RH, Knudson KH, Durand D. Effects of premilitary and military trauma on the development of post-traumatic stress disorder symptoms in female and male active duty soldiers. *Mil Med.* 1998;163:466–470.

53. Martin L, Rosen LN, Durand DB, Stretch RH, Knudson KH. Prevalence and timing of sexual assaults in a sample of male and female U.S. Army soldiers. *Mil Med.* 1998;163:213–216.

54. Merrill LL, Newell CE, Milner JS, et al. Prevalence of premilitary adult sexual victimization and aggression in a Navy recruit sample. *Mil Med.* 1998;163:209–212.

Chapter 19

ENVIRONMENTAL MEDICINE: HEAT, COLD, AND ALTITUDE

ROBERT E. BURR, MD

R. E. Burr; Director of Endocrine Education, Division of Endocrinology; Bayside Medical Center, 3300 Main Street, Suite 3A, Springfield, MA 01199; formerly, Lieutenant Colonel, Medical Corps, US Army; Medical Advisor, Office of the Commander, US Army Research Institute of Environmental Medicine, Natick, MA 01760

INTRODUCTION

Since the beginning of recorded history, there are clear descriptions of the effect of the environment on military campaigns. The armies of Alexander in Central Asia, Hannibal in the Alps, and Napoleon in Russia all suffered the consequences of harsh climate. American military personnel, too, have had ample experience with cold and heat from Valley Forge to the Persian Gulf. And there does not seem to be a reduction in the requirement for military forces to deploy and operate in these places. Just in the 1990s, military conflict has appeared in the altitude of the Himalayan and Andean mountains, in the heat of African and Asian deserts, and in the cold of Central Europe and Central Asia.

This chapter is concerned with three terrestrial environments: hot, cold, and high altitude. Each is characterized by a dominant physical stressor: heat, cold, or hypobaric hypoxia. These three are military occupational stressors that produce measurable physiological or psychological strain, which is a necessary first step on the path to illness (Exhibit 19-1). Although the incidence of illness and injury is a stochastic process and predictable only in population terms, strain is universally present in deployed populations. These stressors are not novel or exotic but everyday, so we

---

EXHIBIT 19-1

MILITARY OCCUPATIONAL STRESSORS

Environmental Toxic Hazards

Dehydration

Weight Loss

Physical Stress

Physical Fatigue

Emotional Fatigue

Cognitive Fatigue

Climatic Extremes

Protective Uniforms

---

assume that their management is within everyone's experience and competence. That is not necessarily the case, to the detriment of service members deployed or training in these environments around the world.

GENERAL PRINCIPLES

There are several important principles concerning the relationship of these environmental stressors and illness. The first of these is that all these stressors are interactive and synergistic. The strain each produces cumulates with the strains produced by all the others to cause a general reduction in physical and psychological performance and to increase the likelihood of illness and injury. Typically, military deployments expose service members to several of these stressors simultaneously. These exposures are an inescapable effect of the psychological, physiological, and social dislocations of military operations.

The clinical illnesses consequent on these exposures usually reflect the net effect of several stressors. For example, dehydration, exercise-related heat exposure, and sleep loss all independently contribute to heat illness. Moderating any one of these three factors will reduce the risk. So, in circumstances where sleep loss

cannot be mitigated, efforts to guarantee adequate hydration and to control work rates in the heat become even more important preventive medicine tools.

It is important to remember, though, that a particular exposure does not result exclusively in any particular clinical illness. For example, trauma from a vehicular accident can be as much a consequence of altitude exposure as acute mountain sickness.

Frequently, one characteristic of an area of operations will be so extreme as to seem to require exclusive attention and intervention. However, the amount that this attention to a single stressor distracts attention from other stressors will prevent the implementation of a successful program of surveillance and prevention. Important and effective strategies to sustain health and performance may be overlooked if medical personnel become too focused on any one stressor.

A MODEL FOR ENVIRONMENTAL STRAIN AND DISEASE

The conceptual model used throughout this chapter expresses the idea that strain is a result of exposure to an environmental stressor moderated both by the capability of the individual to tolerate the stress

and by protective technology. Disease only occurs in the presence of strain. It is important to remember that there are many potential clinical expressions of strain, including psychological stress reactions, accidents

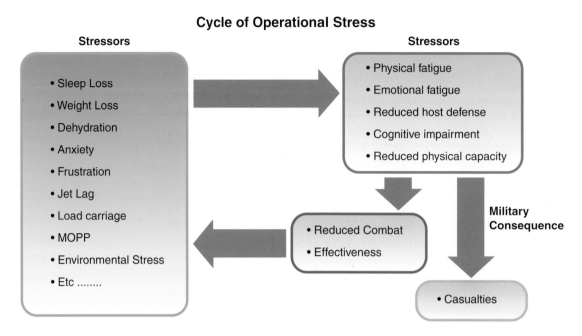

Fig. 19-1. Operational stressors reduce combat effectiveness and increase casualty rates through a variety of mechanisms. Loss of combat forces through stressor-related attrition increases the operational load on those not yet affected which contributes to an acceleration of the loss of combat effectiveness.

and trauma, and environmental illnesses. The individual feels the effect of all the stressors to which he or she is exposed. The cumulated strain will degrade physical and psychological performance, reducing military effectiveness and increasing casualty rates (Figure 19-1). The loss of personnel will take a toll in morale and increase the demands on those who remain, a process that will accelerate the accumulation of strain and further degrade unit effectiveness.

HOT ENVIRONMENTS

Heat and the other threats associated with hot environments are a constant of military training and operations. Acute and chronic heat illnesses have affected the outcomes of military campaigns since there have been military campaigns.[1,2] Heat illnesses continue to be a threat to US forces today.[3,4] Four of the major deployments in the 1990s were to hot environments: Panama, the Persian Gulf, Somalia, and Haiti. Heat stress affected operations in each of these deployments, both as a cause of casualties and as a threat complicating logistics and maneuver.

As the US experience in the Persian Gulf demonstrated, when military forces understand the threat of heat stress, provide appropriate logistic support, and incorporate prevention into the planning and execution of operations, heat illness is almost entirely preventable.[5] Heat illness rates have also fallen in the ordinary day-to-day activities of training and operations, but exertional heat illness, hyponatremia, and rhabdomyolysis continue to be common diagnoses among military populations and remain a cause of death and disability.

The Environment

Hot environments are characterized by a combination of temperature, humidity, and radiant heat; by affecting the rate at which heat energy can be dissipated from the body, these factors are associated with intense heat strain and dehydration during work. These conditions are usually thought of as confined to tropical or desert regions, but hot environments are encountered in every operational setting. In ground operations, the microenvironment of protective uniforms, even when outside temperatures are low, can be tropical and produce considerable heat stress. Military vehicles,[6] aircraft cockpits,[7,8] and mechanical spaces aboard ship[9] expose service members to high radiant and ambient heat loads. The outcomes of exposure to all hot environments are the same: reduced performance and illness.

Hot regions of the world, where heat is a climatic norm, present other threats beside heat stress and heat illness. They include limitations of water supply from either low rainfall or poor water quality, skin disease from sunburn or miliaria, and bronchospasm from dry air and dust.

Physiological Adaptation to Heat Exposure

Humans have well-defined physiological mechanisms to counteract rises in body temperature from either internal heat production or environmental heat stress.[10] These mechanisms support our need to maintain a narrow range of body temperature for optimal function. In response to a rise in body temperature from an internal or external heat source, we increase both cutaneous blood flow and sweating.[11] Heat energy is then dissipated to the environment either directly from the warmed skin surface by conduction-convection and radiation[12] or by evaporation of sweat (Exhibit 19-2).

The rate of direct transfer of heat energy by con-

EXHIBIT 19-2

CORE TEMPERATURE AND THE HEAT BALANCE EQUATION

Core temperature is determined by the balance between heat loss and heat gain from the environment and metabolism. If, on average, the two are equal, core temperature will remain constant, permitting optimum function. If heat gain exceeds heat loss, core temperature rises; conversely, if heat loss exceeds heat gain, core temperature will fall.

Heat balance can be expressed algebraically in the heat balance equation

$$S = M + R + C - E$$

S = Net change in heat content (heat storage)   R = Radiation

M = Metabolic heat production, always positive   C = Conduction/convection

R = Radiation   E = Evaporation, always negative

Metabolic heat production (M) varies with activity. On average, an adult male at rest generates about 80 to 90 kcal per hour (roughly equivalent to a 100 W bulb). Maximum aerobic exercise increases metabolic heat production to about 10 times the resting rate. Individuals performing sustained hard physical work (eg, digging, marching under a load) who can control the rate of exertion will usually work at no more than four to five times their resting metabolic rate. Shivering can increase metabolic rate up to seven times resting level.

Radiation (R) is the loss or gain of heat in the form of electromagnetic energy. The direction of heat energy transfer is from warmer to cooler objects. The warming sensed standing in direct sun or near a hot surface is produced by radiative heat gain. We are warm objects in a cool environment and so radiate heat energy. Radiant heat gain and loss can be moderated by material barriers, which are considered either "shade" or "insulation" depending on the direction of the radiant heat energy flow.

Conduction and convection (C) are the mechanisms of heat energy transfer when there is physical contact between two materials of different temperatures. Conductive heat transfer occurs between two surfaces of different temperature. Conductive heat gain or loss is particularly significant when lying on hot or cold ground. Convection occurs between a surface and a fluid, such as air or water. The change in fluid density due to heat transfer causes the fluid to move and tends to maintain the thermal gradient. Wind and water currents add to the heat transfer process of natural convection and are significant components of heat gain and loss in extreme environments.

Evaporation (E) of water on the body surface causes heat loss. Each liter evaporated transfers 540 kcal to the environment. Sweat evaporation does not depend on the relative humidity but rather on the difference between the vapor pressure of sweat on the skin and the vapor pressure of water in the air adjacent to the skin. Even in cool-wet environments of high relative humidity, sweat on warm skin can evaporate into the air because the vapor pressure of the sweat exceeds that of the water vapor in the air. Sweating is an important form of heat loss in cold environments.

Adapted from: United States Army Research Institute of Environmental Medicine. *Medical Aspects of Cold Weather Operations: A Handbook for Medical Officers.* Natick, Mass: USARIEM; 1993: 4–5. Technical Note 93-4.

duction-convection and radiation depends on the difference in temperature between the body surface and ambient and radiant temperatures of the environment. The two routes of direct energy exchange (radiation and conduction-convection) between the body surface and the environment are two-way streets. If the body surface is warmer than the environment, the body will lose energy to the environment. If the converse is true, the body will gain heat energy from the environment. When the environment is sufficiently hot to cause heat gain by the direct transfer routes, evaporative cooling is the only thermoregulatory mechanism available to control body temperature.

Sweating is primarily controlled by the central nervous system.[13] Core temperature increases detected by thermosensitive neurons in the hypothalamus stimulate increases in skin blood flow and sweating. Sweat production rates can exceed 2 L/h for short periods and can reach 15 L/d. Each liter of sweat evaporated from the body surface removes approximately 540 kcal of heat energy. Under conditions that allow rapid evaporation (eg, the low humidity of deserts), the daily cooling capacity of the sweating mechanism is several thousand kilocalories, adequate to maintain body temperature even during vigorous work in the heat.

Physical work causes an increase in cardiac output and the redistribution of blood flow toward the working muscles and away from the viscera.[10] As exertion elevates core temperature, an additional portion of the cardiac output is directed to the skin for thermoregulation, and visceral flow is further reduced. High sweat rates will quickly compromise blood volume. Therefore, work in the heat requires constant fluid replenishment. Since the maximum rate of water absorption in the gut is about 20 cc/min or 1.2 L/h,[14] compensation for high sweat rates requires rest periods with reduced sweat rates and time for rehydration.

Acclimatization

Acclimatization to heat exposure is a true physiological adaptation that is critical to optimum performance and health in hot environments.[15–17] Both the rate of acclimatization and the degree of acclimatization achieved depend on the thermal stress to which an individual is regularly exposed.[18] Achieving the maximum rate seems to require about 1 to 2 hours of continuous exercise per day. Substantial acclimatization develops in 5 days of daily heat exposure and, for all practical purposes, is complete in 10 to 14 days.[19]

The acclimatization response includes these important physiological adaptations: a lowering of the threshold for the onset of cutaneous vasodilation and sweating,[11] an increase in the rate of sweating for any given core temperature, and a reduction in the concentration of sodium chloride in sweat[13] (Figure 19-2). The combination of a lower threshold and higher sweat rates allows a more vigorous response to heat exposure and increases the opportunity for evaporative cooling. In environments where evaporation contributes to cooling, acclimatized individuals can maintain lower body temperatures for any amount of heat stress. High sweating rates reduce the opportunity for the sweat gland epithelium to conserve salt, so at higher sweat rates, the concentration of salt in sweat rises. Acclimatized sweat glands conserve salt more effectively and produce sweat with a reduced salt concentration for any given flow rate. This conservative phenomenon is an important protection from salt depletion in hot environments. Furthermore, reducing the salt content of sweat increases the proportion of intracellu-

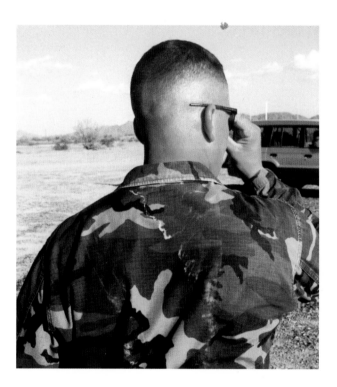

Fig. 19-2. This soldier has just finished his first day of work in a hot desert environment after air travel from a temperate climate. He is not yet acclimatized and has not yet developed salt conserving mechanisms appropriate to his high sweat rates. He has lost enough salt in his sweat to cause a saline crust on his uniform.
Photograph: Courtesy of Dr. Robert E. Burr.

lar water contributing to sweat formation. Consequently, for any given amount of body water lost as sweat, less will be taken from the extracellular fluid, thus conserving plasma volume.

Heat Stress and Heat Strain

Heat stress is the net effect of the metabolic heat load and the environment; it is the force acting to increase core temperature. The heat stress of an encapsulating uniform (eg, MOPP and HAZMAT gear) is much more related to the environment inside the uniform than to the outside environment. Heat stress that does not exceed the ability of the individual to maintain an acceptable range of core temperature is considered compensable. Heat stress that exceeds that level is considered noncompensable.[20] Noncompensable heat stress will produce heat illness if the exposure is long enough. Encapsulating, or occlusive, uniforms are notorious for creating noncompensable heat stress environments because they limit both evaporation and direct heat exchange and are physically demanding to wear.

Heat strain is the change in the individual exposed to heat stress. It includes the physiological and psychological consequences of the rise in core temperature, thermoregulatory load, and dehydration.

PREVENTION OF HEAT ILLNESS

The primary prevention of heat illness depends on a thorough analysis of the factors that affect the likelihood of heat illness and on plans to mitigate those factors that increase risk and maximize those that reduce risk. This section will review the assessment and control of the principal groups of factors in heat illness: heat stress, thermocompetence, and technology. The conceptual relationship between heat stress and heat strain is shown in this equation:

$$(1) \quad \text{Strain} = f \frac{\text{Time} \bullet \text{Heat Stress}}{\text{Thermocompetence} \bullet \text{Technology}}$$

Heat Stress

The heat stress to which service members will be exposed must be known if effective preventive measures are to be taken. Heat stress can be environmental (exogenous) or metabolic (endogenous).

Environmental Factors

There are a number of metrics that are used to measure environmental heat stress.[21] The simplest and most commonly used is ambient temperature, but it does not include allowances for humidity or radiant heat load and can dangerously understate the actual heat stress imposed by an environment. To address that limitation, other metrics have been developed. The Wet Bulb Globe Temperature (WBGT) Index is the most commonly used of these multifactorial indices.[22] It incorporates independent measurements of ambient temperature, radiant heat load, humidity, and wind speed. The measurements of three instruments are combined as a weighted average to calculate the WBGT Index. The wet bulb thermometer estimates humidity and air movement (weighted at 0.7). The black globe thermometer estimates solar load (weighted at 0.2), and the dry bulb thermometer measures ambient air temperature (weighted at 0.1). The high weighting of the wet bulb temperature acknowledges the critical importance of air moisture on evaporative cooling in hot environments (Figure 19-3).

Whatever environmental heat stress metric is used, it should be measured in circumstances as close as possible to those in which the service mem-

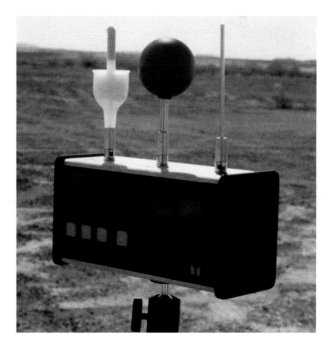

Fig. 19-3. This is an automatic instrument deployed to provide continuous real-time estimates of the Wet Bulb Globe Temperature Index. It should be set up at the spot where the activity is to be conducted.
Photograph: Courtesy of Dr. Robert E. Burr.

bers will be operating. These indices can vary tremendously over short periods of time and distances and in unpredictable ways. For example, on a sunny, calm day, an open field may have greater heat stress than an adjacent forest, but on a windy, cloudy day, the forest may have the greater heat stress. Heat stress indices calculated for a whole installation or region are only general guides. Particularly when conditions seem extreme, on-site measurements are essential. There is no substitute for knowledge of local conditions. Rapid changes in temperature or humidity present increased risk because those exposed are unacclimatized and may not accommodate to the change in weather.

Occlusive uniforms are an important source of heat stress.[23,24] By retarding the transfer of water vapor and heat energy to the environment, they create their own microenvironment. The air trapped in the uniform is warmed by the skin and saturated with water vapor from sweat, so that the service member's immediate environment becomes extremely hot and humid. The only opportunity to moderate the heat and humidity inside the uniform is to transfer water vapor and heat through the fabric—just the

transfer the uniforms are designed to prevent. Protective uniforms that incorporate a mask can interfere with hydration, contributing to the development of heat illness (Figure 19-4). Heat exhaustion is the most common heat illness associated with protective uniforms but exertional heat stroke can also occur.[25]

Metabolic Factors

The metabolic component of heat stress can be estimated from knowledge of the work that is to be performed. Unlike civilian industrial hygiene practice,[26] military work is usually divided into four categories of intensity, and these categories are used instead of specific numeri-

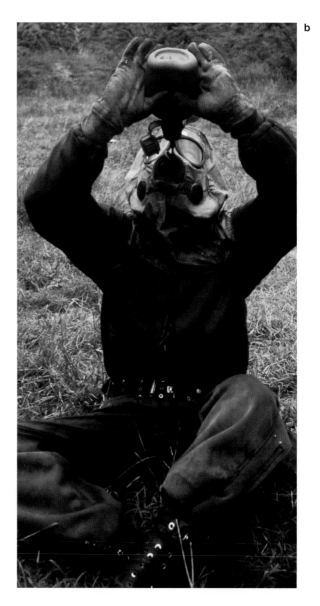

Fig. 19-4. Occlusive uniforms increase the risk of heat injury. These two soldiers in (**a**) are wearing MOPP and have been overcome by heat exhaustion. Protective equipment contributes to heat strain in several ways. Interference with rehydration is one of the more important. (**b**) Prevention of heat casualties depends on successful measures to maintain hydration.
Photographs: Courtesy Commander, USARIEM, Natick, Mass.

EXHIBIT 19-3

WORK INTENSITIES OF TYPICAL MILITARY TASKS

Work Intensity in MOPP* 0–1	Task	Work Intensity in MOPP* 2–4
VERY LIGHT	Sentry duty, Driving a truck Driving a truck	VERY LIGHT
LIGHT	Walking on hard surface (2.25 MPH, 1 m/s): no load Manual of Arms	LIGHT
MODERATE	Walking on hard surface (2.25 MPH, 1 m/s): 30 kg load Walking on loose sand (2.25 MPH, 1 m/s): no load Calisthenics	MODERATE
	Scouting patrol Foxhole digging Crawling with full pack Field assaults	
HEAVY	Walking on hard surface (3.5 MPH, 1.5 m/s): 30 kg load Walking on hard surface (4.5 MPH, 2 m/s): no load Walking on loose sand (3.5 MPH, 1.5 m/s): no load	HEAVY

Adapted from: United States Army Research Institute of Environmental Medicine. *Heat Illness: A Handbook for Medical Officers.* Natick, Mass: USARIEM; 1991: 42. Technical Note 91-3.

---

cal estimates of metabolic rate (Exhibit 19-3). The heat stress associated with running is much higher than that associated with any other military task, typically two to three times the heat generation caused by moderate-to-heavy work. For this reason, work-rest cycles are not applicable to running.

Thermocompetence

Anything that impairs thermoregulatory capacity will reduce performance in the heat and increase the likelihood of heat illness. The most important factors include hydration, acclimatization, physical fitness, skin condition, and fever. Other factors that must be considered include prior heat illness, medications, nutriture, and state of rest. An individual is optimally capable to manage heat stress when he or she is fully hydrated, acclimatized, physically fit, healthy, well nourished, and well rested.

Hydration is essential to maintain blood volume for thermoregulatory blood flow and sweating. Both are reduced by dehydration, and the dehydrated service member has less ability to control body temperature in the heat. Water requirements are not reduced by any form of training or acclimatization. Exercises that attempt to teach personnel to work or fight with less water are fruitless and dangerous.

Service members who are required to deploy on short notice to hot environments will arrive unacclimatized. Adequate acclimatization will require several days to achieve. During the first few days of heat exposure, neither the ability to restrain the rise of core temperature during heat exposure nor the ability to conserve salt in sweat will be adequately developed. Aerobic fitness[17] provides the cardiovascular reserve to maintain the extra cardiac output required to sustain thermoregulation, muscular work, and vital organs in the face of heat stress. In addition, regular, strenuous aerobic physical training will provide a small degree of heat acclimatization.

Fever, whether due to immunization or illness, reduces thermoregulatory capacity by resetting the hypothalamus toward heat conservation rather than heat dissipation. This phenomenon eliminates the beneficial effect of acclimatization. Service members recovering from fever will have increased susceptibility to heat illness even after all clinical evidence of illness has disappeared. Until clearly able to manage normal work rates in the heat, they will require increased command supervision and moderated work schedules. Sunburn[27] and many other skin diseases[28–30] reduce the ability of the skin to thermoregulate. Some medications will effect thermoregulatory adaptations and can increase the risk of heat illness. Prior heat illness also needs to be considered, as it is evidence of reduced heat tolerance in some individuals.

The requirements of military operations frequently mean lack of sleep and missed meals. Both these factors reduce thermoregulatory capacity and increase the risk of heat injury.[31]

Technology

Technology, whether sunshades, fans, air conditioning, or microclimate cooling systems, can be used to reduce heat exposure and to acceler-

ate the removal of endogenous heat generated during exertion. This will allow service members to work longer in environments of high heat stress.

Implementation of a Heat Illness Prevention Program

The approach to the primary prevention of heat illness should include the consideration of ways to mitigate heat stress, to maximize the thermocompetence of the exposed, and to make the best use of available heat stress–control technology[32] (Exhibit 19-4). Primary prevention of heat illness is instituted by using the steps in the exhibit.

EXHIBIT 19-4

HEAT ILLNESS: IMPORTANT PREVENTION POINTS

- A heat casualty in a unit suggests others are at risk—all members of the unit should be evaluated immediately. Service members who are underperforming in the heat (eg, stragglers on a road march) may be incipient heat casualties. It is not safe to assume their underperformance is undermotivation.

- In military operations and training, risk factors for heat illness, all of which reduce thermoregulatory capacity, include:

    -short-notice deployment (service members arrive unacclimatized)
    -fever (from immunization or illness)
    -dehydration
    -fatigue
    -undernutrition

- Acclimatization requires 7 to 10 days, regardless of physical condition. During the acclimatization period, service members who must work vigorously should be provided copious quantities of water and follow carefully supervised work-rest cycles.

- If rations are short or sweating is very heavy, salt supplementation may be needed. Acclimatization should eventually eliminate the need for salt supplementation.

- Service members in hot environments universally demonstrate dehydration of 1% to 2% of body weight. Command-directed drinking is effective in moderating dehydration and must be enforced. Unit leaders must reinforce hydration by planning for elimination as well as consumption.

- Fever reduces thermoregulatory capacity. Service members will have increased susceptibility to heat illness even after all clinical evidence of fever has disappeared. Until clearly able to manage normal work rates in the heat, service members will require increased command supervision and moderated work schedules.

- The requirements of military operations frequently produce lack of sleep, missed meals, and limited availability of water. All these reduce thermoregulatory capacity and increase the risk of heat illness.

- Reducing heat load reduces water requirements, so shade and night hours should be used as much as possible. Planning that ensures there will be enough water when and where needed must not be ignored.

Adapted from: United States Army Research Institute of Environmental Medicine. Medical Aspects of Cold Weather Operations: A Handbook for Medical Officers. Natick, Mass: USARIEM; 1991: 7, 39. Technical Note 91-3.

The service members who will be exposed must be assessed. Their acclimatization, physical fitness, and state of rest, nutrition, and hydration should be considered. Individuals or units at particular risk, such as recruits recovering from a febrile illness or units just beginning training, need to be identified.

The environmental conditions must be measured. Conditions can vary substantially even across short distances and in unpredictable ways. A shaded forest may seem to have less heat stress because of the lower solar load, but may, in fact, have a higher heat stress because of high humidity and lack of wind. Have the environmental conditions become more stressful recently? Sudden increases in environmental heat stress are particularly risky. Service members who have acclimatized to a moderate degree of heat stress will not be tolerant of sudden, more severe heat stress.

The workload must be assessed, especially the plans for work rate and duration. What uniform will be worn during training or while working? Will there be an opportunity to remove or loosen portions of the uniform? Unblousing trousers or removing jackets or helmets can reduce heat stress

considerably but may not be possible.

Technological aids must also be considered. Will there be protection from the solar heat load? Although loosening clothing can permit better evaporative and conductive and convective cooling, the skin and head should be protected from direct sun by shade or light clothing.

Heat Stress Control

Heat stress exposure can be mitigated by reducing either the time or the intensity of exposure. The standard technique for regulating the time of exposure is the work-rest cycle. Other administrative controls that are used include the Threshold Limit Values (developed by the American Council of Governmental Industrial Hygienists),[26] Physiological Heat Exposure Limits (US Navy), and "Flag Conditions" used to regulate military training environments.

Tables of work-rest cycles provide explicit recommendations for the length of alternating periods of work and rest to allow work for an entire shift (Table 19-1). The work-rest tables for the civilian

TABLE 19-1

AN EXAMPLE OF A WORK-REST TABLE THAT GIVES MAXIMUM WORK TIMES IN MINUTES FOR DAYLIGHT OPERATIONS THAT CAN BE SUSTAINED WITHOUT EXCEEDING A GREATER THAN 5% RISK OF HEAT CASUALTIES

		MOPP0				MOPP4 + Underwear				MOPP4 + BDU			
WBGT	T	VL	L	M	H	VL	L	M	H	VL	L	M	H
78	82	NL	NL	NL	65	NL	177	50	33	NL	155	49	32
80	84	NL	NL	157	61	NL	142	49	32	NL	131	48	32
82	87	NL	NL	114	56	NL	115	47	31	NL	110	46	30
84	89	NL	NL	99	53	NL	104	45	30	NL	100	45	30
86	91	NL	NL	87	50	NL	95	44	29	NL	93	44	29
88	94	NL	NL	74	45	NL	85	42	28	NL	83	42	27
90	96	NL	NL	67	43	NL	79	41	27	NL	78	41	27
92	98	NL	NL	60	40	NL	75	40	26	NL	74	40	26
94	100	NL	193	55	37	NL	70	39	25	NL	70	39	25
96	103	NL	101	48	33	203	65	37	23	194	65	37	23
98	105	NL	82	44	31	141	62	36	22	140	62	36	22
100	107	261	70	41	28	118	59	35	21	118	59	35	21

MOPP: mission oriented protective posture
WBGT: wet bulb globe temperature (°F)
T: ambient temperature (°F)

VL: very light work intensity
L: light work intensity
M: moderate work intensity

H: heavy work intensity
BDU: battle dress uniform
NL: No Limitation

Source: United States Army Research Institute of Environmental Medicine. *Heat Illness: A Handbook for Medical Officers*. Natick, Mass: USARIEM; 1991: App E. Technical Note 91-3.

workplace are designed to strictly limit the rise in core temperature. They are more conservative than those available for military use, which are designed to limit heat casualties and are less concerned with specific physiological limits. Techniques that monitor physiological parameters of heat strain, such as temperature and pulse, can be used when work-rest cycles are not available or the exposures are particularly critical or demanding.

The intensity of heat exposure can be mitigated by controlling the rate of work. By slowing metabolic heat generation, the endogenous heat stress in reduced. Factors susceptible to this kind of control are march pace or cargo handling rates. Mechanical assistance (eg, moving by vehicle instead of on foot, using a forklift to move cargo) will also help control this factor.

Environmental heat load can be mitigated by changing the time of day when work is performed. Avoiding times of maximal solar load is one of the oldest techniques for controlling heat stress. Requirements to wear occlusive clothing and equipment should include consideration of the increased risk of heat illness.[33] Use of these items will require adjustment of work-rest guidance and will reduce the amount of work an individual can perform.

Maximizing Fitness for Exposure

In many military situations, the environment and the control technologies available will be dictated by circumstances, so the individual is the principal focus for measures to control heat stress and heat illness.

Some individuals should not be exposed to heat stress. These include those with significant histories of prior heat illness (discussed in more detail later), those with skin diseases that effect thermoregulation (eg, psoriasis, anhidrosis), those requiring medications that impair thermoregulation (eg, anticholinergics, diuretics), and those with illnesses that limit cardiovascular reserve. Sickle cell trait increases the risk of sudden death and exertional rhabdomyolysis during exercise heat stress.[34–37]

Some conditions will transiently limit thermoregulatory capacity. Any febrile response, whether to illness or vaccination, will substantially impair the ability to work in the heat. The duration of this effect is not known but almost certainly depends on a variety of parameters of the inflammatory response that caused the fever. Miliaria and sunburn both reduce the thermoregulatory capacity of the skin and so increase the risk of heat illness.

Hydration is the single most important factor in controlling heat stress and heat illness.[14,38] Training and operations produce many obstacles to maintaining adequate hydration. In hot environments, water losses can reach 15 L/d per individual, and service members do not drink enough water voluntarily to maintain hydration. This phenomenon has been called voluntary dehydration, although there is nothing willful about it. Thirst is not stimulated until plasma osmolarity rises 1% to 2% above the level customarily found in temperate climates. Consequently, if thirst is used as the guide for drinking, service members will maintain themselves at a level that is 1% to 2% dehydrated relative to their usual state. The only solutions to this problem are command-directed drinking and water discipline.

Even in the face of a clear understanding of the importance of water and hydration, other factors will interfere with maintaining hydration. Service members may decide that water drinking creates problems that outweigh its importance. For example, service members may not drink before going to sleep to avoid having to wake up and dress to urinate, or they may not drink before traveling in convoys if no rest stops are planned.

Adequate acclimatization is essential for optimal performance in the heat.[39] During the initial acclimatization period, service members must be provided copious quantities of water and carefully supervised to prevent excessive heat exposure. If possible, work tasks should be regulated using work-rest cycles tailored with the close involvement of unit medical personnel to the service member's physical capacity. Recent immunization, jet lag, and sleep loss, all of which reduce thermoregulation, will increase the risk of heat illness during this initial phase of exposure.

Sunburn must be prevented by adequate clothing, shade, and sunscreens. Skin diseases are best prevented by adequate hygiene. Commanders and logisticians must understand the importance of a functioning skin and provide adequate water for washing.

Salt depletion is a risk if service members are exposed during this time to sufficient heat or work stress to induce high sweating rates (more than several liters per day) if ration consumption is reduced. Salt depletion will contribute to heat exhaustion and heat cramps.[40] Salt supplementation may be necessary.[41]

Technology and Engineering Controls

Overhead shade and heat shields for outdoor workspaces will reduce radiant heat load, sunburn, contact burns, and heat illness. Air circulation by any means facilitates convective cooling and may facilitate evaporative cooling by providing dry air. Air conditioning generates cool, dry air; when possible, it should be provided for indoor spaces to facilitate work and sleep quality. Ice vests and mechanical microclimate cooling systems[42,43] pump cool air or fluid inside occlusive uniforms to extend work times for individuals in high heat stress microenvironments.

Special Considerations: Minimizing Heat Casualties in Recruit Training

Recruits are particularly susceptible to heat illness during basic training in hot weather.[44] A number of reasons for their susceptibility are related to their rapid transition from civilian life to a demanding schedule of physical and military training. Most are neither acclimatized to heat on entry nor as physically fit as fully trained service members. They need to become fit in a short time and so quickly begin strenuous exercise. They also commonly suffer sleep loss and dehydration, and contagious febrile illnesses are common. Compounding their situation is their unfamiliarity with heat illness; they may not recognize early signs of heat illness or understand the importance of early treatment.

Heat illness can occur in any component of basic training. Certain activities, though, are associated with the highest risk: road marches, unit runs (including morning physical training), evening parades, and rifle range marksmanship training. Recruits on road marches and unit runs have very high sustained rates of endogenous heat production and muscular work. They usually develop temperature elevations and after 30 to 60 minutes, significant dehydration. Both temperature elevation and dehydration are aggravated if they begin their exercise dehydrated (eg, if they start just after waking without rehydrating), if they are wearing a heavy uniform that prevents loss of heat to the environment (eg, chemical protective equipment), or if environmental conditions retard heat loss. The combined elevated temperature, muscular work, and dehydration lead to a high risk of heat exhaustion and heat stroke. Heat casualties at evening parades usually result from dehydration developed during a day of vigorous physical training.

Most would not ordinarily associate a significant risk of heat casualties with rifle marksmanship training. The association exists, though, because rifle range training is often done during extreme heat that prohibits other outdoor training. Recruits are exposed for long periods to intense solar and ground-contact heat loads without consideration of the heat-induced water requirement. Under these conditions, recruits develop hyperthermia and dehydration.

Education and Training

The medical officer has an educational role as a unit prepares for operations in hot environments. Service members of every rank must know the steps they can take to minimize the risk of heat illness. They must understand the importance of hydration, nutrition, and skin hygiene. They must know that although thirst means dehydration, dehydration does not necessarily provoke thirst. They must be trained to recognize the signs of heat illness and the basics of buddy aid. Staff must understand the critical importance of water to the unit so they can incorporate adequate water logistics and management into their plans, which must not add impediments to water discipline. Planners must incorporate the degrading effect of heat into their operational schedules by adding rest and hydration stops. Leaders must understand the nature and the magnitude of the threat that heat stress presents to their units so they can emphasize the importance of required countermeasures. Small-unit leaders must know the techniques for managing work in the heat and understand the guidelines for water replacement and work-rest cycles.

Surveillance

Although heat stress modeling is well developed[45,46] and can predict with great accuracy the effects of exercise-heat exposure, the details of living and working in hot environments confound the ability of these models to describe the risks and responses of groups of people through time. Consequently, successful prevention depends on the detection of early evidence of accumulating heat strain. Some of this evidence is seen in day-to-day activities and appears in phenomena such as reduced appetite or physical vigor or deeply colored urine. Some manifests as minor medical complaints such as gastrointestinal disturbances and minor heat illnesses. These all presage both impaired performance and increased incidence of heat illness and dictate intervention.

Specific guidance on work-rest cycles or water requirements depends on assumptions about the population to which it will be applied. These assumptions usually include such factors as age, hydration state, physical fitness, and nutriture. If these assumptions are violated, which is to be expected in many deployments, the guidance may underestimate heat exposure risks. Consequently, experience and formal surveillance of exposures and outcomes are required to develop guidance appropriate to the actual circumstances of the deployment.

HEAT ILLNESSES

Heat illness can be separated into five categories. The first and largest is exertional heat illness, which is itself divided into heat exhaustion, exertional heat injury, and exertional heat stroke. Classic heat stroke, exertional rhabdomyolysis, exertional hyponatremia, and minor heat illnesses are the other categories. Exhibit 19-5 summarizes the salient clinical features of the more serious heat illnesses.

Secondary Prevention

Heat strain and heat illness will worsen if not recognized and managed early. The key to secondary prevention, then, is early recognition followed by extrication, cooling, rehydration, and time for recuperation.

General Considerations in Management and Diagnosis of Heat Illness

There are three important clinical principles that apply to the diagnosis and management of acute illnesses occurring in the heat. First, there are no pathognomonic signs or symptoms of heat illness. Second—and as a consequence of the first—there

---

EXHIBIT 19-5

MILITARILY IMPORTANT HEAT ILLNESSES

Heat Exhaustion
- Occurs during exercise
- Headache, GI symptoms, exhaustion, collapse, syncope
- Rapid recovery with rest and hydration
- Peak CK < 1000
- No abnormal LFT
- No myoglobinuria

Exertional Heat Injury
- Occurs during exercise
- Headache, GI symptoms, exhaustion, collapse, syncope, muscle pain
- Rapid recovery with rest and rehydration except muscle pain
- Peak CK > 1000
- Creatinine: day 2 > day 1
- LFT up to 3 x ULN
- No encephalopathy or coagulopathy

Exertional Heat Stroke
- Occurs during exercise, often early
- May be critically ill from onset
- Encephalopathy
- coagulopathy common
- CK > 5000

- Peak creatinine > 2.0
- LFT > 3x ULN

Exertional Rhabdomyolysis
- Muscle pain after exertion
- CK > 10,000
- Myoglobinuria
- Peak creatinine > 2.0
- No encephalopathy or coagulopathy
- LFT < 3x ULN

Exercise-related Hyponatremia
- Gradual onset
- Symptoms late in the day
- Marked thirst
- Hyponatremia
- No significant change in LFT, renal function, CK, or hemostasis

Dehydration
- After heat exposure
- Headache, nausea, fatigue, constipation
- Heat intolerance, mild orthostasis common
- Mild hemoconcentration
- Concentrated urine

Abbreviations
CK: creatine phosphokinase
GI: gastrointestinal
LFT: liver function test
ULN: upper limit of normal

is always a differential diagnosis. Third, shade and cooling are always appropriate emergency responses to acute illness in the heat.[47]

Management

The initial management of acute illness in the heat should include putting the patient in the supine position; establishing shade and skin cooling; evaluating airway, breathing, and circulation; examining mental status; and measuring temperature. Since the illness may be life threatening (eg, heat stroke) but is hard to diagnose in the field, a rapid decision on disposition should be made.

Diagnosis

The differential diagnosis of acute illness in the heat includes infection (particularly meningococcemia and *P falciparum* malaria), pontine or hypothalamic hemorrhage, drug intoxication (eg, cocaine, amphetamines, phencyclidine, theophylline, tricyclic antidepressants), alcohol or sedative withdrawal, severe hypertonic dehydration, and thyroid storm. Specific questions should be asked about recent immunizations or illnesses and medications taken, including nonprescription medications.[48,49]

The early symptoms of exertional heat illness include fatigue, irritability, headache, and anorexia. Paresthesias and carpopedal spasm can occur in severe heat exposure. As the illness progresses, nausea, vomiting, and, occasionally, diarrhea can develop. Slumping posture and ataxia are signs of impending collapse. Sweating and hyperthermia are characteristic. If the illness progresses beyond its premonitory symptoms and signs, it presents as acute collapse, often with syncope and seizures. Persistence of seizures, delirium, disorientation, or combativeness is presumptive evidence of heat stroke.[47,50]

The most important question to answer in the approach to acute illness in the heat is "Is this heat stroke?" because of the seriousness of that condition. The mental status examination is the key to this determination. Any significant impairment in mental status at the scene of illness is evidence of heat stroke. The mental status examination should be performed quickly but carefully and should evaluate arousal, orientation, interaction, cognition, and memory. Any impairment beyond transient drowsiness and inattention is significant. Other clinical features that may be helpful in the initial field evaluation include exertional heat stroke's frequent presentation as a sudden, severe illness soon after beginning exercise-heat exposure. High temperature immediately after

onset of illness is helpful in narrowing the differential diagnosis but is not diagnostic, as core temperatures in excess of 40°C (105°F) are routinely encountered during vigorous exercise.

While high temperature is not itself diagnostic, accurate and early measurement of body temperature is essential to the diagnosis of heat illness[51]: first, to determine if temperature is elevated and second, to monitor the response to cooling. Core temperature can be effectively measured in any deep body space; the rectum and esophagus are the usual sites.[52] Under field conditions, tympanic temperature is not an accurate reflection of core temperature[53,54] because, among other reasons, it is significantly influenced by the skin and tissue temperature of the neck.

Laboratory evaluation should be directed by the differential diagnosis appropriate for the clinical circumstances and those studies needed to monitor therapy and clinical state. Initial studies for all heat illness should include a complete blood count and measurement of electrolytes, blood urea nitrogen, and creatinine. Individuals suspected of having exertional heat injury or heat stroke should also have baseline studies that include liver function, clotting factors, creatine phosphokinase, myoglobin, calcium, and phosphorus.[55] Patients with heat stroke require serial monitoring of platelets and plasma clotting factors, renal and hepatic function, and electrolyte and acid-base status.

Recurrent heat illness is an indication for a formal evaluation for cystic fibrosis.[56,57] Heat stroke or rhabdomyolysis, particularly if recurrent, is an indication for muscle biopsy and evaluation for primary myopathy.[58–61]

Any patient in whom the diagnosis of heat stroke is possible will need at least 72 hours to complete an adequate period of observation, rest, and rehydration at a second- or third-echelon medical treatment facility. Patients who are clinically well but still being observed can be assigned supervised light duty at the treatment facility if shade and water are plentiful. Under no circumstances should they be reexposed to significant heat stress during this period.

Pathophysiology of Exertional Heat Illness

Exertional heat illness includes three disorders—heat exhaustion, heat injury, and heat stroke—which have in common that they occur acutely during exertion in the heat and are associated with substantial rises in core temperature. Although they are often thought of as degrees of heat illness along a single pathophysiological spectrum, it is not at all clear that they share a common pathophysiology. The clinical effects caused by exertional heat illness range from functional impairment in heat exhaustion to life-threatening organ injury in exertional heat stroke.

The pathophysiological mechanisms of heat exhaustion include an inadequate capacity to maintain cardiac output sufficient to sustain the demands of thermoregulation (ie, skin blood flow), muscular activity, and the viscera.[62,63] Dehydration, high core and skin temperature, and vigorous activity all combine to determine the point at which heat exhaustion occurs. The limitation of blood flow to mesenteric viscera is probably responsible for the gastrointestinal symptoms of heat exhaustion. The limitation of muscular blood flow contributes to the physical collapse. When demands for blood flow are extremely high, the expansion of the vascular bed can lower blood pressure to the point of syncope. Although all the exertional heat illnesses occur in the setting of exercise-heat exposure, it is not clear that heat exhaustion leads to more serious exertional heat illness.

The pathogenesis of exertional heat injury and exertional heat stroke is unclear. In both conditions measurable tissue injury occurs. In exertional heat injury, the tissue primarily affected is muscle, although there is usually evidence of mild injury to liver and kidney tissue. Exertional heat stroke, in contrast, is characterized by serious injury to multiple organs systems, including the central nervous system, and to clotting mechanisms. A variety of hypotheses have been proposed for the mechanisms of the tissue and organ damage of these two more serious forms of exertional heat illness. These include gastrointestinal endotoxin release from mesenteric vasoconstriction,[64–66] cellular energy depletion,[67] potassium depletion,[68] direct effects of hyperthermia,[69] and primary myopathies.[58,59] Dehydration is not as important a component in these two conditions as it is in heat exhaustion. Other factors that contribute to the pathogenesis of exertional heat illness include skin disease, medications that influence sweating or skin blood flow,[49] and the effects of inflammation on central thermoregulation.[70]

Heat Exhaustion

Heat exhaustion is the most commonly encountered form of heat illness.[3] Heat exhaustion, by definition, is a "functional" illness and is not associated with evidence of organ damage. Classically, heat exhaustion has been divided into salt-depletion heat exhaustion and water-depletion heat exhaustion.

Salt depletion in hot environments develops from increased salt loss in sweat (particularly among the unacclimatized) and reduced salt intake due to anorexia. Salt depletion develops over several days, so the contraction of extracellular fluid is gradual and symptoms develop slowly. The reduced extracellular fluid volume produces symptoms of fatigue and orthostatic dizziness. Because salt depletion does not produce intracellular hypertonicity, thirst is not prominent until the extracellular fluid volume has contracted enough to cause volumetric stimulation of thirst. Nausea and vomiting are common but of unknown mechanism. Hemoconcentration occurs due to the contraction of extracellular fluid. Muscle cramps are a common accompaniment of salt depletion (see "Heat Cramps" below). Potassium depletion commonly accompanies salt depletion due to diminished intake and mineralocorticoid-driven kaliuresis. Frank hypokalemia is uncommon.

Water depletion in hot environments develops from sweat rates sufficiently in excess of water replacement rates to produce hypertonic dehydration. Even though the loss of water occurs from both intracellular and extracellular compartments, the rate of dehydration is usually quite rapid and symptoms evolve quickly. Thirst is prominent and is caused by the hypertonicity. Oliguria, clinical dehydration, tachycardia, and tachypnea with symptomatic hyperventilation are all prominent clinical features.

In practice, neither heat exhaustion is encountered in a "pure" form; rather, classic heat exhaustion always includes elements of both water and electrolyte depletion. Rest, cooling, and adequate rehydration with hypotonic saline solutions are common elements of the therapy of both forms of heat exhaustion.

The management of heat exhaustion is directed to correcting the two pathogenic components of the illness: excessive cardiovascular demand and water and electrolyte depletion.[47,71] The load on the heart is reduced by rest and cooling. Water and electrolyte depletion is corrected by administering oral or parenteral fluids. Heat-exhausted patients do not require active cooling measures; removal of heavy clothing and rest in a shaded and ventilated space provides an adequate opportunity for spontaneous cooling. If available, cool water can be used to cool the skin. The consequent cutaneous vasoconstriction will rapidly reduce circulatory demand and improve venous return. Intravenous fluids replenish the extracellular volume quickly. Oral fluids suffice for those patients who can take fluids without risk of vomiting. However, clinical observation suggests parenteral fluids produce more rapid recovery than oral fluids, probably because oral fluids are absorbed more slowly.

Patients with heat exhaustion experience rapid clinical recovery[72] but need at least 24 hours of rest and rehydration under first-echelon or unit-level medical supervision to reverse their water and electrolyte depletion. A single episode of heat exhaustion does not imply any future predisposition to heat injury. An attempt should be made to determine the reason for the heat exhaustion (eg, insufficient work-rest or water discipline, coincident illness or medication). Repeated episodes of heat exhaustion require thorough evaluation.

Exertional Heat Injury

Exertional heat injury is an exertional heat illness that causes significant tissue damage from exercise heat exposure but does not develop into encephalopathy or organ failure. Exertional heat injury can present acutely as collapse during exercise, but some cases present many hours after exercise with prominent muscle pain and marked elevations in creatine phosphokinase and mild evidence of liver and kidney injury. Lack of conditioning and acclimatization appear to be risk factors for this type of exertional heat illness but do not account for all the cases.

Diagnosis is based on the evidence of tissue injury after exercise heat exposure in the absence of progression to heat stroke. Clinical recovery requires rest and restriction from further exercise in the heat. Recovery, defined as the resolution of pain and laboratory abnormalities, takes 7 to 10 days. The risk of recurrence is not known.

Exertional Heat Stroke

Exertional heat stroke is distinguished from exertional heat injury by the degree of organ injury and the appearance of encephalopathy and coagulopathy.[47,73–75] The degree of injury appears to relate to both the degree of temperature elevation and duration of exposure. Five organ systems (ie, the central nervous system, the hemostatic system, the liver, the kidneys, and muscle) are the principal foci of injury in exertional heat stroke. Encephalopathy is the sine qua non of heat stroke. Its presentation ranges from syncope and confusion to seizures or coma with decerebrate rigidity. Disseminated intravascular coagulation is common.[76] The principal causes of disseminated intravascular coagulation seem to be thermal damage to endothelium,[77] rhabdomyolysis, and direct thermal platelet activation causing intravascular microthrombi. Fibrinolysis is secondarily activated. Hepatic dysfunction and thermal injury to megakaryocytes slows the repletion of clotting factors. Hepatic injury is common and may progress to frank hepatic failure. Renal failure following heat stroke can be caused by several factors, including myoglobinuria from rhabdomyolysis, acute tubular necrosis due to hypoperfusion, glomerulopathy due to disseminated intravascular coagulation, direct thermal injury, and hyperuricemia. Rhabdomyolysis is a frequent complication of exertional heat stroke. Acute muscular necrosis releases large quantities of potassium, myoglobin, phosphate, and uric acid and sequesters calcium in the exposed contractile proteins. Adult respiratory distress syndrome complicates heat stroke occasionally and is associated with a high rate of mortality.[78]

The clinical outcome of patients with heat stroke is primarily a function of the magnitude and duration of temperature elevation. Mortality is rare in settings prepared to treat heat casualties with immediate cooling. Therefore, the most important therapeutic measure is rapid reduction of body temperature.[79] Any effective means of cooling is acceptable. While many techniques have been used, none has been unequivocally demonstrated to be superior. Immersion in cool or iced water with skin massage is a classic technique for cooling heat stroke patients. Ice water produces the most rapid cooling,[80] but cool water is less demanding logistically and less uncomfortable for the medical attendants. In hot, dry environments, field-expedient immersion baths that will keep water cool can be constructed by digging pits in the shade and lining them with plastic or by rigging shallow canvas tubs in well-ventilated, elevated frames (Figure 19-5).

Although not as effective at cooling as immersion, wetting the body surface and accelerating evaporation by fanning can also work.[81] The water can be applied by spraying or by application of thin conforming cloth wraps (eg, sheets, cotton underwear). Cooling blankets will also lower body temperature but are unlikely to be available in the field. Although cooling blankets have the advantage of maintaining a dry working environment, their limited contact surface provides slower cooling than

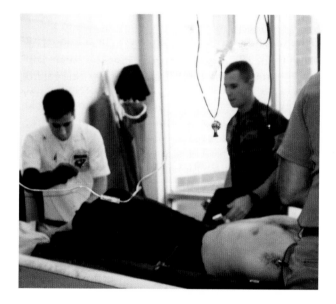

Fig. 19-5. The area for treatment of heat casualties at the USMC Training Base at Parris Island, SC. The tub is filled with ice. The casualty is placed on a litter above the ice and towels cooled in the ice water are placed on the body surface. Cooling comparable to immersion is achieved while preserving access to the torso and extremities for monitoring and emergency medical measures.
Photograph: Courtesy of Colonel John Gardner, Medical Corps, US Army, Uniformed Services University of the Health Sciences, Bethesda, Md.

immersion or surface-wetting techniques. Invasive cooling techniques have been tried, including ice water lavage or enemas and peritoneal lavage with cool fluids. These techniques do not provide faster cooling and have the additional disadvantages of potential complications and inappropriate fluid loads.

After cooling and hemodynamic stabilization, continuing care is supportive and is directed at the complications of heat stroke as they appear. Patients with heat stroke frequently have impaired temperature regulation for several days, with alternate periods of hyperthermia and hypothermia. Prognosis is worse in patients with more severe degrees of encephalopathy. Permanent neurological sequelae can develop after heat stroke, including cerebellar ataxia, paresis, seizure disorder, and cognitive dysfunction.[82,83]

Patients with heat stroke will require prolonged convalescence.[84] Heat stroke has been considered evidence for constitutional heat intolerance, but a recent study[85] demonstrates measurable heat intolerance in only 1 of 10 individuals after recovery from heat stroke. That same study also demonstrates that full heat tolerance was not achieved for up to a year even in those with eventual full recovery of thermoregulation.

Classic Heat Stroke

Classic heat stroke occurs in individuals, frequently those with impaired thermoregulation due to illness or medication, exposed passively to heat and dehydration.[86–88] It is principally an episodic affliction of young children in confined spaces, such as automobiles in the sun,[89] or an epidemic affliction in the elderly during urban heat waves.[90] Classic heat stroke differs in several ways from exertional heat stroke. Classic heat stroke evolves slowly, usually over a few days of continuous heat exposure. (Children in cars are exposed to much higher temperatures and are injured much more quickly.) Dehydration is a prominent feature. There is no exertional component, so rhabdomyolysis is less common, which reduces the likelihood of renal failure.[91] Mortality rates tend to be high because the patients often are alone and unable to summon help as the illness develops.

Heat Cramps

The specific pathophysiological mechanism of heat cramps is not known.[92–94] Heat cramps typically occur in salt-depleted individuals during a period of recovery after working in the heat[95] but are also a common component of salt-depletion heat exhaustion. Salt depletion is thought to be associated with muscle contraction of heat cramps.[40] Supporting that hypothesis is the efficacy of sodium chloride in treating heat cramps and the reduction of heat cramp incidence after salt supplementation

in industrial populations.[96]

Patients with heat cramps present with extremely painful tonic contractions of skeletal muscle.[47,50,95] The cramp in an individual muscle is usually preceded by palpable or visible fasciculation that lasts 2 to 3 minutes. Cramps are recurrent and may be precipitated by manipulation of muscle. The cramps involve the voluntary muscles of the trunk and extremities. Smooth muscle, cardiac muscle, the diaphragm, and bulbar muscles are not involved. In individuals with only heat cramps, there are no systemic manifestations except those attributable to pain. The cramps can begin during work or many hours after work.

The diagnosis of heat cramps is usually straightforward.[95] The differential diagnosis includes tetany due to alkalosis (eg, hyperventilation, severe gastroenteritis, cholera) or hypocalcemia, strychnine poisoning, black widow spider envenomation, or abdominal colic. These entities should be distinguishable on clinical examination. Replenishment of salt orally or parenterally resolves heat cramps rapidly. The response to therapy is sufficiently dramatic to be valuable in the differential diagnosis. The route of administration should be determined by the urgency of symptom relief.

Patients with heat cramps usually have substantial salt deficits (15–30 g, 2–3 days of usual dietary intake). These individuals should be allowed 2 to 3 days to replenish salt and water deficits before resuming work in the heat. No significant complications have been reported from heat cramps except muscle soreness. An episode of heat cramps does not imply any predisposition to heat injury. As with any heat illness, an attempt should be made to determine the reason for the episode so that appropriate advice can be given to the service member and the chain of command to avoid future episodes.

Prevention of heat cramps depends on the recognition of populations at risk and intervention to assure adequate water and salt intake. Sudden changes in weather or sudden exposure to unaccustomed work in the heat combined with inadequate intake of salt in the diet will produce in 2 to 3 days the salt depletion required for heat cramps. Military rations contain sufficient salt to maintain adequate body stores if they are fully consumed. In situations where rations are unavailable or not being consumed completely, salt supplementation from snack foods or salt solutions is appropriate. Environmental controls to reduce heat stress will also reduce salt depletion and reduce the incidence of heat cramps.

Exertional Rhabdomyolysis

Rhabdomyolysis that occurs as a result of exercise-heat exposure but without any other characteristics of exertional heat illness (eg, encephalopathy, hepatic injury) is considered exertional rhabdomyolysis.[47,97] It usually develops in a setting of heavy work with significant muscular loads.[98,99] Its specific pathophysiological mechanism is not known, but high muscle temperature and relative ischemia probably contribute. Some individuals with exertional rhabdomyolysis may have an underlying metabolic myopathy, which only manifests under extreme circumstances.[61,100]

Exertional rhabdomyolysis presents as collapse with marked muscle pain and tenderness during exercise heat exposure.[101,102] Systemic symptoms and signs, except the usual accompaniments of work in the heat, are not prominent initially.[98] As myonecrosis proceeds, however, acute renal failure, metabolic acidosis, and hypocalcemia develop. The diagnosis is established by myoglobinuria, marked elevation of creatine phosphokinase concentrations in blood, and renal injury in the absence of evidence of significant injury to other tissues or organs. Treatment is directed to minimizing renal injury and managing the acute metabolic consequences of the myonecrosis.

Although the circumstances under which exertional rhabdomyolysis develops are well known, it is an uncommon, sporadic illness. Although data are lacking about whether those who have had an episode of exertional rhabdomyolysis are susceptible to it again or to other heat illnesses, prior episodes should preclude future exposure. Prevention will depend on recognizing the circumstances in which it occurs, avoiding extreme muscular loading, and ensuring opportunities for rest and recovery during very strenuous work.

Exertional Hyponatremia

Exertional hyponatremia is a recently recognized heat illness.[103–107] It is a form of water intoxication, which produces dilutional hyponatremia.[107,108] It was originally recognized in elite athletes specializing in long-distance events but is found commonly among military training populations in hot climates. Since the illness requires sufficient water intake to cause hyponatremia, it is possible its recent appearance is related to increased water consumption during exercise-heat exposure in an effort to prevent dehydration and heat illness. Most cases of symptomatic exertional hyponatremia are sporadic, but at least one epidemic has occurred in a military unit required to drink too much water during training.[109]

The manifestations of exertional hyponatremia are thirst, fatigue, and anorexia. The illness develops over a number of hours. The symptoms usually limit work capacity, so hyperthermia is not a common clinical sign. If the water consumption continues, hyponatremia can progress beyond mild symptoms to frank seizures and rhabdomyolysis.[110–112] Hyponatremia responds to the usual measures for water intoxication, including water restriction and seizure control. Exertional hyponatremia resolves quickly, usually with full recovery.[107] The risk of recurrence is not known.

The prevention of exertional hyponatremia depends on the recognition that excessive water consumption can be as dangerous as inadequate water consumption. Guidance about water consumption should provide both a minimum and a maximum amount.[104,113–115]

Minor Heat Illnesses

Miliaria Rubra, Miliaria Profunda, and Anhidrotic Heat Exhaustion

Miliaria rubra is a subacute pruritic, inflamed, papulovesicular skin eruption that appears in actively sweating skin exposed to high humidity.[116] In dry climates, miliaria is confined to skin sufficiently occluded by clothing to produce local high humidity[117] (Figure 19-6). Each miliarial papulovesicle represents a sweat gland whose duct is occluded at the level of the epidermal stratum granulosum by inspissated organic debris.[118,119] Sweat accumulates in the glandular portion of the gland and infiltrates into the surrounding dermis. Pruritus increases with increased sweating. Miliarial skin cannot fully participate in thermoregulation, and therefore the risk of heat illness is increased in proportion to the amount of skin surface involved.[28,29,120,121] Sleeplessness due to pruritus and secondary infection of occluded glands have systemic effects that further degrade optimal thermoregulation.[122]

Miliaria is treated by cooling and drying affected skin, avoiding conditions that induce sweating, controlling infection, and relieving pruritus. Eccrine gland function recovers when the affected epidermis desquamates, which takes 1 to 3 weeks.

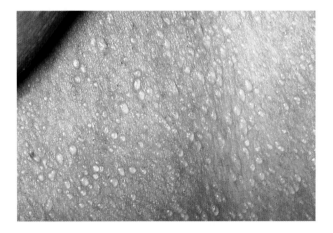

Fig. 19-6. In cases of miliaria crystaluna, sweat is trapped in the ducts of the sweat glands by inspissated material. The trapped sweat produces the appearance of small vesicles on the skin, such as in this photograph.
Photograph: Courtesy of Commander, USARIEM, Natick, Mass.

Miliaria that becomes generalized and prolonged (miliaria profunda) can cause an uncommon but disabling disorder: anhidrotic heat exhaustion, which is also known as tropical anhidrotic asthenia. The lesions of miliaria profunda are presumed to develop from pre-existing miliaria rubra lesions by a superimposed inflammatory obstruction of the eccrine duct. The lesions are truncal, noninflamed, and papular, with less evidence of vesiculation than the lesions of miliaria rubra. They may only be evident during active sweat production. Sweat does not appear on the surface of affected skin. The lesions are asymptomatic, which may explain why the patient does not seek medical evaluation early in the course.

Miliaria profunda causes a marked inhibition of thermoregulatory sweating and heat intolerance similar to that of ectodermal dysplasia. Symptoms of heat exhaustion and high risk of heat stroke occur under conditions well tolerated by other individuals. Management of miliaria profunda requires evacuation to a cooler environment for several weeks to allow restoration of normal function of the eccrine glands.

Heat Syncope

Syncope occurring while standing in a hot environment has been called heat syncope, but it is probably not a discrete clinical entity. Rather, thermal stress increases the risk of classic neurally mediated (vasovagal) syncope by aggravating peripheral pooling of blood in dilated cutaneous vessels.[47,123] No special heat-related significance should be assigned to syncope occurring in these circumstances. Clinical evaluation and management should be directed toward the syncopal episode, not potential heat illness. However, syncope occurring during or after work in the heat or after more than 5 days of heat exposure should be considered evidence of heat exhaustion.

Heat Edema

Mild dependent edema ("deck legs") is occasionally seen during the early stages of heat exposure while plasma volume is expanding to compensate for the increased need for thermoregulatory blood flow. In the absence of other disease, the condition is of no clinical significance and will resolve spontaneously. Diuretic therapy is not appropriate and may increase the risk of heat illness.

Heat Tetany

Heat tetany is a rare condition, which occurs in individuals acutely exposed to overwhelming heat stress.[124] Extremely severe heat stress induces hyperventilation, which appears to be the principal pathophysiological process. The manifestations of heat tetany are characteristic of hyperventilation. They include respiratory alkalosis, carpopedal spasm, and syncope. Management requires removal from the heat and control of hyperventilation. Dehydration and salt depletion are not prominent features.

Chronic Dehydration

Chronic dehydration,[125] also known as voluntary dehydration, is associated with several disabling conditions, including nephrolithiasis,[126] hemorrhoids, fecal impaction, and urinary tract infection. Prevention requires the establishment of water consumption targets and command enforcement of those targets.

COLD ENVIRONMENTS

Cold and Military Campaigns

Casualties from cold exposure occur in all types of operations. Cold can be an effective offensive weapon. Forces including the US Army, the Russians, and the Finns have used cold in this way by displacing their opponent from shelter and allowing the environment itself to force surrender. Rapidly paced operations, though, can outrun supply trains and expose leading elements to unexpected cold weather bivouacs and risk of cold injury. It should not be surprising that the US military has suffered cold weather casualties in almost all of its conflicts, from the American Revolution to the Korean War.[127,128] Cold injuries remain a problem in military operations and training exercises today.[129–136]

Physiological Effects of Cold Exposure

Humans have evolved two physiologic mechanisms to maintain core temperature during cold exposure: (1) reducing skin temperature, which reduces the differential between the skin temperature and the environment and slows heat loss and (2) increasing heat production by shivering.[137]

When the body is exposed to cold, blood is diverted away from the skin and extremities to the trunk by vasoconstriction. Consequently, a layer of relatively hypoperfused tissue is formed between the environment and the viscera. Deprived of the heat from the metabolically active core, this "shell" of tissue cools, thereby reducing the gradients for heat loss from the skin surface by radiation, conduction, and evaporation. This tissue insulation has been estimated to be about the same as that provided by wearing a wool business suit. In contrast, heavy arctic clothing provides six to eight times as much insulation.

Cold sensory receptors in the skin respond to both absolute temperature and the rate of temperature change. Consequently, sudden exposure to cold, such as walking from a warm building into a cold wind, will trigger an acute response with vasoconstriction and even transient shivering. As cold exposure continues, the skin equilibrates at the new colder temperature. As skin temperature stops changing, the response to the cold stimulus moderates and the acute shivering passes. The skin gradually (over a period of 2 to 3 hours) accommodates to the cold, and the sensation of cold becomes less uncomfortable. Conversely, if cold skin is warmed, the reflex response will reduce the insulating vasoconstrictive response, increase heat loss from skin and extremities, and inhibit shivering. This may be the explanation for Baron Larrey's observation during Napoleon's retreat from Moscow during the winter of 1812 that people near campfires were more likely to die during sleep than those sleeping further away.[138] As a consequence of reducing blood flow and volume in skin and extremities, peripheral vasoconstriction causes an expansion in central blood volume that can induce diuresis and dehydration.

If the insulating effect of vasoconstriction is insufficient to protect the core temperature, the continuing fall in temperature triggers the onset of heat production by muscle. Initially, muscle tone increases, which increases metabolic rate 2-fold. However, if core temperature falls further, the muscular activity changes to cycles of contraction and relaxation, producing visible shivering.[139] Maximal shivering increases heat production up to seven times the resting level. It is essential to remember that a fall in core temperature has already occurred when sustained shivering appears.

Although vasoconstriction is beneficial and protects core temperature because it reduces the flow of blood from the core to the periphery, it places the metabolically inactive acral regions of the body at risk of severe cooling and injury. Cold-induced vasodilation (CIVD) is a physiological mechanism that appears to reduce the risk of injury when the hands or feet are exposed to water below 10°C (50°F) and air below 0°C (32°F). As the hands or feet cool, vasoconstriction initially reduces blood flow and volume. After some minutes of low digital temperature, arteriovenous anastomoses in the distal phalanx open and allow a rapid increase in digital blood flow by bypassing the constricted precapillary arterioles.[140] While the anastomoses remain open, the digits remain warm. The phenomenon is usually cyclic, producing alternating periods of vasoconstriction and vasodilation 10 to 20 minutes long. Individuals vary in the magnitude of their CIVD response.[141] The magnitude and duration of the CIVD depend on core temperature. When core temperature is low, the phenomenon is substantially less.

Physiological adaptation to cold is not a phenomenon of the same significance as adaptation to heat or high terrestrial altitude.[142] Indeed, the successful use of clothing and shelter in cold environments prevents much of the cold stress that might induce adaptation or habituation. Consequently, there appear to be no practical means of significantly enhancing physiological cold tolerance through training or predeployment exercises. The principal mechanisms through which cold tolerance develops are familiarization and habituation (Exhibit 19-6).

EXHIBIT 19-6

IMPORTANT PHYSIOLOGICAL POINTS OF COLD EXPOSURE

- Humans cannot sense core temperature.

- Skin is sensitive to cold and will be painful until it cools to 10°C (50°F).

- Skin accommodates to cold; exposure reduces the sensation of both cold and pain.

- Skin is numb below 10°C. The disappearance of pain in an extremity during cold exposure may indicate serious cold injury. Immediate visual inspection for frostbite is mandatory.

- Cold exposure causes diuresis, which aggravates the routine dehydration in field settings.

- Extremities below 10°C are paralyzed.

- The most important adaptation to cold is proper training and equipment.

Adapted from: United States Army Research Institute of Environmental Medicine. *Medical Aspects of Cold Weather Operations: A Handbook for Medical Officers.* Natick, Mass: USARIEM; 1993: 45. Technical Note 93-4.

PREVENTION OF ILLNESS AND INJURY IN THE COLD

It is useful to analyze the risk of environmental cold injury as an interaction of three components: the environmental stress, the thermocompetence of the service member, and the protective technology available. This is an equation that shows this interaction:

$$(2) \quad \text{Strain} = f \frac{\text{Time} \bullet \text{Cold Stress}}{\text{Thermocompetence} \bullet \text{Technology}}$$

Environmental Cold Stress

Cold land environments are generally classified as either wet-cold or dry-cold. Wet-cold environments have ambient temperatures from above freezing to about 18°C (65°F), with wetness ranging from fog to heavy rain. They are associated with nonfreezing peripheral cold injuries, such as trench foot. Usually, many hours to days of exposure are required to cause injury. Dry-cold environments have ambient temperatures below freezing (0°C, 32°F). Precipitation, if present, is in the form of snow. Dry-cold environments are associated with freezing peripheral injuries, which can develop in a few minutes to hours.

Certain exposures carry a high risk of rapid, severe freezing injury. Aircrew exposed to the airstream around a flying aircraft through an open hatch or port in the fuselage can incur serious freezing injuries in seconds. Exposure to fluids at subfreezing temperatures, such as gasoline or propane and butane propellants, will also cause immediate, severe freezing injury.[143]

A quantitative index of risk to exposed skin, the Wind-Chill Index, was developed in the 1940s and has been revised many times.[144,145] If used carefully, it is a useful tool for judging the risk of cold exposure. It is important to remember that the Wind-Chill Index does not provide an index either of hypothermic risk or of risk to covered skin. Effective cover will protect skin even in conditions of very "cold" wind chill. Predictive models for risk assessment and management of other types of cold exposure are being rapidly developed.[143,146]

Changing weather conditions are associated with an increased risk of cold injury. Exhaustion hypothermia classically occurs when individuals are caught in unexpected rain or snow. They may have to bivouac without adequate shelter or become lost or delayed in cross-country movement, any of which leads to prolonged cold exposure. Freezing injuries commonly occur at the conclusion of a period of bitter cold when the slightly warmer, but still cold, temperatures do not produce their usual sensation of cold. Thawing causes wet-cold conditions and increases the risk of nonfreezing cold injury.

Combat conditions often reduce the options for mitigating cold exposure and are the military circumstances associated with the highest risk of cold injury. It is in these circumstances that cold injury control relies on maintaining the highest level of cold tolerance and protection.

Thermocompetence

Characteristics of service members that are generally accepted to be risk factors for cold injury include prior cold injury, predisposing conditions, fatigue, dehydration, weight loss, lack of cold weather training and experience, lower rank, origin in a warm climate, black skin, and tobacco use.[147] The medical officer must be completely familiar with the unit and monitor it carefully to judge when particular risk factors are of sufficient magnitude to require intervention.

Previous cold injury is an important risk factor and should be considered in the predeployment assessment of each unit member.[148] Cold injuries, even of mild degree, are good predictors of the likelihood of another cold injury. The risk of reinjury is extremely high if the cold injury occurred in the same cold season but even years later remains significantly above the risk of others who have not had a cold injury. Military experience is consistent in showing the inability of service members with clinically healed cold injury to return successfully to their units in a cold environment. The rates of reinjury are so high that military medical officers have always eventually realized that these casualties must be accommodated by modified duty assignments.[149]

Predisposing conditions include neuropathic and vascular diseases, such as Raynaud's disease[150] (Figure 19-7) or diabetes mellitus. Increased age and sickle cell trait may increase the risk of peripheral cold injury.[37,151] Many cold injury risk factors are inevitable accompaniments of military operations and become more prevalent and severe as time passes. Among these are

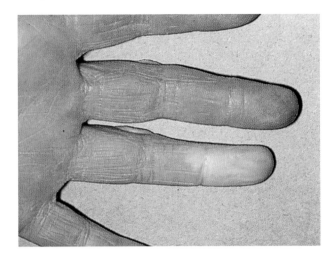

Fig. 19-7. Raynaud's phenomenon in the distal segment of the ring finger. Raynaud's disease is a predisposing factor for cold injury.
Photograph: Courtesy of Commander, USARIEM, Natick, Mass.

dehydration, weight loss,[152,153] and fatigue[154] (Figure 19-8). An increasing incidence of cold injuries is one way these factors will be expressed. Successful primary prevention will depend on con-

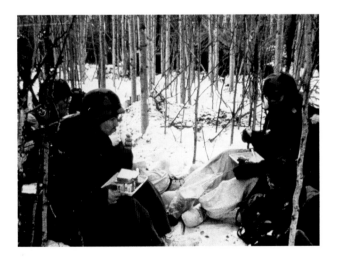

Fig. 19-8. Operations in cold environments increase calorie requirements. Palatability is an important factor in maintaining adequate food intake to meet the increased needs. However, the circumstances of cold weather operations makes the provision of war food difficult. This meal is being consumed in ambient temperatures of –30°F and will freeze in a few minutes.
Photograph: Courtesy of Colonel Wayne Askew, MS, US Army (Ret), USARIEM, Natick, Mass.

tinuous monitoring for these conditions and on actions to mitigate them.

Experience is consistent in showing an increased risk of cold injury among individuals from warm climates and individuals with black skin.[131] The reason of the increased risk is not known but the phenomenon must be addressed by the unit preventive medicine program.

Successful cold injury prevention ultimately rests on the skill and knowledge of the service members conducting operations in cold environments and, consequently, on the training they receive. The unit medics should be thoroughly trained in the signs, symptoms, prevention, and management of cold injuries and how to survey aggressively for illness and injury. They must understand that early recognition of cold injuries is essential to minimize their consequences. Unit leaders must understand the causes and manifestations of cold injury, both for their own benefit and for that of their unit. They should understand the importance of hydration, adequate rations, the "buddy" system, and clean, dry, properly used cold weather clothing and footgear on preserving unit function in the field. They should understand the importance of adequate predeployment preparation for cold by conducting cold weather training, inspecting cold weather clothing and equipment, and assuring appropriate health maintenance and medical screening measures.

In World War II, hospitalized cold injury casualties were twice as likely (about 2/3 to 1/3) to say they had never received training in cold injury prevention than casualties with similar cold exposures hospitalized for other injuries.[149] All unit members should know the signs and symptoms of cold injury in themselves and their buddy and know what to do if they suspect a cold injury. They should be alert to the consequences of dehydration, weight loss, fatigue, tobacco use, and alcohol consumption. They must understand and implement the established techniques for foot care in the cold (Exhibit 19-7).

Technology

The ability of a military force to train and operate in a cold environment is critically dependent on the technology they have to protect themselves from the climate (eg, shelters, heaters) and to transport themselves and food and water.[155,156] Technological failures, inappropriate or unskilled use of the available technology, or contingencies that disrupt the function or supply of this equipment will lead to outbreaks of cold injury.[149,157,158]

EXHIBIT 19-7

FOOT CARE IN COLD ENVIRONMENTS

- Assure the best possible fit of the boots with heavy socks.

- Keep the body as warm as possible, avoid chilling.

- Remove boots and socks at least twice a day; wash, dry, massage, and move the feet to restore circulation and feeling; allow enough time and provide appropriate shelter to complete this task; after massaging and warming feet, put on clean, dry socks, or, if dry socks are not available, remove as much water from the wet socks as possible before putting them back on.

- Do not sleep with wet footgear; remove wet boots and socks for sleep; protect the feet with as much dry cover as possible to keep them warm.

- Dry wet socks by keeping them in the sleeping bag during sleep or placing them inside the field jacket against the chest or across the shoulders.

- In fixed positions, stand on rocks, boards, or brush to keep the feet out of water and mud.

- Keep the feet and legs moving to stimulate warming circulation; instead of crouching all the time to keep low in a fixed position, try to sit or lie back periodically with the feet slightly elevated to reduce swelling of the feet and ankles.

- Watch carefully for numbness or tingling—these are early symptoms of injury; if these develop, immediately take measures to warm the feet.

- Keep the clothing and footgear loose enough to permit easy circulation.

Source: United States Army Research Institute of Environmental Medicine. *Medical Aspects of Cold Weather Operations: A Handbook for Medical Officers.* Natick, Mass: USARIEM; 1993: 12. Technical Note 93-4.

Implementing a Cold Injury Prevention Program

Cold injury prevention starts before exposure, with screening and identification of service members at increased risk (Exhibit 19-8). In some circumstances risk can be reduced, such as by stopping tobacco use or providing extra protective clothing (Exhibit 19-9). Occasionally individuals will not be able to be accommodated, and they should not be assigned to duties requiring cold exposure. In addition, appropriate equipment and training must be provided before exposure. The unit command group should establish standard cold weather operating procedures that incorporate guidelines for sustaining overall fitness and health (eg, hydration, nutrition, rest), limiting exposure times (eg, work-warming cycles, intervals for inspection and rewarming of face and extremities), and assuring the timely maintenance and replacement of personal equipment. Military medical personnel should develop their own policies and procedures for medical monitoring and rapid reporting of cold injuries.

The most important control measure for preventing cold injury is a command requirement to inspect and rewarm the face and extremities periodically. The interval between rewarming should be determined by the immediate circumstances of the unit and may be as frequent as every 20 or 30 minutes in very cold weather.

Medical surveillance should be performed in an organized fashion by all military medical personnel. Regular written reports are an essential part of the discipline that successful medical surveillance requires. Without organized data collection, surveillance becomes anecdotal and loses a significant amount of its sensitivity for early detection and successful intervention (see Exhibit 19-9).

ILLNESS AND INJURY DUE TO COLD

Freezing Injury (Frostbite)

Frostbite is currently the most common cold injury encountered in US forces and has always been a particular problem for the Army. Isolated episodes are usually associated with an episode of carelessness or sudden weather change, either warming or cooling. Clusters of frostbite injuries occur in exer-

---

EXHIBIT 19-8

COLD INJURY: IMPORTANT PREVENTION POINTS

- The best prevention against cold injury is a healthy, trained, equipped, well-fed, and hydrated service member with alert and conscientious leaders.

- In military operations and training, risk factors for freezing injuries include

  - dehydration,

  - weight loss,

  - unplanned or unduly prolonged exposures to cold,

  - undertrained or overtired service members,

  - previous cold injury, and

  - poor or insufficient equipment.

- When one freezing injury has occurred in an operation, remember that everyone in the unit was exposed to the same conditions. Inspect everyone immediately.

- Loss of sensation in the feet (they feel like "blocks of wood" or "like walking on cotton") is an ominous symptom and must be immediately evaluated by direct inspection of the feet.

- Cold injuries during operations usually occur in clusters.

- A service member who is shivering is already too cold.

- No one in whom hypothermia is suspected should be left alone.

- Exercise is dangerous if significant hypothermia is present.

Adapted from: United States Army Research Institute of Environmental Medicine. *Medical Aspects of Cold Weather Operations: A Handbook for Medical Officers.* Natick, Mass: USARIEM; 1993: 45–46. Technical Note 93-4.

---

cises and operations and are frequently the result of poor planning or inattention to control measures. Fortunately, most frostbite injuries occurring during training do not result in permanent tissue loss.[159] The long period of recovery, however, usually means the loss of the injured service member to field duties for the remainder of the cold season. In cold regions, this can mean months of limited duty. For that reason, a unit that suffers a cluster of freezing injuries may become ineffective.

Most freezing injuries will be recognized and initially managed by unit medics and other nonphysician medical providers. Because optimal treatment of the freezing injury depends on early detection and immediate, appropriate management, ultimately the clinical outcome will depend on the successful training and skills of the unit medics.

Pathogenesis

Frostbite injury results when tissue is cooled sufficiently to freeze.[160] Tissues with large surface-to-mass ratios (eg, ears) or with restricted circula-

---

EXHIBIT 19-9

COLD INJURY PREVENTION PROGRAM

- Screen, select, immunize, and train service members before exposure.

- Provide appropriate equipment and training in its use.

- Establish unit exposure-control SOPs.

- Establish medical SOPs for medical monitoring, first aid, and rapid reporting of cold injuries.

- Obtain supplies for casualty management and evacuation in cold environments.

- Predict and monitor exposure.

- Monitor unit members' thermocompetence.

- Maintain and replace equipment.

- Inspect periodically the entire unit for injury.

- Respond to cold injuries with modification in policy and procedure as needed.

SOP: standard operating procedure

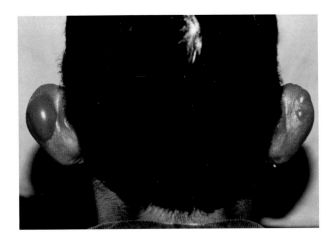

Fig. 19-9. This is a case of second-degree frostbite. The ears are commonly affected by frostbite.
Photograph: Courtesy of Commander, USARIEM, Natick, Mass.

tion (eg, hands, feet) are particularly susceptible to freezing, but any tissue exposed to severe cold can freeze (Figure 19-9).

Tissue does not freeze at 0°C (32°F); the high concentration of electrolytes and other solutes prevents freezing until tissue is cooled below –2°C (28°F). At that point, ice crystals form, which segregate some tissue water and cause concentration of the remainder into a progressively more hypertonic and harmful solution. Once solidly frozen, tissue injury is probably arrested. Additional injury to frozen tissue occurs during and after thawing, probably in two phases. First, on restoration of blood flow, reperfusion tissue injury occurs.[161] Second, marked endothelial swelling develops in the thawed tissue, causing secondary loss of perfusion, ischemia, and infarction of tissue. Despite freezing and reperfusion injury, some frostbitten tissue is able to recover. Refreezing of injured tissue, however, causes irredeemable injury, a phenomenon used therapeutically in cryosurgery.

Clinical Manifestations and Classification

Initially, all frozen tissue has the same characteristics: it is cold, hard, and pale.[162] Except in minor and severe cases, the degree of injury will usually not become clear for 24 to 72 hours. Most significant injuries include areas with different degrees of frostbite, with the distal areas usually more severely affected. Digits, ears, and exposed facial skin are the most commonly injured areas.

Frostbite is classified by depth of injury, which determines both the prognosis and speed of recovery.

Superficial injuries are categorized as first- and second-degree frostbite. Deep injuries are categorized as third- and fourth-degree frostbite. The depth of the injury depends on both the duration and the intensity of the cold exposure. Very intense cold for a few seconds will produce a superficial injury whereas prolonged exposure to moderate freezing cold can freeze an entire extremity.

First-degree frostbite is an epidermal injury. The affected area is usually limited in extent, involving skin that has had brief contact with very cold air or metal (eg, touching an outside door handle). The frozen skin is initially a white or yellow plaque. It thaws quickly, becoming wheal-like, red, and painful. Since deep tissues are not frozen (though they may be cold), mobility is normal. The affected area may become edematous but does not blister. Desquamation of the frostbitten skin with complete clinical healing follows in 7 to 10 days (Figure 19-10).

Second-degree frostbite involves the whole epidermis and may also affect superficial dermis. The initial frozen appearance is the same as a first-degree injury. Since the freezing involves deeper layers and usually occurs in tissue with prolonged cold exposure, some limitation of motion is present early. Thawing is rapid, with return of mobility and appearance of pain in affected areas. A blister, with clear fluid, forms in the injured area several hours after thawing. Usually, the upper layers of dermis are preserved, which permits rapid re-epithelialization. Second-degree injuries produce no permanent tissue loss. Healing is complete but takes at least 3 to 4

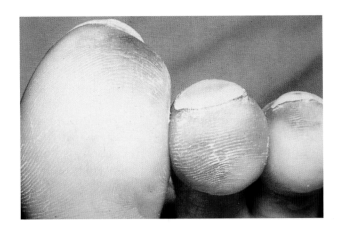

Fig. 19-10. First-degree frostbite ("frostnip") is the most common military cold injury. The affected area is susceptible to deeper injury until healed so cold exposure needs to be curtailed for even this apparently modest injury.
Photograph: Courtesy of Commander, USARIEM, Natick, Mass.

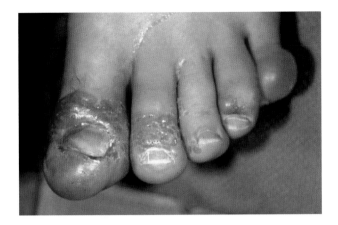

Fig. 19-11. Second-degree frostbite is a severely disabling injury and is likely to affect the service member's ability to remain on active duty. Urgent evacuation is required. Recovery will take many weeks to months.
Photograph: Courtesy of Commander, USARIEM, Natick, Mass.

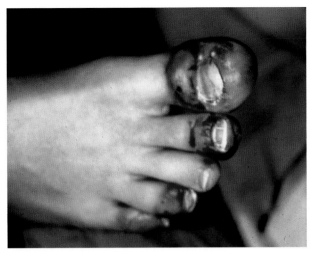

Fig. 19-12. Significant tissue loss and long-term cold sensitivity is to be expected after third-degree frostbite. This is likely a career-ending injury.
Photograph: Courtesy of Commander, USARIEM, Natick, Mass.

weeks. First-degree injury is frequently present in the immediate vicinity of second-degree frostbite. Frostbite should be looked for on all other exposed areas of skin. Following second-degree frostbite, cold sensitivity may persist in the injured area (Figure 19-11).

Third-degree frostbite involves the dermis to at least the reticular layer. Initially, the frozen tissue is stiff and restricts mobility. After thawing, mobility is restored briefly, but the affected skin swells rapidly and hemorrhagic blisters develop due to damage to the dermal vascular plexus. Significant skin loss follows slowly through mummification and sloughing. Healing is also slow, progressing from adjacent and residual underlying dermis. There may be permanent tissue loss. Residual cold sensitivity is common (Figure 19-12).

Fourth-degree frostbite involves the full thickness of the skin and underlying tissues, even including bone. Initially the frozen tissue has no mobility. Thawing restores passive mobility, but intrinsic muscle function is lost. Skin reperfusion after thawing is poor. Blisters and edema do not develop. The affected area shows early necrotic change. The injury evolves slowly (weeks) to mummification, sloughing, and autoamputation. Whatever dermal healing occurs is from adjacent skin. Significant, permanent anatomic and functional loss is the rule.

Basic Principles of Management

Since many frostbite injuries result in formal investigations, careful records should be made from the outset, including at least a complete description of the circumstances of the injury, its initial extent and appearance, and the first steps of management.

The first essential step in cold injury management is detection. Frostbite injuries are insidious. Injured tissue, which is painful initially while it is getting cold, is anesthetic when frozen and is often covered by a glove or boot. Detection requires direct inspection of at-risk tissue, including the hands, feet, ears, nose, and face.

Active warming of frozen tissue should be deferred until there is absolutely no risk that the injured tissue can be reexposed to freezing cold. This recommendation does not mean that the injured part should be deliberately kept frozen by packing in snow or continuing the cold exposure. If refreezing can be prevented during evacuation, then frozen tissue can be immediately warmed by contact with warm skin. Once tissue has thawed, it is essential that it be protected from reexposure to cold. The tissue must not be exposed to temperatures in excess of 40°C (104°F–105°F), which will aggravate the injury. Exposure to exhaust manifolds, open flames, stovetops, incandescent bulbs, or hot water is particularly dangerous. Frostbitten tissue is vulnerable to trauma and should be carefully protected from physical injury during evacuation.

Digits or entire hands or feet can be warmed in a temperature-monitored water bath kept from 39°C to 41°C (102°F–105°F). Facial tissue or the ears can be thawed with warm, wet towels. Warming should be continued until no further improvement in the return of circulation and mobility is noted. The time required will depend on the initial temperature and size of the injured part and can take more than an hour in severe cases. After warming, the frostbitten tissue should be carefully and atraumatically dried, completely covered in bulky, dry dressings, and kept slightly elevated to moderate swelling.

After the necessary emergency stabilization is accomplished and warming has begun, early management includes tetanus prophylaxis as appropriate and analgesics. During warming, pain appears and is often intense. Nonsteroidal antiinflammatory drugs and narcotics should be provided as needed.

Freezing injuries should always be considered serious. Military medical practice is to evacuate all cold-injured casualties to rear echelons for discharge or reassignment to modified duty without cold exposure. The continuing care of freezing injury is intended to minimize the loss of tissue by providing the optimum environment for healing, avoiding additional injury and infection, and permitting spontaneous evolution of tissue loss.

The principal late complications of frostbite include tissue loss, contractures, persistent pain, cold sensitivity, susceptibility to reinjury, and hyperhidrosis. After healing, cold exposure of any portion of the skin may precipitate symptoms in the area of a previous injury. Relocation to a warm climate may be required if cold intolerance is intractable. Tissues that have suffered a frostbite injury are probably more susceptible to cold injury and should receive extra protection and attention when exposed to cold. Hyperhidrosis of the feet can increase the incidence of dermatophyte infection and maceration.

Nonfreezing Cold Injury

Nonfreezing cold injury (NFCI) is the result of prolonged (many hours) exposure of the extremities to wet-cold of between 0°C and 18°C (32°F–65°F).[163] The feet are the most common area of injury, which is reflected in the common names of the two principal types of nonfreezing injury: trench foot and immersion foot. Trench foot occurs during ground operations and is caused by the combined effects of sustained cold exposure and restricted circulation. Immersion foot is caused by continuous immersion of the extremities in cold water and usually occurs in survivors of ship sinkings. Trench foot is rare outside of military operations, but immersion injury is a risk of any maritime venture.

Pathogenesis

Prolonged cooling produces some damage to all the soft tissues, but peripheral nerves and blood vessels suffer the greatest injury.[164–166] The vascular injury causes secondary ischemic injury, which aggravates the direct effect of cold on other tissues. Wet conditions increase the risk and accelerate the injury both because wet clothing insulates poorly and because water itself cools more effectively than air at the same temperature. Factors that reduce circulation to the extremities also contribute to the injury. In military operations, these factors include constrictive clothing and boots, prolonged immobility, hypothermia, and crouched posture. Maceration of the wet skin can complicate NFCI and predisposes the service member to infection.

Clinical Manifestations and Classification

When first seen, the injured tissue is pale, anesthetic, pulseless, and immobile but not frozen.[167] Trench foot or immersion foot (depending on the environmental medium causing the injury) is likely when these signs do not change immediately after warming. Like freezing injury, the degree of the injury is usually not apparent early.

The course of NFCI is classically divided into preinflammatory, inflammatory, and postinflammatory phases.[168] In the preinflammatory phase, despite rest and warmth, the injured part remains pale, anesthetic, and pulseless. After several hours (occasionally as long as 24-36 hours), the inflammatory phase begins with the appearance of a marked hyperemia associated with burning pain and the reappearance of sensation proximally but not distally. The hyperemia represents a passive venous vasodilation and blanches with elevation. Edema, often sanguineous, and bullae develop in the injured areas as perfusion increases. Skin that remains poorly perfused after hyperemia appears is likely to slough as the injury evolves. Persistence of pulselessness in an extremity after 48 hours suggests severe deep injury and high likelihood of substantial tissue loss. The hyperemia lasts a few days to many weeks, depending on the severity of the injury (Figure 19-13).

Recovery from NFCI is slow due to its neuropathic component. Except in minor injuries, deep aching develops that is associated with sharp, intermittent "lightning" pains in the second week after injury. Improved sensitivity to light touch and pain in the area of anesthesia within 4 to 5 weeks suggests reversible nerve injury and less likelihood of persistent symptoms. Persistence of anesthesia to touch beyond 6 weeks suggests neuronal degeneration. Injury of this degree takes much longer to resolve and has a greater likelihood of persistent disabling symptoms.

Hyperhidrosis is a common and prominent late feature of NFCI and seems to precede the recovery of sensation. A distinct advancing hyperhidrotic

and introduces a vicious cycle of hypoxia worsening edema and edema worsening hypoxia. The incidence of HAPE, like that of AMS and HACE, depends on the intensity of the hypoxic exposure. In the 1990 Fuertos Caminos exercise at 4,200 m, it was 3.8% (Exhibit 19-10). The risk is substantially increased by exertion,[275] particularly in the first 3 to 4 days of altitude exposure, but physical exertion is not required to precipitate HAPE.[276]

The manifestations of HAPE include breathlessness, cyanosis, orthopnea, rales, chest pain, cough, frothy sputum, hemoptysis, and tachycardia. Fever is occasionally present. An individual with AMS or HACE can also develop HAPE; this complicates the management of the casualty.

Mild degrees of HAPE can be resolved with treatment at altitude,[277] but it can be lethal and is generally more fulminant than HACE. Severe cases die within a few hours of presentation if not treated. Treatment includes descent, portable hyperbaric chambers,[266] (Figure 19-17) oxygen, nifedipine and other pulmonary vasodilators,[252,278] expiratory positive airway pressure,[258] and dexamethasone. With proper treatment, clinical recovery is usually rapid, but severe acute respiratory distress syndrome that requires assisted ventilation can occur. Subtle abnormalities in pulmonary function can persist for a number of weeks after recovery.[279] Although nifedipine can be used for prophylaxis against recurrence of HAPE, an episode of HAPE should preclude future altitude deployment for the service member.

Other Medical Issues at Altitude

Thromboembolic Disease

Thromboembolic disease is more common at altitude.[280–283] Its increased incidence seems related to hemoconcentration, dehydration, alteration in clotting mechanisms, and enforced inactivity during bad weather. The types of thromboembolic disease include (*a*) thrombosis of the deep veins of the legs complicated by pulmonary embolism (which may present like HAPE[284]) and cerebral thrombosis and (*b*) stroke. Although epidemiological data are very sparse, the risk seems small at moderate altitudes (< 3,000 m) and increases with the duration and intensity of altitude exposure.

High Altitude Retinal Hemorrhage

High altitude retinal hemorrhage (HARH) is a usually benign condition with startling ophthalmoscopic findings. HARH is caused by hemorrhage from retinal vessels that dilate in response to hypoxia.[285,286] The hemorrhages can interfere with vision if they involve the macula. One case of central retinal vein occlusion with marked visual loss and retinal hemorrhage has been described.[287] As a

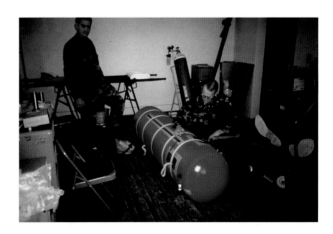

Fig. 19-17. A portable hyperbaric chamber (a Gamov bag) used to treat high altitude pulmonary edema during Operation Fuertos Caminos in Potosi, Bolivia.
Photograph: Courtesy of COL Eugene Iwanyk, Medical Corps, US Army, USARIEM, Natick, Mass.

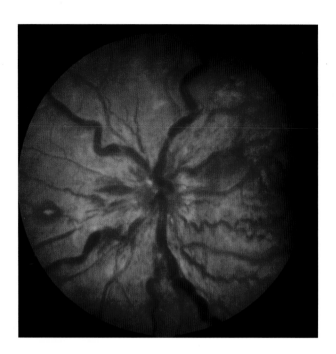

Fig. 19-18. A photograph of a radiograph of high altitude retinal hemorrhage.
Photograph: Courtesy of COL Paul Rock, Medical Corps, US Army, USARIEM, Natick, Mass.

rule, HAPH resolves spontaneously on return to lower altitude, with no permanent visual effects (Figure 19-18).

Chronic Mountain Sickness

Chronic mountain sickness (Monge's disease) appears in some individuals after long residence at altitude.[288] It is rare below 3,000 m. It manifests as extreme secondary polycythemia and hyperviscosity, cor pulmonale, and reduced exercise tolerance. Individuals who are affected either have some additional pulmonary risk factor (eg, smoking, pneumoconiosis) or an abnormality in the regulation of ventilation that aggravates altitude hypoxia (eg, sleep apnea). Premenopausal women are almost never affected, presumably due to the stimulatory effects of progesterone on ventilation.[289] Treatment is directed at correcting hypoxia or polycythemia by relocating to lower altitude, oxygen therapy, respiratory stimulants (medroxyprogesterone), or venesection.

Exposure to Extreme Altitudes

Residence at altitudes over 5,100 m (17,000 ft) leads to a gradual physical and mental deterioration in addition to the debilitating effects of dehydration, fatigue, and weight loss.[290–293] The mechanism is unknown but may be a direct consequence of chronic hypoxia. Descent is required to ameliorate the process. Several studies have shown that exposure at these extreme altitudes has demonstrable neuropsychological sequelae.[294,295]

SUMMARY

Soldiers and campaigns have been victims of hot, cold and high altitude environments for as long as civilizations have conducted military campaigns. These three environments are encountered in all parts of the world and are still major obstacles to the successful conduct of military operations and significant causes of casualties. Casualties are due to the additive effects of climate and the entire suite of physiological and psychological stresses encountered in military operations.

There is a common pathophysiologic mechanism of illness and injury, which, if understood, permits a broader and more effective approach to preservation of unit effectiveness and prevention of casualties in the field. The risk of disease and injury is a strong correlate of the physiological and psychological strain experienced by deployed service members. Any measures to mitigate that strain will reduce the risk of illness and injury.

Hot environments expose service members to the threats of high ambient temperature and humidity, dehydration, sunburn, and acute heat illnesses, among others. Mitigation of these threats requires attention to heat and sun exposure by implementation of work schedule controls and technologies to reduce heat strain. In addition to direct approaches to moderating heat strain, heat tolerance can be increased by provision of adequate nutrition, rest, and other measures to optimize physiological and psychological hygiene. Service members are at risk for a wide spectrum of heat illnesses, from heat exhaustion to life-threatening conditions such as heat stroke or rhabdomyolysis. Experience has shown that most of these conditions are preventable, but medical officers still need to be prepared to manage them competently if they occur.

Cold environments expose service members to low ambient temperatures, wet conditions, long nights, intense ultraviolet radiation, difficult terrain, toxic exposure from carbon monoxide, and the burden of cold-weather clothing. Unlike hot environments, where a reduced pace of operations reduces risk, in the cold, passivity is dangerous. Consequently, effective mitigation of the threat is challenging and depends on careful planning, robust logistics, and well-trained and experienced personnel. Cold injuries are generally insidious and epidemic. They are disabling and slow to heal, usually requiring evacuation for clinical care and recovery.

High altitude environments are infrequent settings for US operations and training. In addition to their dominant environmental characteristic, hypobaric hypoxia, they present threats of heat, cold, rough terrain, dehydration, and cognitive dysfunc-tion. The most common altitude illness, acute mountain sickness, can disable an entire unit soon after deployment to altitude. The other two altitude illnesses, pulmonary edema and cerebral edema, are fatal if not successfully managed.

Because of their ubiquity, potential for causing casualties, and susceptibility to intelligent intervention, environmental stresses must be a core part of the skill and knowledge repertoire of medical officers.

REFERENCES

1. Whayne TF. History of Heat Trauma as a War Experience. Walter Reed Army Medical Center. Lecture Notes.

2. Ellis FP. Heat illness, 1: Epidemiology. *Trans R Soc Trop Med Hyg.* 1977;70:402–411.

3. Dickinson JG. Heat illness in the services. *J R Army Med Corps.* 1994;140:7–12.

4. Bricknell MC. Heat illness—a review of military experience (Part 1). *J R Army Med Corps.* 1995;141:157–166.

5. Epstein Y, Sohar E, Shapiro Y. Exertional heatstroke: A preventable condition. *Israel J Med Sci.* 1995;31:454–462.

6. Henane R, Bittel J, Viret R, Morino S. Thermal strain resulting from protective clothing of an armored vehicle crew in warm conditions. *Aviat Space Environ Med.* 1979;50:599–603.

7. Breckenridge JR, Levell CA. Heat stress in the cockpit of the AH-1G Huey Cobra helicopter. *Aerosp Med.* 1970;41:621–626.

8. Nunneley SA, Stribley RF. Fighter index of thermal stress (FITS): Guidance for hot-weather aircraft operations. *Aviat Space Environ Med.* 1979;50:639–642.

9. Brown JA, Elliott MJ, Sray WA. Exercise-induced upper extremity rhabdomyolysis and myoglobinuria in ship-board military personnel. *Mil Med.* 1994;159:473–475.

10. Rowell LB. Human cardiovascular adjustments to exercise and thermal stress. *Physiol Rev.* 1974;54:75–159.

11. Johnson JM. Exercise and the cutaneous circulation. *Exer Sport Sci Rev.* 1992;20:59–97.

12. Gonzalez R. Biophysics of heat transfer and clothing considerations. In: Pandolf K, Sawka M, Gonzalez R, eds. *Human Performance Physiology and Environmental Medicine at Terrestrial Extremes.* Indianapolis: Benchmark Press; 1988: 45–95.

13. Aoyagi Y, McLellan TM, Shephard RJ. Interactions of physical training and heat acclimation: the thermophysiology of exercising in a hot climate. *Sports Med.* 1997;23:173–210.

14. Sawka MN. Body fluid responses and hypohydration during exercise-heat stress. In: Pandolf K, Sawka M, Gonzalez R, eds. *Human Performance Physiology and Environmental Medicine at Terrestrial Extremes.* Indianapolis: Benchmark Press; 1988: 227–266.

15. Wenger C. Human heat acclimatization. In: Pandolf K, Sawka M, Gonzalez R, editors. *Human Performance Physiology and Environmental Medicine at Terrestrial Extremes.* Indianapolis: Benchmark Press; 1988: 153–197.

16. Terrados N, Maughan RJ. Exercise in the heat: strategies to minimize the adverse effects on performance. *J Sports Sci.* 1995;13(Spec No):S55–S62.

17. Havenith G, van Middendorp H. The relative influence of physical fitness, acclimatization state, anthropometric measures and gender on individual reactions to heat stress. *Eur J Appl Physiol.* 1990;61:419–427.

18. Munro AH, Sichel HS, Wyndham CH. The effect of heat stress and acclimatization on the body temperature response of men at work. *Life Sci.* 1967;6:749–754.

19. Fox RH, Goldsmith R, Hampton IF, Hunt TJ. Heat acclimatization by controlled hyperthermia in hot-dry and hot-wet climates. *J Appl Physiol.* 1967;22:39–46.

20. Montain SJ, Sawka MN, Cadarette BS, Quigley MD, McKay JM. Physiological tolerance to uncompensable heat stress: effects of exercise intensity, protective clothing, and climate. *J Appl Physiol.* 1994;77:216–222.

21. Santee WR, Gonzalez RR. Characteristics of the thermal environment. In: Pandolf K, Sawka M, Gonzalez R, eds. *Human Performance Physiology and Environmental Medicine at Terrestrial Extremes.* Indianapolis: Benchmark Press; 1988: 1–43.

22. Whang R, Matthew WT, Christiansen J, et al. Field assessment of wet bulb globe temperature: Present and future. *Mil Med.* 1991;156:535–537.

23. Holmer I. Protective clothing and heat stress. *Ergonomics.* 1995;38:166–182.

24. Antunano MJ, Nunneley SA. Heat stress in protective clothing: Validation of a computer model and the heat-humidity index (HHI). *Aviat Space Environ Med.* 1992;63:1087–1092.

25. Cole RD. Heat stroke during training with nuclear, biological, and chemical protective clothing: Case report. *Mil Med.* 1983;148:624–625.

26. American Conference of Government Industrial Hygienists, ed. *1996-1997 Threshold Limit Values for Chemical Substances and Physical Agents.* Cincinnati: American Conference of Government Industrial Hygienists; 1998.

27. Kaplan L. Suntan, sunburn and sun protection. *J Wilderness Med.* 1992;3:173–196.

28. Pandolf KB, Griffin TB, Munro EH, Goldman RF. Heat intolerance as a function of percent of body surface involved with miliaria rubra. *Am J Physiol.* 1980;239:R233–R240.

29. Sulzberger MB, Griffin TB. Induced miliaria, postmiliarial hypohidrosis, and some potential sequelae. *Arch Dermatol.* 1969;99:145–151.

30. Johnson C, Shuster S. Eccrine sweating in psoriasis. *Brit J Dermatol.* 1969;81:119–124.

31. Stephenson L, Kolka M. Effect of gender, circadian period and sleep loss on thermal responses during exercise. In: Pandolf K, Sawka M, Gonzalez R, eds. *Human Performance Physiology and Environmental Medicine at Terrestrial Extremes.* Indianapolis: Benchmark Press; 1988: 267–304.

32. Cooper JK. Preventing heat injury: military versus civilian perspective. *Mil Med.* 1997;162:55–58.

33. Reneau P, Bishop P. Relating heat strain in the chemical defense ensemble to the ambient environment. *Mil Med.* 1996;161:210–213.

34. Kark JA, Posey DM, Schumacher HR, Ruehle CJ. Sickle-cell trait as a risk factor for sudden death in physical training. *N Engl J Med.* 1987;317:781–787.

35. Kark JA, Ward FT. Exercise and hemoglobin S. *Semin Hematol.* 1994;31:181–225.

36. Murray MJ, Evans P. Sudden exertional death in a soldier with sickle cell trait. *Mil Med.* 1996;161:303–305.

37. James CM. Sickle cell trait and military service. *J R Nav Med Serv.* 1990:76:9–13.

38. Sawka MN, Greenleaf JE. Current concepts concerning thirst, dehydration, and fluid replacement: overview. *Med Sci Sports Exerc.* 1992;24:643–644.

39. Armstrong L, Pandolf K. Physical Training, Cardiorespiratory physical fitness and exercise heat tolerance. In: Pandolf K, Sawka M, Gonzalez R, eds. *Human Performance Physiology and Environmental Medicine at Terrestrial Extremes.* Indianapolis: Benchmark Press; 1988: 199–226.

40. Shearer S. Dehydration and serum electrolyte changes in South African gold miners with heat disorders. *Am J Ind Med.* 1990;17:225–239.

41. Applegate EA. Nutritional considerations for ultraendurance performance. *Int J Sport Nutr.* 1991Jun;1(2):118–126.

42. Hexamer M, Werner J. Control of liquid cooling garments: Technical control of body heat storage. *Appl Human Sci.* 1996;15:177–185.

43. Shapiro Y, Pandolf KB, Sawka MN, Toner MM, Winsmann FR, Goldman RF. Auxiliary cooling: comparison of air-cooled vs. water-cooled vests in hot-dry and hot-wet environments. *Aviat Space Environ* Med. 1982;53:785–789.

44. Kark JA, Burr PQ, Wenger CB, Gastaldo E, Gardner JW. Exertional heat illness in Marine Corps recruit training. *Aviat Space Environ Med.* 1996;67:354–360.

45. Pandolf K, Stroshein L, Drolet L, Gonzalez R, Sawka M. Prediction modeling of physiological responses and human performance in the heat. *Computers Biology Med.* 1986:319–329.

46. Reardon MJ, Gonzalez RR, Pandolf KB. Applications of predictive environmental strain models. *Mil Med.* 1997;162:136–140.

47. Knochel JP. Heat stroke and related heat stress disorders. *Dis Mon.* 1989;35:301–377.

48. Dinman BD, Horvath SM. Heat disorders in industry: a reevaluation of diagnostic criteria. *J Occ Med.* 1984;26:489–495.

49. Vassallo SU, Delaney KA. Pharmacologic effects on therinoregulation: mechanisms of drug-related heatstroke. *J Toxicol Clin Toxicol.* 1989;27:199–224.

50. Hubbard RW, Gaffin SL, Squires DL. Heat-related illnesses. In: Auerbach PS, ed. *Wilderness Medicine.* 3rd ed. St Louis: Mosby; 1998: 167–212.

51. Assia E, Epstein Y, Shapiro Y. Fatal heatstroke after a short march at night: a case report. *Aviat Space Environ Med.* 1985;56:441–442.

52. Roberts WO. Assessing core temperature in collapsed athletes. *Physician Sports Med.* 1994;22:49–54.

53. Hansen RD, Olds TS, Richards DA, Richards CR, Leelarthaepin B. Infrared thermometry in the diagnosis and treatment of heat exhaustion. *Int J Sports Med.* 1996;17:66–70.

54. Doyle F, Zehner WJ, Terndrep TE. The effect of ambient temperature extremes on tympanic and oral temperatures. *Am J Emergency Med.* 1992;10:285–289.

55. Ahmed A, Sadaniantz A. Metabolic and electrolyte abnormalities during heat exhaustion. *Postgrad Med J.* 1996;72:505–506.

56. Howorth PJ. The biochemistry of heat illness. *J R Army Med Corps.* 1995;141:40–41.

57. Smith HR, Dhatt GS, Melia WM, Dickinson JG. Cystic fibrosis presenting as hyponatraemic heat exhaustion. *BMJ.* 19954;310:579–580.

58. Bourdon L, Canini F. On the nature of the link between malignant hyperthermia and exertional heatstroke. *Med Hypotheses.* 1995;45:268–270.

59. Figarella-Branger D, Kozak-Ribbens G, Rodet L, et al. Pathological findings in 165 patients explored for malignant hyperthermia susceptibility. *Neuromuscul Disord.* 1993;3:553–556.

60. Faigel HC. Carnitine palmitoyltransferase deficiency in a college athlete: a case report and literature review. *J Am Coll Health*. 1995;44:51–54.

61. Figarella-Branger D, Baeta Marchado AM, Putzu GA, Malzac P, Voelckel MA, Pellissier JF. Exertional rhabdomyolysis and exercise intolerance revealing dystrophinopathies. *Acta Neuropathol (Berl)*. 1997;94:48–53.

62. Hubbard RW, Armstrong LD. The heat illnesses: biochemical, ultrastructural and fluid electrolyte considerations. In: Pandolf K, Sawka M, Gonzalez R, eds. *Human Performance Physiology and Environmental Medicine at Terrestrial Extremes*. Indianapolis: Benchmark Press; 1988: 305–359.

63. Nielsen B, Hales JR, Strange S, Christensen NJ, Warberg J, Saltin B. Human circulatory and thermoregulatory adaptations with heat acclimation and exercise in a hot, dry environment. *J Physiol (Lond)*. 1993;460:467–485.

64. Moore GE, Holbein ME, Knochel JP. Exercise-associated collapse in cyclists is unrelated to endotoxemia. *Med Sci Sports Exerc*. 1995;27:1238–1242.

65. Bouchama A, Parhar RS, el-Yazigi A, Sheth K, Al-Sedairy S. Endotoxemia and release of tumor necrosis factor and interleukin I alpha in acute heatstroke. *J Appl Physiol*. 1991;70:2640–2644.

66. Chang DM. The role of cytokines in heat stroke. *Immunol Invest*. 1993;22:553–561.

67. Hubbard RW. Heatstroke pathophysiology: the energy depletion model. *Med Sci Sports Exerc*. 1990;22:19–28.

68. Knochel JP, Dotin LN, Hamburger RJ. Pathophysiology of intense physical conditioning in a hot climate, 1: mechanisms of potassium depletion. *J Clin Invest*. 1972;51:242–255.

69. Gader AM, al-Mashhadani SA, al-Harthy SS. Direct activation of platelets by heat is the possible trigger of the coagulopathy of heat stroke. *Br J Haematol*. 1990;74:86–92.

70. Delaney KA. Heatstroke: underlying processes and lifesaving management. *Postgrad Med*. 1992;91:379–388.

71. Henderson A, Simon JW, Melia WM, Navein JF, Mackay BG. Heat illness: a report of 45 cases from Hong Kong. *J R Army Med Corps*. 1986;132:76–84.

72. Richards R, Richards D. Exertion-induced heat exhaustion and other medical aspects of the City-to-Surf fun runs, 1978–1984. *Med J Aust*. 1984;141:799–805.

73. Aarseth HP, Eide I, Skeie B, Thaulow E. Heat stroke in endurance exercise. *Acta Med Scand*. 1986;220:279–283.

74. Malamud N, Haymaker W, Custer RP. Heat stroke. *Mil Surg*. 1946;99:397–449.

75. Barthel HJ. Exertion-induced heat stroke in a military setting. *Mil Med*. 1990;155:116–119.

76. al-Mashhadani SA, Gader AG, al Harthi SS, Kangav D, Shaheen FA, Bogus F. The coagulopathy of heat stroke: alterations in coagulation and fibrinolysis in heat stroke patients during the pilgrimage (Haj) to Makkah. *Blood Coagul Fibrinolysis*. 1994;5:731–736.

77. Ang C, Dawes J. The effects of hyperthermia on human endothelial monolayers: modulation of thrombotic potential and permeability. *Blood Coagul Fibrinolysis*. 1994;5:193–199.

78. el-Kassimi FA, Al-Mashhadani S, Abdullah AK, Akhtar J. Adult respiratory distress syndrome and disseminated intravascular coagulation complicating heat stroke. *Chest*. 1986;90:571–574.

79. Vicario SJ, Okabajue R, Haltom T. Rapid cooling in classic heatstroke: effect on mortality rates. *Am J Emerg Med*. 1986;4:394–398.

80. Armstrong LE, Crago AE, Adams R, Roberts WO, Maresh CM. Whole-body cooling of hyperthermic runners: comparison of two field therapies. *Am J Emerg Med*. 1996;14:355–358.

81. Costrini A. Emergency treatment of exertional heatstroke and comparison of whole body cooling techniques. *Med Sci Sports Exerc.* 1990;22:15–18.

82. Biary N, Madkour MM, Sharif H. Post-heatstroke parkinsonism and cerebellar dysfunction. *Clin Neurol Neurosurg.* 1995;97:55–57.

83. Royburt M, Epstein Y, Solomon Z, Shemer J. Long-term psychological and physiological effects of heat stroke. *Physiol Behav.* 1993;54:265–267.

84. Lee RP, Bishop GF, Ashton CM. Severe heat stroke in an experienced athlete. *Med J Aust.* 1990;153:100–104.

85. Armstrong LE, DeLuca JP, Hubbard RW, Christensen EL. *Exertional Heatstroke in Soldiers: An Analysis of Predisposing Factors, Recovery Rates and Residual Heat Intolerance.* Natick, Mass: US Army Research Institute of Environmental Medicine; 1989. Report T5–90.

86. Faunt JD, Wilkinson TJ, Aplin P, Henschke P, Webb M, Penhall PK. The effete in the heat: heat-related hospital presentations during a ten day heat wave. *Aust N Z J Med.* 1995;25:117–121.

87. Tucker LE, Stanford J, Graves B, Swetnam J, Hamburger S, Anwar A. Classical heatstroke: clinical and laboratory assessment. *South Med J.* 1985;78:20–25.

88. Weiner JS, Khogali M. A physiological body-cooling unit for treatment of heat stroke. *Lancet.* 1980;1:507–509.

89. King K, Negus K, Vance JC. Heat stress in motor vehicles: a problem in infancy. *Pediatrics.* 1981;68:579–582.

90. Dixit SN, Bushara KO, Brooks BR. Epidemic heat stroke in a midwest community: risk factors, neurological complications and sequelae. *Wis Med J.* 1997;96:39–41.

91. Hart GR, Anderson RJ, Crumpler CP, Shulkin A, Reed G, Knochel JP. Epidemic classical heat stroke: clinical characteristics and course of 28 patients. *Medicine (Baltimore).* 1982;61:189–197.

92. Bentley S. Exercise-induced muscle cramp: proposed mechanisms and management. *Sports Med.* 1996;21:409–420.

93. McGee SR. Muscle cramps. *Arch Intern Med.* 1990;150:511–518.

94. Schwellnus MP, Derman EW, Noakes TD. Aetiology of skeletal muscle "cramps" during exercise: a novel hypothesis. *J Sports Sci.* 1997;15:277-285.

95. Talbott JH. Heat Cramps. *Medicine.* 1935;14:323–376.

96. Bergeron MF. Heat cramps during tennis: a case report. *Int J Sport Nutr.* 1996;6:62–68.

97. Hamer R. When exercise goes awry: exertional rhabdomyolysis. *South Med J.* 1997;90:548–551.

98. Gardner JW, Kark JA. Fatal rhabdomyolysis presenting as mild heat illness in military training. *Mil Med.* 1994;159:160–163.

99. Bolgiano EB. Acute rhabdomyolysis due to body building exercise: report of a case. *J Sports Med Phys Fitness.* 1994;34:76–78.

100. Knochel JP. Mechanisms of rhabdomyolysis. *Curr Opin Rheumatol.* 1993;5:725–731.

101. Sinert R, Kohl L, Rainone T, Scalea T. Exercise-induced rhabdomyolysis. *Ann Emerg Med.* 1994;23:1301–1306.

102. Soni SN, McDonald E, Marino C. Rhabdomyolysis after exercise. *Postgrad Med.* 1993;94:128–132.

103. Backer H, Shopes E, et al. Hyponatremia in recreational hikers in Grand Canyon National Park. *J Wilderness Med*. 1993;4(4):391–406.

104. Noakes TD. The hyponatremia of exercise. *Int J Sport Nutr*. 1992;2:205–228.

105. Noakes TD, Norman RJ, Buck RH, Godlonton J, Stevenson K, Pittaway D. The incidence of hyponatremia during prolonged ultraendurance exercise. *Med Sci Sports Exerc*. 1990;22:165–170.

106. Noakes TD. Hyponatremia during endurance running: a physiological and clinical interpretation. *Med Sci Sports Exerc*. 1992;24:403–405.

107. Irving RA, Noakes TD, Buck R, et al. Evaluation of renal function and fluid homeostasis during recovery from exercise-induced hyponatremia. *J Appl Physiol*. 1991;70:342–348.

108. Armstrong LE, Curtis WC, Hubbard RW, Francesconi RP, Moore R, Askew EW. Symptomatic hyponatremia during prolonged exercise in heat. *Med Sci Sports Exerc*. 1993;25:543–549.

109. Gastaldo E, USN. Preventive Medicine Officer, Beaufort Naval Hospital, Parris Island. Personal Communication, 1996.

110. Rizzieri DA. Rhabdomyolysis after correction of hyponatremia due to psychogenic polydipsia. *Mayo Clin Proc*. 1995;70:473–476.

111. Putterman C, Levy L, Rubinger D. Transient exercise-induced water intoxication and rhabdomyolysis. *Am J Kidney Dis*. 1993;21:206–209.

112. Zelingher J, Putterman C, Ilan Y, Dann EJ, Zveibil F, Shvil Y, Galun E. Case series: hyponatremia associated with moderate exercise. *Am J Med Sci*. 1996;311:86–91.

113. Galun E, Tur-Kaspa I, Assia E, et al. Hyponatremia induced by exercise: a 24-hour endurance march study. *Miner Electrolyte Metab*. 1991;17:315–320.

114. Gisolfi CV, Duchman SM. Guidelines for optimal replacement beverages for different athletic events. *Med Sci Sports Exerc*. 1992;24:679–687.

115. Convertino VA, Armstrong LE, Coyle EF, et al. American College of Sports Medicine position stand: exercise and fluid replacement. *Med Sci Sports Exerc*. 1996;28:i-vii.

116. Feng E, Janniger CK. Miliaria. *Cutis*. 1995;55:213–216.

117. Lillywhite LP. Investigation into the environmental factors associated with the incidence of skin disease following an outbreak of Miliaria rubra at a coal mine. *Occup Med (Oxf)*. 1992;42:183–187.

118. Holzle E, Kligman AM. The pathogenesis of miliaria rubra: role of the resident microflora. *Br J Dermatol*. 1978;99:117–137.

119. Shuster S. Duct disruption, a new explanation of miliaria. *Acta Derm Venereol*. 1997;77:1–3.

120. Griffin TB, Mailbach HI, Sulzberger MB. Miliaria and anhidrosis, II: the relationships between miliaria and anhidrosis in man. *J Invest Dermatol*. 1967;49:379–385.

121. Pandolf KB, Griffin TB, Munro EH, Goldman RF. Persistence of impaired heat tolerance from artificially induced miliaria rubra. *Am J Physiol*. 1980;239:R226–R232.

122. Bouchama A, el-Yazigi A, Yusuf A, al-Sedairy S. Alteration of taurine homeostasis in acute heatstroke. *Crit Care Med*. 1993;21:551–554.

123. Smolander J, Ilmarinen R, Korhonen O, Pyykko I. Circulatory and thermal responses of men with different training status to prolonged physical work in dry and humid heat. *Scand J Work Environ Health*. 1987;13:37–46.

124. Iampietro PF, Mager M, Green EB. Some physiological changes accompanying tetany induced by exposure to hot, wet conditions. *J Appl Physiol*. 1961;16:409–412.

125. Sohar E, Kaly J, Adar R. The prevention of voluntary dehydration. In: United Nations Educational, Scientific, and Cultural Organization, ed. *Environmental Physiology and Psychology in Arid Conditions*. Paris: UNESCO; 1963: 129–135.

126. Prince C, Scardino P, Wolan C. The effect of temperature, humidity and dehydration on the formation of renal calculi. *J Urol*. 1956;75:20–29.

127. Whayne TF. Historical note. In: Whayne TF, DeBakey ME, ed. *Cold Injury: Ground Type*. Washington, DC: Office of the Surgeon General, United States Army; 1958: 29–56.

128. Schechter DC, Sarot IA. Historical accounts of injuries due to cold. *Surgery*. 1968;63:527–535.

129. Barat AK, Puri HC, Ray N. Cold injuries in Kashmir, December 1971. *Ann R Coll Surg Engl*. 1978;60:332–335.

130. Marsh AR. A short but distant war—the Falklands campaign. *J R Soc Med*. 1983;76:972–982.

131. Orr K, Fainer D. Cold injuries in Korea in the winter of 1950–51. *Medicine*. 1952;31:177–220.

132. Tek D, Mackey S. Non-freezing cold injury in a Marine infantry battalion. *J Wilderness Med*. 1993;4:353–357.

133. Sampson JB, Barr JG, Stokes JW, Jobe JB. Injury and illness during cold weather training. *Mil Med*. 1983;148:324–330.

134. Dembert ML, Dean LM, Noddin EM. Cold weather morbidity among United States Navy and Marine Corps Personnel. *Mil Med*. 1981;146:770–775.

135. Vaughn PB. Local cold injury—menace to military operations: a review. *Mil Med*. 1980;145:305–311.

136. McCarroll JE, Jackson RE, Traver CA, et al. Morbidity associated with cold weather training. *Mil Med*. 1979; 144:680–684.

137. Toner M, McArdle W. Physiological adjustments of man to the cold. In: Pandolf K, Sawka M, Gonzalez R, ed. *Human Performance Physiology and Environmental Medicine at Terrestrial Extremes*. Indianapolis: Benchmark Press; 1988: 305–399.

138. O'Sullivan ST, O'Shaughnessy M, O'Connor TP. Baron Larrey and cold injury during the campaigns of Napoleon. *Ann Plast Surg*. 1995;34:446–449.

139. Mercer JB. The shivering response in animals and man. *Arctic Med Res*. 1991;50(Suppl 6):18–22.

140. Edwards MA. The role of arteriovenous anastomoses in cold-induced vasodilation, rewarming, and reactive hyperemia as determined by 24Na clearance. *Can J Physiol Pharmacol*. 1967;45:39–48.

141. Chen F, Liu ZY, Holmer I. Hand and finger skin temperatures in convective and contact cold exposure. *Eur J Appl Physiol*. 1996;72:372–379.

142. Young A. Human adaptation to cold. In: Pandolf K, Sawka M, Gonzalez R, ed. *Human Performance Physiology and Environmental Medicine at Terrestrial Extremes*. Indianapolis: Benchmark Press; 1998: 401–434.

143. James NK, Moss AL. Cold injury from liquid propane. *BMJ*. 1989;299(14):950–951.

144. Osczevski RJ. The basis of wind chill. *Arctic*. 1997;48:372–382.

145. Holmer I. Work in the cold: review of methods for assessment of cold exposure. *Int Arch Occup Environ Health*. 1993;65:147-155.

146. Tikuisis P. Prediction of survival time at sea based on observed body cooling rates. *Aviat Space Environ Med*. 1997;68:441–448.

147. Craig RP. Military cold injury during the war in the Falkland Islands 1982: an evaluation of possible risk factors. *J R Army Med Corps*. 1984;130:89–96.

148. Arvesen A, Rosen L, Eltvik LP, Kroese A, Stranden E. Skin microcirculation in patients with sequelae from local cold injuries. *Int J Microcirc Clin Exp*. 1994;14:335–342.

149. Whayne TF. Epidemiology of cold injury. In: Whayne TF, DeBakey ME, ed. *Cold Injury: Ground Type*. Washington, DC: Office of the Surgeon General, United States Army; 1958: 363–453.

150. Jobe JB, Goldman RF, Beetham WP Jr. Comparison of the hunting reaction in normals and individuals with Raynaud's disease. *Aviat Space Environ Med*. 1985;56:568–571.

151. Sawada S. Cold-induced vasodilatation response of finger skin blood vessels in older men observed by using a modified local cold tolerance test. *Ind Health*. 1996;34:51–56.

152. McCarroll JE, Goldman PF, Denniston JC. Food intake and energy expenditure in cold weather military training. *Mil Med*. 1979;144:606–610.

153. Takano N, Kotani M. Influence of food intake on cold-induced vasodilatation of finger. *Jpn J Physiol*. 1989;39:755–765.

154. Livingstone SD. Changes in cold-induced vasodilation during Arctic exercises. *J Appl Physiol*. 1976;40:455–457.

155. Anttonen H. Occupational needs and evaluation methods for cold protective clothing. *Arctic Med Res*. 1993;52(Suppl 9):1–76.

156. Bean WB. The ecology of the soldier in World War II. *Perspect Biol Med*. 1968;11:675–686.

157. Lehmuskallio E, Lindholm H, Koskenvuo K, Sarna S, Friberg O, Viljanen A. Frostbite of the face and ears: epidemiological study of risk factors in Finnish conscripts. *BMJ*. 1995;311:1661–1663.

158. Tipton MJ, Stubbs DA, Elliott DH. The effect of clothing on the initial responses to cold water immersion in man. *J R Nav Med Serv*. 1990;76:89–95.

159. Rosen L, Eltvik L, Arvesen A, Stranden E. Local cold injuries sustained during military service in the Norwegian Army. *Arctic Med Res*. 1991;50:159–165.

160. Purdue GF, Hunt JL. Cold injury: a collective review. *J Burn Care Rehabil*. 1986;7:331–342.

161. Killian H, Graf-Baumann T. *Cold and Frost Injuries, Rewarming Damages: Biological, Angiological, and Clinical Aspects*. Vol 3. In: *Disaster Medicine*. New York: Springer-Verlag; 1981.

162. McCauley PL, Smith DJ, Robson MC, Heggers JP. Frostbite and other cold induced injuries. In: Auerbach PS, ed. *Wilderness Medicine*. 3rd ed. St Louis: Mosby; 1995: 129–145.

163. Francis TJ. Non freezing cold injury: a historical review. *J R Nav Med Serv*. 1984;70:134–139.

164. Francis TJ, Golden FS. Non-freezing cold injury: the pathogenesis. *J R Nav Med Serv*. 1985;71:3–8.

165. Irwin MS. Nature and mechanism of peripheral nerve damage in an experimental model of non-freezing cold injury. *Ann R Coll Surg Engl*. 1996;78:372–379.

166. Thomas JR, Shurtleff D, Schrot J, Ahlers ST. Cold-induced perturbation of cutaneous blood flow in the rat tail: a model of nonfreezing cold injury. *Microvasc Res.* 1994;47:166–176.

167. Mills WJ Jr, Mills WJ III. Peripheral non-freezing cold injury: immersion injury. *Alaska Med.* 1993;35:117–128.

168. Simeone FA. Trenchfoot in the Italian Campaign, 1945. Report to the Surgeon, Fifth US Army. As cited in: DeBakey ME. Clinical picture and diagnosis. In: Whayne TF, DeBakey ME, ed. *Cold Injury: Ground Type*. Washington, DC: Office of the Surgeon General, United States Army; 1958: 259–305.

169. Guttman L. Topographic studies of the disturbances of sweat secretion after complete lesions of the peripheral nerves. *J Neurol Psychiatry.* 1940;3:197–210.

170. Edwards J, Shapiro M, Ruffin J. Trench foot: report of 351 cases. *Bull US Army Med Dept.* 1942;83:58–66.

171. Webster A, Woolhouse F, Johnston J. Immersion foot. *J Bone Joint Surg.* 1942;24:785–794.

172. Ungley C. The immersion foot syndrome. In: Andrus W, ed. *Advances in Surgery*. New York: Interscience Publishers; 1949: 269–336.

173. Danzl DF, Pozos RS. Accidental hypothermia. *N Engl J Med.* 1994;331:1756–1760.

174. Danzl D, Pozos RS, Hamlet M. Accidental hypothermia. In: Auerbach PS, ed. *Wilderness Medicine*. 3rd ed. St Louis: Mosby; 1995: 51–103.

175. Ferguson J, Epstein F, van de Leuv J. Accidental hypothermia. *Emerg Med Clin North Am.* 1983;1:619–637.

176. Jolly BT, Ghezzi KT. Accidental hypothermia. *Emerg Med Clin North Am.* 1992;10:311–327.

177. Paton BC. Accidental hypothermia. *Pharmacol Ther.* 1983;22:331–377.

178. Granberg PO. Human physiology under cold exposure. *Arctic Med Res.* 1991;50(Suppl 6):23–27.

179. Delaney KA, Howland MA, Vassallo S, Goldfrank LR. Assessment of acid-base disturbances in hypothermia and their physiologic consequences. *Ann Emerg Med.* 1989;18:72–82.

180. Gould L, Gopalaswamy C, Kim BS, Patel C. The Osborn wave in hypothermia. *Angiology.* 1985;36:125–129.

181. Herr RD, White GL Jr. Hypothermia: threat to military operations. *Mil Med.* 1991;156:140–144.

182. Fischbeck KH, Simon RP. Neurological manifestations of accidental hypothermia. *Ann Neurol.* 1981;10:384–387.

183. Lloyd EL. Hypothermia: the cause of death after rescue. *Alaska Med.* 1984;26:74–76.

184. Lloyd EL. Accidental hypothermia. *Resuscitation.* 1996;32:111–124.

185. Okada M. The cardiac rhythm in accidental hypothermia. *J Electrocardiol.* 1984;17:123–128.

186. Mills WJ. Field care of the hypothermic patient. *Int J Sports Med.* 1992;13(Suppl 1):S199–S202.

187. Kornberger E, Mair P. Important aspects in the treatment of severe accidental hypothermia: the Innsbruck experience. *J Neurosurg Anesthesiol.* 1996;8:83–87.

188. Iversen RJ, Atkin SH, Jaker MA, Quadrel MA, Tortella BJ, Odom JW. Successful CPR in a severely hypothermic patient using continuous thoracostomy lavage. *Ann Emerg Med.* 1990;19:1335–1337.

189. Giesbrecht GG, Schroeder M, Bristow GK. Treatment of mild immersion hypothermia by forced-air warming. *Aviat Space Environ Med.* 1994;65:803–808.

190. Lloyd E. Airway warming in the treatment of accidental hypothermia: a review. *J Wilderness Med.* 1990;1:65–78.

191. Gentilello LM, Cobean RA, Offner PJ, Soderberg RW, Jurkovich GJ. Continuous arteriovenous rewarming: rapid reversal of hypothermia in critically ill patients. *J Trauma.* 1992;32:316–325.

192. Gregory JS, Bergstein JM, Aprahamian C, Wittmann DH, Quebbeman EJ. Comparison of three methods of rewarming from hypothermia: advantages of extracorporeal blood warming. *J Trauma.* 1991;31:1247–1251.

193. Iserson KV, Huestis DW. Blood warming: current applications and techniques. *Transfusion.* 1991;31:558–571.

194. Kaufman JW, Hamilton R, Dejneka KY, Askew GK. Comparative effectiveness of hypothermia rewarming techniques: radio frequency energy vs. warm water. *Resuscitation.* 1995;29:203–214.

195. Foulis AK. Morphological study of the relation between accidental hypothermia and acute pancreatitis. *J Clin Pathol.* 1982;35:1244–1248.

196. Hakim EA, Chiverton N, Hossenbocus A. Rhabdomyolysis with renal dysfunction in a hypothermic man. *Br J Clin Pract.* 1990;44:778–779.

197. Goette DK. Chilblains (perniosis). *J Am Acad Dermatol.* 1990;23(2 Pt 1):257–262.

198. Page EH, Shear NH. Temperature-dependent skin disorders. *J Am Acad Dermatol.* 1988;18(5 Pt 1):1003–1019.

199. Spittell JA Jr, Spittell PC. Chronic pernio: another cause of blue toes. *Int Angiol.* 1992;11:46–50.

200. Rustin MH, Newton JA, Smith NP, Dowd PM. The treatment of chilblains with nifedipine: the results of a pilot study, a double-blind placebo-controlled randomized study and a long-term open trial. *Br J Dermatol.* 1989;120:267–275.

201. Weinberg A, Hmnlet M, Paturas J, McAninch G, White R. *Cold Weather Emergencies: Principles of Patient Management.* Branford, Conn: American Medical Publishing; 1990.

202. Pearn JH. Cold injury complicating trauma in subzero environments. *Med J Aust.* 1982;1:505–507.

203. Granberg PO. Alcohol and cold. *Arctic Med Res.* 1991;50(Suppl 6):43–47.

204. West JB. Respiratory and circulatory control at high altitudes. *J Exp Biol.* 1982;100:147–157.

205. Muscular exercise at high altitude. *Int J Sports Med.* 1990;11(Suppl 1):S1–S34.

206. Bailey DM, Davies B. Physiological implications of altitude training for endurance performance at sea level: a review. *Br J Sports Med.* 1997;31:183–190.

207. Kobrick JL. Effects of prior hypoxia exposure on visual target detection during later more severe hypoxia. *Percept Mot Skills.* 1976;42:751–761.

208. Leber LL, Roscoe SN, Southward GM. Mild hypoxia and visual performance with night vision goggles. *Aviat Space Environ Med.* 1986;57:318–324.

209. Wohns RN, Colpitts M, Colpitts Y, Clement T, Blackett WB. Effect of high altitude on the visual evoked responses in humans on Mt. Everest. *Neurosurgery.* 1987;21:352–356.

210. Kramer AF, Coyne JT, Strayer DL. Cognitive function at high altitude. *Hum Factors.* 1993;35:329–344.

211. Mackintosh JH, Thomas DJ, Olive JE, Chesner IM, Knight RJ. The effect of altitude on tests of reaction time and alertness. *Aviat Space Environ Med.* 1988;59:246–248.

212. Eichenberger U, Weiss E, Riemann D, Oelz O, Bartsch P. Nocturnal periodic breathing and the development of acute high altitude illness. *Am J Respir Crit Care Med.* 1996;154(6 Pt 1):1748–1754.

213. Fujimoto K, Matsuzawa Y, Hirai K, et al. Irregular nocturnal breathing patterns high altitude in subjects susceptible to high-altitude pulmonary edema (HAPE): a preliminary study. *Aviat Space Environ Med.* 1989;60:786–791.

214. Masuyama S, Kohchiyama S, Shinozaki T et al. Periodic breathing at high altitude and ventilatory responses to O_2 and CO_2. *Jpn J Physiol.* 1989;39:523–535.

215. Miller JC, Horvath SM. Sleep at altitude. *Aviat Space Environ Med.* 1977;48:615–620.

216. Nicholson AN, Smith PA, Stone BM, Bradwell AR, Coote JH. Altitude insomnia: studies during an expedition to the Himalayas. *Sleep.* 1988;11:354–361.

217. Reite M, Jackson D, Cahoon RL, Weil JV. Sleep physiology at high altitude. *Electroencephalogr Clin Neurophysiol.* 1975;38:463–471.

218. Weil JV. Sleep at high altitude. *Clin Chest Med.* 1985;6:615–621.

219. Goldenberg F, Richalet JP, Onnen I, Antezana AM. Sleep apneas and high altitude newcomers. *Int J Sports Med.* 1992;13(Suppl 1):S34–S36.

220. Kryger M, Glas R, Jackson D, et al. Impaired oxygenation during sleep in excessive polycythemia of high altitude: improvement with respiratory stimulation. *Sleep.* 1978;1:3–17.

221. Malconian M, Hultgren H, Nitta M, Anholm J, Houston C, Fails H. The sleep electrocardiogram at extreme altitudes. *Am J Cardiol.* 1990;65:1014–1020.

222. Hackett PH, Rennie D, Grover RF, Reeves JT. Acute mountain sickness and the edemas of high altitude: a common pathogenesis? *Respir Physiol.* 1981;46:383–390.

223. Coote JH. Medicine and mechanisms in altitude sickness: recommendations. *Sports Med.* 1995;20:148–159.

224. Sugarman J, Samuelson WM, Wilkinson RH Jr, Rosse WF. Pulmonary embolism and splenic infarction in a patient with sickle cell trait. *Am J Hematol.* 1990;33:279–281.

225. Claster S, Godwin MJ, Embury SH. Risk of altitude exposure in sickle cell disease. *West J Med.* 1981;135:364–367.

226. Hultgren H. Effects of altitude upon cardiovascular diseases. *J Wilderness Med.* 1992;3:301–308.

227. Graham WG, Houston CS. Short-term adaptation to moderate altitude. Patients with chronic obstructive pulmonary disease. *JAMA.* 1978;240:1491–1494.

228. Bircher H, Eichenberger U, et al. Relationship of mountain sickness to physical fitness and exercise intensity during ascent. *J Wilderness Med.* 1994;5:302–311.

229. Edwards J, Askew EW. Nutritional intake and carbohydrate supplementation at high altitude. *J Wilderness Med.* 1994;5:20–33.

230. Fenn CE. Energy and nutrient intakes during high-altitude acclimatization. *J Wilderness Med.* 1994;5:318–324.

231. Simon-Schnass IM. Nutrition at high altitude. *J Nutr.* 1992;122(3 Suppl):778–781.

232. Srivastava KK, Kumar R. Human nutrition in cold and high terrestrial altitudes. *Int J Biometeorol.* 1992;36:10–13.

233. Kayser B. Nutrition and high altitude exposure. *Int J Sports Med.* 1992;13(Suppl 1):S129–S132.

234. Alexander D, Winterbom M, et al. Carbonic anhydrase inhibition in the immediate therapy of acute mountain sickness. *J Wilderness Med.* 1994;5:49–55.

235. Acetazolamide for acute mountain sickness. *FDA Drug Bulletin.* 1983:13:27.

236. Bradwell AR, Wright AD, Winterborn M, Imray C. Acetazolamide and high altitude diseases. *Int J Sports Med.* 1992;13(Suppl 1):S63–S64.

237. Dickinson JG. Acetazolamide in acute mountain sickness. *Br Med J (Clin Res Ed).* 1987;295:1161–1162.

238. Ellsworth AJ, Meyer EF, Larson EB. Acetazolamide or dexamethasone use versus placebo to prevent acute mountain sickness on Mount Rainier. *West J Med.* 1991;154:289–293.

239. Meyer BH. The use of low-dose acetazolamide to prevent mountain sickness. *S Afr Med J.* 1995;85:792–793.

240. Pines A. Acetazolamide in high altitude acclimatisation. *Lancet.* 1980;2:807.

241. Iwanyk E, US Army Research Institute of Environmental Medicine. Personal communication, 1991.

242. Dexamethasone and acute mountain sickness. *N Engl J Med.* 1990;322:1395–1396.

243. Bernhard AN, et al. Dexamethasone for prophylaxis against acute mountain sickness during rapid ascent to 5334 m. *J Wilderness Med.* 1994;5:331–338.

244. Ellsworth AJ, Larson EB, Strickland D. A randomized trial of dexamethasone and acetazolmnide for acute mountain sickness prophylaxis. *Am J Med.* 1987;83:1024–1030.

245. Rock PB, Johnson TS, Cymerman A, Burse RL, Falk LJ, Fulco CS. Effect of dexamethasone on symptoms of acute mountain sickness at Pikes Peak, Colorado (4,300 m). *Aviat Space Environ Med.* 1987;58:668–672.

246. Rock PB, Johnson TS, Larsen RF, Fulco CS, Trad LA, Cymerman A. Dexamethasone as prophylaxis for acute mountain sickness: effect of dose level. *Chest.* 1989;95:568–573.

247. Singh MV, Jain SC, Rawal SB, et al. Comparative study of acetazolamide and spironolactone on body fluid compartments on induction to high altitude. *Int J Biometeorol.* 1986;30:33–41.

248. Larsen RF, Rock PB, Fulco CS, Edelman B, Young AJ, Cymerman A. Effect of spironolactone on acute mountain sickness. *Aviat Space Environ Med.* 1986;57:543–547.

249. Hackett PH, Roach RC, Wood RA, et al. Dexamethasone for prevention and treatment of acute mountain sickness. *Aviat Space Environ Med.* 1988;59:950–954.

250. Bartsch P. [Who gets altitude sickness?]. *Schweiz Med Wochenschr.* 1992;122:307–314.

251. Bartsch P, Maggiorini M, Ritter M, Noti C, Vock P, Oelz O. Prevention of high-altitude pulmonary edema by nifedipine. *N Engl J Med.* 1991;325:1284–1289.

252. Oelz O, Maggiorini M, Ritter M, et al. Prevention and treatment of high altitude pulmonary edema by a calcium channel blocker. *Int J Sports Med.* 1992;13(Suppl 1):S65–S68.

253. Hultgren HN. High-altitude pulmonary edema: current concepts. *Ann Rev Med.* 1996;47:267–284.

254. West JB. Oxygen enrichment of room air to relieve the hypoxia of high altitude. *Respir Physiol.* 1995;99:225–232.

255. Kasic JF, Yaron M, Nicholas RA, Lickteig JA, Roach R. Treatment of acute mountain sickness: hyperbaric versus oxygen therapy. *Ann Emerg Med.* 1991;20:1109–1112.

256. Kayser B, Jean D, Herry JP, Bartsch P. Pressurization and acute mountain sickness. *Aviat Space Environ Med.* 1993;64:928–931.

257. Bartsch P, Merki B, Hofstetter D, Maggiorini M, Kayser B, Oetz O. Treatment of acute mountain sickness by simulated descent: a randomised controlled trial. *BMJ.* 1993;306:1098–1101.

258. Schoene RB, Roach RC, Hackett PH, Harrison G, Mills WJ Jr. High altitude pulmonary edema and exercise at 4,400 meters on Mount McKinley: effect of expiratory positive airway pressure. *Chest.* 1985;87:330–333.

259. Roberts MJ. Acute mountain sickness—experience on the roof of Africa expedition and military implications. *J R Army Med Corps.* 1994;140:49–51.

260. Hackett PH, Rennie D. The incidence, importance, and prophylaxis of acute mountain sickness. *Lancet.* 1976;2:1149–1155.

261. Honigman B, Theis MK, Koziol-McLain J, et al. Acute mountain sickness in a general tourist population at moderate altitudes. *Ann Intern Med.* 1993;118:587–592. Published erratum appears in *Ann Intern Med* 1994;120:698.

262. Sampson JB, Cymerman A, Burse RL, Maher JT, Rock PB. Procedures for the measurement of acute mountain sickness. *Aviat Space Environ Med.* 1983;54(12 Pt 1):1063–1073.

263. Savourey G, Guinet A, Besnard Y, Garcia N, Hanniquet AM, Bittel J. Evaluation of the Lake Louise acute mountain sickness scoring system in a hypobaric chamber. *Aviat Space Environ Med.* 1995;66:963–967.

264. Kobrick JL, Sampson JB. New inventory for the assessment of symptom occurrence and severity at high altitude. *Aviat Space Environ Med.* 1979;50:925–929.

265. Roeggla G, Roeggia M, Podolsky A, Wagner A, Laggner AN. How can acute mountain sickness be quantified at moderate altitude? *J R Soc Med.* 1996;89:141–143.

266. Bartsch P. Treatment of high altitude diseases without drugs. *Int J Sports Med.* 1992;13(Suppl 1):S71–S74.

267. Porcelli MJ, Gugelchuk GM. A trek to the top: a review of acute mountain sickness. *J Am Osteopath Assoc.* 1995;95:718–720.

268. Hamilton AJ, Cymmerman A, Black PM. High altitude cerebral edema. *Neurosurgery.* 1986;19:841–849. Published erratum appears in *Neurosurgery* 1987;20:822.

269. Severinghaus JW. Hypothetical roles of angiogenesis, osmotic swelling, and ischemia in high-altitude cerebral edema. *J Appl Physiol.* 1995;79:375–379.

270. Koyama S, Kobayashi T, Kubo K, et al. The increased sympathoadrenal activity in patients with high altitude pulmonary edema is centrally mediated. *Jpn J Med.* 1988;27:10–16.

271. West JB, Colice GL, Lee YJ, et al. Pathogenesis of high-altitude pulmonary oedema: direct evidence of stress failure of pulmonary capillaries. *Eur Respir J.* 1995;8:523–529.

272. West JB, Mathieu-Costello O. High altitude pulmonary edema is caused by stress failure of pulmonary capillaries. *Int J Sports Med.* 1992;13(Suppl 1):S54–S58.

273. Hultgren RN. High altitude pulmonary edema: hemodynamic aspects. *Int J Sports Med.* 1997;18:20–25.

274. Rabold M. High-altitude pulmonary edema: a collective review. *Am J Emerg Med.* 1989;7:426–433.

275. Houston C. Acute pulmonary edema of high altitude. *N Engl J Med.* 1960;263:478–480.

276. Menon N. High altitude pulmonary edema: a clinical study. *N Engl J Med.* 1965;273:66–73.

277. Foulke GE. Altitude-related illness. *Am J Emerg Med.* 1985;3:217–226.

278. Hackett PH, Roach RC, Hartig GS, Greene ER, Levine BD. The effect of vasodilators on pulmonary hemodynamics in high altitude pulmonary edema: a comparison. *Int J Sports Med.* 1992;13(Suppl 1):S68–S71.

279. Guleria J, Pande J, Khana P. Pulmonary function in convalescents of high altitude pulmonary edema. *Dis Chest.* 1969;55:434–437.

280. Cucinell SA, Pitts CM. Thrombosis at mountain altitudes. *Aviat Space Environ Med.* 1987;58:1109–1111.

281. Dickinson J, Heath D, Gosney J, Williams D. Altitude-related deaths in seven trekkers in the Himalayas. *Thorax.* 1983;38:646–656.

282. Song SY, Asaji T, Tanizaki Y, Fujimaki T, Matsutani M, Okeda R. Cerebral thrombosis at altitude: its pathogenesis and the problems of prevention and treatment. *Aviat Space Environ Med.* 1986;57:71–76.

283. Fujimaki T, Matsutani M, Asai A, Kohno T, Koike M. Cerebral venous thrombosis due to high-altitude polycythemia: case report. *J Neurosurg.* 1986;64:148–150.

284. Nakagawa S, Kubo K, Koizumi T, Kobayashi T, Sekiguchi M. High-altitude pulmonary edema with pulmonary thromboembolism. *Chest.* 1993;103:948–950.

285. Lubin JR, Rennie D, Hackett P, Albert DM. High altitude retinal hemorrhage: a clinical and pathological case report. *Ann Ophthalmol.* 1982;14:1071–1076.

286. Wiedman M. High altitude retinal hemorrhage. *Arch Ophthalmol.* 1975;93:401–403.

287. Butler FK, Harris DJ Jr, Reynolds RD. Altitude retinopathy on Mount Everest, 1989. *Ophthalmology.* 1992;99:739–746.

288. Monge C, Arregui A, Leon-Velarde F. Pathophysiology and epidemiology of chronic mountain sickness. *Int J Sports Med.* 1992;13(Suppl 1):S79–S81.

289. Leon-Velarde F, Ramos MA, Hemandez JA, et al. The role of menopause in the development of chronic mountain sickness. *Am J Physiol.* 1997;272(l Pt 2):R90–R94.

290. Rupwate RU, Chitaley M, Kamat SR. Cardiopulmonary functional changes in acute acclimatisation to high altitude in mountaineers. *Eur J Epidemiol.* 1990;6:266–272.

291. Butterfield GE, Gates J, Fleming S, Brooks GA, Sutton JR, Reeves JT. Increased energy intake minimizes weight loss in men at high altitude. *J Appl Physiol.* 1992;72:1741–1748.

292. Rose MS, Houston CS, Fulco CS, Coates G, Sutton JR, Cymerman A. Operation Everest, II: nutrition and body composition. *J Appl Physiol.* 1988;65:2545–2551.

293. Zamboni M, Armellini F, Turcato E, et al. Effect of altitude on body composition during mountaineering expeditions: interrelationships with changes in dietary habits. *Ann Nutr Metab.* 1996;40:315–324.

294. Hornbein TF, Townes BD, Schoene PB, Sutton JR, Houston CS. The cost to the central nervous system of climbing to extremely high altitude. *N Engl J Med.* 1989;321:1714–1719.

295. Hornbein TF. Long term effects of high altitude on brain function. *Int J Sports Med.* 1992;13(Suppl 1):S43–S45.

Chapter 20

ENVIRONMENTAL HEALTH

ROY D. MILLER, PhD; and WELFORD C. ROBERTS, PhD

R. D. Miller; Department of Preventive Medicine and Biometrics, Uniformed Services University of the Health Sciences, 4301 Jones Bridge Road, Bethesda, MD 20814-4799

W. C. Roberts; Department of Preventive Medicine and Biometrics, Uniformed Services University of the Health Sciences, 4301 Jones Bridge Road, Bethesda, MD 20814-4799

INTRODUCTION

People continually interact with their environment, consciously and unconsciously, voluntarily and involuntarily. These interactions can affect health and performance, and performance is critical to successful mission accomplishment. Therefore, military leaders and those who advise them must be aware of how environmental factors affect performance and how adverse effects on performance can be reduced or eliminated.

The field of environmental health is diverse. This chapter addresses its broad aspects from both a general and a military perspective. The general topics provide basic background information for many physicians, nurses, and others with little or no formal training in the field. The military topics provide useful information to all those with responsibilities for environmental health in military situations, including those trained in this field but who are making the transition from a civilian to a military workplace.

Environmental health concerns occur in all phases of military operations—whether in garrison or during mobilization, deployment, sustainment, and redeployment. They encompass deployments aboard ship, to highly industrialized air bases, and to primitive field settings. And although the traditional focus of environmental health on acute effects is still with us in the age of Agent Orange and Persian Gulf illness, chronic effects are now also quite relevant. Environmental health is a continuum of great breadth, and practices within each area need to be explicitly linked. This is also increasingly appropriate for the military because the military mission is evolving to encompass operations other than war, which often involve the military preventive medicine professional in issues well beyond those of traditional field sanitation. Knowledge of the enduring principles, which are relevant to all the services, will help prepare military public health professionals for their ever-expanding role. Military personnel have to appreciate the diversity and complexity of environmental health topics and functions, and the need for a team approach to prevent or solve environmental problems. The expertise of environmental health professionals, who often work as a multidisciplinary team, is truly needed to help plan and execute health and environmental protection for all military operations.

OVERVIEW OF ENVIRONMENTAL HEALTH

Definition

There are dozens of definitions of environmental health that reflect acceptance of basic concepts but show a lack of consensus about all aspects of the field. One that was developed by 75 federal, state, and local environmental health and protection leaders is:

> ...the art and science of protecting against environmental factors that may adversely impact human health or the ecological balances essential to long term human health and environmental quality. Such factors include, but are not limited to air, food and water contaminants; radiation; toxic chemicals; wastes; disease vectors; safety hazards; and habitat alterations.[1(p29)]

Alternate definitions for environmental health may encompass subject areas that are not included in this chapter or elsewhere in this text. The reader should consult other references for these topics.[2–7]

In the US Department of Defense (DoD), the working definition of environmental health is the science and practice of anticipating, recognizing, evaluating, and controlling environmental factors to prevent adverse health effects. Environmental factors include biological, chemical, and physical (including radiological) matter or phenomena.

Environmental Health Paradigm

To affect the environment or human health, a series of events must occur. A model for looking at these events is called the environmental health paradigm or chain (similar to the chain of infection) and includes a contaminant or environmental agent source, a mediation process, and a susceptible receptor (Figure 20-1).

Sources of environmental agents are ubiquitous in the natural environment, workplace, and home. Environmental agents may be anthropogenic or they may exist naturally in the environment, either at acceptable concentrations or at concentrations harmful to people (eg, radon, fluorides, arsenic, and nitrates in water sources). Examples of environmental agents and health threats are listed in Table 20-1. Some agents are released intentionally in quantities believed to be safe. Examples of these are incinerator emissions and wastewater treatment plant effluents. Accidental and deliberate unlawful releases also may occur.

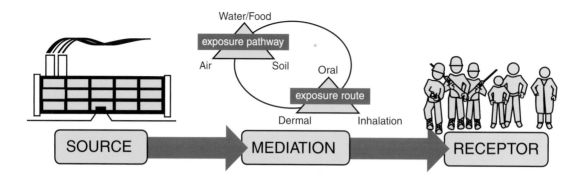

Fig. 20-1. The *Environmental Health Paradigm* depicts the movement of environmental contaminants from a pollution source to an ultimate receptor. This process involves contaminant movement through any or all environmental media (air, water, soil). People ultimately are exposed to pollution by ingestion, inhalation, skin absorption, or any combination of these. Understanding this process allows preventive medicine and environmental health professionals to intervene to mitigate or prevent adverse health effects.

Mediation is the process through which environmental agents travel by means of the exposure pathway (ie, air, soil, water) to susceptible receptors, whether human or some other form of life. The receptor can be challenged through dermal, inhalation, and ingestion routes. These agents may contact receptors directly, or they may successively pass through plants and animals and may increasingly concentrate at each level (bioaccumulation). Toxicity can increase or decrease due to chemical changes as substances pass through the environment or organisms (biotransformation). The exposure routes—inhalation, ingestion, skin absorption—provide an external exposure to the receptor. The nature and the concentration of the agent, the route of absorption, and other factors will determine the receptor's external dose.[8]

TABLE 20-1

EXAMPLES OF ENVIRONMENTAL AGENTS AND HEALTH THREATS

Parameter	Examples
Physical	
Ionizing Radiation	Alpha-, beta-, gamma-, and X-rays
Nonionizing Radiation	Radio frequency radiation, microwaves, lasers
Temperature Extremes	Heat, cold
Noise	Gun shot, aircraft engine
Chemical	
Heavy Metals	Lead, mercury
Solvents	Benzene, toluene, methylethyl ketone
Biological	
Viruses	Rabies (rhabdovirus), viral hepatitis
Rickettsia	Rocky Mountain spotted fever (*Rickettsia rickettsii*)
Chlamydia	Ornithosis (*Chlamydia psittaci*)
Bacteria	Plague (*Yersinia pestis*), food poisoning (*Clostridium botulinum*)
Fungi	Candidiasis (*Candida albicans*), histoplasmosis (*Histoplasma capsulatum*)
Parasites	Hookworm disease (*Necator americanus, Ancylostoma duodenale*), ascariasis (nematodes)

Scope

Based on the DoD's working definition, the scope of environmental health includes all topics that are considered environmental factors with the potential to cause adverse health effects. Science and practice are components; environmental health professionals must understand the relevant science and apply it in practice to protect human health, by both preventing and solving problems. In this approach, the practice of environmental health includes critical functions of setting standards, implementing controls, conducting monitoring, and setting policy.

Standards by definition are "accepted measures of comparison for quantitative or qualitative value."[9(p1131)] Environmental health standards are really consensus standards—they result from collective opinion or general agreement and are a compromise of conflicting opinions. These consensus standards are advocated by an organization (eg, the US Environmental Protection Agency [USEPA], the American Conference of Governmental Industrial Hygienists, the World Health Organization, individual countries, and groups of countries such as the North Atlantic Treaty Organization) for health and economic reasons and reflect minimally acceptable performance. Standards are also dynamic. Standards change because of (a) new knowledge and technology, such as improved analytical methods, and (b) changing social values, such as greater concern for human health and protection of the environment.

Standards and the standard-setting process contain four major components: science, economics, legal issues, and policy. Scientific aspects of environmental standards include basic science, toxicology, epidemiology, and modeling. The economic component addresses economic loss and potential profit caused by a standard. The legal component includes the ability to prosecute those who violate standards. The policy component involves such questions as whether or not there should be certain standards and when, where, and how the standard will be applied. Social values, scientific knowledge, and public opinion compete and often have quite diverse positions in the standard setting process.

The next critical function of environmental health is implementing controls. Environmental health professionals use three categories of control or control methods: engineering controls, administrative controls, and personal protective equipment. These control methods should generally be used in the order presented. That is, one should routinely try first to apply engineering controls to achieve a qual-ity environment or meet standards or other desired conditions. An exception to this order would be to use administrative methods to remove or eliminate potential contaminants. The second choice should normally be administrative controls, such as reducing the work hours to limit total exposure. The last choice should be personal protective equipment because it is the most difficult to enforce.[10] Examples of controls include the following:

- Substituting less harmful material,
- Changing or altering a process,
- Using zoning to limit selected activities,
- Treating to remove specific contaminants, and
- Cleaning up past contamination.

To monitor by definition is "to check systematically or scrutinize for the purpose of collecting specified categories of data."[9(p765)] The categories of environmental monitoring are usually given as operational monitoring and health monitoring, although some might add regulatory monitoring as a third category. Operational monitoring is that surveillance done by managers and operators to ensure that facilities and processes are operating within design expectations. It consists of walk-through surveys, sampling and analysis, and decision making. Operational monitoring is conducted frequently, such as each shift or each day, but only a few parameters are analyzed.

In contrast, health monitoring is that surveillance done by health professionals. It consists of sanitary surveys, sampling and analysis, and interpretation or decision-making concerning the information and situation. One or more sanitary surveys should be conducted for each topical area on a periodic basis, such as initially, monthly, quarterly, or annually based on professional judgment. Sanitary surveys help environmental health professionals anticipate, recognize, evaluate, and control environmental factors that might adversely affect health. Sampling and analysis are also conducted for the same purpose and on a similar periodic basis. Often, many more parameters are analyzed than with operational monitoring but on a much less frequent basis, and certified laboratories are used if possible. Monitoring is not complete until interpretation or decision making has occurred. Primary decisions may be that the situation presents no significant threat (eg, water is safe to drink) or that specific actions need to occur to reduce risks of adverse health effects. Health decisions must be made by health professionals and not left to operational personnel by default.

Regulatory monitoring is a combination of operational and health monitoring. The regulator, the EPA for example, requires that certain monitoring or sampling and analysis be conducted and reported on a specified basis. Health professionals should not be satisfied with results from regulatory monitoring only because it often does not give the complete picture.

Policy is a selected course of action to achieve a desired result. The desired result is often expressed best by use of a vision statement, goals, and objectives. Policy studies should be conducted to help achieve better policy. A policy study is an assessment of the current situation, plus a vision for the more ideal situation, and an implementation plan for options to achieve the vision. Trying to see current reality clearly is the first step (Exhibit 20-1). Personal and organizational values, potential, and opportunities can help formulate a vision; setting goals and objectives helps communicate the vision more specifically to others. Making a commitment to create the desired results requires an awareness

of obstacles and the available options and an implementation plan. Finally, it should be noted that any new choice will create a new situation with new problems.

Managing the Risk Process

The military medical community may be required to recommend how to implement environmental health standards or assist in developing militarily unique standards or to determine the applicability of standards to special populations (eg, refugees, prisoners of war, local nationals). In any of these situations, it is important for the medical community to understand how health-based criteria and standards are developed. Strategies to prevent or mitigate adverse environmental factors can be developed to manage risk by focusing on the environmental health paradigm.

There are three main phases in the development of health-based environmental standards: risk assessment, risk management, and risk communica-

---

EXHIBIT 20-1

POLICY STUDY PROCESS

---

1. Where are we now and where are we headed? ⟶ PROBLEM STATEMENT

   Problems

   Attitudes, perceptions, behavior

   Institutions and infrastructure

   Resources

2. Where do we want to go? ⟶ VISION

   Our values   Goals

   Our potential   Objectives

   Opportunities

3. What are the obstacles? ⟶ ISSUES

                                           Dilemmas

4. What are the best routes to get us to the objectives? ⟶ POLICY OPTIONS

   Framework or map

   Criteria for success

5. How do we take and hold the objective? ⟶ IMPLEMENTATION PLAN

   Problems

   Attitudes, perceptions, behavior

   Institutions and infrastructure

   Resources

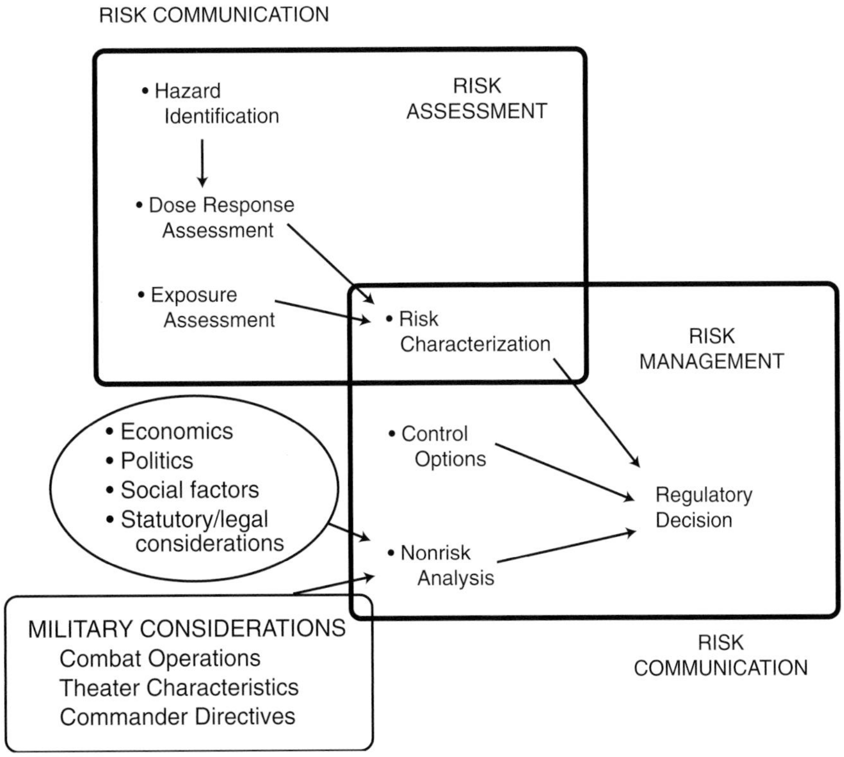

RISK COMMUNICATION

Fig. 20-2. The relationship between Risk Assessment, Risk Management, and Risk Communications. Risk assessment is the scientific determination of the potential health outcome that contaminants may inflict on people and the environment. Risk assessment, however, is only one component of risk management, which also includes a variety of other socioeconomic and technological factors and militarily specific concerns. Controlling risks typically is successful when major stakeholders are informed (risk communication) and involved in the process.

tion.[11] Their relationships to each other are illustrated in Figure 20-2. The risk assessment precedes the risk management process, but both involve several steps. Risk communication should occur throughout the process. Both the National Academy of Sciences[12] and the Presidential/Congressional Commission on Risk Assessment and Risk Management[13,14] describe and define issues associated with risk assessment and management and the necessary role stakeholders play to influence successful outcomes.

Risk Assessment

Risk assessment is the phase of the process in which health effects are identified and evaluated. The National Academy of Sciences[12] has identified four components of the risk assessment process— hazard identification, dose-response assessment, exposure assessment, and risk characterization. It defines each of these steps as follows:

- Hazard identification is the "process of determining whether exposure to an agent can cause an increase in the incidence of a health condition (cancer, birth defect, etc.)."[12(p19)]
- Dose-response assessment is "the process of characterizing the relationship between the dose of an agent administered or received and the incidence of an adverse health effect in exposed populations and estimating the incidence of the effect as a function of human exposure to the agent."[12(p19)]
- Exposure assessment is the "process of measuring or estimating the intensity, frequency, and duration of the human exposure to an agent currently present in the environment or of estimating the hypothetical exposure that might arise from the release of new chemicals into the environment."[12(p20)]
- Risk characterization is "the process of estimating the incidence of a health effect

under the various conditions of human exposure described in exposure assessment. It is performed by combining the exposure and the dose-response assessments. The summary effects of the uncertainties in the preceding steps are described in this step."[12(p20)]

Risk characterization is the final step in the risk assessment paradigm, and it overlaps with the risk management process. Even though it is an integral part of risk management, the risk assessment must not be influenced by the management factors. It is important for the risk assessor to communicate the estimated risk to the risk manager, and the method of expressing risk is critical. Typically the risk characterization is both qualitative and quantitative.[11] A qualitative risk characterization may be a narrative that describes the elements of the risk assessment and express hazard, exposure, and risk potential with terms such as "negligible," "minimal," "moderate," and "severe." Risk may be compared to common hazards expressed with comparative terms such as "less than," "equal to," or "greater than." A quantitative risk characterization expresses hazard and risk numerically by indicating a finite hazard measure per unit dose or exposure of an agent. An example is the percent change in response for each milligram of agent per kilogram of animal body weight.

It is reasonable to expect military preventive medicine practitioners to be health risk assessors and to advise risk managers, who may be commanders and makers of military doctrine or policy, on potential health outcomes associated with military activities. Therefore, it is important for the military preventive medicine practitioner to understand risk assessment and the factors that contribute to the process, especially issues of exposure duration and exposed population characterization. These factors may affect the magnitude of a federal or state standard and may not be applicable to military populations and scenarios. For example, the USEPA typically produces risk assessments that assume a lifetime of exposure and a broadly characterized exposed population to include sensitive subgroups, very young and very old people, and diseased individuals, which are not appropriate for active duty military members. For example, field military drinking water standards differ from their USEPA counterpart (see Field Drinking Water). The reasons for these differences become obvious when the MCLG (maximum contaminant level goal) formula's assumptions about the general United States population are compared with facts about service members in field environments. Active duty military typically serve from 2 to 30 years and only a small portion of that time is in the field; USEPA exposure standards are based on exposure duration of 70 years. Most military people are young, healthy adults; therefore, the age and health status range is smaller than that of the general population. Depending on environmental factors (eg, temperature) and activity, drinking water consumption for military individuals in the field may be much greater than the 2 L per day assumed for the general population. Various quantitative risk and exposure formulas and their bases can be found elsewhere.[15–19]

Risk Management

During the risk management phase, policy alternatives are weighed and the most appropriate regulatory action is selected. The risk characterization is integrated with engineering data and social, economic, and political concerns to reach a decision[12] (see Figure 20-2). Risk management may simply be deciding what to do about a problem, which requires the integration of a broad spectrum of scientific and nonscientific disciplines. It combines risk assessment with regulatory directives and with social, economic, technical, political and other considerations.[20] In the military, combat operations, theater characteristics (to include considerations for special populations such as prisoners of war, refugees, local nationals, and other civilians), and command directives also may influence this process. Sometimes a standard or criterion may be based on management factors rather than health. For example, a drinking water standard may be based on the current available technology for analyzing or treating a contaminant and thus may be higher than that suggested by the risk characterization.

Risk Communication

Throughout the risk assessment and risk management process there should be interaction between the risk assessor, the risk manager, and the affected community. This interaction, known as risk communication, encourages participation in the risk assessment and management process by all interested and affected parties. Risk communication is a method for informing the public and other stakeholders about the risks associated with hazards and the control strategies that are being considered.[11,13] It helps explain technical information to the general public and entails informing the community early, involving them in the decision-making process, using the media, and presenting truthful and frank information.[17,21] Military examples of those who should be informed include commanders, decision and policy makers, combat developers, and materiel developers. Service members are normally informed by their commanders or combat developers.

Managing the Environmental Health Program

Disciplines

Environmental health consists of a number of specialized areas that span a variety of related health, science, and engineering disciplines (Exhibit 20-2).

Typically, environmental health situations are multifaceted and so assessments and problem solving require an integrated approach. Thus, a team of environmental health professionals with varied specialties and a sufficient depth of knowledge may be required. Exhibit 20-3 lists the military environmental health specialties that exist in the US Army, Navy, and Air Force.

EXHIBIT 20-2

ENVIRONMENTAL HEALTH DISCIPLINES

- Environmental Quality

    Water Quality

        Drinking Water

        Wastewater

    Air Quality

        Ambient air (air pollution)

    Soil Science

- Waste Management

    Municipal Waste

    Hazardous Waste

    Medical and Infectious Waste

- Health Physics, Radiation Sciences

- Occupational Health and Medicine

- Bioacoustics

    Occupational Noise

    Environmental Noise

- Toxicology

    Mechanic

    Regulatory

    Forensic

EXHIBIT 20-3

UNIFORMED MILITARY ENVIRONMENTAL HEALTH AND RELATED OCCUPATIONS

US Army

    Environmental Science Officer

    Environmental Engineer

    Entomologist

    Health Physicist

    Epidemiologist

    Audiologist

    Veterinarian

    Biochemist (Environmental Chemist)

    Medical Laboratory Specialist (Environmental Chemistry)

    Preventive Medicine Specialist

    Veterinarian Technician

    Preventive Medicine Physician

    Occupational Medicine Physician

US Navy

    Environmental Health Officer

    Industrial Hygienist

    Audiologist

    Preventive Medicine Technician

    Industrial Hygiene Technician

    Preventive Medicine Physician

    Occupational Medicine Physician

US Air Force

    Public Health Officer

    Bioenvironmental Engineer

    Public Health Technician

    Bioenvironmental Technician

    Flight Surgeon

    Preventive Medicine Physician

    Occupational Medicine Physician

Installation Versus Field Environmental Health Considerations

Environmental health practices and programs on military installations are similar to those of civilian health departments. The goal of an installation environmental health program is to maintain the health of service members so that they remain able to perform their military mission. Also, because the installation caters to military families and, usually, a nonmilitary workforce, environmental health standards and monitoring should be at a level to protect those groups.

Deployment Environmental Health Considerations

Because of the complexity of moving units to other geographical regions and often to a harsher environment, there are additional environmental health considerations that are associated with military operations. These are the planning, execution, and follow-up activities associated with military deployments, which may include war or humanitarian operations. Preventive medicine considerations in planning for such operations are discussed in Chapter 13, Preventive Medicine and the Operation Plan, and Chapter 41, The Challenge of Humanitarian Assistance in the Aftermath of Disasters, and they also apply to environmental health concerns. The basis for both preventive medicine and environmental health planning is the medical threat, which classically includes temperature extremes (eg, heat and cold injury) and infectious disease, whether transmitted by humans, arthropod vectors, food, or water. There also may be other threats specific to the geographical area, the local culture and customs, and the military mission. Countermeasures can be taken to prevent casualty loss from these conditions in the following areas: field sanitation practices, personal hygiene, immunizations, drinking water, field food service sanitation, waste disposal, and insect and rodent control.

Military field environmental health considerations can be organized into the three phases of predeployment, deployment, and postdeployment. Table 20-2 lists some environmental health areas that

TABLE 20-2

ENVIRONMENTAL HEALTH CONSIDERATIONS DURING PREDEPLOYMENT, DEPLOYMENT, AND POSTDEPLOYMENT

Action	Examples of Considerations
Predeployment	
Staff Coordination	Personnel, intelligence, operations, logistics, civil affairs
Operational Scenario	Operations plan, mission, deployment location, units, timetable, transportation, logistics, food and water supply, waste disposal, host-nation requirements, Status of Forces Agreement
Medical Intelligence	Weather, disease, health of supported populations, potable water, vectors, terrain and hydrography, plant and animal threat
Preventive Strategies	Prophylaxis, personal protection measures, education, supplies and equipment, checklists, written directives
Reconnaissance	Potential sites, threat assessment, local liaison, water sources, vector types, sampling and analytical needs, contaminant and pollution sources
Deployment	
Advance Party Actions	Site selection, threat assessment, local liaison, water quality, air quality, soil contamination, vector surveillance
Sustainment	Disease surveillance, environmental health surveillance monitoring, recommendations, training
Redeployment	Retrograde/Agriculture inspections, terminal prophylaxis, health record documentation
Postdeployment	
Deployment Summary	After action report, lessons learned
Postdeployment Briefs	Chain of command, commanders, deploying units
Medical Followup	Epidemic and sexually transmitted disease, medical surveillance
Equipment Preparation	Order new supplies, maintain and replace deployment equipment for next deployment

Adapted with permission from Chardon WX. Presentation at the Navy Occupational Health and Preventive Medicine Workshop, Virginia Beach, Va, 1996.

should be addressed during each of these phases. During predeployment, the environmental health planner should acquire information about the mission and help identify and plan activities that protect the health of the deploying service members. The planner should learn about the prospective operation through continuous interaction with other staff organizations as they answer the who, what, when, where, and why of the mission. This information can be acquired by interacting with the command staff: Personnel (S1, G1, J1), Intelligence (S2, G2, J2), Operations (S3, G3, J3), Logistics (S4, G4, J4), and Civil Affairs (S5, G5, J5). Medical preparation against environmental health hazards includes educating service members about the potential hazards and use of personal protective measures (eg, repellents, appropriate clothing, sufficient water consumption), checking health status to ensure it meets a deployment standard, and giving immunizations. As part of the predeployment process, the environmental health planner should determine environmental sampling and analysis requirements and identify the resources to support the need. The planner should participate in area reconnaissance operations to aid in specific environmental health preparation; conditions may require, for example, on-site analysis (with its special techniques and equipment) or containers and procedures for sending samples to a particular laboratory. There are centers of environmental expertise in all the services (Exhibit 20-4).

When the units are deployed into a theater of operations, environmental health professionals should continuously monitor health indicators that could show a breakdown in environmental health and sanitation. This may include monitoring disease rates and trends, food preparation practices, water quality, and the use of personal protective measures. Problems and deficiencies should be presented to commanders with recommendations for corrective action. Training and education should continue during the deployment to emphasize field sanitation practices and to assist with preventing disease and solving problems.

Before units leave a theater of operations, environmental health personnel may be involved with, if only in an assisting role, performing retrograde inspections of equipment and supplies to determine that cleaning has removed potential insects and plants that could cause disease or agricultural problems in another country. When units return to their home station, an important postdeployment environmental health activity is to replenish environmental health supplies and replace, repair, and maintain equipment to prepare for the next deployment. Environmental health trends, accomplishments, problems, and solutions should be documented in after-action reports. They should cite lessons learned and recommendations in addition to doctrinal and equipment deficiencies and needs.

Managing Environmental Sampling and Analysis

The actual or potential impact of environmental agents on health can only be determined if the offending agent is known, as well as how much of it is present, as is reflected in the risk assessment paradigm's hazard identification and the exposure assessment processes. To address these concerns, samples of the environment must be gathered and analyzed to determine information (eg, qualitative, quantitative; chemical, biological, radiological, physical) for decision making. Data from sampling and analysis efforts are useful to assess public health threats, exposures, and contaminations; to assess remediation effectiveness; and to satisfy regulatory requirements. There are numerous published sampling and analytical procedures for environmental agents.[22–33]

General Methods

There are two broad categories of methods for environmental sampling and analysis. One category is the use of direct-reading instruments, which capture a sample of the soil, water, or air; perform the analysis within the instrument; and provide an im-

---

EXHIBIT 20-4

SELECTED MILITARY ENVIRONMENTAL HEALTH ORGANIZATIONS

- US Army Center for Health Promotion and Preventive Medicine, 5158 Blackhawk Road, Aberdeen Proving Ground, MD 21010-5422

- US Navy Environmental Health Center, 2510 Walmer Avenue, Norfolk, VA 23513-2617

- US Air Force Human Systems Center; Institute for Environment, Safety and Occupational Health Risk Analysis; 2513 Kennedy Circle, Brooks Air Force Base, San Antonio, TX 78235-5123

- Armed Forces Medical Intelligence Center, Fort Detrick, Frederick, MD 21702-5004

---

mediate reading of the concentrations of a contaminant on a display, such as a meter or digital readout. To provide accurate readings, direct-reading instruments must be calibrated, but even then they can be affected by rugged conditions in the field. Direct-reading instruments are only available for limited applications, and their data generally are not accepted by regulatory authorities. However, such instruments provide immediate results for decision makers. Environmental samples can also be obtained at the site of interest, packaged for transportation, and sent or taken to a laboratory for analysis. Disadvantages of this method include the potential sample degradation or contamination when transported to the laboratory and the delay between sample collection and analysis, which denies the decision maker immediate results.

Sampling Versus Analysis

Both the sampling events and the analytical events must be well planned and controlled to provide accurate, useful information that will result in meaningful public health decisions. The sampling and analytical process should produce data that are both scientifically valid and legally defensible.[34] The following paragraphs highlight considerations that should be addressed to enhance the quality of the information acquired.

Very precise procedures must be followed because the analytical results are only as good as the starting materials. Poor sampling can produce data that are inaccurate, inconsistent, and unexplainable; require repeat sampling, which then may delay decision making and mission completion; result in poor decision making, which may affect health; and cause unnecessary costs.

To avoid the perils of poor sampling, the following objectives should be considered. The samples should be representative of the area of interest. Thus, the sampling plan should be site-specific, and the sampling pattern should be statistically based (eg, random, grid, or judgment sampling).[34] The samples should be free of contaminants and substances that may alter or interfere with the analytical procedure. The collection procedure (eg, sample quantity, quality, frequency, matrix) should be appropriate for the analysis that will be performed, and this is best assured by coordinating with the laboratory in advance. Many contaminants must be preserved at the time of sampling to prevent them from degrading (thus giving a false result) before arrival at the laboratory. The sampling process should be fully documented (eg, date, time, location, number of samples, sample number, meteorological conditions, collector's name, activities, unusual circumstances). Other considerations include developing standard operating procedures (eg, equipment use, collection and handling procedures), specifying standard cleaning procedures between samples, collecting quality assurance samples (eg, blanks, duplicates or split samples, background samples), and performing quality assurance audits in the field.[34]

The desired outcome from laboratory analysis is to produce accurate and complete data when it is needed, in a form that can be understood, and at a reasonable price. The data that are produced should be of sufficient quality to allow decision making and problem solving. A laboratory may not be proficient merely because it routinely performs a given analysis or is certified.

Quality environmental laboratory analysis has multiple facets. When samples are received, there should be an accountability and documentation process that records the receipt event (eg, date, time, sample condition) and follows the sample through the laboratory to final disposition, which may include destruction, disposal, archiving, or passage to another laboratory. The data produced by the analysis may not be in a format that is useful or required by the requester, so it may need to be processed. For example, mass data may need to be converted to concentrations. Finally, the data should be reviewed for accuracy, reported to the requestor, and archived. Quality control samples must be analyzed with regular samples, and results must fall within acceptable limits. There should be a quality review that includes statistical control schemes of all the analytical phases.[35,36]

There are several factors to consider when determining the ability of a laboratory to analyze environmental samples properly. There is great variability in environmental samples (eg, drinking water, wastewater, soils, air, industrial products), and they frequently contain high levels of chemicals, called interferences, that can either obscure target contaminants or produce false-positive results. Competent laboratories recognize these facts and have well-developed systems in place to ensure that quality results are obtained and reported. The American Association for Laboratory Accreditation (A2LA) assesses testing laboratories for compliance with International Standardization Organization Guide 25, *General Requirements for the Competence of Calibration and Testing Laboratories, 1990*. This association accredits individual methods and procedures and not entire laboratories; a lab that is A2LA accredited to test for lead in paint may not be accredited to test for lead in water. It is important, therefore, that the accrediting certificate be examined to ensure that the desired testing is covered by the accreditation. Inserting blind (unknown to the analyst) quality control samples, reviewing data, and performing onsite laboratory visits are some of the effective techniques for monitoring laboratory performance.

Summary

The military preventive medicine practitioner frequently serves as a planner and staff advisor to provide medical opinions concerning potential health threats associated with military operations. Both environmental health standards and command emphasis are required to protect the military force from adverse health effects. However, military threats and operational scenarios may require modification of established standards and policy, which also may change the potential health risk. To advise commanders adequately, the preventive medicine practitioner should be familiar with the scope of environmental health, the nature of the science, the availability of environmental health professionals, and aspects of managing risks and programs.

ENVIRONMENTAL HEALTH TOPICS

The basic approach to environmental health practice—the discussion of the subject matter in term of standards, control, monitoring, and policy—will be applied here to fundamental environmental health topics. Drinking water, the first topic, is allotted more space than other topics to explain more fully how these principles apply.

Drinking Water

Municipal drinking water systems are used by the military to the extent possible for military bases and for civilian populations. The health functions with respect to drinking water are to set standards (or at least lead the effort), declare water potable or nonpotable (ie, make a decision based on standards, controls, monitoring, and policy), and provide advice for meeting standards.

Drinking Water Standards

Water standards in general depend on intended use, and municipal drinking water is only one use and results in one type of standard. Other standards exist for other uses. For example, industrial water standards might be more (or less) stringent than standards for drinking water, depending on the specific use. Other categories of water that have their own standards include military field drinking water, water for injection, recreational water, and shower or bathing water. Standards are dynamic; they change as knowledge, technology, and values change.

Drinking water standards can be classified according to the organization that sponsors them. Examples include World Health Organization (WHO) standards for international situations, USEPA standards for the United States, individual state standards within the United States, specific country standards for locations outside the United States, country-group standards in some locations (eg, standards of the Council of European Communities), and military standards for military field situations. Drinking water standards include the total package of requirements for the finished product, not just a specific parameter and its limitation. Therefore, one of the first questions to ask about drinking water is "Which standards apply?" For a civilian population outside the United States (eg, indigenous populations, refugees, migrants), appropriate standards could be WHO standards or the country's standards but not US military field standards.

Considerations for those drafting drinking water standards include safety factors, ability to analyze for a particular contaminant, duration of exposure, sensitive populations, protection of water sources, treatment processes, and policy. For example, some contaminant limitations have safety factors of 1,000 while others (eg, nitrates) have no safety factor. Some contaminants and specific limitations are listed in the standards—or omitted from the standards—because of our ability to analyze for them. As knowledge and capability improve, new parameters are added to the standards. Recent examples include synthetic organic compounds and trihalomethanes. Some contaminants might be too difficult to analyze for routinely, but treatment techniques have been found to control them. An example is *Giardia lamblia*. Therefore, some treatment techniques have been added to the standards, such as filtering surface water.

Drinking water standards are divided into primary and secondary standards. Primary (or health) standards relate to those contaminants that cause acute or chronic health effects at the limitations established and affect the water's potability. Secondary (or aesthetic) standards relate to those contaminants that cause the water to appear unpleasant and unacceptable at the limitations established, such as unsightly appearance, bad odor, and bad taste and adversely affect the water's palatability. Secondary standards are important because if people find drinking water aesthetically unacceptable, they might seek unapproved sources that appear better but are nonpotable or they might become dehydrated because they are not drinking sufficient water. Other factors addressed in drinking water standards include physical contaminants such as pH, turbidity (or cloudiness caused by colloid particles), and color (caused by decaying vegetation); chemical contaminants, such as salts and heavy metals; biological contaminants, such as indicators for pathogenic microorganisms; and radiological contaminants. Military standards include a category for chemical warfare agents. Finally, within the United States, the USEPA develops health advisories for compounds that are a potential threat but for which there is no consensus to include them in the standards. See Table 20-3 and refer to the USEPA

TABLE 20-3

A SUMMARY OF DRINKING WATER STANDARDS WITH SELECTED EXAMPLES

Contaminants	Limitation*	Goal[†]
Microbiological		
Cryptosporidium	Not set	Not set
Giardia lamblia	Treatment (filtration)	Zero
Legionella	Treatment technique	Zero
Standard plate count	Treatment technique	Not set
Total coliforms	< 5% positive samples	Zero
Turbidity	< 0.5 NTU[‡]	Not set
Viruses	Treatment technique	Zero
Chemical—Inorganic		
Fluoride	4 mg/L	4 mg/L
Heavy metals	Specific for each	Specific
Nitrate	10 mg/L	10 mg/L
Chemical—Organic		
Acrylamide	Treatment technique	Zero
Benzene	0.005 mg/L	Zero
Endrin	0.002 mg/L	0.002 mg/L
Trihalomethanes	0.1 mg/L	Zero
Radionuclides		
Radium 226	20 pCi/L	Zero
Radon	300 pCi/L	Zero
Aesthetic		
Chloride	250 mg/L	NA
Color	15 color units	NA
Copper	1.0 mg/L	NA
Corrosivity	Noncorrosive	NA
Fluoride	2.0 mg/L	NA
Iron	0.3 mg/L	NA
Manganese	0.05 mg/L	NA
pH	6.5 - 8.5	NA
Sulfate	250 mg/L	NA
Total dissolved solids	500 mg/L	NA
Zinc	5 mg/L	NA

*Limitation refers to the Maximum Contaminant Level (MCL) or treatment technique
[†] Goal refers to the Maximum Contaminant Level Goal (MCLG) for health impact
[‡] NTU: nephalometric turbidity unit
NA: not applicable, goals have not been set for aesthetic contaminants
Adapted from United States Environmental Protection Agency. *Drinking Water Regulations and Health Advisories.* Washington, DC; EPA: 1996.

for an example of current drinking water standards.[37] Meeting current standards, however, will not necessarily guarantee potable and palatable drinking water.

Controls for Drinking Water

Controls to help achieve high quality for drinking water should be implemented at the source, during treatment to remove contaminants or achieve desirable quality, and during distribution and storage.

The most common sources of drinking water are surface water (eg, streams, lakes) and groundwater. Additional sources include rainfall, the oceans, and glaciers. How the source affects water quality and what possible controls can be put in place should be the focus of preventive medicine personnel. Categories of contamination include fecal contamination, other natural contamination, and industrial contamination. Fecal contamination comes from humans and both wild and domestic animals. Pathogenic microorganisms are the primary and continuous threat. The source of contamination can be a point source, such as an outfall or discharge of wastewater, or it can be a nonpoint source, such as a wooded area or pasture. Other natural sources of contamination include growth and death of algae, decay of other vegetation, erosion, and natural deposits of minerals that dissolve in the water. Industrial contamination may include point and nonpoint discharges, runoff, acid rain, leaking tanks, and use of industrial products in homes and on farms.

The conventional treatment for groundwater is disinfection, and the most common disinfectant is chlorine. Many groundwaters are well protected, and disinfection is sufficient treatment. However, natural or industrial contamination of groundwater can make more extensive treatment necessary. For example, natural deposits of fluoride or radium might dissolve into the groundwater and need to be removed.

Conventional treatment for surface water is coagulation (including chemical addition, rapid mixing, flocculation by slow mixing, and sedimentation), filtration, and disinfection. Figure 20-3 shows a design of a typical water treatment plant. Primary contaminants removed during coagulation are turbidity and color. Turbidity is caused by colloid particles such as clay and bacteria. Color-causing substances are macromolecules that result from decaying vegetation. The coagulation process creates conditions that destabilize charges on discrete particles and allow them to form flocs and settle out of suspension. Color-causing substances are precipitated by the coagulation process. In addition, other contaminants can be acted on by the coagulation process. For example, heavy metals often will be precipitated, depending on the pH of the water; some organic matter may be enmeshed with the floc. The coagulation process can be viewed as pretreatment before filtration, and it allows filters to operate longer and with fewer problems.

Filtration is used to remove remaining particles. It will remove much but not all of the turbidity, to include microorganisms. Rapid sand or multimedia filtration is normally used, but filtration is sometimes used without coagulation. Examples are slow-sand filtration and direct filtration of relatively clear surface waters, such as mountain streams or lakes. Other forms of filters include diatomaceous earth filters and synthetic membranes. Pressure filters use pumps instead of gravity to force the water through

Coagulation Process

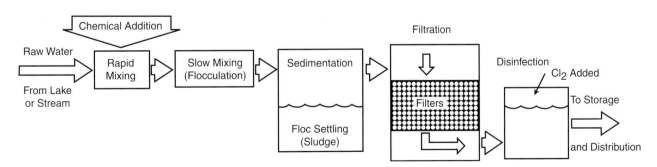

Fig. 20-3. Schematic of a Typical Water Treatment Plant. Generally, the treatment of drinking water involves unit processes to remove contaminants by causing them to coagulate and settle (they will be removed as sludge), to filter out additional contaminants, and to disinfect the final product to further reduce microbes.

the filter. Regardless of the type of filter, the purpose of filtration is to remove particulate matter, especially microorganisms, and make the disinfection process more effective.

Disinfection should always be used to inactivate pathogenic microorganisms. Various chemicals can be used; the more common ones are chlorine and ozone. Chlorine normally comes in the form of a gas or one of two salts [NaOCl or $Ca(OCl)_2$]. The active component in water is the same regardless of the form initially used:

$$HOCl \longleftrightarrow H^+ + OCl^-$$

The effectiveness depends on pH (low pH is best), contact time (preferably 30 minutes or more), temperature (cold temperatures can require higher doses of chlorine), clarity and interferences (particles and compounds can make disinfection less efficient), and concentration of other chlorine-demanding substances, such as ammonia, in the water. Chlorine combines with ammonia to form chloramines, which are also disinfectants but are less efficient than free chlorine. Most public health officials prefer disinfection with free available chlorine rather than combined chlorine residual.

There are a variety of other treatment processes to remove specific contaminants or to condition the water. Drinking water is often conditioned to prevent or control corrosion during storage and distribution. Adjustment of pH with lime [$Ca(OH)_2$] is common practice for corrosion control. Fluoridation is used in many water systems to help prevent dental caries. Water softening can be used at the treatment plant or at the point of use to remove or reduce the level of hardness caused by calcium and magnesium. Reverse osmosis can be used to remove essentially all dissolved solids, such as salts; this process can treat brackish water, seawater, or water contaminated with high levels of nitrates, fluorides, and radium. Aeration can be used to oxidize minerals such as iron and allow them to precipitate or allow volatile organic compounds to transfer from water to air. Adsorption, for example using activated carbon, can remove selected organic compounds. Levels of pH can be adjusted to get optimum conditions for the coagulation process and disinfection. Because chemicals added for treatment are not pure, contaminants can enter the water along with any chemical. Also, contaminants can enter from materials such as plumbing fixtures because of corrosion and leaching.

Contaminants can and do enter the system during storage and distribution. Contaminants can enter by cross connections between drinking water mains or plumbing and sources of wastewater by direct contamination of open reservoirs, by corrosion or leaching of materials in contact with water (eg, lead, copper, and zinc in plumbing fixtures). Significant levels of lead in water at the point of use has motivated professionals since the 1970s to consider the building plumbing as part of the distribution system. The main significance of the decision to make plumbing part of the distribution system is that water must be treated by the purveyor so that dangerous levels of contaminants do not corrode or leach from the plumbing materials.

Some additional considerations for storage and distribution systems include disinfection, fire demand, and treatment at point of use. There should be a continuous residual of chlorine to show that water has not become contaminated with fecal matter. When water mains break or new mains are installed, the procedure is to disinfect with chlorine at high levels (ie, 50 mg/L for 24 hours) while the main is off line. Water mains are looped in distribution systems to keep water flowing and avoid dead ends; this replenishes chlorine and helps prevent biological growth. Fire demand can require oversized mains that result in low flows, loss of chlorine residual, and buildup of precipitation from corrosion.

Drinking Water Monitoring

Operational monitoring for drinking water is that monitoring conducted by plant operations personnel to help ensure that both treatment processes and equipment work correctly. Operational monitoring serves as a quality check on the potability and aesthetics of treated water. It consists of observations, sampling and analysis, and decision making by plant operators. Only a few parameters are analyzed but on a frequent basis (ie, daily or each shift). Specific analyses depend on the treatment processes and chemicals added. An example of drinking water operational sampling and analysis might be daily or every-shift analysis of turbidity, color, pH, chlorine residuals, fluoride, and even coliforms on raw and treated water. Operational analysis would probably not include pesticides, heavy metals, synthetic organic compounds, radioactivity, or microorganisms other than an indicator organism. Operations personnel must decide if a problem exists and when to adjust chemical feed rates or call health personnel or regulators.

Health monitoring for drinking water consists of a sanitary survey, sampling and analysis, and interpretation of results. The main question to be answered concerns the safety and potability of the water. A sanitary survey of the sources of municipal drinking water, the treatment plant, and the storage and distribution system should be done at least annually by a qualified health professional and should focus on detecting and eliminating sources of contamination from spills, poor design and operations, cross connections, and other such problems. Sampling must be done using correct containers, preservatives, holding conditions, and holding time. Analyses should consider requirements for onsite analyses versus analyses in a certified laboratory. Tests for most parameters listed in USEPA standards should be conducted before a water source is put into operation and then annually in the United States for surface water sources and once each 3 years for groundwater sources. Results showing high contaminant levels or suspected contamination are reasons to sample more often. Microbiological sampling and analysis must be conducted quite frequently—daily, weekly or monthly depending on the size and specific processes of the water system. Selected parameters should be tracked with microbiological indicators to give a true picture of the situation (eg, turbidity, pH, chlorine residuals). Finally, a health professional must consider data and other information and make a decision concerning water potability and palatability.

Policy

Policy issues for drinking water include goals, objectives, and resources, all of which affect the comprehensiveness of standards, controls, and monitoring. The goal may be to provide a sufficient quantity of drinking water at low cost while expecting consumers to use point-of-use devices or bottled drinking water to get quality taste. Or the goal may be to provide a safe and high quality drinking water regardless of cost. Policy questions for standards include which parameters or treatment techniques should be included as part of the standards. Policy issues for controls include how well the source is protected and whether to filter surface water, even if clear mountain lakes or streams are used as the source. One policy issue for monitoring is the frequency and specific parameters required for sampling and analyses during operational and health monitoring.

Drinking water is vital to maintaining human health; therefore, its sanitary quality is also vital.

Managing drinking water production and distribution can be complex, and much of the science and technology is beyond the scope of this chapter but can be found elsewhere.[2–4]

Military Field Water

Water supply to service members in field situations is crucial to accomplishing the mission. Water must be both safe to drink and aesthetically pleasing. To prevent dehydration, service members must drink sufficient quantities of water. In addition, water is needed for food preparation and cooking, personal hygiene, medical treatment, laundry, cleaning equipment, and more. Total water needs for US personnel in desert environments are 76 L (20 gal) per person per day, with 15 L (4 gal) of that needed for drinking water.[38,39]

A team of military specialties is necessary to address all aspects of water supply, including standards, controls, monitoring, and policy. Health professionals play a vital role in the water supply team. Responsibilities for providing safe drinking water are divided among military staff. It is the role of logistics to purify, store, and distribute potable water and to develop equipment, but allied military forces often give responsibility for water purification to the engineers. The engineers' role in the US military is to develop water sources, including drilling wells. The medical role is to set health standards, certify water as potable, and provide technical advice for meeting standards. This includes health monitoring to certify water as potable and making recommendations for controls and policy to meet standards. The units are responsible for obtaining drinking water from only approved sources and ensuring that the water does not become contaminated. With these divided responsibilities, it is essential that all the parties coordinate so that essential tasks are not left undone.

Contaminants and Standards

Standards for field drinking water are regulated by two international agreements: the North Atlantic Treaty Organization's STANAG 2136 (Standardization Agreement 2136) and ABCA's QSTAG 245 (American, British, Canadian, and Australian's Quadripartite Standardization Agreement 245). QSTAG 245 was promulgated in 1985 and STANAG 2136 in 1994 with amendments added in 1995. Parameters and specific limitations listed are fairly consistent between the two standards; differences are minor. Sixteen contaminants are regulated under

TABLE 20-4

STANDARDS AND ROUTINE ANALYSIS FOR FIELD WATER

| Contaminants* (listed under QSTAG 245) | Requirements of QSTAG 245 | | Personnel Performing Analysis[†] |
	Short Term (< 7 d)	Long Term (> 7 d, < 1 yr)	
Microbiological			
Coliform	1 CFU/100 mL	1 CFU/100 mL	Health
Viruses	1 PFU/100 mL	1 PFU/100 mL	NA
Spores/Cysts	1 CFU/100 mL	1 CFU/100 mL	NA
Physical			
pH	5 to 9.2	5 to 9.2	Operational, Health
Temperature	2°C to 35°C	15°C to 22°	Operational, Health, Unit
Turbidity	5 NTU	1 NTU	Operational, Health
Total dissolved solids	1,500 mg/L	1,500 mg/L	Operational, Health
Color	NA	15 color units	Operational, Health
Chemical			
Arsenic	2 mg/L	0.05 mg/L	NA
Cyanides	20 mg/L	0.5 mg/L	NA
Mustard	0.2 mg/L	0.05 mg/L	NA
Nerve agents	0.02 mg/L	0.005 mg/L	NA
Chloride	NA	600 mg/L	Health
Magnesium	NA	150 mg/L	Health
Sulphates	NA	400 mg/L	Health
Radiological			
Mixed fission products	NA	0.06 µCi/L	NA

*In addition to contaminants listed in standards, disinfectants (eg, chlorine residual), when added for treatment, should be analyzed by operational, health, and unit personnel and compared to levels set by the command surgeon.
[†]As recommended in Miller R, Phull K, Smith E. An overview of military field water supply. *J US Army Med Dept*. 1991:9–13.
QSTAG: Quadripartite Standardization Agreement
CFU: colony forming unit
PFU: plaque forming unit
NTU: nephalometric turbidity unit
Sources: Department of the Army. *Quadripartite Standardization Agreement 245: Minimum Requirements for Water Potability*. 2nd ed. Washington, DC: DA; 1985. Miller R, Phull K, Smith E. An overview of military field water supply. *J US Army Med Dept*. 1991:9–13.

QSTAG 245 (Table 20-4). US military regulations for field water supply must be at least as stringent as those of QSTAG 245 and STANAG 2136.[40–43] For example, US military regulations allow 1,000 mg/L for total dissolved solids, 1 NTU (nephalometric turbidity unit) for turbidity, 600 mg/L for chloride, 30 mg/L for magnesium, and 100 mg/L for sulfates, when consuming 15 L per day.[43,44]

Differences between drinking water standards in the United States and the QSTAG 245 and STANAG 2136 standards are due to different assumptions. QSTAG 245 and STANAG 2136 standards assume a healthy adult population consuming the water for no more than 1 year and a water consumption of 5 to 15 L per person per day. Long-term effects are ignored by QSTAG 245 and STANAG 2136. Field drinking water is assumed to be the only source of fluids available to service members. The best available source of raw water should be selected for field water. Field water standards are not truly appropriate for refugees or otherwise susceptible individuals, although water purified under field conditions might meet the standards set to protect susceptible persons. For example, QSTAG and STANAG standards do not list levels for heavy metals, nitrates, fluorides, pesticides, or synthetic organic compounds. Also, field water standards should not be used in situations where assumptions are no longer valid (eg, reuse of wastewater as a source for drinking water or shower water).

Controls

Sources should be selected not only to give flexibility to the forces but to limit contamination. Therefore, the best available source should be selected, and sources should be protected from further contamination. The treated drinking water should be protected from contamination during storage and distribution until it is actually consumed.

The US military uses Reverse Osmosis Water Purification Units (ROWPUs) to treat drinking water (Figure 20-4). The ROWPU uses processes of filtration, reverse osmosis, and disinfection. Allied countries use either ROWPUs or conventional surface water treatment processes such as coagulation, filtration, and disinfection or other filtration processes (eg, diatomaceous earth filtration). On land the US military uses chlorine, usually in the form of calcium hypochlorite, as the disinfectant.[43] The reverse osmosis process allows brackish water and sea water, in addition to fresh water lakes and streams, to be used as a source. Also, reverse osmosis is more likely to remove chemical warfare agent contaminants than more conventional treatments. ROWPUs come as 600 gallon-per-hour units (operating 20 hours per day) and 3,000 gallon-per-hour units. A limited number of ROWPUs with larger capacity are available. The capacity of ROWPUs can be a limitation when large

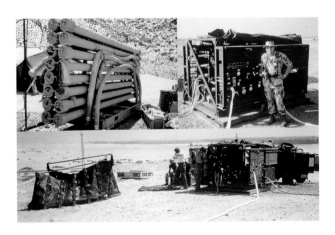

Fig. 20-4. Reverse Osmosis Water Production Unit. This drinking water treatment unit employs reverse osmosis technology to remove chemical and microbial contaminants and is used by the military to produce potable water from raw water sources or public water systems of unknown quality. Bottom view: a distance view of treatment unit and water tank. Top right: a close up view of treatment unit. Top left: Membrane filters that have been separated from the unit for display.

quantities of treated water are needed, such as during some humanitarian assistance efforts.

Monitoring

Operational monitoring is the surveillance, sampling and analysis, and decision making performed by personnel to ensure that water purification equipment is working properly. Analysis does not include all contaminants listed in the standards (see Table 20-4) because extensive testing was conducted during research and development to determine the efficiency of the equipment and it is understood that health monitoring will be conducted.

Health monitoring consists of sanitary surveys, sampling and analysis, and interpretation of data and other information. Since contaminants can enter at the source of water, during treatment, and during storage and distribution, sanitary surveys should be conducted initially and periodically to assess and mitigate likely contamination. Sanitary surveys help water treatment professionals select among alternative sources, identify possible contamination, verify proper treatment, verify safe storage and distribution, and check on water discipline.

Sampling and analysis for health monitoring is conducted to help select among alternative sources and to verify the safety and palatability of treated water, including water in storage and distribution, by comparing analytical results to accepted standards. Routine health analysis concentrates on turbidity, chlorine residual, and an indicator for microbiological quality. A standard will dictate the analytical procedure, which in turn defines sampling and preservation techniques. Sampling and more extensive analyses should be conducted periodically (eg, initially, annually, when a significant change occurs, when problems are reported) by a qualified laboratory using prescribed analytical techniques.

Regardless of the standards and frequency of sampling and analysis, we can never be certain that water is absolutely safe. Some contaminant could enter the water after treatment or be present initially but not identified. Standards, controls, and monitoring provide information and data, but education and experience are needed to make a judgment. Other decisions about water potability and palatability include selecting sources, selecting treatment processes, and determining how to identify and solve problems. Since judgment is a large factor, a professional with expertise in water supply should routinely interpret data, assess information, and make decisions.

Policy

Important policy issues include allocation of sufficient resources to water supply and quality, maintenance of water discipline, need for bottled water, and certification of water as safe to drink. Coordination of responsibilities and having one person in charge overall are essential, both in a theater of operations and within each of the military services.

Using bottled drinking water can be appropriate at times in the field. Possible uses are in the initial phases of deployment when water treatment equipment is not present, not yet operational, or broken. It may also be useful temporarily for personnel in small, remote locations. Bottled water can contain the same contaminants as the source of water and should not be considered safe for consumption until tested; only approved bottled water should be consumed.

To assist health professionals in certifying that water is safe to drink, policy should specify the minimum water treatment requirements, such as treatment processes and chlorine residual. Other factors that may be addressed in policy include use of approved chemicals, equipment, and materials; use of approved raw water sources; restrictions on the use of nonapproved containers (eg, fuel tanks) to store or haul drinking water; maintenance of water containers; water surveillance at the unit and Field Sanitation Team (FST) level; and appropriate training for water equipment operators and health professionals.

Swimming Pools and Bathing Areas

Service members will participate in recreational swimming activities even in a theater of operations, but the morale benefits of swimming should not override environmental health considerations. Since many health concerns of swimming and bathing are similar to those for drinking water, this section primarily will compare waters for human contact with those for drinking.

Both safety and health problems exist for recreational waters. Diseases are transmitted through both ingestion and contact. For service members in field situations (especially outside the United States), contact with surface water could result in exposure to such diseases as leptospirosis; schistosomiasis; skin infections; eye, ear, nose, and throat ailments; and primary amebic meningoencephalitis.

Swimming Pools

In the United States, water used to fill swimming pools is assumed to be drinking water or water of equal quality. Therefore, standards for swimming pools concentrate on contaminants introduced by humans through use of the pool or from the treatment process. Standards for pools usually include total (or fecal) coliform and the standard plate count, chlorine (or other disinfectant) residual, pH level, alkalinity, color, turbidity, and temperature. Microbiological requirements are essentially the same as those for drinking water. The chlorine level is required to be high enough to be effective but not high enough to cause eye irritation. Turbidity levels are usually more stringent than those for drinking water, not just because the particles can interfere with disinfection but because turbid waters can hinder visibility. A drowning swimmer might go unnoticed in turbid water. Within the United States, states or local health authorities set standards and criteria for swimming pools. The military services have likewise established their own requirements for pools on installations (eg, the Army's TB MED 575[45]).

Swimming pool water is normally treated by filtration and disinfection. Filters are often rapid sand, multimedia, or diatomaceous earth. Typically, the pool water is pumped through the filter at a rate to result in three turnovers of the pool volume per day. If microbiological or turbidity problems occur, turnover rate and disinfection levels can be increased. Swimming should be temporarily prohibited if contaminant levels are considered excessive. Other controls for swimming pools include designing pools so that storm water does not enter the pool, having swimmers bathe before entering the pool area, and limiting the number of swimmers. For more details, see the services' technical bulletins on swimming pools or a current text such as Salvato.[2]

Health monitoring of public swimming pools should include a sanitary survey by a qualified health professional before the pool is placed in operation and periodically (such as weekly or monthly) afterwards, sampling and analysis of critical parameters such as those discussed above for standards, and a decision concerning safe use of the pool. The sanitary survey should include review of design, operational monitoring, pool rules and regulations, qualifications of operators, and safety and industrial hygiene considerations. Operational monitoring is concerned with keeping the pool safe on an hour-to-hour basis. Preventive medicine personnel should identify any "field expedient" swimming venues, which may lack attention to many of these force protection issues.

Policy for swimming pools include design considerations, rules and regulations for swimmers, and responsibilities for oversight. Managers of public pools generally must obtain a permit for their design and operation. Health authorities have responsibility to ensure that public pools are safe for users, and they should not hesitate to close pools if they are deemed unsafe. Those responsible for the health of service members should be similarly vigilant.

Natural Bathing Areas

Limitations for bacteriological quality of water used for natural bathing areas (eg, lakes, beaches, streams) are much less stringent than for drinking water or swimming pool water. For fresh and marine waters, a logarithmic mean of 200 CFU (colony-forming unit) per 100 mL for fecal coliform over a 30-day period is the current accepted limitation.[45] The reason for accepting poor quality water is that historically there have been very few reported disease outbreaks where the natural water was not highly contaminated. Caution still is warranted, however, and sanitary surveys are an important factor in deciding to open or close natural bathing areas. The bathing area should be free from obvious industrial, natural, and fecal contamination. The site should also be physically safe for swimmers, and water should be essentially free of turbidity so that swimmers remain clearly visible to lifeguards. Other health concerns for natural bathing areas are similar to those for swimming pools.

Wastewater Management

The practice of environmental health as it applies to wastewater management is the focus of this section; a more detailed discussion of wastewater technological and management issues can be found elsewhere.[2–4,46] Wastewater management procedures are opposite to those of drinking water. Instead of looking at source, treatment, and distribution, wastewater management professionals look at collection, treatment, and disposal. Disposal of wastewater and sludge has health implications. Options for disposal of wastewater are to streams or lakes, to the ocean, to land, or to reuse (no direct discharge). Options for disposal of sludge include to land, to sanitary landfill, and to reuse, but sludge must be tested to ensure that it is not hazardous. Hazardous wastewater sludge must be handled as hazardous waste. Problems from inappropriate disposal or management of wastewater and sludge include diseases spread by drinking water, by recreational water, or through eating contaminated fish and shellfish; nuisances (eg, unsightly situations, odors); and eutrophication (the accelerated degradation of lakes caused by the presence of excessive nutrients).

Wastewater Standards

Within the United States, wastewater standards are implemented through permits granted by the USEPA or state agencies under the National Pollutant Discharge Elimination System (NPDES) of Public Law 92-500. The discharger, whether a municipality, installation, or industry, must apply for a point-source discharge permit. Each permit is site-specific, but there are national minimum treatment requirements and specific toxic compounds can be listed.

The two bases for wastewater standards are identified minimum treatment requirements and specific use of receiving waters. Minimum treatment requirements in the United States are secondary treatment or its equivalent for domestic wastewater and best available technology for industrial wastewater. The USEPA determines treatment standards for specifically identified pollutants. States, local authorities, or interstate commissions can be more stringent than the USEPA to protect selected bodies of water. These stream quality requirements can result in standards that require advanced wastewater treatment or zero discharge and cost twice as much or more than minimum requirements. It is possible to negotiate with authorities on requirements beyond minimum treatment either to decrease costs or to better protect human health. Wastewater standards for overseas areas during deployment may be somewhat equivalent to US requirements.

Characteristics for typical raw or untreated domestic wastewater are shown in Table 20-5. In wastewater, the particles are normally suspended (as opposed to colloid particles in drinking water) and settle rapidly. Volatile suspended solids give an estimate of the organic content, or biodegradable portion, of suspended particles. Human and animal feces are present in domestic wastewater and must be treated or properly disposed of so that disease outbreaks are prevented. Organic matter in wastewater is measured as (*a*) biochemical oxygen demand (BOD), which is the amount of oxygen used by microorganisms to oxidize organic matter into carbon dioxide and water, normally measured after 5 days (BOD_5) of incubation time; (*b*) as chemical oxygen demand (COD); or (*c*) as total organic carbon (TOC). The rate of dissolved oxygen depletion during biodegradation indicates the likelihood of fish kills in receiving streams or lakes due to depleted oxygen levels if proper treatment is not carried out. Phosphorus and nitrogen are essential to biological growth during degradation of organic matter, but these compounds also contribute to eutrophication. Ammonia is toxic to fish. Nitrates can cause methemoglobinemia in people; infants are more susceptible. Extremes of

TABLE 20-5

TYPICAL RAW OR UNTREATED DOMESTIC WASTEWATER IN THE UNITED STATES

Particles		Microorganisms		Dissolved Solids		Priority Pollutants	
Total suspended solids	200 mg/L	Bacteria[*] Viruses[†]	300 x 10⁶/L 7 x 10³/L	Organic BOD COD TOC	150 mg/L 220 mg/L 70 mg/L	Organic Heavy metals	Unknown Unknown
Volatile suspended solids	140 mg/L			Inorganic Phosphorus Nitrogen pH	8 mg/L 20 mg/L 6.0 to 8.0		

BOD: biological oxygen demand
COD: chemical oxygen demand
TOC: total organic carbon
[*]Salvato J. *Environmental Engineering and Sanitation.* Somerset, NJ: John Wiley and Sons; 1992: 479.
[†]Salvato J. *Environmental Engineering and Sanitation.* Somerset, NJ: John Wiley and Sons; 1992: 339.

pH can kill aquatic life. Priority pollutants, as listed by the USEPA, are often poured down drains, and are present in some concentration in most domestic and industrial wastewater. These pollutants can adversely affect biological treatment facilities, end up in receiving waters, or end up in wastewater sludge.

A typical NPDES permit or standard for domestic wastewater is shown in Table 20-6. Note that "secondary treatment" is reasonably well defined in terms of pollutants and their levels. More stringent requirements are considered "tertiary treatment" or advanced wastewater treatment. Also, note that significant nutrient removal is considered to be "tertiary treatment," whether it is for one nutrient or several. Treatment processes will be discussed in more detail later.

TABLE 20-6

TYPICAL DOMESTIC WASTEWATER STANDARD (NPDES PERMIT)

Parameter	Secondary Wastewater Treatment	Tertiary/Advanced Wastewater Treatment
Flow	Volume/d	Volume/d
Total suspended solids	30 mg/L	< 10 mg/L
BOD₅	30 mg/L	< 10 mg/L
pH	6.5 to 8.5	6.5 to 8.5
Fecal coliform	200 MPN/100 mL	< 1 MPN/100 mL
Dissolved oxygen	> 5.0 mg/L	> 5.0 mg/L
Oil and grease	2.0 mg/L	1.0 mg/L
Total phosphorus	–	1.0 mg/L
Ammonia-nitrogen	–	1.0 mg/L
Total nitrogen	–	2.0 mg/L
Total residual chlorine	< 1.0 mg/L	< 1.0 mg/L
Temperature	–	+5°F of receiving water
Priority pollutants	–	< MCL
Toxicity tests	–	Quarterly/annually

BOD₅ biological oxygen demand after 5 days of incubation
MPN: most probable number
MCL: Maximum contaminant level

TABLE 20-7

POLLUTANTS REMOVED OR REDUCED DURING TREATMENT

Treatment Process	Main Pollutant	Other Pollutants
Primary (settling)	Suspended solids	BOD (and more)
Secondary (biological)	BOD	SS (and more)
Tertiary (depends on requirements)	May be BOD, N, NH^3, P, priority pollutants	May be SS, BOD, N, P and more
Disinfection	Pathogens	Fecal coliform

BOD: biologic oxygen demand
N: nitrogen
NH^3: ammonia

P: phosphorus
SS: suspended solids

Wastewater Controls

For municipalities and installations, the three methods for collecting wastewater have been sanitary sewers (which collect only wastewater), storm sewers (which should collect only storm water runoff), and combined sewers (which collect both domestic and industrial wastewater plus storm water runoff). Treatment processes and the main pollutants removed are listed in Table 20-7. A schematic of a typical domestic wastewater treatment plant is shown in Figure 20-5. Wastewater treatment for domestic wastewater consists of primary treatment (ie, settling of most suspended solids) and secondary treatment (ie, biological degradation of most organic matter or the equivalent chemical treatment). Tertiary treatment, also called advanced wastewater treatment, is used for additional deg-

radation of organic matter, significant nutrient removal, or removal of priority pollutants. Biological treatment is normally aerobic and uses intentionally grown microorganisms suspended as flocs in an aeration basin or attached to surfaces. Chemical precipitation is normally used to remove phosphorus. Sludge produced by primary settling and during wasting of biological floc in secondary treatment is often further treated using anaerobic biological organisms or using chemicals such as lime, which conditions sludge to a pH of about 11. Wastewater is often but not always disinfected before disposal. If chlorine is the disinfectant, then dechlorination must be used at times to meet standards and prevent harm to aquatic life. The purpose of disinfection is to inactivate pathogenic microorganisms, and fecal coliforms are used as the indicator organism.

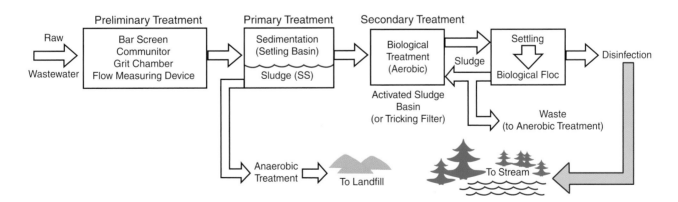

Fig. 20-5 Schematic of a Typical Wastewater Treatment Plant. Minimally, wastewater should receive primary (physical removal/settling) and secondary (biological) treatment, which can be followed by disinfection before discharge. More advanced processes (advanced or tertiary treatment) may be required for special wastes.

Treatment of small flows and individual homes is often by use of septic tank systems. These systems consist of collection (often within the home), treatment (the tank combines settling and anaerobic treatment), and disposal (to an underground drain field). Venting is essential since anaerobic treatment produces methane gas, hydrogen sulfide, and carbon dioxide. Sludge accumulates in the tank and must be disposed of periodically (every 3 to 5 years for individual homes), normally to the local wastewater treatment plant. Otherwise, sludge will eventually clog the drain field.

Industrial wastewater characteristics can be similar to domestic wastewater or present problems such as extremely high BOD (eg, diaries, meat processing plants), nutrient-deficient wastewater, fluctuations of pH, and discharge of priority pollutants (eg, synthetic organic compounds, heavy metals). Treatment can be for direct discharge or for discharge into a municipality's sanitary sewer. Proper treatment or pretreatment should occur before discharge. Treatment processes previously described are often used, plus chemical processes to control specific compounds. However, high BOD waste might be treated by the anaerobic process, nutrients might need to be added, and compounds might need to be removed and conditions adjusted to allow optimum growth of microorganisms for biological treatment. Sludge might need to be handled as a hazardous waste.

Wastewater can be recycled within a process (such as using rinse water effluent for initial wash water) or reused after treatment (such as for irrigation of golf courses). Indirect reuse occurs routinely by use of surface water from streams that have received wastewater discharges. This indirect reuse can be for potable or nonpotable purposes. Potable direct reuse, however, is not routinely acceptable practice although exceptions exist (eg, the National Aeronautics and Space Administration's space station program). Water reuse will require new standards to be developed for the particular situation because drinking water standards assume the source is of relatively high quality.

Wastewater Monitoring

Health monitoring for wastewater management consists of a sanitary survey, sampling and analysis, and interpretation of results. Wastewater must be collected and disposed of in a manner that does not harm human health and the environment. The professional conducting the sanitary survey looks at actual and potential sources of wastewater to decide if water from all sources is properly collected, at treatment to determine if it is proper, and at disposal to ensure it is properly done. When looking at sources, items to consider are individual systems versus the municipal or installation system, characteristics of surrounding industries, pretreatment versus treatment for discharge, proposed projects or developments that affect wastewater management, and pollution prevention. When looking at treatment, items to consider are the standards (eg, NPDES permit or equivalent), treatment processes used, chemicals added, and operations' adequacy for achieving standards. When looking at disposal, items to consider are the standards, the receiving water, the ultimate use of wastewater, and the disposal of sludge.

Sampling and analysis must be appropriate for decision making to help protect human health and the environment. Operational data are not sufficient. Periodic sampling and analysis for health concerns should be conducted separately from operational requirements and include all parameters listed in the standards plus priority pollutants and toxicity testing if industrial wastes could be present. Analysis should be conducted by a certified laboratory or equivalent military laboratory during deployment.

The main question to ask about interpretation of results is if wastewater collection and disposal is safe to humans and the environment. If not, then what must be done in terms of standards, controls, monitoring, and policy needs to be determined. A second questions is if health monitoring for wastewater management is adequate. Health monitoring is not complete until these questions are answered with affirmatives.

Operational monitoring by plant personnel helps serve as quality control for wastewater management, and it partially documents compliance with standards for some routine analyses that are best conducted onsite. Only a few parameters are analyzed but on a frequent basis (eg, daily or each shift). Specific analyses depend on the treatment processes and chemicals added. Typical factors for analysis would be pH, dissolved oxygen, suspended solids, chlorine residual, BOD_5, and flow. Analyses not likely to be performed by plant personnel include toxicity testing and testing for priority pollutants and nutrients. The decisions that plant personnel make include that there are no problems, that chemical feed rates or pump rates need adjusting, and that regulators or health personnel need to be called.

In addition to operational monitoring, regulatory sampling and analysis specifically listed in the NPDES permit are required in the United States. Some of it can be conducted by personnel on-site, but some sampling and much of the analysis are often conducted by a state-certified laboratory. Regulatory sampling and analysis alone do not fulfill requirements for health monitoring.

Policy

Policy issues for wastewater management include the degree of stringency for standards, controls, and monitoring, plus who makes which decisions. Wastewater standards may have been established through negotiation, but health professionals may or may not have been a major party to the negotiation. That is crucial because regulators might not care about the cost of compliance, and they might not be knowledgeable about health effects or environmental effects. But the standards set will greatly affect cost containment and risk management. Health professionals may interpret results from health monitoring and make decisions about adequacy of wastewater management but have sometimes left that decision to others (eg, plant operators) by default. Health professionals may also advocate pollution prevention and good management practices beyond mere compliance to contain costs and better manage risks. An additional issue for deployment is whether or not US forces should meet adequate standards for discharge of wastewater and sludge even though the host nation might not.

Managing Hazardous Materials

As countries industrialize and incorporate the use of new and advanced technology, they increase their use of potentially hazardous chemicals and radioactive substances. There is the potential of increases in incidents that expose people, including deployed US forces, to uncontrolled and dangerous quantities of such materials. One example occurred in Bhopal, India, in 1984 when 30 tons of methyl isocyanate were released accidentally from a chemical plant and caused 3,000 deaths and 200,000 injuries.[8] During the years 1953 to 1961, inorganic mercury was discharged from a plastics factory into the bay by the town of Minimata, Japan.[5] Bacteria in the water converted the inorganic mercury into an organic form, methyl mercury, which is more soluble and toxic. Passively absorbed by microscopic algae, the methyl mercury moved through the food chain—algae to zooplankton to fish—and became more concentrated at each level. Many people who consumed the contaminated seafood developed neurotoxicity and some died.

A more recent example with direct relevance to a US military operation is the massive oil well fires that occurred in 1991 associated with the Persian Gulf War

when Iraqi forces purposely set the wells on fire. There was a potential for the occurrence of adverse health effects in US and allied military forces that were exposed to the oil combustion products. Even if the wells had not burned, their presence was a potential environmental health concern and should have been identified during the medical intelligence assessment for their potential to pollute water and food sources and to expose military forces to harmful vapors.

Military operational planners and intelligence analysts would be concerned about an area that military forces had to pass through or occupy if it recently had been sprayed with sarin (GB; O-isopropyl methylphosphonofluoridate), a chemical warfare nerve agent. They should be equally concerned about the area if it was an agricultural field recently sprayed with the insecticide Parathion (O,O-diethyl-O-p-nitrophenyl phosphorothioate[NB]). Both are organophosphate cholinesterase inhibitors, which adversely affect the nervous system. Potential threats that hazardous chemicals may pose for military forces and operations need to be assessed.

This section provides some simple definitions of hazardous material to allow the reader to recognize and identify them. It identifies various US laws and regulations that also offer some specific definitions and plans and programs to manage hazardous materials. The emphasis in this chapter is on chemical substances. For detailed information concerning radiation hazards please refer to chapter 29, Medical Response to Injury from Ionizing Radiation.

What Are Hazardous Materials?

A hazardous material is a substance that can cause an adverse effect, such as injury or death, to the body, the environment, or both. Whether there is an actual risk of such outcomes depends on other factors, such as the amount of the hazardous material (ie, exposure concentration), exposure time, dose-response relationship, and susceptibility of the final receptor. Several other similar terms that are sometimes used synonymously with hazardous material but may be referred to in specific laws and regulations include hazardous substances, toxic agents, and hazardous wastes. The term "hazardous substance" is synonymous with hazardous material and includes both chemicals and radioactive materials. Toxic agents are chemicals only. Eaton and Klaassen[8] differentiate between toxin, a naturally produced toxic substance, and toxicant, a toxic substance that is produced by or is a by-product of anthropogenic activities. Because this part of the chapter focuses only on chemicals, the terms hazardous material, hazardous substances, and toxic agents will be considered synonymous. Hazardous waste is discussed later in this chapter and refers to hazardous and toxic materials that are no longer used for their original purpose and must be disposed of.

There are numerous environmental laws and regulations that identify and address hazardous materials. Table 20-8 presents information concerning these regulations and the types of hazardous materials they address. Some of the regulations contain lists of chemicals that are considered hazardous.

Classifications (Chemicals)

There are various ways to classify hazardous materials. The method selected reflects the needs and interests of the classifier.[8] They may be classified according to chemical state (eg, organic, inorganic, acid, base, solvent), physical state (eg, solid, liquid, gas, vapor, particulate), type of toxicity (eg, systemic, carcinogenic, target organ), or industrial use (eg, catalyst, primer, explosive, denaturant, preservative). Another type of classification scheme that is based on physiological effect may have more military relevance because outcomes of exposure may affect an individual's ability to perform his or her mission. For example, some shoulder-fired missile weapon systems use perchlorate-based propellants that produce acid gases in their combustion product. These gases irritate the eyes and respiratory mucosa and may temporarily hinder the user and adversely affect a mission. Examples of physiological classes include the following.[47]

- Irritants (eg, ozone, hydrochloric acid, sulfuric acid),
- Asphyxiants (eg, carbon monoxide, hydrogen cyanide),
- Anesthetics (eg, cleaning solvents, alcohols, aldehydes),
- Systemic poisons (eg, mercury, lead, other heavy metals),
- Pneumoconiosis-producing dusts (eg, cotton dust, coal dust),
- Inert and nuisance dusts (eg, sawdust),
- Sensitizing agents (eg, toluene diisocyanate),
- Carcinogens (eg, asbestos, coal tar, benzene),
- Reproductive hazards (eg, dinitrotoluene), and
- Others (eg, mutagens, teratogens).

Hazardous Materials Management—United States

In the United States, there are various levels of controls designed to minimize the occurrence of adverse health or environmental events due to haz-

ardous materials. Such controls are embodied in the types of laws that were presented earlier and are listed in Table 20-8. It is beyond the scope of this chapter to address the details of all the environmental laws that address hazardous materials. General hazardous materials management concepts that can be derived collectively from all of the laws are within the scope of this chapter. Important management concepts include regulatory requirements for registration and testing, design and planning, tracking and documentation, training, transporting, storing, use and handling, and disposal.

Laws like the Federal Insecticide, Fungicide, and Rodenticide Act (FIFRA) and the Toxic Substances Control Act (TSCA) require that when new chemicals are proposed for the market, they must be assessed for their toxicity potential to people and the environment before they are approved or registered. If sufficient studies and tests have not been conducted, they must be done specifically for the assessment. Based on the assessment, the chemical may be approved for use as proposed, receive approval for limited use, or be banned from use. These laws also require that when significant new information is available or if there is a significant new use of the chemical, a new health assessment, and possibly additional testing, is required.

It is important to address hazardous material issues in the early stages of project concept and design. History has shown that trying to control pollutants as emissions or effluents can be costly and prone to accidents. Efforts are now directed to identifying hazardous materials during the design of a process and, ideally, eliminating them, whether by substituting nonhazardous materials or modifying the process to eliminate their use totally. This concept is known as pollution prevention, or P2. If the hazard cannot be completely eliminated, then it should be minimized as much as possible (eg, substitution with a less hazardous chemical or an engineering design that reduces the probability of accidental release). This process is a component of hazard minimization (HAZMIN).

When a hazardous chemical is procured by an organization, the chemical generally comes to a receiving point, is issued to the using activity, and is used by that activity. The used chemical, excess chemical, or outdated chemical is discarded as hazardous waste. The Resource Conservation and Recovery Act (RCRA) requires that hazardous waste be tracked and documented on a manifest from its point of generation to its point of final disposal—a concept frequently called "cradle-to-grave" tracking. Even though this process is required only when a substance is deemed to be a waste, hazardous

TABLE 20-8

SELECTED ENVIRONMENTAL HEALTH LEGISLATION AND GUIDELINES THAT ADDRESS HAZARDOUS MATERIALS

Statute	Federal Agency	Codes	Type of Hazardous Material
Clean Air Act (CAA)	USEPA	40 CFR 50/80	Priority and hazardous air pollutants
Clean Water Act (CWA)	USEPA	40 CFR 100-140, 400-470	Hazardous substance spills, toxic pollutants
Comprehensive Environmental Response, Compensation, and Liability Act (CERCLA)	USEPA	40 CFR 300	"Superfund" sites, hazardous substances
Consumer Product Safety Act (CPSA)	CPSC	16 CFR 1015-1402	Injury or illness to consumers from products
Emergency Planning and Community Right to Know Act (EPCRA)	USEPA	40 CFR 350, 355 370, 372	Superfund Amendment Reauthorization Act, Title III
Federal Food, Drug, and Cosmetic Act (FFDCA)	FDA	21 CFR 1-1300	Food additives and nonadditives, cosmetics
Federal Hazardous Substances Act (FHSA)	CPSC	16 CFR 1500-1512	Labeling requirements (eg. toxics, corrosives)
Federal Insecticide, Fungicide, Rodenticide Act (FIFRA)	USEPA	40 CFR 162-180	Pesticides
Hazardous Materials Transportation Act (HMTA)	DOT	49 CFR 106-107, 171-179	Hazardous materials shipping
Marine Protection, Research, and Sanctuaries Act (MPRSA)	USEPA	40 CFR 200-238	Controls ocean dumping of sewage sludge/toxic substances, "Ocean Dumping Act"
Flammable and Combustible Liquids Code	NFPA	National Fire Code (NFPA 30)	Flammable and combustible liquids
Occupational Safety and Health Act (OSHA)	OSHA/DOL	29 CFR 1910, 1915, 1918, 1926	Workplace toxic chemicals
Oil Pollution Control Act	USEPA	40 CFR 112	Waste oil
Poison Prevention Packaging Act (PPPA)	CPSC	16 CFR 1700-1704	Hazardous household products packaging
Resource Conservation and Recovery Act (RCRA)	USEPA	40 CFR 240-271	Hazardous waste management
Safe Drinking Water Act (SDWA)	USEPA	40 CFR 140-149	Maximum Contaminant Levels (MCLs)
Toxic Substances Control Act (TSCA)	USEPA	40 CFR 700-799	New chemical hazard assessment and testing

USEPA: US Environmental Protection Agency; CPSC: Consumer Product Safety Commission; FDA: Food and Drug Administration; DOT: Department of Transportation; OSHA: Occupational Safety and Health Administration; NFPA: National Fire Prevention Association, DOL: Department of Labor

Adapted with permission from: Derelanko M. Risk assessment. In: Derelanko M, Hollinger M, eds. *CRC Handbook of Toxicology.* Boca Raton, FL: CRC Press; 1995, Copyright CRC press, Boca Raton, Florida.

Adapted by permission of Waveland Press from: Nadakavukaren A. *Our Global Environment, A Health Perspective.* 4th ed. Prospect Heights, Ill: Waveland Press; 1995.

Adapted with permission from The McGraw Hill Companies from: Eaton D, Klaassen C. Principles of toxicology. In: Klaassen C, Amdur M, Doull J, eds. *Casarett and Doull's Toxicology: The Basic Science of Poisons.* New York: McGraw-Hill; 1996.

chemical users are increasingly tracking the chemical from the time it enters their premises through its use to its final disposal.

Individuals who use, transport, or handle hazardous materials are required to be trained in the kinds of hazards and toxic effects that the material can produce. They also must be aware of emergency and cleanup procedures in case of accidents and spills. The Occupational Safety and Health Act requires initial and annual training for individuals who work with hazardous materials. They are to be aware of specific personal protective measures and be knowledgeable about the content, availability, and location of Material Safety Data Sheets (MSDSs). MSDSs are information papers, developed by manufacturers of hazardous materials, that provide details about chemical contents, health effects, personal protective measures, and fire, storage, and transportation safety.

Military Relevance

When US military forces deploy to foreign nations, they should be aware of potential harm to which they could be exposed from the hazardous materials practices of the host nation. Less-developed nations may have either no hazardous materials management program or a poorly enforced one. Also, they may not frequently use hazardous materials. All of these could increase service members' risk of being exposed to hazardous substances. It is important that chemical use and controls be a part of the medical intelligence estimate and assessment. Selected situations of interest follow.

Some agriculture chemicals may have toxicities similar to chemical warfare agents. For example, organophosphates and chlorinated hydrocarbon insecticides also adversely affect the human nervous system. Herbicides are toxic to people as well as plants. Paraquat, a nonselective contact herbicide, is severely debilitating and life-threatening, with the lung being the most susceptible target organ.[48] Also, some pesticides that are banned in the United States because of demonstrated toxicity to humans or the environmental or both are available in other nations. Examples include the neurotoxicants DDT (dichlorodiphenyltrichloroethane) and chlordecone (Kepone).[48,49]

Less-developed countries may not have stringent laws that control hazardous materials and wastes and forbid them from being dumped into the environment. This situation, among others, may allow hazardous materials and wastes to be exported from other countries, either legally or illegally, into less-

developed areas for disposal. Thus, there may be a greater potential for air, water, and soil pollution than would be expected, given the industrial capabilities of the host nation.

Another consideration with hazardous materials is that areas with little or no control of these materials may increase the access of hazardous materials to terrorists, who may contaminate military water sources or create acute exposure situations that could result in acute, delayed, or chronic health effects on US forces.

Concerns for the Preventive Medicine and Environmental Health Planner

There is some information that may be useful to the preventive medicine and environmental health planner concerning the potential for deploying military forces to encounter hazardous materials in a theater of operations. Figures 20-1 and 20-2 provide a conceptual frame for the types of questions that should be pursued and information acquired to develop a risk estimate. Examples of questions that may be considered are presented in Exhibit 20-5. Also, the planner should consider the history of recent hazardous materials incidents (eg, spills, air or water releases), occupational exposure history, terrorist activities, and any other unusual chemical incident. There may be a need to determine the composition of unknown substances or quantitate known ones; therefore, the planner should determine the availability of theater or local laboratory analytical capability.

Managing Waste

Integral to daily life is the generation of various types of waste. One form, wastewater, has been addressed previously and will not be addressed in this section. The other waste types discussed in this section, though, do have some common characteristics with wastewater. They may also consist of a mixture of potentially harmful chemical, biological, and physical agents, and they can have adverse public health effects if not handled properly. The forms of waste that are discussed in this section include solid waste, hazardous waste, and medical and infectious waste.

Solid Waste

Solid waste may consist of a variety of materials, to include "any garbage, refuse, sludge...and other discarded material, including solid, liquid,

---

EXHIBIT 20-5

HAZARDOUS MATERIALS CONSIDERATIONS FOR THE PREVENTIVE MEDICINE AND ENVIRONMENTAL HEALTH PLANNER

- What are the types of hazardous materials?
  - General use chemicals (eg, household items, commercial items)
  - Industrial chemicals (ie, large quantity substances that are used as reactants or are by-products of manufacturing processes)
  - Agricultural chemicals (eg, insecticides, herbicides, fungicides)
  - Other pesticides (eg, rodenticides, molluscacides)
  - Other, special chemicals (eg, munitions, propellants, explosives)
- Who uses the hazardous materials?
- Why are they using the hazardous materials?
- Where are the hazardous materials?
- When are the hazardous materials used?
- How are the hazardous materials used?
- Are there hazardous materials management controls (eg, laws and regulations)?
- Are hazardous materials management controls enforced?
- What is the recent history of hazardous materials incidents (eg, accidents, spills, air releases)?
- What are the known areas of air, water, and soil contamination?
- What is the recent history of occupational exposures?
- What is the recent history of terrorists events?
- Is there an unusually high use of particular chemicals other than in industry?
- What are the theater, in-country, and regional capabilities to analyze chemical substances?

---

semi-solid, or contained gaseous material resulting from industrial, commercial, mining, and agricultural operations and from community activities."[2(p665)] In the United States, each person generates approximately 4 to 6 lbs of waste per day and more than 90% of it is paper, glass, metal, plastics, food, and yard waste.[2,5]

Proper solid waste management is important from a public health perspective. Improper disposal can result in groundwater being contaminated by chemical or radioactive substances or by pathogenic microorganisms. Uncontrolled wastes also attract insects, rodents, and other vermin that may become vectors for disease organisms. Improperly managed wastes also can be a nuisance by being aesthetically unpleasant, emitting foul odors, and attracting other types of animals. In addition to public health criteria, there are a variety of other

factors not related to health that are considered in the design of recycling programs and solid waste collections and disposal systems. These include waste composition and volume, economics, collection frequency (also a public health factor), collection point (eg, curb versus alley), work rate of the collection crew, efficiency of the refuse truck routing, distance to the sanitary landfill or incinerator, time of year, habits, education, economic status, and commercial or industrial activity.[2] A local study is usually required to design a system to meet local requirements.

The major federal regulation that addresses solid waste management practices is the Resource Conservation and Recovery Act (Public Law 94-580, Subtitle D: Non-hazardous Waste). It provides federal money for approved solid waste plans, established design and permitting requirements for sanitary landfills, requires open dumps to be closed or upgraded to landfills, establishes protective measures for groundwater, and prohibits the open burning of solid waste. The criteria for municipal solid waste landfills are found in the Code of Federal Regulations (40 CFR 258).

The current focus of solid waste decision makers is on development of integrated solid waste management programs. This involves using a combination of approaches to handle targeted portions of the waste stream. The Pollution Prevention Act of 1990 established a hierarchy for integrated solid waste management. Source reduction is followed by recycling and reuse, which is followed by disposal. This management sequence is geared toward the goal of reducing the amount of waste that ultimately is disposed.

Source reduction may involve changing a process to result in less material used or the generation of less waste material or both. It may also involve using a different type of product that inherently produces less waste material, has less disposable packaging, or has a longer useful life. Lastly, efficient procurement to avoid over-ordering or ordering items that may not be used is a form of source reduction.

The reuse, recycling, and composting of materials also serve to reduce the waste stream and are the next options in the hierarchy. Basic reuse of materials is self-explanatory. Reuse can also involve procuring reusable rather than disposable products. Recycling involves the separation and collection of postconsumer materials. The materials are then reprocessed or remanufactured into usable products. The loop is closed when the recycled products are used. Composting is the controlled decay of organic matter in a warm, moist environment by aerobic microbial activity. The two major types of composting are of yard waste and municipal solid waste. The resulting humus or compost product can then be used, thus closing the circle.

The last solid waste management technique in the hierarchical succession is disposal. The two disposal methods are incineration (waste combustion) and landfilling. Incineration is a controlled combustion process for burning wastes to gases and ash. For combustion to occur, there must be adequate time to eliminate moisture, proper temperature at the ignition point, and sufficient turbulence to mix resultant gases with oxygen.[2] When compared to the landfill option, incineration offers several advantages. These include a minimal land requirement, a short hauling distance, no weather limitation, and the possibility that wastes may serve as an energy source. Disadvantages include initial high equipment costs and incinerator-generated air pollution.

Most solid waste, approximately 90% as of 1990, is disposed of in sanitary landfills.[50] Sanitary landfills are engineered and controlled methods of solid waste disposal that are distinctly different from open dumps. Open dumps typically are holes dug in the ground where people deposit waste with few or no controls. An open dump can also be trash heaped on top of the ground. RCRA now prohibits the use of open dumps and requires that existing ones be closed or converted to sanitary landfills. In contrast, sanitary landfills are designed precisely to prevent the public health and nuisance problems presented earlier in this section. They usually consist of a series of cells or trenches that are lined with low-permeability clay or a synthetic material to prevent leachate (ie, precipitation that percolates through the landfill) from reaching the groundwater. Other typical design features may include a leachate collection system of pipes that diverts leachate flow away from and further protects groundwater; a leachate treatment system; a system to collect or vent gas (eg, methane and hydrogen sulfide from anaerobic decomposition; this is the same process illustrated in Figure 20-6); and a system of wells (called groundwater monitoring wells) to monitor groundwater and determine the leachate's migration pattern and whether it reaches the groundwater.[2] Daily solid waste deposits are compacted by a bulldozer or similar type of equipment and are covered daily with earth or an artificial cover to discourage vermin and other animals from digging into the landfill. When a cell is full, it is covered with a multilayer cap that may consist of synthetic material or low-permeability clay overlain by a final cap of topsoil and vegetation. Usually only one cell at a time actively receives waste.

Operational and health monitoring are important components of a solid-waste management program. Health monitoring is a responsibility of public health professionals. During the sanitary survey, the health professional should assess storage, collection, and disposal procedures to determine if they are conducted in a sanitary manner. Operational records, methane gas production and migration, and well-monitoring data should be reviewed. There should be a visual inspection of waste sources and wastes that are delivered to the landfill to ensure that the waste is acceptable and suitable for disposal by this method. During the survey, the health professional should determine if there are any specially designated wastes (eg, asbestos, sludge) and that they are handled as required by permit. Sampling and analysis of the monitoring wells around a landfill detects contamination if it

Biochemical Reactions during Treatment

Secondary Treatment

$$\text{Organic Compounds} \xrightarrow[\text{O}_2, \text{P, N}]{\text{Microorganisms}} CO_2 + H_2O + \text{Microbes}$$

Example:

$$\text{Dextrose (C}_6\text{H}_{12}\text{O}_6) \xrightarrow[\text{O}_2, \text{NH}_3, \text{P}]{\text{Microorganisms}} CO_2 + 4H_2O + \underset{\text{(Microbes)}}{C_5H_7NO_2}$$

Nitrification

$$NH_3 \xrightarrow{\text{Nitrifiers}} NO_3 + \text{Nitrifiers}$$

[Conditions: O_2, pH, alkalinity, low BOD, temperature, others]

Biochemical Reactions during Anaerobic Treatment

Nonmethanogenic

$$\text{Organic Compounds} \xrightarrow{\text{Microorganisms}} CH_4 + CO_2 + H_2S + \text{Microbes}$$

Biochemical Reactions during Anoxic Conditions for Denitrification

$$NO_3 + \text{Organic C} \xrightarrow{\text{Denitrifiers}} N_2(g) + \text{Microorganisms}$$

[Conditions: anoxic, P, others]

Fig. 20-6. This simple view of the biochemical reactions that are involved in aerobic and anaerobic wastewater treatment shows that the products differ due to the presence or absence of oxygen and nitrogen compounds. Such conditions require specific types of microbes (eg, aerobes, anaerobes, nitrifiers, denitrifiers, methanogenic microbes, nonmethanogenic microbes) to react with the organic matter in wastewater.

occurs. Unless otherwise specified by the regulator, sampling and analysis should be conducted quarterly to monitor the concentrations of the chemical constituents stipulated by the permit or applicable regulation. Incinerator ash also should be analyzed to determine what is deposited into a landfill. Sampling and analysis should be conducted at least annually (or more frequently if required by the operating permit) by a certified laboratory. The health professional should assess the sanitary survey and monitoring results to determine if the solid waste management process is effective and protective of public health.

Operational monitoring of solid waste management is similar to health monitoring, but it tends to be done more often and not in as much detail. It is done by the operations personnel. They should make frequent observations of storage, collection, disposal, recycling, and composting operations and seek ways to reduce the amount of solid waste generated. Adjustments in operations or equipment should be made as necessary to maximize efficiency and safety and protect human health. Routine monitoring should include sampling and analysis of monitoring wells around the landfill and periodic inspection of refuse truck loads for the presence of recyclable items, special wastes not accepted in landfills, and hazardous wastes. Ultimately the operations personnel decide if they will accept certain wastes and handle them in a special manner based on state and federal regulations and permit requirements. Resolution of solid waste management problems, particularly those involving a regulatory violation, should be coordinated with supervisors and regulatory officials as appropriate.

Hazardous Waste

Hazardous waste is a type of solid waste that requires special handling and disposal. Waste is considered to be hazardous when it can cause or significantly contribute to an increase in adverse health outcomes or environmental effects.[2] Hazardous waste may exist as a solid, liquid, or gas and can include chemical, biological, and radioactive materials. Explosive and flammable materials also can be hazardous wastes. Factors that contribute to the hazardous condition of waste include its quantity, its concentration, and its physical, chemical, or infectious nature. Handling methods, use, storage, and disposal also may contribute to the hazard potential.

There are several federal environmental laws that address hazardous materials management. One of the major ones is the RCRA and its amendment the Hazardous and Solid Waste Act. The RCRA defines hazardous waste as "any material that may pose a substantial threat or potential danger to human health or the environment when improperly handled."[5(p667)] It identifies three classes of hazardous waste: listed, characteristic, and generator identified.[5,51] Listed wastes are found in Title 40 in the *Code of Federal Regulations*, Part 261.31–33. Characteristic wastes are those, not otherwise listed, that are toxic, ignitable, corrosive, or reactive. The generator may simply declare a waste to be hazardous and thus avoid the expense of having a laboratory analyze the waste. However, once declared as hazardous, such waste must be managed in accordance with the RCRA. The RCRA does not address several hazardous or potentially hazardous wastes, to include domestic sewage, industrial discharges (subject to the Federal Water Pollution Control Act), nuclear materials (subject to the Atomic Energy Act), toxic and hazardous household waste (usually not regulated), mining wastes, certain agricultural wastes (excluding pesticides), and medical and infectious waste.[2,5] Most states regulate medical and infectious waste and may have specific local requirements for any hazardous waste. Businesses and activities that generate less than 220 lbs of hazardous waste monthly are not required to comply with RCRA; however, as a good management practice, they may elect to follow the hazardous waste management principles to promote environmental stewardship and reflect concern for public and environmental health.

There are various disposal options for hazardous wastes that range from completely eliminating the need (eg, pollution prevention) to altering the wastes, and perhaps eliminating or reducing their hazards, through chemical, physical, and biological processes. Griffin[52] identifies the principles of hazardous waste treatment and disposal as being detoxification, volume reduction, and isolation from the environment. He specifies treatment and disposal types as being physical, chemical, biological, thermal, and fixation and encapsulation. Other examples of these processes, expanded to include pollution prevention options, in descending order of pubic health desirability, are process modification to eliminate the hazardous waste; waste reduction at the point of generation; recovery, segregation, recycling, reuse, and exchange; treatment by methods such as incineration, detoxification, biological breakdown, immobilization, and physical destruction; "secure" land burial (secure chemical landfill); deep well disposal (injection); and aboveground storage until an acceptable solution can he found. See Salvato[2] and Nadakavukaren[5] for more detailed discussion about these and other disposal options for hazardous waste. In comparison to the sanitary landfill discussed in the solid waste section, a hazardous waste landfill is required to have a double liner, a leak-detection system, a leachate collection system, an impervious cap, and groundwater monitoring wells.[5]

Both operational and health monitoring of hazardous waste management practices are very similar to that described earlier for solid waste. There are additional regulatory requirements for hazardous wastes due to the manifesting, tracking, and documentation requirements of the RCRA.

Medical and Infectious Waste

Solid waste that comes from medical or research facilities includes medical waste, infectious waste, biomedical waste, regulated medical waste, and hospital waste. During the mid- to late-1980s, medical waste was found washed up on beaches and in regular solid waste containers.[2] There was public concern that such waste could transmit disease to people. The ensuing regulations focused on controlling infectious agents, regardless of the term used to describe this waste. This discussion will use the "phrase medical and infectious waste."

Medical waste is defined in the RCRA even though there is not a federal regulation that requires management of medical and infectious waste. Most states, however, have established their own regulations. The RCRA definition for medical waste is "any solid waste that is generated in the diagnosis, treatment, or immunization of human beings or animals, in research pertaining thereto, or in the production or testing of biologicals."[2(p685)] The regulated categories are cultures and stocks of infectious agents and associated biologicals, human blood and blood products, pathological waste, isolation waste, used and contaminated sharps, and contaminated animal carcasses.[2,6] Specific examples are listed in Exhibit 20-6.

The goals of medical and infectious waste management are to control disease, optimize safety, and address public concerns. To accomplish these goals, a medical and infectious waste management program should have the following components: designation and identification, segregation at point of origin, packaging and labeling, storage, transport, treatment, and disposal.[6] Categories and specific items of medical and infectious waste should be identified and written in organizational operating procedures.

Medical and infectious waste should be segregated from other waste streams to allow special packaging and identification that will alert and enhance the safety of people who collect, transport, and dispose of the waste. Also, segregation directs the medical and infectious waste into a waste stream that requires distinctly different handling and disposal procedures from that of other wastes.

Packaging should be impervious to leakage and punctures, and appropriate for the waste type. For example, solid and semisolid items can be put in plastic bags, liquids in capped or stoppered bottles, and sharps in puncture-resistant containers. The universal biohazard sign (see Figure 20-7) or other

---

EXHIBIT 20-6

SPECIFIC EXAMPLES OF MEDICAL WASTE

- Specimens from medical and pathological laboratories

- Wastes from the production of biologicals

- Discarded live and attenuated vaccines

- Waste blood, serum, plasma, and blood products

- Pathological tissues, organs, body parts, blood and body fluids removed during surgery, autopsy, or biopsy

- Used and contaminated needles, syringes, surgical blades, pipettes, and pointed and broken glass

- Contaminated animal body parts and bedding if it was exposed to pathogens

- Soiled dressings, sponges, drapes, lavage tubes, drainage sets, underpads, and gloves from surgery and autopsy

- Miscellaneous laboratory waste, such as specimen containers, slides and coverslips, disposable gloves, lab coats, and aprons

- Waste from dialysis procedures

- Contaminated equipment

Source: Koren H, Bisesi M. *Handbook of Environmental Health and Safety, Principles and Practices.* Vol II. 3rd ed. Boca Raton, Fla: Lewis Publishers; 1996: 1–76, 187–192.

---

accepted clear marking identifying the contents as medical and infectious waste must be on the container. Typically, packages of medical and infectious waste are color-coded (eg, red or bright orange).

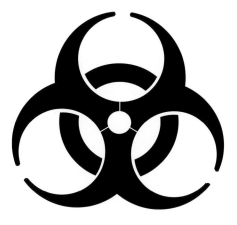

Fig. 20-7. The universal biohazard sign should be placed on any container, room, or vehicle that contains medical and infectious waste.

Storage time should be as short as possible. Medical and infectious waste storage areas should have limited access, should have the universal biohazard sign posted at entry points, and should not be used simultaneously for other purposes.

Carts used to move medical and infectious waste within the facility should be cleaned and disinfected frequently. When the waste is transported from the facility, it first must be put in rigid or semirigid containers and then transported in closed, leakproof dumpsters or trucks. Trucks that are transporting medical and infectious waste should not carry anything else simultaneously and should be cleaned and disinfected before being used for other purposes.

Medical and infectious waste treatment is any method, technique, or process designed to change the biological character or composition of the waste. The treatment process can either render the waste noninfectious or render it unrecognizable. Treatment processes vary with the type of waste. Some examples include incineration, autoclave or steam sterilization, gas-vapor sterilization, thermal inactivation, chemical disinfection, irradiation, and discharge to sanitary sewer. Rendering medical and infectious waste unrecognizable, as by grinding, reduces the potential anxiety, fear, and misperception of a public health threat people may have if they encounter the treated waste. After treatment, medical and infectious waste can be disposed of in the same manner as regular, noninfectious solid waste.

Military Considerations of Waste Management

The preceding discussion about the various forms of waste management presented management principles and controls from the perspective of the United States. This level of detail was presented to demonstrate the complexity, both technological and regulatory, involved in managing waste in a manner that will protect public health. It also gives the reader a context for the following discussions concerning expectations in less-developed and underdeveloped countries and in the field that the military may experience in a theater of operations.

In less-developed and underdeveloped countries, there are a variety of conditions that may affect the process of waste disposal. Information about these conditions should be acquired as part of the medical intelligence gathering process. They should then be considered during the preventive medicine and environmental health planning process. Less-developed and underdeveloped countries will probably differ from the United States in aspects of culture, government, economics, and infrastructure. These factors have a direct effect on waste management practices. For example, the host country's government may choose to enact or enforce laws that govern waste management or it may not. Poor countries may have economic priorities (eg, feeding, clothing, and housing their people) that do not allow sufficient or any funding for waste disposal programs or construction and maintenance of a waste disposal infrastructure (eg, sanitary landfills, incinerators). Other situations that could affect waste management in such countries include overpopulation, relatively little living space, no or poor urban planning, poverty, a small tax base, and a fragile infrastructure.

Given these types of conditions, the environmental health planner might expect the following situations:

- minimal to no waste stream segregation,
- minimal to no disposal infrastructure and technology,
- individual and neighborhood disposal sites, with the most probable disposal method for

all wastes being dumping (above and below ground) and open burning,
- minimal to no vermin control at storage and disposal sights, and
- scavenging through waste sites to find items that poverty-stricken people can sell or use.

When US military units deploy to such areas, they face the risk of increased exposure to hazardous and infectious waste materials and waste-contaminated water sources.

When US military forces deploy into a foreign country to conduct military or humanitarian operations, waste management is an important logistical consideration. The public health concerns associated with solid waste, hazardous waste, and medical and infectious waste can affect the health of deployed forces and adversely affect the military mission. Both logistical and preventive medicine planning should address waste management to prevent potential adverse health conditions. Host-nation requirements, Status of Forces Agreements, Final Governing Standards Related to the Department of Defense Overseas Environmental Baseline Guidance Document, and other agreements should be considered, especially concerning hazardous and medical and infectious waste disposal.

Waste handling procedures in a theater of operation depend on the tactical or operational scenario and the local resources available in the host nation. Using the local infrastructure and contracting waste services with local nationals may be the best and easiest way to manage waste. Such services may include solid waste and special waste (eg, hazardous, medical, and infectious) collection and disposal. However, if there is not a supporting infrastructure or contracting possibilities, if units are not located near such support, or if other tactical considerations prohibit such arrangements, then field disposal methods must be employed. Generally, the options are burial, incineration, or a combination of these two methods. Examples of these methods are presented in the section on field sanitation later in this chapter.

Food Safety and Sanitation

The multifaceted process that brings food from its producer to its consumer requires foods to be handled several times before they reach their final destination and thus provides multiple opportunities for contamination. This section discusses the agents and sources of foodborne disease and contamination and the controls that exist to prevent foodborne disease outbreaks.

Sources of Foodborne Disease and Contamination

There are several types of contaminants that can adulterate foods. These include biological (eg, microorganisms, parasites, seafood toxins, insects, rodents), chemical (eg, pesticides, cleaning agents), and physical (eg, broken glass, metal shavings) hazards. Improper storage, transportation, handling, preparation, and serving practices can provide the opportunity for contamination. Other examples of opportunities for contamination include spills and leaks (eg, sanitizers stored above bags of flour) and inappropriate handling and storage practices (eg, spraying pesticides in the air during food preparation and service).

Some foods may have spoiled or have pathogenic microorganisms on them when they arrive in a food establishment. For example, beef can contain *Clostridium perfringens* and fowl may have *Salmonella*. Allowing uncooked meat to come into contact with ready-to-eat cooked foods or foods that are not cooked before serving (eg, vegetables, fruits) is a means of cross-contamination. Allowing cooked or ready-to-eat foods to contact unsanitized surfaces that previously were in contact with raw meat is another example of cross-contamination.

In addition to physical contact, other factors are required for chemical and biological contaminants to cause illness. A toxic quantity of chemical substances must be consumed. In some cases, as with heavy metals leached from containers, this may be a cumulative phenomenon. Microbes must be present in sufficient quantities to produce disease, which is a function of the ability of the food to support growth (eg, its pH, water content, and nutrients), the temperature, and the contact time. Other factors that favor microbial growth include time and temperature abuse, improper cooking, acquisition from a nonapproved source, additives, and moisture.

Biological Hazards

The types of microorganisms that can cause foodborne illness are bacteria, viruses, and fungi. Detailed discussions concerning various microbial diseases spread by food are presented in Chapter 32, Outbreak Investigation. Given the proper environment (eg, moisture, nutrients, adequate temperature, oxygen for aerobes, lack of oxygen for anaerobes), microorganisms multiply at an exponential rate and can reach disease-producing concentrations in relatively short periods of time. For example, a typical bacterial growth curve, as seen in Figure 20-8, has four phases. Sanitation and other

public health measures seek to prevent contamination or, if contamination occurs, reduce or eliminate microbial growth. Temperature and time control is one important way of limiting the log phase or extending the lag phase of the bacterial growth curve. The food service sanitation industry tries to keep hot foods hot (> 60°C, 140°F) and cold foods cold (≤ 5°C, 41°F). The so-called "danger zone" is between 5°C (41°F) and 60°C for a cumulative time of 3 to 4 hours. However, variances to this temperature range can be found in the latest edition of the *Model Food Code*, published biannually by the US Food and Drug Administration.

Bacterial pathogens can be classified, based on their mechanism of producing illness. Infective bacteria are vegetative cells that cause disease after ingestion (eg, *Salmonella*, *Escherichia coli*). Toxin-pro-

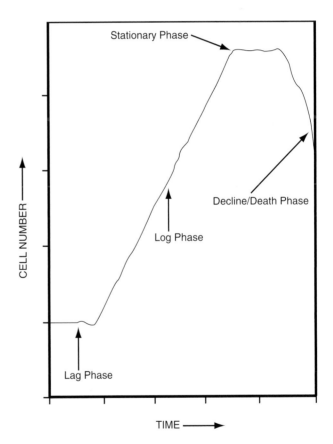

Fig. 20-8. Bacterial Growth Curve. When bacteria are introduced to a new environment, they go through several growth phases. As they adapt to the environment, there is little or no increase in population size (lag phase). Once adapted, the organisms reproduce at a logarithmic rate (log phase) until there is an equilibrium between the population size and available nutrients (stationary phase). When nutrients are depleted and can no longer support the organisms, the population dies (death phase).

ducing bacteria produce a toxin that causes disease when ingested (eg, *Staphylococcus*). Spore-forming bacteria (eg, *Clostridium botulinum, Bacillus cereus*) develop into a thick-walled, resistant spore when environmental conditions are harsh, such as when temperatures are extreme or there are insufficient nutrients, and become viable when favorable growth conditions resume. Thus, if foods come into contact with bacteria, measures taken to prevent foodborne illness must do more than kill vegetative cells. They must also be able to inactivate spores and denature toxins. Some bacterial toxins are heat labile, but others are heat stable and thus require higher temperatures and pressures for longer contact times to denature.

Hepatitis A and Norwalk viruses are examples of viruses that can cause foodborne illness. Both are associated with water and foods contaminated with human feces. Fungi such as *Aspergillus flavus* and *A parasilicas* produce an aflatoxin that is a hepatocarcinogen and may contaminate grains and nuts. Mushrooms (eg, *Amanita*, containing the neurotoxin ibotenic acid) also are fungi that can be deadly if ingested.[53]

Some pathogens that can contaminate foods are parasitic and include organisms that range in size from microscopic protozoa to macroscopic nematodes and tapeworms. *Toxoplasma gondii* is a protozoan disease agent found in cat feces and can contaminate a variety of raw meats. *Giardia lamblia* is another protozoan that frequently contaminates water, but it can also contaminate food. Nematodes (eg, *Trichinella)* and cestodes (tapeworms such as *Taenia*) can be found in beef and pork, and worms of the *Anasakis* genus are sometimes found in marine fish used for sushi.

Certain types of seafoods may be contaminated with toxins that can cause illness or death.[54] Certain large fish (eg, red snapper, grouper) and shellfish may bioaccumulate several toxins from dinoflagellates, the benthic algae that are food sources for some marine animals. The toxins are neurotoxic, may affect the gastrointestinal tract, and can produce cardiovascular effects. These include ciguatoxin. Scombroid poisoning is associated with mackerel, tuna, bonito, and skipjack and rarely is fatal. The musculature of improperly preserved or refrigerated fish degrades and releases histamine and another toxic factor, saurine, that causes nausea, vomiting, diarrhea, epigastric distress, and other food poisoning symptoms.

Insects can cause foodborne illness by mechanical transmission or as stored product pests. The common housefly (*Musca domestica*) and several cockroaches are examples of insects that can transmit disease-causing organisms by mechanical

means. Some insects may infest foods stored in warehouses and kitchens. These pests eat and contaminate stored food so that it cannot be consumed by people.[7] Examples of these type of insects include the confused flour beetle, saw-tooth grain beetle, flour grain beetle, and cabinet beetle. Some leave body parts that when swallowed may choke or irritate people, and others excrete harmful substances.

Rats, mice, and other rodents can transmit foodborne diseases by mechanical transmission and directly through their own urine and feces. They can carry microbes and introduce contaminants such as hair and larvae casings. Three types of rodents typically infest food facilities in the United States: the roof rat (*Rattus rattus*), the Norway rat (*Rattus norveticus*), and the house mouse (*Mus musculus*).

Chemical Hazards

Chemical food contamination can cause adverse health effects that range from discomfort through incapacitation to death. The types of possible health effects are as numerous as the variety of chemicals that exist. Effects may be acute, chronic, or cumulative and typically are dose dependent. Chemicals in foods that may cause adverse effects are both endogenous and exogenous. Endogenous chemicals are those that occur naturally in foods (eg, vitamins, minerals, enzymes, micronutrients including heavy metals). Some of these, if ingested in sufficient quantities, can be toxic. Exogenous chemicals are those that are applied to foods either intentionally or accidentally. Intentional exogenous chemicals include additives (eg, colorants, antioxidants, flavor enhancers, preservatives) and pesticide. Even though these chemicals can be toxic, they are not the focus of this section. Further information on these types of chemical hazards can be found elsewhere.[55]

This section focuses on exogenous chemicals that become food contaminants because of an accident (eg, a spill) or neglect (eg, improper storage practices or mislabeled containers). Typical chemicals that may be found in food operations depend on the location and operation. For example, warehouses and distribution points may have fuels and oils to run forklifts; they may also have household chemicals, such as detergents and pesticides, collocated with foods. Vehicles may transport food items along with household chemicals when they transfer items to markets or restaurants. Food preparation and service facilities usually have cleaning chemicals (eg, detergents, sanitizers) and pesticides (eg, insecticides, rodenticides) on hand.

Some types of food storage and service containers may cause chemical contamination. High-acid foods (eg, citrus fruits, sauerkraut, fruit punches) may cause certain metals to leach out of the container and contaminate the food. This can occur with copper, brass, and galvanized containers; enamelware can leach antimony and cadmium and glazed pottery can leach lead.[7]

Physical Hazards

Foods can be contaminated by physical agents during processing, storage, transportation, preparation, and service. The types of agents that are considered here are items that accidentally may be mixed with foods. Examples may include broken glass, metal or wood shavings, dirt, and other debris.

Food Service Risks

In the retail industry, specific events have been reported to cause foodborne disease outbreaks more frequently than others. These include improper cooling of foods; lapse of a day or more between preparing and serving; infected persons handled non–heat-treated foods; inadequate time-temperature exposure during processing; temperature not kept high enough during hot storage; inadequate time-temperature exposure during reheating; and ingestion of contaminated raw ingredients or foods.[56]

Standards

There are several US federal government agencies that participate in food safety activities.

- The US Food and Drug Administration (FDA) is responsible for the safety, sanitation, nutrition, wholesomeness, and labeling of domestic and imported foods except meat, poultry, and some egg products. It is responsible for the Federal Food, Drug, and Cosmetic Act, which regulates food production, manufacturing, composition, quality, container amounts, and additives.
- The US Department of Agriculture (USDA) is responsible for the safety and quality of meat, poultry, eggs, egg products, and grain products. It promulgates and enforces the Federal Meat Inspection Act, Poultry Products Inspection Act, Egg Products Inspection Act, and the US Grains Standard Act.
- The USEPA regulates the manufacture, labeling, and use of all pesticides sold or dis-

tributed in the United States through a registration program authorized by the Federal Insecticide, Fungicide, and Rodenticide Act. It also establishes the maximum permissible levels of pesticide residue that may remain in or on food and animal feed and evaluates health and environmental information related to pesticide use.
- The National Marine Fisheries Service (National Oceanic and Atmospheric Administration, US Department of Commerce) conducts the National Seafood Inspection Program, a voluntary program to inspect vessels, processing plants, and retail facilities for sanitation and evaluate the quality of seafood products. This program served as the model for FDA legislation on seafood quality and safety.

States and local governments also enact regional food safety laws and regulations. Most states and local communities develop their food service sanitation regulations based on the FDA Model Food Code. The Food Code provisions include detailed time, temperature, and humidity charts for the cooking of meat; recommendations to ensure food service workers' health (eg, restricting infected employees) and hygiene practices (eg, cleaning, sanitizing, and maintaining utensils, equipment, and facilities); time limits for holding cooked foods safely outside of controlled temperatures; and provisions for shellfish safety.

Controls

The public health goal is to deliver foods to the consumer that are free from biological, chemical, and physical adulterants and thereby prevent the occurrence of foodborne illness. This goal is accomplished by applying both engineering and administrative controls throughout the production and distribution process. Generally, food safety regulations will specify the types of controls that must be implemented and followed.

Engineering controls in food safety practice include the design and construction of equipment that is used to process, store, transport, prepare, dispense, and serve foods. For example, the National Sanitation Foundation and the Underwriters[3] Laboratory publish criteria for the sanitary design of food-related equipment and will test equipment to determine if it meets the established criteria. Items that have been tested and certified by these organizations will bear their label. Food service sanitation regulations may require that equipment be approved by either of these organizations or meet similar design guidelines that are approved by local health authorities.

Time-temperature controls, employee health status checks, and food handling practices are considered administrative controls for food sanitation and safety.

Monitoring

Daily operational monitoring should be conducted by food service managers and workers. Managers should perform frequent inspections of workers to ensure that they are healthy (eg, no cold or influenza symptoms, no open sores) and perform their duties in a sanitary manner (eg, no direct hand contact with cooked food, washes hands after using the bathroom or handling raw meats), that raw products are not diseased or contaminated, that equipment operates properly and is sanitized frequently, that proper serving and storage temperatures are maintained, and that storage practices segregate potential contaminates, such as chemicals, from foods.

Health monitoring is performed by a health professional, traditionally a sanitarian or veterinarian. In the US military, Army veterinarians are responsible for approving and monitoring all food procurement sources and activities for all of the military services (see Chapter 30, The Role of Veterinary Public Health and Preventive Medicine During Mobilization and Deployment). Sanitarians (and the military equivalents) are the professionals that monitor the public health aspects of facilities that serve food. Public health monitoring is performed less frequently than operational monitoring.

Health monitoring frequency sometimes is established based on hazard potential factors such as operation size, food types, past inspection performance, and disease outbreak history. The Hazard Analysis Critical Control Point (HACCP) process can be a tool for determining appropriate monitoring frequency.[57] It involves identifying and monitoring the critical and more-hazardous points in food preparation by analyzing each food process; identifying the critical control points (CCP) of each process; establishing critical limits that should not be exceeded as preventive measures of each CCP; monitoring CCPs; correcting deficiencies; and maintaining records to document the system.

An extensive discussion of the numerous areas that are evaluated during a food service sanitation inspection is not possible within this chapter, but Exhibit 20-7 shows some areas that are reviewed during a typical inspection. Additional detail concerning these and other inspection areas, other aspects of food safety and sanitation, and foodborne illnesses can be found elsewhere.[2–5,58]

Field Food Sanitation

Sanitary food practices during military field and combat operations can be vital to the success of a unit's mission. Some foodborne illnesses can completely incapacitate service members or substantially decrease their overall ability to perform. Either is undesirable in a tactical situation. All of the principles and most of the practices applied to installation and civilian food service operations are applicable to field food service operations. The goal is the same in field, installation, or civilian food operations: to prevent foodborne illness.

Food must be protected from adulterants (biological, chemical, and physical) during transportation, storage, preparation, and service. Time-temperature control also remains important. In a theater of operations, health monitoring of these processes is performed by Army veterinarians and preventive medicine personnel. Army veterinarians are responsible for approving and monitoring food procurement sources. They also monitor storage and processing facilities, such as warehouses and food ration points. Environmental health and preventive medicine personnel monitor unit-level food service operations.

Dining facility managers should perform daily operational monitoring in the same manner as described earlier. Unit field sanitation personnel also should provide daily monitoring and frequently advise the commander on the sanitary conditions of the local food service operation.

Generally, the same areas of interest shown in Exhibit 20-7 are applicable to field food service operations; however, there are a few requirements that are applicable specifically to the field situation. These are discussed in an Army technical bulletin[58] and include prohibition of the use of potentially hazardous foods as leftovers; use of Meals-Ready-to-Eat when there is no or inadequate refrigeration; guidance on sanitizing local produce and fruits grown with human excrement fertilizer; and use of field-expedient methods for handwashing, waste disposal, and cleaning and sanitizing utensils and food preparation equipment. An Army field manual[59] has diagrams of these devices.

Ambient Air Quality and Pollution

Air contaminated with harmful substances has a direct entrance to the body. Vapors and gases can diffuse across the alveolar membranes, through capillary cells, and quickly enter the bloodstream to be carried to various regions of the body. Irritant vapors and gases also can react directly with and damage lung tissue. Particulates can lodge in lung tissue and elicit local responses such as fibrosis. The harmful effects that chemicals may exert when inhaled makes air quality a major public health concern and a concern for the military when deploying to a theater of operations.

Selected Health Concerns

Air pollutants can cause significant adverse health effects resulting in acute or chronic illness and death. This discussion presents selected air contaminants that may be of concern during military operations, as reviewed by Costa and Amdur,[60] to exemplify the range of physiological and toxic events that can occur.

EXHIBIT 20-7

FOOD SERVICE SANITATION INSPECTION AREAS

Food Protection

Sanitary quality	Product protection	Food storage
Food preparation	Leftovers	Transportation
Personal medications		First-aid supplies

Food Service Personnel

Employee health	Medical examinations	Personal cleanliness
Employee practices	Training	

Equipment and Utensils

Materials	Sealing compounds	Design and fabrication
Installation	Cleaning and sanitizing	Handling
Location	Maintenance and replacement	Storage

Sanitary Facilities and Controls

Water supply	Steam	Sewage
Plumbing	Toilet facilities	Linens
Garbage, refuse	Handwashing facilities	Pest management

Construction and Maintenance of Food Service Facilities

Floors	Ceilings	Lighting
Ventilation	Premises	Utility lines
Cleaning facilities	Cleaning equipment	Dressing rooms
Lockers	Walls	Service lines

Mobile Food Units

Beverages	Ice	Water system
Waste retention	Retention tank flushing	Storage units
Training	Operations	Construction
Potable water	Servicing facility	Servicing operations
Single-service articles	Special requirements	

Temporary Food Service

Equipment	Single-service articles	Water
Sewage	Handwashing	Floors
Walls	Food preparation areas	Ceilings

Vending Machine Operations

Food supplies	Equipment location	Special requirements

Administrative Procedures of the Food Service Sanitation Program

Inspection reports	Sanitizer effectiveness	Disease outbreaks

Adapted from: US Department of the Army. *Food Service Sanitation*. Washington, DC: DA; 1991. TB MED 530.

Sulfur Dioxide. Sulfur dioxide is a criteria pollutant under provisions of the Clear Air Act that is associated with emissions from fossil fuel combustion and industrial facilities such as coal-burning power plants, metal smelters, boilers, and oil refineries.[5] It can affect the body or the environment directly as sulfur dioxide or as sulfuric acid.[60] Sulfur dioxide is water soluble and thus can irritate the upper airway, cause bronchoconstriction by inhibiting the cervical vagosympathetic nerve, increase mucus secretion by goblet cell proliferation, and increase air flow. The increased airflow also increases the dose received and allows sulfur dioxide and other contaminants to penetrate to the deep lung. When sulfur dioxide is oxidized by photochemical processes or catalyzed by metals, it can form sulfuric acid, a respiratory irritant, and can affect pulmonary function.[60] Metal smelting or fossil fuel combustion can produce small metal oxide particles that may adsorb the acid and transport it long distances. Sulfuric acid may cause respiratory irritation due to its acidity and increase flow resistance because of bronchoconstriction. Its toxicity is associated with both concentration and particle size because smaller particles penetrate deeper into the lung. Acute effects from sulfuric acid exposure include biphasic alterations in mucociliary clearance (ie, concentrations less than $250 \ \mu g/m^3$ increase clearance but greater than $1,000 \ \mu g/m^3$ decrease clearance) and impaired macrophage function at $500 \ \mu g/m^3$. Daily exposure to sulfuric acid at concentrations of $100 \ \mu g/m^3$ or greater may impair clearance (also a biphasic response) and cause chronic bronchitis.

Particulate Matter. Particulate matter is a mixture of organic and inorganic materials that vary in composition and toxicity.[60] It may be composed of metals, gases, and other substances. Even though practically all metals can be found in particulate matter, the most common ones are those associated with fossil fuel combustion (eg, transition and heavy metals) and those common to the earth's crust (eg, iron, sodium, magnesium). Gases and vapors may interact with particulate matter to enhance delivery to the lungs and cause adverse health effects. For example, sulfuric acid adsorbed to metal particles with a mean aerodynamic diameter of 0.1 μm distribute the acid wider and deeper in the lung, causing irritation greater than that expected from the acid alone. When sulfur dioxide absorbs into sodium chloride droplets in the presence of a transition metal, it can oxidize to sulfate to form sulfuric acid, which can cause pulmonary irritation.

Particle size is related to where and how deep particulate matter can deposit in the respiratory system. Generally, particulate matter with a mean aerodynamic diameter of less than 10 μm is considered sufficiently small to deposit at lung levels that adversely affect health. Chemicals that are water soluble can have enhanced toxicity because of increased bioavailability and pulmonary residence time. Diesel exhaust in urban areas has been shown to contain a significant amount of particulate matter and is an example of a chronic health concern because it is considered to be a potential human carcinogen.[60]

Ozone. Ozone is a photochemical air pollutant that can irritate the lungs and can cause death by pulmonary edema.[60] Its effects are cumulative and depend on concentration and time. A substantial portion of inhaled ozone penetrates into the deep lung due to its poor water solubility. Its greatest deposition occurs in the acinar region from the terminal bronchioles to the alveolar ducts (the proximal alveolar ductal region). Exercise increases the dose received because of the increased lung tidal volume and air flow rate. Some of the effects caused by exposure to ozone include epithelial cell injury along the entire respiratory tract, inflammation, and altered permeability of the blood-air barrier; these are reversible. Pulmonary function effects include concentration-related decrements in forced exhaled volumes and increased nonspecific airway reactivity. In animals such as rats, mice, and hamsters, exposure to ozone before challenges with aerosols of infectious agents (eg, *Streptococcus, Klebsiella pneumoniae*) produced a higher incidence of infection than in control animals. Studies of ozone mixed with other air pollutants (eg, nitrogen dioxide and sulfuric acid) suggest that there may be potentiation or additive effects.

Carbon Monoxide. Carbon monoxide concentrations in the atmosphere originate from both natural (eg, forest fires) and humanmade (eg, automotive vehicles) sources.[3] Between 1988 and 1995, carbon monoxide concentrations in the ambient atmosphere ranged between approximately 5 and 7 ppm (parts per million); however, in urban areas they reach levels as high as 70 to 100 ppm due to vehicular traffic.[2,3] Carbon monoxide is a chemical asphyxiant that produces carboxyhemoglobin, which has a 220-times greater affinity for hemoglobin than oxygen. Thus, carboxyhemoglobin prevents systemic transport of oxygenated blood, resulting in characteristic hypoxic signs and symptoms. The brain and heart are most sensitive to hypoxia because of their high oxygen demands. Acute carbon monoxide poisoning may cause subendocardial infarction, cerebral edema, and congestion and hemorrhages in all organs. In addition to exposure from ambient air pollution, heavy cigarette smoking (two packs a day) and occupational exposure to methylene chloride also can produce carboxyhemoglobin.

There are numerous other atmospheric contaminants that can cause adverse health effects in humans. For example, in addition to criteria air pollutants, the Clean Air Act Amendments of 1990 specifically list 189 hazardous air pollutants. A few additional examples are listed in Table 20-9.

Contaminants and Standards

In the United States, the first federal law for air quality was established in 1955 as the Clean Air Legislation and amended in 1960 and 1962. The Air Quality Act of 1967 replaced the 1955-based legislation and subsequently was amended in 1970, 1977, and 1990 as the Clean Air Act. Some collective features the various laws share are control of emissions from both stationary and mobile sources, including vehicles, and the recognition that states have primary responsibility for air quality, monitoring requirements, and application of control technologies. The Clean Air Act obligates the USEPA to develop air quality criteria, standards for sources of

hazardous air pollutants, and regulations for accidental release of extremely hazardous chemicals to protect public health.[2,3,5] The Clean Air Act of 1990 has eleven parts (or titles) that address criteria and control of specific contaminants, research, training enforcement, and other issues.

Salvato[2] identifies several other federal laws that affect air quality, to include the Resource Conservation and Recovery Act; the Comprehensive Environmental Response, Compensation, and Liability Act (CERCLA or Superfund); and the Emergency Planning and Community Right-to-Know Act, also called Superfund Amendment and Reauthorization Act Title III (SARA Title III).

Controls

Air pollution control strategies and treatment options are designed either to control emissions at the source or to dilute them after they are released. Since the emissions contain both gases and particulates, controls and treatments must be designed to address each. Specific examples of control technologies can be found elsewhere.[2,6]

Monitoring

Koren and Bisesi[6] cite three reasons for monitoring air pollution: (1) to provide an early warning

TABLE 20-9

EXAMPLES OF CLEAN AIR ACT CRITERIA POLLUTANTS AND HAZARDOUS AIR POLLUTANTS AND THEIR MAJOR HEALTH EFFECTS

Contaminant	Health Effects
Lead	Retardation and brain damage, especially in children
Nitrogen dioxide	Respiratory illness and lung damage
Asbestos	Asbestosis, cancer
Beryllium	Lung diseases; also affects liver, spleen, kidney, and lymph glands
Mercury	Affects brain, kidneys, and bowels
Vinyl chloride	Lung and liver cancer
Arsenic	Cancer
Benzene	Leukemia
Radionuclides	Cancer
Formaldehyde	Irritates mucous membranes, increased airway resistance
Acrolien	Irritates mucous membranes, increased airway resistance and tidal volume

system for potential health effects, (2) to assess air quality and compare it to standards, and (3) to track trends and specific polluters. Air pollution monitoring consists of both operational monitoring and health monitoring.

Operational monitoring usually is performed by site workers and consists of frequent observation, testing, and assessment of equipment, conditions, and processes to determine if air pollution controls are functioning properly. This may consist of inspecting waste streams or chemicals to ensure that the appropriate types and quantities of substances are being processed, because inappropriate substances may cause or increase air pollution. Also, production and processing equipment and pollution control equipment should be evaluated to determine if they are operating within design specifications. Testing may consist of reviewing the output from continuous monitors or data from grab samples used to determine if air emissions exceed permit and other regulatory requirements. When observations or testing reveal that conditions are not normal, then operational monitors should alert the appropriate health or regulatory agency to allow an assessment of health implications and implementation of corrective measures.

As discussed with other environmental health concerns (eg, drinking water, wastewater) health monitoring for air pollution also includes a sanitary survey, sampling and analysis, and interpretation.

Policy

Generally, policy issues for air quality concerns include economic, political, and technological considerations. Specific examples are the degree of stringency for standards, interstate (eg, acid rain) and international (eg, ozone depleting substances) issues, and control technology. Air quality statutes require establishment of primary standards to protect public health and secondary standards to protect public welfare. Secondary standards relate to "effects on soils, water, crops, vegetation, manmade materials, animals, wildlife, weather, visibility and climate, damage to and deterioration of property, and hazards to transportation, as well as effects on economic values and on personal comfort and well-being."[61(p65640)]

Military Significance

Air quality issues may affect military operations and should be considered by the preventive medicine and environmental health planner. The information in the hazardous material management section and in Exhibit 20-5 is applicable for considering potential air pollution sources. Air pollution's potential to cause acute effects obviously can hinder the ability of military personnel to perform their mission. Potential longer-term and delayed effects also should be considered. For example, the combustion products from the Kuwait oil well fires during the Persian Gulf War could have resulted in acute and chronic adverse health conditions to exposed US and allied military forces and affected tactical capabilities. A health risk assessment of air sampling data showed that ground level concentrations of selected contaminants were negligible and not expected to cause adverse health effects.[62]

Another example of a military-related air quality situation occurred in Ploce, Croatia, in 1996 during Operation Joint Endeavor.[63] A brake-lining facility was located next to the billeting office, motor pool, and administrative spaces of French units involved with port operations and transportation. Also on the site was an Italian compound with military police and medical personnel. There was an unknown odor around the factory, possibly from the matrix material used to contain the asbestos in the brake linings. Commanders were considering moving the units to other locations if there was a demonstrated or potential health hazard. Air sampling for asbestos fibers did not produce any observable fibers, and there were no abnormal cases of lung distress nor increased incidence of respiratory illnesses. A number of service members were questioned about their health, and none expressed any respiratory concerns. The units did not relocate. The importance of air quality in Bosnia-Herzegovina is emphasized further because it is a component of environmental exposure surveillance.[62] When coupled with geographic information system technology, exposure of US force personnel to air contaminants can be monitored as a proactive public health approach to protect US forces from environmentally related disease.

FIELD SANITATION

Introduction and Definition

Environmental health concerns during military operations are different from those of a civilian health department or fixed military installation. The differences can be attributed to the nature of field operations, which tend to be in more environmentally hostile and often more primitive environments.

To reduce and minimize disease and nonbattle injuries, measures of preventive medicine and environmental health are integrated into military operations and doctrine. Also, throughout a theater of operations there are a variety of preventive medicine and environmental health organizations and professionals who provide advice and services to commanders and units (see Exhibit 20-3; Chapter 12, Preventive Medicine Considerations in Planning Multiservice and Multinational Operations; and Chapter 13, Preventive Medicine and the Operation Plan). However, the number of preventive medicine personnel in a theater of operations is not sufficient to assign a preventive medicine professional to each company or similarly sized unit. For example, an Army division, which may have 100 or more companies and up to 21,000 soldiers, is authorized 6 preventive medicine professionals: one Preventive Medicine Officer, one Environmental Science Officer, one Preventive Medicine Noncommissioned Officer, and three Preventive Medicine Specialists. This relatively small number of preventive medicine personnel and the large geographic area over which a division may be spread makes it impossible to provide direct environmental health support to each company-sized unit. To compensate for this shortfall, unit leaders and individual service members must learn environmental health practices that prevent disease and injury and incorporate them into daily practices, operations, and missions. These measures are called field sanitation.

The principles of field sanitation should be practiced in all of the military services; however, the following discussion is based on the US Army model, as described in the Army Regulation *Preventive Medicine*[64] and Field Manual *Field Hygiene and Sanitation*.[59] Other publications that describe various field sanitation practices are listed in Exhibit 20-8.

Command Responsibility and the Unit Field Sanitation Team

Field sanitation is a command responsibility. Commanders at all levels have the overall responsibility for maintaining optimum health conditions. Any condition that is less than optimal can potentially interfere with the ability of a unit to conduct its mission. Commanders are responsible for planning for unit field sanitation efforts before deployment (eg, training, acquiring and maintaining equipment, developing standard operating procedures) and implementing field sanitation practices when deployed. Army doctrine[62] requires commanders of a company or similarly sized field unit (ie, Table of Organization and Equipment units) to appoint and train a Field Sanitation Team (FST) to perform specific environmental health monitoring, testing, and training. This team will consist of a minimum of two soldiers and at least one should be a noncommissioned officer; generally, this is an additional duty.

Typically, unit FSTs are trained by environmental health or preventive medicine professionals from a Division Preventive Medicine Section or a Corps- or theater-level preventive medicine organization. Other medical personnel assigned to unit aid stations (eg, physician assistants and medical corpsman) or other medical units also may provide training. Several of the references listed in Exhibit 20-8 provide the technical information that the FST should be taught. The Field Manual *Unit Field Sanitation Team*[65] contains guidance for training FSTs in aspects of maintaining safe drinking water (eg, evaluating the container, chlorinating, testing chlorine residual), field food service sanitation, arthropod and rodent control, waste disposal, heat and cold injury prevention, and personal hygiene.

The unit FST is an essential line of defense against disease and preventable injury and therefore should continually advise the commander concerning sanitation indicators. Many of the activities that the FST monitors have been discussed earlier in this chapter (eg, field drinking water, field food service sanitation) or elsewhere in this text. Exhibit 20-9 lists some examples of the FST's functions.

Improvised Field Sanitation Devices

As is shown in Exhibit 20-9, the unit FST may recommend the types of and monitor the construction of waste disposal, shower, and handwashing facilities. If the area of operations is in a town or city and the tactical situation permits, an existing infrastructure may supply the necessary facilities. If there are no or limited facilities or the tactical situation does not allow access to existing facilities, however, field sanitation devices must be fabricated. The devices selected for use depend on a variety of conditions, such as the tactical scenario (eg, smoke from a burn-out latrine or from burning trash may give away a unit's location), the amount of time the unit will remain in a particular location, and the environmental conditions (eg, digging holes for sewage and solid waste disposal may not be possible if the ground is frozen or has a shallow rock layer).

The complexity of an improvised sanitation de-

EXHIBIT 20-8

SELECTED MILITARY FIELD SANITATION REFERENCES

Regulations

Immunizations and Chemoprophylaxis (AR 40-562, AFJI 161-13, BUMEDINST 6230.15, CGCOMDINST M6230.4E)

Pest Management (AR 420-76)

Preparation for Oversea Movement of Units (POM) (AR 220-10)

Preparation of Replacements for Oversea Movement (POR) (AR 612-2)

Preventive Dentistry (AR 40-35)

Preventive Medicine (AR 40-5)

Veterinary/Medical Food Inspection and Laboratory Service (AR 40-657)

Field Manuals

Army Food Service Operations (FM 10-23)

Brigade and Division Surgeons' Handbook (FM 8-10-5)

Combat Stress Control in a Theater of Operations (FM 8-51)

Control of Communicable Diseases Manual (FM 8-33)

Field Hygiene and Sanitation (FM 21-10)

Food Sanitation for the Supervisor (FM 8-34)

Management of Skin Diseases in the Tropics at Unit Level (FM 8-40)

Preventive Medicine Technician (FM 8-250)

Unit Field Sanitation Team (FM 21-10-1)

Water Supply in Theaters of Operations (FM 10-52)

Combat Health Support in Stability Operations/Support Operations (FM 8-42)

Planning for Health Services Support (FM 8-55)

Technical Bulletins—Medical

Cold Injury (TB Med 81)

Food Service Sanitation (TB Med 530)

Medical Problems of Man at High Terrestrial Elevations (TB Med 288)

Prevention, Treatment, and Control of Heat Injury (TB Med 507)

Sanitary Control and Surveillance of Field Water Supplies (TB Med 577)

Other Publications and Resources

Commander's Guide to Combat Health Support (DA Pam 40-19)

Disease and Environmental Alert Reports (Armed Forces Medical Intelligence Center, Fort Detrick, Md)

Disease Occurrence—Worldwide (Armed Forces Medical Intelligence Center, Fort Detrick, Md)

Manual of Naval Preventive Medicine (NAVMED P-5010, Bureau of Medicine and Surgery, Washington, DC)

Personal Protective Techniques Against Insects and Other Arthropods of Military Significance (US Army Environmental Hygiene Agency Technical Guide 174, Aberdeen Proving Ground, Md)

Soldier's Handbook for Individual Operations and Survival in Cold-Weather Areas (Department of the Army Training Circular 21-3)

Armed Forces Medical Intelligence Center Medical Environmental Disease Intelligence and Countermeasures CD-ROM (Armed Forces Medical Intelligence Center, Fort Detrick, Md)

Adapted with permission from Withers BJ, Erickson RL, Petruccelli BP, Hanson RK, Kadlec RP. Preventing disease and nonbattle injury in deployed units. *Mil Med*. 1994;159:39–43.

EXHIBIT 20-9

SOME OF THE FUNCTIONS OF THE FIELD SANITATION TEAM

- Assists in the selection and layout of bivouac sites to avoid insect infestations and pollution sources

- Recommends the types of and monitors the construction of facilities for waste disposal, showering, and hand washing

- Monitors the disposal of liquid and putrescible wastes to prevent mosquito breeding and fly breeding (human waste, sometimes referred to as black water, should not be mixed with liquid waste from showers, handwashing stations, and food service facilities, referred to as gray water)

- Monitors drinking water acquisition and consumption; checks chlorine levels and disinfects if necessary

- Monitors the transport, storage, handling, preparation, and service of food to prevent contamination

- Issues iodine tablets

- Issues insect repellent and assists personnel in treating uniforms and bednetting with permethrin; encourages use of personal protection measures

- Issues powders, dusts, and uniform impregnants as appropriate

- Provides limited pest control for insects and rodents

- Trains unit members in aspects of personal hygiene and individual field sanitation measures

---

vice will depend on the availability of building materials and construction support. A decision matrix to select appropriate devices is shown in Exhibit 20-10. Examples of improvised field sanitation devices and some construction criteria are contained in Army field manuals for field hygiene and sanitation[59] and unit field sanitation teams.[65]

Personal Hygiene

In addition to the commander's responsibility and the duties of the FST, the individual service member is the first line of defense for combating disease and must perform certain personal functions to remain healthy in the field environment. The individual is responsible for his or her own personal hygiene and individual field sanitation measures. Some examples are:

- maintaining cleanliness by bathing and brushing and flossing teeth as frequently as possible,
- keeping the feet clean and dry and using foot powder,
- maintaining a clean living area,
- wearing clean clothes,

- wearing clothing properly to prevent heat and cold injuries, insect bites, and injury,
- using insect repellents,
- using bed netting and insect sprays,
- drinking water and eating properly, and
- maintaining proper immunizations.

Standards, Controls, and Monitoring

The environmental health topics in the other sections of this chapter have been presented in terms of applicable standards, controls, and monitoring. Field sanitation also can be discussed in this manner. For example, the Army's preventive medicine regulation,[64] field manual,[59] and field sanitation technical references (see Exhibit 20-8) can loosely be considered the "standards" for field sanitation even though they do not fit the criteria for standards as discussed in this chapter's introduction. Field sanitation practices, field sanitary devices, and FST equipment may be considered as controls. FST surveillance and inspections constitute operational monitoring and visits by division or other theater preventive medicine personnel may be considered health monitoring.

EXHIBIT 20-10

DECISION MATRIX TO DETERMINE FIELD DISPOSAL REQUIREMENTS

	Highly Mobile	Short Bivouac	Extended Bivouac
CAT-HOLE	X		
Cover with dirt after use			
STRADDLE TRENCH		X	
• Enough for 4% of males and 6% of females			
• Cover with dirt after each use			
DEEP PIT			X
• Enough for 4% of males and 6% of females			
• Add urinals to protect seats			
CHEMICAL TOILETS		X	X
• Use where field sanitation devices are prohibited			
GARBAGE PIT		X	X
• Locate near dining facility, but not closer than 30 yards			
• One pit per 100 soldiers served per day			
• Cover with dirt after each meal, close daily			
SOAKAGE PIT (Food Service)		X	X
• Locate near dining facility alternate daily use			
• Fill with loose rocks			
• Add grease trap for dining facility waste			
SOAKAGE PIT (Other)			X
• Provide pit for urinals, shower, or other locations where water collects			
MESS KIT LAUNDRY		X	X
• Dig soakage pit to provide good drainage			
HANDWASHING DEVICES		X	X
• Dig shallow soakage pit			
• Collocate with latrine and food facilities			
SHOWERS			X
• Dig soakage pit			
URINALS			X
• Trough			
• Pipe			
• Urinoil			

Adapted from US Department of the Army. *Field Hygiene and Sanitation*. Washington, DC: DA; 1988. Field Manual 21-10.

SPECIAL TOPICS

Indoor Air

Ambient air quality was discussed earlier in this chapter, but indoor air quality (to include the air in office buildings) and workplace air quality (ie, atmospheres generated by typical industrial work activities, such as welding fumes and solvents) are also important issues.[68–72] Common indoor air agents include gases (eg, nitrogen dioxide, carbon monoxide, and sulfur dioxide from gas stoves and heaters or garaged-vehicle exhaust), volatile organics (eg, formaldehyde from tobacco smoke and glues), reactive chemicals (eg, isocyanates from paints and structural supports), and biological particulates (eg, allergens from dust mites, animal dander, fungi, toxins).[66] In industrial workplaces, contaminants are identified as those substances that are regulated under the Occupational Safety and Health Act (29 CFR 1910) and include a variety of vapors, gases, and particulates that have permissible exposure limits (PELs). The American Conference of Governmental Industrial Hygienists (ACGIH) also recommends exposure limits for hazardous workplace air contaminants.[67] Some military systems generate air contaminants (eg, vehicles and weapons systems) that can cause both acute and chronic effects if excessive exposure occurs.

Confined Space

In both civilian and military settings, confined spaces can be deadly, so precautions and safe practices must be followed to prevent fatal events. Confined spaces are defined as spaces that by design have limited openings for entry and exit and unfavorable natural ventilation that could contain or produce dangerous air contaminants; they are not intended for continuous employee occupancy.[73] Examples include but are not limited to storage tanks, ship compartments, process vessels, pits, silos, vats, degreasers, reaction vessels, boilers, ventilation and exhaust ducts, sewers, tunnels, underground utility vaults, and pipelines. The military preventive medicine or environmental health practitioner should be especially vigilant of such areas at military field, installation, and depot maintenance operations. Examples of other places of military interest include railheads, marine terminals, and ports.

Hazards that may exist in a confined space include oxygen deficiency due to displacement by simple asphyxiants (eg, carbon dioxide, nitrogen) or oxidation reactions (eg, welding, rusting); hazardous atmospheres (eg, flammable, explosive, irritant, or corrosive gases, vapors, fumes, or particulates); and engulfment from fill materials, (eg, grain or stones in a rail car, hopper, or silo).

Federal regulations (OSHA; 29 CFR Part 1910.126) require workplaces to identify confined spaces and institute specific practices to minimize or preclude accidental injury, illness, or death associated with such areas. These spaces must be tested and monitored before and during occupancy, and specific safety and health precautions must be followed to preclude accidental injury or death. Examples of these precautions include sampling the atmosphere, dilution ventilation, use of personal protective equipment (eg, respirators, harnesses), training, and positioning a trained worker outside of the workspace in sight of the person inside.[74,75]

There is another category of similar spaces that also could be harmful. These, identified as enclosed spaces, would normally not be considered confined spaces. During certain conditions (eg, during maintenance and repair work), though, they warrant an evaluation to determine if precautions for entry into confined space are required.[75] Examples of military enclosed spaces include mobile vans, shelters, crew compartments, and vehicle cabs.

Global Issues and Department of Defense Environmental Activities

The environmental health issues presented in this chapter primarily draw on experiences in the United States, with some emphasis on the impact to US military forces. Outside of the United States, however, some issues may have to be looked at from a different perspective because of different social, economic, and political dynamics. For example, in the United States the emphasis in drinking water quality is on controlling chemical contaminants, especially carcinogens. In lesser-developed countries, though, the emphasis on microbial control is greater,[76] presumably because infectious diseases are more prevalent than in the United States. Adverse environmental conditions and subsequent effects on human health can lead to destabilization and cause social, economic, and political unrest in a country. Such conditions may affect how countries interact with each other and lead to regional and global conflicts. Conflicts may be avoided if environmental conditions are sustained in a manner that supports and enhances human health. Thus, if the United States assists other nations in resolving environmental problems, then the possibility of conflicts may be reduced. This concept was addressed by Secretary of Defense William J. Perry in 1997, who described it as "Preventive Defense" which "creates the conditions which support peace, making war less likely and deterrence unnecessary."[77(pW-13)] This also is one of the goals of the Department of Defense's thrust in international environmental activities.[78]

SUMMARY

We strive to interact with the environment in ways that are not harmful to our health but enhance our lives. Environmental health is a public health specialty that promotes a healthy relationship between people and their environment. This chapter presents several perspectives for medical and public health professionals, particularly those in the military, to consider concerning environmental health. Environmental factors need to be anticipated, recognized, evaluated, and controlled to prevent adverse health effects. The critical functions performed in the practice of environmental health—standards, controls, monitoring, and policy—can be applied to specific subjects that occur during and can affect deployments. The subjects introduced in the chapter—drinking water, military field water, swimming pools and bathing areas, wastewater management, managing hazardous materials, managing waste, food safety and sanitation, ambient air quality and pollution, field sanitation—are as important to the health and efficiency of military personnel on deployment as they are on permanent installations in the United States.

Acknowledgment

The authors would like to recognize and thank the following individuals for their reviews, professional expertise, and overall support to the development of this chapter: Ms. Linda Baetz, USACHPPM; Captain (Retired) George Burns, MPH, US Public Health Service; Captain Marlene N. Cole, DVM, MPH, US Public Health Service; Mr. David Daughdrill, PE, USACHPPM; Ms. Kris Durbin, USACHPPM; Colonel (Retired) Joel C. Gaydos, MD, MPH, US Army; Ms. Veronique Hauschild, USACHPPM; Lieutenant Commander James N. Hudson, MPH, US Navy; Colonel (Retired) Fred Leonard, MD, MPH, US Air Force; Ms. Beth A. Martin, USACHPPM; Mr. Patrick R. Monahan, PE, USACHPPM; Colonel Kotu K. Phull, PhD, PE, US Army; Commander Carol Pickerel, CIH, US Navy; Lieutenant Colonel Douglas Rinehart, US Army, Mr. Ed D. Smith, PhD, US Army Construction Engineering Research Laboratory.

REFERENCES

1. Gordon LJ. Environmental health and protection: Century 21 challenges. *J Environ Health*. 1995;56:28–34.

2. Salvato J. *Environmental Engineering and Sanitation*. Somerset, NJ: John Wiley and Sons; 1992.

3. Moeller D. *Environmental Health*. Revised ed. Cambridge, Mass: Harvard University Press; 1997.

4. Last J, Wallace R, ed. *Maxcy-Rosenau-Last Public Health and Preventive Medicine*. 13th ed. East Norwalk, Conn: Appleton and Lange; 1992.

5. Nadakavukaren A. *Our Global Environment, A Health Perspective*. 4th ed. Prospect Heights, Ill: Waveland Press; 1995.

6. Koren H, Bisesi M. *Handbook of Environmental Health and Safety, Principles and Practices*. Vol 2. 3rd ed. Boca Raton, Fla: Lewis Publishers; 1996.

7. Koren H, Bisesi M. *Handbook of Environmental Health and Safety, Principles and Practices*. Vol.1. 3rd ed. Boca Raton, Fla: Lewis Publishers; 1996.

8. Eaton D, Klaassen C. Principles of toxicology. In: Klaassen C, Amdur M, Doull J, eds. *Casarett and Doull's Toxicology: The Basic Science of Poisons*. NY: McGraw-Hill; 1996.

9. *Webster's II New Riverside University Dictionary*. Boston, Mass: Houghton Mifflin; 1984.

10. Salter L. *Mandated Science*. Norwell, Mass: Kluwer Academic Publishers; 1988.

11. Roberts W, Abernathy C. Risk assessment: Principles and methodologies. In: Fan A, Chang L, eds. *Toxicology and Risk Assessment, Principles, Methods, and Applications*. New York: Marcel Dekker; 1996.

12. National Academy of Science. *Risk Assessment in the Federal Government: Managing the Process*. Washington, DC: NAS/National Research Council; 1983.

13. The Presidential/Congressional Commission on Risk Assessment and Risk Management. *Final Report: Framework for Environmental Health Risk Management*. Washington, DC: Government Printing Office; 1997.

14. The Presidential/Congressional Commission on Risk Assessment and Risk Management. *Final Report: Risk Assessment and Risk Management in Regulatory Decision-Making*. Washington, DC: Government Printing Office; 1997.

15. Barnes D, Dourson M. Reference dose (RfD): Description and use in health risk assessments. *Regulat Toxicol Pharmacol*. 1988;8:471–486.

16. Derelanko M. Risk assessment. In: Derelanko M, Hollinger M, eds. *CRC Handbook of Toxicology*. Boca Raton, FL: CRC Press; 1995.

17. US Environmental Protection Agency. *Risk Assessment Guidance for Superfund*. Washington, DC: USEPA; 1989. EPA 5401/1-89/002.

18. US Environmental Protection Agency. *Exposure Factors Handbook*. Washington, DC: USEPA; 1989. EPA 600/8-89/043.

19. Hallenbeck W, Cunningham K. *Quantitative Risk Assessment for Environmental and Occupational Health*. Chelsea, MI: Lewis Publishers; 1987.

20. US Environmental Protection Agency. *Analysis for Polychlorinated Dibenzo-p-Dioxins (PCDD) and Dibenzofurans (PCDF) in Human Adipose Tissue: Method Evaluation Study*. Washington, DC: USEPA; 1986. EPA 560/5-86/020.

21. US Environmental Protection Agency. *Seminar Publication: Risk Assessment, Management and Communication of Drinking Water Contamination*. Washington, DC: USEPA; 1990. EPA 625/4-89/024.

22. American Water Works Association, American Public Health Association, Water Environment Federation. *Standard Methods for the Examination of Water and Wastewater*. 19th ed. Washington, DC: American Public Health Association; 1995.

23. Eller P, Cassinelli M. *NIOSH Manual of Analytical Methods (NMAM)*. Washington, DC: Department of Health and Human Services, National Institute of Occupational Safety and Health; 1994. NIOSH Publication 94-113.

24. Occupational Safety and Health Administration. *OSHA Technical Manual (OTM)*. Washington, DC: OSHA; 1996.

25. US Environmental Protection Agency. *EPA 100–400 Series—Methods for Chemical Analysis of Water and Wastes*. Washington, DC: USEPA; 1983. EPA 600/4-79/020.

26. US Environmental Protection Agency. *EPA 500 Series—Methods for the Determination of Organic Compounds in Drinking Water*. Washington, DC: USEPA; 1988. EPA 600/4-88/039.

27. US Environmental Protection Agency. *EPA 600 Series—40 CFR, Subchapter D (Water Programs), Part 136 (Guidelines Establishing Test Procedures for the Analysis of Pollutants)*. Washington, DC: USEPA; 1988.

28. US Environmental Protection Agency. *EPA 500 Series—Methods for the Determination of Organic Compounds in Drinking Water*. Supplement I. Washington, DC: USEPA; 1990. EPA 600/4-90/020.

29. US Environmental Protection Agency. *EPA 200 Series—Methods for the Determination of Metals in Environmental Samples*. Washington, DC: USEPA; 1991. EPA 600/4-91/010.

30. US Environmental Protection Agency. *EPA 500 Series—Methods for the Determination of Organic Compounds in Drinking Water*. Supplement II. Washington, DC: USEPA; 1992. EPA 600/R-92/129.

31. US Environmental Protection Agency. *EPA 100-400 Series—Methods for the Determination of Inorganic Substances in Environmental Samples*. Washington, DC: USEPA; 1993. EPA 600/R-93/100.

32. US Environmental Protection Agency. *EPA 200 Series—Methods for the Determination of Metals in Environmental Samples*. Supplement I. Washington, DC: USEPA; 1994. EPA 600/R-94/111.

33. US Environmental Protection Agency. *Test Methods for Evaluating Solid Waste: Physical/Chemical Methods*. Washington, DC: USEPA; 1995. EPA 530/SW-846.

34. Adolfo N, Rosecrance A. QA and environmental sampling. *Environ Testing Analysis*. 1993;May/June:26–33.

35. Burkart JA, Eggenberger LM, Nelson JH, Nicholson PR. A practical statistical quality control scheme for the industrial hygiene chemistry laboratory. *Am Ind Hyg Assoc J*. 1984;45:386–392.

36. Keith L, Crummett W, Deegan J, Libby R, Taylor J, Wentler G. Principles of environmental analysis. *Anal Chem*. 1983;55:2210–2218.

37. US Environmental Protection Agency. Drinking Water Regulations and Health Advisories. Washington, DC: USEPA; 1996.

38. US Army Combined Arms Support Command. *Water Consumption Planning Factors Study*. Fort Lee, Va: USACASCOM; 1983. CAN 82888.

39. US Army Training and Doctrine Command. *US Army Operational Concepts Near Term Water Resources Management*. Fort Monroe, Va: USTRADOC; 1981. Pamphlet 525-11.

40. Department of the Army. *Quadripartite Standardization Agreement 245: Minimum Requirements for Water Potability*. 2nd ed. Washington, DC: DA; 1985.

41. North Atlantic Treaty Organization Military Agency for Standardization. *Standardization Agreement 2136: Minimum Standards of Water Potability in Emergency Situations*. 3rd ed. Brussels: NATO; 1994.

42. North Atlantic Treaty Organization Military Agency for Standardization. *Standardization Agreement 2136, Amendment 1. Minimum Standards of Water Potability in Emergency Situations*. 3rd ed. Brussels: NATO;1995.

43. US Department of the Army. *Occupational and Environmental Health: Sanitary Control and Surveillance of Field Water Supplies*. Washington, DC: DA; 1986. Technical Bulletin MED 577.

44. Miller R, Phull K, Smith E. An overview of military field water supply. *J US Army Med Dept*. 1991:9–13.

45. US Department of the Army. *Occupational and Environmental Health: Swimming Pools and Bathing Facilities*. Washington, DC: DA; 1993. Technical Bulletin MED 575.

46. US Environmental Protection Agency. *Environmental Pollution Control Alternatives*. Cincinnati, Oh: USEPA; 1979. EPA 625/5-79/012.

47. Smith R, Olishifski J. Industrial toxicology. In: Olishifski J, ed. *Fundamentals of Industrial Hygiene*. 2nd ed. Chicago: National Safety Council; 1971: 465–500.

48. Ecobichon D. Toxic effects of pesticides. In: Klaassen C, Amdur M, Doull J, eds. *Casarett and Doull's Toxicology: The Basic Science of Poisons*. NY: McGraw-Hill; 1996: 673–676.

49. Saunders D, Harper C. Pesticides. In: Hayes A, ed. *Principles and Methods of Toxicology*. NY: Raven Press; 1994: 389–415.

50. US Environmental Protection Agency. *Characterization of Municipal Solid Waste in the United States: 1990 Update*. Washington, DC: USEPA; 1990.

51. Campbell R, Langford R. *Fundamentals of Hazardous Materials Incidents*. Chelsea, Minn: Lewis Publishers; 1991: 69–80.

52. Griffin R. *Principles of Hazardous Materials Management*. Chelsea, Minn: Lewis Publishers; 1988: 135–169.

53. Norton S. Toxic effects of plants. In: Klaassen C, Amdur M, Doull J, eds. *Casarett and Doull's Toxicology: The Basic Science of Poisons*. NY: McGraw-Hill; 1996: 841–853.

54. Russel F. Toxic effects of animal toxins. In: Klaassen C, Amdur M, Doull J, eds. *Casarett and Doull's Toxicology: The Basic Science of Poisons*. NY: McGraw-Hill; 1996: 801–839.

55. Kotsonis F, Burdock G, Flamm W. Food toxicology. In: Klaassen C, Amdur M, Doull J, eds. *Casarett and Doull's Toxicology: The Basic Science of Poisons*. NY: McGraw-Hill; 1996: 909–949.

56. The Educational Foundation of the National Restaurant Association. *Applied Foodservice Sanitation*. 4th ed. Dubuque, Ia: Kendall/Hunt Publishing; 1995.

57. Collins B. Risk assessment for foodservice establishments. *J Environ Health*. 1995;57:9–12.

58. US Department of the Army. *Occupational and Environmental Health: Food Service Sanitation*. Washington, DC: DA; 1991. Technical Bulletin MED 530.

59. US Department of the Army. *Field Hygiene and Sanitation*. Washington, DC: DA; 1993. Field Manual 21-10.

60. Costa D, Amdur M. Air pollution. In: Klaassen C, Amdur M, Doull J, eds. *Casarett and Doull's Toxicology: The Basic Science of Poisons*. NY: McGraw-Hill; 1996: 857–882.

61. National ambient air quality standards for particulate matter: Proposed rule. *Fed Register*. 1996;61:65637–65713.

62. Hutchens B, Pate BA. Environmental exposure surveillance, Operation Joint Endeavor, Bosnia-Herzegovina. Presented at the American Defense Preparedness Association Conference; 1997; New Orleans, La.

63. Langford RE. Chief of Preventive Medicine, NATO MEDCC, Personal Communication; 1997.

64. US Department of the Army. *Preventive Medicine*. Washington, DC: DA; 1993. Army Regulation 40-5.

65. US Department of the Army. *Unit Field Sanitation Team*. Washington, DC: DA; 1993. Field Manual 21-10-1.

66. Zummo S, Karol M. Indoor air pollution. *J Environ Health*. 1996;58:25–29.

67. American Conference of Governmental Industrial Hygienists. *1996 TLVs and BEIs: Threshold Limit Values for Chemical Substances and Physical Agents and Biological Exposure Indices*. Cincinnati, Oh: American Conference of Governmental Industrial Hygienists; 1996.

68. Yasalonis J. Industrial hygiene in the U.S. Army. In: *Occupational Health: The Soldier and the Industrial Base*. In: *The Textbook of Military Medicine*. Washington, DC: Office of the Surgeon General, The Borden Institute; 1994: 93–128.

69. Herr G, McDiarmid M, Testa M, Caldwell D. Health hazards to health care workers. In: *Occupational Health: The Soldier and the Industrial Base*. In: *The Textbook of Military Medicine*. Washington, DC: Office of the Surgeon General, The Borden Institute; 1994: 129–163.

70. McFee D. Solvents. In: Olishifski J, ed. *Fundamentals of Industrial Hygiene*. 2nd ed. Chicago: National Safety Council; 1971: 133–169.

71. Alpaugh E. Particulates. In: Olishifski J, ed. *Fundamentals of Industrial Hygiene*. 2nd ed. Chicago: National Safety Council; 1971: 171–200.

72. Gross R, Broadwater W. Health hazard assessments. In: *Occupational Health: The Soldier and the Industrial Base*. In: *The Textbook of Military Medicine*. Washington, DC: Office of the Surgeon General, The Borden Institute; 1994: 165–205.

73. National Institute of Occupational Safety and Health. *Criteria for a Recommended Standard, Working in Confined Spaces*. Washington, DC: Department of Health and Human Services, NIOSH; 1979. NIOSH Publication 80-106.

74. 29 CFR. Part 1910, Occupational Safety and Health Standards.

75. US Army Center for Health Promotion and Preventive Medicine. *US Army Health Hazard Assessor's Guide*. Aberdeen Proving Ground, Md: USACHPPM; 1996.

76. World Health Organization. *Guidelines for Drinking Water Quality: Recommendations*. Vol 1. 2nd ed. Geneva: WHO; 1993:188.

77. Perry W. Fulfilling the role of preventive defense. *Defense Issues*. 1997;11(44):W-1–W-4.

78. Vest G. DOD international environmental activities. *Federal Facilities Environ J*. 1997:7–18.

Chapter 21

ARTHROPODS OF MILITARY IMPORTANCE

RAJ K. GUPTA, PhD; LEON L. ROBERT JR., PhD; AND PHILLIP G. LAWYER, PhD

R. K. Gupta; Colonel, MS, US Army; Research Area Director, Research Plans and Programs, US Army Medical Research and Development Command, Fort Detrick MD 21702-5012; formerly, Department of Entomology, Division of Communicable Diseases and Immunology, Walter Reed Army Institute of Research, Silver Spring, MD 20910-7500

L. L. Robert Jr.; Lieutenant Colonel, MS, US Army; Department of Preventive Medicine and Biometrics, Division of Tropical Public Health, Uniformed Services University of the Health Sciences, 4301 Jones Bridge Road, Bethesda, MD 20814

P. G. Lawyer; Colonel, MS, US Army, (Retired); Associate Professor, Department of Preventive Medicine and Biometrics, Uniformed Services University of the Health Sciences, 4301 Jones Bridge Road, Bethesda, MD 20814; formerly, Entomology Consultant, Office of US Army Surgeon General

INTRODUCTION

Until the latter half of the 20th century, military casualties due to disease and nonbattle injuries (DNBI) usually outnumbered those directly related to combat. Historically, arthropods have been a leading cause of DNBI. The direct effects of arthropods include tissue damage due to stings, bites, and exposure to vesicating fluids, infestation of tissue by the arthropods themselves, annoyance, and entomophobia (an uncontrolled fear of arthropods). The indirect effects on human health include disease transmission and allergic reactions due to bites and stings and to arthropod skins or emanations. Arthropods also destroy property and materiel used by the military, and there is even some concern that arthropods could potentially be used as biological weapons. The importance of naturally occurring arthropod-borne disease is well documented, as is the direct injury, annoyance and material damage caused by nuisance arthropods. During World War II, it is estimated that more than 24,000,000 man-days were lost due to arthropod associated disease and injury.[1]

Arthropods are of greatest importance to military operations when they act as vectors of disease. A vector is an organism that transmits a pathogen to a susceptible host. Arthropods serve as vectors in a number of different ways, from simple mechanical transmission of pathogenic organisms on the arthropod body, as when house flies carry dysentery bacilli from infected feces to food, to the more complicated process of biological transmission, where the pathogens must spend part of their life cycle in the body of the arthropod before humans can be infected. A fundamental activity of military medical entomologists is to establish the role that certain arthropod species or populations play in the transmission of a particular infectious disease to service members. There are primary and secondary vectors. Primary vectors are those that are mainly responsible for transmitting a pathogen to humans or animals; secondary vectors are those that play a supplementary role in transmission but would be unable to maintain disease transmission in the absence of the primary vector.[2] The criteria that must be satisfied to declare with reasonable

certainty that a particular arthropod is a vector of human disease are:

- Demonstration that members of the suspected arthropod population commonly feed upon vertebrate hosts of the pathogen, or otherwise make effective contact with the hosts under natural conditions,
- Demonstration of a convincing biological association in time and space between the suspected vectors and clinical or subclinical infections in vertebrate hosts,
- Repeated demonstration that the suspected vectors, collected under natural conditions, harbor the identifiable, infective stage of the pathogen, and
- Demonstration of efficient transmission of the identifiable pathogen by the suspected vectors under controlled experimental conditions.[3]

To minimize adverse effects caused by arthropods, military entomologists must be able to identify vector and pest species accurately and then prescribe appropriate countermeasures. This begins with a basic knowledge of arthropod morphology and classification. Members of the phylum Arthropoda have segmented bodies with paired, segmented appendages, bilateral symmetry, a dorsal heart, a ventral nerve cord, and an exoskeleton. The arthropods are divided into five classes: Insecta (insects), Arachnida (mites, ticks, spiders and scorpions), Crustacea (crabs, lobsters, shrimps, water fleas), Chilopoda (centipedes), and Diplopoda (millipedes). Two of these classes, the Insecta and the Arachnida, are especially important to war fighters because of the potential effect they can have on military operations (Table 21-1). The other three classes are of minor significance. The identification of the arthropods by class, order, family, genus, and species is achieved by matching their morphological characteristics or features to couplets on a published dichotomous key. The class Insecta is the largest arthropod class and the one that includes the majority of the arthropods of military importance.

CLASS INSECTA

Insects can be differentiated from other arthropods by the presence of three distinct body regions (head, thorax and abdomen), and three pairs of legs (Figure 21-1). Insects are the only arthropods that possess wings and most, but not all, have them. Insects also

have only one pair of antennae.

Insects transmit diseases either mechanically or biologically. Mechanical vectors include cockroaches and filth flies. These insects may pick up pathogens on their feet or other parts of their body

TABLE 21-1

SYSTEMATIC LIST OF ARTHROPODS NAMED. ALL FALL WITHIN THE PHYLUM ARTHROPODA.

Scientific name	Common name
Class Arachnida	Arachnids
Order Araneae	Spiders
Family Theridiidae	Comb-footed spiders
Lactrodectus mactans	Black widow spider
Family Loxoscelidae	Recluse spiders
Loxosceles reclusa	Brown recluse spider
Order Acari	Mites and Ticks
Family Trombiculidae	Chigger mites
Leptotrombidium deliense	
Leptotrombidium fletcheri	
Leptotrombidium pallidum	
Trombicula alfreddugesi	Harvest mite
Trombicula autumnalis	
Family Pyroglyphidae	House dust mites
Dermatophagoides farinae	American house dust mite
Dermatophagoides pteronyssinus	European house dust mite
Euroglyophus maynei	
Family Glycyphagidae	
Glycyphagus destructor	
Family Macronyssidae	Fowl mites
Ornithonyssus bacoti	Tropical rat mite
Ornithonyssus bursa	Tropical fowl mite
Ornithonyssus sylviarum	Northern fowl mite
Family Dermanyssidae	
Dermanyssus gallinae	Chicken mite
Liponyssoides sanguineus	House mouse mite
Pyemotes tritici	Straw itch mite
Family Sarcoptidae	Scab or itch mites
Sarcoptes scabiei	Scabies mite
Trixacarus sp.	
Family Demodicidae	Follicle mites
Demodex brevis	Lesser follicle mite
Demodex folliculorum	Follicle mite
Family Argasidae	Soft ticks
Ornithodoros hermsii	
Ornithodoros parkeri	
Ornithodoros turicata	Relapsing fever tick
Family Ixodidae	Hard ticks
Amblyomma americanum	Lone star tick

Scientific name	Common name
Amblyomma maculatum	Gulf Coast tick
Dermacentor andersoni	Rocky Mountain wood tick
Dermacentor variabilis	American dog tick
Ixodes dammini	Northeastern deer tick
Ixodes scapularis	Black-legged tick
Ixodes pacificus	Western black-legged tick
Ixodes persulcatus	
Ixodes ricinus	European castor bean tick
Class Insecta	Insects
Order Anoplura	Sucking lice
Family Pediculidae	Head and body lice
Pediulus humanus capitis	Human head louse
Pediculus humanus humanus	Human body louse
Family Pthiridae	Crab lice
Pthirus pubis	Human crab louse
Order Siphonaptera	Fleas
Family Pulicidae	
Xenopsylla cheopis	Oriental rat flea
Order Hemiptera	True bugs
Family Cimicidae	Bed bugs
Cimex hemipterus	Tropical bed bug
Cimex lectularius	Common bed bug
Family Triatomidae	Assassin bugs
Triatoma infestans	
Triatoma dimidiata	
Triatoma barberi	
Triatoma gerstaeckeri	
Triatoma proctata	
Triatoma sanguisuga	Blood sucking conenose
Panstrongylus megitus	
Rhodnius prolixus	
Order Hymenoptera	Bees, wasps, and ants
Family Apidae	Bees
Apis mellifera mellifera	European honey bee
Apis mellifera scutellata	Africanized honey bee
Family Formicidae	Fire ants
Solenopsis invicta	Imported fire ant

TABLE 21-1 *continued*

Scientific name	Common name	Scientific name	Common name
Order Diptera	True flies	*Culex tritaeniorhynchus*	
Family Ceratopogonidae	Biting midges	*Culex vishnui*	
Culicoides spp.		*Culiseta melanura*	
Family Simuliidae	Black flies	*Deinocerites* spp.	
Simulium spp.		*Eremapodites* spp.	
Family Psychodidae	Sand flies	*Haemagogus* spp.	
Brumtomyia spp.		*Mansonia annulata*	
Chinius spp.		*Mansonia annulifera*	
Lutzomyia spp.		*Mansonia bonneae*	
Phlebotomus papatasi		*Mansonia dives*	
Sergentomyia spp.		*Mansonia uniformis*	
Werileya spp.		*Psorophora columbiae*	Dark rice field mosquito
Family Culicidae	Mosquitoes	*Psorophora confinnis*	
Aedes aegypti	Yellow fever mosquito	*Psorophora discolor*	
Aedes albopictus	Asian tiger mosquito	*Psorophora ferox*	
Aedes fulvus		*Sabethes chloropterus*	
Aedes leucocelaenus		Family Glossinadae	Tsetse flies
Aedes lineatopennis		*Glossina morsitans*	
Aedes niveus		*Glossina palpalis*	
Aedes poicilius		*Glossina swynnertoni*	
Aedes polynesiensis		*Glossina tachinoides*	
Aedes scutellaris		Family Tabanidae	Deer and horse flies
Aedes serratus		*Chrysops dimidiata*	
Aedes sollicitans	Salt marsh mosquito	*Chrysops distinctipennis*	
Aedes taeniorhynchus		*Chrysops silacea*	
Aedes thelcter		*Tabanus* spp.	
Aedes togoi		Family Chloropidae	Eye gnats
Aedes tongae		*Hippelates flavipes*	
Aedes triseriatus		Family Muscidae	Filth flies
Aedes vexans	Inland floodwater mosquito	*Fannia* spp.	
Aedes vigilax		*Musca domesticus*	Common house fly
Anopheles campestris		Family Calliphoridae	Blow flies
Anopheles darlingi		*Auchmeromyia luteola*	Congo floor maggot also called a filth fly
Anopheles donaldi		*Calliphora* spp.	
Anopheles funestus		*Cordylobia anthropophaga*	Human bot fly
Anopheles gambiae		*Lucilia* spp.	
Anopheles minimus		*Chrysomyia bessiana*	
Anopheles punctulatus group		*Cochliomyia hominivorax*	
Culex gelidus		Family Oestridae	Robust bot flies
Culex neavei		*Dermatobia hominis*	Torsalo
Culex pipiens quinquefasciatus	Southern house mosquito	Family Sarcophagidae	Flesh flies
Culex pseudovishnui		*Sarcophaga* spp.	
Culex tarsalis			

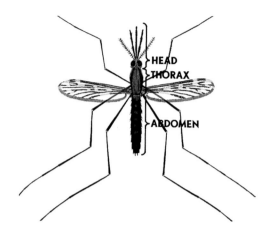

Fig 21-1. The three major divisions of an insect body are shown on this drawing of a mosquito.
Source: Letterman Army Institute of Research, Presidio of San Francisco, Calif.

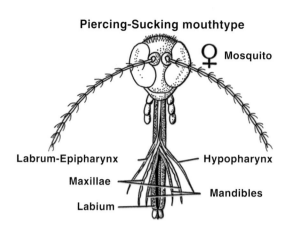

Fig 21-2. The sucking-piercing mouth parts of a female mosquito.
Source: Letterman Army Institute of Research, Presidio of San Francisco, Calif.

while feeding on fecal material or organic waste, or they may ingest the pathogens and later contaminate food consumed by the humans. Some examples of important mechanically transmitted diseases that have plagued military operations are typhoid fever, cholera, and dysentery. However, the insects that are of greatest importance to the military are those that serve as biological vectors of human pathogens. Pathogens transmitted in this manner must pass through part of their life cycle in the vector, where the pathogens multiply, change form, or do both before being passed on to a susceptible host. The host is usually infected via the bite of the vector or by having the excretions or body fluids of the vector rubbed into the skin.

Many of the vector insects discussed in this chapter are members of the order Diptera, the two-winged or true flies. Approximately 80,000 to 100,000 species in about 140 families have been described, and new ones are being added constantly. This order contains more insects involved in transmission of human and animal pathogens than any other. The Diptera are relatively small and soft-bodied insects; all winged members possess only one pair of wings and a pair of short, knob-like structures called halteres. Conspicuous compound eyes are usually present, and most species possess an additional three simple eyes, called ocelli, that are set in a triangle at the top of the head. The Dipteran mouthparts, while subject to great morphological variation, are all adapted for sucking fluids, as opposed to chewing solids, and are either piercing or nonpiercing. They can be divided into three subtypes as follows: (1) mosquito subtype (piercing/

sucking), (2) horse fly subtype (piercing/cutting), and (3) house fly subtype (nonpiercing/sponging) (Figure 21-2). All Diptera are holometabolus, meaning they undergo complete metamorphosis, passing through egg, larva, and pupa stages before becoming adults. The larvae of most medically important Diptera species require high humidity and are aquatic, semi-aquatic, endoparasitic, or live in wet or moist terrestrial habitats. The mosquitoes, sand flies, black flies, horse flies, stable flies, midges and filth flies are examples of Diptera that are serious pests of humans and animals.[2]

Mosquitoes

Mosquitoes are the foremost nuisance insects and disease vectors in most regions of the world and the sole vectors of several pathogens that cause diseases of military importance, including malaria, yellow fever and dengue. They also play a significant role in transmitting filariasis and forms of viral encephalitis.[2,3] Mosquitoes belong to one of the more primitive families of Diptera, the Culicidae. The blood-sucking behavior of female mosquitoes and some other Dipterans predisposes them to acquiring pathogens and parasites from an infected host and depositing them in the skin of a susceptible host.

Life Cycle

The immature stages of all mosquitoes develop only in water, but adaptation to and preference for particular types of water and water locations vary

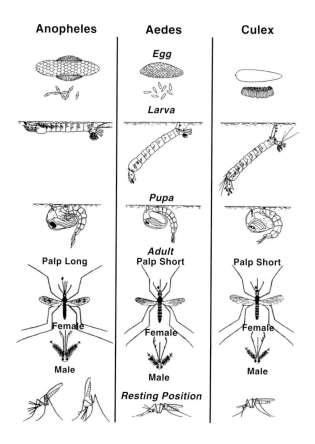

Anopheles   **Aedes**   **Culex**

Egg

Larva

Pupa

Adult

Palp Long   Palp Short   Palp Short

Female   Female   Female

Male   Male   Male

Resting Position

Fig. 21-3. Characteristics of anopheline and culicine mosquitoes.
Source: Centers for Disease Control and Prevention. *Vector-borne Disease Control Self-study Course 3013-G.* Manual G. *Mosquitoes of Public Health Importance and Their Control.* Atlanta: CDC; 1994: 14.

widely among species. The larvae are anatomically different from the adults, live in different habitats, and eat different types of food. Transformation to the adult stage takes place during a nonfeeding pupal stage (Figure 21-3).

Egg. Female mosquitoes may lay several hundred eggs, depositing them on the water's surface or on sites that will be flooded by water later. Each egg is encased in a protective shell. Depending on the species, eggs may be laid singly, in clusters, or in rafts.[2,4]

Larva. Mosquito larvae, also known as "wigglers," can be found in permanent ponds and marshes, temporary flood waters, or in water that has accumulated in tree holes, leaf axils, or other natural and artificial containers. They are very active and feed on minute aquatic animal and vegetable life and on decaying organic matter, coming to the surface to breathe through a respiratory siphon at the posterior end of the body. The larval stage includes four developmental instars. Mos-

quito larvae are affected by light and water conditions (eg, temperature, water movement), predators, and other living organisms in their habitat. When fully grown, a larva changes to a pupa.[2]

Pupa. The pupa, or "tumbler," is active but does not feed. This is the resting stage from which the adult is formed. The pupa rests on the surface of water unless disturbed, then it quickly moves towards the bottom. It breathes through two respiratory trumpets on the thorax. When the adult is ready to emerge, the pupal skin splits, and the adult pulls itself up and out of the floating skin, on which it rests until it is ready to fly.[2]

Adult. Adult mosquitoes are distinguishable from other Diptera by the long, filamentous antennae comprising 14 to 15 segments, a long proboscis adapted for blood sucking, and scales on the fringes of the wings and wing veins. The rounded head bears large compound eyes that almost touch in the middle. Males can usually be separated from the females by their bushy antennae. Adult mosquitoes display great diversity with regard to resting and oviposition habits, biting preferences, vector competence, dispersion, and flight range. Although breeding sites vary by species, mosquitoes can be divided into three major groups based on where they deposit their eggs: permanent water breeders, floodwater breeders, and artificial container or treehole breeders. Because each of these groups contains important vector species, breeding sites should always be considered when investigating a mosquito-borne disease outbreak or when implementing surveillance and control programs. *Anopheles* (including malaria vectors) and *Culex* mosquitoes usually select permanent bodies of water, such as swamps, lakes, ponds, streams and ditches. On the other hand, floodwater mosquitoes lay their eggs on the ground in depressions that are subject to flooding. During heavy rains or after snow melt, eggs deposited in these sites are inundated with water and hatch within minutes or hours. Included in the floodwater group are *Aedes vexans* (inland floodwater mosquito), *Aedes solicitans* (salt marsh mosquito), and *Psorophora columbiae* (dark rice field mosquitoes). Artificial container or treehole breeders include *Aedes aegypti* (the yellow fever mosquito), *Aedes albopictus* (the Asian tiger mosquito), *Aedes triseriatus*, and others.[2,5]

Both male and female mosquitoes feed on plant sugars, such as floral nectars, to obtain nourishment for basic metabolism and flight. In addition, most females will take a blood meal from birds, reptiles, amphibians, or mammals for egg development (Figure 21-4). Biting behavior may be very important

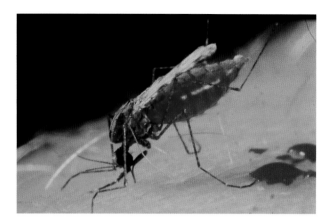

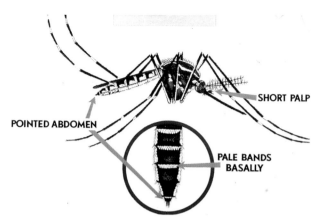

Fig. 21-4. A blood-engorged *Anopheles stephensi* mosquito, which transmits malaria in Asia.
Photograph: Courtesy of Ed Rowton, Walter Reed Army Institute of Research, Silver Spring, Md.

Fig. 21-5. Distinctive characteristics of *Aedes aegypti*
Source: Letterman Army Institute of Research, Presidio of San Francisco, Calif.

in the epidemiology of disease transmission. Many mosquito species bite humans to obtain their bloodmeals, and some feed on humans preferentially. Some will enter houses to bite humans (endophagic), while others bite their human hosts outside (exophagic). Other mosquitoes prefer to feed on non-human hosts, and many species do not bite people at all.[2]

Whereas wind-assisted dispersion records of up to 100 km have been recorded, in control programs and epidemiological studies it is usually safe to say that mosquitoes will not fly more than 2 km from their emergence site.[6] This is an important point to remember when surveying for potential vector breeding sites.

More than 3,000 mosquito species have been described. They are found throughout the world except in places that are permanently frozen. Three quarters of all mosquito species live in the tropics and subtropics, where warm, humid weather favors their rapid development. Mosquitoes may be found at elevations as high as 4,300 m above sea level, such as in Kashmir, India, and 1,160 m below sea level, as in the gold mines of south India.[2] Descriptions of the biology and physiology of mosquitoes can be found in Bates,[7] Christophers,[8] Clements,[9] Gillett,[10,11] and Horsfall.[12]

From a medical perspective, the three most important mosquito genera are *Anopheles*, *Aedes* and *Culex*. These are contained in two subfamilies, the Anophelinae (*Anopheles*) and the Culicinae (*Aedes* and *Culex*). The following characteristics serve to separate *Anopheles* mosquitoes from the other mosquito genera (Figure 21-5). *Anopheles* eggs are laid

singly on the surface of the water and are boat-shaped, possessing a pair of lateral floats. *Aedes* lay their eggs singly on damp litter or moist areas near the water's edge. *Culex* deposit their eggs grouped in rafts of 100 or more on the water's surface. *Anopheles* larvae lack a breathing siphon and lie parallel to the surface. Culicines all have a prominent respiratory siphon at the posterior end of the body and are usually found suspended at a 45° angle beneath the water surface. When at rest and when feeding, adult *Anopheles* hold their bodies at a 45° to 75° angle to the surface, with the proboscis and abdomen in a straight line. *Aedes* and *Culex* rest and feed with the body held parallel to the surface. The most reliable way to distinguish between adult Anophelines and Culicinae is by examination of their heads. The *Anopheles* possesses palpi that are about as long as the proboscis, male palpi that are paddle-shaped at the tip, and an evenly rounded scutellum. The palpi of *Aedes* and *Culex* are much shorter than the proboscis.[6]

Parasitic Diseases Transmitted by Mosquitoes

Malaria. Malaria is the most important arthropod-borne disease of humans. Essentially a disease of the tropics and subtropics, it is present in 102 countries and infects up to 500 million people and causes 2.5 million deaths annually, primarily in the tropics.[13,14] In Africa, malaria is one of three infectious diseases that contribute most significantly to the burden of disease as estimated by DALY (disability adjusted life years).[15]

Malaria is caused by four species of protozoan parasites of the genus *Plasmodium*: *Plasmodium falciparum, P vivax, P ovale,* and *P malariae*. Although *P vivax* causes the most malaria infections worldwide, the most serious, and often fatal, form of malaria is caused by *P falciparum*. In many parts of the world, infected people may carry large numbers of parasites without showing signs or symptoms of the disease, thus serving as reservoirs of infection for blood-feeding mosquitoes. Malaria parasites enter the human host through the bite of an infected female *Anopheles* mosquito. The life cycle of the malaria parasite takes place in two separate cycles: one in the human or vertebrate host and the other in the mosquito. (See chapter 36 for details of the malaria parasite cycle.)

Malaria heads the list of arthropod-borne diseases of importance to the military. It has had tremendous impact on military operations in the past and continues to threaten the health and effectiveness of today's war fighters when they are deployed to malaria-endemic areas. In these areas, native human populations often appear healthy, but a large portion of the people may be carriers of or semi-immune to malaria to which they have been exposed repeatedly since birth. The malaria pathogens are maintained at low levels by the hosts' immune systems. These inapparent infections can be passed quickly to nonimmune newcomers by mosquitoes. US forces deployed to malarious areas lack immunity to the pathogen and if they are bitten by infected mosquitoes, they readily contract the disease. The results include loss of manpower, increased burden on the military health support system, and decreased unit morale. All of these factors reduce the commander's ability to execute the directed mission.

The malaria threat to force readiness that has confounded commanders in the past still confronts our forces today. In 1993, a number of Marines (106) and soldiers (70) in certain units participating in Operation Restore Hope in Somalia developed malaria.[16,17] The reasons for this, the largest outbreak of malaria in US military since the Vietnam War, are a complex mixture of incomplete medical intelligence regarding the malaria threat, lack of command emphasis on and compliance with personal protection measures, and the complex life cycle of the malaria parasite. Medical surveillance revealed that one half of all malaria and dengue cases during Operation Restore Hope occurred in a single Marine battalion located in the Baardera area. A subsequent investigation of these outbreaks found that the Marine commander did not enforce recommended countermeasures. Fortunately, the ill Marines recovered and the unit was not involved in any tactical engagements while in this weakened condition. A resurgence of malaria in South Korea in the late 1990s, particularly around the Demilitarized Zone, underscores malaria's importance to US military forces today.[18]

Filariasis. Lymphatic filariasis is another important mosquito-borne parasitic disease distributed throughout tropical and subtropical areas of the world. Currently, an estimated 146 million people are afflicted with this debilitating and disfiguring disease, which is caused by three species of filarial worms: *Wuchereria bancrofti, Brugia malayi*, and *Brugia timori. Wuchereria bancrofti* is the most widely distributed species, and its infections are the most prevalent.[19,20] An estimated 115 million people are infected with the parasite. It occurs in large sections of sub-Saharan Africa, parts of South and Central America and the Caribbean region, parts of India, China, Bangladesh, Burma, Thailand, Malaysia, Laos, Vietnam, Indonesia, the Philippines, Papua New Guinea, and island groups in the south Pacific Ocean. *Brugia malayi* has a more limited distribution, occurring in China, India, the Republic of Korea, and Southeast Asia, including Indonesia and the Philippines. *Brugia timori* is confined to certain southern islands of Indonesia in the Savu Sea. The number of people infected with the latter two species has not been estimated, although humans in endemic areas have infection rates as high as 30%.[2]

The worms may infest and block human lymphatic channels and cause enormous and debilitating swelling, resulting in much human suffering. Besides their physical and psychological impact, the filariases exact an enormous toll in terms of decreased economic production in nations where such decreases can be ill afforded. The filariases generally cause morbidity but not mortality in infected humans and so normally do not have an immediate effect on military operations. It can, however, cause a significant loss of personnel and resources in units stationed in endemic areas. In World War II, a survey of two units stationed in the South Pacific showed that they had infection rates of 65% and 55%. Both units were returned to the United States without having entered combat.[21]

The vector mosquito acquires the microfilariae from an infected person while obtaining a blood meal. The filariae shed their sac-like sheath and travel quickly through the midgut of the mosquito to the thorax where they develop in the large indirect flight muscles. After a number of internal changes and two molts, infective third-stage larvae develop. The infective larvae find their way into the hemocoele (body cavity) of the vector and eventually to the proboscis, from which they are transmitted to a new host during blood feeding.[22]

Depending on the species, vectors of filarial pathogens may be active during day or night. *Culex pipiens quinquefasciatus* is the main vector responsible for filarial transmission in urban areas; in rural areas, the vectors may be *Anopheles, Aedes,* or *Mansonia* species that inhabit the forests. The main vectors of *Wuchereria bancrofti* in the tropics are *An gambiae, An funestus, An darlingi, An minimus, An campestris, An punctulatus* group, *Aedes niveus, Ae poicilius, Ae polynesiensis, Ae tongae, Ae vigilax,* and *Culex pipiens quinquifasciatus. Brugia malayi* occurs in rural populations in the Far East between 75° and 140° East longitude in small endemic foci. Specific known vectors of this pathogen are *Mansonia annulifera, M dives, M bonneae, M annulata, M uniformis, An campestris,* and *An donaldi.*[2]

Viral Diseases Transmitted by Mosquitoes

Approximately 100 arthropod-borne viruses (arboviruses) are known to produce disease in humans. The best-known examples of human arboviral pathogens are in the following genera and families: *Flavivirus* (Flaviviridae), *Bunyavirus* and *Phlebovirus* (Bunyaviridae) and *Alphavirus* (Togaviridae). The flaviviruses are either mosquito- or tick-borne, the bunyaviruses and other closely related viruses in the family Bunyaviridae may be transmitted by mosquitoes, ticks, sand flies, or midges; the phleboviruses are transmitted by mosquitoes and sand flies, and all but one of the alphaviruses are mosquito-borne. These pathogens cause infections in humans and livestock resulting in febrile illnesses ranging from mild discomfort to severe influenza-like symptoms and can cause encephalitis, encephalomyelitis, and hemorrhagic fevers. Mortality rates can be relatively high, especially in infections with central nervous system involvement or hemorrhagic symptoms.[2] Arboviral diseases are often characterized by sudden onset and periodic epidemics involving thousands of cases, which could seriously affect combat effectiveness in military operations. The following mosquito-borne viral diseases are discussed in order of relative medical significance.

Yellow Fever. Historically, yellow fever virus, a flavivirus, is probably the most important and most dangerous of the mosquito-borne viruses. It was first recognized in humans in the 17th century, but mosquito transmission of yellow fever virus was not demonstrated until the landmark studies by Major Walter Reed, Dr. Carlos Finlay, and their colleagues in Cuba in 1900.[23] Yellow fever has two transmission cycles, a sylvatic or jungle cycle and

an urban cycle. The sylvatic cycle involving forest canopy mosquitoes as the vectors (*Haemagogus* species in Central and South America and *Aedes* species in Africa) and forest primates, mainly monkeys, as the hosts. The urban cycle involves *Ae aegypti* as the vector and humans as the hosts (see Figure 36-10). The urban cycle begins when humans become infected in the sylvatic cycle by entering forest habitats and being bitten by infected sylvatic vectors. People infected in this way return to their villages or cities, thereby initiating urban transmission. Yellow fever originated in Africa and was brought to the New World during the 1500s by slave trade ships. These ships maintained their own colonies of *Ae aegypti* in fresh-water storage containers. The virus and urban vector became established in the Caribbean region, on the east coast of South and Central America, and in the southern United States. During 1741, the British lost 20,000 to 27,000 men to an epidemic of "black vomit" while on an ill-fated expedition to conquer Mexico and Peru. The British and Spanish forces suffered heavy losses on Cuba in the 1760s, and the French lost 29,000 in 1802 while in Haiti and the Mississippi Valley.[3]

In 1900, a US Army Yellow Fever Commission under the direction of Major Walter Reed was established in Cuba, where its studies demonstrated that a filterable agent present in the blood of acute phase patients could be transmitted by *Ae aegypti* mosquitoes (Figure 21-6).[24] Jungle yellow fever in the Western Hemisphere is transmitted chiefly among monkeys, marmosets, and other animals and

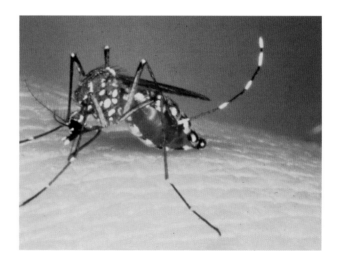

Fig. 21-6. *Aedes aegypti*
Photograph: Courtesy of Colonel Raj Gupta, MS, US Army, and the Letterman Army Institute of Research, Presidio of San Francisco, Calif.

causes fatal infections in these animals. The reported vectors of the forest canopy are *Haemagogus* species, *Ae leucocelaenus*, *Sabethes chloropterus*, and possibly *Ae fulvus*.[25] Many cases of yellow fever have been reported in recent years from South America, the vast majority of these were in males over 15 years of age who were presumably infected while working in the jungle. In the last 30 years, *Ae aegypti* has reinfested Central and South America and brought with it the potential threat to transmit yellow fever in an urban cycle. Because of a very efficacious vaccine, yellow fever is no longer a threat to the US military.

Dengue. Dengue is a viral disease transmitted from person to person by mosquitoes throughout the tropics and subtropics. It is an acute, nonfatal disease of particular importance to military operations because of its rapid spread and its ability to incapacitate large numbers of personnel at critical periods. Dengue fever is caused by any one of four closely related dengue virus serotypes (dengue 1-4) of the Flaviviaridae family.[26] The virus is transmitted primarily by *Aedes* mosquitoes, particularly *Ae aegypti,* an urban species that lives in close association with humans, and is distributed throughout the tropics.[27] Secondary vectors include *Ae albopictus* (the Asian Tiger mosquito, which was introduced into the United States from Asia in the late 1980s), *Ae scutellaris,* and *Ae polynesiensis* (Figure 21-7).[2]

The first epidemics of dengue fever were reported simultaneously in 1779 from Egypt and Indonesia and in 1780 from the United States. The first recognized epidemic of dengue hemorrhagic fever occurred in Manila in 1953 and 1954.[28] In the ensuing 20 years, dengue hemorrhagic fever spread to other parts of southeast Asia, and today it is one of the leading causes of hospitalization and death among children in southeast Asia.[29] Dengue fever was not considered a public health problem in the Americas until the latter part of the 20th century. During the 1970s and 1980s, dengue serotypes 1, 2, and 4 were introduced into the Americas.[30] The increased incidence of dengue and dengue hemorrhagic fever worldwide has resulted in an increased number of cases being imported into the United States. Additional details can be found in chapter 36.

Japanese Encephalitis. Japanese encephalitis is

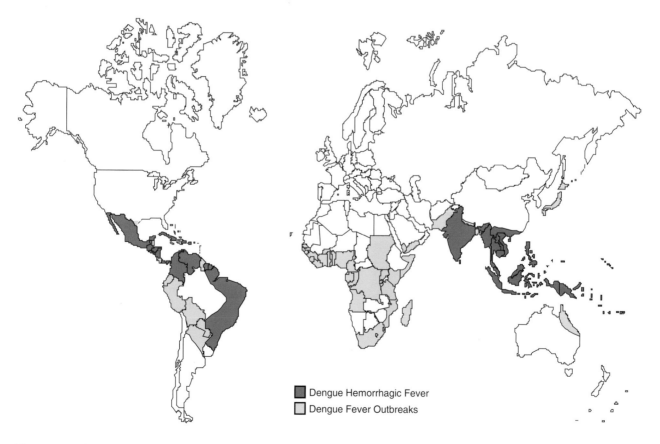

Fig. 21-7. The distribution of dengue fever outbreaks and dengue hemorrhagic fever. Map: Courtesy of Colonel David Vaughn, Walter Reed Army Institute of Research, Silver Spring, Md.

one of the major public health problems in Asia.[31] Outbreaks have been reported from Japan, Korea, Taiwan, Siberia, China, Okinawa, Thailand, Malaysia, and Singapore. They occur in warm weather in temperate regions and throughout the year in the tropics. Japanese encephalitis is principally a disease of rural agricultural areas, where vector mosquitoes breed in close association with pigs, birds, and ducks. Japanese encephalitis virus is a flavivirus and is maintained in mosquitoes and hosts other than humans. The principal vector of Japanese encephalitis is *Cx tritaeniorhynchus,* which feeds primarily on animals and birds. *Cx vishnui, Cx gelidus, Cx pseudovishnui,* and related species are the primary vectors in Thailand and India.[31] These mosquitoes breed in ground pools and especially in rice

paddies flooded with water. Studies have shown that the number of Japanese encephalitis cases is directly proportional to the density of the vector when an epizootic in pigs is in progress.[32] Transovarial transmission has been reported in *Ae albopictus* and *Ae togoi* (Figure 21-8). There have been occasional isolations from Anopheles mosquitoes.[2]

A vaccine affording excellent protection (> 90%) against Japanese encephalitis was licensed by the Food and Drug Administration in 1992 and is available for military personnel deploying to endemic areas. It is widely used in parts of Asia, such as South Korea.

West Nile Fever. West Nile fever (WNF) is probably one of the most common arbovirus infections of humans, considering its broad geographical distribution. It is still considered a disease of unknown origin, however, because of its infrequent epidemics. WNF virus, a flavivirus, has been implicated in outbreaks since 1950, but the largest known outbreak occurred in South Africa in 1974. Infection usually occurs in early childhood and produces only a mild febrile illness. In 1998, an outbreak of WNF occurred in New York City with 9 deaths.[33] WNF could have significant impact on military operations. For example, in an earlier outbreak in Israel, 636 cases of clinical disease were reported in a population of approximately 1,000 at a military camp.[34]

WNF virus has been isolated from humans and wild birds, but isolates also have been recovered from animals, including lemurs, chimpanzees, chickens, ducks, geese, horses, mules, donkeys, pigs, and cows. WNF virus has been isolated in 17 countries from three different zoo-geographic regions: the Palearctic, the Ethiopian, and the Oriental. The transmission activity of WNF virus indicates a seasonal pattern limited to summer months. All of the recorded outbreaks in Israel occurred from July through early September; reported outbreaks in South Africa occurred from December through April.[35]

In nature, WNF virus has been isolated from mosquitoes and ticks, but mosquitoes are considered the major vectors. Studies in Egypt, Israel, and South Africa have implicated *Cx univittatus* as the main vector in these countries.[35] *Cx neavei* has been identified in South Africa. *Cx vishnui* complex, containing *Cx tritaeniorhynchus, Cx vishnui,* and *Cx pseudovishnui,* has been implicated in India and Pakistan.

Rift Valley Fever. Rift Valley fever (RVF) is an acute, febrile, arthropod-borne yet contagious zoonotic disease caused by a bunyavirus of the genus *Phlebovirus*[36] (Table 21-2). Most arboviruses

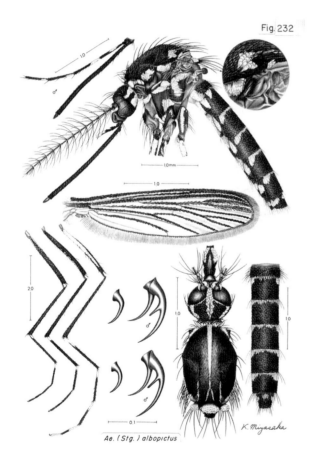

Fig. 21-8. Distinguishing features of *Aedes albopictus* Source: Walter Reed Biosystematics Unit, Department of Entomology, Walter Reed Army Institute of Research, Silver Spring, Md. Art by K. Miyasaka.

are associated with either a single species of mosquito or a closely related group of mosquitoes, except for RVF virus. RVF virus has been associated with numerous flood-water mosquito species, including members of the genera *Aedes, Culex, Anopheles,* and *Eremapodites.*[37] Other incriminated vectors include a biting midge (*Culicoides* species), a black fly (*Simulium* species), and a tick (*Rhipicephalus* species).[36]

RVF virus has been reported in 24 African countries. In 2000, it appeared for the first time outside of Africa when it caused a major epidemic in Saudi Arabia and Yemen.[38,39] A major epidemic and epizootic in Egypt from 1977 to 1979 caused an estimated 200,000 human infections and 598 reported deaths.[40] In May 1993, RVF virus was responsible for an outbreak in Aswan Governorate, Egypt.[41] RVF epizootics follow periods of excessive seasonal rain, which bring an increase in mosquito population. Outbreaks of RVF have occurred in areas of Africa as diverse as the dry low-rainfall climate of Egypt, the wet forested areas of Uganda and the Central African Republic, and the relatively dry, high veld areas of South Africa where winter temperatures frequently drop below freezing.

RVF virus may be maintained transovarially in flood-water mosquitoes, as demonstrated by the recovery of RVF virus from both male and female

TABLE 21-2

ARTHROPODS FOUND NATURALLY INFECTED WITH RIFT VALLEY FEVER VIRUS

Species	Locality	Species	Locality
Aedes		*antennatus, simpsoni,* and	Kenya 1982 Madagascar
aedimorphus		*vansomereni*	1979
cumminsii	Burkina Faso 1983	*theileri*	Kenya 1982 South Africa
dalzieli	Kenya 1982 Senegal 1975, 1983		1953, 1970, 1975
dentatus	Zimbabwe 1969		Zimbabwe 1969
tarsalis	Uganda 1955	*zombaensis*	Kenya 1982
durbanensis	Kenya 1937	*Eumelanomyia*	
Neomelaniconion		*rubinotus*	Kenya 1982
circumluteolus	Uganda 1955 South Africa	*Eretmapodites*	
lineatopennis	Zimbabwe 1969 South Africa	*quinquevittatus* spp.	South Africa 1971
	1975 Kenya 1982, 1984		Uganda 1948
palpalis	Central African Republic 1969	*Coquillettidia*	
Ochlerotatus		*fuscopennata*	Uganda 1960
caballus	South Africa 1953	*grandidieri*	Madagascar 1979
juppi	South Africa 1978	*Mansonia*	
Stegomyia		*uniformis*	Madagascar 1979
africanus	Uganda 1956	*Mansonioides*	
dendrophilus	Uganda 1948	*africana*	Uganda 1959, 1968
furcifer	Burkina Faso 1983		Central African Republic
Anopheles			1969
anopheles		*uniformis*	Uganda 1960
coustani	Zimbabwe 1969		
coustani and *fusicolor*	Madagascar 1979	Other Diptera	
Cellia		*Culicoides* spp.	Nigeria 1967
pauliani and	Madagascar 1979	*Simulium*	South Africa 1953
squamosus			
christyi	Kenya 1982		
pharoensis	Kenya 1982		
Culex			
antennatus	Kenya 1982 Nigeria 1967, 1970		
antennatus, annulioris gp,	Madagascar 1979		
simpsoni, and *vansomereni*			

Reprinted with permission from: Meegan JM, Bailey CL. Rift Valley fever. In: Monath TP, ed. *The Arboviruses: Epidemiology and Ecology.* Vol 4. Boca Raton, Fla: CRC Press; 1989: 51–76.

Ae lineatopennis collected from larvae in the field and reared to adults in the laboratory.[42]

The Equine Encephalitides. The Togaviridae include two genera, only one of which, *Alphavirus* (or Group A virus) is arthropod-borne. All but one of the 15 *Alphavirus* species are transmitted by mosquitoes.[3] The major Alphaviruses transmitted by mosquitoes are eastern equine encephalitis (EEE) virus, Venezuelan equine encephalitis (VEE) virus, and western equine encephalitis (WEE) virus.

EEE virus has been isolated in equine and human cases from Canada to Argentina along the eastern seaboard of the Americas and in the Caribbean region, southeast Asia, and eastern Europe. The main vectors associated with transmission of EEE are *Culiseta melanura, Ae taeniorhynchus, Ae sollicitans,* and *Ae vexans.* EEE virus generally causes a severe and often fatal encephalitis; its mortality ranges from 30% to 60%. Between 1961 and 1985, however, only 99 human cases were reported.[43]

EEE virus was first isolated in 1933 from the brains of horses and in 1938 was identified as causing an epidemic in Massachusetts. The viruses isolated from outside the New World have not been associated with human or equine cases. *Culex pipiens* is known to circulate this virus in bird–mosquito enzootic cycles in Europe.[44] The ecology is poorly understood, and the mechanism of spread to humans remains speculative. Research investigations suggest that EEE virus is maintained in North America in an enzootic bird–mosquito cycle. The main enzootic vector is a fresh water swamp mosquito, *Cs melanura,* which rarely bites horses or humans. Epidemics in humans and equines occur when the amount of virus in hosts living in swamp environments becomes high and it is carried by mosquitoes to birds and mammals outside of the swamp environment (Figure 21-9).

VEE is caused by a number of serotypes and causes fatalities in horses, mules, donkeys, and humans. In 1971, an outbreak of the 1B serotype of VEE virus occurred in Texas in association with a similar outbreak in Mexico.[45] Primary vectors during this outbreak in South Texas were *Psorophora columbiae, Ps discolor, Ae sollicitans,* and *Ae thelcter.* Other species of the genera *Culex, Anopheles, Mansonia,* and *Deinocerites* were also found infected in Texas and may be important vectors in other countries. Twenty major outbreaks of VEE between 1935 and 1971 have occurred in 11 countries but have mainly been centered in Colombia and Venezuela. VEE virus isolations from mosquitoes have mainly involved *Ae serratus, Ae taeniorhynchus, Ps confinnis,* and *Ps ferox.* A study[46] showed that VEE

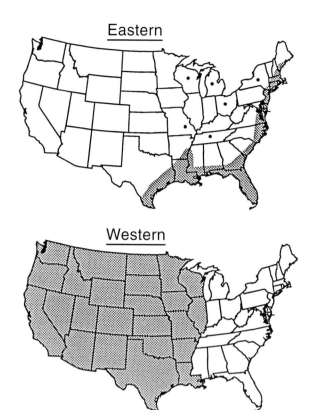

Fig. 21-9. The distribution of eastern and western equine encephalitis in the United States.
• Sporadic or focal infection reported
Source: Centers for Disease Control and Prevention. *Vector-borne Disease Control Self-study Course 3013-G.* Manual G. *Mosquitoes of Public Health Importance and their Control.* Atlanta: CDC; 1994: 4.

virus in *Ae aegypti* invaded many of the mosquito's tissues, with the highest levels in the salivary glands.

WEE is found in the United States west of the Mississippi River and in Wisconsin, Illinois, and Canada. It is also present along the eastern seaboard of North and South America and in eastern Europe. There were many major outbreaks in horses in the 1930s, with thousands of cases and many deaths. The largest human epidemic, involving approximately 3,000 cases, occurred in the western United States in 1941. Another large epidemic was reported in 1990 in the central valley of California.[47]

Culex and *Culiseta* mosquitoes are known vectors of this virus. In western endemic areas, *Cx tarsalis* is the most important vector of WEE because of its suitability for propagating and retaining WEE virus[48] (Figure 21-10). WEE has been isolated from *Cs melanura* in the eastern United States.[49] Isolations

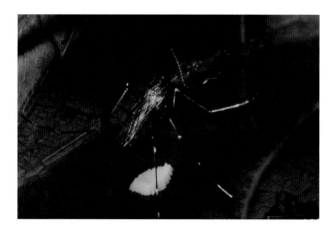

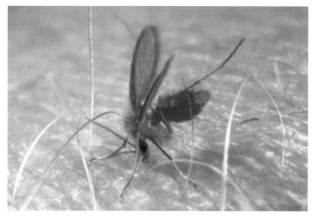

Fig. 21-10. *Culex tarsalis*, a major vector of western equine encephalitis.
Source: The Ken Gray Image Collection, Oregon State University Department of Entomology, Corvallis, Ore.

Fig. 21-11. *Phlebotomus papatasi*, a phlebotomine sand fly vector of Old World cutaneous leishmaniasis.
Photograph: Courtesy of Ed Rowton, Walter Reed Army Institute of Research, Silver Spring, Md.

of WEE virus have also been made from many other species of mosquitoes and from birds.[50]

Flies

Sand Flies

Sand flies are Diptera of the family Psychodidae. Nonbiting moth flies in the genus Psychoda are also in this family, but only the sand flies are medically important. Sand flies occur mainly in the tropics and subtropics, with a few species ranging into temperate zones of the northern (to 50° N) and southern (to 40° S) hemispheres. Distribution is limited to areas that have temperatures above 15.6°C for at least three months of the year. There are no sand flies in New Zealand or on Pacific Islands. The genera *Phlebotomus, Chinius* (represented by a single species in China), and *Sergentomyia* occur in the Old World and the genera *Brumtomyia, Warileya*, and *Lutzomyia* occur in the New World. Anthropophilic sand flies in the Old World are distributed mostly in the subtropics, with a few human-biters south of the Sahara and none in Southeast Asia. In the New World, they are limited mainly to the tropics.[3]

Characteristics. Sand flies are small (2–4 mm in length), delicate flies with long, thin legs and narrow, pointed wings with parallel venation (Figure 21-11). They are small enough to pass through the mesh of a standard mosquito net. At rest, the wings are held erect over the abdomen at a 45° angle. The proboscis of the sand fly is short, and the antennae are long. Only the females bite and suck blood, thus acting as disease vectors. The bite

of the female sand fly is typically sharp and painful and often causes considerable irritation. Extensive reviews of the biology and vector associations of New World[51] and Old World[52] sand flies have been published. There are over 700 species of sand flies that are found in a wide range of habitats.

Female sand flies require vertebrate blood for maturation of their eggs. Some species feed once between ovipositions; others may take multiple blood meals during a single oviposition cycle. Most human-biters feed at dusk and during the evening, but some species will bite during the daytime as well if they are disturbed in their resting site. Windless or nearly windless, dark conditions may suddenly induce great numbers of sand flies to seek hosts. The majority of anthropophagic sand flies are also exophagic, biting persons outside their houses. However, some species are endophagic, readily entering human dwellings, where they bite the occupants and either leave or rest inside.

The type of resting site used by adult sand flies varies according to species, availability of microhabitat, season, and amount of moisture present. In the New World, most species prefer the tropical rain forest. The forest has many microhabitats used by resting sand flies, such as on the underside of leaves; on or under tree bark, on tree trunks, and in animal burrows; in hollow trees; and in rock crevices and caves. In the Old World, sand flies tend to breed and rest in drier habitats. They can be found associated with termite mounds, cracks and fissures in the soil, animal burrows, piles of rubble, cracks in stone or brick walls, and caves. In peridomestic situations in both the New and Old World they may be found resting on walls inside human or animal dwellings.

Diseases Transmitted by Sand Flies

The Leishmaniases. The public health impact of the leishmaniases has been grossly underestimated due mainly to lack of public awareness. Only during the last 2 decades has it become increasingly apparent that most forms of leishmaniasis are much more prevalent than previously expected.[53] The leishmaniases are endemic on four continents in 22 New World and 66 Old World countries; 16 are developed countries, 72 are developing countries, and 13 are among the least-developed countries. Major epidemics of visceral leishmaniasis are in progress in Brazil, India, and the Sudan. In Bihar State in eastern India, it is believed that 200,000-250,000 people contracted the disease in 1993. In southern Sudan 15,000 cases were treated and 100,000 deaths occurred in a 5-year period (1991-1996). Cutaneous leishmaniasis is on the rise in many countries with epidemics ongoing in newly settled areas of the Amazon basin, North Africa and the Middle East.[53,54]

Among the more than 500,000 service members deployed to the Persian Gulf region during the Persian Gulf War, 28 cases of leishmaniasis were identified in personnel after their return from the theater of operations. Of these, 11 were identified as viscerotropic, and 17 presented with cutaneous lesions.[55] The causative agent of the visceral form, the protozoa *Leishmania tropica*, was previously thought to cause only cutaneous disease.[56]

Although not a war stopper, leishmaniasis is a persistent health threat to US military personnel because they are deployed or conduct military exercises in locations where the disease is endemic and its overall potential to compromise mission

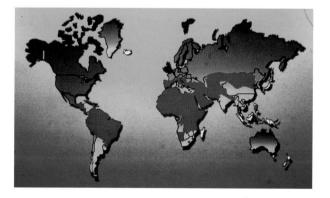

Fig. 21-12. The geographic distribution of leishmaniasis. Courtesy of Colonel Raj Gupta, MS, US Army, and the Walter Reed Army Institute of Research, Washington, DC.

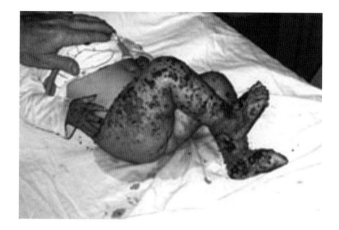

Fig. 21-13. Verruga peruana lesions on a child in Peru. This extreme case resolved after treatment.
Photograph: Courtesy of Richard Andre, Uniformed Services University of the Health Sciences, Bethesda, Md.

objectives is significant (Figure 21-12). Patients seen at Walter Reed Army Medical Center, Washington, DC, have included both active duty and reserve service members from all three branches of the US military, as well as personnel temporarily or permanently assigned to endemic areas. The number of units represented by this relatively small number of patients suggests that many more service members were at risk.[57]

Bartonellosis. Bartonellosis (Carrion's disease), also believed to be transmitted by sand flies, is caused by the bacterium *Bartonella bacilliformis* and only occurs in rural areas in the Andes mountains of South America. The disease causes two distinct clinical manifestations in humans: Oroya fever and verruga peruana. The former condition is characterized by severe hemolytic anemia, joint pains, pallor, fever, and jaundice. Mortality rates range as high as 40% if untreated. *Salmonella* infections are serious concomitant complications of Oroya fever.

The other, less life-threatening form of bartonellosis, verruga peruana, is named for the warty appearance of the skin of infected persons (Figure 21-13). These lesions usually develop following recovery from Oroya fever and may last for up to a year. The number and appearance of the painless nodules varies considerably. *Lutzomyia* sand flies are the suspected vectors of both forms of this disease.[58] Humans are thought to be the only known host.

Sand Fly Fever. Viruses in three families and three genera are transmitted to humans and other vertebrates by sand flies. Symptoms of human illness usually resemble influenza, with fever, retro-orbital pain, myalgia, and malaise. Complete recovery within a week is the norm, but encephalitis has been reported in at least two patients infected with vesiculovirus. Sand fly fever (also known as 3-day fever or papataci fever), the best known example, occurs in the Mediterranean region, the Middle East, Pakistan, and northern India where *Phlebotomus* vectors exist. Stiff neck and limbs, red face, severe headache, and painful neck muscles may occur. Long-lasting immunity is conferred after the first attack. The disease has been considered of military importance because up to 75% of nonimmune adults arriving in an endemic area can be affected.[59]

In the Mediterranean area, the sand fly *Phlebotomus papatasi* is the suspected vector of sand fly fever in humans. Although little if anything is known about transmission cycles, it is suspected that vertebrates, rather than insects, serve as reservoirs of the viruses.[2]

Black Flies

Black flies are blood-sucking Diptera of both public health and economic importance. Besides being disease carriers, they are annoying to humans and domestic animals because of their biting and crawling habits. Black flies belong to the family Simuliidae, which contains several genera but only one of which, *Simulium*, is an important human-biting fly. These are small, stoutly built, hump-backed flies. Only the female feeds on blood and is a daytime feeder. These flies have a worldwide distribution where suitable conditions exist; there must be well-oxygenated water for the immature stages to develop. The larvae feed by filtering particles from the water and brushing microorganisms into the mouth using a pair of prominent mouth brushes. Adults emerge from the water, often attacking in large numbers. In the tropics, there are multiple generations each year. The mouthparts of the female are short and broad. When feeding, they tend to stab the tissue and wait for the ruptured capillaries to ooze blood rather than sucking neatly like mosquitoes do. *Simulium* bites cause considerable pain and irritation and frequently become infected (Figure 21-14). The punctum heals by forming a characteristic black scab.

The parasitic round worm, *Onchocerca volvulus*, which causes onchocerciasis, is transmitted by *Simulium* species. Of the 18 million people infected with this parasite, more than 95% live in Africa.[60] The clinical manifestations of the disease include dermal nodules and lymphatic and systemic complications due to vessel blockage by the microfilariae. This causes severe itching, papule formation in the skin, and thickening and loosening of the skin, which subsequently hangs in folds. The most severe complications are onchocercal lesions of the eye, which may lead to blindness ("river blindness"). This affects

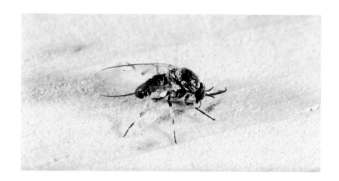

Fig. 21-14. A black fly (*Simulium* sp).
Photograph: Courtesy of Colonel Philip Lawyer, MS, US Army.

40,000 new victims each year. The 1990s, however, saw a decline in the prevalence of onchocerciasis infection and morbidity due to the remarkable success of vector control programs in West Africa.

Black flies also act as mechanical vectors of myxomatosis and certain arboviruses, such as Venezuelan equine encephalitis. However, this mode of transmission is normally of minor importance.

Tsetse Flies

There are at least 23 species of tsetse flies belonging to the genus *Glossina*.[61] These flies are found only on the continent of Africa south of the Sahara desert and infest an area of approximately 12 million square kilometers. They are larger than a house fly and can easily be recognized by the wings, which extend beyond the abdomen when the fly is at rest and lie one over the other like a crossed pair of scissors. The wings also have characteristic venation, with a discal medial cell shaped like a hatchet or cleaver (Figure 21-15). Both sexes of tsetse suck blood and feed

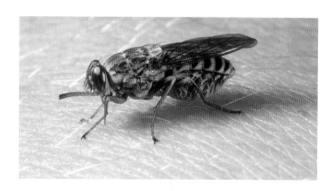

Fig 21-15. The tsetse fly (*Glossina morsitans*) after taking a blood meal.
Photograph: Courtesy of Ed Rowton, Walter Reed Army Institute of Research, Silver Spring, Md.

exclusively by day.

Two groups of *Glossina* are involved in the transmission of African trypanosomiasis or "sleeping sickness" to humans. Other species transmit the trypanosome causing nagana in cattle. The riverine areas of West Africa, mainly the Niger River and Congo River basins, are the habitat of *G palpalis*, vector of the chronic Gambian form of the disease caused by *Trypanosoma brucei gambiense*. Further inland, where the rivers shrink into pools in the dry season, the vector is the smaller species *G tachinoides*.[2,3]

In the dry bush country of East Africa, species of tsetse occur that do not require the humid conditions of river bank vegetation. *G morsitans* is found in wooded savanna where rocks and trees provide the shade that protects the fly from desiccation. *G swynnertoni* inhabits much more open terrain where the only shade is provided by large animals. Both species are associated with the Rhodesian form of the trypanosome found in wild game and infective to humans, *T brucei rhodiesiense*.

Deer Flies and Horse Flies

Although of only minor importance to military operations, deer flies and horse flies can be a nuisance in localized areas. Deer flies (genus *Chrysops*) and horse flies (genus *Tabanus*) are the two most common genera in the family Tabanidae. They are robust flies varying in length from 5 to 30 mm and have clear or mottled wings. The bite of female deer flies and horse flies can cause a severe reaction in a sensitized host, with considerable edematous swelling, pain, and irritation (Figure 21-16).

Species of *Chrysops* known as mango flies, *C silacea* and *C dimidiata* in tropical west Africa (from Sierra Leone to Ghana and Nigeria) and *C distinctipennis* in central Africa (southern Sudan and Uganda), transmit the filarial worm, *Loa loa*, which causes loiasis in humans. The microfilariae are taken up by the female fly from the peripheral blood of an infected human host during the day. The parasite is passed to the susceptible host during a subsequent blood meal. Adult worms live under the skin and migrate around the body, causing allergic "Calabar" swellings and abscesses at the site of the dead worms. The adult worm becomes visible to the patient if it crosses the anterior chamber of the eye, but it does not cause serious ocular damage. Occasionally, worms invade the brain, causing meningoencephalitis. Some tabanids, particularly certain species of *Chrysops*, are known to serve as mechanical vectors of tularemia, anthrax, and possibly other diseases.[62]

Filth Flies

The term filth fly is generally applied to flies that live in close association with humans (synanthropes) and which feed readily on human feces and other decomposing organic matter, as well as food intended for human consumption.[63] These flies are of medical importance because they act as mechanical vectors of pathogenic organisms, especially those causing enteric diseases.

The fly genera *Musca*, *Fannia*, and *Calliphora* all contain important filth fly species. These flies are medium-to-large, burly flies with conspicuous compound eyes and a well-developed thorax and abdomen (Figure 21-17). They lay eggs on feces or other decaying organic matter. The maggot-like larvae subsequently develop and consume the organic matter. The adult fly consumes only liquid food. The fly regurgitates fluid from its crop onto a food source to liquefy the material, and then sucks it up.

Throughout history, military personnel have suspected the association between flies and enteric

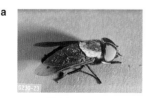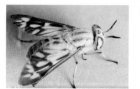

Fig. 21-16. (**a**) a horse fly (*Tabanus punctifer*) and (**b**) a deer fly (*Chrysops discalis*).
Source: The Ken Gray Image Collection, Oregon State University Department of Entomology, Corvallis, Ore.

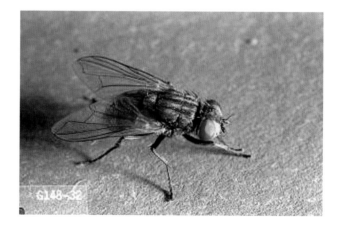

Fig. 21-17. A female filth fly (*Musca domestica*).
Source: The Ken Gray Image Collection, Oregon State University Department of Entomology, Corvallis, Ore.

diseases. They have observed that a rise in enteric disease follows a rise in fly populations. Greenburg discusses evidence that *Shigella*, *Salmonella*, infectious hepatitis virus, and typhoid fever virus are transmitted and spread by a variety of filth fly species. Effective fly control programs have demonstrated on many occasions that fly control can reduce the incidence of enteric disease.[63] However, there are many examples that caution against an exclusively entomological approach to the epidemiology of enteric diseases. There are many potential vehicles for transmission of such diseases, and their importance depends in part on the habits and lifestyle of the people involved. Thus, field sanitation and personal hygiene are as important today as they always have been.

Eye Gnats

Hippelates eye gnats of the family Chloropidae are an important group of synanthropes that frequent the face and eyes, as well as the mucous and sebaceous secretions and the wounds, pus, and blood of humans. Certain species have long been suspected as possible vectors of conjunctivitis and pinkeye or sore eye of humans and animals.[63] In Jamaica, *Hippelates flavipes*, which feeds avidly on humans, has been implicated in yaws transmission.

Adult eye gnats fly throughout the day. These flies are nonbiting but may produce minute incisions with their labellar spines. They feed on exudates of sores and cuts and around natural orifices.

Blow Flies, Bot Flies, and Flesh Flies

Myiasis is the term given to an infestation of living tissue by dipterous larvae. Some species of fly are

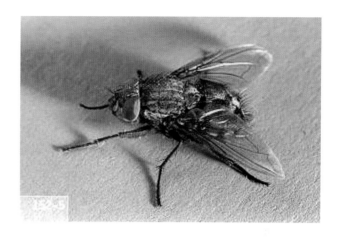

Fig. 21-19. *Calliphora vicina*, the flesh fly.
Source: The Ken Gray Image Collection, Oregon State University Department of Entomology, Corvallis, Ore.

unable to develop through their immature stages except on living tissue. This condition is known as specific or obligatory myiasis and is restricted to tropical species. Examples include the Old World screwworm (*Chrysomyia bessiana*), the tumbu fly *(Cordylobia anthropophaga)* and the Congo floor maggot (*Auchmeromyia luteola*) in Africa, and the New World screwworm (*Cochliomyia hominivorax*) and the human bot fly *(Dermatobia hominis)* in Central and South America. Specific myiasis occurs when fly larvae invade the skin. The infection presents as multiple painful blind boils in which secondary infection may occur (Figure 21-18). The head of the boil shows the black spiracles of the fly larvae. Treatment involves the suffocation of the larvae with an oily ointment, after which they can be removed with forceps; care must be taken to ensure that the larvae are removed intact.[5] Another method that seems effective and less likely to result in infection or other complications is commonly used in endemic areas of South and Central America. A slab of raw meat is placed over the boil and held there overnight. When the fly larva surfaces to breathe, it crawls between the surface host's skin and the meat, or it may burrow into the slab of meat and can then be removed. The presence of larvae can be psychologically distressing, but they are not usually life threatening.

Some larvae of *Calliphora*, *Lucilia*, and *Sarcophaga* (the flesh fly) species that normally develop on decaying organic matter will readily feed on wounds or other live, damaged, or contaminated tissue (Figure 21-19). This condition is known as semi-specific or facultative myiasis and can sometimes occur in the anal and genital regions. Accidental myiasis occurs when fly eggs or larvae are swallowed in food, and it results in intestinal disturbances.

a 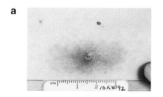 b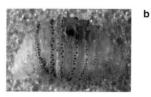

Fig. 21-18. A warblelike lesion produced by the larva of the human bot fly, *Dermatobia hominis*, is shown in photograph (**a**). A *Dermatobia hominis* larva is shown in photograph (**b**). The adult fly lays her eggs on the abdomen of a blood-sucking insect, such as a mosquito (and sometimes a tick). When the mosquito bites a host, the proximity of the *Dermatobia* eggs to the host causes the eggs to hatch and the bot larvae burrow into the skin.
Photographs: (a) Courtesy of Colonel Philip Lawyer, MS, US Army. (b) Armed Forces Institute of Pathology, Washington, DC.

Fleas

Fleas are small, wingless insects that can be important vectors of disease and often are serious pests. Their bodies are flattened laterally, are usually brown, heavily sclerotized, and generally possess bristles. The legs are well developed for jumping. The oriental rat flea, *Xenopsylla cheopis*, found on commensal rats in many parts of the world, is the most important vector of bubonic plague and murine typhus. The plague bacilli and murine typhus rickettsiae are ordinarily acquired by the flea during feeding on infected rats. Then the pathogens may be transmitted to humans in the absence of the flea's normal hosts, as when the rats are dying of plague in an epizootic. Plague exists in a sylvatic form in widespread parts of the world, and many of the 2,000 species of fleas are vectors of this disease.[2] Fleas can be very annoying, and their bites may produce itching and dermatitis in sensitive individuals.[5]

There are identification keys for most common fleas of public health importance. Fleas are generally discussed by families, which are based on the fleas' morphological characteristics and their ability to serve as vectors. The families are Ceratophyllidae, Leptopsyllidae, Pulicidae, and Tungidae. Family Pulicidae includes a significant number of species that are pests of humans, domestic fowl, and pets; are vectors of the plague pathogen; and are putative vectors of murine typhus to humans.

Fleas have piercing and sucking mouthparts and feed exclusively on blood. They lay their eggs on or among the hairs or plumage of the host or on debris on the ground. Eggs hatch into yellowish white, maggot-like larvae. The flea larva usually has one or two rows of sparse but well-developed bristles on most of its segments. The larva usually lives in the nest of the host and feeds on host-associated organic debris including food particles, dried skin, dried blood, or excreta. Larvae of some medically important species undergo three molts in 2 to 3 weeks. It may take a few months in other species. The larva spins a silken cocoon around itself, thus entering the pupal stage. The pupa develops into an adult in a few days. Adult emergence from the cocoon may be triggered by vibrations resulting from host movements. Adults may live for weeks or months, sometimes even without food. If environmental conditions are unfavorable, or if hosts are not available, developing adult fleas may remain inactive within the cocoon for extended periods.

Lice

Lice are small (1-4 mm long), wingless insects with elongated or discoidal bodies that are compressed or flattened dorso-ventrally. Three kinds of bloodsucking lice infest humans: body lice, head lice, and crab (pubic) lice. The head louse and body louse are somewhat elongated and similar in appearance, but the head louse is the smaller of the two. The crab louse is much smaller and has a nearly round, hairy body. The life cycles of these three species vary slightly, but all take place on the body or clothing of the host. The body louse confines its feeding to the host's body and remains on the clothing next to the skin. The head louse lives in the hair of the head and the crab louse among the hairs of the pubic region. The crab louse can also be found on the hairs of the legs, the chest, the armpits, and occasionally the beard and eyebrows.

The genera *Pediculus* and *Pthirus* contain the lice that normally infest humans (Figure 21-20). *Pediculus humanus*, containing both the head louse (*P humanus capitis*) and body louse (*P humanus humanus*—no longer *P humanus corporis*) of humans, is one of the three or four species included in genus *Pediculus*. Ferris[64] has discussed the nomenclature in detail. The genus *Pthirus* includes the crab louse, *Pthirus pubis*.

The most important member of this group is the human body louse. Historically, it has had a more profound effect on the history of humanity than has any other insect.[65] Lice have always been associated with wars because they thrive when sanitary conditions are poor and human populations are homeless and dislocated.

Head Lice

The head louse is gray but tends to resemble the color of the hair of the host. Head lice remain mostly

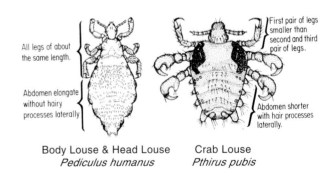

Fig. 21-20. The body louse, head louse, and crab louse. Source: Centers for Disease Control and Prevention. *Vector-borne Disease Control Self-study Course 3013-G*. Atlanta: CDC; 1994: 11.

on the scalp. Head lice have been pests of human-kind throughout history and pose no health threat to infested persons. However, the infestation may lead to embarrassment and social ostracism. Head lice are small (1–3 mm long), elongate, wingless insects that occur on the head and around the ears and occiput, but heavy infestations may move on to other parts of the body. The female lays the eggs on the hair. The eggs are glued to the hair and take about 5 to 10 days to hatch. The nymphal stage includes three molts before changing into the adult stage. The entire life cycle takes about 3 weeks.

Body Lice

The body louse looks almost identical to the head louse, but it usually stays on clothing and makes contact with the body while feeding. In heavy infestations, some lice may remain on the human body even when all clothing has been removed. Eggs are deposited in the seams of clothing. The incubation period varies from 5 to 7 days when eggs are laid near the body; it is longer at lower temperatures. After hatching, the young lice begin to suck blood at once and feed frequently throughout the nymphal stage. Like the head lice, the body lice nymphs go through three molts before becoming adults and the egg-to-egg cycle takes about 3 weeks. The optimum temperature for development is similar to normal human body temperature. The louse does not leave the body unless the body becomes too cold (death) or too hot (high fever). New louse infestations mainly occur during contact with louse-infested persons or their clothing.

Crab Lice

Crab lice are only found on humans and die within 24 to 48 hours if forced to leave the host.[66] The eggs are laid mainly on the coarse hairs of the pubic area. Nymphs pass through three molts before becoming adults. The total life cycle takes about 3 to 4 weeks. Pubic lice are transmitted from person to person, most often by sexual contact.

Diseases Transmitted by Lice

Three diseases of public health importance that are associated with lice are louse-borne (epidemic) typhus, trench fever, and epidemic relapsing fever. *Pediculus humanus humanus* is probably the sole vector of the organisms that cause these diseases. Louse-borne (epidemic) typhus has been recognized since ancient times and occurs mainly in Europe; the African highlands, especially Burundi, Rwanda, and Ethiopia; Asia; and the higher altitudes of Mexico, Central America, and South America.[2] The causative organism is *Rickettsia prowazekii.*

Trench fever is a nonfatal disease, and the causative agent is *Bartonella quintana.* This organism multiplies freely in the lumen of the louse's digestive tract and is not pathogenic to the louse. Epidemic relapsing fever has occurred in many parts of the world. The pathogen is a spirochete, *Borrelia recurrentis.* The insect can acquire the pathogen by a single feeding on an infected person but cannot directly pass it on to a second person. It is transmitted by crushing the louse and so releasing its infected hemolymph onto the skin.[67]

Bugs

The true bugs may be winged or wingless, but they always have a proboscis or beak suitable for piercing and sucking that is attached anteriorly and kept flexed under the head when not in use. The two bugs of medical importance belong to the families Cimicidae (bedbugs) and Reduviidae (assassin and kissing bugs).

Assassin and Kissing Bugs

These bugs are commonly called cone nose bugs because of their elongate (cone-shaped) head (Figure 21-21). Most Reduviids "assassinate" or kill other insects, but a small group of reduviids belonging to subfamily Triatominae exclusively feeds on the blood of vertebrates.[2] They are also called kissing bugs because occasionally they take the blood meal from around the lips of the host. The bites of these bugs are

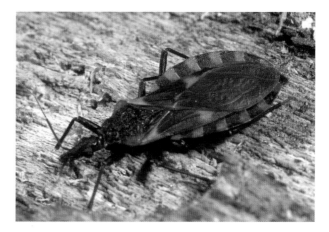

Fig. 21-21. An assassin or kissing bug (Family Reduviidae), which is the vector of American trypanosomiasis. Photograph: Courtesy of Ed Rowton, Walter Reed Army Institute of Research, Silver Spring, Md.

usually painless but may cause urticaria if the host becomes sensitive to the injected saliva. Chagas' disease, or American trypanosomiasis, is one of the most important arthropod-borne diseases in tropical America; it is caused by *Trypanosoma cruzi*, which is transmitted by various species of Triatominae. The four principal vectors of Chagas' disease in Central and South America are *Panstrongylus megitus, Rhodnius prolixus, Triatoma infestans,* and *Triatoma dimidiata.* The most important vector in Mexico is *T barberi,* while *T gerstaeckeri* and *T proctata* are important species in the southwestern United States, and *T sanguisuga* is found throughout the United States.[68] The victims of this disease are mainly humans, dogs, and to a varying extent other domestic and wild animals. The infection mainly occurs in rural areas of the tropics and subtropics, but may occur in suburban and urban areas around poorly constructed houses.

Both sexes of triatomid bugs bite, and they take their blood meal at night and hide in any cracks or crevices when not feeding.[3] The pearl-like eggs are laid singly around the adult habitat. The incubation period varies, depending on the species and temperature. The nymphs typically go through five developmental instars. Nymphs camouflage themselves with dust particles or other debris. In temperate regions, some species overwinter in the egg stage, others as adults, and still others as nymphs.

Bedbugs

Bedbugs have been associated with humans for centuries. Bedbugs have been occasionally found infected with anthrax, plague, and typhus disease organisms, but they are not considered an important vector of these diseases.[5] They are extremely annoying; their bites produce small hard swellings or wheals that are often confused with flea bites. The bedbug's principal medical importance is the itching and inflammation associated with its bite. Two bedbug species attack humans: *Cimex lectularius* (in temperate regions) and *Cimex hemipterus* (in tropical areas).[2]

Bedbugs are dorso-ventrally flattened, reddish brown, wingless insects approximately 5 mm long. They lay eggs in wall cracks, furniture, bedding, and other sheltered places. The eggs hatch in about 6 days, and if a suitable host is available, the young bugs begin feeding on blood. Immature bedbugs look like adults except they are yellowish white. The nymphs mature into adults in 30 to 45 days. Adults live for 6 to 8 months and may survive for several days without food. The adults lack hind wings, and the forewings are reduced to two small pads.

Stinging Insects

Allergic reactions to insect stings are a common and often a serious medical problem: estimates of anaphylaxis in the general population range from 0.3% to 3%.[69] Insects that sting are members of the order Hymenoptera. There are two major subgroups: vespids (eg, yellow jacket, hornet, wasp) and apids (eg, honeybee, bumblebee); ants belong to a third subgroup. In most parts of the United States, yellow jackets are the principle cause of allergic reactions to insect stings.

The stinging apparatus originates in the abdomen of the female insect. It consists of a sac containing venom attached to a barbed stinger. A sting occurs when the stinger is inserted into tissue, the sac contracts, and venom is deposited into tissue.

Bees and Wasps

Although Africanized honeybees *(Apis mellifera scutellata),* the so-called "killer bees," have received much publicity, their venom is no more allergenic or toxic than that of European honeybees *(Apis mellifera mellifera).*[69] However, Africanized bees are much more easily provoked and more aggressive than European honeybees. This behavior can lead to massive stinging incidents. These bees are expected to keep moving northward in the United States, although they do not survive well in colder areas.

Reaction to honeybee stings range from slight pain and swelling to much more serious symptoms, including anaphylaxis. In the United States, deaths from all hymenopterous insects (bees, wasps, yellow jackets, and ants) average between 40 and 50 per year.[70] A single bee sting is seldom fatal unless its victim is hypersensitive and has a severe allergic reaction. All persons should know whether or not they are hypersensitive to bee and wasp stings (Figure 21-

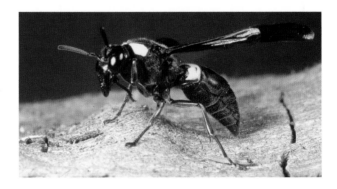

Fig. 21-22. A wasp. Photograph: Courtesy of Ed Rowton, Walter Reed Army Institute of Research, Silver Spring, Md.

22). Hypersensitive persons should carry insect sting kits when frequenting an area where interaction with bees and wasps may occur.

Honeybees are often encountered in swarms, which can remain in an area a few hours or days. Bee swarms are only temporary and will move away as soon as the bees find a new location to colonize. However, situations may occur that require the immediate elimination of bee swarms. Swarms may be eliminated with approved insecticides or by using high-volume sprays of a 5% solution of liquid dishwashing soap.[70]

Fire Ants

The fire ant, *Solenopsis invicta*, is a nonwinged hymenopteran. It is responsible for an ever-increasing number of allergic reactions in the United States and throughout its range in North and South America. With its jaws, the fire ant attaches itself to a person. It then pivots around its head and stings with the abdominal stinger at multiple sites in a circular pattern. Within 24 hours, a sterile pustule develops that is diagnostic of a fire ant sting.

CLASS ARACHNIDA

The class Arachnida includes such diverse forms as ticks, mites, spiders, and scorpions and is found almost exclusively in terrestrial habitats throughout the temperate and tropical regions of the world. The most important of the arachnids—ticks, mites, and spiders—lack distinct body segmentation; scorpions, pseudoscorpions, and a few others are obviously segmented. The body is divided into two parts, the cephalothorax (composed of the combined head and thorax) and the abdomen. In ticks and mites, the cephalothorax and abdomen are strongly fused, giving the body a sac-like form. These arthropods have four pairs of legs, at least in the adult stage; larval ticks and mites have only three pairs of legs. None of the arachnids possess antennae or wings. The mouthparts lack mandibles and usually consist of a pair of piercing chelicereae and the pedipalpi, and

in ticks and some mites, a hypostome. In general, arachnids are predatory or parasitic, although many mites are plant feeders or scavengers.

Like many of the medically important insects, ticks and some mites are important as mechanical and biological vectors of bacteria, rickettsia, viruses, and protozoa, which they transmit to humans and other animals by their bites.

Ticks and Mites

Ticks

There are three families of ticks, of which two contain species capable of transmitting pathogens to humans: the hard ticks (family Ixodidae) and the soft ticks (family Argasidae) (Figure 21-23). Hard ticks are

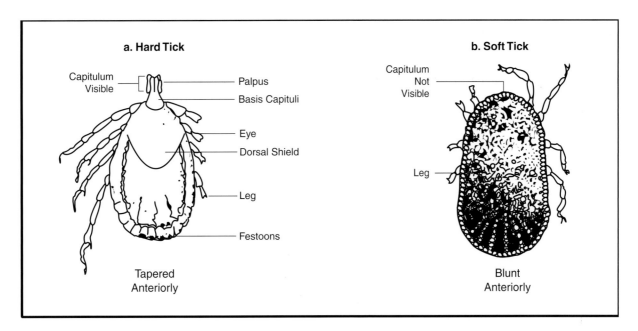

Fig. 21-23. The characteristics of female hard and soft ticks.
Source: Centers for Disease Control and Prevention. *Vector-borne Disease Control Self-study Course 3013-G.* Atlanta: CDC; 1994: 14.

oval with a sac-like body and vary in length from 2 to 10 mm when unfed, although the engorged female may be at least twice this size. They possess a hard dorsal plate called a scutum (hence the name "hard ticks"), and their mouthparts point anteriorly and are visible from above. Soft ticks are leathery and nonscutate. They are about the same size as the hard ticks. Their mouthparts point downward and are not visible from above.

Ticks feed by using their mouthparts to cut a small hole in the host epidermis; they insert the hypostome into the cut, thereby attaching themselves to the host. Blood flow is presumably maintained with the aid of an anticoagulant from the tick's salivary glands. Some hard ticks also secrete a "cement" to secure their attachment to the host. Blood-fed female ticks are capable of enormous expansion.

In the United States, more vector-borne diseases are transmitted by ticks than by any other arthropod.[71] Documented cases of ticks and tick-borne diseases affecting military personnel are increasing.[72] Ticks generally affect military operations in two ways: (1) directly, by tick bite and the accompanying psychological stress, and (2) indirectly, by disease transmission. Various bacteria, rickettsiae, viruses, and protozoa are transmitted to people via tick bites.

Lyme Disease. Lyme disease or Lyme borreliosis has emerged as the most common vector-borne disease in the United States. It also occurs in Eurasia and Australia. In the United States, 16,273 cases were reported in 1999[73] and nearly 50,000 cases were reported from 1982 through 1992.[74] Most human infections of *Borrelia burgdorferi* in the United States occur during the months of May through August, when tick activity is at its peak.

The causative agent of Lyme disease is the spirochete *B burgdorferi,* and it is transmitted by Ixodes ticks.[75] *Ixodes scapularis* (previously known as *I dammini*) (Figure 21-24) in the East and upper Midwest and *I pacificus* in the West are the primary vectors of this disease in the United States. *Ixodes ricinus* is the vector in eastern, central, and western Europe and *I persulcatus* in Japan, eastern Russia, and China.[76]

Tick-borne Relapsing Fever. Tick-borne relapsing fever is caused by *Borrelia* species other than *B burgdorferi* and is the one significant disease transmitted by soft ticks. In the United States, the geographic distribution of this disease is limited to remote, undisturbed natural areas in the West. The tick *Ornithodoros hermsi* transmits *B hermsi* in forested mountain areas, generally above an elevation of 900 m. In semi-arid plains areas, *Borrelia turicatae* is transmitted by *O turicata* ticks and *B parkeri* is transmitted by *O parkeri* ticks.[77] In general,

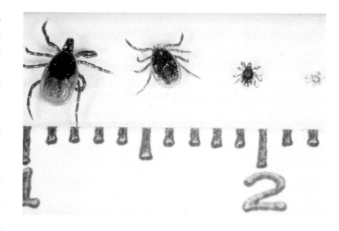

Fig. 21-24. Various life stages of the *Ixodes scapularis* tick. The larva has six legs and the nymph and adult have eight. The scale is in millimeters.
Photograph: Courtesy of Colonel Philip Lawyer, MS, US Army.

only sporadic cases of tick-borne relapsing fever are diagnosed, but isolated epidemics have occurred in such places as the Grand Canyon.[78]

Tick-borne relapsing fever has an incubation period of 4 to 18 days, after which the illness characteristically begins abruptly with high fever, chills, tachycardia, headache, myalgias, arthralgias, abdominal pain, and malaise. If the disease is untreated, the primary fever breaks in 3 to 6 days and is followed by an afebrile interval of approximately 8 days. Without treatment, 3 to 5 relapses typically occur. The severity of illness generally decreases with each relapse. Death is rare and limited mainly to infants and the elderly. Antibiotics are an effective treatment.

Tularemia. Tularemia is caused by the bacillus *Francisella tularensis*. The most important reservoirs for *F tularensis* are rabbits, hares, and ticks. The many modes of transmission include tick bite, direct contact with infected animal tissues, inhalation of aerosolized organisms, ingestion of contaminated meat or water, and bites of infected mammals, deer flies, or mosquitoes.[77] The three major tick vectors of tularemia in the United States are *Amblyomma americanum* (Figure 21-25) in the southeastern and south central United States, *Dermacentor andersoni* in the West, and *D variabilis* in many parts of the country. Tick bites account for about 50% of the tularemia cases in the United States. The incubation period of this disease is usually 3 to 5 days. The severity of tick-borne tularemia is highly variable and ranges from mild, afebrile, self-limited disease to cases of fulminating septic shock.[79]

Rocky Mountain Spotted Fever. Rocky Mountain spotted fever is caused by *Rickettsia rickettsia*

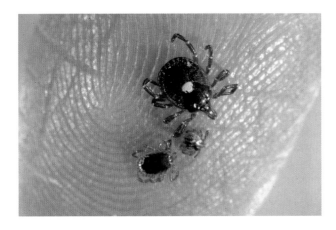

Fig. 21-25. *Amblyomma americanum*, the tick that transmits tularemia and human monocytic ehrlichiosis. The large tick at the top of the slide with the white spot is the female, the nymph is in the middle, and male is at the bottom. Photograph: Courtesy of James Occi, Biological Sciences, 195 University Avenue, Newark, NJ 07102.

and is transmitted by *Dermacentor variabilis* (Figure 21-26) in the eastern United States and *D andersoni* in the western United States. Although Rocky Mountain spotted fever is widely distributed across the United States, most infections are now acquired in the south Atlantic coastal region and the western and south-central states.[80] Three hundred sixty-five cases were reported in the United States in 1998.[81] This disease, if properly diagnosed, is easily treated with appropriate

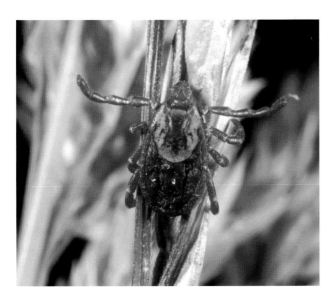

Fig. 21-26. *Dermacentor variabilis*, the dog tick. Photograph: Courtesy of Ed Rowton, Walter Reed Army Institute of Research, Silver Spring, Md.

antimicrobial agents. Death is usually associated with missed or delayed diagnosis and mistreatment.

Human Monocytic Ehrlichiosis. *Ehrlichia chaffeensis* is the sole causative agent of human monocytic ehrlichiosis in the United States.[82] This disease was first described in 1987 in a middle-aged man in Arkansas.[83] An outbreak of this disease also occurred in an Army Reserve unit.[84] Most of the 250 reported cases have occurred in the central and south Atlantic states. Recently, the ticks *D variabilis* and *Am americanum* have been identified as potential vectors.[77]

Ehrlichiosis generally presents as a nonspecific febrile illness that resembles Rocky Mountain spotted fever without the rash. Approximately 90% of patients have a history of a tick bite in the 3-week period preceding the onset of illness. Characteristic clinical features include high fever and headache, and other common symptoms include malaise, nausea, vomiting, myalgia, and anorexia. Acute complications, including acute renal failure, encephalopathy, respiratory failure, and death, are rare. Tetracycline (or its analogues) is an effective treatment.

Colorado Tick Fever. Colorado tick fever ("mountain fever") is caused by an RNA virus and is presumably transmitted by the tick *D andersoni*. Ground squirrels are the main vertebrate reservoir for this disease. The disease occurs in 11 Rocky Mountain states.[85] Most human infections are caused by tick bites, but the virus has also been transmitted by blood transfusion.[77]

Babesiosis. Babesiosis is a malaria-like illness caused by a protozoan parasite that invades erythrocytes. *Babesia microti* has been implicated in babesiosis acquired in the northeastern United States, and *B equi* is thought to be the causative agent of the disease in California.

Babesiosis is usually transmitted by the bite of *I scapularis* and *I pacificus* ticks. The white-footed mouse, *Peromyscus leucopus*, is the principal reservoir for *B microti* in the northeastern United States.

Tick Paralysis. Five tick species (*D andersoni*, *D variabilis*, *Am americanum*, *Am maculatum*, and *I scapularis*) can cause tick paralysis in humans. A neurotoxin that is produced in the tick's salivary glands is believed to cause the paralysis.[86] This toxin, which is usually transmitted by an engorged, gravid female tick, either blocks the release of acetylcholine at the synapse or inhibits motor-stimulus conduction.[77]

Diagnosis is made by finding an embedded tick, usually on the scalp. After removal of the tick, symptoms generally resolve within several hours or days. If untreated, tick paralysis can be fatal.

Boutonneuse Fever. An outbreak of boutonneuse fever in US Army personnel deployed to Botswana was reported in 1996.[87] More than 30% of the 169 deployed soldiers sought medical attention for boutonneuse fever symptoms. Subsequent serological tests indicated that 39 soldiers had boutonneuse fever. This disease is caused by *Rickettsia conori* and other rickettsia species and is believed to be transmitted by ticks. This disease has previously been reported from travelers returning from Morocco, Kenya, Botswana, and South Africa.

Mites

There are many free-living and predaceous mites, but some groups and families are exclusively parasitic. More than 200 families of mites are recognized in the entomological literature, but only a few contain species that affect humans. Some mites are vectors of organisms that cause human disease, and others cause dermatitis and allergic reactions in humans. Most species of mites are so small that they are barely visible to the naked eye. Their life cycles are often short (2 to 3 weeks), so mites can increase their numbers very rapidly under favorable conditions. For simplicity, the mites discussed here are grouped into five categories: chigger mites, house-dust mites, human biting mites, scabies mites, and follicle mites.[5]

Chigger Mites. Larvae of mites belonging to the family Trombiculidae are called "chigger mites" (Figure 21-27). There are approximately 20 different species in the family that are known to cause

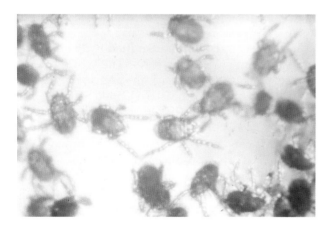

Fig. 21-27. Chiggers, which are trombiculid mites, are vectors of scrub typhus.
Source: Walter Reed Army Institute of Research, Silver Spring, Md.

dermatitis or transmit diseases. The larval body is less than 1 mm long and more or less round. As adults, they are about 1 mm long, oval or, more often, hour-glass shaped. They are most often bright red. Larvae are six-legged and the only parasitic form. The adults and nymphs are eight-legged and free-living. Chigger larvae do not burrow into the skin or feed primarily on blood. The formation of a feeding tube, or stylostome, at the site of chigger attachment is characteristic of chigger attack. It is presumably the action of the mite's digestive fluid that causes the attachment site to itch after a few hours.

The life cycle of chigger mites is very complex and includes six stages.[88] The female lays eggs singly on soil or litter, and the eggs hatch in about a week, exposing the six-legged larvae. The larval stage is the only parasitic stage. Larvae may attach themselves to many species of vertebrates. Engorged larvae leave the host and pass through a quiescent stage before they become nymphs and finally adults. The nymphs and adults are eight-legged and free living; they feed on insect eggs and other small soil invertebrates. The total life cycle takes about 60 days.

From a public health perspective, chiggers deserve attention because they are known to cause dermatitis and, more important, serve as vectors of scrub typhus. Chigger mites are found worldwide. Among the chigger mites that cause dermatitis is the European species *Trombicula autumnalis*, also known as the harvest mite, and *T alfreddugesi*, which occurs in the United States and parts of Central and South America. The chigger mite species that transmit scrub typhus, *Leptotrombidium deliense* and *L fletcheri*, are prevalent from New Guinea and the coastal fringe of Queensland, Australia, through the Philippines and China and westward through Southeast Asia to Pakistan.[2] *L pallidum* is reported as the vector of scrub typhus in parts of Japan, Korea, and the Primorye region of the former USSR.

Scrub typhus has caused significant casualties in Asian-Pacific military operations.[89] The American 6th Army in World War II lost more than 150,000 man-days during their operations in and around Schouten Islands and Sansapor beach head in Netherlands New Guinea.[90] The causal organism is *Rickettsia tsutsugamushi*. The disease has an incubation period of 6 to 21 days and is discussed in detail in Chapter 36.

House Dust Mites. House dust mites, in the family Pyroglyphidae, do not feed directly on living tissue but can be found in skin dander, stored food products, furniture, debris in household carpets, and areas that provide a variety of organic materials. Mites in the genus *Dermatophagoides* have been associated with house dust allergy and climate allergy.[91] The European house dust mite, *D pteronyssinus*, was implicated as an allergenic component of house dust to which most asthmatics are sensitive and that elicits the strongest responses.[2,92] The American house dust mites *D farinae*, *Euroglyphus maynei*, and *Glycyphagus destructor* have also been reported to cause allergies.[93]

Adult mites are plump and have well developed chelicerae and suckers. Their color varies from white to light tan. The life cycle takes about a month to complete, and adults may survive up to 2 months under optimum conditions. They are most abundant in home environments that are warm with high humidity.[94]

Biting Mites. The majority of the human-biting mites belong to the families Dennanyssidae, Macronyssidae, and Sarcoptidae. They are generally ectoparasites of poultry, wild birds, and rodents but may also attack humans, causing skin disorders and discomfort. The more medically important mites are the scabies mite and the hair follicle mite, which are discussed separately.

The tropical rat mite, *Ornithonyssus bacoti*, has been associated with debilitation, retarded growth, and high mortality in colonies of research mice. When the rats die or abandon their nests, the mites can travel considerable distances and bite humans, causing a sharp itching pain that may lead to development of dermatitis in sensitive individuals. The tropical fowl mite, *Ornithonyssus bursa*, is primarily an ectoparasite of poultry (it cannot exist for more than 10 days apart from its avian host), but it may bite humans. The bite causes only slight, temporary irritation.[2] *Ornithonyssus sylviarum*, the northern fowl mite, is a widespread parasite of poultry in New Zealand and Australia. The crawling of these mites is known to cause itching in personnel working on heavily infested farms. The chicken mite, *Dermanyssus gallinae*, commonly found on domestic fowl, pigeons, English sparrows, starlings and other birds, is considered one of the most common species causing dermatitis in humans, especially those working in poultry houses and on farms.

The house mouse mite, *Liponyssoides sanguineus*, is primarily an ectoparasite of mice but has been reported to feed on rats and other rodents and will readily attack humans. This mite is known to transmit the rickettsial pox pathogen to humans.

The etiologic agent is *Rickettsia akari*, which is primarily found in the house mouse, *Mus muscularis*, but may be transmitted to humans by accident.

The straw itch mite, *Pyemotes tritici*, belongs to the family Pyemotidae. It commonly attacks a variety of stored-grain insects and is highly toxic to humans. Dermatitis associated with *P tritici* is known as straw, hay, or grain itch. The infestation generally occurs after sleeping on straw mattresses, working in grain fields during harvesting, or coming in contact with various grains or materials infested with the mites.

Scabies Mites. The scabies mites belong to the family Sarcoptidae. The family includes the genera *Sarcoptes*, *Notoedres*, and *Trixacarus*, each producing a particular type of dermatosis (Figure 21-28). *Sarcoptes scabiei* causes scabies, also known as 7-year itch or Norwegian itch. The mite most often is found on skin between the fingers, at the bend of knees and elbows, on the penis, on the breasts, and on the shoulder blades. Rash and itching are not experienced in newly infested persons for up to a month after infestation. The rash and itching are directly associated with the burrowing of mites into the skin. Human scabies occurs worldwide.

Follicle Mites. Follicle mites, *Demodex folliculorum* and *Demodex brevis*, live in hair follicles and sebaceous glands, respectively.[95] They are mainly found around the eyelids, nose, and other facial areas. Most commonly, the infestation is benign but may result in the loss of eye lashes or in granulomatous

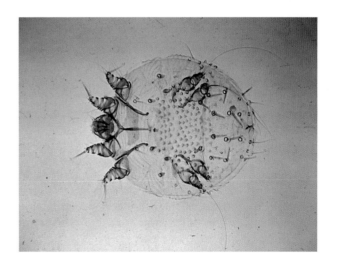

Fig. 21-28. A scabies mite.
Photograph: Courtesy of Richard G. Robbins, PhD, Defense Pest Management Information Analysis Center, Armed Forces Pest Management Board.

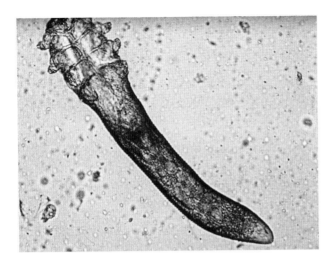

Fig. 21-29. The ventral view of the follicle mite *Demodex folliculorum.*
Source: Uniformed Services University of the Health Sciences, Bethesda, Md.

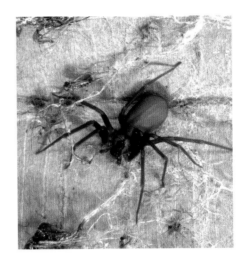

Fig. 21-30. The brown recluse spider (*Loxosceles reclusa*)
Photograph: Courtesy of Ed Rowton, Walter Reed Army Institute of Research, Silver Spring, Md.

acne.[96] The follicle mite is an elongated species (Figure 21-29).

Spiders and Scorpions

There are several thousand species of spiders worldwide and the size range is considerable, the smallest being a few millimeters in length and the largest having a leg span of up to 20 cm. Spiders use their mouthparts to capture their prey and sometimes cause paralysis by injecting venom. The venom of a few species is particularly toxic to humans.

Large, hairy tarantulas found in many tropical and Mediterranean countries are rarely dangerous, although their large size is commonly frightening. In contrast, the small widow spiders (ie, *Lactrodectus* species, which includes *L mactans*, the black widow spider) found in most temperate, tropical, and subtropical regions, can be particularly toxic and sometimes fatal. Other species (eg, the brown recluse spider, *Loxosceles reclusa*, Figure 21-30) can cause considerable necrosis at the site of the bite. The bite of almost any large spider, although not necessarily poisonous, may be contaminated with pathogenic bacteria and may result in extensive and dramatic secondary infection.

Scorpions are found in many parts of the tropics and warm temperate regions. They are found in both humid and arid areas. Adults have eight legs, large pedipalps, and a flexible tail with a needle-like stinger. They typically exhibit cryptic behavior, sheltering under rocks, logs, and other debris. All scorpions inject a paralyzing poison into their prey and feed on the fluid content. All these animals should be presumed to be dangerous and are to be avoided.

SUMMARY

Arthropods and the diseases they transmit have had devastating effects on US and foreign military forces in the past and there is great potential for these effects to be felt in the future. Arthropod-borne disease and injury can severely affect training and can render entire units temporarily or permanently ineffective. Deployed military personnel are particularly vulnerable to arthropods and often are immunologically naïve to the diseases they carry. One of the maxims of war is to know your enemy. This applies to arthropod enemies as well at to human enemies. The more preventive medicine professionals know regarding arthropods of military medical importance, the more likely they are to be able to implement countermeasures to protect service members.

Acknowledgment

The authors wish to thank Major (retired) Louis Rutledge, Dr. (Captain) Pollie Rueda, Dr. Michael Turell, Dr. Curtis Hayes, Colonel (retired) William Bancroft, Lieutenant Colonel Jeffrey Gambel, and Colonel (retired) Don Johnson for their insightful review of the chapter. Dr. Edgar Rowton, Dr. Richard Wilkerson, and Medical Audio-Visual Services personnel from the Letterman Army Institute of Research and the Walter Reed Army Institute of Research were very helpful with photographs and illustrations.

REFERENCES

1. Peterson RKD. Insects, disease, and military history. *Am Entomologist*. 1995;41:147–161.

2. Harwood RF, James MT, eds. *Entomology in Human and Animal Health*. 7th ed. New York: MacMillan Publishing Co; 1979.

3. Eldridge BF, Edman JD, eds. *Medical Entomology: A Textbook on Public Health and Veterinary Problems Caused by Arthropods*. Boston, Mass: Kluwer Academic Publishers; 2000.

4. Clements AN. *Development, Nutrition and Reproduction*. Vol 1. In: *The Biology of Mosquitoes*. London: Chapman and Hall; 1992.

5. Goddard J. *Physician's Guide to Arthropods of Medical Importance*. 2nd ed. Boca Raton, Fla: CRC Press; 1996.

6. Service MW. *Medical Entomology for Students*. London: Chapman and Hall; 1996.

7. Bates M. *The Natural History of Mosquitoes*. New York: MacMillan Publishing; 1949.

8. Christophers SE. Aedes aegypti *(L.) the Yellow Fever Mosquito: its Life HistoryBionomics, and Structure*. London: Cambridge University Press; 1960.

9. Clements AN. *The Physiology of Mosquitoes*. Oxford: Pergamon Press; 1963.

10. Gillett JD. *Mosquitoes*. London: Weidendield and Nicolson; 1971.

11. Gillett JD. *The Mosquito: Its Life, Activities, and Impact on Human Affairs*. Garden City, NY: Doubleday; 1972.

12. Horsfall WR. *Mosquitoes: Their Behavior and Relation to Disease*. New York: Ronald Press; 1955.

13. Oaks SC Jr, Mitchell VS, Pearson GW, Carpenter CCJ, eds. *Malaria: Obstacles and Opportunities*. Washington, DC: Institute of Medicine, National Academy Press; 1991.

14. World Health Organization. World malaria situation in 1992, I. *Weekly Epidemiol Rec*. 1994;69:309–314.

15. World Bank. *World Development Report 1993: Investing in Health*. New York: Oxford University Press; 1993.

16. Newton JRA, Schnepf GA, Wallace MR, Lobel HO, Kennedy CA, Oldfield EC III. Malaria in US Marines returning from Somalia. *JAMA*. 1994;272:397–399.

17. Centers for Disease Control and Prevention. Malaria among US military personnel returning from Somalia, 1993. *MMWR*. 1993;42:524–526.

18. Feighner BH, Pak SI, Novakoski WL, Kelsey LL, Strickman D. Reemergence of *Plasmodium vivax* malaria in the Republic of Korea. *Emerg Infect Dis*. 1998;4(2):295–297.

19. Otteson EA. Filarial infections. *Infect Dis Clin N Am.* 1993;7:619–633.

20. Michael E, Bundy DAP. Global mapping of lymphatic filariasis. *Parasitol Today.* 13:472–476.

21. Swartzwelder JC. Filariasis bancrofti. Coates JB Fr, Hoff EC, Hoff PM, eds. *Communicable Diseases: Arthropodborne Diseases Other Than Malaria.* Vol 7. In: *Preventive Medicine in World War II.* Washington, DC: Office of the Surgeon General, Department of the Army; 1964.

22. Zeilke E. Studies on the mechanism of filarial transmission by mosquitoes. *Z Tropenmed Parasitol.* 1973;24:32–35.

23. Sosa O, Carlos J. Finlay and yellow fever: A discovery. *Bull Entomol Soc Am.* 1989:35:23–25.

24. Reed W, Carroll J, Agramonte A, Lazear JW. Etiology of yellow fever, preliminary note. *Philadelphia Med J.* 1900;6:790.

25. Kumm HW, Novis O. Mosquito studies on Ilha de Margio, Para, Brazil. *Am J Hyg.* 1938:27:498.

26. Gubler DJ. Dengue. In: TP Monath, ed. *Epidemiology of Arthropod-borne Viral Diseases.* Vol 2. Boca Raton, Fla: CRC Press; 1988.

27. Gubler DJ, Trent DW. Emergence of epidemic dengue/dengue hemorrhagic fever as a public health problem in the Americas. *Infect Agents Dis.* 1993;2383–2393.

28. Hanimon W, Rudnick A, Sather G, Rogers KD, Morse LJ. New hemorrhagic fevers of children in the Philippines and Thailand. *Trans Assoc Am Physicians.* 1960;73:140–155.

29. World Health Organization. *Dengue Haemorrhagic Fever: Diagnosis, Treatment and Control.* Geneva: WHO Press; 1986.

30. Trent DW, Manske CL, Fos GE, Chu MC, Kliks SA, Monath TP. The molecular epidemiology of dengue viruses: Genetic variation and microevolution. In: Kurstak E, Marusyk RG, Murphy FA, Van Regenmortel MH, eds. *Virus Variability, Epidemiology, and Control.* Vol 2. In: *Applied Virology Research.* New York: Plenum Press; 1990.

31. Burke DS, Leake CJ. Japanese encephalitis: In: Monath TP, ed. *The Arboviruses: Epidemiology and Ecology.* Vol 3. Boca Raton, Fla: CRC Press; 1988: 63–92.

32. Fukumi H, Hayashi K, Mifune K, Shichijo A, Matsuo S, Omori N. Ecology of Japanese encephalitis virus in Japan, I: mosquito and pig infection with the virus in relation to human incidence. *Trop Med.* 1975;17:97–110.

33. Update: West Nile Virus activity—Eastern United States, 2000. *MMWR.* 2000;49: 1044–1047.

34. Klingberg MA, Jasinska-Klingberg W, Goldblum N. Certain aspects of the epidemiology and distribution of immunity of West Nile virus in Israel. *Proc 6th Intl Congr Trop Med.* 1959:5:132.

35. Hayes CG. West Nile fever. In: Monath TP, ed. *The Arboviruses: Epidemiology and Ecology.* Vol 5. Boca Raton, Fla: CRC Press; 1989.

36. Meegan JM, Bailey CL. Rift Valley fever. In: Monath TP, ed. *The Arboviruses: Epidemiology and Ecology.* Vol 4. Boca Raton, Fla: CRC Press; 1988:51–76.

37. Turell MJ, Presley SM, Gad AM, et al. Vector competence of Egyptian mosquitoes for Rift Valley fever virus. *Am J Trop Med Hyg.* 1996;54:136–139.

38. Update: Outbreak of Rift Valley fever—Saudi Arabia, August–November, 2000. *MMWR.* 2000;49:982–985.

39. Outbreak of Rift Valley fever—Yemen, August–Ocotber, 2000. *MMWR.* 2000;49:1065–1066.

40. Laughlin LW, Meegan JM, Strausbaugh LJ, Morens DM, Watten RH. Epidemic Rift Valley fever in Egypt: observations on the spectrum of human illness. *Trans R Soc Trop Med Hyg.* 1979;73:630–633.

41. Arthur RR, el-Sharkaway MS, Cope SE, et al. Recurrence of Rift Valley fever in Egypt. *Lancet*. 1993;342:1149–1150.

42. Linthicum KJ, Davies FG, Kairo A, Bailey CL. Rift Valley fever virus: isolations from Diptera collected during an inter-epizootic period in Kenya. *J Hyg (Lond)*. 1985;95:197–209.

43. Morris CD. Eastern equine encephalomyelitis. In: Monath TP, ed. *The Arboviruses: Epidemiology and Ecology*. Vol 3. Boca Raton, Fla: CRC Press; 1988.

44. Ising E. Zoological aspects of the epidemiology of EEE in Europe. *Angew Zool*. 1975;62:419–434.

45. Zehner RB, Dean PB, Sudia WD, Calisher CH, Sather GE, Parker RL. Venezuelan equine encephalitis epidemic in Texas, 1971. *Health Surv Rep*. 1974;89:278–282.

46. Larsen JR, Ashley RF. Demonstration of Venezuelan equine encephalomyelitis virus in tissues of *Aedes aegypti*. *Am J Trop Med Hyg*. 1971;20:754–760.

47. Reeves WC. Epidemiology and control of mosquito-born arboviruses in California. *Cal Mosq Vector Control Assoc*. 1990;XIV:508.

48. Thomas LA. Distribution of the virus of western equine encephalomyelitis in the mosquito vector, *Culex tarsalis*. *Am J Hyg*. 1963;78:150–165.

49. Saugstad ES, Dalrymple JM, Eldridge BF. Ecology of arboviruses in a Maryland freshwater swamp, I: population dynamics and habitat distribution of potential mosquito vectors. *Am J Epidemiol*. 1972;96:114–116.

50. Reisen WK, Monath TP. Western equine encephalitis: In: Monath TP, ed. *The Arboviruses: Epidemiology and Ecology*. Vol 3. Boca Raton, Fla: CRC Press; 1988.

51. Young DG, Duncan MA. *Guide to the Identification and Geographic Distribution of Lutzomyia Sand Flies in Mexico, the West Indies, Central and South America (Diptera: Psychodidae)*. Gainesville, Fla: Associated Publishers; 1994.

52. Killick-Kendrick R. Phlebotomine vectors of the leishmaniases: a review. *Med Vet Entomol*. 1990;4:1–24.

53. Desjeux P. Leishmaniasis, public health aspects and control. *Clinic. Dermatol*. 1996; 14:417–423.

54. Magill AJ. Epidemiology of the leishmaniases. *Clinic. Dermatol*. 1995; 13:505–523.

55. Kreutzer RD, Grogl M, Neva FA, Fryauff DJ, Magill AJ, Aleman-Munoz MM. Identification and genetic comparison of leishmanial parasites causing viscerotropic and cutaneous disease in soldiers returning from Operation Desert Storm. *Am J Trop Med Hyg*. 1993;49:357–363.

56. Magill AJ, Grogi M, Gasser RA Jr, Sun W, Oster CN. Visceral infection caused by *Leishmania tropica* in veterans of Operation Desert Storm. *N Engl J Med*. 1993;328:1383–1387.

57. Martin S, Gambel J, Jackson J, et al. Leishmaniasis in the United States military. *Mil Med*. 1998;163:801–807.

58. Hertig M. Phlebotomus and Carrion's disease. *Am J Trop Med*. 1942;22(Suppl):1–80.

59. Lane RP. Sandflies. In: Lane RP, Crosskey RW, eds. *Medical Insects and Arachnids*. London: Chapman and Hall; 1993.

60. Greenberg B. *Flies and Diseases*. Vol 1. In: *Ecology, Classification, and Biotic Associations*. Princeton, NJ: Princeton University Press; 1971.

61. World Health Organization. *Control and Surveillance of African Trypanosomiasis: Report of a WHO Expert Committee*. Geneva: WHO; 1998. WHO Technical Report Series No. 881.

62. Lehane MJ. *Biology of Blood-sucking Insects*. London: Harper Collins Academic; 1991.

63. Greenberg B. *Flies and Diseases*. Vol 2. Ecology, Classification, and Biotic Association. Princeton University Press, NJ; 1973.

64. Ferris GF. *Contributions Toward a Monograph of the Sucking Lice*. Stanford, Calif: Stanford University; 1935.

65. Zinsser H. *Rats, Lice and History*. New York: Bantam Books; 1967.

66. Fisher I, Morton RS. *Phthirus pubis* infestation. *Br J Vener Dis*. 1970;46:326–329.

67. Kettle DS. *Medical and Veterinary Entomology*. New York: John Wiley and Sons; 1987.

68. Ochs DE, Hnlica VS, Moser DR, Smith JH, Kirchhoff LV. Postmortem diagnosis of authochthonous acute chagasic myocarditis by polymerase chain reaction amplification of a species-specific DNA sequence of *Trypanosoma cruzi*. *Am J Trop Med Hyg*. 1996;54:526–529.

69. Reisman RE. Insect stings. *N Engl J Med*. 1994;331:523–527.

70. Armed Forces Pest Management Board. *Bee Resource Manual with emphasis on the Africanized Honey Bee*. Washington, DC: AFPMB; 1995. Technical Memorandum No. 34.

71. Centers for Disease Control. Lyme Disease—United States, 1987 and 1988. *MMWR*. 1989;38:668–672.

72. Goodard J. *Ticks and Tickborne Diseases Affecting Military Personnel*. San Antonio, Tex: Brooks Air Force Base; 1989. USAFSAMSR-89-2.

73. Centers for Disease Control and Prevention. Lyme disease—United States, 1999. *MMWR*. 2001;50:181–185.

74. Centers for Disease Control and Prevention. Lyme disease—United States, 1991–1992. *MMWR*. 1993;42:345–348.

75. Burgdorfer W, Barbour AG, Hayes SF, Benach JL, Grunwaldt E, Davis JP. Lyme disease—a tick bome spirochetosis? *Science*. 1982;216:1317–1319.

76. US Department of Defense. Lyme disease: Vector surveillance and control. Washington, DC: Armed Forces Pest Management Board; 1990. Technical Information Memorandum No. 26.

77. Spach DH, Liles WC, Campbell GL, Quick RE, Anderson DE Jr, Fritsche TR. Tick-borne diseases in the United States. *N Engl J Med*. 1993;329:936–947.

78. Horton JM, Blaser MJ. The spectrum of relapsing fever in the Rocky Mountains. *Arch Intern Med*. 1985;145:871–875.

79. Evans ME, Gregory DW, Schaffner W, McGee ZA. Tularemia: A 30-year experience with 88 cases. *Medicine (Baltimore)*. 1985;64:251–269.

80. Centers for Disease Control. Lyme disease—United States, 1987 and 1988. *MMWR*. 1990;38:668–672.

81. Centers of Disease Control and Prevention. Summary of notifiable diseases, United States, 1998. *MMWR*. 1999;47:1–92.

82. Anderson BE, Dawson JE, Jones DC, Wilson KH. *Ehrlichia chaffeensis*, a new species associated with human ehrlichiosis. *J Clin Microbiol*. 1991;29:2838–2842.

83. Maeda K, Markowitz N, Hawley RC, Ristic M, McDade JE. Human infection with *Ehrlichia canis*, a leukocyte rickettsia. *N Engl J Med*. 1987;316:853–856.

84. Petersen LR, Sawyer LA, Fishbein DB, et al. An outbreak of ehrlichiosis in members of an Army Reserve unit exposed to ticks. *J Infect Dis*. 1989;159:562–568.

85. Emmons RW. An overview of Colorado tick fever. *Prog Clin Biol Res*. 1985;178:47–52.

86. Kaire GH. Isolation of tick paralysis toxin from *Ixodes holocyclus*. *Toxicon*. 1966;4:91–97.

87. Smoak BL, McClain B, Brundage JF, et al. An outbreak of spotted fever rickettsiosis in U.S. Army troops deployed to Botswana. *J Emerging Infect Dis.* 1996;2:217–221.

88. Sasa M. Biology of chiggers. *Ann Rev Entomol.* 1961;6:221–244.

89. Philip CB. Tsutsugamushi disease (scrub typhus) in World War II. *J Parasitol.* 1948;34:169–191.

90. Philip CB. Scrub typhus and scrub itch. Coates JB Fr, Hoff EC, Hoff PM, eds. *Communicable Diseases: Arthropodborne Diseases Other than Malaria.* Vol 7. In: *Preventive Medicine in World War II.* Washington, DC: Office of the Surgeon General, Department of the Army; 1964.

91. Lang JD, Chariet LD, Mulla MS. Bibliography (1864–1974) of house dust mites *Dertnatophagoides* spp. (Acarina: Pyroglyphidae), and human allergy. *J Sci Biol.* 1976;2:62–83.

92. Fain A. Le genre Dermatophagoides Bogdanov 1864, son importance dans les allergies respiratoires et cutainees chez l'homme (Psoroptidae: Sarcoptiforines). *Acarologia.* 1967;9:179–225.

93. Wharton GW. House dust mites. *J Med Entomol.* 1976;12:577–621.

94. Murton JJ, Madden JL. Observations on the biology, behavior and ecology of the house dust mite, *Dermatophagoides pteronyssinus* in Tasmania. *J Aust Entomol Soc.* 1977;16:281.

95. Desch C, Nutting WB. *Demodex folliculorum* (Simon) and *D. brevis akbulatova* of man: redistribution and reevaluation. *J Parasitol.* 1972;58:169–177.

96. Grosshans EM, Kremer M, Maleville J. [*Demodex folliculorum* and the histogenesis of granulomatous rosacea.] *Hautarzt.* 1974;25:166–177.

Chapter 22

PERSONAL PROTECTION MEASURES AGAINST ARTHROPODS

RAJ K. GUPTA, PhD; JEFFREY M. GAMBEL, MD, MPH, MSW; and BERNARD A. SCHIEFER, MS

R. K. Gupta; Colonel, MS, US Army; Research Area Director, Research Plans and Programs, US Army Medical Research and Materiel Command, Fort Detrick, Frederick, MD 21702-7581; formerly, Department of Entomology, Division of Communicable Diseases and Immunology, Walter Reed Army Institute of Research, Silver Spring, Md.

J. M. Gambel; Lieutenant Colonel, MC, US Army; Staff Physiatrist, Walter Reed Army Medical Center; formerly, Chief, Field Studies, Division of Preventive Medicine, Walter Reed Army Institute of Research, Silver Spring, MD 20910-7500

B. A. Schiefer; Colonel, Medical Service, US Army (Retired); formerly, Entomology Consultant, Office of The Surgeon General, US Army

INTRODUCTION

Proper use of a system of personal protection measures (PPMs) can be very effective in preventing disease transmission and reducing nuisance bites by biting or blood-sucking arthropods. The US military's system of PPMs includes the application of insect repellents on skin and field clothing and proper wearing of the field uniform. Operational doctrine supports the use of PPMs whenever the risk of receiving insect bites is significant, including the relatively few instances when vaccines (eg, yellow fever and Japanese encephalitis vaccines) or chemoprophylaxis (eg, anti-malarial pills) are also available to prevent arthropod-borne diseases. A medical threat assessment performed before deployment is essential in defining the risk that insect bites pose to deployed personnel. In addition to PPMs, unit-level preventive medicine and field sanitation teams in each service play a crucial role in vector control. In many tactical field situations involving combat or rapid troop movements, use of PPMs may be the only practical option to prevent arthropod-related casualties. Even in those tactically stable situations where pesticide application may be possible, widespread use of pesticides may be impractical because of the time, personnel, and equipment needed to perform area pesticide application, plus the hazard to the environment and the contribution to increasing vector resistance. Service members must be capable of using and adhering to the US military's system of PPMs when they are at significant risk of becoming arthropod-related casualties (Figure 22-1).

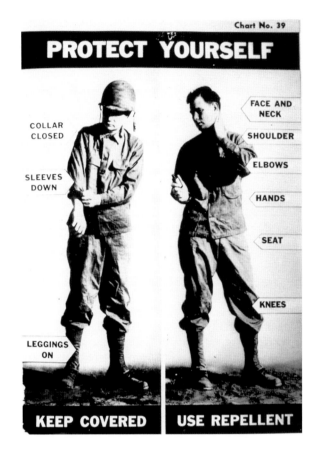

Fig. 22-1. Personal protection measures have protected US forces in the past and their correct usage continues to protect today's service members.
US War Department poster, 1945. From the Letterman Army Institute of Research, Presidio of San Francisco, Calif.

THE ARTHROPOD THREAT

The arthropod threat to a military force includes contact with disease vectors and nuisance factors. Arthropods can inflict severe physiological stress, and their bites can be painfully distracting and lead to devastating secondary infections, dermatitis, and allergic reactions. Arthropods can cause serious erosions in individual and unit performance. A study[1] in the Karelian Republic, Russia, showed that use of an insect repellent (dimethyl phthalate) increased the efficiency of workers in logging camps by 25%. In military terms, this could be the equivalent of several extra battalions in every division. The diseases transmitted by insects are equally important. Four of the most important parasitic diseases of humans are arthropod-borne. Of the 80 diseases important to military operations, more than two thirds are transmitted by arthropods.[2] Both indi-

vidual and unit adherence to PPMs is essential if arthropod-related casualties are to be minimized.

There are many examples that illustrate the detrimental affect of arthropod-borne disease and nonbattle injuries on military campaigns. One of the most striking examples depicts the tremendous losses suffered by Napoleon's army during his campaign of 1812. In June 1812, Napoleon invaded Russia with 422,000 men. In September, the army reached Moscow, but by this time, he had lost seven of every ten soldiers to epidemic louse-borne typhus[3] (Figure 22-2). With the force already reduced by disease, cold injuries on the retreat from Moscow completed the rout. Dysentery and pneumonia together with typhus reduced the Grande Armee further and by June 1813, fewer than 3,000 of the original force were alive.[4]

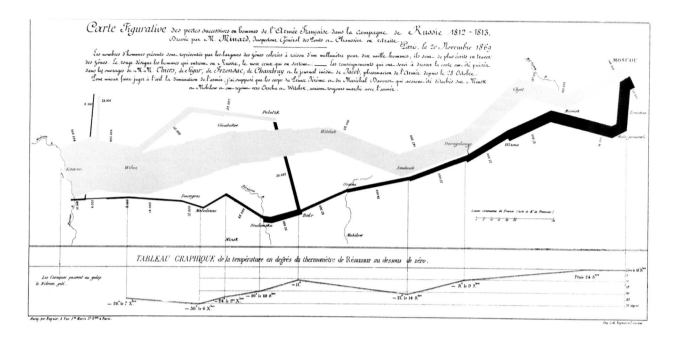

Fig. 22-2. Normally, Napoleon's campaign in Russian in 1812 is given as a classic example of the effects of environmental injury of an army. It is also an example of the effects arthropod-borne disease can have. As described by Robinson* in June 1812, Napoleon invaded Russia entering from the Polish-Russian border near the Nieman River with 422,000 men. The width of the band indicates the size of the army at each place on the map. The movements of auxiliary troops are also shown, as they sought to protect the rear and the flank of the advancing army. The path of Napoleon's retreat from Moscow is depicted by the darker, lower band, which is linked to a temperature scale and dates at the bottom of the chart. Typhus struck down seven in ten of the Grand Armee on its march into Russia. With the force already reduced by disease, cold injuries completed the devastation. It was a particularly cold winter, and many froze to death on the march out of Russia. After a disastrous crossing of the Berezina River, the army finally struggled back to its starting point with only 10,000 men remaining.
* Robinson AH. The thematic maps of Charles Joseph Minard. *Imago Mundi.* 1967;21:95–108. Map reproduced with permission from Edward R. Tufte. *The Visual Display of Quantitative Information.* Cheshire, Conn: Graphics Press; 1983.

Historically, malaria has been and still remains one of the most serious arthropod-borne disease threats for the US military, particularly the Army, in strategic parts of the world. During World War I, an estimated 2 million man-days were lost to the debilitating effects of malaria.[5] Nearly 695,000 cases occurred during the 4 years the US fought in World War II, with an estimated 12 million man-days lost to the US forces during that period.[6] During the Korean War, US forces reported 390,000 cases of malaria, and during the Vietnam War, more than 50,000 cases occurred among US military personnel.[7] Malaria, as well as dengue fever, has been reported during more recent deployments, such as Operation Restore Hope in Somalia.[8–10]

Future US military operations will continue to expose military personnel to region-specific biting arthropods and the vector-borne diseases they carry. The degree of exposure will largely depend on environmental factors and operational intensity. Success of high-intensity field operations in regions of significant arthropod biting may be associated with service members' adherence to an effective system of PPMs. One lesson to be learned from the medical management of disease casualties from past wars is that the military must prepare during peacetime to meet the emergencies of war.[11]

PROPER AREA CONTROL AND SANITATION

Minimizing the impact of arthropod bites and related diseases in the field begins with proper area control and sanitation. A careful decision regarding where to establish bivouac sites can greatly aid the effectiveness of field sanitation activities. For example, exposure to arthropods can be avoided or reduced if operational field sites and bivouac areas are established on high, well-drained ground away from arthropod habitats and breeding areas.[12] It may be important to clear environments of underbrush that support arthropod-resting sites or animal hosts. Clearing may take the form of raking and cutting grass. If controlled burning is to be used, considerable environmental expertise and planning is essential. Mosquito breeding areas—usually standing water sites or discarded containers such as tires and 55-gallon drums—should be eliminated by draining, filling, or relocating discarded containers where they can be destroyed using methods approved by environmental authorities. Standing water should not be created or allowed around water points, laundry facilities, and other military operations. Area application of pesticides, which must only be done by trained personnel, should be

considered by preventive medicine professionals only if other interventions do not achieve the needed level of control. Service members normally should not enter pesticide-treated areas until residual pesticide has completely dried.

Some arthropod species and their animal hosts are attracted to decaying food and waste. Therefore, it is essential that all deployed personnel follow excellent field sanitation practices ("stash your trash") to minimize materials that might attract pests and vermin. Although Army field sanitation teams and their equivalents in the other services play key roles in managing effective area control and field sanitation programs, persistent command emphasis mandating the participation of each individual is vital to unit success.[13,14]

DEPARTMENT OF DEFENSE PERSONAL PROTECTION MEASURES SYSTEM

The most effective personal protection system is a combination of three elements: controlled-release deet (*N,N*-diethyl-1,3-methylbenzamide) as a topical repellent, permethrin-treated field uniforms, and proper wearing of the field uniform (Figure 22-3). This system of overlapping protection is necessary because it is usually necessary to defend against several types of biting arthropods simultaneously under changing field conditions and each component of the system has its own limitations. Sand flies and biting midges cannot bite through clothing, so proper wearing of the uniform plus insect repellents will be effective against them. Clothing impregnation with repellents may be necessary to provide protection from mosquitoes, tsetse flies, deer flies, and many other insects that can bite through the field uniform. Ticks and other insects attempt to crawl under clothing; therefore, routine buddy checks may be indicated.

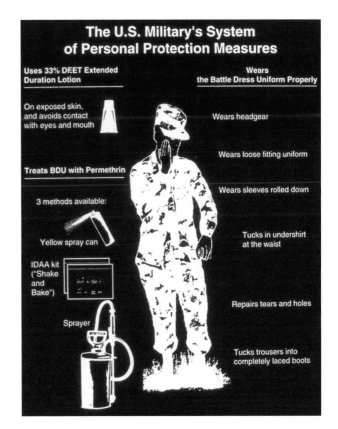

Fig. 22-3. To be most effective, adherence to all three components of the US military's system of personal protection measures is essential.
Graphic courtesy of Kathleen Huycke, Walter Reed Army Institute of Research, Silver Spring, Md.

INSECT REPELLENTS

Along with proper area control and sanitation, use of insect repellents is a vital countermeasure in reducing arthropod-related casualties. Dethier[15] defines a repellent as a chemical that causes the insect to make oriented movement away from its source. Repellents may be classified based on their site of application or their mode of action. The two

important types of insect repellents are topical repellents and clothing repellents. Based on the mode of action, insect repellents can be further classified as vapor (or olfactory or spatial) repellents and contact (or gustatory) repellents. Repellents such as deet, dimethyl phthalate, and ethyl hexanediol depend on their vapors to keep insects at a distance,[16] but the contact repellents, such as Indalone, are slightly volatile so that the insect must touch the treated surface before being repelled.[17,18] Permethrin, which functions as a contact repellent and contact insecticide, as well as a short-range olfactory repellent, has largely replaced every other repellent in the military system for use on clothing and other fabric items.

The identity of the first repellents used by humans is lost in prehistory, but they were no doubt similar to those in use as folk remedies today. In the Jeypore and Madras regions of India, women and girls apply turmeric (*Curcuma longa*, Family Zingiberaceae) in vegetable oil daily for protection against mosquitoes.[19] In some areas of Mexico, the women apply anatto (*Bixa orellana*, Bixaceae) in vegetable or animal oil to the men to protect them against mosquitoes and other insects when they go to hunt, fish, or work.[20] The first recorded use of repellents has not been determined, but Pliny (23–79 AD) and Dioscorides (fl. 60 AD) described use of wormwood juice (*Artemisia absinthium*, Compositae) to repel gnats and fleas.[21] Pliny also described use of the leaves and fruits of citron (*Citrus medica*, Rutaceae) to repel insects from stored clothing.[22]

In the early years of the 20th century, an assortment of natural products, both inorganic and botanical, were still being used to repel insects. Sulfur was dusted on skin and clothing to repel chiggers.[23] Application of a 1:10 solution of Epsom salts (hydrated calcium sulfate) was prescribed by the US Army Medical Field Service School in the 1930s to repel mosquitoes.[24] The preeminent botanical materials were pyrethrum (*Chrysanthemum cinerariaefolium*, Compositae) and citronella (*Cymbopogon nardus*, Gramineae). Sulfur, pyrethrum, and citronella are still in use today in some commerical products.[25]

Topical Repellents

Repellents for topical use are available in a wide variety of forms. These include lotions, creams, foams, soaps, aerosols, sticks, and towelettes. In general, formulations containing greater concentrations of active ingredient provide more effective and long-lasting protection. Aesthetic acceptance of the repellent by the user, though, has a major impact on the amount used and the frequency of use of the various products.

The first synthetic repellents to gain wide acceptance were dimethyl phthalate and dibutyl phthalate, which was patented in 1929.[26] By the end of World War II, dimethyl phthalate, ethyl hexanediol (also called Rutgers 612), and Indalone (butyl-3,3-

dihydro-2,2-dimethyl-4-oxo-2H-pyran-6-carboxylate) had been identified as superior mosquito repellents.[27] These were recommended for military use. Dimethyl pthalate is effective against *Anopheles* mosquitoes but less effective against *Aedes* species, whereas the reverse is true with ethyl hexanediol. After the war, combinations of repellents were developed to exploit the respective advantages of these individual components in a single product. The 6-2-2 repellent contained dimethyl phthalate, ethyl hexanediol, and Indalone in the proportion 6:2:2. Dimethyl phthalate and Indalone are still in limited use in 2001, but in 1991 the US Environmental Protection Agency (EPA) canceled all registrations of ethyl hexanediol at the request of its manufacturers because of new information on possible adverse fetal developmental effects.[28]

Deet

Perhaps the single most important event in the evolution of repellents was the discovery of deet in 1954.[29] It has virtually eclipsed other repellents for topical use, and it remains the principal repellent in use today, more than 40 years after its discovery. Deet was initially marketed commercially in 1956, and 75% deet in alcohol was adopted as the standard topical and clothing repellent by the US military in 1957[30] (Figure 22-4). Even though deet is an effective repellent against a broad spectrum of arthropods, it has several drawbacks. Under warm, humid conditions, the application lasts for only 1 to 2 hours. It is a strong plasticizer, has a disagreeable odor, and feels "oily" to some service members. Results from a survey conducted in 1983 indicated that 62% of more than 1,500 troop respondents thought that the Army needed a better repellent.[31] The Armed Forces Pest Management Board has endorsed development of more effective insect repellents for military use.

In the early 1980s, research at Letterman Army Institute of Research (Presidio, San Francisco, Calif) demonstrated the feasibility of various extended-duration mechanisms to release deet at a predetermined rate that was sufficient to prevent insect bites. Subsequently the US Army Medical Materiel and Acquisition Activity (Fort Detrick, Md) worked with private industry to formulate an effective extended-duration deet repellent for topical application to meet the following operational specifications: (*a*) provide at least 12 hours of protection against a wide variety of arthropods, (*b*) be nonirritating and nonallergenic, (*c*) be odorless at a distance of 10 feet, (*d*) have no objectionable oily

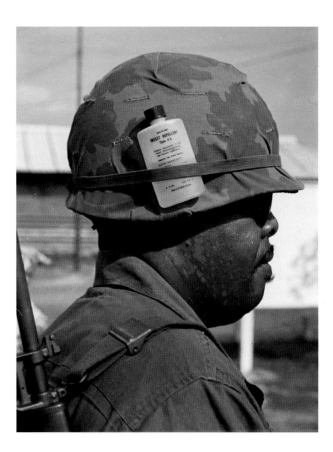

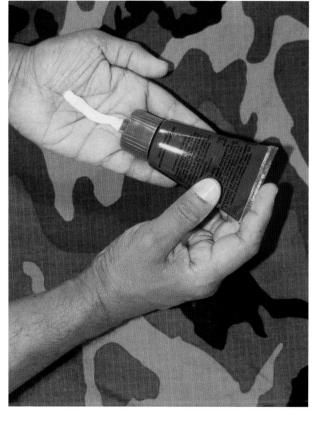

Fig. 22-4. 75% deet in the bottle was the military-issue topical and clothing repellent during the Vietnam Conflict. Photograph: Courtesy of the Walter Reed Army Institute of Research, Silver Spring, Md.

Fig. 22-5. The standard military insect repellent now in use. Photograph: Courtesy of the Walter Reed Army Institute of Research, Silver Spring, Md.

appearance or feel on the skin, (*e*) be inert to commonly used plastics, and (*f*) have a shelf life of at least 2 years. Prototype repellent formulations from various manufacturers were tested in a variety of laboratory and field conditions. An extended-duration topical arthropod repellent formulation of deet produced by 3M Company was selected in 1989 as the standard military insect repellent, personal application (NSN 6840-01-284-3982). This multipolymer, extended-duration repellent formulation contains 33% deet and forms a thin film over the surface of skin that slows the absorption and evaporation of deet and provides long-term protection (6 to 14 hours) against a wide variety of militarily relevant arthropods under varying environmental conditions.[32–35]

The extended-duration formulation of deet is the best repellent developed to date (Figure 22-5). It provides long-lasting protection at a much lower percentage of the active ingredient (33%) than past formulations and so is more cosmetically acceptable. Nevertheless, the intrinsic repellency of deet

is inadequate against biting midges and black flies and only marginally adequate against some anopheline mosquitoes.

Progress in the development of new repellents has been limited. One important reason for the lack of success in this area is the limited understanding of the repellents' mode of action on the target organisms. The general assumption that all repellents affect all arthropods in the same way is incorrect. It has been shown that even strains of the same species differ significantly in their tolerance to the same repellent. Therefore, selection of appropriate repellents for personal protection greatly depends on the species to be repelled. Also, a certain minimum effective evaporation rate of repellent is required to effectively repel insects.[36] Repellent applied on the skin decays exponentially with time, and evaporation and absorption rates account for a substantial fraction of the loss.[35] In addition, it is believed that abrasion (loss of topical repellent due to mechanical action such as rubbing) plays a significant role in repellent loss from skin. It has been shown that the clothing abrasions of repellent-treated skin affected the efficacy of the extended-duration formulation of deet.[37] An increase in the number of repetitions of skin abrasion by clothing resulted in a reduced duration of protection against mosquito bites. To maximize repellent effectiveness, it is important to test new repellent formulations under the conditions that service members experience in the field.

An active, joint-service research program is directed toward discovering new repellent materials for future use. Efforts have begun at the Walter Reed Army Institute of Research (Silver Spring, Md) to create multipurpose insect repellent formulations, such as sunscreen insect repellent and camouflage face paint repellent combinations, to improve repellent effectiveness, ease of application, and user adherence (Figure 22-6). Recent advances in the delivery mechanisms and formulation of insect repellent with camouflage face paint may increase insect repellent use because camouflage skills are taught as an integral part of basic training. Laboratory[38] and field studies have proven that a camouflage face paint repellent formulation is feasible and effective. An added advantage of this product would be the visible indication that it had been applied to exposed skin.

Montemarano and colleagues[39] have shown that sequential use of sunscreen and insect repellent results in reducing the sun protection factor (SPF) by 28%. A successful sunscreen insect repellent that provides protection against both sun rays and insect bites has shown efficacy under laboratory and field conditions. Moreover, it uses only 20% deet and provides similar protection from insect bites as the extended duration repellent formulation containing 33% deet (R.K.G., unpublished data, 1996).

Deet Side Effects

It is estimated that 50 million to 100 million persons use deet each year, and few cases of adverse reactions have been reported.[40] It has been associated with allergic and toxic effects in some people, especially when used repeatedly on the skin in high concentrations. A report in 1976 showed regular applications of deet on the skin of white rats was gonadotoxic and embryotoxic.[41] Deet is partially absorbed through skin and has been used to enhance transdermal delivery of drugs.[42] In human studies, variable penetration into the skin from 9% to 56% of a topically applied dose and absorption into the circulatory system of approximately 17% has been reported. Urinary excretion of deet, which accounted for most of the absorbed repellent, occurred primarily in the first 24 hours in animal models.[30] Deet has been associated with bullous eruptions in the antecubital fossa and contact urticaria, and rare cases of toxic encephalopathy have occurred with excessive or prolonged use, particu-

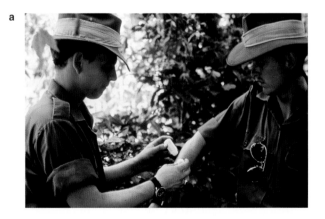
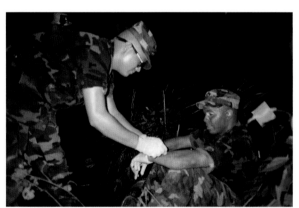

Figure 22-6. Field trials of insect repellents are vital to evaluate how the repellents perform under real-world conditions and how the products are perceived by the intended users: military personnel. (**a**) A field trial of three experimental controlled-release topical insect repellents was conducted by the US and Australian militaries at the Joint Tropical Trials Research Establishment, Australian Department of Defense, near Innisfail, Queensland, Australia. Two Australian soldiers are collecting biting insects after applying one of the assigned treatments including test formulations. (**b**) US soldiers are participants in a field study of camouflage-face paint-insect repellent formulations in Panama in 1997.
Photographs: Courtesy of Colonel Raj Gupta, MS, US Army; Walter Reed Army Institute of Research, Silver Spring, Md.

larly in infants and children.[43] To minimize possible adverse reactions to deet, only products containing less than 35% concentrations of deet should be used and the skin should be cleaned as soon as the risk of arthropod biting is over.

Of 9,086 human exposure cases reported to poison control centers involving deet-containing insect repellents, two thirds had no adverse effects or experienced only minor symptoms.[44] The majority of the people exposed to deet-containing repellents went home after an evaluation and therapy in emergency departments. Sixty-six patients had moderate effects, and the majority of these cases had ocular symptoms. Deet generally is of low acute toxicity, and, based on the available toxicological data, the EPA has concluded that the normal use of deet does not present a health concern to the general US population. Deet has been classified as a Group D carcinogen (not classifiable as a human carcinogen). Although deet's use has been implicated in seizures among children, the incident data are insufficient to establish deet as the cause of the reported effects. However, the EPA required improved label warnings and restrictions on all deet product labels.

Clothing Repellents

History

Many repellents can be applied to field clothing for protection against militarily important arthropods, especially those that crawl or hop (eg, mites, ticks, fleas, body lice). Repellents that are or have been widely used for clothing impregnation include sulfur, dimethyl phthalate, dibutyl phthalate, benzyl benzoate, deet, and permethrin. These materials are also effective when applied to bed nets, curtains, window screens, ground cloths, tents, and protective overgarments.

The need for clothing repellents came into prominence during World War II, with the high incidence of scrub typhus in the Pacific Theater. The value of repellent-impregnated clothing was observed when comparing three similarly sized patrols operating in the same area in the South Pacific in 1944. The first and third patrols were not protected by repellent-impregnated clothing. The first had 53 cases of scrub typhus and the third had 23 cases. In contrast, dimethyl phthalate was liberally applied to the clothing and gear of the second patrol. No member of this second group developed disease; two individuals acquired a single mite bite.[45]

The major problem with dimethyl phthalate was that it became ineffective after a single rinsing in cool water. As the war ended, benzyl benzoate was adopted by the US Army as its standard clothing repellent. It was shown to be effective through at least two soap-and-water washings. The US Department of Agriculture continued to search for clothing repellents for military use that were more persistent and more effective against a wider range of species. In 1951, a new mixture of compounds, M-1960, was found and adopted as the standard clothing repellent for the military.[46]

Clothing repellent M-1960 contained 30% 2-butyl-2-ethyl-1,3-propanediol for protection against mosquitoes and biting flies, 30% N-butylacetanilide for ticks, 30% benzyl benzoate for chiggers and fleas, and 10% of an emulsifier, Tween 80 (polyoxyethylene ether of sorbitan monooleate). Clothing treated with M-1960 was proven 100% effective against chiggers and more than 90% effective against mosquitoes, ticks, and fleas, but clothing had to be retreated after each washing. M-1960 repellent was widely used by US forces during the Korean War to reduce mite bites then thought to transmit epidemic hemorrhagic fever. Both M-1960 and benzyl benzoate had a number of undesirable qualities, such as causing skin irritation, having a disagreeable odor, and being a plasticizer; they were poorly accepted by military personnel and are no longer used.

Permethrin

Permethrin (3-phenoxybenzyl(±)-3-(2,2-dichlorovinyl-2,2-dimethylcyclopanecarboxylate) is a synthetic pyrethroid insecticide and repellent first synthesized in England in 1972. Starting in 1977, it was studied by the US Department of Agriculture for the Department of Defense for use as a clothing treatment to protect the wearer from biting arthropods. But in 1983, the Program Manager for Arthropod Repellents, US Army Medical Materiel and Development Activity (Fort Detrick, Md), organized an advanced development program for permethrin that involved the Letterman Army Institute of Research; the US Army Natick Research Development, Test, and Evaluation Center (Natick, Mass); the Walter Reed Army Institute of Research; the Uniformed Services University of the Health Sciences (Bethesda, Md); and the US Department of Agriculture (Gainesville, Fla).

Permethrin has no noticeable odor, is nonirritating, has low mammalian toxicity, is biodegradable, and provides excellent protection against many different species of biting arthropods. Clothing treated at 0.125 mg/cm^2 has excellent permethrin retention in spite of wear and wash abrasion, weathering, and light-induced chemical breakdown. Persistence of permethrin in fabrics far exceeds that of any previously available repellent. A further advantage of permethrin and other pyrethroids is that they act as insecticides as well as repellents.

Eight to ten different methods for permethrin application of field uniforms were investigated and the following methods were found to be economical, efficient, and effective in providing long-term protection against militarily-important arthropods (Figure 22-7). Four impregnation methods were registered for US Army use by the EPA: (1) the Individual Dynamic Absorption (IDA) Application,

(2) the 2-gallon sprayer, (3) the aerosol can, and (4) the Pad Roll. A new method of treating finished uniforms has completed user-acceptance trials and will be available for us in the future.

The IDA kit ("shake and bake") contains two small containers of 40% permethrin, treatment bags, twine, disposable gloves, and a marking pen. The kit is designed for use by the individual service member; and one kit treats one field uniform (shirt and pant). The shirt and pant are separately rolled and tied in the middle by twine. Three-quarters of a canteen cup of water is poured into each treatment bag along with contents of one of the containers. The

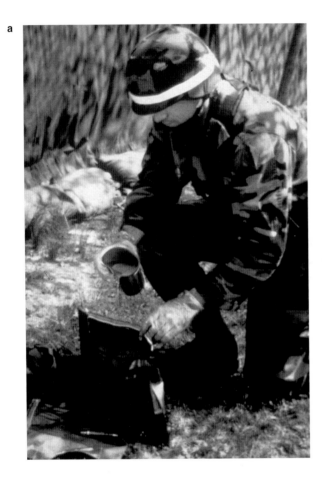

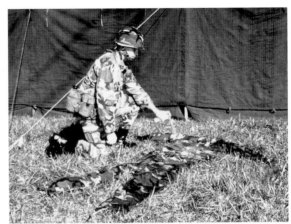

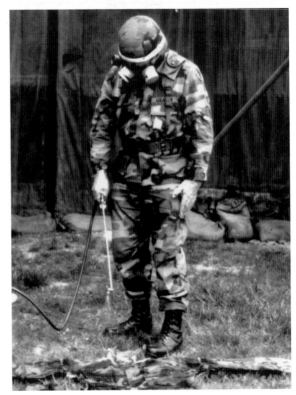

Fig. 22-7. Soldiers treating field uniforms with permethrin using (**a**) the IDA (Individual Dynamic Absorption) method, (**b**) a spray can, and (**c**) a 2-gallon sprayer.
Source: Walter Reed Army Institute of Research, Silver Spring, Md.

bag is shaken to mix the water and permethrin, the rolled shirt or pant is placed inside its own bag, and the fastener is closed. Then the bag is left undisturbed for 2.5 hours while the liquid is being absorbed by the cloth. The shirt or pant is then hung and allowed to dry thoroughly. During field trials, this method was shown to be simple and effective.

The 2-gallon treatment method is used to treat field uniforms and tents. The 40% permethrin from the 5.1-ounce (151 mL) bottle is mixed in a sprayer containing 2 gallons of water, and the sprayer is brought to a pressure of 55 psi. The 2-gallon field sprayer can treat nine sets of field uniforms per 5.1-ounce bottle. The field uniforms are placed flat on the ground and sprayed evenly until all the material is thoroughly wet. They are then hung to dry. Two-gallon compressed air sprayers are required equipment of company-sized Army unit field sanitation teams and are used by all the services. This is a simple and effective method if properly done.

Aerosol spray cans containing 0.5% permethrin may also be used for treatment. The application to the field uniform is made by holding the spray can 6 to 8 inches from the clothing. The uniform is laid flat on the ground and the outer surface is treated. This method is simple but is not as efficient and effective as the other methods.[18,47]

The Pad Roll method for impregnation involves pretreating field uniform cloth during the manufacturing process. The fabric is passed through a permethrin and water bath and is then sent through squeeze rollers. After it is dried, the cloth is then made into uniforms.[48] The last method, factory treatment of finished uniforms, involves treatment of individual uniforms during the manufacturing process.

Permethrin treatment—using the IDA kit, 2-gallon sprayer, Pad Roll application, and factory treatment of finished uniforms methods—provides effective protection against insects for up to 50 washings; the aerosol can method lasts for six washings. Starching field uniforms does not affect the treatment but certain dry cleaning processes may remove it. Underwear and caps should not be treated with permethrin. Tentage should be re-treated after 9 months in temperate climates and after 6 months in tropical climates. Preventive medicine personnel should monitor the level of protection achieved after treatment of clothing.

OTHER PROTECTIVE MEASURES AUTHORIZED FOR MILITARY PERSONNEL

The Uniform

One of the most practical means of reducing arthropod bites that is often overlooked, neglected, or not enforced is the proper wearing of the field uniform. Most insects cannot bite through its material unless it is tightly stretched against the skin. Service members must remember to wear a loosely fitted uniform and minimize the amount of skin exposed to blood-sucking or biting arthropods. Shirts should be worn with collars closed and sleeves rolled down from dusk until dawn or whenever mosquitoes or biting flies are present. The bottom of trousers should be tucked inside the tops of boots, and undershirts should never be worn as the outer garment when the threat of vector-borne disease exists.[48] Service members should shake out all clothes before putting them on, wear socks and shoes whenever walking, and look closely before reaching into concealed areas. Tears or holes in the field uniform should be repaired. Individuals should use a buddy system frequently to check for ticks on body areas that cannot easily be personally surveyed and to remove ticks that are found safely. Protection against insect bites is of paramount importance during off-duty hours when service members may let down their guard and wear shorts, sandals, and t-shirts. Exposed skin should be protected with deet repellent if biting arthropods are present. National Stock Numbers and costs of some of the items mentioned here are listed in Table 22-1.

Head Nets

The head net is a fine-mesh, olive-drab, nylon screen that is designed to fit over headgear (Figure 22-8). The cloth top piece has an elastic suspension that fits over the kevlar helmet or other headgear. Metal rings hold the net away from the face and neck. It is worn over the collar in back and is held in place in the front by two elastic loops that can be attached to the pocket buttons of the shirt. Properly worn head nets will protect against biting insects and are particularly useful in areas where biting flies and mosquitoes are so numerous that they overwhelm repellents, as in the Arctic during summer.[48]

Bed Nets

Bed nets, or insect bars, have long been used to protect people from mosquitoes and sand flies. The bed net is a canopy usually made from finely woven nylon mesh (Figure 22-9). It may be used with the folding cot, steel bed, shelter-half tent, or ham-

TABLE 22-1

NATIONAL STOCK NUMBERS AND COSTS OF SOME PERSONAL PROTECTION ITEMS AVAILABLE THROUGH THE MILITARY SUPPLY SYSTEM AS OF JULY 2000

Item	NSN	Units of Issue	Cost ($)
33% Deet Repellent, Extended Duration	6840-01-284-3982	12 2-oz tubes/box	34.32
0.5% Permethrin, Clothing Application	6840-01-278-1336	12 6-oz cans/box	38.41
40% Permethrin, Clothing Application	6840-01-345-0237	12 IDA kits/box	42.77
2-Gallon Sprayer, Pressure Type	3740-00-641-4719	Each	140.11
40% Permethrin, Clothing Application	6840-01-334-2666	12 151-mL bottles/box	159.30
Pole, Folding Cot, Insect Net Protector	7210-00-267-5641	Set	4.05
Insect Net Protector	7210-00-266-9736	Each	27.20
Insect Bar, Head Net	8415-00-935-3130	Each	5.15
Parka, Insect Repellent, small	8415-01-035-0846	Each	16.60
Parka, Insect Repellent, medium	8415-01-035-0847	Each	16.60
Parka, Insect Repellent, large	8415-01-035-0848	Each	16.60
Jacket, Bug-Out outer wear, small	01-483-2988	Each	37.60
Jacket, Bug-Out outer wear, medium	01-483-3002	Each	37.60
Jacket, Bug-Out outer wear, large	01-483-3004	Each	37.60
Jacket, Bug-Out outer wear, extra large	01-483-3007	Each	37.60
Jacket, Bug-Out outer wear, extra extra large	01-483-3008	Each	42.50

IDA: Individual Dynamic Absorption
Source: Department of Defense Pest Management Materiel List (Other Than Pesticides). May 1, 2001. Maintained by the Armed Forces Pest Management Board, Forest Glen Section, Walter Reed Army Medical Center, Washington, DC 20307-5001.

mock. Poles to help suspend the bed net over the folding cot are available. The net must be suspended so that there is clearance between it and the sleeping person. While bed nets not treated with permethrin performed well, numerous studies[49] indicate that treated bed nets, even those with holes, were far superior to untreated bed nets. Research efforts are underway to develop a bed net that has better air flow and is lightweight, self-supporting, easily collapsible, and impregnated with a quick-acting insecticide. The newer design must also be useable with the military cot and on the bare ground.

The new bed net incorporates a self-supporting, low-profile design; a "no-see-um" polyester mesh with factory impregnated insecticide (permethrin); and an integral support frame with canopy. The bed net can be folded into a flat circular package (12 inches in diameter and weighing approximately 2 lbs) and can be carried in the military rucksack or a civilian backpack. When released, the bed net instantaneously springs into a complete and fully deployed bed net. It has a water resistant floor that is also treated with insecticide. It can be used with a military field folding cot, a field hospital bed, or alone.

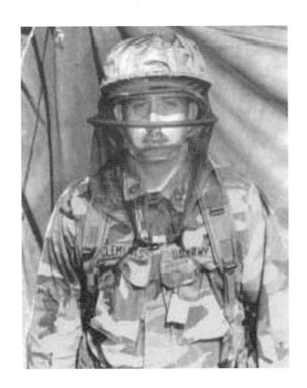

Fig. 22-8. The standard-issue head net.
Source: Defense Pest Management Information Analysis Center. *Personal Protective Techniques Against Insects and Other Arthropods of Military Significance.* Washington, DC: Armed Forces Pest Management Board; 2000: 16. AFPMB Technical Memorandum 36.

Other Clothing

An insect repellent parka or overjacket made of wide-mesh polyester-cotton netting is worn over outer clothing after being treated with a full 2-ounce bottle of 75% deet (NSN 6840-00-753-4963). The insect repellent parka, fabric mesh (deet jacket) is available in small, medium, and large sizes (see Table 22-1). The waist length parka with extra long sleeves and hood is stored in a plastic bag when not in use. After being treated with 2 ounces of 75% deet and if properly stored and not washed, the parka should remain effective against mosquitoes, biting midges, and biting flies for about 6 weeks before retreatment is necessary.[50]

a

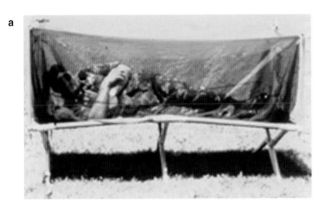

b

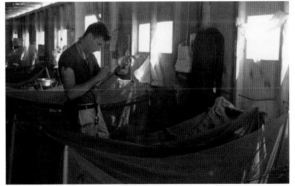

c

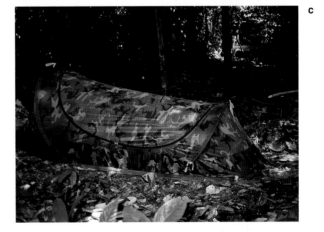

Fig. 22-9. Bed nets, especially if properly treated with permethrin, offer additional protection against nuisance and disease-carrying insects. Photograph (**a**) shows a soldier demonstrating the use of a bed net with a standard issue cot. Photograph (**b**) shows a Navy Hospitalman 3rd class in the 1st Medical Battalion Field Hospital in Mogadishu, Somalia in 1993. The patients are all in bed under bed nets. This not only protects them from biting arthropod and the diseases they transmit, but it also keeps those personnel with arthropod-borne diseases from becoming sources of nosocomial infections. Photograph (**c**) shows the new self-supporting, low profile bed net design. It is compatible with standard issue cots and hospital beds.

Photograph sources: (a) Defense Pest Management Information Analysis Center. *Personal Protective Techniques Against Insects and Other Arthropods of Military Significance.* Washington, DC: Armed Forces Pest Management Board; 2000: 18. AFPMB Technical Memorandum 36. (b) DoD Joint Combat Camera Center. *US Forces in Somalia.* CD-ROM. March AFB, Calif: DoD JCCC. Image 189. (c) Colonel Raj Gupta, MS, US Army.

A new, smaller mesh jacket that is durable, effective and does not need to be treated with Deet is being introduced into the military supply system. The new jacket, Bug-Out outer wear, will be available in small, medium, large, extra large, and extra extra large. Both jacket systems may be used by those personnel who remain stationary (eg, sentries, forward observers, combat vehicle drivers).

Area Repellents

Area repellents, also referred to as space repellents, are generally applied to a limited area and are designed to reduce or eliminate arthropod biting in the treated area. Space repellents fill the void between personal topical repellents and large-scale area insecticidal control of arthropod vectors. Area repellents have been available from commercial sources for decades; however, none of the systems tested have proven effective enough for inclusion in the Department of Defense supply system.[51,52] Although not an area repellent, d-phenothrin (NSN 6840-01-412-4634) is an aerosol spray insecticide that can be used to spray inside of enclosed spaces such as bed nets and tents immediately before entry.

USE OF UNAUTHORIZED PRODUCTS BY SERVICE MEMBERS

Although many service members use them to repel arthropods, certain commercial repellents and other products are not authorized for military use. Therefore, commercial repellents, even if they contain deet, are not to be substituted for standard military-issue 33% deet extended-duration lotion or permethrin formulations. Some service members have reported satisfaction using the Avon bath oil Skin-So-Soft during recreation or training. However, Skin-So-Soft has been shown to provide protection against insect bites for at most 30 minutes,[53,54] and its continual application is not practical during military operations. In 1994, another Avon Skin-So-Soft product containing sunscreen (SPF 15) and insect repellent (0.05% oil of citronella) became available. It should never be considered as a substitute for the standard military-issue 33% deet extended-duration lotion. Other items, such as flea and tick collars, have been associated with severe skin damage when used by humans. The use of garlic, sulfur (from matchsticks), diluted turpentine, high doses of B vitamins, talc, vinegar, or the like have not been shown to be effective insect repellents and can be toxic. These items are not to be added to or substituted for military-issue repellents. Questions or concerns regarding military-issue insect repellents or other items that might be used to repel insects should be directed up the chain of command. Written medical permission is required before substitution is authorized. Available for consultation are the Executive Director or the Contingency Liaison Officer of the Armed Forces Pest Management Board (Silver Spring, Md) and the entomology consultants to the three Surgeons General.

ADHERENCE TO THE US MILITARY'S SYSTEM OF PERSONAL PROTECTION MEASURES

Although the current system of PPMs is the most effective ever fielded, outbreaks of arthropod-borne disease continue to occur during field operations when service members do not properly implement PPMs. For example, there were approximately 200 cases of malaria[8,9,55] among US military personnel who served in Somalia during Operation Restore Hope. In addition to dengue virus infections in Somalia,[10] at least 29 dengue virus infections[56] occurred among US military personnel during the initial phase of Operation Uphold Democracy in Haiti. No effective vaccines exist for malaria, dengue, and many other arthropod-borne diseases so their prevention requires consistent use of PPMs and environmental control of insect populations. (In the case of malaria, adherence to an appropriate chemoprophylactic regimen is also required.) Investigations of both outbreaks led predictably to a recommendation that service member adherence to PPMs be enforced more vigorously to prevent additional cases.

Arthropod-borne disease outbreaks also occur during training. Four cases of cutaneous leishmaniasis were identified among 51 US Army Rangers who attended the French Foreign Legion's Jungle Training Course in French Guiana in 1993. Of 34 Rangers who completed a questionnaire, 27 (79%) reported using insect repellent, but the majority preferred to use commercial repellents they had purchased. Among the four cases, one reported not using any repellent and the remaining three reported using commercial repellents exclusively.[57] The costs to the individual Ranger, the unit, and the military appear excessive given the relatively low cost of available prevention measures.[58]

More than 550 US Army soldiers (approximately

half in combat arms) who were deployed either to Kuwait (Operation Vigilant Warrior, 1994), Haiti (United Nations Mission in Haiti, 1995), and Bosnia (Operation Joint Endeavor, 1996) participated in a survey regarding their use of PPMs to prevent insect bites. Survey results[59,60] revealed that:

- 41% of respondents reported that they received insect bites either daily or almost daily.
- 69.5% of respondents felt that they had adequate knowledge about the US military's system of PPMs.
- Less than half (40.3%) of respondents were able to identify the current standard US military-issue insect repellent for skin application (33% deet extended-duration lotion), and 35.6% were uncertain. A smaller proportion of respondents (39%) was able to identify permethrin as the contact insecticide for application to the field uniform.
- Regarding insect repellents applied to the skin, 29.2% of respondents reported using commercial repellents exclusively, 33.8% used both military-issue and commercial repellents, while only 9.9% used military-issue repellents exclusively.
- Field uniforms were treated before deployment by only 7.6%.
- 51.5% of respondents felt that their commanders emphasized the use of military-issue insect repellents in general either some but not enough or not at all.

These survey results and related data[61] suggest that in the mid-1990s many service members were relatively unfamiliar with military doctrine regarding PPMs and did not routinely practice it in the field. Although military-issue repellents appeared to have been largely available, approximately half of respondents felt that their commanders did not sufficiently emphasize their use during deployment.

When implemented in 1991, the US military's system of PPMs was known to be a highly effective tool in preventing insect bites. Future missions during war and peace will continue to expose service members to insect bites and related diseases depending on the time of year, geographic location of deployment, and other factors. In some situations, units in the field may be the targets of very intense insect biting activity or bites that transmit disease. As history has shown, infectious diseases, including those transmitted by insect bites, can change the outcome of vital field operations. Military readiness requires an aggressive field preventive medi-

cine capability, including service members' proper use of the US military's system of PPMs.

Data gathered from deployed US Army soldiers suggest that there is a basic lack of knowledge about the system and, not surprisingly, widespread nonadherence to it. No one likes to get bitten by insects, so many service members needlessly spend their own money to purchase commercial insect repellents for use in the field rather than use the standard military-issue repellents, despite their effectiveness. It is likely that these findings are generalizeable to other units in the US military. As with cold-weather or hot-weather injuries, preventable illnesses associated with insect bites must be considered largely command failures. Commanders are responsible for the health of their personnel, including their appropriate use of PPMs to prevent insect bites.

How can adherence to the US military's system of PPMs by service members be increased to acceptable levels? Greater adherence will only occur when service members develop confidence in the effectiveness of the system to significantly reduce insect bites and in their ability to use the system properly under realistic training and operational conditions. To help personnel build sufficient confidence, commanders must have a working knowledge of the system, practice its use in regular unit training for deployment, and strictly enforce its use in the field (with the help of the unit's field sanitation team).[12] More specifically, commanders must provide leadership[59-63] regarding PPMs in the following areas:

- Training and testing their service members at the unit level; common task testing reinforces the importance of the task and assures regular testing to standards.
- Treating bed nets with permethrin before deployment, as is done with field uniforms, when such measures can be expected to add significantly to the prevention of insect bites in the field.
- Requesting that current doctrine about the use of PPMs be included in field manuals, training materials, and other relevant military publications.
- Using knowledgeable personnel (eg, field sanitation teams) in a timely manner to address service members' attitudes, myths, and memories (eg, of 75% deet) that undermine the current system an encourage commercial repellent use, sporadic repellent use, or no repellent use.
- Including PPM doctrine in their unit's standards of operation, budgeting for and pro-

curing adequate supplies of standard military-issue personal protection items (see Table 22-1), and enforcing the system's use in the field during the entire period units are at risk of receiving insect bites.[64]

- Ensuring that each company-sized unit has a fully functional field sanitation team that is responsible for teaching the system of PPMs, monitoring its use among unit members, providing timely feedback regarding adherence to their commander, and coordinating their activity with division or corps preventive medicine assets, as indicated.

- Providing repellent researchers and doctrine developers with information from the field about what works well and what must be improved in the system so it can become even more practical, effective, and user-friendly.[65]

SUMMARY

The US military's system of PPMs has no equal. It is a command responsibility to ensure that every soldier, sailor, airman, and Marine at risk of receiving insect bites or acquiring an arthropod-borne disease in the field uses PPMs properly. As an important part of their knowledge about deployment medicine, unit commanders must lead their service members in countering the significant threats to health posed by biting insects. This is a vital task that is part of training for deployment. Apathy, negligence, or poor adherence can lead to preventable casualties. As British Lieutenant General Sir William J. Slim wrote in his World War II memoirs, "Good doctors are no use without good discipline. More than half the battle against disease is fought not by doctors, but by regimental officers."[66p180]

Acknowledgment

The authors wish to thank Colonel Donald Driggers, Colonel (Retired) Phillip Lawyer, Lieutenant Colonel Stephen B Berté, Lieutenant Colonel Mustapha Debboun, Major (Retired) Louis Rutledge, and Dr. Edward Evans for their insightful review of the chapter. Colonel (Retired) Moufied Moussa and Ms. Sandy Evans were very helpful with illustrations.

REFERENCES

1. Lutta AS; Karelo, Trans. Individual protection against blood sucking flies in logging areas in the Karelian Finnish S.S.R. [Russian]. *Finnish Filiala Ascad Nauk S.S.S.R.* 1956;4:150.

2. Defense Intelligence Agency. *Handbook of Diseases of Military Importance.* Washington, DC: Government Printing Office; 1982: 135.

3. Robinson AH. The thematic maps of Charles Joseph Minard. *Imago Mundi.* 1967;21:95–108.

4. Peterson RKD. Insects, disease, and military history. *Am Entomologist.* 1995;141:147–160.

5. Navy Environmental Health Center. *Navy Medical Department Guide to Malaria Prevention and Control.* Norfolk, Va: NEHC; 1991.

6. Bunn RW, Knight KL, Lacasse JC. The role of entomology in the preventive medicine program of the armed forces. *Mil Med.* 1955;116:119–123.

7. Navy Environmental Health Center. *Navy Medical Department Guide to Malaria Prevention and Control.* Norfolk, Va: NEHC; 1984.

8. Centers for Disease Control and Prevention. Malaria among U.S. military personnel returning from Somalia, 1993. *MMWR.* 1993;42:524–526.

9. Newton JA Jr, Schnepf GA, Wallace MR, Lobel HO, Kennedy CA, Oldfied EC III. Malaria in US Marines returning from Somalia. *JAMA.* 1994;272:397–399.

10. Sharp TW, Wallace MR, Hayes CG, et al. Dengue fever in U.S. troops during Operation Restore Hope, Somalia, 1992–1993. *Am J Trop Med Hyg.* 1995;53:89–94.

11. Ognibene AJ. Medical and infectious diseases in the theater of operations. *Mil Med.* 1987;152:1–14.

12. Department of the Army. *Unit Field Hygiene and Sanitation Team.* Washington, DC: DA; 1989. Field Manual 21-10-1.

13. Withers BG, Erickson RL. Good doctors are not enough. *Mil Rev.* 1994;March:57–63.

14. Withers BG, Erickson RL, Petruccelli BP, Hanson RK, Kadlec RP. Preventing disease and non-battle injury in deployed units. *Mil Med.* 1994;159:39–43.

15. Dethier VG, Browne LB, Smith CN. The designation of chemicals in terms of the responses they elicit from insects. *J Econ Entomol.* 1960;53:134–136.

16. Garson LR, Winnike, ME. Relationship between insect repellency and chemical and physical parameters—a review. *J Med Entomol.* 1968;5:339–352.

17. Kennedy JS. The excitant and repellent effects on mosquitoes of sub-lethal contacts with DDT. *Bull Entomol Res.* 1947;37:593–607.

18. Gupta RK, Rutledge LC, Reifenrath WG, Gutierrez GA, Korte DW Jr. Resistance of permethrin to weathering in fabrics treated for protection against mosquitoes (Diptera: Culicidae). *J Med Entomol.* 1990;27:494–500.

19. Philip MI, Ramakrishna V, Rao VV. Turmeric and vegetable oils as repellents against anopheline mosquitoes. *Indian Med Gaz.* 1945;80:343–344.

20. Mom AM. El empleo de la proteccion antisolar y de los repelentes de insectos en los indigenas latinoamericanos. *Rev Argentina da Dermatosifilologia.* 1948;32:303–306.

21. Arnold WN. Absinthe. *Sci Am.* 1989;260:112–117.

22. Rice EL. *Pest Control with Nature's Chemicals: Allelochemics and Pheromones in Gardening and Agriculture.* Norman, Okla: University of Oklahoma Press; 1983.

23. Ewing HE. Sulphur-impregnated clothing to protect against chiggers. *J Econ Entomol.* 1925;18:827–829.

24. US Army Medical Field Service School. *Essentials of Field Sanitation for the Medical Department, United States Army.* Carlisle Barracks, Penn: US Army Medical Field Service School; 1933.

25. Gupta RK, Rutledge LC. Role of repellents in vector control and disease prevention. *Am J Trop Med Hyg.* 1994;50(Suppl):82–86.

26. Moore W, Buc HE. Insect repellent. 1929. United States Patent 1,727,305.

27. Stage HH. Mosquitoes. In: Stefferud A, ed. *Insects: The Yearbook of Agriculture.* Washington, DC: US Government Printing Office; 1952: 476–486.

28. US Environmental Protection Agency. 2–Ethyl-1,3-hexanediol; receipt of requests to cancel. *Fed Reg.* 1991;8:43767–43768.

29. McCabe ET, Barthel WF, Gertler SI, Hall SA. Insect repellents, III: N,N-diethylamides. *J Org Chem.* 1954;9:493–498.

30. Robbins PJ, Cherniack MG. Review of the biodistribution and toxicity of the insect repellent N,N-diethyl-m-toluamide (DEET). *J Toxicol Environ Health.* 1986;18:503–525.

31. Hooper RL, Wirtz RA. Insect repellent used by troops in the field: Results of a questionnaire. *Mil Med.* 1983;148:34–38.

32. Gupta RK, Rutledge LC. Laboratory evaluation of controlled-release repellent formulations on human volunteers under three climatic regimens. *J Am Mosq Control Assoc.* 1989;5:52–55.

33. Gupta RK, Rutledge LC. Controlled-release repellent formulations on human volunteers under three climatic regimens. *J Am Mosq Cont Assoc.* 1991;7:490–493.

34. Gupta RK, Sweeney AW, Rutledge LC, Cooper RD, Frances SP, Westrom DR. Effectiveness of controlled-release personal-use arthropod repellents and permethrin-impregnated clothing in the field. *J Am Mosq Control Assoc.* 1987;3:556–560.

35. Sholdt LL, Schreck CE, Qureshi A, Mammino S, Aziz Z, Iqbal M. Field bioassays of permethrin-treated uniforms and a new extended duration repellent against mosquitoes in Pakistan. *J Am Mosq Control Assoc.* 1988;4:233–236.

36. Rutledge LC, Reifenrath WB, Gupta RK. Sustained release formulations of the US Army insect repellent. *Army Science Conference Proceedings.* 1986;3:343–357.

37. Rueda LM, Rutledge LC, Gupta RK. Effect of skin abrasion on the efficacy of the repellent deet against *Aedes aegypti*. *J Am Mosq Cont.* 1998;14:178–182.

38. Hoch AL, Gupta RK, Weyandt TB. Laboratory evaluation of a new repellent camouflage face paint. *J Am Mosq Control Assoc.* 1995;11(2 Pt 1):172–175.

39. Montemarano AD, Gupta RK, Burge JR, Kline K. Insect repellents and the efficacy of sunscreens. *Lancet.* 1997;349:1670–1671.

40. Centers for Disease Control. Seizures temporally associated with use of DEET insect repellent—New York and Connecticut. *MMWR.* 1989;38:678–680.

41. Gleiberman SE, Volkova AP, Nikolaev GM, Zhukova EV. [Experimental study of the long-term effects of using repellents, report 1: An experimental study of the long-term effects of the repellent Diethyltoluamide (DETA).] *Med Parazitol (Mosk).* 1976;45:65–69.

42. Windheuser JJ, Haslam JL, Caldwell L, Shaffer RD. The use of N,N-diethyl-m-toluamide to enhance dermal and transdermal delivery of drugs. *J Pharm Sci.* 1982;71:1211–1213.

43. Are insect repellents safe? *Lancet.* 1988:2:610–611.

44. Veltri JC, Osimitz TG, Bradford DC, Page BC. Retrospective analysis of calls to poison control centers resulting from exposure to the insect repellent N,N-diethyl-m-toluamide (DEET) from 1985–1989. *J Toxicol Clin Toxicol.* 1994;32:1–16.

45. US War Department. Impregnation of clothing with insect repellent (dimethyl phthalate). Washington, DC: USWD: 1944. TB MED 121.

46. Gilbert IH, Gouck HK. All purpose repellent mixtures as clothing treatments against chiggers. *Florida Entomologist.* 1953;36:47–51.

47. Gupta RK, Rutledge LC, Reifenrath WG, Gutierrez GA, Korte DW Jr. Effects of weathering on fabrics treated with permethrin for protection against mosquitoes. *J Am Mosq Control Assoc.* 1989;5:176–179.

48. Armed Forces Pest Management Board. *Personal Protective Measures Against Insects and Other Arthropods of Military Significance.* Washington, DC: AFPMB: 2001. Technical Information Memorandum 36. Available at http://www.afpmb.org.

49. Curtis CF, Myamba J, Wilkes TJ. Comparison of different insecticides and fabrics for anti-mosquito bed nets and curtains. *Med Vet Entomol.* 1996;10:1–11.

50. Lindsay IS, McAndless JM. Permethrin-treated jackets versus repellent-treated jackets and hoods for personal protection against black flies and mosquitoes. *Mosq News.* 1978;38:350–356.

51. Rutledge LC, Wirtz RA, Semey HG, Gupta RK. Tests of area mosquito repellents. *Insecticide Acaricide Tests.* 1991;16:327.

52. Wirtz RA, Turrentine JD, Fox RC. Mosquito area repellents: Laboratory testing of candidate materials against *Aedes aegypti* (L.). *Mosq News.* 1981;40:432–439.

53. Rutledge LC, Wirtz RA, Buescher MD. Repellent activity of a proprietary bath oil (Skin-So-Soft®). *Mosq News.* 1982;42:557–559.

54. Schreck CE, McGovern TP. Repellents and other personal protection strategies against *Aedes albopictus. J Am Mosq Control Assoc.* 1989;5:247–250.

55. Wallace MR, Sharp TW, Smoak B, et al. Malaria among United States troops in Somalia. *Am J Med.* 1996;100:49–55.

56. Centers for Disease Control and Prevention. Dengue fever among U.S. military personnel—Haiti, September-November, 1994. *MMWR.* 1994;43:845–848.

57. Brundage J. Preliminary epidemiology consultation (EPICON) report: Cutaneous leishmaniasis outbreak among US Army Rangers returned from French Guiana. Washington, DC: Walter Reed Army Institute of Research; 9 Sept 1993. Memorandum.

58. Grogl M, Gasser RA Jr, Magill A, et al. Cutaneous leishmaniasis in US Rangers and Marines associated with jungle warfare training in French Guiana during 1992–1993. Presented at the American Society of Tropical Medicine and Hygiene Meeting, November 1993; Atlanta, Ga. Abstract No. 619.

59. Gambel J. Debugging the battlefield: Winning the war against insect bites and related diseases. *Mil Rev.* 1996;6:51–57.

60. Gambel JM, Brundage JF, Kuschner RA, Kelley PW. Deployed US Army soldiers' knowledge and use of personal protection measures to prevent arthropod-related casualties. *J Travel Med.* 1998;5:217–220.

61. Gambel JM, DeFraites RF, Brundage JF, Smoak BL, Burge RJ, Wirtz RA. Survey of US Army knowledge, attitudes, and practices regarding personal protection measures to prevent arthropod-related diseases and nuisance bites. *Mil Med.* 1998;163:695–701.

62. Gambel J. Preventing insect bites in the field: A key force mulitiplier. *US Army Med Dept J.* 1995;May-Jun:34–40.

63. Gambel J, Aronson N. Bugs mug soldiers: NCOs key to implementing personal protection measures. *NCO J.* 1997:Spring:22–23.

64. Department of the Army. *Standing Logistics Instructions.* Washington, DC: DA; 1993. US Army FORSCOM Regulation 700-2.

65. Ledbetter E, Shallow S, Hanson KR. Malaria in Somalia: Lessons in prevention. *JAMA.* 1995;273:774–775. Published erratum: *JAMA,* 1995;273:1836.

66. Slim W. *Defeat Into Victory.* London: Cassell and Company, Ltd; 1956.

Chapter 23

DEPLOYMENT INJURIES

JAMES V. WRITER, MPH

J. V. Writer; Environmental Monitoring Team, US Department of Agriculture Animal and Plant Health Inspection Service, 4700 River Road, Riverdale, MD 20737; formerly, Epidemiologist Division of Preventive Medicine, Walter Reed Army Institute of Research, Silver Spring, MD 20910-7500

INTRODUCTION

Injuries are a major cause of morbidity and mortality during deployments.[1–3] They adversely affect personal and unit readiness and can affect the success of a mission by consuming both limited manpower and available medical resources. During the Persian Gulf War, nearly 5,000 US Army soldiers were admitted to medical treatment facilities in Southwest Asia for injury-related conditions from 1 August 1990 through 31 July 1991.[3]

An injury is the result of an energy transfer from one medium to another—a human being.[4] For an injury to occur, the amount of energy transferred must exceed the individual's ability to absorb it.[4,5] Injury control is the science of preventing the energy transfer, reducing the amount transmitted to safer levels, and repairing the damage inflicted.

Health care providers, to a large extent, become involved in injury control only after the injury occurs. The focus of physicians and others has been to limit damage through treatment and rehabilitation of the injured patient. During deployment, however, such factors as mission success, access to medical care, and availability of replacements require that injury prevention be a primary focus of those responsible for medical readiness. On deployment, injury prevention is a force multiplier. Physicians and other providers must be involved in primary, secondary, and tertiary injury prevention (Table 23-1). A key part of that involvement is the management of comprehensive injury surveillance systems that permit the evaluation of medical care in the field for combat[6] and noncombat casualties. Reducing the number and severity of injuries is, however, a multidisciplinary undertaking (Exhibit 23-1). It involves safety professionals, equipment designers, commanders, small unit leaders, and medical personnel. Interactive and effective communication between the myriad players is essential.

A comprehensive discussion of injury prevention techniques and strategies is beyond the scope of this chapter. Injuries are a broad and diverse diagnostic category with many causes. Even when the focus is narrowed to unintentional blunt and penetrating trauma, which is what this chapter will concentrate on (eliminating battle injuries, homicide, and suicide from the discussion), there are a multitude of injury types, causes, and preventive strategies. This chapter will provide a framework of historical and epidemiologic information that demonstrates the impact of injuries on deployments, followed by an overview of available methods for identifying, managing, and eliminating high-risk situations.

MAGNITUDE OF THE PROBLEM

Historical Perspective

Traumatic unintentional injuries can have a significant effect on operations during deployment. Relative to other nonbattle casualties, unintentional nonbattle injuries have been increasing in importance since the early 20th century.

Through the first World War, illnesses were the greatest threat to a US soldier's health.[7] In the second World War, as the US Army became increasingly mechanized and as advances in the sanitary and medical control of infectious diseases were made, nonbattle injuries became the leading cause of death in US soldiers.[8] In the US Navy and Marine Corps, injuries were the fourth leading type of casualty, fatal and nonfatal, in World War I.[1] They were the third leading cause during World War II and the Korean War. In the Vietnam War, they had become the leading type of casualty. During Navy and Marine Corps deployments in the 20th century, injury casualty rates (both battle and nonbattle) have remained constant while disease casualties have declined dramatically.[1]

Several studies have examined the epidemiology of injuries, mainly musculoskeletal injuries, in soldiers at basic training facilities and in garrison.[9–11] But good published deployment injury data are few, and most are available only years or even decades

TABLE 23-1

INJURY PREVENTION SYSTEMS AND THEIR PURPOSES

System Level	Purpose
Prevention System (Primary Prevention)	Prevent occurrence Reduce incidence Be a force multiplier
Acute Care System (Secondary Prevention)	Recognize injuries early Treat injuries early Minimize severity
Rehabilitation System (Tertiary Prevention)	Optimize patient's function Minimize disability

EXHIBIT 23-1

INJURY PREVENTION PARTNERS DURING DEPLOYMENTS

- Safety Center/Safety Command/Safety Officers

- Commanders, noncommissioned officers, and supervisors

- Service members

- Military schools

- Preventive and occupational medicine care providers

- Other medical care providers

- Technology and equipment developers

- Engineers

- Data system managers

after the deployment. Comprehensive Army statistics on injuries in World War II and the Korean War were not published until the 1970s.[8,12] Reports of disease and nonbattle injuries (DNBIs) in the Vietnam War were not available until the 1980s and 1990s.[13,14] Other reports have not separated diseases and nonbattle injuries from all casualties.[15]

Deaths During Recent Deployments

During the Persian Gulf War, 183 of 225 (81.3%) unintentional nonbattle deaths among all deployed US military personnel were due to injuries, as opposed to 30 (13.3%) deaths due to illnesses. Suicides accounted for 10 (4.4%) deaths and homicides for 1 (0.4%) death; one death was reported as cause unknown.[2] In contrast, among the nondeployed force, unintentional injuries accounted for 56.1% of the total deaths. This difference clearly illustrates the relative importance of unintentional injuries during deployments.

Among the deployed, motor vehicle accidents were the leading mechanism of death (62 deaths, 33.9%), followed by aircraft accidents (47 deaths, 25.7%). Motor vehicles accidents were also the leading cause of death in the nondeployed forces: 439 of 784 deaths (56.0%). Death by explosion was rare in nondeployed forces (1 death, 0.05/100,000 person-years) but was a significant cause of death in Southwest Asia (18 deaths, 6.8/100,000 person-years). Table 23-2 compares the causes of unintentional trauma death for service members who deployed to the Persian Gulf War and those who did not.

Hospital Admissions During Recent Deployments

Admissions of soldiers to US Army hospitals during the Persian Gulf War, August 1990 through July

TABLE 23-2

NUMBER, RATE, AND RATE RATIO OF UNINTENTIONAL TRAUMA DEATHS IN US MILITARY PERSONNEL DEPLOYED TO THE PERSIAN GULF REGION AND NONDEPLOYED FORCES, 1 AUGUST 1990 THROUGH 31 JULY 1991

Cause of Death	Nondeployed		Deployed		
	No.	Rate*	No.	Rate*	Rate Ratio
All DNBI†	1,397	73.38	225	84.95	1.16
Unintentional trauma	784	41.18	183	69.09	1.68
Motor vehicle	439	23.06	62	23.41	1.02
Aircraft	104	5.46	47	17.74	3.25
Explosions	1	0.05	18	6.80	136.00
Other	175	9.19	56	21.14	2.30

*per 100,000 person-years
†DNBI: disease and nonbattle injury
Data source: Writer JV, DeFraites RF, Brundage JF. Comparative mortality among US military personnel in the Persian Gulf region and worldwide during Operations Desert Shield and Desert Storm. *JAMA*. 1996;275:118–121.

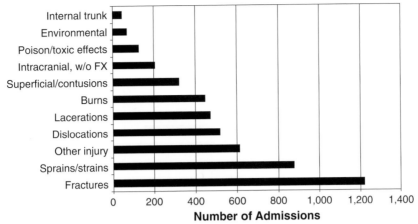

Fig. 23-1. Primary Discharge Diagnosis for US Army Soldiers Hospitalized in Southwest Asia, 1 August 1990 to 31 July 1991

1991, have been analyzed.[3] During the deployment, 19,926 US soldiers were admitted to hospitals in Southwest Asia. Acute nonbattle injuries (4,940, 24.8%) were the primary reason for admission during the conflict. Figure 23-1 summarizes the leading types of injuries reported. The highest number and rate of nonbattle injury admissions were reported during the ground and air war and in the month following cessation of hostilities (Figure 23-2).

Of the available computerized admissions records of nonbattle injury, only 2,632 (53.3%) were coded to indicate the cause of injury. Among these, motor vehicles accidents were the leading cause of admission during the deployment (494, 18.8%). Falls (491, 18.7%) were second, followed by sports

and athletics injuries (450, 17.1%). The mechanisms of injury are summarized in Figure 23-3. Sports injuries are a significant contributor to nonbattle injuries.

Outpatient Visits During Recent Deployments

A concerted tri-service effort to collect and report outpatient surveillance data is a recent development. During the Persian Gulf War, the US Army had no theater-wide surveillance program. In 1993, the Joint Staff mandated medical surveillance with weekly reporting of DNBI on all joint deployments. A uniform, theater-wide program for collecting outpatient data was in place during deployments to

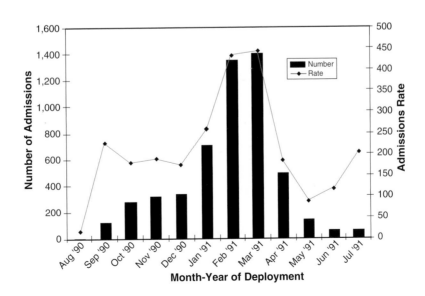

Fig. 23-2. Rate and Number of US Army Soldiers Hospitalized in Southwest Asia, 1 August 1990 to 31 July 1991, by Month

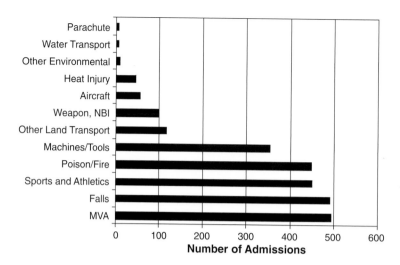

Fig. 23-3. Reported Mechanisms of Injury for US Army Soldiers Hospitalized in Southwest Asia, 1 August 1990 to 31 July 1991

Somalia and Haiti and the 1994 Bright Star training exercise in Egypt.[16] Yet information from these deployments still has been incomplete or nonspecific. For example, the Somalia data listed injuries and orthopedic conditions as a single category and did not describe what the injury or condition was. Improvements and refinements were implemented in the mid-1990s during deployments to Haiti and Bosnia.

During Operation Restore Hope in Somalia, 32 outpatient facilities reported injury surveillance data. Each week, 2.5% to 3.5% of the force was seen for an injury or orthopedic problem. However, no more specific information about the encounter was reported. Similar rates were seen during Operation Uphold Democracy in Haiti.[16] In the 1994 Bright Star exercise in Egypt, 146 (25%) of outpatient visits were injury related during the 19-day deployment. Sprains and strains were the leading cause of injury and resulted in restricted duty in 70% of cases.[16]

Who Is at Risk

Military populations are by their nature (mostly young, healthy men) at high risk for injuries, whether deployed or at their home installations. Studies in civilian populations show that young men are more likely to be hospitalized or die as a result of an unintentional traumatic injury than any other US population subgroup.[17,18] Young men are more likely to be risk takers and may have jobs that place them at risk.

The hospital admissions data from the Persian Gulf War have been analyzed to create a profile of who is at risk of being admitted for an injury.[3] US Army men were 30% more likely to be admitted for an injury than Army women. Being younger than 25 years of age conferred an 18% to 21% higher risk than being in the older age groups. Rank is also associated with higher risk: enlisted soldiers were 70% more likely than officers to be admitted for an injury. Reserve component soldiers were at a 20% higher risk of admission than the active duty Army troops.

While the above data were not analyzed by occupation, risk should also vary by military occupation. For example, truck drivers are likely to be at a higher risk of injury in motor vehicle accidents, dock workers of being crushed, and helicopter pilots of being involved in an aircraft crash than other military personnel.

EVALUATING THE PROBLEM

Surveillance and Reporting

Physicians and other health care providers are an important part of the injury prevention and control process. Through medical surveillance and clinical impressions, they can gather important information and report it to risk managers. Such information could significantly alter the level of danger believed to be present in an operation. Good, solid surveillance data combined with accurate and timely reporting have been effective in identifying dangerous products and activities.

GROUND SAFETY DATA SHEET

Name: _____ Injury date: ____ ____ ____ Time: _____
(last, first, m.i.)   (mm/dd/yy)

SSAN: ____ / ___ / ___ Sex: _____ Age: _____

Organization: _____ Grade/rank: _____ Job series/AFSC: _____

Injured on duty: ☐ yes ☐ no ☐ unknown

Illness: *report to Public Health*

1. Injury (*check all that apply*)
- ☐ needle stick
- ☐ contusion/bruise
- ☐ laceration/cut
- ☐ puncture
- ☐ abrasion/scrape
- ☐ fracture
- ☐ sprain/strain
- ☐ inhalation/ingestion
- ☐ burn/blisters
- ☐ environmental (heat, cold, altitude, depth)*
- ☐ electrical shock/electrocution
- ☐ rupture/avulsion
- ☐ amputation
- ☐ foreign body
- ☐ overexertion
- ☐ other:

2. Part of body (*check all that apply*)
- ☐ eye
- ☐ head
- ☐ neck
- ☐ arm
- ☐ hand
- ☐ chest/shoulder
- ☐ spine/back
- ☐ abdomen
- ☐ pelvis
- ☐ knee
- ☐ ankle
- ☐ foot
- ☐ eg (other part)
- ☐ other:

3. Event type (*check 1*)
- ☐ military aircraft (form ____)
- ☐ parachute – *go to a*
- ☐ motor vehicle – *go to b*
- ☐ other transport – *go to c*
- ☐ march/drill –*go to d*
- ☐ sport/recreation – *go to e*
- ☐ other fall/jump – *go to f*
- ☐ slip/trip/stumble – *go to g*
- ☐ lift/push/pull – *go to h*
- ☐ immersion/diving – *go to i*
- ☐ struck by – *go to j*
- ☐ thermal - *go to k*
- ☐ poisoning – *go to l*
- ☐ electromag/radiation – *go to m*
- ☐ machinery – *go to n*
- ☐ electricity/lightning – *go to o*
- ☐ fighting – *go to p*
- ☐ gun/explosion – *go to q*
- ☐ other: _____

4. Intent (*check 1*)
- ☐ unintentional
- ☐ in battle
- ☐ non-battle assault (intentional)
- ☐ self-inflicted
- ☐ unknown

5. Place (*check 1*)
- ☐ on maneuvers
- ☐ military property (non-maneuver-able)
- ☐ private residence
- ☐ sports area
- ☐ street/highway
- ☐ commercial area
- ☐ industrial/construction area
- ☐ farm
- ☐ other specified: _____
- ☐ unspecified

6. Disposition
- ☐ return to regular duty
- ☐ return to limited duty: ____ days
- ☐ sent home for rest of shift (military: quarters, no duty)
- ☐ sent home for _____ days (military: quarters, no duty: _X_ days)
- ☐ admitted to hospital
- ☐ died before admission
- ☐ died after admission
- ☐ other: _____

Returned to duty

Date: ____ ____ ____
(mm/dd/yy)

Time: _____

*Additional injury information: _____

Describe circumstances: _____

(**Fig. 23-4** *continues*)

529

a. Parachute
- ☐ impact with aircraft
- ☐ chute failure
- ☐ opening shock
- ☐ ground impact
- ☐ dragged by chute
- ☐ other: _____

b. Motor Vehicle
(1) <u>Vehicle:</u>
- ☐ military
- ☐ personally owned vehicle
- ☐ unknown

(2) <u>Person:</u>
- ☐ driver
- ☐ passenger
- ☐ pedestrian
- ☐ other/unknown

(3) <u>Seatbelt/Helmet:</u>
- ☐ yes
- ☐ no
- ☐ unknown

(4) <u>Vehicle type:</u>
- ☐ car
- ☐ truck
- ☐ sport utility
- ☐ tracked vehicle
- ☐ private aircraft
- ☐ commercial aircraft
- ☐ other: _____

c. Other transport
- ☐ watercraft
- ☐ motorcycle
- ☐ bicycle
- ☐ pedestrian
- ☐ other: _____

d. March/drill
- ☐ ceremony-related
- ☐ long-distance march
- ☐ training

e. Sports/recreation
- ☐ baseball/softball
- ☐ basketball
- ☐ boxing
- ☐ football
- ☐ golf
- ☐ gymnastics
- ☐ hockey
- ☐ horsemanship
- ☐ racquet sport
- ☐ running/track
- ☐ hunting/shooting
- ☐ skiing
- ☐ soccer
- ☐ swimming
- ☐ volleyball
- ☐ weight training
- ☐ wrestling
- ☐ other: _____

f. Fall/jump *(not parachute)*
- ☐ on same level
- ☐ on/from steps
- ☐ from ladder/scaffold
- ☐ from building
- ☐ from tree/cliff
- ☐ other: _____

g. Slip/trip/stumble
- ☐ due to obstacle
- ☐ on slippery surface
- ☐ while lifting
- ☐ other: _____

h. Lift/push/pull/twist without falling
- ☐ cargo handling
- ☐ flightline activity
- ☐ warehousing
- ☐ medical/patient
- ☐ outdoor maintenance
- ☐ other exertion: _____

i. Immersion/diving
- ☐ immersion
- ☐ diving
- ☐ other: _____

j. Struck by...
- ☐ falling object
- ☐ projected object

k. Thermal effect
- ☐ scald/steam
- ☐ hot object
- ☐ fire/flame
- ☐ heat, unspecified
- ☐ cold
- ☐ other: _____

l. Poisoning
- ☐ therapeutic drug
- ☐ illegal drug
- ☐ vehicle exhaust
- ☐ other ingestion
- ☐ other inhalation
- ☐ unknown, other: _____

m. Electromagnetic/radiation
- ☐ ultraviolet light
- ☐ laser
- ☐ microwave
- ☐ ionizing radiation (radioactive)

n. Machinery
- ☐ vehicle (non-road)
- ☐ fixed
- ☐ for lifting
- ☐ hand tool
- ☐ other: _____

o. Electricity/lightning
- ☐ electric appliance
- ☐ other 110/220
- ☐ high tension wire
- ☐ lightning strike
- ☐ other: _____

p. Fighting
- ☐ fists/teeth/feet, etc
- ☐ other weapon: _____

q. Gun/explosion
- ☐ military rifle or shotgun
- ☐ military sidearm
- ☐ mounted machine gun
- ☐ mine, bomb
- ☐ exploding gas
- ☐ personal rifle/shotgun
- ☐ personal handgun
- ☐ other: _____

Fig. 23-4. A sample Injury Surveillance Form

Because deployed service members are at a greater risk of suffering a serious injury (eg, death, hospital admission) than those not deployed, reasonably accurate predictions of the number of losses and type of injuries expected on a mission need to be made to determine required troop strengths and medical assets. Ultimately this information can be used to develop injury prevention measures.

To make accurate and useful predictions, medical surveillance during deployments needs to be an essential part of the field preventive medicine program. This need has been recognized, and programs have been developed for the missions in Haiti and Bosnia. Accurate and timely data delivered to medical and line commanders in the field can lead to appropriate responses to higher-than-anticipated injury rates or unusual injury types. Figure 23-4 shows a prototype injury surveillance form, developed under the auspices of the Armed Forces Epidemiological Board, that could be adapted for use during deployments.

The medical surveillance system should work in concert with the existing accident reporting systems managed by the safety professionals. In the Army, that system requires the reporting of any accident that causes a lost workday.[19]

Medical surveillance identifies an injury only after it has occurred, and many systems have recorded only the medical diagnosis in general terms. Often missing from the data are the pre-injury, during-injury, and post-injury events that contribute to the occurrence and severity of the injury. An injury surveillance system that captures and reports the type, the mechanism, and, if possible, the circumstances surrounding the injury event is needed to allow risk managers and others, such as commanders, to fully understand the evolution of an unintentional trauma casualty.[4]

The effectiveness of surveillance is demonstrated by a civilian example: the National Electronic Injury Surveillance System (NEISS), operated by the Consumer Product Safety Commission.[20] This surveillance system uses a probability sample of emergency rooms throughout the United States to collect injury incidence data and is a model of how reports from the field (in this case, the general US population) can be used to reveal dangerous consumer products and lead to the implementation of control measures. For the Consumer Product Safety Commission, these could include better hazard labeling, product recall, or product reengineering. The same principles can and should be applied during deployments of military personnel.

Tracking of specific types of injuries by researchers and clinicians has led, in one example, to better automotive design.[21,22] Using crash tests and reports from emergency rooms and other settings, automotive developers have been able to pinpoint specific problem areas in the design of automobile passenger compartments. Reengineering based on these reports has made automobiles safer and reduced the severity of injuries following a crash. The Army has used this type of reporting in its MANPRINT[23] and Health Hazard Assessment programs[24] to assess the health risks and human performance issues of military equipment at any stage in its life cycle. An ankle brace developed in the late 1980s and early 1990s for service members in airborne units to reduce the risk of jump injuries is an example of how medical surveillance, safety professionals, product developers, and line units can work together to produce an intervention that reduces injury risk and aids the mission.[25] Postmarketing surveillance of the brace continues to evaluate its safety, effectiveness, and efficacy.

Risk Assessment

Injury prevention is a five-step process (Exhibit 23-2). The Army Safety Center defines the process in a similar way.[26] Although risk of injury is inherent in all military operations, risk managers must find ways to reduce or eliminate unnecessary risks (Figure 23-5). In the military, successfully implementing this process allows a commander to accomplish the mission. The scope of the safety program, its general direction, and the responsibilities of all involved are made clear by regulation (eg, AR 385-15[26]) and, in the Army, the commanding general of US Army Forces Command establishes safety policy,

---

EXHIBIT 23-2

THE FIVE-STEP PUBLIC HEALTH APPROACH TO INJURY PREVENTION

1. Identify the problem and its magnitude

2. Determine the causes of the problem

3. Know what works to prevent the problem and develop a plan

4. Implement the plan

5. Evaluate the results

Effect		Hazard Probability				
		Frequent A	Likely B	Occasionally C	Seldom D	Unlikely E
Catastrophic	I	Extremely high	Extremely high	High	High	Medium
Critical	II	Extremely high	High	High	Medium	Low
Moderate	III	High	Medium	Medium	Low	Low
Negligible	IV	Medium	Low	Low	Low	Low

Fig. 23-5. This matrix shows how risk managers classify the level of danger inherent in an operation. The resultant score, the risk assessment code, is based on a hazard's likelihood of occurring and its potential for doing damage. It is used to prioritize the need for and timing of interventions.

standards, and guidelines during operations, exercises, and maneuvers.

A civilian model that may be useful in conducting a risk assessment is shown in Figure 23-6.[27] The operational, political, epidemiologic, and managerial elements of identifying and controlling an injury problem are given equal weight in an unbroken circle. This is a good visual analogy of how risk assessment can be approached. The assessor can enter the circle at any point and travel in any direction but often must address each of the elements to identify and control risk successfully.

PREVENTION AND CONTROL STRATEGIES

Injuries do not just happen; in injury control science, there are no such things as accidents. Leading up to every injurious event are a series of actions or inactions and conditions that combine to produce the injury.[4] Making sense of these complex interactions is key to anticipating and countering them. Simply providing education and training materials and issuing recommendations will not effectively prevent injuries.[25,28]

Injury Event Modeling

There are two important models that evaluate causes and effects of unintentional injuries: the classic epidemiologic model of agent–host–environment interaction and the Haddon matrix. The epidemiologic model is applicable to injury prevention,[29] and Haddon incorporated it into his matrix because the three points of this triangular model represent the elements that must interact to produce an injury.

The agent in unintentional trauma is usually mechanical or kinetic energy transferred from an object to a human being. The mechanical impact or impulse could be from the sudden and unexpected deceleration of one motor vehicle striking another, a falling crate, or a human body hitting another during a football game. Other energy transfers, such

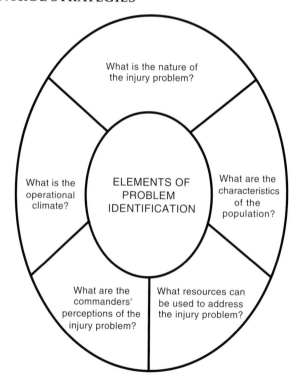

Fig. 23-6. Risk Assessment Model. Source: The National Committee for Injury Prevention and Control. Injury prevention: Meeting the challenge. *Am J Prev Med.* 1989;5(3 suppl):23. Adapted by permission of Oxford University Press.

as thermal, chemical, and radiological, also play a role. The environment can facilitate or reduce an energy transfer (eg, driving conditions, guardrails, other barriers), the amount of energy transferred (eg, shock absorbing material, availability of safety equipment), and ultimately the damage done by an injury (eg, emergency medical response, available medical care). The host is the individual receiving the transferred energy. Factors related to hosts include their chance of exposing themselves to danger (eg, fatigue, other impairment), their ability to tolerate the amount of energy transferred (eg, muscle mass, bone density), their behaviors (eg, using seat belts, wearing a helmet), and their ability to heal (eg, age, physical condition).

In the 1960s, Haddon developed a matrix that includes the three points of the epidemiologic triangle and adds the preevent, during-event, and postevent phases of an injurious event.[30,31] The matrix has been used most often for motor vehicle injuries but can be applied to almost any potentially hazardous situation. The resulting 3 x 3 matrix (Figure 23-7) is a comprehensive model that serves as a framework for developing and evaluating control programs. But it is not, as Haddon himself warned, a formula or guide that needs to be strictly followed.

The matrix does not focus as much on the causes of injuries as on the means available to reduce morbidity and mortality by helping the user identify where interventions may be effective.[32]

The figure shows a Haddon matrix that could be applied in a deployment situation. As the prevention officer moves through the model, he or she can identify possible places for intervention. In reality, many of the elements are beyond the control of medical and safety personnel, but by thinking through the possible cause of injuries, thinking of interventions to counteract them, and either applying or lobbying for the doable interventions, the burden of injuries can be reduced.

Developing an Injury Prevention Program

Haddon later proposed a 10-point system for reducing the risk of injury.[32] It addresses preevent, during-event, and postevent interactions. These include eliminating, reducing, or modifying the amount and type of energy available for transfer; reducing an individual's absorbed dose; increasing the individual's threshold for injury; and countering and repairing the damage when an injury does occur (Exhibit 23-3). These 10 points clearly illus-

	Human	Vehicle	Environment
Preevent	Fatigue Alcohol/drugs Anxiety	Speed Cargo (eg, explosives) Vehicle condition	Road conditions Time of day Speed limit Blackout conditions Operational tempo
During event	Bone density Muscle mass Helmet or seat belt use	Speed Site of impact Severity of impact Explosion Vehicle design (eg, occupant protection)	Road design (eg, barriers, breakaway light poles)
Postevent	Preexisting medical condition Age Severity of initial injury	Dissipation of energy Postcrash fire	First aid Emergency medical response Time to medical care Level of care available Temperature

Fig. 23-7. A Haddon Matrix for a Military Convoy

trate the complexity of designing effective preventive programs. Like Haddon's matrix, they provide a way to systematize the process of defining countermeasures to a potentially dangerous situation. They also reinforce the fact that successful injury control strategies require input, support, and cooperation from many diverse professionals.

Baker has developed a four-point outline for interventions to reduce injuries.[33] The general guidelines suggest modifying the environment (including the social environment), providing training and education, strengthening the individual, and providing an emergency medical response capability.

A simpler way to approach development of preventive strategies may evolve from the model used by occupational health professionals called the hierarchy of controls.[34] It separates preventable on-the-job illness and injury into three broad areas of interventions in descending order of effectiveness: engineering changes, personal protective equipment, and administrative controls. This triad can

be discussed in the context of reducing the hazards associated with motor vehicles through safer roads and more crashworthy motor vehicles (engineering changes), providing seat belts (personal protective equipment), and establishing and enforcing speed limits (administrative controls). In the field, these controls can translate into building safety into equipment and processes; using seat belts, flak jackets, and helmets when required; and following established safety procedures and orders. It should be noted that safety guidelines and education are most effective when there is the threat of legal punishment if they are not followed.[27]

Unlike civilian injury prevention strategies, military approaches must take into account the potential limits placed on any intervention by operational requirements. These requirements may also create hazards. In a very simplistic example, the dangers of driving at night without headlights are well known; in fact, it is illegal to do so in the United States. Mission success may, however, require night driving under

---

EXHIBIT 23-3

HADDON'S TEN-STEP INJURY PREVENTION SYSTEM

1. Prevent the creation of the hazard in the first place (eg, ban certain sports activities, such as tackle football).

2. Reduce the amount of hazard brought into being (eg, transport explosives in smaller quantities).

3. Prevent the release of a hazard that already exists (eg, enforce no-smoking rules around fuel dumps).

4. Modify the rate of release or spatial distribution of a hazard (eg, build military vehicles to better absorb energy during a crash, thus reducing the amount of energy transferred to the occupants; require the use of seat belts even in tactical vehicles, when possible).

5. Separate in time or space the hazard and that which is to be protected (eg, store fuel and ammunition away from living quarters).

6. Separate the hazard and that which is to be protected by imposition of a barrier (eg, require the use of appropriate personal protective equipment such as helmets and cut-resistant gloves).

7. Modify basic, relevant qualities of the hazard (eg, make explosives more stable).

8. Make what is to be protected more resistant to the hazard (eg, encourage "safe" physical training activities).

9. Begin to counter the damage already done by the environmental hazard (eg, train all personnel in emergency first aid, establish an emergency medical response capability).

10. Stabilize, repair, and rehabilitate the object of the damage (eg, deploy the right mix of medical specialists and equipment to provide effective acute and rehabilitative care).

Source: Haddon W Jr. Advances in the epidemiology of injuries as a basis for public policy. *Public Health Rep.* 1980;95:411–421.

blackout conditions. Accepting this as a necessary hazard means looking for other ways to reduce the hazards created by this operational requirement. Options to consider (though they still may not be possible given the operational tempo) could include ensuring drivers are well rested, spacing vehicles at a greater distance than normal, requiring the use of seat belts and helmets, providing sufficient traffic controls, and providing an increased level of emergency medical support. Ultimately, however, it will be the commanders who will decide what necessary risks must be assumed to ensure the success of a mission.[26]

Often, simple solutions to serious problems work well. During the Allied buildup in England for the Normandy invasion in World War II, football was banned in US camps to reduce the risk of injury and loss of soldiers from the invasion force.[35] Soldiers were provided with bats and balls instead.

Haddon's matrix and 10-point system and other models allow the injury-control professional, whether medical or safety, to see and evaluate the full spectrum of contributors to an injurious event. Selecting what interventions are possible and where to attempt them becomes easier using this somewhat structured approach.

EFFECTING CHANGE

On deployment, safety and injury prevention is the responsibility of the commander and everyone else down through the chain of command to the individual service member.[36] Prevention and control of injuries is a partnership among many people. The responsibility of the medical community is to understand the process of injury causation and prevention, track the kinds and severity of injuries, inform the commanders of the magnitude and nature of the injury problem, and work closely with commanders and safety professionals to reduce the risk.

The primary injury control function of preventive medicine is the collection, analysis, and reporting of complete and accurate surveillance data. Solid and detailed injury epidemiology is essential for identifying hazards, determining their potential impact on the mission, influencing commanders and the deployed community, and evaluating control measures. But while surveillance and epidemiology may be the primary contribution to injury control, physicians and other health care providers must use their medical, epidemiologic, political, and managerial skills to define and effect the changes needed to reduce hazards within the context of the military mission. Commanders and others must be kept informed of the injury burden in their units and what steps can and should be taken to maintain readiness. Prevention and control are an ongoing process. Interventions must be continuously reviewed and evaluated, and surveillance is the key to determining effectiveness.

SUMMARY

Safety in working, playing, and living should not be the first casualty of a deployment. Given the limits on personnel and medical resources and the increase in potential hazards during a military operation, injury prevention becomes a mission-essential responsibility for everyone. Health care personnel, and especially those in preventive medicine, are key players in reducing the burden of unintentional trauma casualties.

Medical personnel need to be strong advocates for primary, secondary, and tertiary injury prevention during deployments. This is accomplished first through routine, detailed, and accurate surveillance to define the magnitude of the problem, persons at risk, and type and mechanisms of injury. This is followed by timely reporting of this essential information. Medical personnel need to communicate and work with the prevention partners identified above, at times forcing injury prevention onto commanders' and others' agendas, to define problems and seek out solutions based on the strategies discussed in this chapter. Next, appropriate solutions should be implemented and evaluated continually to determine the effectiveness of the intervention. The proposed solution may need to be adjusted or discarded and other solutions tried. The models and methods presented here are guidelines to developing successful injury prevention programs, because injury prevention is both a science and an art.

REFERENCES

1. Hoeffler DF, Melton LJ 3rd. Changes in the distribution of Navy and Marine Corps casualties from World War I through the Vietnam conflict. *Mil Med.* 1981;146:776–779.

2. Writer JV, DeFraites RF, Brundage JF. Comparative mortality among US military personnel in the Persian Gulf region and worldwide during Operations Desert Shield and Desert Storm. *JAMA.* 1996;275:118–121.

3. Writer JV. Hospitalization for non-battle injuries among US soldiers in Southwest Asia, August 1990–July 1991. *Am J Epidemiol.* 1995;141(supp):S7. Abstract.

4. National Research Council. *Injury in America.* Washington, DC: National Academy Press; 1985.

5. Haddon W. A note concerning accident theory and research with specific reference to motor vehicle accidents. *Ann N Y Acad Sci.* 1963;107:635–646.

6. Carey ME. Learning from traditional combat mortality and morbidity data used in the evaluation of combat medical care. *Mil Med.* 1987;152:6–13.

7. Beebe GW, DeBakey ME. *Battle Casualties: Incidence, Mortality and Logistic Considerations.* Springfield, Ill: Charles C Thomas; 1952.

8. Lada J, Reister FA, eds. *Medical Statistics of World War II.* Washington, DC: Office of the Surgeon General, US Department of the Army; 1975.

9. Jones BH. Overuse injuries of the lower extremities associated with marching, jogging, and running, a review. *Mil Med.* 1983;148:783–787.

10. Reynolds KL, Heckel HA, Witt CE, Martin JW, et al. Cigarette smoking, physical fitness, and injuries in infantry soldiers. *Am J Prev Med.* 1994;10:145–150.

11. Jones BH, Cowan DN, Tomlinson JP, Robinson JR, Polly DW, Frykman PN. Epidemiology of injuries associated with physical training among young men in the Army. *Med Sci Sports Exerc.* 1993;25:197–203.

12. Reister FA. *Battle Casualties and Medical Statistics: US Army Experience in the Korean War.* Washington, DC: The Surgeon General, US Department of the Army; 1973.

13. Palinkas LA, Coben P. Disease and non-battle injuries among US Marines in Vietnam. *Mil Med.* 1988;153:150–155.

14. Blood CG, Anderson ME. The battle for Hue: casualty and disease rates during urban warfare. *Mil Med.* 1994;159:590–595.

15. Blood CG, Jolly R. Comparisons of disease and nonbattle injury incidence across various military operations. *Mil Med.* 1995;160:258–263.

16. Writer JV, DeFraites RF, Keep LW. Casualties during deployments due to non-battle injuries. In: Jones B, ed. *Injuries in the Military: A Hidden Epidemic, A Report for the Armed Forces Epidemiologic Board.* Washington, DC: The Injury Prevention and Control Work Group of the Armed Forces Epidemiological Board; 1996.

17. Hall MJ, Owings MF. *Hospitalizations for Injury and Poisoning in the United States, 1991.* Hyattsville, Md: National Center for Health Statistics : 1994. Pamphlet 252.

18. Baker SP, O'Neill B, Ginsberg MJ, Li G. *The Injury Fact Book.* 2nd ed. New York: Oxford University Press; 1992: 211–227.

19. Department of the Army. *Accident Reporting and Records.* Washington, DC: DA; 1990. Army Regulation 385-40.

20. Multiple tube mine and shell fireworks device: advance notice of proposed rule making: request for comments and information. *Fed Register.* July 5, 1994;59.

21. Robertson LS. Reducing death on the road: the effects of minimum safety standards, publicized crash tests, seat belts, and alcohol. *Am J Public Health.* 1996;86:31–24.

22. Waller JA. Reflections on a half century of injury control. *Am J Public Health.* 1994;84:664–670.

23. Department of the Army. *Manpower Personnel Integration in the Materiel Acquisition Process* (MANPRINT). Washington, DC: DA; 1990. Army Regulation 602-2.

24. Department of the Army. *Health Hazard Assessment Program in Support of the Army Materiel Acquisition Decision Process*. Washington, DC: DA; 1991. Army Regulation 40-10.

25. Amoroso PJ, Ryan JB, Bickley BT, Taylor DC, Leitschuh P, Jones BH. *The Impact of an Outside the Boot Ankle Brace on Sprains Associated with Military Airborne Training*. Natick, Mass: US Army Research Institute of Environmental Medicine; 1994. USARIEM Report T95-1.

26. Department of the Army. *The Army Safety Program*. Washington, DC: DA; 1988. Army Regulation 385-10.

27. The National Committee for Injury Prevention and Control. Injury prevention: Meeting the challenge. *Am J Prev Med*. 1989;5(3 suppl):1–303.

28. Loimer H, Guarnieri M. Accidents and acts of God: A history of terms. *Am J Public Health*. 1996;86:101–107.

29. Mausner JS, Kramer S. *Mausner and Bahn, Epidemiology: An Introductory Text*. 2nd ed. Philadelphia: W.B. Saunders; 1985: 33.

30. Haddon W Jr. The changing approach to the epidemiology, prevention and ameliorization of trauma: The transition to approaches etiologically rather than descriptively based. *Am J Public Health Nations Health*. 1968;58:1431–1438.

31. Haddon W Jr. A logical framework for categorizing highway safety phenomena and activity. *J Trauma*. 1972;12:193–207.

32. Haddon W Jr. Advances in the epidemiology of injuries as a basis for public policy. *Public Health Rep*. 1980;95:411–421.

33. Baker SP. Determinants of injury and opportunities for intervention. *Am J Epidemiol*. 1975;101:98–102.

34. Olishifski JB. Methods of controls. In: Plog BA, ed. *Fundamentals of Industrial Hygiene*. 3rd ed. Chicago: National Safety Council; 1988: 457.

35. Ambrose SE. *D-Day, June 6, 1944: The Climatic Battle of World War Two*. New York: Simon and Schuster; 1994: 43.

36. Department of the Army. *Operations*. Washington, DC: DA; 1993. Field Manual 100-5.

Chapter 24

SELECTED TOPICS IN DEPLOYMENT OCCUPATIONAL MEDICINE

PAUL D. SMITH, DO, MPH; DOUG OHLIN, PhD; STEVE SMITH, MD, MPH; AND WILLIAM A. RICE, MD, MPH

P. Smith, Colonel, Medical Corps, US Army, Occupational Environmental Medicine Staff Officer, Proponency Officer for Preventive Medicine, Office of The Surgeon General, 5109 Leesburg Pike, 6 Skyline Place, Falls Church, VA 22041-3258

D. Ohlin, Occupational and Environmental Medicine, Hearing Conservation Program, US Army Center for Health Promotion and Preventive Medicine, 5158 Blackhawk Rd., Aberdeen Proving Ground, MD 21010

S. Smith, Site Medical Director, Umatilla Chemical Agent Demilitarization Facility, Umatilla Chemical Depot, 78068 Ordnance Road, Hermiston, OR 97838; formerly, Major, Medical Corps, US Army, Command Surgeon, US Army Industrial Operations Command, ATTN: AMSIO-SG, Rock Island IL 61299-6000

W. Rice, Lieutenant Colonel, Medical Corps, US Army; currently, Division Surgeon, 1st Armored Division, Germany; formerly, Director, Occupational Medicine, US Army Center for Health Promotion and Preventive Medicine-Europe, APO AE 09180

HEALTH EFFECTS OF REPEATED IMPACT AND WHOLE-BODY VIBRATION

With the dawn of the industrial age, human exposures to vibration changed dramatically. Machines of the industrial revolution resulted in vibration exposure to the individual that continues today. Vibration transmitted to humans may be classified into several common types. Whole-body vibration consists of waves of mechanical energy transmitted throughout the human body. It is differentiated from segmental vibration, which is mechanical energy generally concentrated in a segment of the body, such as an arm or leg. Vibration may be further classified by the nature of the mechanical waves. Sinusoidal vibration is characterized by a smooth repetitive cycle, such as we see in the vibrations of an electric motor. Diagrammatically, this type of vibration may be represented by a sine wave. Repeated impact vibration, also known as bump and jolt vibration, is characterized by markedly abrupt accelerations and decelerations that occur in a random and chaotic manner.

Vibration exposure is particularly pronounced in the military setting.[1] Occupants of aircraft are usually exposed to sinusoidal vibration produced by the aircraft's engines. Occupants of military ground vehicles experience a "bump and jolt" vibration as the vehicle crosses rough terrain. Tactical ground vehicles, such as armored personnel carriers and tanks, greatly exceed published exposure limits to vibration according to Griffin's *Handbook of Vibration*.[2] Vibration should be kept in mind when evaluating soldiers who operate equipment such as tanks, trucks, and armored engineering equipment. Patients may present with a variety of symptoms related to vibration exposure. Vibration as a cause of fatigue, pain, and other complaints should also be considered for aircrew members, particularly those flying modified or new aircraft. Unfortunately, vibration in military ground vehicles has not been adequately studied. The following section presents a review of the signs, symptoms, and health effects of vibration exposure.

Vibration-Related Illnesses

General Effects

It should be noted that nearly all illness and injury seen in vibration-exposed patients are not unique to vibration alone. Vibration is felt to be a cofactor in the development of certain diseases or is believed to accelerate certain disease processes, such as low back degenerative disease. This is well

reviewed by Dupuis.[3] Such conditions are classified as an occupational illness in some European nations and by the International Labor Organization.

Vibration affects multiple body systems (Table 24-1). The effects of vibration on the musculoskeletal and gastrointestinal systems are well documented, with large-scale epidemiologic studies demonstrating increases in low back pain and esophageal dismotility.[2–6] The cardiovascular and nervous systems are also affected. Whole-body vibration, including the bump and jolt variety common in the Army and Marine Corps, acts as a general body stressor. Exposed subjects experience an overall increase in adrenaline levels.[7] In addition, there is a general activation of the sympathetic nervous system with continued vibration exposure.[7,8] These result in sustained muscular and cardiovascular activity with concomitant fatigue. Cortisol excretion is also increased during vibration exposure, further indicating that this exposure acts as a general body stressor and perhaps results in reduced immunity.[9–11]

Musculoskeletal System

The human spine and supporting structures are sensitive to vibration. The spine itself may be damaged by repeated impact or from vibration that matches the spine's resonant frequencies. The lumbar spine, for instance, resonates at approximately 4 to 6 Hz.[12] These frequencies of vibration are commonly encountered in all vehicles. Vibration causes reduced disc nutrition and elevations in hydroxyproline that indicate damage to cartilage and vertebral end plates.[2,3,13–16] Electromyography of vibration-exposed subjects reveals increases in motor activity until fatigue ensues.[17–19] Back pain has been documented in truck drivers and train operators. This is, presumably, related to fatigue from the increase in motor activity during vibration exposure. It is likely that the same effect exists in troops using tactical ground vehicles, although this remains to be studied.

Vibration and repeated impact should be considered when seeing troops with back injury who are operators of tactical ground vehicles and truck drivers.[4,5,20–22] In one instance, back pain and hematuria were associated with testing of the rapid response vehicle, a dune buggy modified for military use.[23] Back pain and hematuria in exposed personnel should bring vibration exposure to mind after ruling out ureterolithiasis. These symptoms and signs

TABLE 24-1

PHYSIOLOGICAL AND HEALTH EFFECTS OF REPEATED IMPACT AND WHOLE-BODY VIBRATION BY MAJOR SYSTEM

Body System	Physiological/Health Effect	References
Whole-body	Increased adrenaline cortisone	a–d
Musculoskeletal	Vertebral end plate, vertebral disc deterioration, back pain	e–r
Cardiovascular	Increased blood pressure, increase heart rate, hand-arm vibration syndrome, increased blood lipids	a,e,s
Hematological	Increased hematocrit, decreased hemoglobin, increased haptoglobin, pooling in extremities	a,b,e
Gastrointestinal	Esophageal dysmotility, peptic ulcer disease, gastrointestinal bleeding	e,p,q,t–w
Nervous System	Altered neurotransmitters, dorsal root ganglia	x–cc
Reproductive	Abortion, altered menses	dd,ee

Sources:

a. Johanning E. Back disorders and health problems among subway train operators exposed to whole body vibration. *Scand J Work Environ Health.* 1991;17:414–419.

b. Johanning E, Wilder DG, Landrigan PJ, Pope MH. Whole-body exposure in subway cars and review of adverse health effects. *J Occup Med.* 1991;33:605–612.

c. Daleva M, Piperova-Dalbokova D, Hadjiolova I, Mincheva L. Changes in the excretion of corticosteroids and catecholamines in tractor drivers. *Int Arch Occup Environ Health.* 1982;49:345–352.

d. Kamenskii YN, Nosova IM. Effects of whole body vibration on certain indicators of neuro-endocrine processes. *Noise Vibration Bull.* 1989;Sept:205–207.

e. *Initial Health Hazard Assessment Report on the Fast Attack Vehicle (FAV).* Aberdeen Proving Ground, Md: Environmental Hygiene Agency; 1984.1. Griffin MJ. *Handbook of Human Vibration.* London: Academic Press Ltd; 1988. RCS Med 388.

f. Dupuis H. Medical and occupational preconditions for vibration induced spinal disorders: Occupational disease number 2110 in Germany. *Int Arch Occup Environ Health.* 1994;66(5):303–308.

g. Nakamura R Moroji T, Nohara S, Nakamura M, Okada A. Activation of cerebral dopaminergic systems by noise and whole-body vibration. *Environ Res.* 1992;57(1):10–18.

h. Barron JL, Noakes TD, Levy W, Smith C, Millar RP. Hypothalmic dysfunction in overtrained athletes. *J Clin Endocrinol Metab.* 1985;60:803–806.

i. Ariizumi M, Okada A. Effect of whole body vibration on the rat brain content of serotonin and plasma corticosterone. *Eur J Applied Physiol Occup Physiol.* 1983;52:15–19.

j. Granjean E. *Fitting the Task to the Man.* New York: Little Brown; 1989.

k. Pope MH, Hansson TH. Vibration of the spine and low back pain. *Clin Orthop.* 1992;279:49–59.

l. Pope MH, Kaigle AM, Magnusson M, Broman H, Hansson T. Intervertebral motion during vibration. *Proc Inst Mech Eng [H].* 1991;205(1):39–44.

m. Ishihara H, Tsuji H, Hirano N, Ohshima H, Terahata N. Effects of continuous quantitative vibration on rheologic and biological behaviors of the intervertebral disc. *Spine.* 1992;17(3 suppl):S7–S12.

n. Hansson T, Holm S. Clinical implications of vibration-induced changes in the lumbar spine. *Orthop Clin North Am.* 1991;22:247–253.

o. Kaji H, Sato E, Nagatsuka S, et al. Evaluation of sensory disturbances using short latency somatosensory evoked potentials (SSEPs) in vibration-exposed workers. [Japanese]. *Sangyo Igaku.* 1991;33:605–612.

p. DeLuca CJ. Myoelectrical manifestations of localized muscular fatigue in humans. *Crit Rev Biomech Eng.* 1985;4:251–278.

q. Klein AB, Snyder-Mackler L, Roy SH, DeLuca CJ. Comparison of spinal mobility and isometric trunk extensor forces with electromyographic spectral analysis in identifying low back pain. *Physical Therapy.* 1991;71(6):445–454

r. USAARL Contract Reports No. CR 95-1,CR 95-2, CR 95-3, CR 95-4.

s. Boshulzen HC, Bongers PM, Hulshof CT. Self-reported back pain in fork-lift truck and freight-container tractor drivers exposed to whole-body vibration. *Spine.* 1992;17:59–65.

t. Chatterjee S, Bandyopadhyay A. Effect of vibrating steering on the grip strength in heavy vehicle drivers. *J Human Ergology.* 1991;20(1):77–84.

u. Gow BS, Legg MJ, Yu W, Kukongvlrlyapan U, Lee LL. Does vibration cause post-stenotic dilatation in vivo and influence atherogenesis in cholesterol-fed rabbits? *J Biomech Eng.* 1992;114(1):20–25.

v. Nakamura H, Katoh A, Nohara S, Nakamura M, Okada A. Experimental studies on the pathogenesis of the gastric mucosal lesions induced by whole-body vibration. *Environmental Research.* 1992;58(2):220–229.

w. Katoh A, Nakamura H, Nohara S, Ohmura K, Munemoto Y, Oda M. Experimental studies on the development of acute gastric lesions induced by vibration stress in rats and its pathogeneitc mechanisms. *Japanese J Gastroenterol.* 1992;89:469–476.

x. Kabacinska-Knapikowa D, Paradowski L, Kwiatkowski S. Esophageal motility in personnel operating heavy self-propelled mining machines. *Materia Medica Polona.* 1992;24(3):153–155.

y. Mecel H, Wozniak H, Sun L, Frazier E, Mason HC. Effects on rats of exposure to heat and vibration. *J Applied Physiol.* 1962;17:759–762.

z. Nakamura H, Moroji T, Naaase H, Okazawa T, Okada A. Changes of cerebral vasoactive intestinal polypeptide- and somatostatin-like immu-noreactivity induced by noise and whole-body vibration in the rat. *Eur J Appl Physiol Occup Physiol.* 1994;68(1):62–67.

aa. McLain RF, Weinstein JN. Nuclear clefting in dorsal root ganglion neurons: A response to whole body vibration. *J Comp Neurol.* 1992;322(4):538–547.

bb. McLain RF, Weinstein JN. Ultrastructal changes in the dorsal root ganglion associated with whole body vibration. *J Spinal Disord.* 1991;4(2):142–148.

cc. McLain RF, Weinstein JN. Effects of whole body vibration on dorsal root ganglion neurons: Changes in neuronal nuclei. *Spine.* 1994;19:1455–1461.

dd. Nakamura H, Moroji T, Nohara S, Nakamura M, Okada A. Activation of cerebral dopaminergic systems by noise and whole-body vibration. *Environ Res.* 1992;57(1):10–18.

ee. Bartsch C, Meihe B. The effect of vibrations in the early stages of embryogenesis on the postnatal motor and physical development of Wistar rats [German]. *Anat Anz.* 1991;173(4):239–242.

should clear once the patient's exposure to vibration has stopped.

Cardiovascular System

The cardiovascular response to vibration is well studied. This system reacts to vibration as it does to any stress, with an increase in heart rate and blood pressure. Several limited Scandinavian studies indicate a rise in blood lipids.[3,24] Additionally, vibration results in hand-arm vibration syndrome, in which segmental vibration results in endothelial damage to the small arterioles. Patients present with vasospasm of the digits, especially in response to cold.

Gastrointestinal System

Studies reveal an increase in motility disorders in vibration-exposed workers. The prevalence of gastroesophageal reflux disease increases, and in experimental animals gastrointestinal bleeding is produced by vibration exposure.[5,6,25–27] In troops presenting with symptoms of reflux esophagitis, gastroesophageal reflux, or intestinal bleeding, the differential diagnosis should include repeated impact vibration in the field. Although not proven by studies, reducing that exposure where practical may result in a reduction or cessation of the symptoms.

Neurological System

The peripheral and central nervous systems are both affected by vibration. Animal research has demonstrated an increase in vasointestinal peptide and a decrease in substance P, possibly caused by a pain response.[28] In the dorsal root ganglia, nuclear clefting is noted after vibration exposure, denoting injury to the peripheral nervous system.[29–31] In the central nervous system, alterations of dopamine levels are described in experimental animals, although this has not been studied in humans.[32]

Female Reproductive System

The reproductive system may be adversely affected by vibration exposure. Case studies dating to the 1950s and 1960s report spontaneous abortions in women exposed to vibration in their work. Menstrual abnormalities may be increased in vibration-exposed women.[33,34] No studies are available at present to support or refute this effect in female service members exposed to vibration.

Future Studies and Guidelines

Adequate guidelines for vibration exposure in military ground vehicles are under development. Sinusoidal vibration is of heightened concern to the Air Force and is studied at Wright Patterson Air Force Base, Ohio. Repeated impact vibration in ground vehicles is of concern principally to the Army and Marine Corps and is actively being investigated by the US Army Aeromedical Research Lab, Fort Rucker, Ala. These efforts should result in better guidelines for controlling vibration exposure in troops by providing needed information on health effects and relating these effects to vibration levels.[34]

[Paul D. Smith]

HEARING CONSERVATION

Scope of the Problem

Hazardous noise pervades the military environment. Moreover, the increasing demand for greater range, firepower, and speed all translate into higher and more hazardous noise levels. In 1994, among US Army enlisted combat arms (infantry, artillery, and armor), 25.5% of soldiers with more than 17.5 years of service had a significant hearing loss. Of those with 12.5 to 17.5 years, it was 15.3%. Among soldiers with less than 2.5 years, only 5.4% had a hearing loss.[35] Although still a problem of sizable concern, this is significant progress since 1974 when, for the same lengths of service, the prevalences of hearing loss were 54.2%, 47.8%, and 11.5%, respectively.[36]

One training session on a firing range can wreak havoc on unprotected ears. It is possible for a soldier to emerge from basic training with a significant hearing loss. Since the majority of noise exposure over a soldier's career is the result of routine training exercises, most noise-induced hearing loss is preventable by implementing protective measures during training.

Importance of Hearing to the Mission

Acute hearing (in both ears) is a 360° warning sense, whereas vision is only slightly better than 180°. Soldiers can identify an enemy's location by certain sounds: closing rifle bolts, loading cartridges, engaging or disengaging safety locks, clipping barbed wire, and footsteps[37] (Figure 24-1).

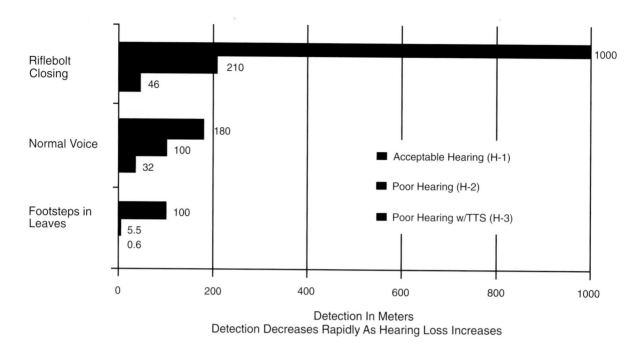

Fig. 24-1. Detection of Sound by Hearing Ability
Data source: Price GR, Kalb JT, Garinther GR. Toward a measure of auditory handicap in the Army. *Ann Otol Rhinol Laryngol Suppl.* 1989;140:42–52.

Good hearing also enables soldiers to discriminate between friendly and enemy fire: the different acoustic signatures of M-16 and AK-47 rifles, for example. In addition, soldiers with good hearing have less trouble understanding radio transmissions over noisy communication systems. The Army Research Laboratory, Aberdeen Proving Ground, Md, has produced convincing data that have linked communication ability to performance among experienced tank crews.[38]

Program Implementation

Hearing conservation program requirements and procedures are outlined in Department of the Army Pamphlet 40–501.[39] Detailed implementation procedures and technical guidance are included in various technical guides available from the US Army Center for Health Promotion and Preventive Medicine (USACHPPM), 5158 Blackhawk Road, ATTN: MCHB-TS-CHC, Aberdeen Proving Ground, MD 21010–5403.[40-44]

Noise Hazard Identification

For the purposes of administering the Hearing Conservation Program, a steady noise of 85 decibels (dB)A3 or greater is considered hazardous regardless of duration of exposure. Examples of

steady-state noise include generators, tracked vehicle interiors and exteriors, and aircraft. In the absence of noise data or hazard posting, there is a simple rule of thumb for determining the presence of a steady-state noise hazard if one has to raise one's voice to be heard at a distance of 1 m.

All small- and large-caliber weapons (including blanks) exceed the peak (P) impulse noise criteria of 140 dB peak (dBP). The use of hearing protection in the vicinity of weapon systems must take into account the requirement to use hearing protection within a 140 dBP contour. For small arms, this contour will extend back from the firer's position approximately 15 m. Larger-caliber weapons and shoulder-fired rockets will have much larger contours behind the firing point, depending on type of round, level of charge, and firing elevation.[44]

A direct, positive correlation has been observed between the posting of hazard signs and the use of hearing protection. At no time, however, should the exteriors of tactical weapon systems be posted.

Noise Controls

Engineering controls can reduce or eliminate the noise hazard and the need for other hearing conservation measures. Although such intervention opportunities are rare in the military, exploiting them can offer tactical advantages, as well as a reduction or elimination of a noise hazard. For example, the blast attenuating device on the end of the large-caliber mortar not only reduces the noise level at the crews' ears, but the device also makes the mortar easier to load and adds approximately 1,000 m to its range. The tactically quiet generator affords the advantages of hazard elimination and reduced detectability[37] (Figure 24-2).

Administrative controls are employed when hearing protection cannot protect personnel from a given exposure. Weapons system operator manuals should be consulted for any limitations on the number of rounds permitted and any time limits on noise exposure.

Hearing Protective Devices

Hearing protective devices are issued to US military personnel. The user is given a choice from among approved protectors unless there is a medical or environmental contraindication. Approved hearing protectors are listed in Department of the Army Pamphlet 40–501.[39]

Noise muffs are a safety item and may be purchased using a National Stock Number (NSN) or as a local purchase item. Earplugs, however, are a medical item. Choices are limited to two types of preformed (triple- and single-flange) and a hand-formed foam. Two exceptions to the restricted use of earplugs are custom-molded earplugs for individuals who cannot be properly fitted with approved devices and musician's earplugs for band members.

Single- and triple-flange earplugs must be fitted under medical supervision. The hand-formed earplugs can be stocked in noise-hazardous areas (eg, firing ranges, airfields) for transient personnel or for other personnel without their issued protectors. Local commanders can authorize wearing earplugs and

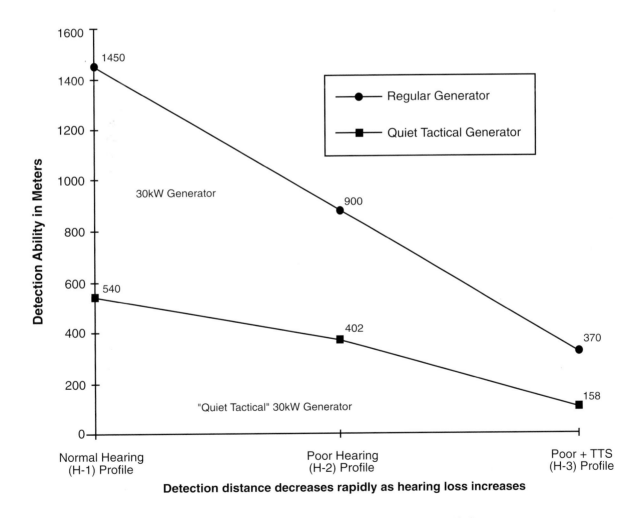

Fig. 24-2. Detectability of Generator Noise as a Function of Design and Hearing Ability
Data source: Army Research Laboratory, Aberdeen Proving Ground, Md.

the earplug carrying case on the Battle Dress Uniform and are strongly encouraged to do so.[45] The military-approved earplugs have been thoroughly tested for their noise reduction capabilities and freedom from toxic effects. Not all earplugs can make such claims. The approved foam earplug is made of a polyvinyl, closed-cell foam. Polyvinyl foam will stay rolled down long enough for proper insertion even in humid environments.

The earplug carrying case also has unique features for military applications. The olive-drab translucent color and matte finish is designed not to reflect light while allowing the contents of the case to be seen. Seating and insertion devices for the single- and triple-flange plugs are incorporated into the case lid.

Hearing Protector Use in the Field

Measures for protection against steady-state noise are the same as for impulsive noise. Hearing protection devices should be worn when the steady-state noise is above 85 dB and when impulse noise exceeds 140 dBP sound pressure level. All small arms used in the military produce impulse noise above this level. Therefore, hearing protection must always be worn on firing ranges and during field firing exercises and other forms of weapons training practice or evaluation.

Hearing protection can significantly degrade communication ability when protection is needed the most, that is, during weapons firing. During the relatively quiet periods between high-level impulse noise exposures, hearing protection can interfere with communication. Loud speaker systems at fixed firing points are designed to overcome the sound attenuation of the hearing protectors and ensure that voice signals are received at sound levels no lower than those of conversational speech. For best results, loud speakers must be spaced at appropriate intervals to maximize the benefits of amplification.

Such amplification is also effective on close combat courses and grenade ranges when standard commands and instructions are used.[46,47] These recommendations are limited to operations in wind speeds of less than 25 miles per hour. On grenade ranges, hearing protection can be waived for pit noncommissioned officers if they insert their fingers into their ears as soon as the tower announces "frag out."[46]

A new earplug has been developed in partnership with the French Army that addresses these communication issues for the dismounted soldier or Marine. The combat arms earplug affords protection from weapons fire over a wide range (up to 190 dBp) while marginally interfering with voice communications and the detection and localization of environmental (combat) sounds.

The filter inserted in the stem of the earplug is "nonlinear." Noise reduction capability increases with the noise level of the weapons fire. At low sound levels, however, there is little or no sound reduction and speech is understood without shouting. A detection model, developed at the Army Research Laboratory predicts that a normal-hearing soldier can detect a truck at the same distance (800 m) with or without the combat arms earplug. That detection capability is cut in half (400 m) with conventional foam plugs. The double-plug design includes a solid linear earplug that can be used for steady-state noise, such as in helicopters or armored personnel carriers.

Blank rounds fired from M-16 rifles, although not as noise-hazardous as live ball ammunition, are still hazardous to hearing. Blank suppressors attached to rifle muffles can reduce noise levels 4 to 7 dB, for example, from to 147 to 143 dBP.

This does not imply that hearing protection should be worn when actually in combat, except where weapons are fired from positions out of the immediate zone of fighting. Even in the immediate zone of fighting, however, hearing protection may sometimes be advantageous. The effective loss of hearing produced by use of a hearing protector can be quickly eliminated by removal of the protector. On the other hand, the loss of hearing produced by the action of noise on the unprotected ear could be permanent or, at best, can require many hours, sometimes even days, before recovery of hearing sensitivity.

The use of hearing protection during transport in tracked-wheeled personnel carriers, trucks, helicopters, or other aircraft should be enforced as a practical and feasible procedure for enhancing communication during transport and for preserving hearing for both training or wartime missions. The flight surgeon responsible for medical planning on the Son Tay prison camp raid in Vietnam insisted that all troops wear earplugs while being airlifted.[42] The result was that the troops arrived at the prison camp, removed their earplugs, and found their hearing unimpaired from the noise of the helicopters. This is not an isolated example. Most soldiers appreciate that under these conditions, earplugs function like sunglasses that cut down excess glare. First Lieutenant Clarence Briggs told of the Panama fight:

> Our CH-47 [helicopter] descended rapidly, the ramp dropped open and we charged out... Suddenly we stopped. Troops were quickly coming up behind us, and I could barely hear Crittenden yelling! "They landed in pairs!" He was trying to tell me that the two Hueys had landed 10 minutes before us instead of just 30 seconds, as had been the plan. I couldn't

hear. My ears were deafened by the noise of the CH-47's engines. "Next time we'll wear earplugs," I thought. "This craziness might get us killed." Before I knew it, CPT Dyer was kneeling next to me. We yelled at each other, unable to hear anything. Somehow we started to move toward the edge of the golf course, where 1st Platoon was securing the linkup site. Talking on the radio was useless. We blundered into them and moved into the bush just before the railroad tracks.[48]

Monitoring Audiometry

Through detection of small decrements in hearing sensitivity, individuals susceptible to noise can be identified before their hearing loss becomes a social or occupational handicap. All monitoring audiometry in the Army's Hearing Conservation Program is conducted through the Defense Occupational and Environmental Health Readiness System in Hearing Conservation (DOEHRS-HC) application, which will be integrated into the Composite Health Care System II (CHCS II). The DOEHRS-HC provides automated

hearing testing, as well as data for installation and Army-wide program management.

Health Education

Since noise-induced hearing loss is a relatively painless and bloodless process, an individual will not always be aware of the damage incurred until the loss has reached moderate-to-severe levels. Effective health education is essential to reinforce the faithful and proper use of hearing protection. The widespread use of earplugs presents a special challenge. Unless an expert performs a visual inspection of the earplug in the ear canal and tests the earplug stem or tab for tension, only the user knows whether or not the earplugs are properly inserted. Hence, there is an imperative that the user be convinced that hearing protection must be used and know how to maintain and insert them properly. Training aids, unique to the military and designed for this purpose, are available through publication and audiovisual support centers.[39]

[Doug Ohlin]

CARBON MONOXIDE

Carbon monoxide's high toxicity and extensive exposure potential have made it one of the most widespread poisons in the world, the most significant toxic gas in the workplace, and another element of danger for the service member. Carbon monoxide is toxic by several mechanisms, though principally by carboxyhemoglobin formation—an affinity for hemoglobin well known since the last century. Manifestations of its toxicity run from mild headaches to coma and death (Table 24-2).

Carbon monoxide poisoning has manifested itself in every modern armed conflict. In World War I, the French identified propellants, combustion engines, and explosives as CO sources that created casualties in enclosed spaces. In World War II, carbon monoxide policy in the US Army started at the Armored Medical Research Laboratory, Fort Knox,[49] when scientists developed an infrared gas analyzer to study carbon monoxide levels in armored vehicles. World War II also saw the first study incriminating low levels of carbon monoxide as a cause of neurobehavioral defect.[50]

Operational Exposures in the Military

Today, the army is literally "an army on wheels." Armored fighting vehicles move more soldiers, have bigger engines, burn more propellant throwing bigger projectiles faster, and are sealed against the external environment, allowing fumes and gases to accumulate. Improved bore extraction and ve-

hicle ventilation systems have reduced the incidence of carbon monoxide intoxication, but there continue to be intermittent occurrences.

The foot soldier is not immune from carbon monoxide intoxication. He or she may be exposed to it while in transport, whether in a "HumVee," "Bradley Fighting Machine", "deuce and a half," Blackhawk, Chinook, or US Air Force transport; while operating weapon systems including machine guns, rocket launchers, and recoilless rifles; and even while sleeping in tents, buildings, or vehicles heated with combustion heaters or charcoal. There is additional risk in enclosed spaces. Service members cannot smell it. It has no color. Chemical masks will not protect against it. Only a knowledge of its sources and continuous vigilance may preserve the service member from intoxication or demise.

Clinical Presentation and Treatment

In the initial evaluation, mild effects are often incorrectly attributed to mild viral syndromes or food poisoning. Failure to identify the carbon monoxide source may lead to more serious presentations or even fatalities. Unexpected symptoms of "inebriation" may actually be advanced carbon monoxide intoxication, requiring immediate intervention to prevent further or permanent injury to the service member or loss of an entire weapon sys-

TABLE 24-2

MANIFESTATIONS OF CARBON MONOXIDE TOXICITY

Carboxyhemoglobin Saturation (%)	Signs and Symptoms
0–10	none
0–20	tightness across forehead, possibly slight headache, dilation of cutaneous blood vessels
20–30	headache, throbbing in temples
30–40	severe headache, weakness, dizziness, dimness of vision, nausea and vomiting, collapse
40–50	worsening symptoms, increased possibility of collapse and syncope, increased respiration and pulse
50–60	syncope, increased respiration and pulse, coma with intermittent convulsions, Cheyne-Stokes' respiration
60–70	coma with intermittent convulsions, depressed heart action and respiration, possibly leading to death
70–80	weak pulse, slowed respiration, respiratory failure and death

Source: Weyandt TB, Ridgeley CD Jr. Carbon monoxide. Deeter DP, Gaydos JC, eds. *Occupational Health: The Soldier and the Industrial Base.* Part III, Vol 3. In: *Textbook of Military Medicine.* Washington, DC: Office of The Surgeon General; 1993: 412.

tem. When available, carboxyhemoglobin determinations (or breath carbon monoxide measurement) should be made if carbon monoxide intoxication is even remotely suspected.[51]

Intervention begins with recognition of the hazard and removal from the exposure. In the absence of hyperbaric capabilities, supplemental oxygen will assist in recovery. Hyberbaric oxygen is preferred to reduce the incidence of late sequelae, recognized as a problem in serious incidents of carbon monoxide intoxication and even with apparently less-severe intoxications. Sequelae can range from minor psychoneural deficits (eg, slight memory loss, fine tremors) to visual, hearing, IQ, and motor deficits. Hyperbaric therapy also reduces recovery time to a fraction of that required for supplemental oxygen therapy. Although its availability is limited in battlefield situations, it is increasingly available for treatment of intoxication resulting from peacetime training activities in the United States and even overseas.

While there is still disagreement as to what levels of carboxyhemoglobin first lead to measurable impairment, current Army policy (first established in 1981) calls for aviators to be below 5% and the general Army population to be below 10%.[52] Military vehicles and weapon systems are usually designed with this in mind. Evidence in the literature suggests that the majority of the force would experience no measurable impact at levels of up to 15% to 20%.[53] Unfortunately, there may be subpopulations who experience impairment at levels below 5%.[54] What the PM community should do with this information is undecided. To date, the 5% and 10% standards remain in effect, and there is no initiative to change them.

Carbon monoxide has been a significant problem for 20th century armies. A more complete account of the US Army and carbon monoxide appears in another volume of the *Textbooks of Military Medicine* series.[55] That chapter provides a detailed history of carbon monoxide experiences of modern armies. The chapter also reports an important equation—the Coburn-Forster-Kane equation—used by engineers designing weapon systems for estimating carboxyhemoglobin values from known concentrations of carbon monoxide. The reader is cautioned to consult the article by Smith and colleagues,[56] before attempting to use this equation.

[Steve Smith]

SMOKE AND OBSCURANTS

On perceived or actual attack by a predator, an octopus will release a cloud of ink into the water to conceal it from its attacker, while it escapes. Humans have developed a tactic that is similar to that of the octopus by the use of smoke on the battlefield. Since the 1930s, the US Army has extensively used smokes and obscurants during training and combat. Smokes are products produced by burning or vaporizing substances such as oils and organic fuels. Obscurants are suspended particles, such as fog, mist, and dust, that block or weaken transmission of a part or parts of the electromagnetic spectrum, such as infrared and visible radiation or microwaves.[57] Their uses have included obscuration, screening, deception, identification, and signaling. During World War II, the strategic and tactical use of smoke was advanced to a point never before attained in warfare. Using newly developed smoke devices, it was possible to screen whole cities from the sight of enemy aircraft for the first time in history. Laying down smoke in strategic areas was effective in keeping down the number of casualties and in greatly reducing the effectiveness of enemy air operations.[58]

Throughout the modern battlefield, forces acquire and engage targets based on visual, infrared, and millimeter wave technologies. To disrupt these engagements, several types of smokes and obscurants have been developed; each targets particular portions of the electromagnetic spectrum to disrupt enemy surveillance, target acquisition, and weapons guidance systems. The effectiveness of each smoke depends on its ability to reflect, refract, and scatter light rays to obscure visibility. For this reason, all military smokes consist of aerosols with particle dimensions approximating the wavelength of the portion of the magnetic spectrum that they are designed to obscure.[59] The list of smokes and obscurants is long and includes hexachloroethane, fog oil, diesel oil, white and red phosphorus, colored smokes, brass, graphite, titanium dioxide, and terephthalic acid. Depending upon the smoke or obscurant being used and its intended purpose, these may be delivered by projectiles, grenades, smoke pots, or smoke generators.

Tactical Uses

Smokes and obscurants can be used in either hasty or deliberate operations. Hasty smoke covers a small area for a short period of time. Deliberate smoke is usually employed over large areas for extended periods and is planned at the brigade level or higher.[60]

Smoke is used in four ways: to obscure, to screen, to deceive, and to identify or signal. Smoke that is referred to as "obscuring" smoke is used on enemy positions to degrade their sighting capabilities and their command and control. In contrast to this, "screening" smoke is used in friendly operational areas or between friendly and enemy forces. Smokes can also be used to deceive the enemy; this is especially useful in defensive retrograde troop movements. Colored smokes, to include white smokes,

are used for signaling and identification purposes only, such as marking a landing zone or communicating pre-arranged signals (Figure 24-3).

There are three types of smoke screens: smoke blankets, smoke hazes, and smoke curtains. A smoke blanket is a dense and horizontal development of smoke in friendly operational areas or between friendly and enemy forces. It is used to screen friendly forces from enemy ground and aerial observation. However, the high density of smoke used in a smoke blanket can hamper friendly operations (Figure 24-4). In contrast to a smoke blanket, a smoke haze is only a light concentration of smoke. It is used to restrict the accuracy of enemy observation and fire but it is not dense enough to disrupt friendly operations. A smoke curtain is a dense, vertical development placed between enemy and friendly forces. It restricts ground observation but not aerial observation (Figure 24-5).

US forces will use smokes and obscurants whenever the tactical advantage to be gained outweighs the potential degradation to friendly operations. When smoke is used in the above manner, the smoke will deny information to the enemy, reduce the enemy's effectiveness in target acquisition, create conditions to surprise the enemy, deceive the enemy, disrupt organized enemy movement, operations, and command and control, and restrict nap-of-the-earth (NOE) and contour approaches by enemy aircraft. NOE flights occur when pilots fly as close to the terrain as the speed and performance contours of the aircraft will allow.

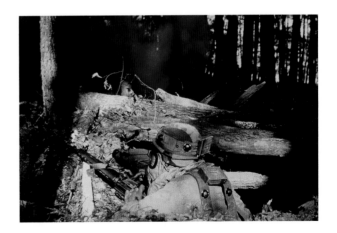

Fig. 24-3. In conditions where verbal communication is difficult, such as when being masked, colored smokes such as the violet seen here are sometimes used for communicating prearranged signals.
Photograph: Courtesy of Commander, US Center for Health Promotion and Preventive Medicine, Aberdeen Proving Ground, Md. Photographer: W. Ben Bunger III.

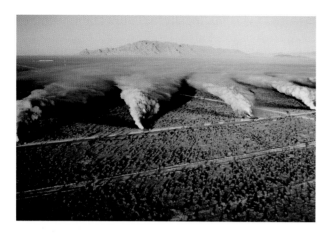

Fig. 24-4. This is an example of a smoke blanket being produced by HMMWV-mounted smoke generators vaporing fog oil. Over a friendly area, this would prevent observation by the enemy from both the ground and the air. A lighter density of smoke—a smoke haze—would make operations within the smoke easier.
Photograph: Courtesy of Commander, US Center for Health Promotion and Preventive Medicine, Aberdeen Proving Ground, Md.

Delivery Systems

There are several ways in which to employ smoke on the battlefield. These include projectiles, smoke grenades, smoke pots, smoke generators, vehicle engine exhausts. Smoke can come via air and sea. Methods of projectile employment include mortars,

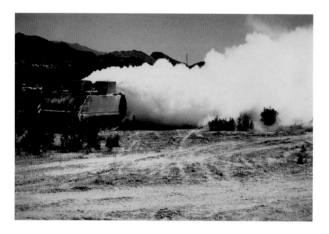

Fig. 24-5. This is an M113 track vehicle with smoke generators mounted on it. It can quickly develop a long smoke curtain.
Photograph: Courtesy of Commander, US Center for Health Promotion and Preventive Medicine, Aberdeen Proving Ground, Md.

field artillery, tank guns, and grenade launchers. Grenade launchers can be mounted on armored vehicles. These grenade launchers fire eight or twelve grenades simultaneously, with firing arcs of 90° to 110°. The vehicle commander launches the grenades as soon as the enemy fires on the vehicle. The individual smoke clouds from each of the eight or twelve grenades quickly coalesce into one continuous smoke curtain. Evasive action may then be taken behind that curtain (Figure 24-6).

The smoke grenades are classified according to the color of their smokes. The M8 grenade contains hexachloroethane and so produces a white smoke. The M18 grenades produce red, green, yellow, and violet smokes.

There are several types of smoke pots, and each has different capabilities. The M1 and M5 smoke pots differ only in their weights and thus their burn times. The M1 smoke pot weighs 10 lbs and lasts 5 to 8 minutes, while the M5 smoke pot weighs 30 lbs and has a burn time of 12 to 22 minutes. The M4A2 and the M207A1 smoke pots weigh 30 lbs and have fuzes so that they can be delivered by helicopter. The M4A2 smoke pot floats, so that it can be used in water operations.

The M3 smoke generator, which is for use over large areas, vaporizes fog oil. The generator burns about 40 gallons of fog oil per hour. The M56 turbine generator is under development. It can be mounted on a HMMWV (High Mobility Multipurpose Wheeled Vehicle). It will be able to produce a cloud that will obscure both outside and within the visible spectrum by burning fog oil and grinding and blowing graphite particles out of an ejector (Figure 24-7).

The vehicle engine exhaust smoke system is mounted on M1 and M60 series tanks. The engine's fuel pump injects about 1 gallon of diesel fuel per minute into the hot engine exhaust system, causing the fuel to flash-vaporize and exit with the engine's exhaust gases. However, the Army has switched to JP8 as the standard vehicle fuel, and it produces inadequate obscuration due to its high volatility. To overcome this problem, the Army has developed a bolt-on reservoir for fog oil that mounts on the rear of the M1 Abrams tank. Fog oil is pumped from the reservoir using existing VEESS hardware into the M1's exhaust.

Hexachloroethane Smoke

The hexachloroethane-based smoke munition is referred to as "HC smoke." The precursor to the HC smoke munition was developed by Captain E.F. Berger of the French Army. Berger's mixture con-

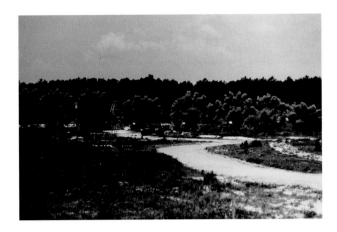

Fig. 24-6. This is a smoke curtain being developed by a grenade launcher mounted on an armed vehicle. These eight clouds will quickly coalesce into one continuous smoke curtain.
Photograph: Courtesy of Commander, US Center for Health Promotion and Preventive Medicine, Aberdeen Proving Ground, Md.

tained carbon tetrachloride, powdered zinc, and zinc oxide. When ignited, it produced an aerosol of zinc chloride and sooty carbon particles. Between the two world wars, the US Army's Chemical Warfare Service made several refinements of Berger's mixture. The first refinement replaced the volatile

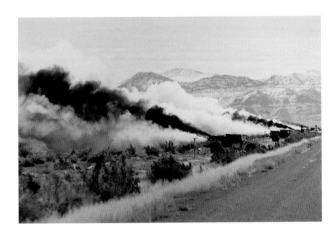

Fig. 24-7. This is a ground-level view of the smoke blanket shown in Figure 24-4. The blanket is being developed by a HMMWV-mounted M56 turbine generator. This generator is under development and will be able to produce a multispectral cloud by burning fog oil and grinding and blowing graphite particles out of an ejector.
Photograph: Courtesy of Commander, US Center for Health Promotion and Preventive Medicine, Aberdeen Proving Ground, Md.

liquid carbon tetrachloride with hexa-chloroethane, which is a solid at room temperature. Later changes in the chemical mixture were made to overcome difficulties caused by the limited availability of some of the chemical ingredients and the explosive nature of others, leading to the Type C composition widely employed today in HC smoke–producing devices.[59]

HC smoke pots are ordinarily used to provide screens for small areas, to supplement other smoke sources by filling holes in screens, and to help rapidly establish screens. HC smoke pots were used extensively in World War II to provide preliminary screens during the approximately 5 minutes needed to set up large thermo-mechanical fog oil smoke generators. In addition, HC smoke pots were used by the US Army and Navy to cover harbors in Italy and North Africa and in both the European and Pacific theaters. They were used on land and water to screen supply routes, bridge construction, amphibious operations, tanks, ammunition dumps, troop concentrations, and ground operations. They were also used to hide mortar flash.[59] In the assault on Salerno, Italy, on September 9, 1943, the first infantry waves burned HC smoke pots, and a chemical smoke unit landed with the mission of concealing the beaches from aerial observation. For the first few days, until the mechanical generators arrived, the screens were made and maintained only with smoke pots. Although the Salerno beaches were under constant enemy air attack and observed artillery fire for nearly 2 weeks, the German fire could not be directed accurately to a single target on or off the beach. Priceless lives and vital equipment were saved, and smoke as an instrument of assault had proved itself.[58]

Although fog oil is the most widely used smoke, the smoke munition that has caused the most service member morbidity and mortality is the HC smoke munition. Between 1945 and 1993, many individuals have been hospitalized and have died due to exposure to HC smoke.[61] These cases have involved the use of HC smoke in enclosed spaces or in extremely close proximity. The morbidity and mortality have been largely caused by pulmonary edema or secondary bronchopneumonia. Zinc chloride, a combustion product of the HC smoke munitions, is the most likely cause of these health effects.

The health hazards to the service member using the HC smoke munitions can be disastrous, and physicians practicing acute care near military installations need to be aware of the importance of taking a good exposure history, the time course to the development of symptoms and pathology, and the acute treatment.

Uncombusted Type C composition HC munitions contain approximately 7% grained aluminum and roughly equal parts of hexachloroethane and zinc oxide. The HC munition is ignited by a pyrotechnic starter and is then self-perpetuating. Below is the ideal combustion equation in which the aluminum, hexachloroethane, and zinc oxide are converted into zinc chloride, aluminum oxide, and particulate carbon in an exothermic reaction[62]:

$$2Al + C_2Cl_6 + 3ZnO \longrightarrow 3ZnCl_2 + Al_2O_3 + 2C + heat$$

Zinc chloride, which constitutes approximately two thirds of the smoke and accounts for the acute toxic effects, is hydroscopic and becomes coated with water molecules, which in turn produce the smoke effect.

The chemical equation for HC smoke combustion is merely an ideal equation. In reality and so that the rate of combustion can be controlled, there is stoichiometrically not enough aluminum to balance this equation. Therefore, there are side reactions that produce additional combustion products as chlorinated vapors (Table 24-3 and Exhibit 24-1). The proportion of the various side-products depends on atmospheric conditions, especially relative humidity. For example, hydrochloric acid at lower humidities only is produced at much higher levels than the other additional combustion products.[62] HC smoke munitions produce both severe respiratory irritants, an asphyxiant, and known or suspected carcinogenic substances.

The uncombusted HC smoke munition contains several impurities: lead, cadmium, arsenic, and mercury. Lead and cadmium are present at higher levels than arsenic and mercury. The impurities, though, are present in relatively small amounts compared with the other munition ingredients. They are present at levels of less than 0.2%.[63] The impurities are also present in the smoke cloud as oxides and are likewise present in low levels.

In training and in combat, the service member may be exposed to HC smoke through the skin, through the gastrointestinal tract, and through open wounds. However, by far the most significant route of exposure is inhalation. The acute health effects from HC smoke are thought to be due to zinc chloride, which makes up two thirds of the resultant smoke from a combusted HC smoke munition. Zinc chloride is a corrosive astringent compound that is highly soluble in water. Its water-solubility results in easy deposition in the upper airways. In lower doses, zinc chloride will deposit primarily in the nasal passages and the pharynx. In higher doses,

zinc chloride molecules will deposit in lower respiratory anatomical sites, to include the alveoli in extremely high doses.

Pathological changes are variable but are largely dose-dependent. Pathologic changes reported in the literature include laryngeal tracheal, and bronchial mucosal edema and ulceration; interstitial edema; interstitial fibrosis; alveolar obliteration; bronchiolitis obliterans; and subpleural emphysematous blebs complicated by pneumothorax.[61,64,65]

TABLE 24-3

APPROXIMATE COMPOSITION OF HC SMOKE

Constituent	Estimated Mass Fraction, %
Total particulate phase	89.2
Zinc chloride	62.5
Zinc oxide	9.6
Iron oxide	10.7
Aluminum oxide	5.4
Lead oxide	1.0
Chlorinated vapors*	10.8

*chlorinated vapors are listed in Exhibit 24-1
Source: DeVaull GE, et al. Analysis Methods and Results of Hexachloroethane Smoke Dispersion Experiments Conducted as Part of Atterbry-87 Field Studies. Fort Detrick, Md: US Army Medical Research and Development Command; 1989. Contract No. 84PP-4822.

EXHIBIT 24-1

ADDITIONAL CHLORINATED VAPOR COMBUSTION PRODUCTS OF HC SMOKE MUNITIONS

HCl (hydrochloric acid)
$COCl_2$ (phosgene)
CCl_4 (carbon tetrachloride)
C_2Cl_4 (tetrachloroethane)
C_2Cl_6 (hexachloroethane)
C_6Cl_6 (hexachlorobenzene)
CO (carbon monoxide)

Source: Katz SA, et. al. Physical and Chemical Characterization of Fog Oil Smoke and Hexachloroethane Smoke. 1980. Final Report. Contract DAMD17–78–C–8085. NTIS: AD A080936.

Most extremely high doses are a result of exposures to HC smoke in confined spaces, such as in tunnels during MOUT (military operations in urbanized terrain) training. There have been many instances in which individuals have died from high-dose acute exposure to HC smoke. In Malta during World War II, 70 people were exposed to HC smoke after enemy bombs ignited a store of 79 smoke munitions located 80 yards into a 200-yard tunnel. Thirty-four of the exposed people passed through the nearby first-aid station and one other was taken on board a ship in the harbor where he died within a few minutes. Of the 34 treated at the first-aid station, 2 died there; 15 were sent to a nearby general hospital, of whom 6 died; 17 were sent to their homes. Of the 17 sent home, 3 were subsequently admitted to the general hospital, and 1 of these died, making the total number of deaths from this exposure 10.[61]

This case illustrates several points. First, exposure to HC smoke in an enclosed space is life-threatening. Second, serious pulmonary complications can appear in a delayed fashion. Three of the seventeen people who were sent home after an initial medical evaluation were subsequently admitted to the hospital and one of these died. It is extremely important for clinicians to ascertain an estimate of the dose of inhaled HC smoke. The exposure history should include the location of exposure (eg, confined space, distance from munition), approximate visibility, duration of exposure, respiratory protection used (eg, M17 mask), and the elapsed time since exposure. Given this information, the clinician is better able to decide whether someone who appears to have only mild respiratory symptoms may later develop life-threatening respiratory distress.

Treatment of the HC smoke–exposed casualty begins on the battlefield or training site. The service member should be removed from exposure; masking the casualty may be necessary if the smoke cloud is large and removal from exposure may be prolonged. Humidified supplemental oxygen (100%) should be administered with assisted ventilation as required. Exposed skin and eyes should be copiously flushed with water. Respiratory tract irritation, if severe, can progress to pulmonary edema, which may be delayed in onset for up to 72 hours. Therefore, the HC smoke–exposed patient should be closely monitored for respiratory symptoms and signs for at least 48 hours. Adequate ventilation and oxygenation should be maintained, with close monitoring of arterial blood gases. If pO_2 cannot be maintained above 50 mmHg with inspiration of 60% oxygen by face mask or mechanical ventilation, then positive end-expiratory pressure in intubated patients or continuous positive airway pressure in non-intubated patients may be necessary. Crystalloid solutions must be administered carefully to avoid a net positive fluid balance. Central hemodynamic monitoring should be considered for ascertaining current fluid status. Morphine is not recommended since respiratory depression may occur. Antibiotics are indicated only when there is evidence of infection. Finally, although corticosteroids may prolong the onset of noncardiogenic pulmonary edema, it is unclear whether early administration of corticosteroids can prevent its eventual development.[66]

Another smoke munition, terephthalic acid smoke is being fielded as a training replacement for HC smoke. Although it is considered to be much safer than HC smoke, it does contain respiratory irritants. Unfortunately, the quality of the smoke is not sufficient to produce the desired amount of obscuration for actual combat, so the terephthalic acid smoke munition will only be used in training.

Other Smokes and Obscurants

Fog Oil

The smoke generated by injecting mineral oil into a heated manifold is termed fog oil. The oil is vaporized when heated and condenses when exposed to the atmosphere to produce an opaque mist. Fog oil is produced from naphthenic oils. Such oils have been associated with increased incidence of skin cancer. The military specification for fog oil was changed in 1985 after it was determined that untreated naphthenic oils were carcinogenic. The new specification requires that the oil be processed to remove known carcinogenic and potentially carcinogenic substances.[57]

Diesel Oil

Diesel oil smoke is formed by using the vehicle engine exhaust smoke system described above. The fuel is vaporized, resulting in a suspension in air of 0.5 to 1.0 mm droplets. The vaporized fuel consists mostly of saturated hydrocarbons, substituted benzenes, and 2-3 ring aromatic hydrocarbons. The respiratory tract is the major organ system of concern. Mortality from acute exposures is a function of the duration of exposure in addition to the concentration of the diesel oil smoke. Repeated exposure studies have shown that pulmonary toxicity is dependent on the frequency of exposure. Pulmonary lesions increase when exposure frequency exceeds twice weekly. The pulmonary lesions are largely inflammatory in nature.[57]

Red Phosphorus

Red phosphorus is combined with styrene-buta-diene rubber (butyl rubber) in a 95:5 mixture. The butyl rubber reduces the cloud-pillar effect found with pure red phosphorus. This mixture also contains insulating oil (1.25% by weight) and talc or silica (1% by weight), which is added to improve uniformity of the pattern. Red phosphorus reacts slowly with oxygen and water vapor to produce the highly toxic phosphine gas. However, this reaction is extremely slow at normal temperatures and humidities and is therefore not significant to military operations. The combustion products from red phosphorus in butyl rubber have been characterized. The particles consist primarily of various species of phosphoric acid. Phosphoric acid is an irritant that may result in terminal bronchiolar fibrosis.[57]

Colored Smokes

These smokes come in yellow, green, red, and violet. The colored smokes are to be used for signaling and identification purposes only. Quite often, these smokes are used inappropriately, resulting in unnecessary exposure to personnel. Each color has its unique formulation. (Some of the colored smokes are undergoing product improvement so that old and new compositions exist in the inventory). They commonly contain an anthraquinone dye and other components that are added to effect a controlled combustion of the munition. Soldiers

---

EXHIBIT 24-2

DEPARTMENT OF THE ARMY SAFETY POLICY REGARDING TRAINING IN SMOKE

The following precautions apply to all smoke training:

A. Personnel will carry the protective mask when participating in exercises which include the use of smoke.

B. Personnel will mask:

1) before exposure to any concentration of smoke produced by M8 white smoke grenades or smoke pots (HC smoke) or metallic powder obscurants.

2) when passing through or operating in dense (visibility less than 50 m) smoke such as smoke blankets and smoke curtains.

3) when operating in or passing through a smoke haze (visibility greater than 50 m) and the duration of exposure will exceed 4 hours.

4) any time exposure to smoke produces breathing difficulty, eye irritation or discomfort. Such effects in one individual will serve as a signal for all similarly exposed personnel to mask.

5) personnel will mask when using smoke during military operations in urban terrain (MOUT) training when operating in enclosed spaces. Note: The protective mask is not effective in oxygen deficient atmospheres. Care must be taken not to enter confined spaces where oxygen may have been displaced.

6) smoke generator personnel will mask when it is impossible to stay upwind of the smoke.

C. Showering and laundering of clothing following exercises will eliminate the risk of skin irritation following exposure to smoke. Troops exposed to smoke should reduce skin exposure by rolling down sleeves.

D. Special care must be taken when using HC smoke to ensure that appropriate protection is provided to all personnel who are likely to be exposed. When planning for the use of HC smoke in training, specific consideration must be given to weather conditions and the potential downwind effects of the smoke. Positive controls (observation, control points, communications) must be established to prevent exposure of unprotected personnel.

E. Request applicable publications and standard operating procedures be reviewed to ensure appropriate safety precautions for use of smoke are included in training and employment guidance. Commanders should ensure this policy is widely disseminated.

Source: US Department of the Army, DAPE-HR. *Smoke Safety*. Washington, DC: DA; 1985. Message.

are exposed to the combustion products of these mixtures. The combustion products can include irritants that can result in significant pulmonary effects.[67] The mutagenicity and carcinogenicity of the combustion products of the anthraquinone dyes are variable. A combustion product of the old red smoke grenade, 2-aminoanthraquinone, is classified as a suspected animal carcinogen by the International Agency for Research on Cancer.[68]

Graphite

Graphite flakes are disseminated mechanically into the atmosphere. Graphite dust behaves biologically as a nuisance dust; dust-laden macrophages are seen in the lungs as well as type II pneumocyte proliferation. However, the presence of crystalline silica in graphite may increase fibrogenic potential and result in a pneumoconiosis.[69] Fortunately, the particle sizes being disseminated are typically larger than the alveolar respirable range.[70]

Policies and Controls

The Army's first safety policy on the use of smokes was developed in 1985 in response to sporadic episodes of soldier exposures to HC smoke that resulted in illnesses and deaths[71] (Exhibit 24-2). The safety policy was a common sense approach to minimizing exposures. The policy has been criticized by some as being too conservative with regard to masking conditions. The concern has been that soldiers are less effective when wearing respiratory protection due to decreased visual fields and diminished communication. This diminution of effectiveness can lead to a decreased level of safety from other dangers that outweigh the risks from exposure to the smokes.

To formulate a safety policy that is founded on more objective data, the Army Surgeon General sought the assistance of the National Academy of Science's Committee on Toxicology to formulate exposure guidance levels.[57] The National Academy of Science used existing health data from peer-reviewed scientific literature to formulate the exposure guidance levels using a health risk assessment method.[72] These levels, coupled with industrial hygiene exposure data from the field, may be used to refine the level at which masking must take place to prevent health effects to military personnel. These levels may also be used to determine safe locations for the employment of smoke on training installations and may be used to assess an individual's postexposure risk.

[William A. Rice]

REFERENCES

1. Gaydos JC, Thomas RJ, Sack DM, Patterson R. Armed Forces. In: JM Stellman, ed. *Encyclopedia of Occupational Health and Safety*. 4th ed. Geneva: International Labor Organization; 1998: 95.14–95.17.

2. Griffin MJ. *Handbook of Human Vibration*. London: Academic Press Ltd; 1988. RCS Med 388.

3. Dupuis H. Medical and occupational preconditions for vibration induced spinal disorders: Occupational disease number 2110 in Germany. *Int Arch Occup Environ Health*. 1994:66(5):303–308.

4. Johanning E. Back disorders and health problems among subway train operators exposed to whole body vibration. *Scand J Work Environ Health*. 1991;17:414–419.

5. Johanning E, Wilder DG, Landrigan PJ, Pope MH. Whole-body exposure in subway cars and review of adverse health effects. *J Occup Med*. 1991;33:605–612.

6. Kabacinska-Knapikowa D, Paradowski L, Kwiatkowski S. Esophageal motility in personnel operating heavy self-propelled mining machines. *Materia Medica Polona*. 1992;24(3):153–155.

7. Daleva M, Piperova-Dalbokova D, Hadjiolova I, Mincheva L. Changes in the excretion of corticosteroids and catecholamines in tractor drivers. *Int Arch Occup Environ Health*. 1982;49:345–352.

8. Kamenskii YN, Nosova IM. Effects of whole body vibration on certain indicators of neuro-endocrine processes. *Noise Vibration Bull*. 1989;Sept:205–207.

9. Nakamura R Moroji T, Nohara S, Nakamura M, Okada A. Activation of cerebral dopaminergic systems by noise and whole-body vibration. *Environ Res*. 1992;57(1):10–18.

10. Barron JL, Noakes TD, Levy W, Smith C, Millar RP. Hypothalmic dysfunction in overtrained athletes. *J Clin Endocrinol Metab*. 1985;60:803–806.

11. Ariizumi M, Okada A. Effect of whole body vibration on the rat brain content of serotonin and plasma corticosterone. *Eur J Applied Physiol Occup Physiol*. 1983;52:15–19.

12. Granjean E. *Fitting the Task to the Man*. New York: Little Brown; 1989.

13. Pope MH, Hansson TH. Vibration of the spine and low back pain. *Clin Orthop*. 1992;279:49–59.

14. Pope MH, Kaigle AM, Magnusson M, Broman H, Hansson T. Intervertebral motion during vibration. *Proc Inst Mech Eng [H]*. 1991;205(1):39–44.

15. Ishihara H, Tsuji H, Hirano N, Ohshima H, Terahata N. Effects of continuous quantitative vibration on rheologic and biological behaviors of the intervertebral disc. *Spine*. 1992;17(3 suppl):S7–S12.

16. Hansson T, Holm S. Clinical implications of vibration-induced changes in the lumbar spine. *Orthop Clin North Am*. 1991;22:247–253.

17. Kaji H, Sato E, Nagatsuka S, et al. Evaluation of sensory disturbances using short latency somatosensory evoked potentials (SSEPs) in vibration-exposed workers. [Japanese]. *Sangyo Igaku*. 1991;33:605–612.

18. DeLuca CJ. Myoelectrical manifestations of localized muscular fatigue in humans. *Crit Rev Biomech Eng*. 1985;4:251–278.

19. Klein AB, Snyder-Mackler L, Roy SH, DeLuca CJ. Comparison of spinal mobility and isometric trunk extensor forces with electromyographic spectral analysis in identifying low back pain. *Physical Therapy*. 1991;71(6):445–454.

20. Bovenzi M, Zadini A. Self-reported low back symptoms in urban bus drivers exposed to whole-body vibration. *Spine*. 1992:17:1048–1059.

21. Boshulzen HC, Bongers PM, Hulshof CT. Self-reported back pain in fork-lift truck and freight-container tractor drivers exposed to whole-body vibration. *Spine*. 1992;17:59–65.

22. Chatterjee S, Bandyopadhyay A. Effect of vibrating steering on the grip strength in heavy vehicle drivers. *J Human Ergology*. 1991;20(1):77–84.

23. *Initial Health Hazard Assessment Report on the Fast Attack Vehicle (FAV)*. Aberdeen Proving Ground, Md: Environmental Hygiene Agency; 1984.

24. Gow BS, Legg MJ, Yu W, Kukongvlrlyapan U, Lee LL. Does vibration cause post-stenotic dilatation in vivo and influence atherogenesis in cholesterol-fed rabbits? *J Biomech Eng*. 1992;114(1):20–25.

25. Nakamura H, Katoh A, Nohara S, Nakamura M, Okada A. Experimental studies on the pathogenesis of the gastric mucosal lesions induced by whole-body vibration. *Environmental Research*. 1992;58(2):220–229.

26. Katoh A, Nakamura H, Nohara S, Ohmura K, Munemoto Y, Oda M. Experimental studies on the development of acute gastric lesions induced by vibration stress in rats and its pathogenetic mechanisms. *Japanese J Gastroenterol*. 1992;89:469–476.

27. Mecel H, Wozniak H, Sun L, Frazier E, Mason HC. Effects on rats of exposure to heat and vibration. *J Applied Physiol*. 1962;17:759–762.

28. Nakamura H, Moroji T, Naaase H, Okazawa T, Okada A. Changes of cerebral vasoactive intestinal polypeptide- and somatostatin-like immunoreactivity induced by noise and whole-body vibration in the rat. *Eur J Appl Physiol Occup Physiol*. 1994;68(1):62–67.

29. McLain RF, Weinstein JN. Nuclear clefting in dorsal root ganglion neurons: A response to whole body vibration. *J Comp Neurol*. 1992;322:538–547.

30. McLain RF, Weinstein JN. Ultrastructural changes in the dorsal root ganglion associated with whole body vibration. *J Spinal Disord.* 1991;4(2):142–148.

31. McLain RF, Weinstein JN. Effects of whole body vibration on dorsal root ganglion neurons: Changes in neuronal nuclei. *Spine.* 1994;19:1455–1461.

32. Nakamura H, Moroji T, Nohara S, Nakamura M, Okada A. Activation of cerebral dopaminergic systems by noise and whole-body vibration. *Environ Res.* 1992;57(1):10–18.

33. Bartsch C, Meihe B. The effect of vibrations in the early stages of embryogenesis on the postnatal motor and physical development of Wistar rats [German]. *Anat Anz.* 1991;173(4):239–242.

34. USAARL Contract Reports No. CR 95-1,CR 95-2, CR 95-3, CR 95-4.

35. Ohlin DW. *20 Years Revisited: The Prevalence of Hearing Loss Among Selected U.S. Army Branches.* Aberdeen Proving Ground, Md: US Army Center for Health Promotion and Preventive Medicine; (Draft). Hearing Conservation Special Study No. 51-FK-5367-96.

36. Walden BE, Prosek RA, Worthington DW. *The Prevalence of Hearing Loss Within Selected U.S. Army Branches.* Washington, DC: U.S. Army Medical Research and Development Command; 1975. Interagency IAO 4745.

37. Price GR, Kalb JT, Garinther GR. Toward a measure of auditory handicap in the Army. *Ann Otol Rhinol Laryngol Suppl.* 1989;140:42–52.

38. Garinther GR, Peters LJ. Impact of communications on armor crew performance. *Army Res Development Acquisition Bull.* 1990;January-February:1–5.

39. US Department of the Army. *Hearing Conservation.* Washington, DC: DA; 1991. DA Pamphlet 40–501.

40. US Army Environmental Hygiene Agency. *Hearing Evaluation Automated Registry System (HEARS) Audiometer Operation Manual.* Aberdeen Proving Ground, MD: USACHPPM; 1991. Technical Guide 167A. Available from the USACHPPM, 5158 Blackhawk Road, ATTN: MCHB-DC-CHC, Aberdeen Proving Ground, MD 21010–5422.

41. US Army Environmental Hygiene Agency. *Hearing Evaluation Automated Registration System (HEARS) Manager's Module Operation Manual.* Aberdeen Proving Ground, Md: USACHPPM; 1991. Technical Guide 167B.

42. Ohlin, DW. *Personal Hearing Protective Devices, Fitting, Care and Use.* Aberdeen Proving Ground, Md: US Army Environmental Hygiene Agency; 1975. USACHPPM Technical Guide 041.

43. *Noise Dosimetry and Risk Assessment.* Aberdeen Proving Ground, Md: US Army Environmental Hygiene Agency; 1994. USACHPPM Technical Guide 181.

44. Goldstein J. *Noise Hazard Evaluation, Sound Level Data of Noise Sources.* Aberdeen Proving Ground, Md: US Army Center for Health Promotion and Preventive Medicine; 1975. USACHPPM Technical Guide 040.

45. US Department of the Army. *Wear and Appearance of Army Uniforms and Insignia.* Washington, DC: DA: 1992. Army Regulation 670-1.

46. Ohlin DW. *Evaluation of Communication Abilities with Hearing Protective Devices on a Grenade Range.* Aberdeen Proving Ground, Md: US Army Environmental Hygiene Agency; 1974. Bio-Acoustics Special Study, No. 34–048–75.

47. Ohlin DW. *Evaluation of Communication Devices with Hearing Protective Devices on a Close Combat Course.* Aberdeen Proving Ground, Md: US Army Environmental Hygiene Agency; 1974. Bio-Acoustics Special Study, No. 34–029–74/7s.

48. Briggs CE III. *Operation Just Cause: Panama, December 1989: A Soldier's Eyewitness Account.* Harrisburg, Penn: Stackpole Books; 1990.

49. LTC Hatch, CPT Nelson, CPT Horvath, LT Eickma, LT Walpole. *Control of Gun Fumes in M-4 Series Medium Tanks*. Fort Knox, Ky: US Army Armored Force Medical Research Laboratory; 1943. Project Nos. 3-1 and 3-5, File No. 724.41.

50. McFarland RA, Roughton FJW, Halperin MH, Niven JI. The effects of carbon monoxide and altitude on visual thresholds. *Aviation Med*. 1944;Dec:381–394.

51. Dalton BA. Carbon monoxide in US Army tactical vehicles. *Med Bull US Army Med Dept*. 1988;Feb:11–13.

52. US Department of Defense. *Military Standard: Human Engineering Design Criteria for Military Systems, Equipment and Facilities*. Washington, DC: Government Printing Office: 1989. MIL-STD-1472D.

53. US Environmental Protection Agency. *Air Quality Criteria for Carbon Monoxide*. Washington, DC: EPA; 1991. Document EPA/600/8-90/045F.

54. Benignus VA, Petrovick MK, Newlin-Clapp L, Prah JD. Carboxyhemoglobin and brain blood flow in humans. *Neurotoxicol Teratol*. 1992;14:285–290.

55. Deeter DP, Gaydos JC, eds. *Occupational Health: The Soldier and the Industrial Base*. Part III, Vol 3. In: *Textbook of Military Medicine*. Washington, DC: Office of The Surgeon General; 1993.

56. Smith SR, Steinberg S, Gaydos JC. Errors in derivations of the Coburn-Forster-Kane equation for predicting carboxyhemoglobin. *Am Ind Hyg Assoc J*. 1996:57:621–625.

57. Committee on Toxicology, National Research Council. *Toxicity of Military Smokes and Obscurants*. Vol 1. Washington, DC: National Academy Press; 1997.

58. The Chemical Corps Association. *The Chemical Warfare Service in World War II*. New York: Reinhold Publishing Corporation; 1948.

59. Eaton JC, Lopinto RJ, Palmer WG. Health effects of hexachloroethane (HC) smoke. Fort Detrick, Md: US Army Biomedical Research and Development Laboratory; February 1994. Technical Report 9402.

60. US Department of the Army. *Deliberate Smoke Operations*. Washington, DC: DA; 1984. US Army Field Manual 3-50.

61. Evans EH. Casualties following exposure to zinc chloride smoke. *Lancet*. 1945;2:368.

62. Cichowicz JJ. *HC Smoke*. Vol 4. In: *Environmental Assessment, Programmatic Life Cycle Environmental Assessment for Smoke/Obscurants*. Aberdeen Proving Ground, Md: Chemical Research and Development Center, US Army Armament, Munitions and Chemical Command; 1983. ARCSL-EA-83007.

63. Katz SA, et al. *Physical and Chemical Characterization of Fog Oil Smoke and Hexachloroethane Smoke: Final Report*. 1980. Contract DAMD17–78–C-8085. NTIS: AD A080936.

64. Milliken JA, Waugh D, Kadish ME. Acute interstitial pulmonary fibrosis caused by a smoke bomb. *Canadian Med Assoc J*. 1963;88:36–39.

65. Matarese SL, Matthews JI. Zinc chloride (smoke bomb) inhalational lung injury. *Chest*. 1986;89:308–309.

66. Micromedex Tomes Medical Management System. Zinc chloride. Volume 27. Englewood, Colo: Micromedex Inc; 1996.

67. Rubin IB, Buchanan MV, Moneyhun JH. *Chemical Characterization and Toxicologic Evaluation of Airborne Mixtures: Chemical Characterization of Combusted Inventory Red and Violet Smoke Mixes*. Oak Ridge, Tenn: Oak Ridge National Laboratory; 1982. ORNL/TM-8810, AD A131527.

68. National Institute for Occupational Safety and Health. *Registry of Toxic Effects of Chemical Substances, 1983–84 Supplement to 1981–82 Edition*. Cincinnati, Ohio: US Department of Health and Human Services, Public Health Service, Centers for Disease Control, NIOSH H; 1984.

69. Driver CJ, et al. Environmental and health effects review for obscurant graphite flakes. Aberdeen Proving Ground, Md: Edgewood Research, Development and Engineering Center; 1993. Report CR-056.

70. Guelta MA, Banks DR, Grieb RS. Particle size analysis of graphite obscurant material from an XM56 smoke generator. Edgewood Research, Development and Engineering Center Technical Report 053, 1993.

71. US Department of the Army, DAPE-HR. Smoke safety. 272030Z Nov 85. Message.

72. Committee on Toxicology, National Research Council. *Criteria and Methods for Preparing Emergency Exposure Guidance Level (EEGL), Short-term Public Emergency Guidance Level (SPEGL), and Continuous Exposure Guidance Level (CEGL) Documents*. Washington, DC: National Academy Press; 1986.

Chapter 25

AVIATION MEDICINE

DAVID M. LAM, MD, MPH

D. M. Lam; Colonel, Medical Corps, US Army (Retired), Associate Professor, University of Maryland School of Medicine, National Study Center for Trauma and Emergency Medical Systems and US Army Telemedicine and Advanced Technology Research Center, PSC 79, Box 145, APO AE 09714

INTRODUCTION

Historically, military recruits were selected primarily for their strength and size and, more recently, for a lack of infectious or debilitating medical conditions because soldiers traditionally walked to war carrying their weapons and survival equipment and had to fight hand to hand. In all the services, physical strength was a sine qua non of job performance. The selection of military aviators was among the first deviations from this concept, as it was realized early that flying did not simply require strength but also excellent sensory perception, an agile mind, and quick reaction speed.

Since the early days of military aviation, it has been recognized that the aviator faces most of the same stressors as other service members, plus many more from the aerial operational environment (Exhibit 25-1). (Since at present manned space flight has little direct military utility, this chapter omits the space aspect of aerospace medicine.) Compounding these stresses is the fact that to be combat effective, the aviator must be at the highest possible level of mental and physical capability. To ensure that he or she maintains this peak capability, each US military service has devoted specially trained physicians to this duty—the flight surgeons.

Many of the flight surgeon's duties (Exhibit 25-2) are the same as those of any operational military physician, so the question must be asked, "What makes aviators different from other soldiers, sailors, airmen, and Marines, and why must aviators have their own specially trained physicians?" The answer is that most medicine is concerned with the patient experiencing abnormal physiological function in his or her normal environment; aviation medicine, in contrast, focuses on normal physiological function in an abnormal environment. This short description of aviation medicine will discuss some of the medical aspects of this abnormal environment

and will consider some issues in operational flight medicine. This presentation is only intended to summarize the basics of the field—the information all military physicians should know in the event that they find themselves providing care for aviation personnel. It is not intended as a "short course" in aviation medicine. Numerous references are available for more in-depth information; some are listed at the end of this chapter.

EXHIBIT 25-1

STRESSES OF THE AVIATION ENVIRONMENT

Aircraft crash protection equipment

Aircraft escape systems (eg, parachutes, ejection seats)

Altitude-induced dysbarisms

Cold

Exposure to toxic gases and chemicals

Fatigue

G forces (acceleration)

Heat

Helmet-mounted displays and sighting systems

Hypoxia

Motion sickness

Noise

Operational psychological stress

Simulator sickness

Vertigo

Vibration

Visual and sensory illusions

HISTORY OF AVIATION

Lighter-Than-Air Period

Excluding myths and legends, probably the first human flights took place in balloons, and physicians rapidly became involved in identifying the physiological stresses faced in this new environment. Dr. Jacques Charles made a balloon ascent on 1 December 1783, during which he served both as aeronaut and flight surgeon, suffering from and correctly diagnosing barotitis (which he was unfortunately unable to treat). Soon after the flight of the

Montgolfier brothers in front of the Medical Faculty of Montpelier in 1784, physicians began to discuss the effects of flight on both sick and healthy aeronauts, with one physician recommending that the sick be offered the benefit of flight because of "the purer air encountered at altitude."[1p833] Early balloon flights reached only very low altitudes and thus rarely caused physiological distress in the aeronauts. The major health hazard of balloon flight at low altitude was death from falls. However, higher altitudes reached within a decade of those first

<table>
<tr><td>

EXHIBIT 25-2

DUTIES OF THE FLIGHT SURGEON*

Administrative functions (eg, flight evaluation boards, grounding and ungrounding, waiver actions)

Aircrew physical evaluation (selection and maintenance)

Care of acute trauma

Crash investigation

Diving medicine (in some services)

Emergency care

Evaluation of aircrew survival equipment

Evaluation of crash protection equipment

High-altitude parachuting support (in some services)

Hyperbaric treatment (in some services)

Inflight evaluation of pilots' capabilities

Medical aspects of civic action programs (disaster relief)

Medical intelligence production and evaluation

Medical preparation of unit for deployment

Occupational medicine (eg, hearing conservation, toxic exposures, repetitive stress injury)

Operational planning support

Participation in flight missions

Pre-deployment planning and medical advice

Prevention of combat stress

Primary care (sick call)

Provision of inflight care during medical evacuation

Research and development

Staff advisor to commanders

Training and supervision of medics

Training of aircrew in physiological factors of flight and human factors affecting flight safety

Unit-level preventive medicine

---

*The US Army has trained physician assistants in aviation medicine—the aeromedical physician assistants—and for the purposes of this chapter, they are considered flight surgeons.

</td></tr>
</table>

as the concern was more whether flight other than by balloon was possible. Particularly as balloonists reached higher altitudes, though, basic work on altitude physiology was accomplished. Soon after the manned balloon appeared, it became a military tool. The French used observation balloons in the battle of Fleurus in 1794, and they were used repeatedly by many nations for this purpose during the 19th century. There is no documented evidence of medical problems engendered by these tethered flights at low levels, but one wonders how many potential observers were eliminated due to "fear of flying."

Heavier-Than-Air Period

As with many other medical advances, operational aviation medicine grew out of war. In the first few years of heavier-than-air aviation, flights were low and slow and demanded little more than courage from the aviator. Physical considerations were of much less importance. There was little in the medical literature about altitude physiology, since only after 1910 could airplanes even approach 10,000 ft and the relevance of flight experience in balloons was nearly forgotten. In 1910, there were only about 320 aircraft in the entire world,[2] but during World War I this number climbed to tens of thousands. More important than the numbers, however, was the rapidly developing technology of aviation, as exemplified in the massive changes in aviation from 1913 to 1918. Speeds, altitudes, and military operational necessity soon added a host of stresses to those recognized before the war. No longer would an interest in flight coupled with physical courage be sufficient to qualify for pilot training. Certain physical capabilities began to be sought by the military.

In the earliest days of the war, some officers were reassigned into aviation when they became physically unfit for the infantry or cavalry. However, the necessities of war soon led all participating nations to realize that they needed to pay special attention to the selection and care of the aviator, and studies on the actual physiological and psychological requirements began to be carried out.

In these early days, accident rates were horrendous, largely due to "pilot failure." British studies[3] showed that of every 100 aviators killed, 2% were lost to enemy action, 8% to mechanical failure, and 90% to physical or mental deficiencies. In an attempt to reduce this large number of physical failures, physicians were assigned to aviation units to care for and monitor aviators. As these flight

flights regularly caused medical problems, which are noted in the ballooning reports of Glaisher, Robertson, and Gay-Lussac, among others.

During the 19th century, other means of flight, each with its own risks and stresses, were experimented with, including man-lifting kites, gliders, and powered heavier-than-air craft. There was little interest in the physical effects of flight on humans,

surgeons became more familiar with the flight environment, they began offering aviators and their commanders advice based on practical experience rather than theories. Although it was realized that not everyone should be an aviator, there was no recognition of any valid basis for selection. Each nation developed pilot qualification standards (which varied widely in emphasis) in accordance with its own national medical theories. Some standards were so stringent that few candidates could pass them, severely limiting the number of pilots.

After 1916, there was an outpouring of research on altitude effects, psychophysiological reactions, and cardiocirculatory response to flight stresses, including altitude. Much of this research analyzed the oft-discussed *mal du aviator*, the concept that flying was difficult, exhausting, and destined to wear out the bodies of aviators. Much additional effort was expended on determining individual pilots' tolerance to lowered oxygen tension and whether repeated exposure led to tolerance.

The immediate postwar years were nearly stagnant in technological terms, with little aircraft production or new technology, but aviators continued to push the limits of their aircraft and their bodies. Speeds and altitudes continuously increased, with maximum speeds reaching 575 km/h in 1929 and maximum altitudes reaching 13,100 m in 1930.[4] For the first time,

pilots were routinely experiencing sustained gravity, or G, forces of acceleration. Aviators began intensive study of night flying and blind (instrument) flying, and the few flight surgeons left on active duty were deeply involved in evaluating the physiology involved in these new techniques. Other work led to the elucidation of the causes of decompression sickness. The work from this period proved that aviation itself is not inherently unhealthy (laying to rest the old canard of "aviator's illness") and that it causes no persistent organic or functional changes in aviators.

During World War II, the stresses of flight grew exponentially. Flights at altitudes hitherto record-setting became routine, air-to-air combat increasingly allowed the development of sustained G loads, multiple engines of increased power led to increased problems with vibration, and operational requirements led to aviators flying in the extreme cold of high altitude and the extreme heat of North Africa. As jet aircraft and helicopters entered the inventory, additional stresses were placed on pilots. The military's heavy reliance on the helicopter in Korea and Vietnam and during Operation Desert Storm raised new medical problems, especially vibration and crash survivability. In general, though, the problems were medically the same as during previous wars. Despite these changes in technology, the medical needs of the aviator and the duties of the flight surgeon have not changed.

CLINICAL AVIATION MEDICINE

Routine clinical care for aviation personnel is similar to that for other military personnel. The major distinction is in the degree of impact on mission accomplishment caused by even minor illnesses. Aviation personnel must always be as close to 100% performance as possible. While a combat service support soldier with diarrhea will be miserable and less than optimally functional, he or she usually will be able to carry out the mission; an aviator with severe diarrhea or taking most medicines that control it will be unable to carry out any

aviation mission safely. Some medications exacerbate the various physiological stresses of flight and though perfectly safe in the ground environment may be hazardous in aviation. Thus, the difference in medical mission is not so much in the clinical variations of practice as it is in the knowledge and recognition of the effects of disease and of medications on the body in the abnormal environment of flight. Understanding the physiology of the aviation environment is necessary to understand the medical needs of the aviator.

MAJOR PHYSIOLOGICAL CONCERNS ASSOCIATED WITH FLIGHT

Humans are adapted for life near sea level, where the normal atmospheric pressure is 760 mm Hg. Temperature and pressure decrease with increased altitude, adversely affecting physiological functions. A healthy individual readily adapts to minor variations, but if an organ or system is the site of pathological change or if the environmental change is too great, then adjustment may not occur

and adverse symptoms will develop. If the aviator cannot compensate in some way, body functions will fail, and he or she will not be able to control the aircraft in an operational environment.

Alterations in barometric pressure occurring with altitude changes cause the primary adverse effects of flight on the body's physiological processes. The effects due to increasing altitude are manifested primarily in two forms: a decrease in the partial pressure of oxygen in the inspired air and an expansion of gases.

Hypoxia

Although the composition of the atmosphere remains nearly constant at all flying altitudes (78% N_2, 21% O_2), the amount of oxygen physiologically available does not. In any mixture of gases, the total pressure exerted by the mixture is equal to the sum of the pressures each gas would exert if alone in the same volume. At sea level, the total atmospheric pressure is 760 mm Hg, and the partial pressure attributable to oxygen is 159 mm Hg. This PO_2 is adequate to produce a hemoglobin saturation of 98%, which sustains life. However, the PO_2 is reduced at increased altitude, with consequent reduction in hemoglobin saturation even in normal individuals. At 10,000 ft, the total atmospheric pressure is approximately 523 mm Hg, with only 110 mm Hg provided by O_2. This leads to 60 mm PO_2 in the alveoli, which produces an arterial hemoglobin saturation of only 87% and causes symptoms of insidious hypoxia. But hypoxia simply due to altitude must be differentiated from other types of hypoxia, including pathological hypoxia, hypemic hypoxia, stagnant hypoxia, and histotoxic hypoxia (Table 25-1), because both preventive measures and corrective measures vary depending on the cause.

People differ in their reaction to hypoxia, but there are also many variables that determine the rapidity of onset and the severity of hypoxia symptoms, including:

- altitude reached (which determines the PO_2 in the lungs),
- rate of ascent to altitude (rapid rates of ascent may lead to achievement of high or hypoxic altitudes before the onset of warning symptoms),
- duration of time at altitude (in general, longer exposures lead to increased effects),
- temperature (increased metabolic rates may lead to hypoxic effects at lower altitudes),
- physical activity (increased oxygen demand may lead to the more rapid onset of clinical hypoxia), and
- individual factors, such as inherent individual tolerance, physical fitness, emotional state, acclimatization, and use of cigarettes.

A high external temperature, significant physical exertion, or fear favors the development of symptoms at lower altitudes. Physical fitness and acclimatization to high altitudes (eg, by living at elevations above 10,000 ft) raise the altitude level at which an individual will begin to experience hypoxic symptoms.

As hypoxia develops, the body experiences several stages, which are defined in terms of the degree of incapacity.

Indifferent Stage

This stage occurs at altitudes between sea level and 10,000 ft (39,000 ft if breathing 100% oxygen). The barometric pressure drops from the normal sea level pressure of 760 mm Hg to 523 mm Hg. Healthy individuals are physiologically adapted to this level, and ambient PO_2 is sufficient without the aid of protective equipment. There are no physiological effects except for some deterioration of night vision, which starts at about 5,000 ft. Hemoglobin saturation remains 90% to 100%.

TABLE 25-1

TYPES OF HYPOXIA

Type	Physiology	Common Causes
Hypoxic hypoxia	Inadequate oxygenation of blood in the lungs	Insufficient O_2 in inspired air (eg, at altitude, with contaminated breathing air)
Pathologic hypoxia	Inadequate oxygenation of blood in the lungs	Defects in oxygen diffusion from lungs to bloodstream even in the presence of adequate inspired O_2
Hypemic hypoxia	Reduction of oxygen-carrying capacity of the blood	Anemia, blood loss, carbon monoxide poisoning, drug effects (eg, nitrites, sulfa)
Stagnant hypoxia	Inadequate circulation (oxygen-carrying capacity of blood is normal)	Heart failure, arterial spasm, venous pooling during positive-G maneuvers
Histotoxic hypoxia	Interference with the use of O_2 by the tissues	Alcohol, narcotics, certain poisons (eg, cyanide)

Compensatory Stage

This stage occurs at altitudes between 10,000 and 15,000 ft (39,000 to 42,000 ft if breathing 100% oxygen). At the upper altitudes of this range, the barometric pressure falls to 429 mm Hg and the ambient PO_2 drops to 87 mm Hg. Unless supplemental oxygen and other equipment (eg, pressure regulators at the higher altitudes) are used, noticeable physiologic problems occur. This lowered PO_2 rapidly leads to oxygen deficiency, causing mild altitude hypoxia. Hemoglobin saturation ranges from 80% to 90%, and cardiac output, blood pressure, and pulse rate increase. Respiration increases in depth and sometimes in rate. Physiologic compensation provides some defense against hypoxia so that effects are reduced unless the exposure is prolonged. The healthy aviator functions normally in this stage for approximately 2 or 3 hours.

Disturbance Stage

This stage occurs at altitudes between 15,000 and 20,000 ft (42,000 to 44,000 ft if breathing 100% oxygen), and physiological responses no longer compensate for the oxygen deficiency. Hemoglobin saturation is 70% to 80%. Occasionally there are no subjective symptoms of hypoxia until unconsciousness occurs, but usually symptoms are noted. The aviator becomes drowsy and may make errors in judgment. He or she has difficulty with simple tasks requiring mental alertness or muscular coordination.

Critical Stage

This stage occurs at altitudes between 20,000 and 23,000 ft (44,000 to 46,000 ft if breathing 100% oxygen). Hemoglobin saturation is less than 70%. Within 3 to 5 minutes, judgment and coordination deteriorate and mental confusion, dizziness, and incapacitation occur.

Due to the significant risk of hypoxia during flight, it is imperative that each aviator knows about the symptoms of hypoxia (Exhibit 25-3) so that countermeasures may be taken as soon as possible. Failure to recognize the symptoms and take corrective action has caused numerous aircraft accidents.

Dysbarisms

Dysbarisms are syndromes resulting from the nonhypoxic effects of a pressure differential between the ambient barometric pressure and the pressure of gases within the body. These are of two predominant types, trapped gas and evolved gas dysbarisms.

Trapped Gas Dysbarisms

These dysbarisms are caused by the effects of Boyle's Law, which states that the volume of a gas is inversely proportional to pressure when temperature remains constant. This means that as altitude increases, gas expands. One liter of gas occupies

---

EXHIBIT 25-3

SIGNS AND SYMPTOMS OF HYPOXIA

Special Senses

    Extraocular muscle weakness and incoordination

    Central vision impairment

    Peripheral vision impairment

    Hearing loss (usually one of the last senses to be lost)

    Touch and pain diminished

Personality Traits

    Depression

    Euphoria

    Overconfidence

    Pugnaciousness

Psychomotor Function

    Decreased muscular coordination

    Loss of fine muscular movement

    Stammering

Mental Processes

    Calculations unreliable

    Intellectual impairment (often prevents recognition of hypoxic symptoms by the affected individual)

    Judgment and reaction time slowed

    Memory poor

    Thinking slowed

Subjective Symptoms

    Air hunger

    Apprehension or anxiety

    Dizziness

    Fatigue

    Headache

    Nausea

    Numbness

1.5 L at 10,000 ft, 2 L at 18,000 ft, and 4 L at 34,000 ft. Trapped gas dysbarisms vary, depending on which normal or pathological body cavity contains the gas. Air trapped in the gastrointestinal tract, the middle ear, the sinuses, or under a recent dental filling may cause problems. Perhaps the most common example of this syndrome is barotitis or "ear block." When the barometric pressure is reduced during ascent, the expanding air in the middle ear exits the middle ear through the eustachian[3] tube. The eustachian tube readily permits the exit of air but tends to collapse and resist reentry of air into the middle ear on descent. If the pressure differential becomes too great, it may be impossible to open the eustachian tube. This condition is painful and may lead to tympanic rupture. A similar problem is "sinus block," which occurs with similar physiology if the aeration of the sinus cavities is inadequate. Since two major causes of blockage of both the sinus ostia and the eustachian tube are the common upper respiratory infection and allergies, the significant concern among flight surgeons about aviators flying with a "simple cold" may readily be understood.

Evolved Gas Dysbarisms

Evolved gas dysbarisms are also called decompression sickness (DCS) and are caused by the effects of Henry's Law, which states that the amount of a gas dissolved in a solution is directly proportional to the pressure of the gas on the solution. This situation is exemplified by gas being held under pressure in a soda bottle—when the cap is removed, the liquid inside is exposed to a lower pressure, so gases escape in the form of bubbles. Nitrogen in the bloodstream behaves in the same manner. When an individual is exposed to such a reduction of pressure that he or she becomes supersaturated with nitrogen, nitrogen bubbles form in the blood and tissues, then cause symptoms by exerting pressure on surrounding tissues. Depending on where the bubbles form, the patient may suffer from classic bends (pain in the joints), paresthesias (tingling and itching sensations caused by bubbles formed along the nerve tracts), chokes (bubbles blocking the smaller pulmonary vessels), or central nervous system effects if the brain or spinal cord is affected.

Numerous variables determine whether an individual will develop DCS. The incidence increases with increased altitude. Traditionally 18,000 ft has been felt to be a threshold, but cases have occurred at significantly lower altitudes. Flying within 24 hours after SCUBA diving is extremely hazardous (see Chapter 26, Military Diving Medicine). The

longer the exposure to altitude, the higher the incidence of DCS. The incidence is also increased in older personnel and those with previous injuries.

Mechanisms used to prevent DCS include pressure suits, pressurized cabins, and prebreathing of 100% oxygen for a period of time sufficient to rid the body of dissolved nitrogen before reaching altitude. If DCS occurs, the optimum treatment is pressurization in a compression chamber to reduce the bubble size, then a slow return to sea-level pressure.

Other Medical Concerns Associated With Flight

In addition to the two major potential problems noted above, numerous other stresses of flight may affect aircrew function.

Vibration

Vibration has been a problem in flight ever since heavier-than-air craft were fitted with engines. As multiple reciprocating engines became the norm, multiple nodes of vibration developed in an airframe, having lesser or greater effects depending on where the crewmember was placed. In helicopters, however, vibration is omnipresent, affecting all those inside the aircraft equally. The medical impact of vibration has been debated for years. Current belief is that there is a distinct relationship with the chronic low back pain often experienced by helicopter pilots, though posture and seat design are believed to be greater causative factors. Although vibration has an impact on medical issues (eg, it is a significant contributor to chronic and acute fatigue in operational aircrew), its major effects are operational. For example, the utility of sights and vision-enhancing devices is degraded by severe vibration. Engineering solutions have to date been unsuccessful in eliminating vibration as a stressor, so the flight surgeon must remain alert to the demonstrated effects on aviators of repeated exposure.

Noise

Ever since powered flight became a reality, "aviator's ear," or hearing loss, has been noted. Aircraft engines, weapons systems, and other sources of ambient noise (eg, auxiliary power units) are constant sources of damaging steady state or impulse noise. Noise-induced hearing loss occurs when the receptors on the cochlear hair cells become fatigued and do not return to their normal state or when the ossicular chain is acutely disrupted by overpressure. Sudden noise-induced loss is usually due to impulse noise above 140 dB (eg, explosions, weapons firing). Gradual noise-induced loss is insidious and caused by noises from equipment that abounds in aviation, such as engines, transmissions, and power units. Hearing loss from chronic noise exposure is painless, progressive, permanent, and preventable. It remains, however, a major cause of disability for aviation personnel. Much of the hearing loss induced by noise exposure can be prevented by proper hearing conservation measures, and thus a major part of an aviation medicine program is devoted to hearing protection. Protection is by means of ear plugs, earmuffs, headsets, or helmets.

Problems of Proprioception

Despite modern technological instruments, the basic instruments used by pilots to orient themselves are those that evolved for slow-moving terrestrial beings—vision, vestibular system, and proprioceptive receptors. Unfortunately, these systems were not developed to serve in the airborne environment and can readily be deluded by position or direction changes, especially when coupled with partial loss of some input (as when vision is hindered by weather conditions) or with a lack of reference data (as in the desert or arctic snow fields). In these extreme environments, altitude and distance may be very difficult to judge, and dangerous objects such as crevasses or sand dunes may visually blend with the background and not be seen. The use of modern vision-enhancing devices (eg, night-vision goggles) may actually make these problems worse, since such devices have reduced fields of view, are monochromatic, and provide less than 20/20 visual acuity.

The range of problems that fall into the category of spatial disorientation is huge: visual and vestibular illusions of flight predominate, but psychological phenomena such as "breakoff" (in which the aviator feels a strong sense of unreality and may suffer an "out of aircraft" experience) are relatively common.

Visual System. The eyes can be fooled by many sensory inputs during flight. These illusions result from the pilot's misinterpretation of visual input, often due to conflict between "what is seen" and "what should be seen." For example, runways that are not the expected length or width may make an aviator believe that an approach is perfect, when in fact it may be high or low. The slope of terrain can cause a pilot to misjudge the aircraft's height above the approach path. Multiple visual illusions occur at night, often involving fixed light sources that

appear to move ("autokinesis") or ground lights that may be mistaken for stars, leading to abnormal flight positions.

Vestibular System. The otoliths and semicircular canals of the inner ear make up the vestibular system. They detect acceleration rather than speed, which explains many vestibular illusions. The otoliths detect linear acceleration, while the semicircular canals detect angular acceleration. Just as in the visual system, errors may occur due to failure to detect clues (eg, very slow turns), or active illusions may arise from falsely interpreted input (eg, after stopping a prolonged turn). Vestibular illusions experienced by the aviator include somatogravic and somatogyral illusions and the leans.

A somatogravic illusion is due to failure to correctly interpret otolith movements. Since the greatest continuous linear acceleration humans normally experience is gravity, otolith changes are normally interpreted as a change in the earth's gravitational vector rather than as some alternative acceleration. An example of this illusion is the sense of pitching up during forward acceleration (especially with catapult takeoffs).

Somatogyral illusion, in contrast, is a response to rotation. The vestibular system is unable to recognize prolonged rotation; it detects changes in angular acceleration, not persistent acceleration. Thus, if rotational acceleration turns to constant angular velocity, the sensation of rotation experienced by aviators becomes less and less, until they feel they are no longer rotating. If they then slow the turn and return to straight and level flight, their vestibular systems may interpret the angular deceleration as being acceleration in the direction opposite to the original turn. In simpler terms, a constant slow turn to the right may eventually be perceived as straight and level flight, and stopping that turn may be perceived as a turn to the left.

The illusion known as the leans occurs when a pilot allows the aircraft to make a very slow, subthreshold roll. When the pilot subsequently notices the abnormal attitude and rapidly corrects it, the labyrinthine system senses this second roll, and the pilot believes that he or she is banked in the opposite direction, even if flying straight and level.

Aviation Toxicology

Military aviation operations expose aviation personnel to a wide range of potentially toxic chemicals. Jet fuel, carbon monoxide, and weapons exhaust may be encountered during normal operations of the aircraft. Other exposures may occur only under unusual circumstances, such as an aircraft fire, which may expose the crew to hydrocyanic acid, hydrochloric acid, hydroflouric acid, Halon, or hydrazine. The recent increased use of composite materials in aircraft construction has increased the range of potential exposures. Typical occupational medical surveillance and protection programs have direct applicability in the aviation environment.

G Forces

Flight imposes major effects on the body when acceleration forces are applied during aerial maneuvering. Acceleration is the rate of change in velocity and is measured in G units. As an aircraft accelerates, the occupants experience acceleration forces in the opposite direction. A pilot exposed to 2G is being acted upon with force equal to two times the normal force of gravity in a direction opposite to that of the accelerative force. In many aircraft maneuvers, G forces are applied along the spinal cord toward the feet, causing movement of body components toward the feet. Since blood is the most mobile part of the body, it tends to move the most under the impact of G forces. As G forces are applied, the ability of the automatic regulatory system to ensure a continuous flow of blood to the heart and brain is affected. At some point less than 2.5G, the blood pressure at the level of the eye and

brain stem starts to decrease. As a result, most individuals begin to experience fuzziness of the visual fields (ie, grey-out) at about 3G to 4G. At around 4G to 4.5G, further increase in forces leads to total loss of vision (ie, blackout). At approximately 5G, unconsciousness (G force–induced loss of consciousness or GLOC) occurs. GLOC has caused the loss of many high-performance aircraft and pilots. Unfortunately, the preceding progression of symptoms may not occur in cases of rapid onset G forces; the pilot may progress directly to GLOC without any intervening visual or other symptoms.

The brain and retina are very sensitive to hypoxia; function is lost seconds after the blood supply ceases. Although this theoretically would allow up to 5 seconds of consciousness even after high G exposures, centrifuge studies[5,6] have demonstrated that up to 30 seconds are required before the pilot can function adequately to regain control of the aircraft. Normal G tolerance can be reduced by many factors, including many common to aviators in a field environment: lack of sleep, dehydration, inadequate diet, illness, and medication, among others. Pilots are protected from G forces by training in protective maneuvers (eg, L-1 straining maneuver), development of mission profiles limiting rate of onset of high G forces, pressure suits, seat positioning, weight training, and positive-pressure breathing systems.

SELECTED TOPICS IN OPERATIONAL AVIATION MEDICINE

Medications

Since all medications have an effect on the body, the flight surgeon must be knowledgeable about these effects and their potential interaction with the flight environment to ensure that pilots do not fly when impaired. Normally if a pilot is ill enough to take therapeutic medications, he or she should probably not be flying because of the medical condition rather than the medication. Prophylactic medications pose a risk-benefit question, but when the risk demands them, efforts must be made to minimize the effects. For example, the US Army does not permit pilots to take mefloquine for malaria prophylaxis because of its acknowledged side effects on the central nervous system in some patients; doxycycline is substituted. All services have strict regulations against aviation personnel self-medicating, even for minor illnesses; all care must be under the supervision of a flight surgeon who knows how the medication may affect the aviator in the flight environment.

Crew Rest

Both acute and chronic fatigue are severe threats to aviation safety. The military aviator is constantly stressed in this regard, particularly with military doctrine requiring continuous or sustained operations. Even in combat, crew rest schedules and flight schedules must be carefully monitored to ensure safe operations (see Chapter 15, Jet Lag and Sleep Deprivation). Fatigue, whether due to physical or mental stress, degrades the ability to make rapid decisions. Acute fatigue is relatively common and is caused by excessive mental or physical exertion. It is usually relieved by rest, relaxation, or sleep. Acute fatigue cannot be avoided but can be controlled. Chronic fatigue is both more insidious and more dangerous. It is secondary to unresolved acute stress over a variable period of time and may be unrecognized by the aviator or the chain of command, but it can be prevented. Each service has developed crew rest guidelines based on aircraft and mission types designed to ensure that aircrew have the opportunity to recover from their acute fatigue, thus preventing it from becoming chronic. Signs and symptoms of fatigue may include boredom, headache, chest pain, dyspnea, inability to concentrate, increased rate of errors, acceptance of unnecessary risks, carelessness, irritability, physical exhaustion, and sleep disturbances.

Contact Lenses

The development of new vision-enhancing systems, chemical protective equipment, and instrument display mechanisms has made the use of spectacles in the aviation environment less satisfactory than previously. The use of contact lenses is therefore desirable operationally. All services currently have ongoing projects to evaluate the safety and efficacy of contact lenses in this environment. While the benefits are in many cases obvious, the potential detriments are less so. In addition to the problem of aviators who cannot wear contact lenses, problems of ophthalmologic support and resupply, the incidence of ocular trauma caused by the lenses, and the actual utility of lenses in an operational environment must be considered. Much concern has been raised about the possibility that lenses (especially soft or gas-permeable lenses) may trap toxic fumes or chemicals, thus increasing corneal exposure. Most research to date, however, has shown this to be more of a theoretical than a practical problem. Currently, many aviators have been granted waivers to fly using contact lenses by their services on a case-by-case basis, and blanket approval in at least some services appears imminent.

Surgical Correction of Refractive Problems

Since perfect vision is such a desideratum for pilots, particularly with regard to use of new generation sighting and vision-enhancement equipment, there has been a great deal of interest in ways to achieve 20/20 vision without the use of lenses. Radial keratotomy, laser corneal reshaping, and laser in-situ keratomileusis (LASIK) are the three most commonly discussed modalities. Because of unresolved issues with glare and flare in patients after these procedures and the absence of long-term outcome data, none is currently accepted for flight personnel in any US service. As these techniques become more a part of the mainstream of ophthalmologic care and the incidence of side effects is reduced, it is likely that some version of them will be considered acceptable for flight personnel, but that time is not yet here.

Flight Physicals and Standards

To many aviators and medical personnel, the primary function of the flight surgeon is to perform the routine Flying Duty Medical Examination (FDME), better known as the flight physical. The routine FDME gives the flight surgeon an opportunity to detect future medical problems in their early stages, when they may be prevented or ameliorated, and to emphasize preventive medicine recommendations to their aviators. But the FDME is a more complex issue than it would appear at first glance. Closely intertwined with the actual clinical examination are the issues of what standards should be applied for both selection and retention. Standards and the components of the FDME have changed over the years, based on the results of public health epidemiology, aeromedical experience, and a review of medical factors involved in aviation mishaps. Frequency and content of FDMEs vary between services, and requirements may vary depending on the type of aircraft being flown. Today, major attention is paid to vision, hearing, cardiovascular condition, and psychological status. One of the greatest contributions of the flight surgeon has been in the evaluation of the actual impact of various health conditions on flight safety, which has frequently led to modification of the standards or to the granting of restrictive flight waivers for aviation personnel with various conditions. If an aviator can be safely allowed to fly under restrictions such as "no ejection seat aircraft" or "must fly with another qualified pilot," the aviation community may be able to make continued use of his or her experience and training, which otherwise would be lost to the military.

Aeromedical Evacuation

Providing medical care in flight is in many ways different from providing the same care in a hospital or a ground ambulance. Although aircraft have been used for the movement of critically ill patients since World War I, this modality still poses risks as well as benefits to the patients. Most of the physiological changes noted to affect aviation personnel apply with equal force to patients who already have a deranged physiology. In addition, the stresses of flight have special impact on some types of medical equipment and materiel. Gas, which expands on ascent to altitude, poses a significant threat when it is enclosed in an air cast, the inflated cuff of an endotracheal tube, or MAST (military anti-shock trousers). The vibration of flight makes many pieces of medical equipment fail. Many pieces of medical materiel commonly used on the ground produce electromagnetic radiation, which can interfere with aircraft navigation or flight controls. Capabilities for providing care in flight are constantly expanding, and we now routinely transport patients who would have been considered nontransportable only a few years ago. The knowledge to merge medical care successfully with the in-flight environment is a major contribution of experienced aviation medical personnel.

Crash and Incident Investigation

Although the incidence of military aircraft accidents that involve medical factors reached an all-time low in the late 1990s, the flight surgeon today still plays an important role in accident investigation. Not only does the flight surgeon on an accident board evaluate possible medical causes of the incident, but also he or she plays a major role in analyzing other factors surrounding the situation. Through examination of the injured or dead aircrewmen, the flight surgeon can often identify causes and mechanisms of injury or fatality. Analysis of these factors are frequently used in human factors or safety redesign of aircraft or survival equipment. Analysis of life support equipment, which either worked as designed or failed, allows continuous improvements in protection of aviators against crash stress. Closely associated with this role is the role that flight surgeons play in the human engineering of new airframes and flight equipment. Their knowledge of human factors in the flight environment continuously helps make this inherently dangerous environment safer.

SUMMARY

Aviation has inherent hazards, but these threats can be reduced by appropriate selection of pilots and adequate training. While aviation has changed significantly in the past two centuries, the human part of the equation has not. Aviation medicine for the most part has not been able to change the body's reactions to stress and has had to concentrate on selecting people able to compensate for the stresses of flight and on developing mechanisms to ameliorate those stresses. Each new generation of aircraft stresses aviators in new ways. While the stresses of flight against which the aviator must be protected have changed as aircraft performance has increased (especially in the space operational environment), the basic mission of ensuring optimum performance in an abnormal environment has not changed. Today, flight surgeons in all military services carry out duties little different in concept from those performed by the first flight surgeons in World War I. The mission of aviation medicine—to select, train, and maintain those pilots most capable of dealing with the stresses of flying these aircraft—has not changed and is unlikely to do so.

REFERENCES

1. Dureieux J. Essai sur l'usage des aerostats et ses applications en medecine. *Paris Medical*. 1913;12:833.

2. Sergeyev AF. *Ocherki po Istorii Aviatsiionnoy Meditsiny*. Moscow: USSR Academy of Sciences Publishing House; 1962. Translation: *Essays on the History of Aviation Medicine*. Washington, DC: National Aeronautics and Space Administration; 1965: 30. NASA TT F-176.

3. Anderson HG. The medical aspects of aeroplane accidents. *Br Med J*. 1918;Jan:73–76.

4. Gibbs-Smith C. *Aviation*. London: Her Majesty's Stationery Office; 1985.

5. DeHart R, ed. *Fundamentals of Aerospace Medicine*. 2nd ed. Baltimore: Williams & Wilkins; 1996.

6. Dhenin G, ed. *Aviation Medicine*. London: Tri-Med Books; 1978.

RECOMMENDED READING

1. Conference or Meeting Proceedings

   These are published by the Human Factors and Medicine Panel of the NATO Research and Technology Organisation (previously the Advisory Group for Aerospace Research and Development), 7 Rue Ancelle, 92200 Neuilly-Sur-Seine, France. Full Bibliographic details are available in the "Government Reports Announcements and Index" of the National Technical Information Service, Springfield, VA 22161. Not only are these proceedings quite detailed and topically organized, but they tend to be much more current than any textbook can hope to be. Some specific ones of interest include:

   - CP-492 Ocular Hazards in Flight and Remedial Measures. May 1991.
   - CP-540 The Support of Air Operations Under Extreme Hot and Cold Weather Conditions. Oct 1993.
   - CP-554 Recent Issues and Advances in Aeromedical Evacuation. Feb 1995.
   - CP-588 Selection and Training Advances in Aviation. Nov 1996.
   - CP-599 Aeromedical Support Issues in Contingency Operations. Sep 1998.
   - MP-19 Current Aeromedical Issues in Rotary Wing Operations. Aug 1999.

2. Military Regulations

   - Department of the Army. *Temporary Flying Restrictions Due to Exogenous Factors.* Washington, DC: DA: 1976. Army Regulation 40-8.
   - Department of the Army. *Standards of Medical Fitness.* Washington, DC: DA: 1995. AR 40-501.
   - Department of the Air Force. *Medical Examination and Standards.* Washington, DC: DAF; 1994. Air Force Instruction 48-123.
   - Department of the Navy. *Aeromedical Reference and Waiver Guide.* Pensacola, Fla: Naval Aerospace and Operational Medical Institute; 1998.

3. Other Publications

   - Department of the Air Force. *USAF Flight Surgeon's Manual.* Washington, DC: DAF; 1997. AFP 161-1.
   - US Air Force School of Aviation Medicine. *US Air Force Flight Surgeon's Guide.* Brooks Air Force Base, San Antonio, Tex: USAFSAM; 1999.
   - Naval Aerospace Medical Institute. *US Naval Flight Surgeon's Manual.* Pensacola, Fla: NAMI; 1989.
   - Crowley JS, ed. *United States Army Aviation Medicine Handbook.* 3rd ed. Fort Rucker, Ala: Society of US Army Flight Surgeons; 1993.
   - Federal Aviation Administration Office of Aviation Medicine. *FAA Guide for Aviation Medical Examiners.* Washington, DC: FAA; 1996.
   - Lam D. *Aeromedical Evacuation: A Handbook For Physicians.* Fort Rucker, Ala: Army Aeromedical Center; 1980.
   - *Aviation, Space, and Environmental Medicine.* (The journal of the Aerospace Medical Association)
   - Societies of US Naval, US Air Force, and US Army Flight Surgeons. *The Ultimate Flight Surgeon Reference.* 2nd ed. Fort Rucker, Ala: Societies of US Naval, US Air Force, and US Army Flight Surgeons; 1999.

4. Textbooks

   - Gilles JA. *A Textbook of Aviation Physiology.* London: Pergamon Press; 1965.
   - Rayman R. *Clinical Aviation Medicine.* 3rd ed. New York: Castle Connolly Graduate Medical Publishing; 2000.

Chapter 26

MILITARY DIVING MEDICINE

RICHARD S. BROADHURST, MD, MPH; LELAND JED MORRISON, MD; CHARLES R. HOWSARE, MD; AND ANDREW F. ROCCA, MD

R. S. Broadhurst; Colonel, Medical Corps, North Carolina Army National Guard; Commander, Company C, 161st Area Support Medical Battalion; formerly, Lieutenant Colonel, Medical Corps, US Army, Senior Diving Medical Officer, US Army Special Operations Command, Fort Bragg, NC 28307

L. J. Morrison; Captain, Medical Corps, US Navy (Retired); Chief Physician Naval Forces, United Arab Emirates; formerly, Senior Medical Officer, Naval Diving and Salvage Training Center, 350 S. Crag Road, Panama City, FL 32407

C. R. Howsare; Medical Director, Healthforce; 210 W. Holmes Avenue, Altoona, PA 16602; formerly, Lieutenant Commander, Medical Corps, US Navy, Training Medical Officer, DMO Course Coordinator, Naval Diving and Salvage Training Center, 350 S. Crag Road, Panama City, FL 32407

A. F. Rocca; Lieutenant Commander, Medical Corps, US Navy; Senior Resident, Department of Orthopedics, National Naval Medical Center, Bethesda, MD 20889-5600; formerly, Director of Clinical and Hyperbaric Medicine, Naval Diving and Salvage Training Center, 350 S. Crag Road, Panama City, FL 32407

INTRODUCTION

All services in the Department of Defense have elements actively involved in diving operations. Historically the US military, particularly the US Navy, has been a world leader in the development of diving and undersea technology, including diving medicine.[1] Diving Medical Officers (DMOs), both physicians and physician assistants, and Diving Medical Technicians (DMTs) are specifically trained in military diving medicine and perform fitness-to-dive evaluations, prevent and treat diving-related injuries, and monitor ongoing diving operations for safety. Diving medicine, a specialized type of occupational medicine, considers the medical issues involved in working in the unique conditions of the undersea environment, much as aviation medicine is concerned with similar issues in the hypobaric realm of flight. This chapter will address the issues that military preventive medicine specialists should understand about military diving, including relevant physics and physiology associated with diving, approaches to the prevention of diving illnesses and injuries, and the epidemiology and management of diving medicine problems.

MILITARY DIVING OPERATIONS

Military diving is divided into two general missions, fleet diving (eg, underwater ship's husbandry, salvage, underwater construction) and specialized diving (eg, special operations, explosive ordnance disposal [EOD], saturation). Military diving is generally performed at depths of less than 60 ft, except for some salvage, EOD, and saturation (prolonged duration) diving operations. Fleet diving is conducted throughout the US Navy and by US Army Engineer Corps divers, while specialized diving is performed by all four services in the Department of Defense. Special Operations Forces (SOF) in the Army include Rangers and Special Forces ("Green Berets"). Combat divers in the Special Forces perform inland search and rescue and combat search and rescue, as well as coastal infiltration and exfiltration, reconnaissance, and demolitions. Army Ranger combat divers are currently used only to perform reconnaissance. The SOF elements in the Air Force—Pararescue Teams and Combat Controllers—also must be capable of conducting downed-aircraft recovery and infiltration into denied territory. Navy Sea/Air/ Land (SEAL) forces conduct all aspects of SOF diving, including maritime direct-action operations (eg, ship attacks, ship boardings, harbor penetrations, hydrographic reconnaissance, clearance of beaches for amphibious assaults, shallow-water mine countermeasures). Divers in the Marine Corps Force Reconnaissance Units survey landing beaches and conduct covert underwater insertions. The Coast Guard, a Naval augmentee in time of war, uses divers for ship's husbandry, navigational buoy maintenance, and ocean search and rescue. As part of what is the most extensive diving program in the US military, the Navy operates the Naval Experimental Diving Unit, the Naval Submarine Medical Research Laboratory, and the Naval Medical Research Center. These organizations conduct manned and unmanned testing of military diving equipment, decompression algorithms, and hyperbaric physiology. The Naval Safety Center supports all diving in the Department of Defense by managing diving data, issuing safety messages, inspecting diving lockers, and investigating accidents.[2,3]

HISTORY OF DIVING

Early Diving Endeavors

The first recorded example of military diving was in the 5th century BC when a Greek diver cut the anchor lines of Persian warships to create confusion between vessels and cover his escape.[4] Salvage diving is nearly as old, traceable to the 1st century BC in the eastern Mediterranean. Over time, the use of divers in combat operations has evolved to include reconnaissance, covert infiltration, ordnance disposal, obstacle removal, and demolitions, in addition to underwater sabotage. US divers disposed of ordnance during the Civil War, investigated the sinking of the *USS Maine* in 1898, and performed submarine rescue and salvage in the early part of the 20th century. It was the period during and after the second World War, however, that saw rapid growth in military diving, including the development of all types of specialized diving and significant improvements in fleet diving.[5] All of these advances were made possible by revolutionary improvements in diving technology.

Evolution of Diving Equipment

Humanity's success underwater has always depended on the ability to procure air or oxygen and to survive in the environment. Although the ancients initially relied on simple breath-hold diving, they soon recognized the need to spend greater time working at depth. One solution was the diving bell, an inverted container lowered by rope to provide air at depth and increase bottom time. Alexander the Great is reported to have used one in the 4th century BC.[4] Diving bells were improved and came into widespread use from the 16th to the 19th centuries to support the growing business of salvage diving. Then in 1840, Augustus Siebe improved on existing diving suits, designed to protect divers from temperature and pressure extremes and other hazards, with new technology that allowed air to be pumped from the surface to divers at depth (Figure 26-1). This surface-supplied diving apparatus was the prototype for deep sea diving rigs, which are still used today in situations requiring prolonged bottom time, stationary work, or other specific circumstances.[5]

The next significant technological breakthrough was the development of scuba (self-contained underwater breathing apparatus). In 1878, Fleuss demonstrated the first practical scuba, which was a closed-circuit (no expired gas released into the water), 100% oxygen rebreather rig. This technology was used to develop oxygen rebreather systems for submarine escape and rescue in the early 20th century. The first scuba used to a significant degree in the US was invented in 1940 by Dr. Christian Lambertsen and was a semi-rebreather rig with steady-flow oxygen. This physician was also instrumental in military diver training during and after World War II and was an early authority in diving medicine. In World War II, scuba was used by Navy Underwater Demolition Teams and combat divers from the Office of Strategic Services, both forerunners of today's SOF divers. Finally in 1947, Frenchmen Cousteau and Gagnon developed the first successful open-circuit (releases expired gas into the water) air scuba rig, including a demand regulator, which supplied air only as the diver breathed. This Aqua-Lung rig conserved air

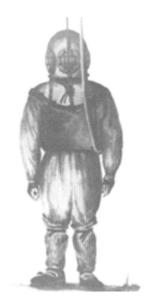

Fig. 26-1. Siebe's Diving Dress and Helmet. Augustus Siebe developed the first practical diving suit. He improved on earlier attempts by attaching the helmet to the rest of the suit and adding an exhaust valve.
Source: US Department of the Navy. *US Navy Diving Manual*. Rev 4. Washington, DC: Naval Sea Systems Command; 1999: 1-5.

and increased diving time, while the use of air as a breathing gas was a safer and cheaper alternative to oxygen. The Aqua-Lung not only provided more opportunities in military diving, it set the scene for the development of diving for sport and recreation.[4]

After World War II, researchers became interested in testing human endurance under the waves. Saturation diving grew out of experiments designed to test whether or not divers could survive at depth for days and weeks with their tissues "saturated" with the gases they breathed. Neither air nor pure oxygen could be used at these extreme depths because they caused nitrogen narcosis and oxygen toxicity, respectively, which are explained later in this chapter. Helium was the principal gas added to combat these conditions. In 1924, the US Navy began to experiment with helium-oxygen breathing mixtures, and this technology was successfully used in the famous salvage of the USS Squalus in 1939. The Navy continued to pioneer advances in mixed-gas diving, which was a necessary step to allow divers to dive longer and deeper. The US Navy performed its saturation diving experiments with personnel in an artificial habitat, SEALAB, which remained at depth for extended periods but required signifi-

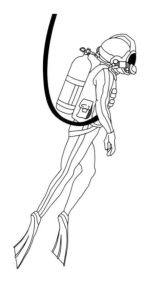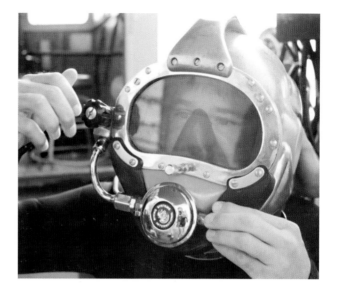

- Principle of Operation:
  1. Self-contained, closed-circuit oxygen system
- Minimum Equipment:
  1. MK-21 Helmet
  2. Harness
  3. Weight belt (if required)
  4. Dive knife
  5. Swim fins or boots
  6. Surface umbilical
  7. EGS bottle deeper than 60 fsw
- Principal Applications:
  1. Search
  2. Salvage
  3. Inspection
  4. Underwater Ships Husbandry and enclosed spamce diving
- Advantages:
  1. Unlimited by air supply
  2. Head protection
  3. Good horizontal mobility
  4. Voice and/or line pull signal capabilities
  5. Fast deployment
- Disadvantages:
  1. Limited mobility
- Restrictions:
  1. Work limits: 190 fsw
  2. Emergency air supply (EGS) required deeper than 60 fsw or diving inside a wreck or enclosed space
  3. Current—Above 1.5 knots requires extra weights
  4. Enclosed space diving requires an Emergency Gas Supply (EGS) with 50- to 150-foot whip and second stage regulator
- Operational Considerations:
  1. Adequate air supply system required
  2. Standby diver required

Fig 26-2. General Characteristics of the MK 21 Diving System.
Source: US Department of the Navy. *US Navy Diving Manual*. Rev 4. Washington, DC: Naval Sea Systems Command; 1999: 6–54.

cant support from the surface. An improved approach, the Deep Diving System, allowed divers to operate at depth out of a tethered capsule, which was then pressurized to that depth and returned to the surface at the completion of the dive. The capsule was mated to a pressurized decompression chamber, which provided a larger living area and was mounted on the deck of a ship where the divers and capsule could be easily monitored.[5]

Since the early 1980s, saturation diving in the Navy has been deemphasized and attention targeted toward missions in shallower water, particularly specialized diving.

Current fleet divers use open-circuit scuba primarily but sometimes dive with surface-supplied rigs, such as the MK 20 and the MK 21 (Figure 26-2), which provide more protection and allow communication with the surface. Combat and EOD divers

- Principle of Operation:

  1. Self-contained, closed-circuit oxygen system

- Minimum Equipment:

  1. Secumar life jacket
  2. Dive knife
  3. Swim fins
  4. Face mask
  5. Dive watch
  6. Depth gauge(0–80 fsw type and/or depth timer)
  7. Whistle
  8. Emergency flare (open water)
  9. Weight belt (as required)

- Principal Applications:

  1. Special warfare operations
  2. Shallow search and inspection

- Advantages:

  1. No surface bubbles
  2. Minimum support
  3. Long duration
  4. Portability
  5. Excellent mobility

- Disadvantages:

  1. Limited to shallow depths
  2. Central nervous system O_2 toxicity hazard
  3. No voice communications
  4. Limited physical and thermal protection

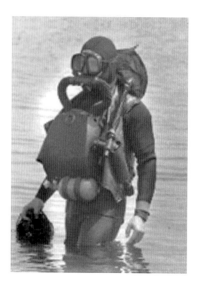

- Restrictions:

  1. Working limits: 190 fsw
  2. Normal—20 ft for 240 min
  3. Maximum—50 ft for 10 min
  4. No excursions are allowed when using Single Depth Dive Limits

- Operational Considerations:

  1. Buddy diver required if diver not tethered
  2. One safety boat required for diver recovery

Fig. 26-3. General Characteristics of the LAR V Diving System.
Source: US Department of the Navy. *US Navy Diving Manual.* Rev 3. Washington DC: Naval Sea Systems Command; 1993: 10-19.

use both open- and closed-circuit scuba. The LAR V (Figure 26-3) is often used for long, shallow, clandestine insertions, while the MK 16, which supplies oxygen at a fixed partial pressure, is used at deeper depths. Both are closed-circuit diving rigs that allow extended operating times, remove or "scrub" carbon dioxide from the exhaled gases and emit no bubbles.[5]

DIVING PHYSICS AND DECOMPRESSION THEORY

Application of Gas Laws to Diving

To function safely in the undersea environment, a diver must possess a fundamental knowledge of basic physics and how its laws predict the behavior of matter under a wide range of temperatures, pressures, and volumes. Pressure is defined as the amount of force applied per unit of area and is commonly expressed in terms of pounds per square inch (psi) or atmospheres (atm). Divers more frequently use feet of seawater (fsw), which is not a pressure measurement in the strict sense but is useful when actually working in the undersea environment. For calculations, feet of seawater can be easily converted to pounds per square inch or atmospheres because 1 fsw exerts a pressure equal to 0.445 psi, and every 33 fsw is equivalent to 1 atm[5,6] (Table 26-1).

TABLE 26-1

PRESSURE CHART

Depth (gauge pressure)	Atmospheric Pressure	Absolute Pressure
0	1 atm	1 ata (14.7 psi)
33 fsw	+ 1 atm	2 ata (29.4 psi)
66 fsw	+ 1 atm	3 ata (44.1 psi)
99 fsw	+ 1 atm	4 ata (58.8 psi)

fsw: feet of seawater
atm: atmosphere
ata: atmosphere-absolute
psi: pounds per square inch
Adapted from US Department of the Navy. *US Navy Diving Manual.* Vol 1 and 2. Rev 3. Washington, DC: Naval Sea Systems Command; 1993.

TABLE 26-2

GAS LAWS

Boyle's Law: P(A)V(A) = P(B)V(B)	Dalton's Law: P(total) = ppA+ppB+ppC	Henry's Law: V(A) = ppA x S(A)
P(X) = pressure of gas X V(X) = volume of gas X	P(total) = total pressure in mixture ppX = partial pressure of gas X	V(A) = volume of gas A ppA = partial pressure of A S(A) = solubility of A

Source: US Department of the Navy. *US Navy Diving Manual*. Vol 1 and 2. Rev 3. Washington, DC: Naval Sea Systems Command; 1993.

At sea level, the absolute pressure on a diver is 1 atmosphere-absolute (ata), and so the absolute pressure exerted on a diver at depth is always equal to the weight of the water plus the weight of the atmosphere. The weight of the water acts as a force on the diver called hydrostatic pressure, which is measured as gauge pressure.

Given this overview of pressure, the basic physics definitions and gas laws attributed to Boyle, Henry, and Dalton (Table 26-2) can be used to explore the behavior of gases and liquids. Boyle's Law states that if the temperature of a fixed mass of gas is kept constant, the volume of the gas will vary inversely with the pressure, such that the product of the pressure and the volume will remain constant. Boyle's Law is important to divers because it relates changes in the volume of a gas to the change in pressure (or to changes in depth) such that when pressure doubles, volume decreases to half its original value (Figure 26-4). This law is most important in the first 33 ft of water because as the diver moves through this pressure differential of 1 ata at the surface to 2 ata at 33 fsw, the volume of gas in the diver undergoes its greatest absolute change in volume. This relationship is integral to appreciating the pathophysiology of both pulmonary over-inflation syndrome and barotrauma.

Dalton's Law, or the "law of partial pressures," dictates that the total pressure exerted by a mixture of gases is equal to the sum of the pressures of each of the different gases making up the mixture, with each gas acting as if it were alone and occupying the entire container. Divers usually use a mixture of gases rather than a single pure gas, so this law enables a diver to calculate the individual pressures exerted by component gases, to predict potential ranges for individual gas toxicity, and to prevent such diving hazards as oxygen toxicity.

Henry's Law states that the amount of any given gas that will dissolve in a liquid at a given temperature is a function of the product of the solubility coefficient for that gas and the partial pressure of the gas in

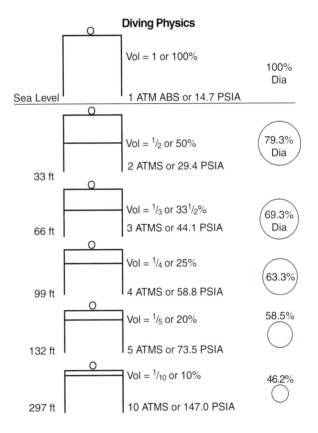

Fig. 26-4. Gas volume and bubble diameter as a function of depth—Boyle's Law.
Reprinted with permission from: Somers LH. Diving physics. In: Bove AA, Davis JC. *Diving Medicine*. 2nd ed. Philadelphia: W.B. Saunders; 1990: 13.

contact with the liquid. Furthermore, the solubility coefficient depends on both the properties of the solute (the gas) and solvent (the liquid—usually plasma) and is different for each combination. Simply stated, since water constitutes such a large portion of the human body, as a person dives deeper, more gas will dissolve in body tissues, which must then be released upon ascent. If a diver remains at depth for enough time, his or her body tissues will ultimately reach equilibrium with the ambient breathing gas such that eventually no more gas can be dissolved, a state known as saturation. When a diver whose body tissues are saturated with a dissolved gas ascends toward the surface, less ambient pressure is exerted on the diver, and there is more release (off-gassing) than acceptance (on-gassing) of the inspired gas. A simple example is removing the cap from a bottle of soda. Carbon dioxide is under pressure, and the liquid is saturated with it. When the cap is removed and the ambient pressure reduced, carbon dioxide comes out of solution as bubbles. If a diver ascends too quickly, he or she may not off-gas fast enough and may transiently enter a supersaturation state where so much gas is dissolved in the tissues that it cannot all naturally escape through exhalation, and gas molecules coalesce to form bubbles. This theory has become the dominant hypothesis in explaining the development of decompression sickness or the "bends." Determining how a diver could avoid this malady and predictably ascend safely to the surface became the impetus for the development of the US Navy Diver Decompression Tables.[5–7]

History and Development of Decompression Procedures

Diving and medicine have been closely linked through history, as is demonstrated by the crucial role physiology has played in the study of decompression sickness (DCS). Pol and Watelle first suggested in 1854 that gas bubbles might be involved in the development of what is now known as DCS and realized that there was a relationship between pressure, duration of exposure, rapidity of decompression, and onset of illness. They also noted that relief of symptoms occurred during recompression. In 1857, Seyler demonstrated that bubbles blocked the pulmonary circulation. Then in 1878, Bert demonstrated bubbles in blood and tissue after decompression and noticed that these bubbles consisted predominately of nitrogen. He recommended using recompression with oxygen as therapy for DCS and also recommended decompression with oxygen, but he did not specify decompression rates.[7,8]

In 1900, Heller, Mager, and Von Schrotter proposed the first decompression procedure, noting that partial pressures of inert gases at depth could be calculated using Dalton's Law and that nitrogen could be assumed to be inert. Using Henry's Law as a guide, they developed a gas elimination equation to describe the movement of an inert gas into and out of solution at varying partial pressures and the movement of this dissolved gas into and out of tissues. Their simple model assumed no additional tissue diffusion barrier for nitrogen but predicted that the

rate of on- or off-gassing of dissolved nitrogen would depend on three factors: (1) the diffusion gradient of nitrogen into the blood, a function of partial pressure and depth, (2) tissue blood flow, and (3) the ratio of inert gas solubility in blood to its solubility in tissue. The model described tissue gas characteristics in terms of half-times and an exponential time constant, as in drug pharmacokinetics. The calculated decompression rate of 20 min/ata, when tested in occupational scenarios, proved adequate for short dives to 5 to 6 ata but not for longer dives.[7]

In 1908, Boycott, Damant, and Haldane, who were evaluating caisson workers, noticed that the incidence of DCS increased as the duration of the dive approached 5 hours, but the incidence appeared to remain constant for exposures longer than 5 hours. Their experiments with goats confirmed these observations.[9] Additionally, the researchers felt that the body should not be considered one compartment but rather a series of tissue compartments, due to the variability in tissue homogeneity and gas solubility. The time it took for half the gas to leave a saturated tissue compartment was termed a half-time. For mathematical convenience, Haldane arbitrarily selected half-times of 5, 10, 20, 40, and 75 minutes to cover the spectrum of possible exchange rates, but these rates were not assigned to specific real tissues. The gas elimination equation demonstrated that the 75-minute tissue would be almost 95% saturated at the 5-hour point.[7,10]

Haldane is also credited with the observation that men could be decompressed to 1 ata after complete saturation at 2 ata without developing symptoms but could not tolerate greater drops in pressure without developing DCS. Experimentally he found that goats could perform a 2:1 drop in ambient pressure without developing DCS and confirmed this in the hyperbaric chamber by observing decompression drops from 2 to 1 ata, from 4 to 2 ata, and from 6 to 3 ata without clinical sequelae. It appeared, therefore, that both men and goats could tolerate a 2:1 pressure drop or a 1.58:1 ratio of P_{N2}/P_B, (where P_{N2} is the partial pressure of nitrogen in tissue and P_B is the absolute pressure) at least to a depth of 3 ata. Based on these data, Haldane and his associates proposed decompression procedures designed to ensure that the ratio of P_{N2} to P_B never exceeds 1.58:1 in any tissue compartment. For convenience, however, decompression stops were proposed in increments of 10 fsw. This was the beginning of "staged decompression," which can be likened to intermittently opening and closing the cap of a shaken soda bottle to avoid the soda's bubbling over. The Royal Navy adopted the Haldane Tables in 1908, and these early tables provided adequate decompression for dives as deep as

200 fsw for as long as 30 minutes, but they were not recommended for exposures at deeper depths.[7,10]

The first tables developed for US Navy use were devised by French and Stillson in 1915 and are called the Bureau of Construction and Repair tables (C and R tables). They used the Haldanian ratio of 1.58:1, employed oxygen decompression for dives between 200 and 300 fsw, and were used successfully in 1915 to salvage the sunken submarine F-4 at a depth of 306 fsw.[11,12] Since 1915, various modifications have been made to these tables by US Navy researchers to extend bottom time while minimizing DCS. Hawkins, Shilling, and Hansen in 1935[13] and Yarborough[14] again in 1937 performed retrospective mathematical analyses of nitrogen uptake and elimination for nearly 3,000 dives. Tissues with short half-times (called fast tissues) appeared to tolerate very high ratios and off-gas quickly during ascent, allowing the decompression stops for these tissues to be deleted. Based on the longer 20-, 40-, and 75-minute half-times, Yarborough calculated new decompression tables, which were issued in 1937 and resulted in an acceptable annual incidence of DCS of only 1.1% in Navy divers.[7,10]

In 1951, while developing surface decompression tables for dives using air, Van der Aue conducted an extensive evaluation of the Yarborough tables on long working dives. For these dive profiles, he discovered that the 5- and 10-minute tissues did sometimes require deep decompression stops for off-gassing, while to achieve adequate decompression at the shallower stops, it was necessary to factor in another hypothetical tissue with a half-time of 120 minutes.[15] This work demonstrated that as dive depth or duration, or both increased, deeper decompression stops were required because of the greater saturation of tissues.

Before revising the Yarborough Tables, DesGranges, Dwyer, and Workman in 1956 analyzed inert gas uptake and elimination during 609 working dives using half-times of 5, 10, 20, 40, 80, and 120 minutes. They confirmed that the Haldanian ratio was not constant but that the ratios for slow and fast tissues differed and that they decreased exponentially with depth. The authors graphed the safe and unsafe nitrogen supersaturation ratios for each decompression stop and constructed a table of safe ratios on the basis of both tissue half-time and depth of stop.[16] Tables based on these concepts were adopted by the US Navy.

Workman in 1957 took a different approach to the decompression table, which previously had focused on time required for off-gassing at certain stops. Since the degree of allowable supersaturation differed for every tissue and every depth, he produced a table that simply stated what the maximum allowable inert gas pressure or saturation was for each tissue at each decompression stop.[17] These maximum values, called M-values, can be used to develop tables for air and mixed-gas diving. After considerable additional research, Workman eventually also added tissue half-times of 160 and 240 minutes and reduced the allowable ratios to provide for adequate decompression on long, deep exposures.[18] Despite extremely limited testing of these final additions, these tables were promulgated for emergency use.

The decompression tables currently used by the US military were developed through careful calculations and were largely verified with human testing. Berghage and Durman[19] evaluated the incidence of DCS in divers using the US Navy Tables from 1971 to 1978. During this period, 16,120 dives involving decompression were reported by the Navy, yielding 202 cases of DCS and an overall incidence rate of 1.25%. The majority of Navy dives are shallow (< 50 fsw) and do not involve decompression, so only 43 of a possible 295 depth/time combinations on the tables had more than 100 dives (data points) that could be used in analysis. On these schedules, the overall incidence of DCS was 1.1%, but it was as high as 4.8% with some schedules, particularly for those dive profiles of 100 fsw for 60 minutes and longer. Recent analysis of Naval Safety Center diving data[20] for more than 600,000 dives during the period 1990 through 1995 demonstrated identical rates for the two types of DCS at 1.3 per 10,000 dives.

Current Decompression Procedures and Tables

The US Navy Diving Decompression Tables (Figure 26-5) have been improved and modified to apply the safest decompression procedures to all types of diving. Specific populations whose dive profiles may be unpredictable (eg, special operations divers) have benefited greatly from these changes. The nature of SOF diving is to spend a considerable period of time at shallow depths with the occasional need to perform deeper excursions. For an extra margin of safety, the standard Navy decompression tables are based on the "square dive" concept, which means if the total dive time is 30 minutes, the table considers that the diver has spent the entire 30 minutes at the deepest depth, even though the diver may have been at that depth for only a few minutes.[5] Using this concept, the decompression obligation for SOF divers was unnecessarily long. So the Combat Swimmer Multilevel Dive decompression procedures were developed by Butler and Thalmann[21] for air diving in 1983 and expanded to include Mark 15 and 16 oxygen rigs in 1985. LAR V divers can also use these procedures, which consider the dive profile as multiple square dive segments and acknowledge off-gassing credit for the long intervals in shallow water, just like off-

Decompression stops (feet/meters)

Depth feet /meters	Bottom time (min)	Time first stop (min:secc)	50 15.2	40 12.1	30 9.1	20 6.0	10 3.0	Total decompression time (min:sec)	Repetitive group
80 **24.3**	40						0	2:40	*
	50	2:20					10	12:40	K
	60	2:20					17	19:40	L
	70	2:20					23	25:40	M
	80	2:00				2	31	35:40	N
	90	2:00				7	39	48:40	N
	100	2:00				11	46	59:40	O
	110	2:00				13	53	68:40	O
	120	2:00				17	56	75:40	Z
	130	2:00				19	63	83:40	Z
	140	2:00				26	69	97:40	Z
	150	2:00				32	77	111:40	Z

Fig. 26-5. A Portion of the US Navy Standard Air Decompression Tables.
Source: US Department of the Navy. *US Navy Diving Manual*. Rev 4. Washington, DC: Naval Sea Systems Command; 1999: 9-56.

gassing credit is awarded during a surface interval in between repetitive diving (multiple dives within 12 hours). The standard air decompression tables for repetitive diving, as developed by DesGranges, are used with the following four exceptions: (1) in place of the 10-minute surface off-gassing time required in normal repetitive diving, a 30-minute "shallow interval" at depths of less than 20 ft can be used, (2) for safety, all segments of the dive at 30 ft or less are rated on repetitive tables in decompression groups that are one group higher than the standard tables, (3) divers cannot move to lower repetitive groups over time, and (4) a diver can stay at depths of 30 ft or less indefinitely without ever exceeding repetitive group "O."[21]

Special Warfare divers currently have an additional option, the Naval Special Warfare Dive Planner, to plan dives and calculate decompression obligations.[22] The Dive Planner was developed because of the perception that the current tables were not equally safe across all depth and bottom-time (approximate duration of on-gassing) combinations, which was supported by the variable DCS rates noted earlier in those using standard decompression tables. Tissue saturation models, which previously had been the focus of decompression theory, contained too many parameters to be determined precisely and simultaneously and could not exactly predict decompression obligation. It was suspected that long, deep dives required substantially more decompression time than the standard tables indicated. Scientists at the Naval Medical Research Institute (now the Naval Medical Research Center, Silver Spring, Md) developed a probabilistic nitrox (nitrogen and oxygen mixture, with more oxygen than normal air) decompression algorithm named

USN-93 that used formal statistical techniques and maximum likelihood modeling to form safe decompression tables. USN-93 is capable of calculating decompression obligations given an endless array of possible depths, bottom times, and travel rates. In addition, the model adjusts for divers who switch breathing mediums between air and constant partial pressure oxygen breathing apparatuses (ie, the MK 16) during the same dive.[23] This statistical model was developed using a large database of well-documented experimental chamber, air, and nitrox dives correlated with cases of DCS. Using the results of these "safe" chamber (or dry) dives, an algorithm for computing decompression schedules in real time was developed and was then successfully validated in a prospective trial of more than 700 "wet" dives, including multilevel dives and dives where the breathing gas was switched between air and a constant partial pressure of oxygen of 0.7 ata during different segments of the same dive. SEALS are equipped with "real-time" depth and time meters capable of recording and downloading very accurate dive profile information. Given a computer with at least a 486-level microprocessor, a math coprocessor loaded with USN-93, and the specific multilevel dive profile, a DMO can calculate a decompression table for almost any dive. This computer is an adjunct to the sources of decompression information already available, including the Combat Swimmer Multilevel Dive procedures and Standard Air Decompression Tables, which are used by the DMO to predict the best possible decompression plan given the specific operational diving scenario.[24,25]

Standard Navy decompression tables are designed for use at altitudes less than 2,300 ft (700 m) above sea level. Diving gauges may not compensate for altitude or for fresh water being less dense than seawater. These two factors contribute to inadequate decompression by divers at altitude who are unfamiliar with the unique decompression requirements there. The Navy Experimental Diving Unit maintains altitude decompression tables for US military use.[26] Civilian divers venturing into bodies of water above 700 m can consult Buhlmann's Swiss dive tables.[27]

GASES AND DIVING

Oxygen Disorders

Oxygen deficiency, or hypoxia, leads to unconsciousness and death. The majority of military diving uses air, the absence of which is easily and quickly recognized by the diver. But unlike sudden strangulation or suffocation, a gradual decrease in oxygen content may not be detected. Unconsciousness can occur without anticipated warning signals. Any diving system that utilizes either surface-supplied mixed gas or rigs that carry their own oxygen (eg, LAR V, MK 16) can produce a hypoxic state due to malfunction or incorrect gas mixing. The treatment of suspected hypoxia in the water is to shift to an alternate gas supply. Incoherent or unconscious divers should be placed on 100% oxygen, if available, from 40 fsw or shallower until the diver reaches the surface and can be monitored appropriately.[5]

Just as too little oxygen can create difficulty for divers, excessive amounts can cause oxygen toxicity, specifically in the tissues most sensitive to high levels of oxygen, including the lung, the eye, and the brain. Pulmonary oxygen toxicity is seen at oxygen partial pressures of 0.5 ata (the equivalent of breathing air at 46 fsw or deeper).[6,7] The symptoms include discomfort or a burning sensation deep in the throat or substernal area, accompanied by cough or burning on inspiration. Findings include a decrease in vital capacity as measured by pulmonary function tests. Pulmonary oxygen toxicity requires several hours or days to develop and may be seen if a stricken diver requires several iterations of recompression treatment. If repetitive treatments are needed for persistent symptoms, pulmonary function tests are required. If there is a decrement in vital capacity of more than 10%, treatment with oxygen must be interrupted and a transition to other treatments considered. After daily exposures to high levels of oxygen (eg, daily treatments for 2 to 4 weeks), ocular oxygen toxicity may produce transient myopia, which will resolve over the course of 4 to 6 weeks if there are no further exposures.[28] Central nervous system (CNS) oxygen toxicity has been observed at oxygen partial pressures above 1.3 ata (the equivalent of breathing air at 171 fsw or breathing 100% oxygen at 9 fsw or deeper).[6,7] During dives with enhanced oxygen rigs and chamber runs that use oxygen, CNS toxicity must be a constant consideration because, unlike pulmonary oxygen toxicity, CNS oxygen toxicity can strike within minutes of exposure.

Sensitivity to oxygen toxicity varies between individuals and within the same individual, making it impossible to predict which divers are at increased risk. The warning symptoms associated with CNS toxicity are taught using the acronym VENTID-C, with convulsions being the most common presentation (Table 26-3). Treatment is straightforward. Since high partial pressures of oxygen created the problem, the goal in therapy is to reduce oxygen tension. This can be done by several methods, including removing the oxygen mask from a chambered diver, ascending a few feet or switching to a gas of lower oxygen content, if available. The seizures of CNS oxygen toxicity are not epilepsy and usually do not require medicinal intervention; they are simply a toxic reaction. There is no increased predisposition for further seizure disorder throughout life. The cold water immersion and hypercarbia seen on long, arduous combat swimmer missions predispose divers to oxygen seizures, which if suffered at depth, place divers at great risk for drowning and developing an arterial gas embolism.[5]

Carbon Dioxide Toxicity

Carbon dioxide is a by-product of human metabolism, and its serum concentration is maintained within

TABLE 26-3

SYMPTOMS OF CENTRAL NERVOUS SYSTEM OXYGEN TOXICITY

Vision	Vision is reported to "tunnel" or close in
Ears	Ringing and increased perception of sound
Nausea	Feeling of vague discomfort in the abdomen
Twitching	Particularly the muscles of the face (cheeks)
Irritable	Sense of agitation and uneasiness
Dizziness	Sense of lightheadedness, vertigo, or both
Convulsions	Tonic-clonic seizures, usually with no warning

Source: US Department of the Navy. *US Navy Diving Manual.* Vol 1 and 2. Rev 3. Washington, DC: Naval Sea Systems Command; 1993.

the relatively narrow range of approximately 35 to 45 mmHg by both lung and tissue functions. Despite the efficiency of these systems, excessive carbon dioxide levels can develop during diving due to overproduction (from increased duration and intensity of exercise), poor ventilation, or failure of carbon dioxide removal systems in rebreather rigs.[5,6] Inadequate ventilation results from missed breathing or breath-holding during a dive, increased breathing resistance in the equipment, or excessive dead space in the breathing system. Hypercapnia, an elevated level of carbon dioxide, can present in a variety of ways. An increased rate and depth of breathing may be noticed first, followed by a nagging frontal headache or such symptoms as nausea, confusion, or unconsciousness. Alternatively, too little carbon dioxide produces painful muscle spasm of the hands and feet (tetany), paresthesias, numbness, lightheadedness, confusion, and, again, loss of consciousness. Low levels of carbon dioxide, or hypocapnia, usually occur secondary to hyperventilation. Treatment is straightforward: efforts should be made to slow the respiratory rate, and, if necessary, abort the dive. In cases of suspected hypercapnia, the diver should stop work and allow time for adequate ventilation. If the cause of the hypercapnia is the equipment, the dive should be aborted.[5,6]

Carbon Monoxide Poisoning

Divers will encounter carbon monoxide poisoning through exposure to a contaminated air supply. Containers of breathing gas, such as scuba tanks, must be pressurized to deliver the gas underwater to divers. Compressor intakes must be distant to any exhaust sources, which typically contain carbon monoxide. A shifting breeze can create a problem if the system is not monitored carefully. Headache, nausea, confusion, and unconsciousness are symptoms of high levels of carbon monoxide, which is tasteless and odorless. If more than one diver complains of symptoms consistent with carbon monoxide poisoning, contaminated gas should be suspected. Treatment involves removal from the gas source and treatment with 100% oxygen at an elevated partial pressure.[5,6,28]

Nitrogen Narcosis

Nitrogen makes up approximately 79% of air and at 1 atm serves essentially as a diluent for oxygen. Nitrogen—as with any of the diluting gases used in diving—will become toxic if the partial pressure is excessive. Humans note an anesthetic or sedating effect associated with nitrogen as partial pressure is increased. At depths much below 50 fsw, alterations in function can be detected by psychological and motor skill testing; below 200 fsw, symptoms progress to loss of fine motor control, inattention to tasks, and poor judgment. Treatment is straightforward: the partial pressure must be decreased by ascending or surfacing.[5–7]

Helium Diving

Helium is used as a breathing gas in saturation diving to reduce breathing resistance at deep depths, as well as to prevent the occurrence of nitrogen narcosis, which otherwise limits diving depth to approximately 200 ft. Helium can present three primary problems when employed in diving operations. The first is hypothermia, because helium has a thermal conductance that is seven times that of air. Divers can become hypothermic quickly at depths, so care must be taken to heat breathing gases, as well as to provide adequate thermal protection from the surrounding water (ie, dry suit or hot water suit). The second potential problem is the distorting effect of helium on oral communication, the so-called "Donald Duck effect," which can make communicating with a diver at deep depths very difficult. Finally, high pressure nervous syndrome is a derangement of central nervous system function that occurs during deep helium-oxygen dives, particularly saturation dives. The cause is unknown, but it is thought to be an effect of depth, not a specific effect of the breathing gas. The clinical manifestations include nausea, fine tremor, imbalance, incoordination, loss of manual dexterity, and loss of alertness. In severe cases, a diver may develop vertigo, extreme indifference to his or her surroundings, and marked confusion. The nervous syndrome is first noted between 400 and 500 ft, and its severity appears to depend on both depth and compression rate. With slow compression, depths of 1,000 ft may be achieved with relative freedom from symptoms. Attempts to make the syndrome less severe have included the addition of nitrogen or hydrogen to the breathing mixture, but no method has been entirely successful below depths of 1,000 ft.[5–7] These gases may influence high pressure nervous syndrome because their narcotic properties may provide a partial anesthetic effect.

ENVIRONMENTAL HAZARDS

The aquatic environment is at once both incredibly beautiful and unforgivingly dangerous to those who do not respect it. Survival here requires an awareness of hazards, such as temperature extremes and animal life, as well as an appreciation of physics to understand the behavior of gases under pressure, the significance of light refraction, and the differences in blast effects and sound conduction in water versus air.

Thermal Dangers

Divers may be exposed to thermal extremes on the surface, in a hyperbaric chamber, and in the water. Heat loss can occur through convection, conduction, radiation, and evaporation, including significant respiratory loss in dehumidified air and in diving gases such as helium. Heat loss in still water is 25 times that in air, while heat loss in moving water increases to a factor of 200.[5,6] Heat is produced by basal metabolism and exercise (shivering) and may be absorbed from environmental sources. Hypothermia is defined as a core temperature of 35°C (95°F) or less, which requires various treatments depending on whether it is mild (35°C–32°C, 95°F–90°F), moderate (32°C–28°C, 90°F–82°F), or severe (< 28°C, < 82°F). Cardiac rhythms degrade into ventricular fibrillation very easily if divers are jostled while severely hypothermic. Unfortunately, the rhythms are also quite refractory to the usual acute cardiac life support protocols.[5,29]

At the other extreme is hyperthermia. A resting diver in a swim suit will remain euthermic in 33°C (92°F) water, but if working in water warmer than 30°C (86°F), he or she may develop hyperthermia. Types of injuries include heat cramps, heat exhaustion, and heat stroke, which may present in the absence of dry, hot skin. Even personnel riding in a chamber can be thermal casualties. The Navy Diving Manual gives guidelines for which treatment tables can be used if the ambient temperature is greater than 29°C (85°F), and the chamber is not equipped with an environmental package to cool the gas inside the chamber.[5]

Acoustic Hazards

Sound is transmitted much more efficiently in water than in air, so sound that would normally be inaudible in the air can be heard at great distance underwater. Unfortunately, this rapid conduction also makes localization of sound underwater more difficult. Humans are able to detect the small difference in the time of arrival of airborne sound (traveling at about 1,000 ft/s) reaching one ear as compared to the other, thus allowing us to localize the source. With waterborne sound (traveling at nearly 5,000 ft/s), however, it is impossible for humans to identify the direction of sound transmission.[5,6] Sonar and low frequency sound have been explored as offensive weapons by which to keep unfriendly divers away from military vessels because injuries, including vestibular disturbances, cardiac arrhythmia, and tissue destruction, occur given certain conditions of frequency and volume. Low-frequency vibration can be perceived by the submerged diver, just as vibration due to sound can be felt by the music lover when touching a stereo speaker.[30,31]

Blast Injuries

Underwater explosions are very dangerous to a submerged diver. The type of the explosive used, the size of the device, its location in the water column, the surrounding seabed topography, and the location of the diver all affect the outcome of the exposure (Figure 26-6). Damage occurs as the shock wave of blast overpressure leaves the dense water and passes through the

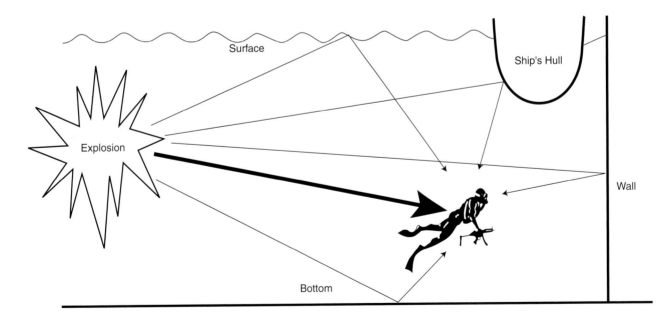

Fig. 26-6. Reflected shock waves can increase or decrease the total effect of the blast on a diver.
Source: Noonburg G. *US Army Special Forces Diving Medicine Manual*. Key West, Fla: Special Forces Underwater Operations School; 1995: SS-1.

diver's less-dense, air-filled compartments (eg, lung, intestine, sinus, middle ear). At this interface, the wave decreases in velocity and shreds the tissue, an effect referred to as "spalling." Hemorrhage, compartment rupture, air embolism, and even bone fractures have been reported in submerged blast victims.[5,32]

Electrical Hazards

Military divers are exposed to electrical hazards in their daily duties. Fleet divers, for example, are required to operate 220-volt equipment manually to cut and weld underwater. Wet divers move about the deck, and the dive station itself is in contact with wet decking, thereby enhancing the potential for inadvertent electrocution. Shipboard systems have both alternating and direct current (AC and DC), as well as high- and low-voltage sources. Dry skin offers approximately 10 times (10,000 ohms) the resistance to electricity afforded by wet skin. Once contact with a wet diver is established, alternating current levels of only about 15 mA are sufficient to produce tetany, manifested by strong and sustained muscle contraction. Direct current does not exhibit this "let go" threshold (also recognized as the inability to let go of an object) but produces heat in tissues instead. Nevertheless, a single, violent contraction may occur, throwing the diver away from the direct current source. Exposure to direct current may cause cardiac asystole, while contact with alternating current may induce ventricular fibrillation, and both may cause respiratory arrest.[5,33]

Radiation Hazards

All US Navy submarines are now nuclear powered, as are many surface ships. Potential radiation exposure is maximized near the bottom of the submarine where shielding is thinnest. Divers must often dive there, examining the submarine for various reasons. The water acts as a very good radiation shield, but divers must wear thermal luminescence dosimeters and be monitored for radiation exposure.[5]

Dangerous Marine Life

Animal Bites

Despite media attention devoted to this subject, bites are rare. Shark encounters are commonplace, but shark injuries are not. It has been stated that humans are far more likely to experience a lightning strike than a shark attack and more likely to survive a shark attack than a lightning strike. Moray eels are found in most tropical and subtropical oceans and are commonly encountered by military divers. Divers fear eels because they move like snakes, bare their many sharp

teeth, and appear threatening. In actuality, the eel is a shy and very near-sighted animal. A military diver must go out of his way to provoke an encounter. Eels do not have fangs and do not envenomate.[5,6,27,34] Barracuda bites likewise are rare for divers, although surface swimmers and boaters with arms dangling in the water may attract undue attention, particularly if they are wearing shiny objects. Barracuda are found in most tropical waters of the world.[5]

Envenomation

Envenomation, in contrast to bites, is commonplace. Numerous creatures capable of inflicting discomfort on humans exist in the sea (Figure 26-7). The majority of these encounters are nonfatal. All are avoidable. The following is a short list of the more notable hazards.

The sea wasp, a member of the Coelenterate family, which includes jelly fish, hydroids, sea anemones, and coral, has a very fatal venom in the thousands of nematocysts aligned on its meter-long tentacles. Reaction is swift, with shock and death possible within 4 to 6 minutes of the encounter. Antivenin is available but often administered too late. These hydroids are found around Australia and the Great Barrier Reef.[27,34]

Sea snakes provoke the same primitive, exaggerated, and unnecessary fear response as their land-bound cousins. Sea snakes are most commonly found in the warm waters of the Pacific and Indian Oceans. One member of the family, *Pelamis platurus*, is found in unusual areas, such as the cooler waters along the west coast of Latin America to just south of California and from southern Siberia to the cold waters off Tasmania. It is doubtful that any venomous snake has yet crossed into the Caribbean waters, though many banded Caribbean eels, often mistaken for sea snakes, offer divers an opportunity to swear to the contrary. Sea snakes are air breathers and are often seen in shallow water or within the protection of a rocky section of beach. They move moderately well on dry beach. They do not hiss but rather create a snoring or gurgling sound. They are often seen as "curious," not aggressive, and are not afraid to approach an unusual object for closer observation. A diver must generally go out of the way to provoke a negative encounter. The sea snake is more venomous than a cobra, but the sea snake's fixed fangs make envenomation more difficult because of the shallower penetration associated with the bite. Antivenin is available.[27,34]

Stone fish are widely distributed, including in cold coastal waters of the United States. Aside from the beautiful, feathered-looking fish found in warm waters and referred to as lionfish, turkeyfish, or zebrafish, the members of this family are really quite ugly. They

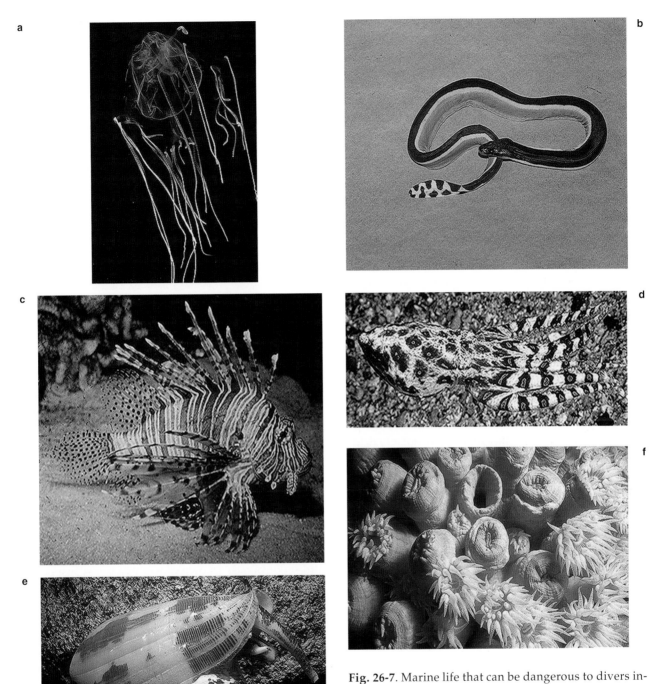

Fig. 26-7. Marine life that can be dangerous to divers includes (*a*) the sea wasp, (*b*) the sea snake, (*c*) the zebrafish, (*d*) the blue-ringed octopus, (*e*) the cone shell, and (*f*) the anemone.
Images from *Envenomations and Poisonings Reference*. Bethesda, Md: Naval School of Health Sciences; 2000. CD-ROM.

are masters of camouflage and are easily stepped on. The dorsal spines can puncture normally protective footwear and inject venom into the wound. In addition to severe pain, tissue destruction can be impressive and death is not uncommon. Antivenin is available.[6,27,34]

The blue-ringed octopus, found in the warm waters of

Australia, is unique within the family of octopi. As with its cousins, it will attempt to defend itself if mishandled by biting with its beak-like mouth. But unlike its larger cousins (this one spans only about 6 inches), the blue-ringed octopus secretes a venom into the usually painless bite. Death can occur.[6,27,34]

Cone shells have a very wide distribution, from US waters off California and Hawaii to the warm waters of the world. Cone shells usually lie buried in the sandy bottom during the day and hunt during the night, crawling about like a garden snail. Cone shells are often beautifully marked and colorful, making them a tempting target for the aesthetically inclined military diver. Unfortunately, they can kill. They extend a proboscis until they touch fingers or skin and then quickly impale the contacted tissue with a small, harpoon-shaped radicular tooth that injects the venom.[5,6,27,34]

Stingrays are found in a wide range of oceans and in a moderate variety of colors, but all are described as flat, disc-shaped animals with "whip" tails, which appear to fly through the water. Military divers encounter them most often while exercising, such as jogging, in the shallow water along sandy beaches. The ray, buried in the warm sand and protected by the few inches of sun-warmed water, feels the force of a human foot landing on its back. In a rapid reflex, the tail strikes the offending human ankle and implants a formidable barb, which tears and envenomates the leg. The diver immediately steps off of the ray's back, and the ray swims away. The human, on the other hand, requires pain medication and surgical debridement of the wound to remove the barb and other foreign material. These envenomations are not lethal, but death has been attributed to freak accidents in which the chest or abdomen, usually of a child, was penetrated by a barb from a large ray. Rays are not aggressive and will do anything they can to avoid a diver. A cousin of the stingray, the torpedo ray, along with the South American eel and the African catfish, produces a nonlethal electric current. The torpedo ray does not frighten away as easily as the stingray, is stockier, and has a more fin-shaped tail.[5,6,27,34]

Sea urchins, the porcupines of the sea, are found in many colors and sizes, are very slow moving, and will not swim into a diver. To effect an injury, the diver must step or kneel on the urchin or grab at an object without noticing the urchin. The spine of an urchin can then penetrate rubber soles, gloves, neoprene, and skin. Because the pain associated with a penetrating spine is greater than can be explained by simple mechanical tissue damage, the discomfort is attributed to a venom. Experts disagree as to whether or not all urchins possess venom, as well as the mechanism of envenomation. The removal of a spine is tedious because the spines, or pedicellariae, crumble like sand. Deaths do not occur.[6,34]

Fire coral, a hard coral, is a ubiquitous organism and a problem for divers. Its appearance varies with locale but generally is brownish with very short, white, hair-like fuzz on the surface. That fuzz penetrates the skin as invisibly as does fiberglass insulation but contains thousands of microscopic nematocysts, which are miniature envenomators. Stinging hydroids are similar to fire coral in effect but appear more like a feather or plume.[5,6,27,34]

Sea anemones are giant versions of the microscopic coral animal itself, but unlike coral, which builds a rock-like calcareous skeleton, the anemone remains soft. Some reach 3 ft across, undulating in the water surge like a huge flower in a breeze. Their colors can vary from pure white to pinks to violet to deep scarlet reds. The sea anemone's tentacles are home to nematocyts, which can sting the careless diver who touches them with bare skin.[34] Divers must maintain respect for the reef as the home of abundant marine life, including anemones. Hundreds of years of work are required for the coral animals to group together and create the stone-like skeletons that remain after their death, forming the base for the next generation of the colony to attach and deposit their own calcareous skeletons. Nature teaches the careless diver to avoid coral contact by way of lacerations and abrasions, which are slow-healing and easily infected wounds.[5,6,34]

Puffer or porcupine fish are rather bulky, awkwardly moving animals, but they are considered delicacies in some Asian countries. When disturbed (a favorite pastime of night divers), they will inflate or puff up, erecting normally flat-lying spines. In this state, the fish has little control over its own movement but is suspended in the water like a huge prickly burr, making it a hazard for its tormentors to handle any further. Puncture wounds result from slow learning.

Bristle worms are underwater caterpillars, amazingly similar in appearance to their cousins on land. The bristle worm's small tufts of fuzz can cause a contact dermatitis reaction in some divers.[6,34]

Sponges are commonplace in warmer waters and are found in several varieties, from huge barrel sponges to iridescent tube sponges. After touching the mucous surface of a marine sponge, some divers develop a contact dermatitis.[5,6,34]

DYSBARIC ILLNESS

Various diving-related maladies are associated with alterations in pressure. These dysbaric illnesses include DCS and barotrauma. In 1991, Francis and Smith[35] advocated altering the classification of dysbaric illness including DCS, to emphasize symptoms rather than assumed phsysiology of injury. The system is not widely accepted, so this chapter will focus on the traditional categorization of dysbaric illness.

Decompression Sickness

DCS probably results from the formation of bubbles in tissues and blood vessels, with resultant ischemia and tissue injury.[36,37] This occurs when a diver ascends from higher to lower pressure at a rate that exceeds the body's ability to eliminate the gas, and the partial pressure of dissolved gas in tissue overcomes the pressure to keep it in solution. Despite the existence of decompression schedules for varying depths and bottom times that describe the limits of "no-decompression" dives, NO dive is risk-free. Tissue responses to pressure vary between divers and even daily within the same diver and are not understood well enough to eliminate all risk. A wide range of signs and symptoms may accompany the initial episode of DCS. Some of these may be so pronounced that there will be little doubt as to the cause, while others may be subtle and easily overlooked in a cursory examination.[5–7] Classifying DCS into Type I or Type II (Table 26-4) permits the treating facility to recognize or anticipate serious, even life-threatening, consequences. Divers at risk for DCS often delay reporting symptoms and wait for them to resolve. While the body is very forgiving, the consequences of misjudging a diving incident can be permanent and costly, so all divers must be advised to report any symptoms. If DCS cannot be eliminated as a potential diagnosis, treatment with recompression is recommended.[5]

Type I Decompression Sickness

Symptoms of Type I, also called "pain-only" or "simple," DCS include skin marbling, lymph node swelling, joint pain, and muscle pain. The most frequent symptom of Type I DCS is joint pain, usually seen in the shoulder, elbow, wrist, hand, hip, knee, or ankle. Type I pain may be excruciating but is usually mild when first noticed and becomes more intense as time passes. It may be located in a muscle group and is usually described as a progressive, deep, dull ache that is often very difficult to localize and unchanged by movement. In contrast, typical mechanical injuries, such as a strain or bruise, are often more painful with movement. Several methods of differentiating DCS pain from mechanical injury have been described, such as applying pressure to the site manually or with a blood pressure cuff (DCS pain reportedly diminishes) or warming the area (DCS pain increases), but none is reliable.[5–7] Medical history is the best way to distinguish DCS Type I pain from trauma, but if confusion exists and circumstances permit, the casualty should be treated presumptively for DCS. Another area of confusion arises when evaluating truncal pain. There is always the possibility that shoulder or hip pain does not originate in that specific joint and may be referred from the CNS. It is important to differentiate the origin of the pain because Type I problems may be treated with a shorter recompression table than Type II DCS.[5] Divers with Type I DCS symptoms, which are not considered life threatening, must be monitored carefully because they may progress to Type II DCS.

Cutis marmorata, a mottling or raised marbling of the skin, is a presentation of Type I DCS, which begins as itching but quickly progresses to redness and then a patchy, bluish discoloration of the skin (Figure 26-8). The condition is uncommon but should be differentiated from simple pruritus, which may be seen in dry (chamber) dives and is not DCS. Cutis marmorata

TABLE 26-4

COMPARISON OF SYMPTOMS IN DECOMPRESSION SICKNESS TYPES I AND II

DCS Type I	DCS Type II
Joint and/or muscle pain ("bends")	Pain in bilateral or multiple joints or muscle groups
Skin itch and rash	Pulmonary symptoms ("chokes")
Cutis marmorata	Inner ear symptoms ("staggers")
Lymph node swelling	Central nervous system symptoms
	Cardiac symptoms
	Pain under pressure

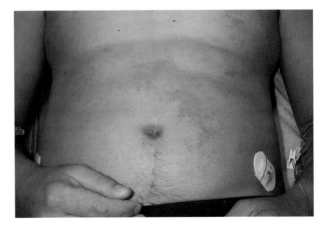

Fig. 26-8. A 27-year-old male with cutis marmorata on his abdomen.
Photograph by permission of the Center for Hyperbaric Medicine and Environmental Physiology, Duke University Medical Center, Durham, NC.

sometimes precedes evidence of neurological deficits. A rare presentation of Type I DCS involves localized pain and swelling of lymphoid tissue. Though recompression may provide symptomatic pain relief, resolution of the swelling may require several days or weeks of watchful waiting after recompression.[5–7]

Type II Decompression Sickness

Type II or "serious" DCS is potentially life threatening and includes symptoms involving the inner ear, the lungs, multiple joints, the brain, and the spinal cord. Inner ear DCS, or the "staggers," results from bubble production in the inner ear (seen almost exclusively when switching breathing gases during saturation or deep mixed-gas diving) and involves symptoms of vertigo, tinnitus, and hearing loss.[6,7] Staggers can sometimes be difficult to distinguish from inner ear barotrauma, which is typically preceded by middle ear barotrauma and a forceful attempt to equalize the pressure in the middle ear (Valsalva maneuver) against a closed Eustachian tube during descent. Inner ear barotrauma is discussed in detail later in this chapter. In addition to neurological symptoms, divers with severe DCS may suffer cardiovascular collapse or other symptoms from profuse venous bubbling, which is analogous to shaking a soda bottle then suddenly removing the cap. Large volumes of intravenous gas disrupt the pulmonary vasculature, causing diffuse pulmonary injury. This pulmonary DCS, referred to as the "chokes," starts as chest pain followed by increasing respiratory rate, dyspnea, and hemoptysis. There is rapid progression to complete circulatory collapse, loss of consciousness, and death. Immediate on-site recompression therapy is the diver's only hope. Finally, divers with Type I symptoms located bilaterally or in more than one joint or muscle group may represent the beginning of serious DCS and therefore should be treated as if they had Type II DCS. Similarly, pain in the chest, spine, or hip requires special evaluation. If a DMO is not immediately available, these symptoms should be regarded as Type II and the afflicted diver should be recompressed accordingly. Additionally, any DCS symptom that occurs during the ascent phase of a dive is considered "pain under pressure," and should be treated as Type II DCS.[5]

In the early stages, CNS symptoms of Type II DCS may not be obvious, and the stricken diver may consider them inconsequential. The diver may feel fatigued or weak and attribute the condition to overexertion. Even as weakness becomes more severe, the diver may not seek treatment until walking, hearing, or urinating becomes difficult. Symptoms must be anticipated during the period after the dive and treated before they become too severe. Many other findings can be attributed to the effects of DCS on the neurological system, including numbness, tingling, feelings of "pins and needles," weakness, frank paralysis, loss of bladder or bowel control, mental status changes, motor performance decrement, ringing in the ears, vertigo, dizziness, hearing loss, vision disturbance, tremors, personality changes, and amnesia. Attempting to differentiate such findings with nondive etiologies from those that are dive-related can be problematic. A diver with a headache has an extensive list of differential diagnoses other than DCS, and fatigue in a diver may reflect only a lack of sleep the previous evening. Divers with unexplained focal neurological symptoms following a dive must be treated with recompression therapy. Expedient delivery of recompression therapy is mandatory for Type II DCS, unless otherwise directed by a DMO.[5]

Aviators and flight crews exposed to the hypobaric environment at altitude may experience symptoms of DCS also, but symptoms usually resolve as they descend (see Chapter 25, Aviation Medicine). To avoid DCS, divers are prohibited from flying above 2,300 ft (commercial airliners are pressurized to 6,000 ft) for a minimum of 12 hours after a dive that requires decompression stops. Patients who are treated for DCS Type I must not fly for 24 hours. Both of these limitations will be extended for more complicated situations, such as aviators who dive (must wait 24 hours to fly) or patients treated on Treatment Table 4 (must wait 72 hours).[32] Treatment tables are reviewed toward the end of this chapter.

Pulmonary Over-Inflation Syndrome

Pulmonary over-inflation syndrome (POIS) is explained by Boyle's Law and can result when gas trapped in the lung expands with decreasing pressure during ascent and forces its way out into the interstitial tissues. This syndrome can be life threatening, depending on where the escaping air travels. POIS can be the most dangerous form of barotrauma because of the possibility of gas embolism. It is separated into four distinct entities for diagnosis and treatment:

1. pneumothorax;
2. mediastinal emphysema;
3. subcutaneous emphysema; and, the most serious,
4. arterial gas embolism (AGE).

A pneumothorax results when air escapes from the ruptured alveoli into the pleural space. If it is severe enough, the lung will be compressed and displaced by the air. The patient may describe sudden chest pain and may experience shortness of breath, rapid, shallow breathing, or a cough. The examination may reveal an absence or diminution of breath sounds. A simple pneumothorax may be transformed into a tension pneumothorax, particularly during the ascent phase of recompression chamber treatments, and medical personnel should be prepared for these emergencies. If a diver complains of sudden chest pain during the ascent phase of the chamber run, the ascent should be stopped and the diver should descend to a depth where he or she has relief of symptoms as a temporary measure. A chest tube should be placed to provide permanent relief.[5] A spontaneous pneumothorax, one that occurs without obvious reason, is permanently disqualifying for dive duty because of its potential for recurrence. Asthma is also disqualifying, since a plug of mucus may create an area of trapped gas distal to it. A traumatic pneumothorax, one associated with rib fracture, gun shot wound, or other trauma, is temporarily disqualifying.[38]

Mediastinal emphysema is caused by gas dissecting into in the tissues behind the sternum. Patients may report a dull ache or tight feeling in the front of the chest, with pain made worse by deep breathing, coughing, or swallowing. The pain may radiate to the shoulder, jaw, or back. Subcutaneous emphysema results when air leaks from lung tissue and accumulates between tissue planes of the upper chest and neck. These patients seldom complain of pain but often note a change in voice, may have a full or bloated look about the neck, and feel a popping or crepitus when the neck is palpated. Recompression is not the recommended treatment for mediastinal emphysema, subcutaneous emphysema, or pneumothorax. Definitive treatments are the same as for injuries not related to diving, except that a diver should have a detailed neurological examination to ensure an AGE is not also present.

An AGE is a bubble that has forced its way out of the alveoli and into the pulmonary venous circulation via an alveolar capillary. It then travels to the heart and is pumped through the arterial system until it reaches a capillary that is too small to accommodate its size. The AGE occludes further blood flow and the necessary delivery of oxygen to the tissues beyond the occlusion, creating an area of ischemia. In divers, AGE may occur while they hold their breath during ascent, following trauma such as blast injury, as a result of occluded airways due to allergies or infections, or in those with venous DCS bubbles that pass through occult or congenital cardiac shunts. AGE is generally dramatic in presentation with obvious, possibly severe, neurological symptoms occurring within seconds to minutes of the injury. Any organ system can be involved, but the most striking are the CNS and the cardiovascular system, where presentations mimic, respectively, classic stroke and myocardial infarction. Treatment requires immedi-

ate recompression in an attempt to diminish the size of the bubble and deliver oxygen to ischemic tissues. If recompression is accomplished before hypoxic damage, hemorrhage, or edema develops, a rapid and complete recovery is likely.[5–7]

Barotrauma

The most common diving-related injury is barotrauma, which results when pressure within a body cavity and the ambient pressure do not equilibrate. To be subject to barotrauma, a cavity must usually meet several criteria: (*a*) be gas filled, (*b*) have relatively rigid walls, (*c*) be enclosed, and (*d*) be subjected to change in the ambient or surrounding pressure. Ambient increases in pressure will cause the gas trapped within a cavity to compress and attempt to occupy less space. This creates a relative vacuum, which draws in the tissue forming the walls of the cavity to equalize pressure and fill the space created by the compressed gas. If the pressure difference continues, vessels in the tissue will engorge and eventually rupture, filling the space with blood and equalizing the vacuum. When this phenomenon occurs in conjunction with descent during a dive, it is termed a "squeeze." A "reverse squeeze" results from tissue damage caused by overpressurization of a cavity during ascent, as with POIS. This pathophysiological model can be applied to any gas-filled cavity, and Table 26-5 is a listing of common forms of squeezes. Prevention of

TABLE 26-5

EXAMPLES OF NEGATIVE PRESSURE BAROTRAUMA ("SQUEEZE") AND CAUSES

Squeeze	Cause
Middle ear	Eustachian tube dysfunction
External ear	Hood or piece of equipment covering the external ear passage
Sinus	Blockage of the duct that normally vents a sinus
Face mask	Failure to equalize air in the mask by nasal exhalation
Tooth	Faulty filling with trapped air beneath
Suit	Pocket of air in a dry suit that becomes trapped under a fold or fitting and pinches the skin
Lung	Extremely rare but seen with deep breath-hold diving
Whole body	Failure of the air supply in a dry suit to balance water pressure

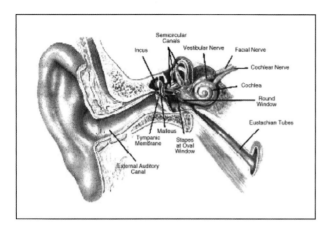

Fig. 26-9. The anatomy of the ear in frontal section. Source: US Department of the Navy. *US Navy Diving Manual.* Rev 4. Washington, DC: Naval Sea Systems Command; 1999: 3-22.

barotrauma is relatively simple and includes not diving with a cold or during a flare-up of allergies, using proper-fitting equipment, and not creating air-filled cavities that cannot be vented, as when using goggles or ear plugs.

The most common site for barotrauma of descent is the middle ear (Figure 26-9). Normally, the only connection between the ambient air and the air inside the middle ear is the Eustachian tube. This tube may not be patent due to inflammation from allergies or an infection or due to compression during the dive from a large pressure gradient that has already developed between the middle ear space and the upper pharynx. As a diver descends, he or she must perform a Valsalva maneuver to equalize the pressure in the middle ear space. If the Eustachian tube is not operating properly, middle ear pressure cannot be increased and there will be a pressure differential across the tympanic membrane, drawing it inward and causing pain. With continued descent, the middle ear may fill with blood from surrounding tissues in an attempt to equalize pressure or the tympanic membrane may rupture. As the largest pressure-volume change occurs within the first additional atmosphere (33 fsw) of descent, once a diver clears that distance, barotrauma of descent becomes uncommon. Symptoms of middle ear squeeze include pain (caused by the extreme tympanic membrane stretch), temporary vertigo, decreased hearing, or tinnitus.

Inner ear barotrauma, although relatively uncommon, usually presents in the context of concomitant middle ear barotrauma and requires medical attention. The majority of these injuries are produced during descent by an excessive Valsalva against a blocked Eustachian tube. When the pressure differential from the middle ear to the environment exceeds 90 mmHg or at a mere 4 fsw, the Eustachian tube will not open regardless of the force of the Valsalva. The relative vacuum in the middle ear will draw the eardrum, and the round and oval windows into the middle ear space. A Valsalva maneuver may raise the intracranial pressure several hundred millimeters of mercury, which is transmitted through the cochlear duct, exploding the round window into the middle ear. This force may cause tears in any of the membranous windows or vestibular apparati or cause inner ear hemorrhage. The trauma often produces a severe vertigo, with sensorineural hearing loss and tinnitus, and may be confused with other ear conditions.[6,7] All persistent symptoms of vertigo or hearing loss in a diver should be meticulously evaluated. If a diagnosis of inner ear barotrauma is suspected, the diver should be placed in a semi-sitting position and kept as still as possible; intravenous diazepam (Valium) may be useful to control vomiting. The patient should be evaluated expeditiously by an otolaryngologist.[5–7]

Sinus squeezes are less common than middle ear barotrauma. The frontal sinuses are the ones most frequently involved, but any air-filled sinus may be injured. Pain in the face over the affected sinus is the most common presentation, but there is sometimes a bloody nasal discharge in the mask. A blocked sinus ostium prevents normal venting of the sinus to release air.

Middle ear oxygen absorption syndrome can present as a middle ear squeeze, but its pathophysiology is different. Ear pain may follow long oxygen dives (as with a LAR V rig) after gas with a very high oxygen percentage enters the middle ear cavity and the oxygen is absorbed through the mucosa of surrounding tissues. If the middle ear space is not actively vented to replace the oxygen with air, a negative pressure relative to ambient may result from the oxygen being absorbed. Without an inert gas such as nitrogen in the middle ear, there will be insufficient volume support to the tympanic membrane. The diver may notice ear fullness the morning after a long oxygen exposure, which may be accompanied by sharp pain with ear-clearing maneuvers and transient hearing loss. Equalizing the pressure will eventually relieve the symptoms, although sometimes a serous effusion persists.[5]

Treatment of barotrauma of descent is straightforward—stop the descent. The diver should be brought up a few feet; if this does not relieve the symptoms, the dive should be terminated. Once on the surface, the patient should be seen by medical personnel to evaluate the degree of trauma. If the diagnosis of a squeeze is confirmed by examination, the diver should be kept out of the hyperbaric environment until the tissue damage heals. This period of time is variable depending on the extent of injury; a ruptured tympanic membrane may require weeks to heal but blood in the middle ear may require only days to resolve. A mild squeeze may not stop a diver from diving the next day, yet a severe squeeze may keep the diver out of the water for weeks. Each case of barotrauma of descent must be individually evaluated, but no form of barotrauma is treated by recompression except AGE.

Dysbaric Osteonecrosis

Dysbaric osteonecrosis is not a diagnosis that is made in the acute setting; it is primarily a chronic disease of career divers and is strongly associated with saturation diving. The pathogenesis for the disease is unknown, but it is suspected to be a result of extreme pressures causing direct damage to bone (ie, gas osmosis) or multiple microinfarctions from asymptomatic DCS.[6,7] The bone lesions present as aseptic necrosis, which can manifest as deep bone pain or be entirely asymptomatic, depending on the location of the lesion. Juxtaarticular lesions are most painful, but midshaft lesions are mild and most commonly discovered on routine radiographs. Treatment is nonspecific, and nonsteroidal anti-inflammatory drugs and, for debilitating conditions, joint arthroplasty are effective. Personnel with juxta-articular lesions are permanently disqualified from diving, while those with asymptomatic lesions are considered on a case-by-case basis.[38]

EPIDEMIOLOGY OF DIVING CASUALTIES AND DECOMPRESSION ILLNESS

AGE and DCS may be difficult to distinguish clinically, due to the similarity of their signs and symptoms. Decompression Illness (DCI) is now used to describe cases which have characteristics of both AGE and DCS. Military diving, when compared with civilian sport diving and commercial diving, is relatively safe, but comparisons are difficult because accurate population-based data on DCI and diving fatalities are difficult to obtain. Military diving medical personnel can gain valuable insights by reviewing underwater accident information from both sport and commercial diving. The Naval Safety Center (NSC) collects diving accident and mishap data for the Department of Defense, which has a known and quantified population at risk.[2,20,39] All mishaps, cases of DCI, and fatalities must be reported. In addition, the computerized Dive Reporting System provides excellent data for population-based analysis of military diving accidents.[2,3]

Civilian Experiences

Sources of Data

Various organizations, including the National Underwater Accident Data Center, Diver Alert Network (DAN), and the Australian Diving Medicine Center, have compiled diving accident statistics since the early 1980s for sport, open-circuit, and air scuba diving.[7] DAN, a nonprofit diving safety association affiliated with Duke University Medical Center, Durham, NC, depends on a network of 247 hyperbaric chambers in the United States and around the world to report DCI and diving fatalities.[7,40] DAN annually solicits participation from hyperbaric facilities and requests standardized DAN forms for each DCI case or diving fatality. All cases must meet strict inclusion criteria to be used in DAN's annual "Report on Diving Accidents and Fatalities."[38] These data are excellent for their characterization of factors leading to recreational scuba fatalities and cases of DCI, but they are not adequate to compute accurate diving accident rates because there is no precise count of either the total number of dives or divers to be used as denominators. In addition, civilian DCI cases are notoriously underreported, and there is no autopsy protocol for diving fatalities that is widely accepted and practiced throughout the United States.

Risk Factors

Most fatalities and DCI cases involve multiple factors that interact as confounders, yet understanding these factors is crucial to the development of risk management strategies. The DAN data suggest a very crude fatality rate of 2 to 4 deaths per 100,000 sport divers annually from 1989 to 1994.[40] Older divers (older than 50 years) and younger divers (younger than 24 years) have higher-than-expected fatality rates. Cardiovascular disease has been a leading cause of death in DAN fatality case reports, especially among older divers. Fatigue as the result of poor physical fitness is an aggravating factor. Inexperience, risk taking, and alcohol use within 12 hours of their fatal dive often are contributing factors in all divers but particularly those younger than 24 years of age. DCI rates were increased in divers doing repetitive daily dives and dives deeper than 80 fsw. Interestingly, over 80% of the 566 cases of DCI reported to DAN for 1994 developed neurological symptoms. This high percentage of more serious decompression sickness may be due to underreporting of pain-only DCS, to more liberal decompression procedures, or to time delays in initiating recompression treatment. Only two thirds of the reported 55 cases of AGE and less than 40% of the 513 cases of DCS were treated with hyperbaric oxygen within 12 hours of surfacing. This represents a significant delay to recompression therapy and adversely affected clinical outcomes. Causes for treatment delays include patient denial of symptoms, failure to recognize the signs and symptoms of DCI, long transportation times from remote diving locations to a chamber, and failure of symptoms to spontaneously resolve with other therapies.[40] Decompression computers and decompression tables increase awareness of the need for slow ascent rates and decompression, but sometimes divers assume that since they follow tables or their computer, DCS will not occur. To the contrary, many DCI cases follow no-decompression dives or those which are not expected to require decompression.[39,40]

Accident Rates

Commercial diving accident rates are more unreliable than sport diving rates. No central data collection organization exists, and commercial diving accident information is often sketchy. There are no accurate estimates of the number of commercial divers at risk, let alone the total number of dives made. Rough estimates from the United Kingdom Department of Energy suggest diving mortality rates in the North Sea are similar to, or better than, the mortality rates in the construction industry.[7] While many sport divers follow US Navy no-decompression limits, commercial divers often do deeper dives, including mixed-gas or saturation dives, and do not follow military decompression tables when they complete their underwater work. Nevertheless, more attention is given to dive planning, equipment selection, and medical screening of divers by industry than by sport divers. The emphasis on safety in industry is driven somewhat by financial considerations because accidents delay completion of work, increase personnel and material costs, and increase insurance premiums. The military has similar concerns.

Military Data

US military diving operations are conducted in a disciplined manner by well-trained divers. The NSC studies all military diving mishaps in the continuing interest of accident prevention and emphasizes investigation procedures, reporting requirements and lines of responsibility for diving mishap and diving fatality inquiries. Unlike sport diving and commercial diving, "near misses" and nonfatal accidents are also evaluated for risk management and corrective action. NSC accident data can be regarded as reasonably accurate but not applicable to diving outside operational military dives.[2,7,39,41]

Table 26-6 shows a comparison of the use of various diving rigs in the US Navy from 1991 through

TABLE 26-6

TOTAL NAVY DIVES BY DIVING APPARATUS, 1991–1995

RIG	1991	1992	1993	1994	1995
SCUBA	55,499	57,133	53,605	44,990	26,324
MK 20	8,488	9,388	13,204	12,420	8,705
MK 21	10,923	13,793	13,865	11,489	9,972
LAR V	16,912	17,458	15,802	15,169	11,474
MK 16	4,862	3,607	4,154	3,450	2,674
CHAMBER	5,625	6,099	5,222	4,913	4,668
OTHERS	12,729	10,152	1,648	730	334
TOTALS	115,038	117,630	107,500	93,161	64,151

Data sources: (a) US Naval Safety Center. *Naval Safety Center Diving Database*. Norfolk, Va: US Department of the Navy; 1997. (b) Butler FK, Thalmann ED. *A Procedure for Doing Multiple Level Dives on Air Using Repetitive Groups*. Panama City, Fla: US Naval Experimental Diving Unit; 1983. NEDU Report 13-83.

1995.[20,42] During this period, 84% of Navy dives were shallow (between 10 and 50 fsw). An even greater percentage of dive profiles in the Army, Air Force, and Marine Corps, where Special Operations diving constitutes a larger share of the total dives, are in this range. Most EOD and Special Operations dives use closed-circuit scuba, either the LAR V or the MK 16 closed-circuit oxygen rebreather rigs. For the 5-year period mentioned, 25% of diving missions were Special Operations, 25% were ship's husbandry, and 20% were EOD. Inspections, searches, and underwater construction each made up 5% of the total number of dives. Salvage operations, which are often at 50 fsw or deeper, constituted only 1.8% of dives during this period, although there was an increase in the total percentage of deeper dives (> 50 fsw) in years when there were deeper salvage jobs or research protocols with deeper dives. These data are representative of the evolution of US military diving away from deeper, mixed-gas, bounce diving, or saturation diving to shallower, open- and closed-circuit scuba diving.[20,39]

The NSC Dive Reporting System maintains a database for epidemiologic studies of military diving. Mandatory reporting requirements, regular safety inspections of diving units, and computerized local data entry were established to collect a reasonably complete set of data.[2,3,39,41] The NSC diving database has logged more than 2.3 million military dives from 1985 through 1995, but good quality injury data were not collected until 1990.[2,3,20,41] During the period 1 January 1990 to 31 December 1995, there were 382 cases of DCI reported to the NSC in divers from the US Naval Services.[39,41] Independent analysis of these reports by DMOs from the Naval Medical Research Center and the Naval Diving and Salvage Training Center report an annual misdiagnosis rate of 23% to 39%.[39,42] Since most recompression treatments in the military are initiated by nonmedical providers, who may be disciplined if they miss a case of DCI or inadequately treat a fellow diver, many nonspecific symptoms are treated and overreporting of DCI is common.[39,41] Supervisors are taught that risk-benefit analyses favor hyperbaric treatment in almost all cases when a diver feels abnormal following a dive.[5] Even given these limitations, reasonably accurate mishap rates can be computed and tracked.[41] All of the 382 DCI cases in Navy or Marine Corps divers from the NSC database were reviewed by DMOs from the Naval Diving and Salvage Training Center for medical merit, resulting in identical adjusted DCI rates of 1.3 per 10,000 dives for AGE, 1.3 per 10,000 dives for DCS Type I, and 1.3 per 10,000 dives for DCS Type II.[39]

During this same 6-year period (1 January 1990 to 31 December 1995), there were 11 diving fatalities in the US Naval Services. The Marine Corps had five fatalities, all of which were off-duty. The Navy's six fatalities were all on duty. The fatality rate for Naval Service operational diving for this period was 0.9 per 100,000 dives. Most operational deaths were primarily from drowning secondary to poor operational planning, underwater hazards, or poor diver judgement. Some fatalities, especially the off-duty ones, were attributable to risk-taking. Five of the six operational fatalities were diving scuba and their final dive was shallower than 50 fsw. In a minority of these, improper use of underwater tools initiated the fatal event.[20,39] A surprisingly high 43% of diving fatalities since 1985 occurred in sailors and Marines while off-duty, and diving ranked 10th for overall cause of death for Naval Service personnel during this period.[43] Considering mortality only, though, military diving is relatively safe as a hazardous duty, and compares well to parachuting. An analysis of data supplied by the Army Safety Center revealed a fatality rate of 1.8 per 100,000 parachutes deployed in fiscal years 1994 through 1996 for static line operations, and a rate of 5 per 100,000 freefall parachutes deployed. There is likely significant underreporting of denominator data (parachutes deployed), and these rates may be closer to 1 in 100,000.[44]

Operational diving involves risks to which the typical service member is not exposed, and it definitely deserves its special duty designation. Good medical screening, diver training, and operational planning are important to avoid underwater accidents. Although data demonstrate that most military diving is conducted in shallow water, there is still a very significant risk of serious injury and death. There is little room for error, and a healthy respect for the hazards of the underwater environment, as well as attention to detail, rigorous continual training, and dedication to preventing accidents, will serve all divers well.

PREVENTION OF DIVING-RELATED ILLNESSES AND INJURIES

Prevention of diving accidents is the single most important task of diving medical personnel. Safety is the primary objective; it is addressed through conscientious and deliberate dive planning, which considers diving equipment, environmental conditions, medical fitness, physical fitness, and training. A safety-conscious organization with a comprehensive program, from the senior leaders down to the newly qualified diver, is essential. Officers and noncommissioned officers must ensure fitness-to-dive evaluations are current, diver training is of high quality, and an active diving research program is supported that provides working divers the best possible equipment and decompression procedures.

The Fit Diver

Fitness-to-dive evaluations in the military are done in several settings. The diver candidate is evaluated with medical standards that are more restrictive than for other service members. Selecting not only the most physically fit divers but also those without preexisting medical conditions minimizes time-consuming evaluations for borderline medical conditions, lessens the administrative burden of waivers, and provides unit commanders medically ready divers to complete mission requirements. Women who meet the medical and fitness standards for military diving are eligible for all diving duty except combat diving. Once the military has invested the time and expense to train divers, decisions regarding fitness to dive must focus on the ability of the divers to dive safely, without undo risk to themselves or their fellow divers, and to complete the mission successfully.[45] Medical conditions may be temporary and require that diving be briefly suspended (eg, upper respiratory infections, nonpulmonary barotrauma, musculoskeletal injuries), they may be chronic and require medications but not significantly affect diving duty (eg, hypertension, hypercholesterolemia, low back pain), or they may be serious and result in permanent disqualification as a diver (eg, DCI with residual symptoms, psychiatric illness, substance abuse, significant trauma with head injury). The same principles and medical insight applied to assessing fitness to dive must be used to determine when a temporarily disqualified diver can return to duty. Women are temporarily disqualified during pregnancy because diving has been associated with an increase in the incidence of birth defects (even in the first trimester) and because DCS can result in stillbirth and other complications.[27] Finally, the immediate predive check by the diving supervisor, asking whether divers are physically and mentally prepared to make a dive, is vital in preventing injury.[5,46] Military divers, however, are typically stoic, confidant, motivated, and, by nature, risk takers. Diving medical personnel, particularly the enlisted DMTs, should be quickly accessible on the dive station and easily approachable on a personal level. It is critical that medical personnel supporting diving operations be divers themselves or be familiar with the hyperbaric environment. Experience and insight are infinitely better than sympathy in assessing diving casualties, and divers tend to trust and confide in one of their own.

Many dysbaric illnesses can be prevented when divers, leaders, and medical personnel understand the general concepts of diving medicine, including recompression therapy. Training for entry-level divers should stress prevention of injuries and avoidance of risk factors for DCS and POIS. The single most important rule to teach is to avoid diving with either lower or upper respiratory congestion. Smoking increases the risk of developing these conditions and is a particularly bad habit for divers. Entry-level divers are taught safe ear clearing techniques to avoid injury from a forceful Valsalva maneuver, prophylaxis for otitis externa, and the basic signs and symptoms of decompression illness. A basic understanding of vertigo and its causes is essential because it is common and a potential cause of disorientation at depth.

Personnel and Their Roles in Prevention

Diving supervisor candidates, typically noncommissioned officers, receive advanced diving medicine training that builds on their initial knowledge base and significant diving experience. Dive operations planning is a crucial part of supervisor training, emphasizing the consideration of environmental conditions, rig selection, diver selection, protective garments selection, and proper scheduling of dives to complete the task safely.[5] Diving supervisors are the most important resource for continuous unit training, and they set the standard for safe practices on all dive stations. When accidents do occur, the supervisor and the team are the first responders and may be the only responders. They initiate the majority of recompression treatments for DCI in the operational setting and sometimes complete the entire treatment without direct physician supervision.[5,20,46] DMTs are corpsmen or medics with advanced diving medicine training, who usually are also divers. They help the diving supervisor make medical decisions and tend patients inside the chamber during most hyperbaric treatments. The DMTs are extremely valuable resources who function as on-site extensions of the DMO, administering neurological examinations and rendering care directed by the DMO during hyperbaric treatments. DMTs are also teachers, assisting the supervisors with unit medical training and monitoring dive station safety. In planning a dive, DMTs help coordinate support from DMOs, evacuation services, and recompression chambers,

---

EXHIBIT 26-1

PRIMARY EMERGENCY KIT FOR DIVERS

Diagnostic Equipment

- Flashlight
- Stethoscope
- Otoscope (Ophthalmoscope)
- Sphygmomanometer (Aneroid type only, case vented for hyperbaric use)
- Reflex hammer
- Tuning fork (128 cps)
- Sterile safety pins or swab sticks which can be broken for sensory testing
- Tongue depressors

Emergency Treatment Equipment and Medications

- Oropharyngeal airways (#4 and #5 Geudel)
- Self-inflating bag-mask ventilator with medium adult mask NOTE: Some of these units do not have sufficient bag volume to provide adequate ventilation. Use a Laerdal Resusci folding bag II (adult) or equivalent.
- Foot-powered or battery-powered suction unit
- Nonflexible plastic suction tips (Yankauer suction tip)
- Large-bore needle and catheter (12 and 14 gauge) for cricothyroidotomy or relief of tension pneumothorax
- Trocar thoracic suction catheter (10F and 24F) or McSwain dart
- Small penrose drain, Heimlich valve, or other device to provide one-way flow of gas out of the chest
- Christmas tree adapter (to connect one-way valve to chest tube)
- Adhesive tape (2-inch waterproof)
- Elastic-wrap bandage for a tourniquet (2 and 4 inch)
- Penrose drain tourniquet
- Bandage scissors
- #11 knife blade and handle
- Curved Kelly forceps
- 10% povidone-iodine swabs or wipes
- 1% lidocaine solution
- #21 ga. 1-1/2" needles on 5 cc syringes
- Cravats
- 200 cc syringe

as needed. Additionally, they prepare a medical kit with equipment required to evaluate and treat diving casualties (Exhibit 26-1). DMOs receive graduate-level diving medicine instruction, and they must qualify as military divers. Their schooling emphasizes accident prevention, safety, and current concepts in hyperbaric physiology and treatment. DMOs are the local diving medicine authorities; they advise commanders, supervise and train DMTs, review diving duty examinations, and treat diving-related illnesses and injuries.[5,46]

Diver Training

In addition to medical topics, diver training must emphasize equipment knowledge, proficiency in emergency and operating procedures, physical endurance and strength, and good judgment. The military diver must be prepared to operate in adverse conditions, such as low or no visibility, cold water, enclosed spaces, contaminated water, high seas, strong currents, and even under ice, if the mission requires it. Unlike the sport diver, the military diver must repeatedly train and perform certain critical skills, such as emergency procedures, because the mission often dictates diving in relatively hazardous conditions where these skills might be needed. The military diver must be able to control anxiety and manage many potential stressors underwater, to include fatigue, equipment failures, unfavorable environmental conditions, and weapons fire.[5] Simple tasks such as clearing a face mask may cause panic in a novice. The most important prophylaxis to panic is ample training and confidence in the diving equipment and procedures. All military divers endure intensive "confidence training" during their initial in-water scuba instruction. Under controlled conditions, they are forced to solve problems with equipment malfunctions, loss of air, loss of equipment, and disorientation in a calm, deliberate manner. Candidates who exhibit panic under these situations are deemed unsuitable for military diving and dropped from training. Candidates are taught equipment preventive maintenance procedures, while diving supervisors receive hyperbaric systems instruction and formal quality assurance training to ensure all diving systems remain reliable. Military divers have ongoing training requirements to maintain their diving qualifications.[5] Divers whose qualifications have lapsed must requalify, which may include a medical fitness-to-dive evaluation, physical fitness screening, demonstrated proficiency in diving

medicine and physics, and successful completion of a requisite number of dives.[45] Inexperience, panic, and human error cause many diving accidents, so there can be no substitute for quality diver training.[20,39,40]

Research

Finally, an active, well-conceived diving research program helps prevent diving injuries by selecting the safest diving equipment, developing reliable decompression procedures, and understanding the psychological, physical, and physiological factors affecting divers. Ideally, researchers are constantly searching and testing new equipment and decompression procedures to improve diving safety continually; they should not merely react to mishaps as they occur. Investigating the basic mechanisms of hyperbaric oxygen, the physiological consequences of water immersion, and the psychological effects of operating in the underwater environment provides precious insights for medical officers, equipment designers, and military commanders, all of whom want to give their divers every chance to be successful. The Navy Experimental Diving Unit, Panama City, Fla; the Naval Submarine Medical Research Laboratory, Groton, Conn; and the Naval Medical Research Center, Silver Spring, Md, carry on the fine tradition of US Navy diving and undersea research, which is among the best in the world.[5]

INJURED DIVER ASSESSMENT

Establishing the differential diagnosis of a diver's complaint requires keen insight. The average military diver is young, male, exceptionally fit, and often given to avoiding physicians. Although trained to report any unusual physical or mental condition, the military diver will often minimize complaints and symptoms. Therefore, the health care provider must not be lulled into a state of complacency. Divers can present with almost any of the complaints of a nondiving patient, so when evaluating the military diver, the medical provider must augment years of medical training with knowledge of diving physiology and the unique conditions associated with the hyperbaric environment to ensure that diving-unique diagnoses are included in the differential diagnosis. For example, a military diver presenting with chest pain would be approached slightly differently than a civilian counterpart. Chest pain of cardiac origin would not be an overwhelming initial concern unless the diver had multiple risk factors for coronary artery disease. Trauma

would be a priority consideration, as would evaluation of possible POIS and pulmonary oxygen toxicity. Even DCS can present with chest pain. Another example is vertigo, which may be viral or be related to a tumor but in a diver is more likely to be occupationally related. Vertigo on descent is seen when the ear is exposed to changing temperatures (caloric vertigo) or barotrauma, while vertigo on ascent is most commonly due to unequal clearing of Eustachian tubes, leading to a pressure difference between middle ear spaces (alternobaric vertigo). Vertigo that worsens after surfacing and was associated with difficulty clearing on descent is probably caused by inner ear barotrauma. Fluctuating or severe vertigo that persists is often associated with inner ear barotrauma and must be evaluated.

The most common injury seen in military divers is barotrauma, particularly barotrauma of the middle ear. Unlike civilian sport divers, a military diver may use various military diving rigs (eg, hard hat, surface-supplied, full face mask) that limit access and make it difficult to perform ear clearing maneuvers that relieve pressure in the middle ear. The diver may be unable to stop or slow the rate of descent to perform a Valsalva maneuver while being lowered on a diving stage. Barotrauma will generally present with ear pain, decreased hearing, vertigo, or any combination of these.

The next most common complaint in military divers is musculoskeletal injuries. Military divers are working divers, risking injury by manually moving hundreds of pounds of equipment each day. Salvage divers must dive using rigs or systems that are very heavy and require great strength and stamina to operate. Fleet divers make underwater repairs, moving heavy objects for extended hours, working in nearly zero visibility and in thermal extremes. Additionally, they handle potentially dangerous hydraulic and electrical equipment.[33] To perform these duties, military divers must maintain a high level of physical readiness through daily physical training, which, ironically, is associated with an increased chance of injury. Overuse injuries are particularly common.[5,46]

Finally, skin injuries, skin infections, and otitis externa are associated with prolonged water and environmental exposure. Treatment is the same as for nondivers.[5,6,46]

The Evaluation

In examining a military diver, as with any patient, the history of the complaint is paramount. The more chronologically distant the diver's complaint is from a dive or hyperbaric exposure, the more unlikely the association. Although exceptions exist, most diving-related illnesses and injuries present within the first few hours following a dive. Since DCS and AGE are the most acutely dangerous nontrauma diving injuries, the DMO or DMT must examine the patient for these conditions quickly and efficiently, emphasizing the thorax and the neurological system, to establish whether AGE and DCS can be eliminated from the differential diagnosis. Radiographic studies can be valuable in confirming diagnoses of POIS, except for AGE, but should never delay recompression in patients with obvious neurological deficits. Since the primary source of injury in POIS is in the lung, a chest roentgenogram should be taken at some point. Laboratory tests are seldom useful in identifying or confirming diving conditions. Clinicians should use these tests to evaluate the differential diagnosis as appropriate. For example, a diver with sharp unilateral chest pain should be evaluated for a pneumothorax. The diver should be treated with the insertion of a chest tube and with other supportive therapy, just as a nondiver with pneumothorax would be treated, but the diver must also receive a thorough neurological exam. Additionally, the dive profile (ie, a detailed description of the dive that includes the depths, time submerged, time at each depth, and decompression steps) is beneficial in establishing a record of the dive's depths and the times spent at each depth. A shallow dive for only few minutes tends to minimize the possibility of DCS but does not eliminate it entirely. Dives of long duration to significant depth are more commonly associated with DCS, particularly if the dives require decompression stops or if they are repetitive dives. Finally, specific diving equipment is associated with specific injuries (Table 26-7). For example, oxygen toxicity is not seen when diving on air scuba, if the dive depth is restricted to shallower than 190 fsw, as is required by Navy regulations. Caustic cocktail occurs only with closed-circuit rigs, which use hydroxide compounds as carbon dioxide absorbents. When

TABLE 26-7

COMMON US MILITARY DIVING RIGS, THEIR USES, AND THE POTENTIAL MEDICAL PROBLEMS ASSOCIATED WITH THEIR USE

Military Diving Rigs	Principal Uses	Potential Medical Problems
Open-circuit scuba	Inspections, searches, ship's husbandry, shallow salvage, insertions	DCS, POIS, nitrogen narcosis, contaminated gas exposure
Closed-circuit scuba (eg, LAR V, MK 16)	Explosive ordnance disposal, combat diver operations, searches	Oxygen toxicity, POIS, hypoxia, hypercarbia, carbon dioxide scrubber failure, caustic cocktail
Surface-supply systems (eg, MK 20, MK 21)	Ship's husbandry, inspections, enclosed-space diving, salvage	DCS, contaminated gas, nitrogen narcosis, POIS, trauma from underwater tools

DCS: decompression sickness
POIS: pulmonary over-inflation syndrome

TABLE 26-8

RELATIONSHIP BETWEEN DIVING INJURIES AND ILLNESSES AND DIVE PHASES

Condition	Predive	Phase I Descent	Phase II Bottom	Phase III Ascent	Phase IV Postdive
Not diving-related	x	x	x	x	x
Trauma	x	x	x	x	x
Fatigue	x		x	x	x
Heat stress	x		x		x
Dehydration	x				x
Immersion hypothermia		x	x	x	x
Marine life trauma		x	x	x	x
Drowning/near drowning		x	x	x	x
Gas contamination		x	x	x	
Hypoxia		x	x	x	
Oxygen toxicity		x	x		
Hypercarbia		x	x		x
Barotrauma/vertigo		x		x	x
Hypocarbia		x			x
Nitrogen narcosis		x	x		
HPNS			x		
DCS				x	x
POIS				x	x

Sources: US Department of the Navy. *US Navy Diving Manual.* Vol 1 and 2. Rev 3. Washington, DC: Naval Sea Systems Command; 1993; Edmonds C, Lowery C, Pennefeather J. *Diving and Subaquatic Medicine.* 3rd ed. Oxford: Butterworth-Heinemann Ltd; 1992; Noonburg G. *US Army Special Forces Diving Medicine Manual.* Key West, Fla: Special Forces Underwater Operations School; 1995.

water leaks into the system and contacts these chemicals, a caustic alkaline solution is produced. If this mix enters the pharynx, it produces painful choking. Although the on-site medical provider certainly can respond quickly to diving emergencies and can treat injuries, he or she is of greatest benefit in anticipating and preventing them.[5,6,27]

Monitoring the Dive

Based on the history of the presenting complaint and the dive profile, a differential diagnosis can be developed. The dive can be broken into phases, with certain injuries more prevalent in each phase (Table 26-8).

Before the Dive

The establishment of a dive site is often time consuming, and safety checks and equipment corrections will often require the diver to be in a "standby" mode for extended periods. The divers may be at risk for heat stress, dehydration, and fa-

tigue. Additionally, since the effects of most drugs in the underwater environment are unknown, drugs are best avoided. The combination of pressure, increased concentration of gases in solution, and alterations in physiology with immersion can all affect the metabolism of pharmaceuticals.[5,6,27]

Descent

Medical personnel should anticipate barotrauma, caloric vertigo, and, if divers are using mixed-gas or surface-supplied equipment, hypoxia and CNS oxygen toxicity.

On the Bottom

Trauma is most likely in this phase, secondary to equipment and work requirements. Carbon dioxide toxicity, carbon monoxide poisoning, nitrogen narcosis, and, for specialized diving, high pressure nervous syndrome are all are more common at depth because of the increased partial pressure of gases. Drowning and difficulty with temperature extremes are also frequent here.

Ascent

POIS (ie, arterial gas embolism, pneumothorax, mediastinal emphysema, and subcutaneous emphysema) is most likely to occur in this phase, particularly if the diver should lose buoyancy control and experience an uncontrolled ascent or "blow-up." Additionally, alternobaric vertigo is most common in this phase.

On the Surface

AGE will generally occur within the first 10 minutes of surfacing, and most DCS symptoms appear within hours. Symptoms of inner ear barotrauma become increasingly easy to separate from other causes of vertigo as time passes. Casualties from heat and cold extremes are common at this point.

Summary

When treating a military diver, the DMO or DMT must immediately explore the possibility of a diving-related illness or injury, specifically DCS and AGE. The evaluation process requires constant awareness, insight into diving, and, ideally, a knowledge of the patient's baseline health status for comparison. Being alert to the oftentimes subtle presentations of these diving injuries can mean the difference between recovery and a permanent deficit.

DIVING ACCIDENT MANAGEMENT

Despite the potential for catastrophe, the vast majority of military dives are conducted safely. Medical problems during or following dives are infrequent and usually minor. Most of the advanced diving medicine training in the military focuses on treating the small percentage of more severe injuries and on prevention of diving-related illnesses. The primary function of medical personnel who support diving operations is prevention of diving accidents. If an injury occurs, however, those personnel must make a quick working diagnosis and render appropriate treatment in a timely fashion.[5,6]

Diving accidents can be grouped several ways. Many diving-related illnesses do not require recompression (eg, ear squeezes, POIS other than AGE and otitis externa). DCS, AGE, and more severe cases of carbon monoxide toxicity require recompression therapy. Extreme fatigue, although not considered a focal neurological symptom, correlates highly with cerebral DCS and is included as an indication for recompression treatment. Neurological symptoms arising after a dive may be caused by DCS or AGE. Symptoms of these disorders occur almost exclusively during the decompression phase of a dive, which includes the time after surfacing.

All cases of AGE are considered serious and all divers with an AGE require immediate recompression. Divers who hold their breath on ascent can suffer an AGE in as little as 4 fsw. Neurological symptoms secondary to AGE usually are obvious and dramatic and occur immediately after surfacing, so any diver developing neurological symptoms within 10 minutes of surfacing should be considered to have an AGE.[5] A diver with an AGE may be debilitated or unconscious in the water, requiring in-water rescue and respiratory support. He or she may also suffer from near drowning, a nonfatal condition resulting from immersion, fluid aspiration, and progressive hypoxemia.[27] A wide range of potential neurological, cardiac, and respiratory sequelae complicate postinjury management of these divers. An AGE may be confused with CNS oxygen toxicity, which may occur at depth with the LAR V oxygen rebreather. Such a diver may appear unconscious on the surface or develop altered consciousness or a seizure in the water. Nevertheless, a diver who surfaces unconscious is considered to have suffered an AGE until proven otherwise.[5]

In contrast to AGE, DCS may occur at varying times after a dive, with 98% of cases occurring within the first 24 hours following a hyperbaric exposure[5] (Table 26-9). However, divers also may experience DCS symptoms during decompression stops in the water or shortly after surfacing. Divers

TABLE 26-9

TIME COURSE OF SYMPTOM PRESENTATION IN DECOMPRESSION SICKNESS

	< 1 h	< 3 h	< 8 h	< 24 h
Time to onset of symptoms				
Percent of divers with symptoms	42%	60%	83%	98%

Source: US Department of the Navy. *US Navy Diving Manual.* Vol 1 and 2. Rev 3. Washington, DC: Naval Sea Systems Command; 1993.

who have uncontrolled ascents or who miss decompression stops are considered at risk for developing DCS or AGE. The risk is even more pronounced if they missed greater than 30 minutes total decompression time or the first decompression stop missed was deeper than 20 fsw. These divers need recompression treatment to reduce their risk of both DCS and AGE even though they may be asymptomatic. The initial symptoms of DCS may be mild and subtle, causing the diver to discount them as overuse injuries or mild trauma. Delays in initial treatment for DCS are very common in sport divers and not infrequent in military divers. Timely recognition of these conditions requires a high index of suspicion, especially in those cases without obvious neurological symptoms.[5,6,40]

Decisions regarding treatment options for DCI depend on the availability of a recompression chamber. If one is not immediately available, patients either must be transported to a chamber or undergo in-water recompression treatment. The latter is generally discouraged, and transport is recommended unless the chamber is more than 12 hours away.[5] In-water recompression treatment, especially with oxygen, is used with success in remote areas of the South Pacific and Australia.[27]

When transporting a patient with DCI, "fast and low" is preferred, taking into consideration availability of aircraft, stability of the patient, and life support requirements. The patient must not be flown above 1,000 ft or, preferably, the aircraft cockpit should be pressurized to 1 atm.[5,6] Ground transport should also travel the lowest possible route, avoiding mountain passes if possible. The referring physician must ensure the pilots understand the importance of pressurizing the aircraft because the patient's condition invariably will worsen if the ambient pressure is reduced. Transportable chambers, such as the Marine Corps' Transportable Recompression Chamber, were developed to bring recompression treatment closer to the theater of operations. This has obvious benefits for early treatment of patients with DCI, especially AGE.

Ideally, all patients requiring transport should have intravenous access, adequate fluids for resuscitation, 100% non-rebreather oxygen, and close monitoring by diving medical personnel. If a long transport of several hours is anticipated, the patient's bladder may need to be drained with a catheter. The goal is to avoid curing the patient's neurogenic bladder via recompression only to permanently lose bladder control from an atonic bladder, which had held a liter of urine the patient could not feel. Tracheal and bladder catheters should be inflated with saline, not air, to avoid compression injury or rupture with pressure changes. Finally, the referring physician should create a clear chain of responsibility for the care of the patient and communicate with the accepting physician.[5,6]

The urgency to initiate recompression therapy depends on several factors. If a chamber is readily available, divers who are suspected of having an AGE should have a complete examination delayed until they are at treatment depth and breathing treatment gas. Tissue injury occurs in a matter of minutes from an AGE, so time delays are associated with poorer recompression treatment outcomes.[5–7,40] The physician must not forget that divers suffering from an AGE have a primary lung injury and may develop other forms of POIS, especially if positive-pressure ventilation is required. If recompression treatment for serious DCI has been delayed longer than 1 hour, a quick examination (3 to 5 minutes) should be done before recompression to begin to map neurological deficits. If the delay is greater than 4 to 6 hours, a more complete examination can be done before recompression.[46] Military diving medical personnel are trained to do relatively complete neurological examinations within 10 minutes. In addition, adequate intravenous access, chest roentgenogram, bladder catheterization, and administration of medications may be performed before recompression if there have been long delays. Divers who present with pain following a dive must receive a complete evaluation at some point to rule out more serious injury or subtle neurological symptoms. The evaluator should assume that the diver has a neurological symptom until proven otherwise by a thorough examination.[5,46]

Rarely, a diver may suffer from cardiac arrest either secondary to DCI affecting the brainstem or from loss of the airway that progresses to cardiac arrest. Although a few civilian chambers are equipped with defibrillators, no military chambers allow defibrillation at depth. Cardiopulmonary resuscitation should be instituted on the surface as soon as possible. Advanced Cardiac Life Support (ACLS) should be initiated immediately because complete recovery rates are dismal if a pulse is not reestablished within 8 to 10 minutes of the arrest.[29] If the diver is resuscitated, it should be assumed he or she suffers from an AGE and should be recompressed appropriately. If ACLS will not be available within 10 to 20 minutes, the diver should be compressed to 60 fsw. If ACLS becomes available within 20 minutes of recompression, the pressure within the chamber

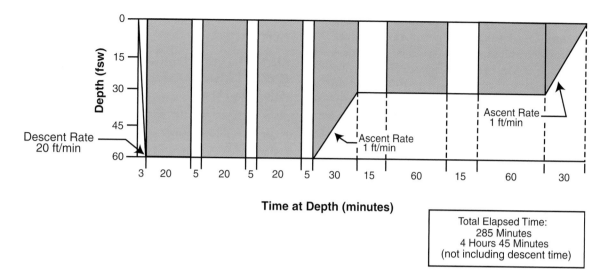

Total Elapsed Time:
285 Minutes
4 Hours 45 Minutes
(not including descent time)

Fig. 26-10. Treatment Table 6.
Source: US Department of the Navy. *US Navy Diving Manual.* Rev 4. Washington, DC: Naval Sea Systems Command; 1999: 21–41.

should be brought to surface levels and ACLS started. If ACLS has been started, the diver must not be compressed or recompressed until a viable rhythm has been established. Diving medical personnel should be able to "call the code" if a pulse has not been established within 20 to 30 minutes.[47]

There are many DCI treatment algorithms used throughout the United States and the world. No treatment regimen has been proven effective for all cases of DCI. A few stricken divers, regardless of the extent or promptness of recompression treatment, will have permanent neurological sequelae. For the most part, however, military diving is standardized and well controlled, with minimal treatment delays for casualties. The US Navy Diving Manual is followed closely and most dives are single, no-decompression dives.[20] These factors greatly improve outcomes when treating DCI. The present Navy treatment algorithms are

efficacious and respected worldwide.[6,7,10,28] Treatment Table 5 (TT-5) and TT-6 in particular, have been used to treat the large majority of DCI cases arising from standard, uncomplicated dives (Figure 26-10). These tables use an initial treatment depth of 60 fsw and a treatment gas of oxygen at 2.8 ata. Occasionally, deeper recompression (usually 165 fsw) may be required, especially for injuries occurring from nonstandard dives. Examples of these injuries are an AGE from an uncontrolled ascent from deeper than 60 fsw, serious DCS from deep, mixed-gas decompression dives, and serious DCS following large amounts (more than 30 minutes) of skipped or shortened decompression.[5] Special Operations dive profiles are typically shallow (less than 40 fsw), and DCI arising from these nonstandard dives usually responds well to standard treatment protocols (Table 26-10). Sport divers will often do multiple, repetitive, no-decompression

TABLE 26-10

A TREATMENT ALGORITHM FOR DECOMPRESSION ILLNESS

Diagnosis	Initial Treatment	Decision Point	Full Treatment
DCS Type 1	Compress to 60 fsw on oxygen	Complete relief within 10 minutes?	Yes, decompress on TT-5 No, decompress on TT-6
DCS Type 2	Compress to 60 fsw on oxygen	Worsening or need for deeper recompression within 20 minutes?	Yes, compress on TT-6A or TT-4 No, decompress on TT-6

dives on consecutive days.[40] Occasionally, they develop serious DCS requiring deeper recompression, but there is no consensus for treatment strategies in these cases. If recompression deeper than 60 fsw is deemed necessary, the best results are seen when high oxygen gas mixtures (nitrox or heliox) can provide treatment gas with oxygen partial pressures similar to those seen with a TT-6 (2.8 ata partial pressure of oxygen).[5,6,7,28] The algorithm in Table 26-10 offers a standard treatment protocol for uncomplicated cases of DCI from standard military dives and suggests a reasonable protocol for cases needing deeper recompression. The initial recompression treatment usually results in the most improvement in neurological function. Additional oxygen breathing periods, termed "extensions," may be added to most treatment tables. A rule of thumb is to strive for one symptom-free oxygen-breathing period before decompression to a shallower treatment depth. For patients with residual neurological symptoms following the initial treatment, neurological examinations should be done every 2 to 4 hours after surfacing, and subsequent retreatments rendered within 12 hours if symptoms worsen significantly. Otherwise, repeat treatments are given daily until clinical improvement plateaus for two consecutive treatments.[5] Usually one TT-6 or two TT-5s are administered within a 24-hour period for sequelae. Pulmonary oxygen toxicity may require the modification of the frequency of retreatments.[5-7,28]

Recompression Chambers

Recompression chambers are rigid-walled structures that are usually spherical or cylindrical to better tolerate the high pressures necessary to treat divers and others requiring recompression and hyperbaric oxygen therapy. According to the predominant theory, the high pressure in the chamber compresses bubbles and facilitates gas return into plasma or interstitial fluid, relieving obstruction and alleviating the tissue effects of AGE and DCS.[5-7,28] Concomitant use of oxygen (100% O_2 at 60 fsw) increases the amount of oxygen dissolved in plasma to levels where life can be sustained without red blood cells, thereby nourishing tissues that are poorly perfused due to an obstruction created by an AGE or DCS.[6,7,28] The same principle underlies hyperbaric oxygen therapy, which is used to treat carbon monoxide poisoning, gangrene, and other conditions of relative hypoperfusion (Exhibit 26-2). Chambers are pressurized with one or more patients

EXHIBIT 26-2

LIST OF DISORDERS FOR WHICH HYPERBARIC OXYGEN THERAPY IS APPROVED

- Air or gas embolism
- Anemia from exceptional blood loss
- Carbon monoxide poisoning (may be complicated by cyanide poisoning)
- Clostridial myositis and myonecrosis
- Compromised skin grafts and flaps
- Crush injury, compartment syndrome, and other acute traumatic ischemias
- Decompression sickness
- Enhancement of healing in selected problem wounds
- Necrotizing soft tissue infections
- Refractory osteomyelitis
- Delayed radiation injury
- Thermal burns
- Intracranial abscess

Adapted with permission from: Hampson NB, ed. *Hyperbaric Oxygen Therapy: 1999 Committee Report.* Kensington, Md: Undersea and Hyperbaric Medicine Society; 1999.

and a medical tender or tenders inside to care for them. The DMO or other provider trained in hyperbaric medicine must never forget the decompression obligations of the tenders inside, especially if deeper recompression or a nonstandard treatment is rendered. In addition, life support requirements, to include chamber temperature control, chamber atmospheric control, and minimum staffing requirements, must be maintained for all hyperbaric treatments. During recompression treatments, DMOs must anticipate potential problems, such as oxygen toxicity, pneumothorax (especially for divers suffering from an AGE), or symptom recurrences on ascent. Consent forms for civilians should be completed before recompression but should not delay timely or appropriate treatment.[5] And liaison with a local medical treatment facility for the immediate care of the patient should be arranged before the end of the treatment. The patient and tenders should remain at the chamber for 2 hours following a TT-5 and 6 hours following a TT-6, and within 1 hour's transport of the chamber for 24 hours. Follow-up evaluation by a medical provider should be done within 12 hours for asymptomatic patients.[3,5]

EXHIBIT 26-3

DIVING EMERGENCY INFORMATION

Divers Alert Network (DAN)	3100 Tower Blvd, Suite 1300 Durham, NC 27707	(919) 684-8111
Navy Experimental Diving Unit (NEDU)	321 Bullfinch Road Panama City, FL 32407	(850) 230-3100 DSN: 436-
Naval Medical Research Center (NMRC)	503 Robert Grant Ave Silver Spring, MD 20910-7500	(301) 319-7699 DSN: 285-
Naval Diving and Salvage Training Center (NDSTC)	350 South Crag Road Panama City, FL 32407	(850) 234-4651 DMO Beeper: (850) 784-6516 DSN: 436-

---

Assistance is available 24 hours a day through the numbers listed in Exhibit 26-3.

Diving Accident Investigation

A diving accident that results in a fatality or serious injury or one in which a piece of equipment is believed to have malfunctioned or contributed to the accident must be investigated and reported. The chain of command, the Naval Safety Center, and the Naval Experimental Diving Unit must be notified as soon as possible with circumstances of the accident. All equipment worn by divers involved in the accident must be secured and shipped in its untampered state to the Naval Experimental Diving Unit for evaluation. Compressed gas cylinders must be shipped in accordance with current Department of Transportation and command guidance. Detailed equipment information sheets, which can be found in the *Navy Diving Manual*, must be completed and forwarded to the Naval Experimental Diving Unit also.[5]

SUMMARY

Military diving medicine is practiced by a small corps of professional DMOs, dedicated to safe and productive diving operations in the armed services. Many of these dives are conducted in remote locales under austere conditions, so DMOs must remain flexible. Additionally, they must rely on Master Divers and DMTs to enforce safe diving practices. Military DMOs often practice alone but must recognize when to contact more experienced practitioners at Navy and civilian institutions. Clinically, DMOs must maintain expertise in physiology and neurology, and they must retain a low threshold for initiating recompression therapy for diving injuries.

REFERENCES

1. US Department of Defense. *Single Manager Responsibility for Joint Service Military Diving Technology and Training*. Washington DC: DoD; 1996. DoD Directive 3224.4.

2. US Department of the Navy. *Dive Reporting*. Washington DC: DN; 1992. OPNAVINST 3150.28A.

3. US Department of the Navy. *Diving Mishap and Hyperbaric Treatment Reporting Procedures*. Washington DC: DN; 1996. OPNAVINST 5100.19C, Change 1.

4. Larson HE. *History of Self-Contained Diving and Underwater Swimming*. Washington, DC: National Academy of Sciences, National Research Council; 1959. Prepared for the Office of Naval Research under the auspices of the Committee on Undersea Warfare.

5. US Department of the Navy. *US Navy Diving Manual*. Vol 1 and 2. Rev 3. Washington DC: Naval Sea Systems Command; 1993. Also published as: US Department of the Army. *Military Diving*. Washington, DC: DA; 1995. Field Manuals 21-11-1 and 21-11-2.

6. Bove AA, Davis JC. *Diving Medicine*. 2nd ed. Philadelphia: W.B. Saunders; 1990.

7. Bennett PB, Elliott DH. *The Physiology of Medicine and Diving*. 4th ed. London: W.B. Saunders; 1993.

8. Bert P; Hitchcock MA, Hitchcock FA, trans. *Barometric Pressure: Research in Experimental Physiology*. Columbus, Oh: College Book Co; 1943.

9. Boycott AE, Damant GCC, Haldane JS. The prevention of compressed air illness. *J Hyg*. 1908;8:342–443.

10. Flynn ET, Catron PW, Bayne CG. *Diving Medical Officer Student Guide*. Washington, DC: Naval Technical Training Command; 1981.

11. Stillson GD. *Report on Deep Diving Tests*. US Bureau of Construction and Repair; 1915.

12. French GRW. Diving operations in connection with the salvage of the USS F-4. *US Navy Med Bull*. 1916;10:74–91.

13. Hawkins JA, Shilling CW, Hansen RA. A suggested change in calculating decompression tables for diving. *US Navy Med Bull*. 1935;33:327–338.

14. Yarborough OD. *Calculation of Decompression Tables*. Washington, DC: US Navy; 1937. US Navy Experimental Diving Unit Report.

15. Van der Aue OE, Kellar RJ, Brinton ES, Barron G, Gilliam HD, Jones RJ. *Calculation and Testing of Decompression Tables for Air Dives Employing the Procedure of Surface Decompression and the Use of Oxygen*. Washington, DC: US Navy Experimental Diving Unit; 1951. NEDU Research Report 1-51.

16. Desgranges M. *Standard Air Decompression Tables*. Washington, DC: US Navy Experimental Diving Unit; 1956. NEDU Research Report 5-56.

17. Workman RD. *Calculation of Air Saturation Decompression Tables*. Washington, DC: US Navy Experimental Diving Unit; 1957. NEDU Research Report 11-57.

18. Workman RD. *Calculation of Decompression Schedules for Nitrogen-Oxygen and Helium-Oxygen Dives*. Washington, DC: US Navy Experimental Diving Unit; 1965. NEDU Research Report 6-65.

19. Berghage TE, Durman D. *US Navy Air Decompression Schedule Risk Analysis*. Bethesda, Md: US Naval Medical Research Institute; 1980. NMRI Technical Report 1-80.

20. US Naval Safety Center. *Naval Safety Center Diving Database*. Norfolk, Va: US Department of the Navy; 1997.

21. Butler FK, Thalmann ED. *A Procedure for Doing Multiple Level Dives on Air Using Repetitive Groups*. Panama City, Fla: US Naval Experimental Diving Unit; 1983. NEDU Report 13-83.

22. US Department of the Navy. *Approval of the Naval Special Warfare Dive Planner*. Washington DC: DN; 1994. NAVSEA ltr 6420 Ser OOC38/3227, 16 May 1994.

23. Weathersby PK, Survanshi SS, Hays JR, MacCallum ME. *Statistically Based Decompression Tables III: Comparative Risk Using US Navy, British, and Canadian Standard Air Schedules*. Bethesda, Md: US Naval Medical Research Institute; 1986. NMRI Report 86-50.

24. US Department of the Navy. *Approval of Naval Special Warfare Dive Planner Version 6.0 with Appendix A*. Washington, DC: DN; 1996. NAVSEA ltr 10560 ser OOC/3264, 14 June 1996.

25. Valaik DJ, Parker EC, Survanshi SS. *Calculating Decompression in Naval Special Warfare SEAL Delivery Diving Operations Utilizing the Real Time Dive Planner*. Bethesda, Md: US Naval Medical Research Institute; 1996. NMRI Report 96-54.

26. US Naval Experimental Diving Unit. *High Altitude Decompression Procedures*. Panama City, Fla: NEDU; 1986. NEDU Ltr 10560/TA86-06 Ser 02/150, 28 Feb 1986.

27. Edmonds C, Lowery C, Pennefeather J. *Diving and Subaquatic Medicine*. 3rd ed. Oxford: Butterworth-Heinemann Ltd; 1992.

28. Kindwall EP. *Hyperbaric Medicine Practice*. Flagstaff, Ariz: Best Publishing; 1994.

29. American Heart Association. *Textbook of Advanced Cardiac Life Support*. Dallas: AHA; 1994.

30. Russell KL, Knafelc ME. *Low-Frequency Waterborne Sound: Manned Dive Series*. Panama City, Fla: US Naval Experimental Dive Unit; June 1995. NEDU Technical Report 10-95.

31. Smith PF, Sylvester R, Baran F, Steevens C. *Development of a General Hearing Conservation Standard for Diving Operations: Experiment 1 Comparison of Temperature Auditory Threshold Shifts Induced by Intense Tone in Air and Water*. Groton, Conn: US Naval Submarine Medical Research Laboratory; 1996. NSMRL Report 1203.

32. Noonburg G. *US Army Special Forces Diving Medicine Manual*. Key West, Fla: Special Forces Underwater Operations School; 1995.

33. Bove AA. Underwater hazards and the physiology of electric shock. In: National Academy of Sciences. *Underwater Electrical Safety Practices*. Washington, DC: NAS; 1976.

34. Halstead BW. *Poisonous and Venomous Marine Animals of the World*. 2nd ed. Princeton: The Darwin Press, Inc; 1988.

35. Francis TJR, Smith DH, eds. *Describing Decompression Illness*. 42nd Undersea and Hyperbaric Medicine Society Workshop. Bethesda, Md: 1991.

36. Hallenbeck JM, Bove AA, Elliott DH. Mechanisms underlying spinal cord damage in decompression sickness. *Neurology*. 1975;25:308–316.

37. Moon RE, Vann RD, Bennett PB. The physiology of decompression illness. *Sci Am*. 1995;273:70–77.

38. US Department of the Navy. *Manual of the Medical Department*. Washington, DC: Bureau of Medicine and Surgery; 1994. NAVMED P-117.

39. Howsare CR, Jackson RL, Rocca AF, Morrison LJ. US Navy decompression illness and fatalities, 1990–1995: patterns and trends. Presented at the 1997 Undersea and Hyperbaric Medical Society Annual Scientific Meeting; June 1997; Cancun, Mexico.3

40. Divers Alert Network. *Report on Diving Accident and Fatalities: The Annual Review of Recreational Scuba Diving Injuries and Deaths Based on 1994 Data*. Durham, NC: DAN; 1996.

41. Howsare CR. Process improvement: an assessment of the US Navy diving database. Presented in poster session at the 37th Annual Navy Environmental Health Conference; February 1997; Virginia Beach, Va.

42. Flynn ET. *Shallow Water Air No-Decompression Limits: Analysis of Naval Safety Center Data*. Notes from the presentation at the Annual Diving Research Conference; Groton, Conn, February 20, 1997.

43. Almond M. Personal Communication; Senior Flight Surgeon, US Naval Safety Center; 1997.

44. Wallace R. Personal Communication; Infantry Safety Officer, US Army Safety Center; 1997.

45. Butler FK. Medical fitness standards for military divers. Presented at the Medical Qualifications for US Military Divers Conference; January 1995; Panama City, Fla.

46. US Department of the Navy. *Medical Department Diving Medical Officer Course Manual*. Pensacola, Fla: Chief of Naval Education and Training; 1996. CIN A-6A-0010.

47. US Department of the Navy. *US Navy Diving Manual*. Revision 4 (Draft). Washington, DC: NAVSEA; 1996.

Chapter 27

CHEMICAL WARFARE AGENTS

FREDERICK R. SIDELL, MD

F. R. Sidell; Chemical Casualty Consultant, Bel Air, MD 21014; formerly, Chief, Chemical Casualty Care Office, US Army Medical Research Institute of Chemical Defense, Aberdeen Proving Ground, Md

INTRODUCTION

Chemical agents have been used in warfare since ancient times. The first use of a chemical weapon, which in a broad sense includes smoke and flame, is generally considered to have been in 423 BC during the Peloponnesian War. Boeotians and their allies attacked Delium and succeeded in taking this village by burning a mixture of coals, sulfur, and pitch and sending the smoke and flame into the village through a hollowed out log. The walls were burned by the flame, the inhabitants were overcome by the smoke, and the village was captured.[1] A thousand years later, the Greeks used a similar mixture, known today as "Greek fire," against their enemies. Throughout the medieval period poisons of various types were used, particularly on crops and in water supplies.

The first modern day, or industrial era, use of chemical agents—and the only time in which US military personnel have been involved—was during World War I. Riot-control agents were used initially in small battles, but the first large-scale use was of chlorine by the Germans in April 1915. Chlorine, phosgene, and other lung-damaging agents were widely used for the next several years. In July 1917, mustard, a compound that damages the skin and the eyes as well as the lungs, was introduced and was the major chemical agent used throughout the remainder of the war. Overall, about a third of US casualties were from chemical agents and about a third of these were from mustard.

Between World War I and World War II, there were several instances in which chemicals were allegedly used, but although both sides had these weapons during World War II, they were not used. In more recent years, alleged uses of these materials against the Hmong in Laos, the Cambodian refugees, and the Afghans have not been proven.

Chemical agents—mostly nerve agents and mustard—were widely used in the Iraq-Iran war (1980–1988). Iraq had a production facility that remained active until the Persian Gulf War (1990–1991). US forces and the military forces of other members of the Coalition were prepared to face these agents at the beginning of the liberation of Kuwait. Fortunately, the agents were not used.

Despite the destruction of Iraq's known chemical agent production facilities and despite the efforts of United Nations inspection teams, it is possible that Iraq still has chemical weapons. Libya has been involved with producing chemical agents.[2] Some people feel that at least 20 other countries possess chemical weapons.[3]

Today, chemical agent use is not confined to the battlefield and to warfare. Chemical agents are not difficult to produce, and it is very possible that future use of chemical agents against US citizens could be on US soil by terrorists rather than against US military personnel on foreign soil.

CHEMICAL WARFARE AGENTS AND THEIR CLINICAL EFFECTS

Nerve Agents

The Agents

Nerve agents are the most toxic chemical agents. They produce biological effects by inhibiting the enzyme acetylcholinesterase and thus preventing the destruction of the neurotransmitter acetylcholine; this excess acetylcholine then causes hyperactivity in muscles, glands, and neurons.

The nerve agents are GA (tabun), GB (sarin), GD (soman), GF, and VX. (The letters are the North Atlantic Treaty Organization designations for these agents.) The United States has large stockpiles of GB and VX and a very small amount of GA. These are in bulk storage containers and obsolete weapons at six depots throughout the continental United States and at an island in the Pacific Ocean, Johnston Atoll, where the agents and weapons are being destroyed.[4] The Soviet Union had large stockpiles of several of these agents, and these stocks are somewhere in the independent states that emerged from that country. Iraq used nerve agents in its war with Iran, and it has been alleged that Iran also retaliated with nerve agents.

In addition to their military potential, these agents have been used as terrorist weapons. In June 1994, sarin was released in the city of Matsumoto, Japan, injuring about 300 civilians and killing seven. A larger attack took place the following year when on March 20, 1995, sarin was released in the subways in central Tokyo. Although 5,510 people sought medical attention after this incident, only about a quarter of these had effects from the agent. Most of the victims had mild effects, although several dozen required intensive care and 12 died. Both attacks were blamed on members of the Aum Shinrikyo Cult.

The first of what we know today as nerve agents was synthesized before World War II by a German scientist. Germany had these agents in munitions during that war but did not use them. The remainder of the weaponized nerve agents were synthesized between World War II and the early 1950s. From the early 1950s until the mid-1960s, the United States manufactured GB and VX; these stockpiles are now being destroyed.[5,6] The only known battlefield use of these agents was in the war between Iran and Iraq. Iraq's widespread use has been well publicized, and Iran may have also used nerve agents but in smaller amounts.

The nerve agents are clear, colorless liquids. Several (eg, GA, GD) have slight, not-well-described odors, but these odors are not characteristic and should not be used for detection or warning. Their freezing points range from –30°C (GF) to –56°C (GB) and their boiling points from 158°C (GB) to 298°C (VX). The most volatile is GB, followed by GD, GA, GF, and VX.[7] The volatility of GB is similar to that of water, whereas that of VX is similar to that of light motor oil.

GA is the least toxic by vapor exposure, followed by, in order of increasing potency, GB, GD, and VX. (Data are not available for GF.) Toxicity on the skin is in the same order, with VX being the most potent. Several of the G agents, (eg, GB, GA) require very large amounts on the skin to produce toxicity because much of these volatile agents evaporates.

Clinical Effects

The nerve agents listed above are not the only compounds that inhibit acetylcholinesterase to produce these biological effects. Drugs used in medicine, such as the carbamates, physostigmine, pyridostigmine, and neostigmine, as well as many carbamate insecticides, such as carbamyl, can also be considered "nerve agents" because of their biological activity. Malathion is the best known organophosphate insecticide with this activity.[8]

The nerve agents cause biological effects by inhibiting, or blocking the activity of, the enzyme acetylcholinesterase. The normal function of this enzyme, which exists at the receptor sites of cholinergic nerves, is to hydrolyze, or break down, the neurotransmitter acetylcholine. When the enzyme is inhibited, the intact acetylcholine accumulates and causes continuing stimulation of the receptor site, which in turn causes hyperactivity in the innervated structure. Cholinergic nerves (nerves with acetylcholine as their neurotransmitter) innervate skeletal muscles, smooth muscles, and exocrine glands; preganglionic fibers to autonomic nerves and some

cranial nerves are also cholinergic. After inhibition of acetylcholinesterase, there is hyperactivity in all of these structures.[8]

Two other forms of cholinesterase are present in blood—the erythrocyte cholinesterase (also known as acetyl-, "true," or red cell cholinesterase) and plasma cholinesterase (also known as serum, pseudo, or butyryl cholinesterase). They are used as markers for tissue cholinesterase when a person has been exposed or is suspected of having been exposed to a cholinesterase inhibitor. Neither is an exact marker for the tissue enzyme, and the erythrocyte enzyme is a better indicator of the tissue enzyme and of resulting clinical effects.[9]

Vapor Exposure

The most common means of exposure to these agents, based on the Japanese experiences in the mid-1990s and on experiences in research and manufacturing accidents in the United States, is by vapor. After vapor exposure, the effects begin almost immediately, reach maximal intensity within minutes, and do not worsen later. The latent period between exposure and onset is seconds to several minutes at most.

Small amounts of vapor produce effects in the exposed sensitive organs of the face: the eyes, the nose, and the mouth/airways. Miosis is almost always present after exposure of unprotected eyes to nerve agent vapor and is often accompanied by conjunctival injection and pain or discomfort in the eye or head. The patient may complain of dimness of vision (because of miosis and of disruption of cholinergic pathways in the visual system) and after a large exposure, blurred vision. Severe miosis may reflexly cause nausea and vomiting; these effects, including the nausea and vomiting, can be relieved by topical atropine.

Rhinorrhea is common after vapor exposure. Because of increased bronchosecretions and bronchoconstriction, the patient may complain of shortness of breath or tightness in the chest; this is usually accompanied by audible pulmonary abnormalities. The dyspnea may be mild and reverse within 15 to 30 minutes or may cause prolonged severe distress, depending on the amount of vapor inhaled.

Inhalation of a large amount of vapor will cause sudden loss of consciousness followed by a short period of seizure activity and finally cessation of respiration and flaccid paralysis. These are accompanied by copious secretions from the nose and mouth and in the airways and by muscular fasciculations throughout the body. The initial effect is within seconds of inhalation of the agent, and cessation of respiration follows within 10 minutes. Under these circumstances, the exposed person may die before there can be medical intervention, as happened with several casualties in Tokyo.

Liquid Exposure

In contrast to vapor exposure, liquid exposure has an asymptomatic latent period between time of exposure and the onset of effects (unless the amount is much greater than the lethal amount), and effects may continue to worsen after their onset as more agent is absorbed through the skin layers.

A droplet of liquid agent on the skin may initially cause fasciculations and sweating in the area of the droplet, and if the amount is small these may be the only effects. A larger amount will produce systemic effects; if it is a sublethal amount, the first effects will be gastrointestinal: nausea, vomiting, and diarrhea. Later, a feeling of muscular weakness may be followed by generalized fasciculations and twitching. These initial effects may occur anytime from 30 minutes to 18 hours after contact with the agent and may appear even though the area has been decontaminated.

A droplet containing a lethal amount of agent will cause, without noticeable preceding effects, the sudden loss of consciousness and seizure activity, followed by cessation of respiration and flaccid paralysis. These may start within seconds to 30 minutes after agent contact, depending on the amount of the liquid on the skin.

Vesicants

Vesicants are substances that cause vesicles, or blisters. There are many of these in the animal and plant kingdoms (eg, poison ivy). The chemical vesicants of concern are sulfur mustard, Lewisite, and phosgene oxime. In addition to causing blisters, these compounds also damage the eyes, airways, and other organs.

Mustard. Sulfur mustard is probably the best known and has been the most widely used chemical warfare agent. Depretz probably first synthesized sulfur mustard in 1822, although he did not recognize its properties. Other historians give credit to Riche or Guthrie in the mid-1800s for its discovery.[10] Later in the 1800s, Mayer developed a production process. Mustard's potential as a chemical warfare agent was recognized by the Germans, who

first attacked with it on July 12, 1917. The Allies soon began using this agent, and it caused more casualties during the last 17 months of World War I than any other chemical agent had during the entire war.[11] It has been used since and gained much notoriety because of Iraq's large-scale use of it during the Iran-Iraq war and the widely publicized photographs of Iranian mustard casualties. Not as well documented are the alleged uses of sulfur mustard by Japan against China in the late 1930s and by Italy against Abyssinia in the 1930s and its use in the Yemenese civil war in the 1960s.[10]

A slightly different form of mustard was synthesized in the pre–World War II period: nitrogen mustard. This contains a nitrogen instead of a sulfur in the molecule, plus some side chains. Nitrogen mustard was found to be unsuitable for warfare use for a variety of reasons. In the early 1940s, however, it was found to be useful as a cancer chemotherapeutic agent,[12] and it remained an important drug for this purpose for several decades. It is no longer considered a chemical warfare agent, and throughout the remainder of this chapter the word mustard will refer to sulfur mustard.

Mustard, also known as H, HD, or HS, is a light yellow to brown oily liquid. It freezes at 14°C (57°F), which makes it unsuitable for cold weather use unless mixed with another compound to lower the freezing point. Its volatility is low, but in warm weather or when there are large amounts of mustard on the terrain, its vapor is a hazard. Most mustard casualties in World War I were injured by the vapor. Mustard has an odor of onions, garlic, or mustard (hence its name).

The biological mechanism by which mustard causes tissue damage is unknown. One hypothesis is that mustard produces DNA alkylation and crosslinking. This produces an inflammatory reaction and death in cells, such as the basal keratinocytes and rapidly dividing cells of the mucosal epithelium and bone marrow. In the skin, protease digestion of anchoring filaments at the epidermal-dermal junction leads to blister formation.[13]

Several known biological activities of mustard are important clinically. Once mustard penetrates skin or mucous membranes, it cyclizes to form a reactive compound. This in turn rapidly attaches to intracellular and extracellular proteins, enzymes, DNA, and other substances. Intact mustard is no longer present and is not present in blood, urine, or blister fluid. A more important consequence is that the biochemical damage takes place within the first minutes after contact with mustard, and decontamination done after this may reduce but not prevent damage. Despite this early biochemical damage, the clinical effects from mustard do not appear until hours later. Contact with mustard liquid or vapor causes no immediate pain or other clinical effect.

The most commonly seen signs of mustard exposure are in the skin, eyes, and airways. Even small concentrations of vapor will cause eye effects. When absorbed systemically in sufficient amounts, mustard also damages bone marrow, the gastrointestinal (GI) tract, and other organs. The LD_{50} (the dose that is lethal to 50% of those exposed) on the skin is about 7 gm of the liquid; the lethal amount of vapor is less than half of the lethal amount of cyanide vapor.

The characteristic effect of mustard on skin is erythema and blistering. On the skin, a droplet of 10 mcg will cause a blister. Between 2 and 24 hours after exposure to mustard vapor (the time is shorter after liquid exposure), erythema appears and is accompanied by pruritis or burning, stinging pain. This may be the extent of the lesion, but more commonly small vesicles develop within the erythematous area. These later coalesce to form bullae, which characteristically are dome shaped and thin walled and filled with translucent yellowish fluid. If the amount of mustard was large, a central zone of coagulation necrosis may develop within the lesion.

Mild conjunctivitis may be the only evidence of eye exposure to mustard vapor, but usually this develops into a moderate-to-severe conjunctivitis with lid edema and inflammation, blepharospasm, and possibly corneal damage. The eye does not blister; instead edema and clouding of the cornea occurs, which may progress to corneal vascularization. Inflammation of the iris and lens may lead to later scar formation. Lesions caused by liquid mustard are generally more severe and may cause perforation of the cornea. Except in severe cases, recovery is complete.

Mustard damage to the airways consists of destruction of the mucosa, and this damage descends in a dose-dependent manner from the nares to the smallest bronchioles. Mild exposure involves the nose, sinuses, and pharynx and causes irritation and pain in these areas. There may be voice changes or total aphonia, along with an irritating nonproductive cough. As mustard descends to the trachea and larger bronchi, the irritation and cough become worse, and smaller airway involvement causes dyspnea and an increasingly severe cough with sputum production. In severe instances, there may be necrosis of the terminal bronchioles and hemorrhagic edema into surrounding alveoli. Except under these circumstances, pulmonary edema is rarely a feature of mustard poisoning. The necrotic mucosa and inflammatory reaction in the airways often lead to the formation of pseudomembranes; these tend to obstruct the airway where they form or sluff off and obstruct lower airways.

The mucosa of the GI tract is very susceptible to damage from absorbed or ingested mustard. After systemic absorption of a large amount of mustard, the mucosa necroses, which leads to large fluid and electrolyte losses. This terminal event resembles radiation damage, and mustard has been called a radiomimetic agent. A small exposure to mustard may cause nausea and vomiting within the first 24 hours of exposure. This is self-limiting, is not related to GI mucosa damage, and is thought to be due to cholinergic stimulation by mustard or to stress.

Large amounts of absorbed mustard damage or destroy the precursor cells of the bone marrow, which leads to leukopenia followed by decreases in circulating erythrocytes and platelets. After an initial leukocytosis in the first day or two after mustard exposure, there may be a decline in leukocytes beginning about 3 to 5 days after exposure. If the exposure was not too large, these will return over the following days, but after a large exposure the leukocyte count may fall to under $200/mm^3$.

Nonspecific psychological problems have been described in people exposed to mustard. These may begin shortly after exposure and have been described a year or two later.[14] Mustard (particularly nitrogen mustard) also has neurological effects; it regularly caused convulsions when large amounts were given intravenously to animals.[15]

Death from mustard vapor exposure is usually the result of airway damage. This invites infection, and this in turn often leads to sepsis, which in the absence of a functioning bone marrow is usually fatal. Occasionally a pseudomembrane will obstruct airways, leading to death. If exposure was only to liquid on the skin with no inhalation of the vapor, tissue damage and death are similar to those caused by radiation: GI damage and massive fluid and electrolyte loss.

Lewisite. Lewisite was synthesized and produced during World War I, but supplies did not reach Europe before the war terminated, so it was not used. Japan allegedly used Lewisite against China in the late 1930s, but otherwise there is no known battlefield use of this agent.

Lewisite is a trivalent arsenic and combines with many thiol groups, but the mechanism by which it produces toxicity is unknown. It is an oily, colorless liquid with a geranium odor, it is more volatile than mustard, and it has a much lower freezing point.

The clinical effects caused by Lewisite are similar to but more severe than those produced by mustard, with skin, eyes, and airways as the main targets. The skin lesions produced by Lewisite are usually deeper with more necrotic tissue. An important clinical distinction between mustard and Lewisite is that Lewisite vapor or liquid is extremely irritating and causes pain on contact with skin or mucous membranes. The casualty knows he or she has been exposed to something and masks or leaves the area and takes steps to decontaminate, whereas with the painless mustard exposure the victim usually does not realize he or she has contacted an agent. The Lewisite lesion appears sooner, with grayish dead epithelium appearing 5 to 10 minutes after Lewisite contacts the skin. Erythema and blisters also follow sooner than for a similar mustard exposure. Pulmonary edema is more likely to occur than with mustard. Lewisite does not damage bone marrow, but it does damage systemic capillaries and makes them permeable to fluid loss. This may lead to hypovolemia, hypotension, and organ damage.

Phosgene Oxime. Phosgene oxime is a urticant or nettle agent. Instead of fluid-filled blisters, it produces solid urticaria. It causes severe tissue necrosis and might be thought of as a corrosive agent. There has been no known battlefield use of this agent, and few investigations of its biological activities have been undertaken.

On the skin, phosgene oxime is extremely irritating and causes immediate pain, followed by blanching and erythema within 30 seconds. A wheal appears in about 30 minutes and is followed by necrosis. Lesions in the eyes and airways are similar to those of mustard and Lewisite except that the pain and tissue damage are more severe. Phosgene oxime can produce pulmonary edema after inhalation or after contact of the liquid with skin.

Cyanide

The Agent

Cyanide is widely used in industry for a variety of purposes (hundreds of thousands of tons are manufactured annually), it occurs in natural products and foods (eg, peach pits and cassava, a food staple in some parts of the world), and it is a product of combustion of many synthetic materials, such as plastics and fibers.[16] But it also has a reputation as a very deadly chemical. This reputation is probably based its rapidity of action; large amounts cause effects within seconds and death within minutes. Cyanide was not a useful agent when it was briefly used in World War I because the amount required to produce effects and lethality is high, because it causes few effects at small amounts, and because hydrogen cyanide—the form used—is lighter than air and tended to leave the area where it was delivered. According to press reports, cyanide was used against the Kurds at Halabja, Iraq, in March 1988, but this was neither proved nor disproved.

Salts of cyanide, specifically the sodium, potassium, and calcium salts, are the forms used for various purposes in industry. When a strong acid is mixed with a cyanide salt, hydrogen cyanide gas is released. This was used by the Nazis in concentration camps and has been used for executions in state "gas chambers." These chemicals were found in restrooms in Tokyo subways in the months following the March 1995 nerve agent release. Cyanide is occasionally used for suicides or homicides. In the 1980s and early 1990s, it was the substance in the grape drink that cult followers of the Reverend Jim Jones used for their mass suicide in Guyana, it was placed in Tylenol bottles, and it was responsible for deaths among people taking Laetrile (cyanide is released when that drug is metabolized).

The military uses two forms of cyanide. Hydrogen cyanide (hydrocyanic acid, AC) has a boiling point of 25.7°C, so in warm weather it is a true gas. It smells like bitter almonds, but half the population cannot smell it because of a genetic deficiency. It is the only agent that in the vapor or gaseous form is lighter than air. Because it rises and blows away quickly, it is not efficient when used outside. Cyanogen chloride (CK) is a nitrile that liberates cyanide during metabolism. This occurs minutes after it enters the bloodstream, so that cyanogen chloride possesses the biological activity of cyanide. It boils at 12.7°C so is a true gas under temperate conditions.

Clinical Effects

Cyanide inhibits one of the enzymes in the intracellular cytochrome system. Cells then cannot use oxygen; they switch to anaerobic metabolism and soon die. Cells of the central nervous system (CNS) are most susceptible to oxygen deprivation, and most signs and symptoms of cyanide toxicity are of CNS origin.[17] Chronic ingestion of cyanide, such as occurs in people who eat large amounts of cassava, can result in tropical ataxic neuropathy.[18] Other diseases (eg, Leber's hereditary optic atrophy) have been associated with chronic ingestion of cyanide.

When ingested, small amounts of cyanide cause a brief hyperpnea followed by feelings of anxiety or apprehension, vertigo, a feeling of weakness, nausea with or without vomiting, and muscular trembling. Consciousness is then lost, respiration decreases in rate and depth, and convulsions, apnea, and cardiac dysrhythmias with eventual cardiac standstill follow. The time of progression of these is dose-dependent but may range from minutes to an hour or longer.[15]

After inhalation of a large amount of cyanide, events occur rapidly. In about 15 seconds, a brief period of hyperpnea occurs. Fifteen seconds later convulsions occur, and these are followed within minutes by a decreasing respiration that stops in 2 to 3 minutes. After dysrhythmias, the heart stops 6 to 8 minutes postexposure.

There are few physical findings. Characteristically, the skin is "cherry-red" because venous blood is still oxygenated; however, the skin may be normal or cyanotic in the late stages. Laboratory findings include a high blood concentration of cyanide (normal is < 0.5 µg/mL), a metabolic acidosis (because cyanide stops aerobic metabolism), and a high oxygen content of venous blood. The latter two findings are not specific for cyanide.

Pulmonary Agents

The Agents

Pulmonary agents damage the peripheral portions of the lung, terminal bronchioles, and alveoli. These agents are in contrast to those agents, such as mustard, that damage primarily the central parts of the lung (eg, the airways). The prototype of pulmonary agents is phosgene, which is not to be confused with phosgene oxime. Phosgene was a major agent in World War I until mustard use began. Other chemicals fall into this category, such as perfluoroisobutylene (PFIB), a pyrolysis product of Teflon that lines some military vehicles including personnel carriers; the oxides of nitrogen released from burning gunpowder; and HC smoke, in which zinc is probably the primary toxic compound, although a solvent that hydrolyzes to phosgene may also contribute. Phosgene (carbonyl chloride; CG), however, is the most thoroughly studied and the following discussion will concentrate on this agent, although most of the discussion can be applied to these other chemicals.

Phosgene is the most volatile of the military chemical agents. It boils at 7.6°C, so it is a true gas in most weather. The gas is much heavier than air and sinks into valleys, ditches, and trenches. Its odor is that of new-mown hay or freshly cut grass.

Clinical Effects

Phosgene causes damage at only one anatomic site, the alveolar-capillary membrane, and this damage is a local effect of the agent contacting the membrane. Unless the amounts of agent are extremely high, phosgene causes no effects by skin application, ingestion, or intravenous administration. Inhalation of the agent with subsequent contact of the agent with the most peripheral airways is the only manner in which phosgene produces biological activity.

When the carbonyl moiety of the phosgene molecule, which remains after the chlorine atoms are hydrolyzed off of the molecule, reaches the alveoli, it reacts with proteins and enzymes of the alveolar-capillary membrane to cause loss of integrity of this membrane. This results in plasma loss from the capillary to the alveolus and pulmonary edema, the severity of which depends on the amount of agent inhaled.

Phosgene may cause a transient irritation of the eyes, nose, or upper airways at time of agent contact because of hydrochloric acid released from the molecule, but otherwise the first effect is an increasing shortness of breath, which starts hours after the exposure. This asymptomatic latent period may last from 2 to 24 hours. The increasing dyspnea is accompanied by cough with clear frothy sputum. The time of onset and severity of the dyspnea are dose-dependent. As more plasma leaks into the alveoli, hypovolemia and hypotension are accompanied by hemoconcentration. The decreased fluid volume and subsequent hypoxia may damage organs such as the brain, liver, and kidneys. In people with hyperactive airways, the auscultatory sounds of bronchospasm accompany those of pulmonary edema.

A common complication is infection in the damaged lung. Pulmonary edema developing within several hours of exposure is a predictor of a fatal outcome. Death is caused by pulmonary failure, hypoxemia, and hypotension or a combination of these factors.

Incapacitating Agents

Incapacitating agents cause temporary inability to function appropriately. They should be safe to use (a large overdose will not kill) and leave no permanent effects. In addition to their military battlefield use, incapacitating agents could be useful to law enforcement officials in other scenarios, such as hostage situations, airline hijackings, or prison riots.

Incapacitation can be produced by interfering with mental or physical processes. A compound that will cause loss of vision will incapacitate an individual for most tasks, as will a compound producing hypotension. The latter might prove to be lethal, and there is no compound to cause the former. A sudden "knock-down" effect with temporary loss of consciousness is produced by certain tranquilizers used in dart guns for animals. There are other means of incapacitation, but most compounds considered to be incapacitating agents affect the central nervous system.

Additional considerations in the selection of a compound for incapacitation are the rapidity of onset and duration of the effects. On a battlefield, the onset may be rapid or prolonged but the duration should be hours or days to give the user time to capture the victims. In a hostage situation, the onset should be rapid and the duration rather short so that the incapacitated casualties are not a burden on medical resources.

In the late 1950s and the 1960s, the United States developed incapacitating agents for military use. One, BZ, which is an anticholinergic compound similar to atropine and scopolamine, was put in munitions, but these munitions were destroyed in the late 1980s. There is no information on the military stockpiles of incapacitating agents in other countries, but these agents are not considered threat agents.

The onset time of BZ is about half an hour, and the effects last several days after an effective dose. BZ causes the same effects as atropine: mydriasis, blurred vision, decreased secretions from glands including salivary and sweat glands and glands in the airways and GI tract, decreased motility in the GI tract, and changes in the heart rate consisting of a brief bradycardia followed by a prolonged tachycardia and then normocardia. Similar compounds are used or have been used therapeutically for diseases of the eye and GI tract because of these properties.

BZ causes the same effects on the CNS as large amounts of atropine: confusion, disorientation, misperceptions (eg, delusions, hallucinations), incoherence in speech, inability to concentrate, and ataxia, all of which make up the syndrome known as delirium.

Riot-Control Agents

The riot-control agents are relatively unimportant as battlefield agents but are used in military training. These agents include CS, used mostly for training in the military and also used by law enforcement agencies; pepper spray; and CN (Mace), used in World War I and now commercially available in devices for self-protection. These compounds are solids and are usually delivered in a solution as an aerosol.

These agents produce burning, erythema, stinging, or pain on exposed skin and mucous membranes. In the eye there is burning, tearing, redness, and blepharospasm; in the nose and mouth there is burning on the exposed surfaces; and in the airways there may be discomfort, coughing, and a sensation of shortness of breath.

Capsaicin, or pepper spray, is a new agent that belongs in this category. It is marketed in self-protection devices, is used by some law enforcement agencies, and has been purchased by the military for limited use.

Capsaicin is a pure, crystalline material from the fruit of certain pepper plants, where it is found with the capsaicinoids, or capsicum oleoresin, an impure material containing over 100 chemicals. Both capsaicin and the oleoresins have been found useful topically for certain painful conditions such as arthritis, but toxicological data are scanty.

Capsaicin has about the same effects as CS and CN in the eyes, on the skin, and in the airways. But capsaicin is effective on those under the influence of alcohol or drugs, it causes more rapid effects, its recovery time is longer, its effects are more severe, it does not cause contamination of objects, and there is no danger of dermatitis, eye injuries, or an allergic reaction.

Severe effects after exposure to any of these agents are unusual. Prolonged eye symptoms may follow impaction of a particle in the cornea or conjunctiva. Skin exposure of a large concentration in a hot, humid environment may cause a delayed reaction with erythema and blistering. A person with hyperactive airways may have an asthma-like reaction after inhaling one of these agents. These compounds have a wide margin of safety, and death has occurred only when large amounts of them have been delivered into an enclosed space.

MANAGEMENT OF CHEMICAL AGENT CASUALTIES

The most important aspect of management of a chemically exposed casualty (or a casualty exposed to any type of toxic substance, including biological agents and radiation) is for the medical care provider to protect himself or herself. Otherwise there will be one more casualty and one fewer medical care provider. This is done by wearing appropriate protective equipment (ie, mask, gloves, suit) or by ensuring that the casualty has been completely decontaminated.

Nerve Agents

The key factor in managing a nerve agent casualty is to block the excess acetylcholine at cholinergic receptor sites and thereby reduce the hyperstimulation of the organs innervated by these nerves. There are many cholinergic-blocking, or anticholinergic, drugs available, but atropine was chosen decades ago because it was effective and produced fewer side effects. Scopolamine is very effective, but its side effects would be devastating in a nonexposed or mildly exposed person who took it unnecessarily.

Atropine is very effective at reducing the clinical effects of nerve agents in those organs with muscarinic receptor sites, such as smooth muscles and exocrine glands. Constriction of the airways and GI musculature is reduced, and secretions from the exocrine glands decrease. Atropine has very little or no effect on those organs with nicotinic receptor sites, namely the skeletal muscles. Thus, after atropine administration the casualty's secretions will dry and he or she will breathe better but will still be fasciculating and twitching.

A second drug that should be used along with atropine is an oxime. Oximes attach to the nerve agent bound to the acetylcholinesterase and remove the agent from the enzyme. The clinical effect of an oxime is seen primarily in those organs with nicotinic receptors, the skeletal muscles. Twitching and fasciculations decrease and strength improves. The oxime used in the United States is pralidoxime chloride (2-PAM Cl; Protopam Chloride).

The two drugs, atropine and oxime, are synergistic when used together. In the military, these are fielded in automatic injectors, one containing 2 mg of atropine and the other containing 600 mg of pralidoxime. These are supplied together in the MARK I kit (Meridian Medical, Columbia, Md).

In the event of mild-to-moderate poisoning by a nerve agent (ie, the casualty is still breathing, is conscious, and has muscular control), one MARK I kit should be self-administered. If the casualty does not improve, additional kits should be given at 5- to 10-minute intervals. Additional atropine should be given after three MARK I kits until there are signs of improvement, but no more than a total of three injectors of oxime should be administered each hour. The ca-

sualty who is unable to self-administer the antidotes, who is unconscious, who is breathing with difficulty or not breathing, or who has poor or no muscular control should be given three MARK I kits initially, followed by additional atropine until there is improvement. Improvement is when (*a*) the secretions are dry or are drying and (*b*) the casualty states that his or her breathing is better or there is less resistance to assisted ventilation.

For a severe casualty who is unable to self-administer the antidotes, the anticonvulsant diazepam should also be given. This is supplied in an automatic injector containing 10 mg of the drug. This should be given whether the casualty is convulsing or not.

One nerve agent, GD or soman, rapidly binds to the enzyme in such a manner that the oxime cannot remove it; the enzyme-agent complex is refractory to oxime reactivation. This process is known as "aging." After GD poisoning, aging occurs in about 2 minutes. Aging occurs after poisoning with other nerve agents also, but the time of aging is many hours after poisoning, and the process is not significant when treating an acutely poisoned casualty. Aging negates the usefulness of an oxime as an antidote and reduces the effectiveness of the standard atropine and oxime therapy.

Because of the rapid aging of the GD-enzyme complex and because GD was felt to be the major chemical threat agent against the US military, decades of research were devoted to a more effective therapy for GD poisoning. The result was the introduction of a pretreatment compound: pyridostigmine, a carbamate.

Carbamates attach to the active site on acetylcholinesterase the same as nerve agents do, but they remain attached only transiently; carbamylation of the enzyme is spontaneously reversible. Once the carbamate leaves the enzyme, or decarbamylation occurs, the enzyme again functions normally. While the carbamate occupies the active site of the enzyme, the nerve agent cannot attach, so in a sense the carbamate "protects" the active site from the nerve agent.

Pyridostigmine given before the agent exposure increases the efficacy of atropine and oxime therapy after GD poisoning and to a lesser extent after GA poisoning. It does not contribute to the therapy of GB, GF, and VX poisoning and should not be used in anticipation of poisoning by these agents. If pyridostigmine is taken after poisoning by GD and GA, it will contribute to the poisoning, not to the therapy. Pyridostigmine provides no benefit unless atropine and oxime are administered after poisoning. The dosing regimen of pyridostigmine is 30 mg every 8 hours. This regimen is started and stopped on order from the commander.

Additional care of the nerve agent casualty includes ventilation, suction of secretions, and correction of acidosis. The usual ABCs of airway management and ventilation will not be beneficial until the antidotes are given to relax the bronchial constriction. So the mnemonic in this case should be AABC, for antidote, airway, breathing, and circulation.

Vesicants

The most important aspect of the management of a vesicant is to prevent infection on the skin, in the eyes, and in the airways. There are no antidotes for mustard and phosgene oxime poisoning.

Skin care includes application of calamine lotion or other soothing material for erythema. Small blisters should be left intact; larger ones should be unroofed and the denuded area irrigated three or four times a day, followed by liberal application of a topical antibiotic. Systemic antibiotics should be started only when there are signs of infection and the organism has been identified.

Eyes should be irrigated at least daily, although the agent will be gone from the eye by the time the casualty is seen in a medical facility. A topical antibiotic along with topical atropine (or other mydriatic) to prevent later scar formation should be applied several times daily. Petroleum jelly or a similar substance should be applied frequently to the eyelid edges to prevent the lids from sticking together. Pain should be controlled with systemic, not topical, analgesics. Some ophthalmologists feel that topical steroids may reduce the inflammatory process if used within the first 24 hours, but steroids should not be used after this period.

Some form of positive-pressure ventilation (CPAP [continuous positive airway pressure] or PEEP [positive end-expiratory pressure]) might be useful if started at the first sign of airway involvement. Assisted ventilation with oxygen will be needed for someone in airway distress. Bronchodilators should be used for signs of airway constriction; steroids might be considered if bronchodilators are not effective. Antibiotics should be started only after an infecting organism has been identified; daily sputum examinations (Gram stain and culture) should be performed in a casualty with airway involvement.

To date there have been no attempts to replace damaged marrow after mustard exposure. However, marrow transplants or transfusions might be considered if facilities are available.

In animal studies, some forms of sulfur (eg, sodium thiosulfate) have elevated the LD_{50} of mustard when administered preexposure or within 15 minutes after exposure. Sulfur compounds have no effect on the topical lesions of the skin, eyes, or airways.

British anti-Lewisite (BAL) is an antidote for Lewisite and for other substances containing certain heavy metals. When the topical ointments are placed in the eyes or on the skin within minutes after exposure and decontamination, they reduce the severity of damage. However, these topical products are not available. BAL-in-oil (given intramuscularly) will reduce the severity of systemic effects. The lesions of phosgene oxime should be treated as lesions from a corrosive substance.

Cyanide

Cyanide casualties who are conscious when they reach a medical facility usually do not need therapy. Those who are unconscious, apneic, seizing, or any combination of these symptoms should immediately receive the antidotes sodium nitrite and sodium thiosulfate (both given intravenously). These are effective in maintaining life as long as they are administered while the circulation is intact.

Nitrites combine with hemoglobin to produce methemoglobin, which has a high affinity for cyanide. By diffusion processes, cyanide will leave the intracellular cytochrome oxidase and attach to methemoglobin. The intracelluar enzyme then reverts to its normal function. Thiosulfate attaches to free cyanide to form thiocyanate, a relatively nontoxic substance that is quickly excreted in the urine. These compounds come prepackaged in ampules, one containing 300 mg of sodium nitrite and the other containing 12.5 gm of sodium thiosulfate.

A compound used in the first aid treatment of cyanide poisoning is amyl nitrite. This is packaged in a perle, and after the perle is crushed the drug is administered by inhalation. If the casualty is not breathing, the drug can be placed in the ventilation apparatus. If the subject is breathing, he or she generally does not need the drug. Amyl nitrite is not in the military field medical system.

Pulmonary Agents

There is no specific antidote for these agents. Assisted ventilation should be begun as soon as effects appear. The intravascular fluid lost into the alveoli must be replaced to reduce hypovolemia, hypotension, and subsequent organ damage. Fluid replacement should be done in a hospital under the management of those skilled in pulmonary disease. The casualty should be monitored for airway infection by daily sputum examinations; antibiotics should be begun only after an infecting organism is identified. Bronchospasm should be treated with systemic bronchodilators or, if these fail, with systemic steroids, but the effectiveness of steroids for parenchymal damage is equivocal.[19]

Incapacitating Agents

Physostigmine (eserine, Antilirium) will produce temporary (about an hour) reversal of delirium in a BZ-intoxicated casualty, and its administration should be continued hourly until the casualty recovers. It should not be administered to a severely poisoned casualty with seizures and acidosis. There are no specific antidotes for the other known incapacitants.

Riot-Control Agents

Medical assistance is not commonly needed for people exposed to riot-control agents. Removal of an impacted particle from the eye and other eye care should be done by an ophthalmologist. A casualty with a bronchospastic episode should receive bronchodilators and assisted ventilation. A delayed-onset dermatitis should be treated as a vesicant lesion.

PERSONAL PROTECTION

Personal protection is provided by service-specific protective garments and masks. The US Army and Marine Corps use an ensemble of jacket and trousers lined with activated charcoal, rubber boots and gloves, and the M40 mask. The mask is smaller than the older M17 series of masks, and it has a single external canister or filter instead of the two internal filters of the M17 series. The Navy and Air Force have similar suits but are less bulky and more fire resistant. The masks for all services are designed to fit the needs of the user. For example, the M24 mask for pilots has an adapter to attach to an oxygen supply and a microphone to permit use of the intercom system.

DECONTAMINATION

Decontamination is the process of removing or reducing contamination. There are three types of decontamination: self-decontamination, casualty decontamination, and decontamination of unit personnel who are not casualties. Decontamination of unit personnel (performed at what is sometimes called the Personnel Decontamination Station or MOPP exchange) is not a medical-specific matter and will not be discussed further.

After exposure to a liquid chemical agent, decontamination is an urgent matter. Nerve agents and vesicants start penetrating the skin within seconds. Skin decontamination done within a minute will not prevent damage from mustard exposure, but the damage from the exposure will be less than if decontamination is done 15 minutes later. Decontamination more than 30 minutes after exposure decreases the size of the lesion negligibly, which is why decontamination of a casualty in a medical facility does not help the casualty, but it does prevent spread of contamination to others, including medical personnel.

Many items might be of use in self-decontamination to remove liquid agent from skin. A popsicle stick can be used to remove a globule. Flushing with copious amounts of water will wash off the contamination. Flour and similar substances will adsorb much of the liquid. None of these actually destroys the agent.

The individual service member carries the M291 kit for self-decontamination. This contains packets of activated charcoal and resins; the charcoal adsorbs the agent as the skin is wiped with the packet, and the resins accelerate the breakdown or destruction of the agent. The destruction takes hours, however, so the major action of this packet is to physically remove the agent by wiping and adsorption.

In the decontamination station (see below), a solution of dilute (0.5%) hypochlorite is used to decontaminate skin. This combines with the agent and oxidizes or hydrolyzes it, but again this process is slow. While the decontaminating solution is placed on the skin and then washed off, the agent continues to penetrate the skin. The most immediate effect is the physical removal of the agent by the decontaminant.

FIELD MANAGEMENT

The Service Member's Role

The management of or care for a chemical casualty on a battlefield begins with the casualty himself. What is done within the first few minutes after exposure to a liquid chemical agent is the most important procedure that can be done. Self-decontamination is necessary because medical personnel will not be present at this time. The service member should immediately decontaminate himself with the M291 kit if he suspects liquid contamination. In addition, self-administration of the nerve agent antidotes immediately after onset of the effects will reduce the illness. Buddy-aid is crucial if the casualty cannot self-administer the antidotes. There are no antidotes for the other agents that can be given by self- or buddy-administration.

What happens to the casualty next depends on the agent. A service member who had a small nerve agent exposure and was able to self-administer the antidotes will be able to continue the mission. A service member exposed to a large amount of nerve agent who did not receive the antidotes will die. A service member exposed to a large amount of nerve agent who received buddy-aid will continue to be symptomatic and will need medical care. A cyanide casualty will either die within minutes or will recover quickly. In neither instance will he or she require medical care. However, in some instances a casualty may present to the medical facility while still alive, and in those cases drug therapy might be useful. The effects from the other agents are delayed in their onset, and the signs and symptoms will begin hours or days later. At that time the casualty will seek medical care.

Echelons of Care

There are echelons of medical care on the battlefield. The first place a service member might turn to for assistance is to echelon I, which is the combat lifesaver, combat medic, or battalion aid station. Resources for care are limited at this echelon. Division level care, or echelon II care, is provided at the clearing station by the treatment platoon of the medical company. Although resources here are greater than at the battalion aid station (they include emergency care, radiology, a laboratory, and limited patient holding), the care needed may be beyond the capability here, and the casualty might need to be evacuated to an echelon III facility.

At echelon III are Mobile Army Surgical Hospitals, Combat Support Hospitals, and Field Hospitals, all of which are staffed and equipped to provide care for all categories of patients. The largest and most completely staffed medical resource within the military theater is the General Hospital at echelon IV.

At the Medical Facility

At the entrance to any medical facility that receives potentially contaminated chemical casualties is a casualty receiving area. The purpose of this area is to sort casualties and to ensure that contamination does not enter the medical facility. This area contains the entry point, a triage station, an emergency treatment station, a decontamination area, and the hot line. Until the casualty crosses the hot line, he or she is considered contaminated, and all personnel in front of the hot line—the contaminated area—must wear protective clothing, including masks.

Staffing at the casualty receiving area depends on the resources of the medical facility. At echelon I, triage and emergency treatment may be performed by a single senior medic or physician's assistant. The physician or physician's assistant will remain in the noncontaminated area. At a hospital in echelon III, a physician in protective gear may triage and may provide emergency care to a casualty also in protective gear. However, even at this echelon, a medic or physician's assistant may be the person in the contaminated area. Augmentees from the supported unit decontaminate the casualties.

The entry point is a clearly demarcated area into which all casualties arrive. Ambulances and other vehicles carrying contaminated casualties unload at this point. Establishing such a point is necessary so that contaminated vehicles will not enter the noncontaminated areas.

At the triage station, the medic, physician's assistant, or physician sorts the casualties according to priority for medical care. The five categories of triage, as listed in the *Handbook of War Surgery*,[20] are (1) urgent, for those needing care within minutes to save life (eg, someone with an airway obstruction or severe nerve agent intoxication), (2) immediate, for someone needing life-saving care within an hour or two, (3) delayed, for someone who has an injury needing further care that can wait without affecting the outcome (this includes almost all casualties with vesicant injuries), (4) minimal, for someone with a minor injury that can be quickly treated and the casualties returned to duty, and (5) expectant, for someone with wounds that are beyond the capabilities of the facility to treat.

In the emergency treatment area, care is limited with both the care provider and casualty in full protective gear. A bandage can be applied, a pressure dressing can be applied to stop bleeding, intravenous fluids can be started, chemical agent antidotes can be administered, and an endotracheal tube can be inserted and assisted ventilation begun. The RDIC (Resuscitation Device, Individual, Chemical, a bag-valve mask with a filter for incoming air) may be used in this area, or the standard bag-valve mask may be used since the vapor hazard would be minimal and the casualty would probably die without ventilation. Before each procedure, both the casualty's skin and the care provider's gloves must be decontaminated.

The decontamination area consists of two areas, one for walking casualties and one for litter casualties. In the ambulatory area, the casualty is walked through several stations and at each station is told what to do and assisted in doing it by either an augmentee or a buddy. In steps, the casualty's hood is decontaminated and removed, he removes his jacket, his gloves are removed, he removes his outer boots and trousers, and he is monitored for contamination (usually with the CAM [Chemical Agent Monitor]), after which he crosses the hot line into

the clean area, where he removes his mask. In the litter decontamination area, augmentees cut off the casualty's mask hood and outer garments, remove the rest of the garments, decontaminate the skin (with 0.5% hypochlorite), and check for contamination (usually with the CAM) before passing the casualty across the hot line into the clean treatment area. The capabilities within this area depend on the facility.

Casualties may be evacuated to a higher echelon either directly from the triage station if the level of care needed is beyond that of the facility or from the clean treatment area after initial treatment. In the former case, a contaminated vehicle would be used, and in the latter a clean vehicle would be used.

SUMMARY

Chemicals have been used as military weapons for more than 2,000 years. From the flame and smoke of ancient Greece to the nerve agents and vesicants of the Iran-Iraq war, theses weapons have killed or incapacitated hundreds of thousands of combatants and innocent civilians. US fighting forces have not been exposed to chemicals on the battlefield since World War I, more than 80 years ago, but the possibility of their use is always present. Many third world countries possess them and are not reluctant to use them. US military forces preparing for Operation Desert Storm had great concern that these weapons might be used.

Nerve agents cause death shortly after exposure, but casualties from this agent can be treated if antidotes and other assistance are begun in time. Mustard, the primary vesicant agent, causes effects that

begin hours after exposure and causes death days after exposure. Cyanide produces death within minutes but has characteristics that make it less than ideal as a warfare agent—there are good antidotes if they can be administered before irreversible changes occur in the casualty. The pulmonary agents, such as phosgene, are less potent and less deadly than nerve agents and generally are excluded from lists of modern-day agents. The incapacitating agents do not produce lethality and might be considered for specific uses. The riot-control agents are used for civil disturbances and are not usually considered for battlefield use. This chapter summarizes the effects of these agents, the management of casualties from them, and the general management of chemical casualties on the battlefield.

REFERENCES

1. Thucydides. *The Peloponnesian War*. Crawley R, trans. New York: The Modern Library; 1951: 262.

2. Waller D. Target Gaddafi, again. *Time*. 1996;April 1:46–47.

3. Orient JM. Chemical and biological warfare: Should defenses be researched and deployed? *JAMA*. 1989;262:644–648.

4. *Chemical Stockpile Disposal Program Final Programmatic Environmental Impact Statement*. Aberdeen Proving Ground, Md: Program Manager for Chemical Demilitarization; 1988. Publication A3.

5. Harris R, Paxman J. *A Higher Form of Killing*. New York: Hill and Wang; 1982: 53.

6. Robinson JP. *The Problem of Chemical and Biological Warfare*. Vol 1. In: *The Rise of CB Weapons*. New York: Humanities Press; 1971: 71.

7. *Potential Military Chemical/Biological Agents and Compounds*. Washington, DC: Department of the Army; 1990. Field Manual 3-9.

8. Koelle GB. Anticholinesterase agents. In: Goodman LS, Gilman A, eds. *The Pharmacological Basis of Therapeutics*. 4th ed. New York: Macmillan; 1970: 448–451.

9. Grob D, Lilienthal JC Jr, Harvey AM, Jones BF. The administration of di-isopropyl fluorodate (DFP) to man, I: Effect on plasma and erythrocyte cholinesterase; general systemic effects; use in study of hepatic function and erythropoieses; and some properties of plasma cholinesterase. *Bull Johns Hopkins Hosp*. 1947;81:217–244.

10. Medema J. Mustard gas: the science of H. *NBC Defense Technol Int*. 1986;1:66–71.

11. Gilchrist HL. Statistical consideration of gas casualties. In: Weed FW, ed. *Medical Aspects of Gas Warfare*. Vol 14. In: *The Medical Department of the United States Army in the World War*. Washington, DC: Government Printing Office; 1926: 273–279.

12. Gilman A. The initial clinical trial of nitrogen mustard. *Am J Surg*. 1963;105:574–578.

13. Papirmeister B, Gross CL, Meier HL, Petrali JP, Johnson JB. Molecular basis for mustard-induced vesication. *Fundam Appl Toxicol*. 1985;5:S134–S149.

14. Balali-Mood M, Navaeian A. Clinical and paraclinical findings in 233 patients with sulfur mustard poisoning. In: *Proceedings of the Second World Congress on New Compounds in Biological and Chemical Warfare*. Ghent, Belgium; 1986: 464–473.

15. Marshall EK Jr. Physiological action of dichlorethyl sulphide (mustard gas). In: Weed FW, ed. *Medical Aspects of Gas Warfare*. Vol 14. In: *The Medical Department of the United States Army in the World War*. Washington, DC: Government Printing Office; 1926: 369–406.

16. Homan ER. Reactions, processes and materials with potential for cyanide exposure. In: Ballantyne B, Marrs TC, eds. *Clinical and Experimental Toxicology of Cyanides*. Bristol, England: Wright; 1987: 1–21.

17. Ballantyne B. Toxicology of cyanides. In: Ballantyne B, Marrs TC, eds. *Clinical and Experimental Toxicology of Cyanides*. Bristol, England: Wright; 1987: 41–126.

18. Hall AH, Rumack BH, Schaffer MI, Linden CH. Clinical toxicology of cyanide: North American clinical experiences. In: Ballantyne B, Marrs TC, eds. *Clinical and Experimental Toxicology of Cyanides*. Bristol, England: Wright; 1987: 312–333.

19. Diller WF, Zante RA. A literature review: Therapy for phosgene poisoning. *Toxicol Ind Health*. 1985;1:117–128.

20. Bowen TE, Bellamy RF, ed. *Emergency War Surgery*. 2nd rev US ed. Washington, DC: Department of Defense, Government Printing Office; 1988.

Chapter 28

BIOLOGICAL WARFARE DEFENSE

JULIE A. PAVLIN, MD, MPH; EDWARD M. EITZEN, JR., MD, MPH; AND LESTER C. CAUDLE III, MD, MTM&H

J. A. Pavlin, Lieutenant Colonel, Medical Corps, US Army; Chief, Department of Field Studies, Division of Preventive Medicine, Walter Reed Army Institute of Research, Silver Spring, MD 20910-7500; formerly, Assistant Chief, Operational Medicine Department, US Army Medical Research Institute of Infectious Diseases, Fort Detrick, Frederick, MD 21702-5011

E. M. Eitzen, Jr., Colonel, Medical Corps, US Army; Commander, US Army Medical Research Institute of Infectious Diseases, Fort Detrick, Frederick, MD 21702-5011

L. C. Caudle III, Lieutenant Colonel, Medical Corps, US Army; Office of The Surgeon General, 5111 Leesburg Pike, Falls Church, VA 22041-3206

INTRODUCTION

Contrary to common beliefs, many preventive medicine measures can protect US forces on the battlefield from biological warfare agents. The importance of these measures gained visibility toward the end of the 20th century. After knowledge surfaced about the Iraqi biological warfare program before and during the Persian Gulf War, which was followed by Boris Yeltsin's 1992 announcement regarding the then-active Russian program, the United States realized the seriousness of the biological warfare threat. By the end of the 1990s, there was increasing awareness of the possibility of a terrorist attack using biological agents against civilians in the United States. The potential for military involvement in such an incident, whether as victims of an attack or as responders with the civilian medical community in a mass casualty situation, has made military preparation for and prevention of any type of biological attack a necessity.

Military medical professionals need to know the epidemiology of a biological warfare or terrorist attack and how to recognize rapidly that an attack has occurred. Timely recognition will allow the prompt institution of available medical countermeasures, which can be very effective against several of the most likely bacteria, viruses, and toxins that might be used against US forces. The public health impact of a biological weapon as well as the role public health and other assets should play in executing a program for defense against biological warfare and terrorism also need to be understood. The importance of knowledge regarding medical biological defense cannot be overemphasized. The threat is serious, and the potential for devastating casualties is high. However, with proper planning, proper surveillance techniques, and appropriate use of medical countermeasures either already developed or under development, casualties can be prevented or minimized, and the fighting strength of US forces can be conserved.

THE HISTORY OF BIOLOGICAL WARFARE

Attempted warfare with biological weapons has occurred many times, dating back to antiquity.[1] The attempts are difficult to document, as epidemiologic and microbiological data are scarce and unreliable and many programs were shrouded in secrecy, but interest in the use of biological agents as weapons has been present for centuries and continues to the present day.[2] The devastating impact that infectious diseases can have on an army has long been known and resulted in the often crude but ingenious use of disease organisms and poor sanitation to weaken the enemy. The use of corpses of humans and animals to pollute wells and other sources of water of the opposing forces was a common strategy. The fouling of water supplies was used in many European wars, in the American Civil War, and into the 20th century.[1,3]

The use of specific disease vectors, such as corpses of plague victims in the siege of Caffa (14th century) and smallpox-laden blankets and handkerchiefs in the French and Indian War (18th century), heralded a new means of disease dissemination against populations.[2] In both cases, it cannot be proven that the attempts were successful, as both diseases can occur naturally. This dilemma is still of importance today as newly emerging diseases can be confused with a biological warfare or terrorism event.

Biological warfare became more sophisticated during the 1900s; the goal was to select agents and delivery methods that could produce desired effects without harming the proliferator.[4] Allegations during World War I that Germany had been working on anti-livestock agents, such as *Bacillis anthracis* (the bacterium that causes anthrax) and *Burkholderia* (formerly *Pseudomonas*) *mallei* (the bacterium that causes glanders), led to the first attempt at an international treaty to ban biological weapons.[5]

On June 17, 1925, the Protocol for the Prohibition of the Use in War of Asphyxiating, Poisonous or Other Gases and of Bacteriological Methods of Warfare was signed. This was the first multilateral agreement that extended prohibition of chemical agents to biological agents.[1,6] A total of 108 nations, eventually including the five permanent members of the United Nations Security Council, signed the agreement, which became known as the Geneva Protocol.

World War II

Events during and after World War II were clouded by charges and countercharges of experimentation with biological warfare agents.[1,6] Probably the only use of biological agents on a large scale in the 20th century was Japan's against China.[7] In October 1940, a Japanese plane allegedly scattered contaminated rice and fleas over the city of Chuhsien in Chekiang province. Reportedly, this event was soon followed by an outbreak of bubonic plague, a disease never previously recorded in Chuhsien. Several other mysterious flights of Japanese aircraft over at least 11 Chinese cities—with the dropping of grain (eg, wheat, rice, sorghum, corn), strange granules containing Gram-negative bacilli, and other materials suspected of being contaminated with the plague bacterium—took place through August 1942. Thousands are estimated to have been hospitalized and 700 died from artificially spread plague bacilli.[6] Despite compelling evidence, testimony, and documents, though, failure to associate directly the isolation of plague bacilli in the laboratory with actual materials dropped by the planes made prosecution difficult.

It is alleged that at least 3,000 prisoners of war were used as experimental subjects by Japan's Imperial Unit No. 731, the notorious "death factory" that conducted what was perhaps the most gruesome series of biological warfare experiments in history.[1,8] Conservatively, more than 1,000 of these prisoners are estimated to have died in experiments with agents causing anthrax, botulism, brucellosis, cholera, dysentery, gas gangrene, meningococcal infection, and plague. Subjects either died in the experiments or were "sacrificed" when they were no longer useful.[9] The Japanese experiments may also have led to the epidemics of plague that occurred in the Harbin area after World War II, possibly due to the release of thousands of infected animals during the Japanese evacuation in 1945.[9] No prisoner left Unit 731 alive.[10]

The British also experimented with biological agents during 1941 and 1942. British trials with *Bacillis anthracis* were held on Gruinard Island off the coast of Scotland. The small-bomb experiments resulted in heavy contamination, with anthrax spores contaminating parts of the island for many years.[11,12] After World War II, the United States, United Kingdom, Canada, and Soviet Union developed large biological warfare programs.[4] These are the countries that have openly admitted to having had a program; other nations have never admitted their work in biological weapons.

The Banning of Biological Weapons

In November 1969, the World Health Organization (WHO) issued a report on chemical and biological weapons. It described the unpredictability of biological warfare weapons and the attendant risks and lack of control when such weapons are used.[13] In that same year, President Nixon declared a ban on the US offensive biological weapons program. It was soon dismantled, and all stocks of bio-

logical warfare weapons and agents were destroyed.[2]

In 1972, the Convention on the Prohibition of the Development, Production, and Stockpiling of Bacteriological (Biological) and Toxin Weapons and on their Destruction, commonly known as the Biological Weapons Convention, was convened.[1,6] Agreement was eventually reached among the 103 signing nations (including the Soviet Union and Iraq) that

> [e]ach State party to this convention undertakes never in any circumstances to develop, produce, stockpile, or otherwise acquire or retain microbial or other biological agents or toxins, whatever their origin or method of production, of types and in quantities that have no justification for prophylactic, protective or other peaceful purposes; and weapons, equipment or means of delivery designed to use such agents or toxins for hostile purposes or in armed conflict.[6p135]

The agreement went into effect in March 1975 and reduced the concerns that some nations had about the development and use of biological agents. However, problems with verification and the interpretation of "defensive" research continued.

Recent Biological Warfare Incidents

Since the signing of the Biological Weapons Convention in 1972, the US intelligence community has identified many significant events and emerging threats in the area of offensive biological warfare. The number and identity of countries engaged in offensive biological warfare work is classified, but it can accurately be stated that the number of state-sponsored programs of this type has increased significantly. In her book entitled *Doomsday Weapons in the Hands of Many—The Arms Control Challenge of the 90's*, Kathleen C. Bailey states that Central Intelligence Agency Director William Webster said in 1988 that at least 10 nations were developing biological weapons, a number the author feels to be almost certainly too low.[14]

W. Seth Carus, in *Bioterrorism and Biocrimes: The Illicit Use of Biological Agents in the 20th Century*,[15] states there are seven confirmed countries that are state supporters of biological terrorism: Cuba, Iraq, Iran, Libya, North Korea, Sudan, and Syria. He also describes 19 confirmed uses of a biological agent in terrorist or assassination attacks during the 20th century. It can be hypothesized that the number of terrorists without state support using biological weapons is significantly higher than those with state support. Evidence of state-sponsored programs of biological agent development and use exists.

Anthrax Outbreak in Sverdlovsk

On April 3, 1979, a mysterious outbreak of anthrax at Sverdlovsk, USSR, the site of the Soviet Institute of Microbiology and Virology (VECTOR, since renamed the Russian State Research Center of Virology and Biotechnology but still known as VECTOR), raised questions about the effectiveness of any weapons control agreements.[6,16] This institute had long been suspected of being a biological warfare research facility. In spite of US accusations, the Soviets maintained for years that this outbreak was not due to an accidental release of anthrax from the military research facility but instead was due to ingestion by the local residents of contaminated animal products. Controversy raged in the lay press over the incident. Ultimately, in 1992, the President of Russia, Boris Yeltsin, admitted that there had, in fact, been an accidental airborne release of anthrax spores from the research facility, confirming the long-held belief of many in the United States.[17] In 1992, researchers from the United States interviewed survivors of the incident and confirmed at least 77 cases and 66 deaths. Human cases occurred as far as 4 km downwind of the release, with animal deaths recorded over 50 km downwind.[18] Ken Alibek, a former top-ranking Soviet biological warfare official who defected to the United States in 1992, offers an excellent detailed account of the incident.[19]

Cold War Assassinations

Toxins were used as weapons during the Cold War. In 1978, a Bulgarian exile named Georgi Markov was attacked in London with a device disguised as an umbrella. This weapon fired a tiny pellet into the subcutaneous tissue of his leg while he was waiting for a bus. He died several days later. On autopsy, the tiny pellet was found and determined to contain the toxin ricin.[20] It was later revealed that this assassination was carried out by the communist Bulgarian government with technology supplied by the Soviet Union.[21] An attempted killing with a ricin pellet occurred in Paris, France, 13 days before the Markov assassination. Similar pellet-firing weapons may have been responsible for at least six assassinations in the late 1970s and early 1980s.[22] Another alleged use of toxin is that of trichothecene mycotoxins ("yellow rain") in Laos, Kampuchea, and Afghanistan in the late 1970s and early 1980s by the Soviets.[2] Because of numerous confounding factors, this allegation is regarded by many to be suspect.[23]

Persian Gulf War

In the Persian Gulf theater during the fall and winter of 1990 to 1991, the United States and the coalition of allies faced the threat of biological and chemical warfare. Fortunately, Iraq did not use unconventional weapons, but the allies believed that Iraq retained this capability after its defeat. This belief was verified in 1995 by the UN Special Commission investigating Iraq's weapons of mass destruction.[24] In fact, Iraq had weaponized large quantities of botulinum toxin, anthrax, and aflatoxins by the time of the Persian Gulf War.[25] No concrete information on the scope of Iraq's biological warfare program was available until August 1995, when Iraq disclosed, after Husayn Kamil's defection, the existence of a biological warfare capability. Iraqi officials admitted that they had produced the biological warfare agents anthrax (8,500 L), botulinum toxin (19,000 L), and aflatoxin (2,200 L) after years of claiming that they had conducted only defensive research. Baghdad also admitted preparing biological warfare–filled munitions, including 25 Scud missile warheads (5 with anthrax, 16 with botulinum toxin, and 4 with aflatoxin), 157 aerial bombs, and aerial dispensers, during the Persian Gulf War, although they were not used. Iraq acknowledged researching the use of 155 mm artillery shells, artillery rockets, an MIG-21 drone, and aerosol generators to deliver biological warfare agents.[26]

THE BIOLOGICAL THREAT

The threat of biological and chemical weapons presents a troubling and difficult challenge to society.[27] In a statement made to the Senate Foreign Relations Committee on March 21, 2000, Director of Central Intelligence George J. Tenet stated:

> The preparation and effective use of biological weapons (BW) by both potentially hostile states and by non-state actors, including terrorists, is harder than some popular literature seems to suggest. That said, potential adversaries are pursuing such programs, and the threat that the United States and our allies face is growing in breadth and sophistication.[28]

The Former Soviet Union

The Soviet Union's extensive program subsequently has been controlled largely by Russia. Russian President Boris Yeltsin stated in 1992 that he would put an end to further offensive biological research;[17] however, the degree to which the program has been scaled back is not known. It has only recently come to public attention that the Soviet government operated a massive open-air test site for studying the dissemination patterns of biological warfare–agent aerosols and methods to detect them, as well as the effective range of aerosol bomblets with biological agents of different types, on Vozrozhdeniye Island in the Aral Sea. Biological warfare agents tested at the site were developed at Ministry of Defense facilities in Kirov, Sverdlovsk (now Yekaterinberg), and Zagorsk and at the Biopreparat center in Stepnogorsk; they included the causative agents of anthrax, tularemia, brucellosis, plague, typhus, Q fever, smallpox, botulism, and Venezuelan equine encephalitis. The experiments were conducted on horses, monkeys, sheep, and donkeys, as well as on laboratory animals such as mice, guinea pigs, and hamsters. In an attempt to ascertain the extent to which the Soviet program had been scaled back, specialists from the US Department of Defense visited Vozrozhdeniye Island in August 1995 and confirmed that the experimental field laboratory had been dismantled, the site's infrastructure destroyed, and the military settlement abandoned.[29]

There is intense concern in the West about the possibility of proliferation or enhancement of offensive programs in countries hostile to the Western democracies because of the potential for these countries to hire expatriate Russian scientists.[30] Substantial numbers of scientists have departed one of the former offensive biological warfare facilities of Biopreparat—VECTOR. It now houses one of the two WHO-sanctioned repositories of smallpox virus, the other being the US Centers for Disease Control and Prevention (CDC). Where the departed scientists have gone is unknown, but Libya, Iran, Syria, Iraq, and North Korea have actively been recruiting such expertise.[31]

In the late 1990s, the United States quietly aided Russia in the opening up of former offensive Russian biological warfare facilities and their conversion to peaceful, legitimate purposes. The Clinton administration informed Congress that VECTOR had rebuffed offers from Iran to buy products, technology, and scientific expertise. As a result, Congress substantially increased the amount of money used to finance these conversions.[32] However, there remains a serious concern despite the successes being seen in the conversion of these former biological warfare facilities. Through 1999, the Rus-

sians had not opened their military biological facilities to international inspection, even though President Yeltsin promised to open those secret military installations for Western inspection in 1992. The facilities of the Ministry of Defense, most notably those at Sergiyev Posad (formerly Zagorsk), Kirov, Yekaterinburg, and Strizhi, remained to be inspected at the end of 1999. Only a few of the facilities managed by the civilian arm of the Soviet/ Russian biological weapons program, Biopreparat, have been inspected but none since 1994. Until there is a full disclosure and accounting of the Russian program, doubt will remain as to its status.[33]

New Technologies, New Threats

Biological warfare agents provide a broader area of coverage per pound of payload than any other weapons system. The proliferation of technology and scientific progress in biochemistry and biotechnology have simplified production requirements in some cases and have provided the opportunity for creation of exotic agents in others.[34] Genetic engineering holds perhaps the most dangerous potential to create novel agents. Pathogenic microorganisms capable of causing a new disease could be tailor-made. If an adversary inserted a gene coding for a virulence factor lethal to humans into a virus or bacterium, that agent could then spread a disease that could overwhelm the diagnostic, therapeutic, and preventive capacity of a country's health service.[35] Genetic warfare, the targeting of specific populations or individuals with specific genotypic characteristics, could theoretically be accomplished. It has been estimated, however, that only 0.1% to 1% of the human genome can clearly be associated with pure ethnic differences. Whether this diversity is sufficient for the development of tailored agents is an open question.[36]

International proliferation of biological weapons programs broadens the range of agents that US forces may encounter. The modernization of many Third World nations, with subsequent development of industrial, medical, pharmaceutical, and agricultural facilities needed to support these advancing societies, also provides the basis for development of a biological weapons program. A biological weapons program can be easily concealed within legitimate research and development and industrial programs.[35] A report issued in 1993 by the Committee on Armed Services, US House of Representatives, on its inquiry into the chemical and biological threat noted that 11 nations possess or could

TABLE 28-1

INTERNATIONAL BIOLOGICAL WEAPONS PROGRAMS

Known	Probable	Possible
Iraq	China	Cuba
Former Soviet Union	Iran	Egypt
	North Korea	Israel
	Libya	
	Syria	
	Taiwan	

Source: Committee on Armed Services, House of Representatives, 102nd Congress. *Countering the Chemical and Biological Weapons Threat in the Post-Soviet World: Report of the Special Inquiry into the Chemical and Biological Threat.* Washington, DC: Government Printing Office: 1993.

develop an offensive biological weapons capability (Table 28-1). While many in government, intelligence, and diplomatic circles express grave concern about the proliferation of biological weapons, there has been relatively little carryover into the general public.

Incentives for the Use of Biological Warfare

An analysis of the incentives associated with a biological weapons program may offer insights into the current proliferation problem. Such a program has military, technical, and economic incentives, as well as political incentives.[37]

Military Incentives

From a military viewpoint, the ability of biological warfare to produce large numbers of casualties makes these weapons highly attractive for long-range targeting of populations. A report from the WHO[13] on the health aspects of use of these weapons details the enormous impact these weapons would have on a population. According to this report, if a biological agent such as anthrax were used on an urban population of approximately 5 million in an economically developed country such as the United States, an attack from a single plane disseminating 50 kg of the dried agent in a suitable aerosol form would affect an area far in excess of 20 km downwind. The report estimates that approximately 100,000 would die quickly and 250,000 would be incapacitated or die within several days

of exposure, assuming unrecognized dissemination with no institution of prophylactic antibiotics. In the same scenario but using a different agent (eg, Q fever), it would be expected to find only several hundred deaths but the same number of people who were temporarily incapacitated.

Technical Incentives

The comparative ease with which many biological warfare agents can be produced is a strong incentive for their use. Virtually all the technology needed to support a biological weapons program is readily obtainable for a variety of legitimate purposes.[38] This technology is very different from nuclear warfare technology, which requires dedicated facilities, or chemical warfare technology, where the agent precursors have few, if any, civilian applications. In addition, both nuclear and chemical technologies require raw materials that are difficult to explain to the international community as being for innocent and legitimate use.

Economic Incentives

The start-up costs of biological weapons programs are not prohibitive, especially when compared with the cost of embarking on a nuclear weapons program.[35] The cost of a biological program is much less than either a nuclear or chemical program: estimates range from $2 billion to $10 billion for a nuclear program, tens of millions for a chemical program, and less than $10 million for a biological program.[39] From an economic standpoint, biological weapons are, according to a famous saying, a poor man's nuclear bomb.[40] Even the weapons used to deliver these agents are relatively cost-effective. A group of chemical and biological experts appearing before a UN panel in 1969 estimated that

> for a large-scale operation against a civilian population, casualties might cost about $2,000 per square kilometer with conventional weapons, $800 with nuclear weapons, $600 with nerve-gas weapons, and $1 with biological weapons.[41(p16)]

Political Incentives

Two distinct political incentives might persuade a country to pursue a biological weapons program: (1) domestic and international status and (2) a favorable risk-benefit ratio. First, a country's ability to threaten its enemies with a weapon capable of inflicting mass casualties offers some tangible advantages.[37] W. Seth Carus, then Director of Defense Strategy on the Policy Planning Staff in the Office of the Secretary of Defense, summarized this political incentive:

> The perceived need for deterrence or compellence [sic] capabilities, a desire to influence the political-military calculations of potential adversaries, the search for national status, and even bureaucratic and personal factors can play a role in the initiation of such programs.[38(p22)]

Second, detecting a clandestine biological warfare program is difficult. The risk is relatively low that biological weapons research and development will be uncovered and confirmed—unlike a nuclear or chemical weapons program. Because virtually all of the equipment associated with biological weapons can be used for legitimate purposes, there is no incriminating, unambiguous evidence.[38] A country can undertake many illicit biological warfare activities toward developing a sophisticated offensive biological warfare program, short of actual use, without provoking inquiries from the international community.[37]

Nations With Biological Warfare Capability

The most likely route for the United States or its allies to become involved in a biological conflict would be in regional conflicts, whether as members of a UN peacekeeping force or through an act of terrorism.[37] Of the nations currently believed to have an offensive biological warfare program, only a few are potential candidates for engaging in a direct armed conflict with the United States. Iraq is one and continues to defy UN resolutions mandating inspection and dismantling of its weapons of mass destruction program. Weapons inspectors and intelligence officials also have reason to fear that Iraq is working on more-sophisticated programs to develop viral agents for use as biological weapons.[42]

North Korea possesses the capability to produce significant quantities and varieties of biological warfare agents. It also possesses the ability to employ such weapons both on the Korean peninsula and, to a lesser degree, worldwide, using unconventional methods of delivery. North Korean biological warfare research is believed to have begun sometime during the early 1960s and to have focused primarily on 10 to 13 different strains of bacteria, including the causative agents of anthrax,

cholera, and typhoid fever. There are also reports that they have worked on smallpox and maintain this agent in their inventory. Not surprisingly, substantive details concerning the North Korean program are lacking but are worrisome nonetheless and need to be taken seriously.[43]

A statement issued in February 1993 by Russia's Foreign Intelligence Service, the successor to the Soviet Union's KGB, stated:

> North Korea is performing applied military-biological research in a whole number of universities, medical institutes and specialized research institutes. Work is being performed in these research centers with inducers of malignant anthrax, cholera, bubonic plague and smallpox. Biological weapons are being tested on the island territories belonging to the DPRK (Democratic Peoples Republic of Korea).[44pA10]

Biological Terrorism

Although biological warfare is most often discussed in terms of weapons of mass destruction and usually in the context of war, foreign and domestic use of biological agents by terrorists or other subversive forces cannot be ignored. Biological warfare agents are, for the most part, inexpensive and relatively readily obtainable, although effective large-scale distribution may be more difficult to achieve. To lethally infect large numbers of people, the terrorist would have to create an agent that remains viable in a respirable cloud and is retained in the airways. Advanced expertise, methods, and equipment are required to achieve this level of sophistication. Even without advanced technology, though, the terrorist can still effectively accomplish the mission. The goals of terrorists include creating fear in the populace. Just the threat of using a biological agent, let alone the creation of even small numbers of actual cases of disease, can have a significant impact and achieve the terrorist's goals.

In November 1995, hearings conducted by the US Senate Permanent Subcommittee on Investigations revealed that the Japanese Aum Shinrikyo cult had worked to produce both botulinum toxin and anthrax, ostensibly for use as terrorist weapons. Since then, the number of hoaxes involving biological warfare agents has increased dramatically in the United States, but actual incidents remain quite rare.[45] There have been only a few instances where subversive groups tried to inflict mass casualties, and only one where they were successful—the 1984 use of *Salmonella* bacteria to contaminate salad bars by the Rajneeshee cult in The Dalles, Oregon. This attack, which was motivated by a desire to test the ability to incapacitate voters and so influence an upcoming election, resulted in 751 cases of food poisoning.[46] The threat that a subversive organization could carry out a successful biological attack is one reason that the US Congress dramatically increased funding for preventive measures against biological terrorism at the end of the 20th century. At the request of President Clinton and with bipartisan support from Congress, $133 million was appropriated in fiscal year 1999 for countering biological and chemical threats, $51 million of which was for an emergency stockpile of antibiotics and vaccines. Most of the funds were allocated to the CDC, primarily for strengthening the infectious disease surveillance network and increasing the capacity of federal and state laboratories.[31]

It seems clear that resolution of this problem should be given the highest priority. If enough cause for concern, though, the recent progress in the biomedical sciences threatens the development of an entirely new class of weapons of mass destruction: genetically engineered pathogens. As George Orwell put it, "Life is a race between education and catastrophe."[27(p75)] Matthew Meselson, a well-known Harvard biochemist who described so well the 1979 Sverdlovsk anthrax outbreak, made the statement:

Every major technology—metallurgy, explosives, internal combustion, aviation, electronics, nuclear energy—has been intensively exploited, not only for peaceful purposes but also for hostile ones.... Must this also happen with biotechnology, certain to be the dominant technology of the coming century?[47(pA14)]

USE OF BIOLOGICAL WEAPONS

Biological warfare agents would in most cases be primarily delivered as small-particle aerosols, and they are silent, odorless, and invisible in such aerosols. Once the particles are of optimal size and condition (the difficult part), they can be delivered by relatively easily available, technologically unsophisticated devices from long distances away. Many cannot be sensed by currently fielded detection devices. The attackers may escape days before the attack is even noticed because of the incubation period necessary for the clinical effects on humans to occur. Use may cause fear and even mass panic in the population attacked. A biological warfare agent need not be highly lethal to be effective, though, because incapacitation and confusion may be all the disruption necessary to cause the intended effects. Biological weapons may also be used in combination with other types of weapons or to add to the disruption produced by conventional weaponry.

Technical Considerations

Initial symptoms resulting from a biological warfare agent may often be similar to those produced by infections endemic to an area, such as influenza. When one member of a unit falls ill, others may still be incubating disease. Service members deployed to foreign lands are known to be at greater risk for exotic endemic disease agents since they may lack natural immunity. Therefore, a biological warfare attack may not be suspected even after the first patients have presented to medical personnel.

Biological agents may enter the human body via several routes:

- entering the lungs as an aerosol (the inhalational route),
- being ingested in food or water (the oral route),
- being injected through the skin (the percutaneous route), and
- being absorbed through the skin or placed on the skin to do damage to the integument (the dermal route).

The inhalational or aerosol route of entry into the body is by far the most important to consider when planning defenses against biological warfare attacks. An ideal biological warfare agent would be of a particle size that would allow it to be carried for long distances by prevailing winds and inhaled deeply into the lungs of unsuspecting victims. Particles that meet both of these conditions are 1 to 20 µm in diameter. Smaller particles would be inhaled and exhaled without deposition in the lungs. Larger particles would either settle onto the ground or be filtered out in the upper respiratory tract of those who inhale them. Particles in the 1-to-20-µm size range also are invisible to the human eye, so a cloud of such particles would not usually be detected by those attacked.

In addition to having the proper particle size, an ideal biological warfare agent might also be dried, which would make it easier to disseminate widely and over long distances. Dry powders composed of very small particles tend to have better dissemination characteristics and have advantages in storage and handling. Dried agents require an increased level of technological sophistication to produce, but the technology to do so has been available in industry for a number of years.

Logistical difficulties mitigate against using toxins of low lethality as open-air weapons, but they could be used on a smaller scale (eg, in an enclosed space such as a building or as an assassination or terrorist weapon). Such uses may become more likely in light of the kinds of limited conflicts and terrorist scenarios facing US forces in the post–Cold War world.

Line Source. Biological warfare agents might be released by an aggressor by means of sprays, explosive devices, and contamination of food and water. Most of these delivery methods use aerosolized agent. The agent can be dispersed by attaching a spray device to a moving conveyance; an industrial insecticide sprayer designed to be mounted on an aircraft is an example. A line of release would then occur while the sprayer is operating. This is known as a *line source*, and the agent is sprayed perpendicular to the direction of the wind upwind of the intended target area. Anyone downwind of such a line source, within a certain range, is theoretically at risk. The range of the infectious or toxic agent depends on a number of factors (eg, wind speed and direction, atmospheric stability, presence of inversion conditions), and on characteristics of the agent itself (eg, stability to desiccation or ultraviolet light).

Point Source. A second type of aerosol source, *point source*, is a stationary device for aerosolization of the agent, such as a stationary sprayer. A modified point source would be a group of spray devices, such as specially designed bomblets dispersed in a pattern on the ground by a missile or artillery shell. Bomblets may be designed to disseminate on impact or at a predetermined altitude above the ground. They may be released from missiles or aircraft and may have special designs to improve their aerodynamics or pattern in the target area. Other types of delivery systems for biological agents have been designed by various countries. These include bombs or bomblets that release the agent by exploding (generally very inefficient delivery systems), land and sea mines, and pipe bombs.[48]

Clandestine Sources. Clandestine means of delivering biological warfare agents are potentially available to terrorists or special forces units; these include devices that penetrate and carry the agent into the body via the percutaneous route, (eg, pellets, flechettes) or means to contaminate food or water supplies so that the agent is ingested.

Physiological Effects

Biological warfare agents are likely to be selected for their ability to either incapacitate or kill the human targets of the attack. An agent such as staphylococcal enterotoxin B (SEB) has the potential to render entire military units ineffective by incapacitating a high percentage of unit personnel. If one of an adversary's aims is to overload field medical care systems, an incapacitating agent such as SEB might be chosen rather than a lethal biological agent, as SEB casualties may require hospitalization for 1 to 2 weeks. If lethality is the goal, agents such as *Bacillus anthracis* (anthrax); the causative agents of Ebola, Marburg, and Crimean-Congo viral hemorrhagic fevers; or *Yersinia pestis* (plague), might be used. Inhalational anthrax, pneumonic plague, and certain viral hemorrhagic fevers have high case-fatality rates once infection is established in nonimmune hosts.

Psychological Effects

An attack using biological weapons may be more sinister than an attack using conventional, chemical, or nuclear weapons, where the effects are immediate and obvious. By the time the first casualty is recognized, the agent may have already been ingested, inhaled, or absorbed by many others, and more casualties may be inevitable despite medical countermeasures. The psychological and demoralizing impact of the use of a lethal infection or toxin should not be underestimated. Use of these agents against command and control infrastructure in the US could result in far-reaching consequences. The ease and low cost of producing an agent; the difficulty in detecting its presence, protecting its intended victims, and treating those who fall ill; and the potential to selectively target humans, animals, or plants conspire to make defense against this class of weapon particularly difficult.[49] An enemy may also be able to deny the use of such a weapon after casualties occur, claiming that a natural outbreak of an endemic disease with similar symptoms is to blame for the occurrence of disease in opposing forces.

By virtue of their invisibility and undetectability, biological agents may be more psychologically disruptive than conventional weapons to an unprepared military unit. Most military organizations have little experience in dealing with casualties of biological warfare, and facing an unknown threat can give rise to considerable anxiety and fear. Even the prospect of facing such a threat can create a great deal of concern. Worry about biocontamination may affect or even halt operations at key bases or facilities. Medical personnel may be even more susceptible to concerns over biological warfare, as they are more likely to understand the challenging circumstances that would follow enemy use of such weapons.

Use Against Civilians

Many characteristics of biological weapons make them particularly attractive for use by subversive forces against civilian populations. Biological weapons may, in fact, be much more effective if used against unsuspecting, unprotected, and nonimmune civilian populations than against a fast-moving, immunized military force. The objectives of a terrorist group may not be typical military objectives, so biological weapons may be better suited to their

purposes.[50] Biological weapons can be employed effectively as a means of terrorism or sabotage, especially in rear-echelon areas, port or staging sites, and industrial and storage areas. The stealth with which these weapons can be employed is a factor, especially if the terrorist wishes to escape detection. Terrorist use of a biological agent could create panic and cause hundreds or even thousands of people to demand medical care. The potential impact on health care facilities in the area of an attack or a threatened attack is tremendous. Emergency departments may be overrun with patients, unfilled hospital beds scarce, intensive care units filled, and antibiotic stocks depleted. The extent of panic may make traditional approaches to triage, which are based on accident scenarios, very difficult to execute. Public health and medical personnel must be prepared to prevent, detect, and treat biological casualties so as to decrease the panic and the morbidity and mortality rates. Beyond the impact on the health care system, panic associated with a biological terrorist attack could lead to large-scale flight and civil unrest.

BIOLOGICAL THREAT AGENTS AND MEDICAL COUNTERMEASURES

There are three basic types of biological agents: bacteria, viruses, and toxins. Other types of advanced biochemical agents, such as bioregulators, are causing increased concern and attention in the Department of Defense. Unfortunately, at the time of publication there are no available, approved medical countermeasures for these new types of agents, and they will not be discussed further. For the traditional biological agents, their characteristics (Table 28-2) and their available vaccines, chemoprophylaxis, and chemotherapy (Table 28-3) are summarized here. More detailed information on anthrax, brucellosis, cholera, tularemia, plague, Q fever, the viral encephalitidies, and the viral hemorrhagic fevers is presented elsewhere in this textbook and will not be duplicated here. Information on smallpox and the most likely toxin agents are included in this chapter.

Smallpox

The last natural case of smallpox occurred in Somalia in 1977; in 1980, the WHO declared the worldwide eradication of the disease.[51,52] Two WHO-approved repositories exist for the agent of smallpox, variola virus, at the CDC in Atlanta and at VECTOR in Russia. However, the extent of clandestine stockpiles of the virus is unknown.[53]

The United States stopped commercial distribution of vaccine to civilians in May 1983 and phased out vaccination of the military at the end of that decade.[4] Most of the population is now susceptible to infection with variola major. It is stable, infectious by aerosol, transmissible from person to person, has a mortality rate of up to 30%, and is a potentially potent biological weapon when combined with an immunologically naïve population. The potential of genetic recombination to produce a modified poxvirus with enhanced virulence increases the threat of smallpox as a weapon.[53]

After an incubation period of from 7 to 17 days, clinical symptoms begin abruptly with malaise, fever, rigors, vomiting, headache, and backache. Fifteen percent of patients develop delirium. Two to three days later, a rash appears on the face, hands, and forearms. Mucous membrane lesions shed infectious secretions from the oropharynx after the first few days of the rash.[54] Eruptions then appear on the lower extremities and spread to the trunk. The lesions start as macules and quickly progress to papules and pustular vesicles. In contrast to varicella, smallpox lesions are more abundant on the extremities and face and remain generally synchronous in their stage of development. After 8 to 14 days, the pustules form scabs, which may leave scars. Although virus in the throat, conjunctiva, and

TABLE 28-2

CHARACTERISTICS OF BIOLOGICAL WARFARE AGENTS

Disease	Transmissible Person to Person	Infective Dose	Incubation Period	Duration of Illness	Lethality	Persistence (aerosol exposure)	Vaccine Efficacy
Inhalation Anthrax	No	8,000–50,000 spores	1–6 d, possibly longer	3–5 d (usually fatal if untreated)	High	Very stable, spores remain viable for years in soil	2-dose efficacy against 200–500 LD_{50}s in monkeys
Brucellosis	No	10–100 organisms	5–60 d	Weeks to months	< 5% untreated	Very stable	No vaccine
Cholera	Rare	10–500 organisms	4 h to 5 d	≥ 1 wk	Low with treatment, high without	Unstable in aerosols and fresh water; stable in salt water	No data on aerosol
Glanders	Low	Assumed low	10–14 d via aerosol	Death in 7–10 d in septicemic form	> 50%	Very stable	No vaccine
Pneumonic Plague	High	100–500 organisms	2–3 d	1–6 d (usually fatal)	High unless treated within 12–24 h	For up to 1 y in soil; 270 d in live tissues	3 doses not protective against 118 LD_{50}s in monkeys
Tularemia	No	1–50 organisms	2–10 d (avg 3–5 d)	≥ 2 wk	Moderate if untreated	For months in moist soil or other media	80% protection against 1–10 LD_{50}s
Q Fever	Rare	1–10 organisms	10–40 d	2–14 d	Very low	For months on wood and sand	94% protection against 3,500 LD_{50}s in guinea pigs
Smallpox	High	Assumed low (10–100 organisms)	7–17 d (avg 12 d)	4 wk	High to moderate	Very stable	Vaccine protects against large doses in primates
Venezuelan Equine Encephalitis	Low	10–100 organisms	2–6 d	Days to weeks	Low	Relatively unstable	TC 83 protects against 30–500 LD_{50}s in hamsters
Viral Hemorrhagic Fevers	Moderate	1–10 organisms	4–21 d	Death between 7–16 d	High for Zaire strain of Ebola, lower for others	Relatively unstable	No vaccine
Botulism	No	0.001 µg/kg is LD_{50} for type A	Variable (hours to days)	Death in 24–72 h; lasts months if not lethal	High without respiratory support	For weeks in non-moving water and food	3 doses give efficacy of 100% against 25–250 LD_{50}s in primates
Staphylococcal Enterotoxin B	No	0.03 µg/person incapacitation	3–12 h	Hours	< 1%	Resistant to freezing	No vaccine
Ricin	No	3–5 µg/kg is LD_{50} in mice	18–24 h	Days; death within 10–12 d for ingestion	High	Stable	No vaccine
T-2 Mycotoxins	No	Moderate	2–4 h	Days to months	Moderate	For years at room temperature	No vaccine

LD_{50}: a dose that is lethal for 50% of the subjects
Source: *Medical Management of Biological Casualties Handbook.* Fort Detrick, Md: US Army Medical Research Institute of Infectious Diseases; 1998.

urine gradually decreases,[55] variola can be recovered from scabs throughout convalescence, and patients should be isolated and considered infectious until all scabs separate.[56]

The disease caused by variola major had a case fatality rate of 3% in the vaccinated and 30% in the unvaccinated.[52] Other forms of variola major infection, such as flat-type and hemorrhagic-type smallpox, had higher mortality rates. Monkeypox, caused by a naturally occurring viral relative from Africa, is associated with greater than 50% mortality if a secondary bacterial pneumonia develops.[57] It can cause disease in humans but has limited potential for person-to-person transmission.[58] Recent reports suggest that declining smallpox immunization may result in sustained person-to-person transmission,[59] raising the concern that smallpox could be weaponized.

Since few practicing clinicians in the US have seen cases of smallpox, distinguishing this disease from other vesicular exanthems, especially initially, may be difficult. It is also possible that close contacts to cases may shed virus from the oropharynx without manifesting signs of disease.[60] Therefore, rapid and accurate diagnosis is urgently needed so that effective quarantine and other countermeasures can be put in place to decrease panic and the spread of disease.

The standard diagnostic method is detection of characteristic virions with electron microscopy or of Guarnieri bodies under light microscopy.[61] Discrimination between variola, vaccinia, monkeypox, and cowpox is not possible with these techniques. In the past, virus isolation on chorioallantoic membrane was performed, but today polymerase chain reaction techniques promise more accurate and rapid methods to distinguish between the poxviruses.[62]

The occurrence of smallpox is an international public health emergency. Any suspected or confirmed case should be isolated and droplet and airborne precautions implemented. Public health authorities must be notified immediately. If confirmed, all persons in direct contact with the patient should be isolated for 17 days, especially unvaccinated personnel. All those exposed to either weaponized variola virus or a clinical case of smallpox should be vaccinated immediately. Nosocomial transmission is thought to require close person-to-person contact, but in two hospital outbreaks, its potential to spread in low-humidity environments was alarming.[63]

Treatment of smallpox is supportive. Some antivirals have demonstrated good in vivo and in vitro activity against *Poxviridae* and may eventually prove useful as treatments.[53]

Stocks of smallpox vaccine (vaccinia virus) were allowed to drop to very low levels following the eradication of naturally occurring disease. In recent years, increasing this stockpile has received significant attention. Smallpox vaccine must be given by scarification. During the WHO eradication program, a clinical "take" (vesicle with scar formation) following vaccination within the past 3 years correlated with protective immunity. Side effects include low-grade fever and axillary lymphadenopathy. More-severe reactions, such as secondary inoculation to other sites or other persons and generalized vaccinia, can also occur but much less frequently. Vaccination is contraindicated in immunocompromised individuals, during pregnancy, and in those with eczema. However, with the exception of significant impairment of systemic immunity, there are no absolute contraindications to vaccination of a person with a confirmed exposure to variola. Since the antibody response after primary vaccination usually occurs 4 to 8 days earlier than after naturally acquired infection, vaccination within a few days after exposure to variola may be effective in preventing disease or decreasing morbidity and mortality.[64]

Biological Toxins

While biological toxins are not usually regarded as the most effective biological weapons agents, they have been used or their use has been threatened by more terrorist groups and individuals than the more traditional replicating agents.[4] Toxins are defined as any toxic substance produced by a living organism—animals, plants, or microbes. They are different from bacteria and viruses in that they do not replicate in the body. Unlike chemical agents, they are not man-made, not dermally active (except for the trichothecene mycotoxins), and are not volatile. Therefore, they require some sort of weapon system to bring them into contact with the human respiratory tract. Because of this trait, they would not be a persistent battlefield threat or produce secondary or person-to-person exposures. Some of the toxins are quite stable, but their utility as a military weapon can be limited by low toxicity or difficulty in producing large enough quantities for battlefield use. Out of the hundreds of biological toxins that occur naturally, only a very small number have the right characteristics to be an effective weapon. Mechanisms of action, clinical syndromes, treatment, and prophylaxis of the three highest threat toxins will be described here.

TABLE 28-3

VACCINES, CHEMOPROPHYLAXIS AND CHEMOTHERAPEUTICS FOR BIOLOGICAL
WARFARE AGENTS

Disease	Vaccine	Chemotherapy
Anthrax	Bioport vaccine (licensed) 0.5 mL SC @ 0, 2, 4 wk, 6, 12, 18 mo, then annual boosters	Ciprofloxacin 400 mg IV q 8–12 h Doxycycline 200 mg IV, then 100 mg IV q 8–12 Penicillin 2 million units IV q 2 h
Cholera	Wyeth-Ayerst Vaccine 2 doses 0.5 mL IM or SC @ 0, 7–30 d, then boosters q 6 months	Oral rehydration therapy during period of high fluid loss Tetracycline 500 mg q 6 h x 3 d Doxycycline 300 mg once, or 100 mg q 12 h x 3 d Ciprofloxacin 500 mg q 12 h x 3 d Norfloxacin 400 mg q 12 h x 3 d
Q Fever	IND 610-inactivated whole cell vaccine given as single 0.5 mL SC injection	Tetracycline 500 mg PO q 6 h x 5–7 d Doxycycline
Glanders	No vaccine available	Sulfadiazine 100 mg/kg in divided doses x 3 wk may be effective, TMP-SMX may be effective
Plague	Greer inactivated vaccine (FDA licensed): 1.0 mL IM; 0.2 mL IM 1-3 mo later; 0.2 mL 5-6 mo after dose 2; 0.2 mL boosters @ 6, 12, 18 mo after dose 3 then q 1-2 y	Streptomycin 30 mg/kg/d IM in 2 divided doses x 10 d (or gentamicin) Doxycycline 200 mg IV then 100 mg IV bid x 10–14 d Chloramphenicol 1 gm IV QID x 10–14 d
Tularemia	IND: Live attenuated vaccine, one dose by scarification	Streptomycin 30 mg/kg IM divided BID x 10–14 d Gentamicin 3-5 mg/kg/d IV x 10–14 d
Brucellosis	No human vaccine available	Doxycycline 200 mg/d PO plus rifampin 600–900 mg/d PO x 6 wk Oflaxacin 400 mg/rifampin 600 mg/d PO x 6 wk
Viral Encephalitidies	VEE DoD C-83 live attenuated vaccine (IND): 0.5 mL SC x 1 dose VEE DoD C-84 (formalin inactivated TC-83 (IND): 0.5 mL SC for up to 3 doses q 2 wks EEE inactivated (IND): 0.5 mL SC at 0 and 28 d WEE inactivated (IND): 0.5 mL SC at 0, 7, 28 d	Supportive therapy, analgesics, and anticonvulsants prn
Viral Hemorrhagic Fevers	AHF Candid #1 vaccine (x-protection for BHF) (IND) RVF inactivated vaccine (IND)	Ribavirin (CCHF/arenaviruses), 30 mg/kg IV initial dose, 15 mg/kg IV q 6 h x 4 d, 7.5 mg/kg IV q 8 h x 6 d Passive antibody for AHF, BHF, Lassa fever, and CCHF
Smallpox	Wyeth calf lymph vaccinia vaccine (licensed): 1 dose by scarification	Cidofovir (effective in vitro)
Botulism	DoD pentavalent toxoid (A-E) (IND) 0.5 mL SC at 0, 2, 12 wk, then yearly boosters	DoD heptavalent equine despeciated antitoxin (A-G) (IND): 1 vial (10 mL) IV CDC trivalent equine antitoxin (A,B, &E) (licensed)
Staphylococcus Enterotoxin B	No vaccine available	Ventilatory support for inhalation exposure
Ricin	No vaccine available	Inhalation: supportive therapy; GI: gastric lavage, superactivated charcoal, cathartics
T-2 Mycotoxins	No vaccine available	

BID: twice a day, CDC: Centers for Disease Control and Prevention, DoD: Department of Defense, EEE: eastern equine encephalitis, GI: gastrointestinal, IM: intramuscularly, IND: investigational new drug, IV: intravenously, q: every, QID: four times a day, SC: subcutaneously, VEE: Venezuelan equine encephalitis, WEE: western equine encephalitis
Source: *Medical Management of Biological Casualties Handbook.* Fort Detrick, Md: US Army Medical Research Institute of Infectious Diseases; 1998.

Chemoprophylaxis	Comments
Ciprofloxacin 500 mg PO bid x 4 wk; if unvaccinated, begin initial doses of vaccine Doxycycline 100 mg PO bid x 4 wk plus vaccination	Potential alternates for Rx: gentamicin, erythromycin, and chloramphenicol Penicillin for sensitive organisms only
	Vaccine not recommended for routine protection in endemic areas (50% efficacy, short term) Alternatives for Rx: erythomycin, trimethoprim and sulfamethoxazole, and furazolidone Quinolones for tetracycline-/doxycycline-resistant strains
Tetracycline start 8–12 d postexposure x 5 d Doxycycline start 8–12 d postexposure x 5 d	Currently testing vaccine to determine the necessity of skin testing before use.
Postexposure prophylaxis may be tried with TMP-SMX	No large therapeutic human trials have been conducted owing to the rarity of disease
Ciprofloxacin 500 mg PO bid x 7 d Doxycycline 100 mg PO bid x 7 d, Tetracycline 500 mg PO qid x 7 d	Plague vaccine not protective against aerosol challenge in animal studies Alternate Rx: TMP-SMX Chloramphenicol for plague/meningitis
Doxycycline 100 mg PO bid x 14 d, Tetracycline 500 mg PO qid x 14 d	
Doxycycline and rifampin x 3 wk	TMP-SMX may be substituted for rifampin, but relapse rate may reach 30%
Not applicable	TC-83 reactogenic in 20%, no seroconversions in 20%, only effective against subtypes 1A, 1B, and 1C C-84 vaccine used for nonresponders to TC-83 EEE and WEE inactivated vaccines are poorly immunogenic, multiple immunizations required
Not applicable	Aggressive supportive care and management of hypotension very important
Vaccinia immune globulin 0.6 mL/kg IM (within 3 d of exposure, best within 24 h)	Preexposure and postexposure vaccination recommended if > 3 y since last vaccine
	Need to skin test before use of antitoxin
Decontamination of clothing and skin	

TABLE 28-4

COMPARATIVE LETHALITY OF SELECTED TOXINS AND CHEMICAL AGENTS IN LABORATORY MICE

Agent	LD$_{50}$ (μg/kg)	Molecular Weight	Source
Botulinum toxin	0.001	150,000	Bacterium
Shiga toxin	0.002	55,000	Bacterium
Tetanus toxin	0.002	150,000	Bacterium
Abrin	0.04	65,000	Plant (Rosary Pea)
Diphtheria toxin	0.10	62,000	Bacterium
Maitotoxin	0.10	3,400	Marine dinoflagellate
Palytoxin	0.15	2,700	Marine soft coral
Ciguatoxin	0.40	1,000	Marine dinoflagellate
Textilotoxin	0.60	80,000	Elapid snake
Clostridium perfringens toxins	0.1–5.0	35,000–40,000	Bacterium
Baltrachotoxin	2.0	539	Arrow-Poison Frog
Ricin	3.0	64,000	Plant (castor bean)
Alpha-Conotoxin	5.0	1,500	Cone snail
Taipoxin	5.0	46,000	Elapid snake
Tetrodotoxin	8.0	319	Puffer fish
Alpha-Tityustoxin	9.0	8,000	Scorpion
Saxitoxin	10.0 (Inhal 2.0)	299	Marine dinoflagellate
VX	15.0	267	Chemical agent
SEB (Rhesus/Aerosol)	27.0 (LD$_{50}$ in pg)	28,494	Bacterium
Anatoxin-A(s)	50.0	500	Blue-green algae
Microcystin	50.0	994	Blue-green algae
Soman (GD)	64.0	182	Chemical agent
Sarin (GB)	100.0	140	Chemical agent
Aconitine	100.0	647	Plant (monkshood)
T-2 Toxin	1,210.0	466	Fungal mycotoxin

Sources: (1) Franz DR. *Defense Against Toxin Weapons*. Ft Detrick, Md: US Army Medical Research and Materiel Command; n.d: Table 2. (2) Sidell FR, Takafuji ET, Franz DR, eds. *Medical Aspects of Chemical and Biological Warfare*. In: *Textbook of Military Medicine*. Washington, DC: Borden Institute and Office of The Surgeon General, US Army; 1997: 607.

Botulinum Toxins

The botulinum toxins are a group of seven related neurotoxins produced by the bacillus *Clostridium botulinum*. These toxins, types A through G, could be delivered by aerosol to concentrations of service members. When inhaled, these toxins produce a clinical picture very similar to foodborne intoxication, although the time to onset of paralytic symptoms may actually be longer than for foodborne cases and may vary by type and dose of toxin. The clinical syndrome produced by one or more of these toxins is known as botulism. Although an aerosol attack is by far the most likely scenario for the use of botulinum toxins, theoretically the agent could be used to sabotage food supplies. Enemy special forces or terrorists might use this method in certain scenarios to produce foodborne botulism in their targets.

The botulinum toxins are among the most toxic compounds known. Table 28-4 shows the comparative lethality in laboratory mice of selected toxins and chemical agents. Botulinum toxin is the most toxic compound per weight of agent, requiring only 0.001 μg per kilogram of body weight to kill 50% of the animals challenged.[65] As a group, bacterial toxins such as botulinum tend to be the most lethal of all toxins. Note that botulinum toxin is 15,000 times more toxic than VX and 100,000 times more toxic than sarin, two of the well-known organophosphate nerve agents.

Botulinum toxins act by binding to the presynaptic nerve terminal at the neuromuscular junction and at cholinergic autonomic sites.[66] These toxins then act to prevent the release of acetylcholine presynaptically and thus block neurotransmission. This interruption of neurotransmission causes both bulbar palsies and the skeletal muscle weakness seen in clinical botulism. Unlike the situation with nerve-agent intoxication, where there is in effect too much acetylcholine because of inhibition of acetylcholinesterase, the problem in botulism is lack of the neurotransmitter in the synapse. Thus, pharmacological measures such as atropine are not helpful in botulism and could even exacerbate symptoms.

The onset of symptoms of inhalation botulism may range from 24 to 36 hours to several days following exposure.[67] Bulbar palsies are prominent early, as are eye symptoms (eg, blurred vision due to mydriasis, diplopia, ptosis, photophobia) and other bulbar signs (eg, dysarthria, dysphonia, dysphagia). Skeletal muscle paralysis follows, with a symmetrical, descending, and progressive weakness that may culminate abruptly in respiratory failure. Progression from onset of symptoms to respiratory failure has occurred in as little as 24 hours in cases of foodborne botulism.

Physical examination usually reveals an alert and oriented patient without fever. Postural hypotension may be present. Mucous membranes may be dry and crusted, and the patient may complain of dry mouth or sore throat. There may be difficulty with speaking and swallowing, the gag reflex may be absent, and the pupils may be dilated and fixed. Ptosis and extraocular muscle palsies may also be observed. Variable degrees of skeletal muscle weakness may be observed depending on the degree of progression in an individual patient. Deep tendon reflexes may be present or absent. With severe respiratory muscle paralysis, the patient may become cyanotic or exhibit narcosis from carbon dioxide retention.

The occurrence of an epidemic of cases of a descending and progressive bulbar and skeletal paralysis in afebrile patients points to the diagnosis of botulinum intoxication. Numbers of cases in a theater of operations should raise at least the possibility of a biological warfare attack with aerosolized botulinum toxin. Foodborne outbreaks are theoretically possible in service members eating meals other than the standard meals-ready-to-eat (MRE) rations.

Individual cases might be confused clinically with other neuromuscular disorders such as Guillain-Barré syndrome, myasthenia gravis, or tick paralysis. The edrophonium (Tensilon) test may be transiently positive in botulism, so it may not distinguish botulinum intoxication from myasthenia. The cerebrospinal fluid in botulism is normal, and the paralysis is generally symmetrical, which distinguishes it from enteroviral myelitis. Mental status changes generally seen in viral encephalitis should not occur with botulinum intoxication.

It may become necessary to distinguish nerve agent or atropine poisoning from botulinum intoxication. Nerve agent poisoning produces copious respiratory secretions and miotic pupils, whereas there is, if anything, a decrease in secretions in botulinum intoxication. Atropine overdose is distinguished from botulism by its central nervous system excitation (eg, hallucinations, delirium) even though the mucous membranes are dry and mydriasis is present. The clinical differences between botulinum intoxication and nerve agent poisoning are listed in Table 28-5.

Laboratory testing is generally not helpful in the diagnosis of botulism. Survivors do not usually develop an antibody response due to the very small amount of toxin necessary to produce clinical symp-

TABLE 28-5

DIFFERENTIAL DIAGNOSIS OF CHEMICAL NERVE AGENT, BOTULINUM TOXIN, AND STAPHYLOCOCCAL ENTEROTOXIN B INTOXICATION FOLLOWING INHALATION EXPOSURE

	Chemical Nerve Agent (Organophosphate)	Botulinum Toxin	Staphylococcal Enterotoxin B
Time to symptoms	Minutes	Hours (12–48)	Hours (1–6)
Nervous system	Convulsions, muscle twitching	Progressive paralysis	Headache, muscle aches
Cardiovascular system	Slow heart rate	Normal rate	Normal or rapid heart rate
Respiratory system	Difficulty breathing, airways constriction	Normal, then progressive paralysis	Nonproductive cough, Severe cases: chest pain, difficulty breathing
Gastrointestinal system	Increased motility, pain, diarrhea	Decreased motility	Nausea, vomiting, diarrhea
Ocular	Small pupils	Droopy eyelids	May see "red eyes" (conjunctival injection)
Salivary system	Profuse, watery saliva	Normal, but swallowing difficult	May be slightly increased quantities of saliva
Death	Minutes	2–3 d	Unlikely
Responds to atropine/2PAM-Cl?	Yes	No	Atropine may reduce gastrointestinal symptoms

2PAM-Cl: pralidoxime chloride
Source: US Army Medical Research Institute of Infectious Diseases. *Medical Management of Biological Casualties Handbook*. Fort Detrick, Md: USAMRIID; 1998.

toms. Detection of toxin in serum or gastric contents is possible with a mouse neutralization assay, but it is the only test available and can be found only in specialized laboratories. If an aerosol attack with botulinum toxin is suspected, serum specimens should be drawn from suspected cases and held for testing at such a facility.

Respiratory failure secondary to paralysis of respiratory muscles is the most serious complication and usually the cause of death. Reported cases of botulism before 1950 had a mortality rate of 60%. With tracheostomy or endotracheal intubation and ventilatory assistance, fatalities should be less than 5%.[68] Intensive and prolonged nursing care may be required for recovery, which may take several weeks or even months.

Circulating toxin is present in isolated cases of foodborne botulism, perhaps due to continued absorption through the gut wall. Botulinum antitoxin (equine origin) has been used as an investigational new drug (IND) in those circumstances and is thought to be helpful. Animal experiments show that after aerosol exposure, botulinum antitoxin can

be very effective if given before the onset of clinical signs.[67] Administration of antitoxin is reasonable if disease has not progressed to a stable state. A trivalent equine antitoxin has been available from the CDC for cases of foodborne botulism. This product has all the disadvantages of a horse serum product, including the risks of anaphylaxis and serum sickness. An "especiated" equine heptavalent antitoxin (against types A, B, C, D, E, F, and G) is under advanced development but is available under IND status. Its efficacy is inferred from its performance in animal studies and compassionate use in infant botulinum intoxication.[4] Disadvantages include rapid clearance by immune elimination, as well as a theoretical risk of serum sickness. Sensitivity testing must be carried out for both products before administration, as is explained in the package insert.

For preexposure prevention, a pentavalent toxoid of *C botulinum* toxin types A, B, C, D, and E is also available under an IND status. This product has been administered to several thousand volunteers and occupationally at-risk workers and induces serum antitoxin levels that correspond to protective levels in experimental animal systems. The currently recommended schedule (ie, 0, 2, and 12 weeks, then a 1-year booster) induces protective antibody levels in greater than 90% of vaccinees after 1 year.[69] Adequate antibody levels are transiently induced after three injections, but decline before the 1-year booster. Contraindications to the vaccine include sensitivities to alum, formaldehyde, and thimerosal or hypersensitivity to a previous dose. Reactogenicity is mild, with 2% to 4% of vaccinees reporting erythema, edema, or induration at the site of injection that peaks at 24 to 48 hours, then dissipates. The frequency of such local reactions increases with each subsequent inoculation; after the second and third doses, 7% to 10% will have local reactions, with a higher incidence (up to 20%) after boosters. Severe local reactions consisting of more extensive edema or induration are rare. Up to 3% report systemic reactions, consisting of fever, malaise, headache, and myalgia. Incapacitating reactions (local or systemic) are uncommon. The vaccine should be stored at refrigerator temperatures and not frozen.

Three or more vaccine doses given by deep subcutaneous injection are recommended only to selected individuals or groups judged at high risk for exposure to botulinum toxin aerosols. There is no current indication for use of botulinum antitoxin prophylactically except under extremely specialized circumstances.

Staphylococcal Enterotoxins

Staphylococcus aureus produces a number of exotoxins, one of which (SEB) was weaponized and tested by the United States as part of its offensive program. SEB is very stable and causes illness with minute amounts of toxin exposure and therefore makes a good biological weapon. Other staphylococcal toxins, such as SEC, could also be weaponized.

SEB is a common cause of food poisoning in humans after ingestion of improperly handled food that has allowed production of toxin by the bacteria. Gastrointestinal manifestations, predominantly nausea and vomiting with occasional diarrhea, are the hallmark of intoxication after ingestion. After inhalation, SEB produces a markedly different clinical syndrome, but either method of intoxication causes significant morbidity. The incapacitating dose is several logarithms lower than the lethal dose and can cause illness and inability to perform the mission for 1 to 2 weeks.

The effects of staphylococcal enterotoxins are mediated by interactions with the host's own immune system. Toxins bind directly to the major histocompatibility complex and stimulate the proliferation of large numbers of T cell lymphocytes.[70] These so-called superantigens stimulate the secretion of various cytokines from immune system cells.[71] These cytokines mediate many of the toxic effects of SEB.

Symptoms of intoxication with SEB begin 3 to 12 hours after inhalation. The sudden onset of fever, chills, headache, myalgia, and nonproductive cough can be followed by dyspnea and retrosternal chest pain in more severe cases. If toxin has been ingested, nausea, vomiting, and diarrhea can occur and may produce significant fluid loss. High fever (39°C to 41°C) with chills and prostration can be present for up to 5 days. The cough can persist for up to 4 weeks, and patients may be incapacitated for 2 weeks.[53]

The diagnosis of SEB intoxication requires clinical and epidemiologic skill. Symptoms can be similar to other respiratory pathogens, such as influenza, adenovirus, and mycoplasma, and they must be included in the differential diagnosis. The physical exam is usually unremarkable, with possible conjunctival injection and postural hypotension if fluid losses have been significant. The chest radiograph is usually normal, but in severe cases may show pulmonary edema or an acute respiratory disease picture. Laboratory findings are not helpful with SEB intoxication. Typical signs of illness, such as a neutrophilic leukocytosis and elevated erythrocyte sedimentation rate, may be seen. While toxin is difficult to detect in serum, a specimen should be drawn for future analysis. Urine samples should also be tested, as toxin metabolites may accumulate in the urine. The toxin can be detected for 24 hours in nasal swabs after an aerosol exposure, and antibody can also be detected in convalescent serum.[53]

Treatment is currently limited to supportive care. Oxygenation and hydration must be monitored, and, in severe cases of pulmonary edema, positive end-expiratory pressure ventilation and diuretics may be needed. Most patients will recover fully in 1 to 2 weeks, although the cough may persist longer. There is no presently available vaccine, although a toxoid and several recombinant vaccines have potential for the future.[72]

Ricin

Ricin is a potent protein toxin derived from the beans of the castor plant (*Ricinus communis*). Its significance as a potential biological warfare toxin relates in part to its wide availability. Worldwide, 1 million tons of castor beans are processed annually in the production of castor oil; the waste mash from this process is approximately 5% ricin by weight. The toxin is quite stable and extremely toxic by several routes of exposure, including the respiratory route.

Ricin can be produced relatively easily and inexpensively in large quantities with fairly simple technology. It is of marginal toxicity in comparison with toxins such as botulinum, so an enemy would have to produce it in larger quantities to cover a significant area on the battlefield. This might limit large-scale use of ricin by an adversary. Ricin can be prepared in liquid or crystalline form, or it can be lyophilized to make it a dry powder. It could be disseminated by an enemy as an aerosol or used by saboteurs, assassins, or terrorists.

Ricin is very toxic to cells. It acts by inhibiting protein synthesis.[4] The clinical picture in intoxicated victims depends on the route of exposure. After aerosol exposure, signs and symptoms depend on the dose inhaled. Accidental sublethal aerosol exposures that occurred in humans in the 1940s were characterized by onset of the following symptoms in 4 to 8 hours: fever, chest tightness, cough, dyspnea, nausea, and arthralgias.[73] The onset of profuse sweating some hours later was commonly the sign of termination of most of the symptoms. Although lethal human aerosol exposures have not been described, the severe pathophysiological changes seen in the animal respiratory tract, including necrosis and severe alveolar flooding, are probably sufficient to cause death if enough toxin is inhaled. Time to death in experimental animals is dose dependent, occurring 36 to 72 hours after inhalation.[74] Humans would be expected to develop severe lung inflammation with progressive cough, dyspnea, cyanosis, and pulmonary edema.

By other routes of exposure, ricin is not a direct lung irritant, but intravascular injection can cause minimal pulmonary perivascular edema due to vascular endothelial injury. Ingestion causes gastrointestinal hemorrhage with hepatic, splenic, and renal necrosis. Intramuscular administration causes severe local necrosis of muscle and regional lymph nodes with moderate visceral organ involvement.[4]

An attack with aerosolized ricin would be diagnosed, as with many biological warfare agents, primarily by the clinical and epidemiologic setting. Acute lung injury affecting a large number of cases in a war zone where an attack could occur should raise suspicion of an attack with a pulmonary irritant such as ricin, although other pulmonary pathogens could present with similar signs and symptoms. Additional supportive clinical or diagnostic features after aerosol exposure to ricin may include the following: bilateral infiltrates on chest radiographs, arterial hypoxemia, neutrophilic leukocytosis, and a bronchial aspirate rich in protein compared to plasma, which is characteristic of high permeability pulmonary edema. Specific enzyme-linked immunosorbent assay testing on serum or immunohistochemical techniques for direct tissue analysis may be used where available to confirm the diagnosis. Ricin is an extremely immunogenic toxin, and acute and convalescent sera should be obtained from survivors for measurement of antibody response.[4]

Management of ricin-intoxicated patients depends on the route of exposure. Patients with pulmonary intoxication are given appropriate treatment for pulmonary edema and respiratory support as indicated. Gastrointestinal intoxication is best managed by vigorous gastric decontamination with lavage and superactivated charcoal, followed by use of cathartics such as magnesium citrate. Volume replacement of gastrointestinal fluid losses is important. In percutaneous exposures, treatment is primarily supportive.

When worn correctly, the military's protective mask is effective in preventing aerosol exposure. Although a vaccine is not currently available, candidate vaccines are under development that are immunogenic and confer protection against lethal aerosol exposures in animals.[4] Prophylaxis with such a vaccine is the most promising defense against a biological warfare attack with ricin.

EPIDEMIOLOGY AS A DETECTION TOOL

The understanding of agent characteristics, diagnosis, and treatment is important in effectively responding to a biological attack. However, the health care provider must also think like an epidemiologist to achieve an advantage over an intentional, or even naturally occurring, outbreak of disease. Through the knowledge and application of basic epidemiologic principles, a biological warfare or terrorist attack can be quickly detected and effective preventive and treatment measures instituted to save lives.

A biological attack can be overt (with an announcement of the release of an agent) or covert (with no notice that an agent has been released). The overt attack, which includes hoaxes, will cause profound, immediate psychological manifestations and raise the questions of how to verify the attack

---

EXHIBIT 28-1

EPIDEMIOLOGIC CLUES FOR A BIOLOGIC WARFARE OR TERRORIST ATTACK

- The presence of a large epidemic with a similar disease or syndrome, especially in a discrete population
- Many cases of unexplained diseases or deaths
- More severe disease than is usually expected for a specific pathogen or failure to respond to usual therapy
- Unusual routes of exposure for a pathogen, such as inhalation anthrax
- A disease that is unusual for a given geographic area or transmission season
- Disease normally transmitted by a vector that is not present in that area
- Multiple simultaneous epidemics of different diseases in the same population
- A single case of disease by an uncommon agent (smallpox, some viral hemorrhagic fevers)
- A disease that is unusual for an age group
- Unusual strains or variants of organisms or antimicrobial resistance patterns differ from those circulating
- Similar genetic type among agents isolated from distinct sources at different times or locations
- Higher attack rates in those exposed in certain areas, such as inside a building if released indoors, or lower rates in those inside a sealed building if released outside
- Disease outbreaks of the same illness occurring in noncontiguous areas
- A disease outbreak with zoonotic impact
- Intelligence of a potential attack, claims by a terrorist or aggressor of a release, and findings of munitions or tampering

---

and what preventive measures to take, such as decontamination, quarantine, vaccination, and prophylaxis. The covert attack presents more difficulties, both in recognizing an attack and in rapidly and effectively responding to it. The covert attack is where the epidemiologic clues are most important. These clues are listed in Exhibit 28-1.

Because the medical effects of biological warfare and terrorism may mimic many endemic diseases, medical personnel will have to be extremely alert to differentiate the initial cases resulting from natural disease. The range of causes of an outbreak needs to be considered. The possibilities include a spontaneous outbreak of a known endemic disease, a spontaneous outbreak of a new or reemerging disease, a laboratory accident, or an intentional attack with a biological agent. Use of the epidemiologic clues can assist in this differentiation.

Once a biological attack or any outbreak of disease is suspected, the epidemiologic investigation should begin. The first step is to confirm that a disease outbreak has occurred. A case definition should be constructed to determine the number of cases and the attack rate. The case definition allows investigators who are separated geographically to use the same criteria when evaluating the outbreak. The use of objective criteria in the development of a case definition is very important in determining an accurate case number, as additional cases may be found and some cases may be excluded, especially as the potential exists for hysteria to be confused with actual disease. The estimated rate of illness should be compared with rates during previous years to determine if the rate constitutes a deviation from the norm.

Once the attack rate has been determined, the outbreak can be described by time, place, and person. These data will provide crucial information in determining the potential source of the outbreak. The epidemic curve is calculated based on cases over time. In a point-source outbreak, which is most likely in a biological attack or terrorism situation, the early parts of the epidemic curve will tend to be compressed compared with propagated outbreaks. The peak may be in a matter of days or even hours. Later phases of the curve may also help determine if the disease appears to spread from person to person, which can be extremely important in instituting effective disease control measures.

Early recognition of a disease outbreak through prior knowledge of disease rates, a good surveillance system, and a quick epidemiologic investigation can allow prompt institution of prophylactic antibiotic therapy (eg, for anthrax, plague) or vaccination (eg, for smallpox), which could save thousands who are still incubating infections and prevent the spread of contagious organisms. It can also help allocate scarce military and public sector resources and enable military and political leaders to reduce panic through disseminating accurate information.

PUBLIC HEALTH PREPAREDNESS

Especially in civilian settings, it will be the physician and the medical facility, probably not the emergency responders, who will face the initial shock of a biological attack. Medical personnel must be prepared for this possibility, just as with any other public health disaster or disease outbreak.

First of all, medical personnel need to be trained to recognize and treat casualties of biological warfare or terrorism. They must be able to apply appropriate preventive measures rationally and without unnecessary panic or alarm. All members of the hospital team need to be trained, including engineering personnel, to establish improvised containment if necessary.

A Bioterrorism Readiness Plan should be prepared for all military and civilian medical facilities similar to the Federal Response Plan for disasters, with details for management of both overt and covert attacks and with phone numbers of both internal and external contacts.[75] Important contacts include the hospital infection control activity, the preventive medicine office, the local and state health departments, the CDC, and the Federal Bureau of Investigation. A plan should also be prepared for field and overseas military situations.

Well before any event, public health authorities must implement surveillance systems so they can recognize patterns of nonspecific syndromes that could indicate the early manifestations of a biological warfare attack. The system must be timely, sensitive, specific, and practical. But it is difficult for medical advisors to know if a disease outbreak is consistent with a biological warfare or terrorism attack or an endemic disease outbreak unless background rates of disease for an area are known. A theater, installation, or municipal epidemiologic surveillance program therefore must be specifically tailored to both the mission and the geographical area and must allow for specific, diagnosable disease entities and syndromes (eg, influenza-like syndromes). Regular and rapid analysis of syndromic epidemiologic surveillance data may provide the first clue that an attack has occurred. These data may be based on standard disease rates or more nontraditional sources such as laboratory test requests, pharmaceutical sales, or emergency services calls (Exhibit 28-2). As medical systems and records become more automated, extraction and rapid analysis of these data should become more routine. Such information can provide invaluable data to focus response activities, allocate scarce resources, and contain panic.

The possibility of psychological consequences and the need for mental health preparedness should not be overlooked. Following a biological attack, potential psychological responses include anger, panic, fear, paranoia, demoralization, and a loss of faith in social organizations.[76] If quarantine or rationing of medical supplies is needed, even more disruption of usual social supports can occur. As medical personnel are not immune to these psychological reactions, they must be prepared. This emphasizes the importance of realistic training. Training of medical responders will need to include rec-

---

EXHIBIT 28-2

POSSIBLE SURVEILLANCE DATA TO DETECT AN EMERGING DISEASE OR BIOLOGICAL WARFARE OR TERRORISM

- Traditional reportable diseases from clinicians
- Unexplained deaths
- Intensive care unit admissions
- Syndromic groupings of diseases not based on specific diagnoses (eg, respiratory, gastrointestinal, neurological, fever)
- 911 or emergency calls for conditions such as respiratory distress
- Pharmaceutical usage rates and use of prescription, over-the-counter, and investigational new drugs
- Laboratory test ordering (eg, stool cultures)
- Laboratory results for specific diseases
- Radiological test ordering (eg, chest radiographs)
- Veterinary surveillance
- School absenteeism
- Billing and insurance data
- Internet access of health websites

ognizing the symptoms of anxiety, depression, and dissociation. Plans should be in place to prevent or mitigate stress for both the affected population and the responders.[76] One important way to decrease fear and panic is effective risk communication, and every hospital should be prepared to provide accurate and timely information to the public. Protocols should be developed covering a broad range of scenarios to prevent panic in the community or the military units affected. Through careful planning and preparation, some of the terror involved in a biological attack can be diminished.

Diagnostic capacities should be determined for each hospital or field location. Most standard hospital laboratories can provide a significant amount of support, especially for bacteriology, with traditional culture, staining, and sensitivity capabilities. However, there are many agents that cannot be identified in routine laboratories. It is important to know where the closest reference laboratory is located, whether it is civilian or military, and how to request its assistance if necessary. Many state health departments have the capability to diagnose many biological threat agents. Specialized laboratories, such as at the CDC and at the US Army Medical Research Institute of Infectious Diseases, Fort Detrick, Md, can also provide confirmatory and reference laboratory services. There has been an increase in handheld and rapid detection and diagnostic devices, but the sensitivity and specificity of these diagnostic tools are still in question, and a sample must be sent to an appropriate laboratory. Any clinical information that can be obtained will assist the laboratory in making a rapid and accurate diagnosis. Advance planning to identify appropriate packaging materials and how to coordinate specimen transport should also be done (see Chapter 34, Laboratory Support for Infectious Disease Investigations in the Field).

Infection control practices in the hospital must be planned before a biological attack occurs. Most traditional agents are not transmitted from person to person, with the two major exceptions being smallpox and pneumonic plague. Both of these diseases will require that the patient be isolated until he or she is no longer infectious. Persons affected by most other traditional agents can be managed by health care providers using standard precautions, to include handwashing, wearing gloves when touching blood or any body fluids, and wearing masks, eye protection, and gowns if splashes may occur.[75]

Decontamination of persons after exposure depends on the suspected agent and in most cases is not necessary. The goal of decontamination is to reduce the contamination and to prevent further spread of the agent. Most biological agents are not dermally active and do not form secondary aerosols so are not likely to be a hazard to the patient or the medical staff once the original aerosol has dispersed. Decisions regarding decontamination of persons should be made in consultation with public health personnel. Depending on the intensity of contamination, clothing of the patient may need to be removed and placed in a sealed biohazard bag. Patients should then shower with soap and water, including washing their hair, to remove any residual agent. Bathing patients with bleach solutions can be harmful and is not necessary. Bleach is an excellent way to decontaminate any grossly contaminated equipment and material or any areas known to have come in contact with the agent.

It is important to remember that preparation for a biological attack is similar to that for any disease outbreak, but the surveillance, response, and other demands on resources would likely be of an unparalleled intensity. A strong public health infrastructure is truly a dual-use way to control diseases from either source, whether they are naturally occurring or otherwise.

ENVIRONMENTAL OR ATMOSPHERIC DETECTION OF BIOLOGICAL WARFARE AGENTS

Adequate and accurate intelligence is required to develop an effective defense against biological warfare. Once an agent has been dispersed, detection of the biological aerosol before its arrival over the target in time for personnel to don protective equipment would be an important way to minimize or prevent casualties. However, not until the late 1990s were interim systems of detecting biological agents fielded in limited numbers. Until reliable detectors are available in sufficient numbers, the first indication of a biological attack in unprotected service members may well be the ill individual.

This is even more likely in a civilian setting.

Detector systems are evolving and represent an area of intense interest with the highest priorities within the military research and development community. One of the first systems fielded was the Biological Integrated Detection System. This is vehicle-mounted and can test environmental air samples by concentrating appropriate aerosol particle sizes in the air samples, then subjecting the sample to both generic and antibody-based detection for selected agents. The Long-Range Standoff Detection System is being developed to provide a biological standoff detection capability and, it is hoped, early warning. It employs an infrared laser to detect aerosol clouds at a distance of up to 30 km, with plans to extend the range to 100 km. This system will be available for fixed-site applications or inserted into various transport platforms, such as fixed-wing or rotary aircraft. The other standoff detection system that is currently in the research and development phase is the Short-Range Biological Standoff Detection System. It will employ an ultraviolet- and laser-induced fluorescence to detect biological aerosol clouds at distances of up to 5 km. The information will be used to provide early warning, enhance contamination avoidance efforts, and cue other detection assets.[77]

The principal difficulties in detecting biological agent aerosols are timeliness, false positives, and differentiating the artificially generated biological warfare cloud from the background of organic matter normally present in the atmosphere. Therefore, the aforementioned detection methods must be used in conjunction with medical protection (eg, surveillance, vaccines, other prophylactic measures), intelligence, and physical protection to provide service members layered primary defenses against a biological attack.

SUMMARY

The threat of a battlefield or terrorist attack with a biological agent is real. It is known that several potential adversaries of the United States have worked on or are continuing to explore the offensive use of biological weapons. All military medical personnel should have a solid understanding of the biological threat, how to recognize an attack, and the medical options for defending against that attack. The potential for devastating casualties is high for certain biological agents. With appropriate use of medical countermeasures either already developed or under development, however, many casualties can be prevented or minimized.

REFERENCES

1. Stockholm International Peace Research Institute. *The Rise of CB Weapons*. Vol 1. In: *The Problem of Chemical and Biological Warfare*. New York: Humanities Press; 1971.

2. Christopher GW, Cieslak TJ, Pavlin JA, Eitzen EM. Biological warfare: A historical perspective. *JAMA*. 1997;278:412–417.

3. Rothschild JH. *Tomorrow's Weapons*. New York: McGraw-Hill; 1964.

4. Franz DR, Zajtchuk R. Biological terrorism: Understanding the threat, preparation and medical response. *Dis Mon*. 2000;46(2):125–190.

5. Robertson AG, Robertson LJ. From asps to allegations: biological warfare in history. *Mil Med*. 1995;160:369–373.

6. Geissler E, ed. *Biological and Toxin Weapons Today*. Oxford, England: Oxford University Press, Stockholm International Peace Research Institute; 1986.

7. Williams P, Wallace D. *Unit 731: Japan's Secret Biological Warfare in World War II*. New York: The Free Press (Macmillan, Inc.); 1998.

8. Hersh SM. *Chemical and Biological Warfare: America's Hidden Arsenal*. Indianapolis, Ind: Bobbs-Merrill; 1968.

9. Harris SH. *Factories of Death*. New York: Routledge; 1994.

10. Tomilin VV, Berezhnoi RV. Exposure of criminal activity of the Japanese military authorities regarding preparation for bacteriological warfare [in Russian]. *Voen Med Zh*. 1985;8:26–29.

11. Cole LA. *Clouds of Secrecy: The Army's Germ Warfare Tests Over Populated Areas*. Totowa, NJ: Rowman and Littlefield; 1988.

12. Manchee R, Stewart W. The decontamination of Gruinard Island. *Chem Br*. 1988;July:690–691.

13. World Health Organization Group of Consultants. *Health Aspects of Chemical and Biological Weapons*. Geneva: WHO; 1970. Report.

14. Bailey KC. *Doomsday Weapons in the Hands of Many: The Arms Control Challenge of the 90's*. Chicago: University of Illinois Press; 1991.

15. Carus WS. *Bioterrorism and Biocrimes: The Illicit Use of Biological Agents in the 20th Century*. Washington, DC: Center for Counterproliferation Research, National Defense University; November 1998 revision. Working Paper.

16. Defense Intelligence Agency. *Soviet Biological Warfare Threat*. Washington, DC: Department of Defense, DIA; 1986. DST-1610F-057–86.

17. Smith JR. Yeltsin blames '79 anthrax on germ warfare efforts. *Washington Post*. June 16, 1992: A1.

18. Meselson M, Guillemin J, Hugh-Jones M, et al. The Sverdlovsk anthrax outbreak of 1979, *Science*. 1994;266:1202–1208.

19. Alibek K. *Biohazard: The Chilling True Story of the Largest Covert Biological Weapons Program in the World: Told from the Inside by the Man Who Ran It*. New York: Random House; 1999.

20. Carus WS. *Bioterrorism and Biocrimes: The Illicit Use of Biological Agents in the 20th Century*. Washington, DC: Center for Counterproliferation Research, National Defense University: July 1999 (revision). Working Paper.

21. Crompton R, Gall D. Georgi Markov: Death in a pellet. *Med Leg J*. 1980;48:51–62.

22. Livingstone NC, Douglass JD. *CBW: The Poor Man's Atomic Bomb*. Cambridge, Mass: Institute for Foreign Policy Analysis, Inc.; 1984.

23. Seeley TD, Nowicke JW, Meselson M, Guilleman J, Akratanakkul P. Yellow rain. *Sci Am*. 1985;253(3):128–137.

24. United Nations Security Council. *Report of the Secretary General on the Status of the Implementation of the Special Commission's Plan for the Ongoing Monitoring and Verification of Iraq's Compliance with Relevant Parts of Section C of Security Council Resolution 687 (1991)*. New York: United Nations; October 11, 1995. Publication S/1995/864.

25. Zilinskas RA. Iraq's biological weapons: the past as future? *JAMA*. 1997;278:418–424.

26. US Government White Paper. *Iraqi Weapons of Mass Destruction Programs*. February 13, 1998.

27. Block SM. Living nightmares: Biological threats enabled by molecular biology. In: Drell SD, Sofaer AD, Wilson GD, eds. *The New Terror: Facing the Threat of Biological and Chemical Weapons*. Stanford, Calif: Hoover Institution Press, Stanford University; 1999.

28. Statement by Director of Central Intelligence George J. Tenet Before the Senate Foreign Relations Committee on the Worldwide Threat in 2000: Global Realities of Our National Security. 21 March 2000. As prepared for delivery.

29. Bozheyeva G, Kunakbayev Y, Yeleukenov D. *Former Soviet Biological Weapons Facilities in Kazakhstan: Past, Present, and Future*. Monterey, Calif: Monterey Institute of International Studies, Center for Nonproliferation Studies; June 1999. Occasional Paper No. 1.

30. US General Accounting Office, National Security and International Affairs Division. Biological Weapons: *Effort to Reduce Former Soviet Threat Offers Benefits, Poses New Risks*. Washington, DC: GAO/NSIAD: 2000. GAO/NSIAD-00-138.

31. Henderson DA. The looming threat of bioterrorism. *Science*. 1999;283:1279–1282.

32. Miller J. U.S. helps Russia turn germ center to peace uses. *New York Times*. January 8, 2000: A3.

33. Alibek K. Statement before the Joint Economic Committee. United States Congress. May 20, 1998.

34. Committee on Armed Services, House of Representatives. *Special Inquiry into the Chemical and Biological Threat: Countering the Chemical and Biological Weapons Threat in the Post-Soviet World.* Washington, DC: US Government Printing Office; 23 February 1993. Report to the Congress.

35. Chemical and bacteriological weapons in the 1980s. *Lancet.* 1984;2:141–143.

36. Takafuji ET, Johnson-Winegar A, Zajtchuk R. Medical challenges in chemical and biological defense for the 21st century. In: Sidell FR, Takafuji ET, Franz DR, eds. *Medical Aspects of Chemical and Biological Warfare.* Part 1, Vol 5. In: *Textbook of Military Medicine.* Washington, DC: Office of the Surgeon General, US Department of the Army, and the Borden Institute; 1997.

37. Spertzel RO, Wannemacher RW, Linden CD. *Biological Weapons Proliferation.* Fort Detrick, Md: US Army Medical Research Institute of Infectious Diseases; 1993. Defense Nuclear Agency Report DNA-TR-92–116.

38. Roberts B. *Biological Weapons: Weapons of the Future?* Washington, DC: The Center for Strategic and International Studies; 1993.

39. Huxsoll DL. The nature and scope of the BW threat. In: Bailey KC, ed. *Director's Series on Proliferation.* Livermore, Calif: Lawrence Livermore National Laboratory; 1994. UCRL-LR-114070-4.

40. Leskov S; Kovan V, trans. Military bacteriological programs in Russia and USA are strictly secretive and represent terrible threat to the world. *Izvestiya.* June 26, 1993: 15.

41. Douglass JD Jr, Livingston NC. *America the Vulnerable: The Threat of Chemical and Biological Warfare.* Lexington, Mass: Lexington Books; 1987.

42. Iraq's growing threat. *Boston Globe.* Feb 13, 2000; E6. Editorial.

43. Bermudez JS. Asia, exposing the North Korean BW arsenal. *Jane's Intelligence Rev.* 1998;10(8):28.

44. Fialka JJ. CIA says North Korea appears active in biological, nuclear arms. *Wall Street Journal.* February 25, 1993: A10.

45. Tucker JB. Historical trends related to bioterrorism: An empirical analysis. *Emerg Inf Dis.* 1999;5:498–504.

46. Torok TJ, Tauxe RV, Wise RP, et al. A large community outbreak of salmonellosis caused by intentional contamination of restaurant salad bars. *JAMA.* 1997;278:389–395.

47. Perlman D. Russia accused of violating pact with secrecy on its germ weapons: Major nations, not terrorists or loonies, called biggest threat. *San Francisco Chronicle.* February 19, 2000: A14.

48. Patrick WC 3d. Biological Warfare: An overview. In: Bailey KC, ed. *Director's Series on Proliferation.* Livermore, Calif: Lawrence Livermore National Laboratory; 1994. UCRL-LR-114070-4.

49. Department of the Army. *NATO Handbook on the Medical Aspects of NBC Defensive Operations: Biological.* Washington, DC: DA; 1996. Field Manual 8-9.

50. Zilinskas RA. Terrorism and biological weapons: Inevitable alliance? *Perspect Biol Med.* 1990;34(1):44–72.

51. Arita I. Virological evidence for the success of the smallpox eradication programme. *Nature.* 1979;279:293–298.

52. Fenner F, Henderson DA, Arita I, Jezek Z, Ladnyi ID. *Smallpox and Its Eradication.* Geneva: World Health Organization; 1988.

53. Franz DR, Jahrling PB, Friedlander AM, et al. Clinical recognition and management of patients exposed to biological warfare agents. *JAMA.* 1997;278:399–411.

54. Downie AW, St Vincent L, Meiklejohn G, et al. Studies on the virus content of mouth washings in the acute phase of smallpox. *Bull World Health Organ.* 1961;25:49–53.

55. Sarkar JK, Mitra AC, Mukherjee MK, De SK, Mazumdar DG. Virus excretion in smallpox. *Bull World Health Organ.* 1973;48:517–522.

56. Mitra AC, Sarkar JK, Mukherjee MK. Virus content of smallpox scabs. *Bull World Health Organ.* 1974;51:106–107.

57. Zdenek J. *Human Monkeypox.* Basel, Switzerland: S Karger; 1988.

58. Jezek A, Fenner F. Human monkeypox. *Virol Monogr.* 1988;17:93–95.

59. Human monkeypox—Kasai Oriental, Zaire 1996–1997. *MMWR.* 1997;46:304–307.

60. Sarkar JK, Mitra AC, Mukherjee MK, De SK. Virus excretion in smallpox, 2: Excretion in the throats of household contacts. *Bull World Health Organ.* 1973;48:523–527.

61. Kato S, Takahashi M, Kameyama S, Kamehora J. A study on the morphological and cyto-immunological relationship between the inclusions of variola, cowpox, rabbitpox, vaccinia (variola origin) and vaccinia IHD and consideration of the term "Guarneri body." *Biken J.* 1959;2:353–363.

62. Ibrahim MS, Esposito JJ, Jahrling PB, Lofts RS. The potential of 5' nuclease PCR for detecting a single-base polymorphism in orthopoxvirus. *Mol Cell Probes.* 1997;11:143–147.

63. Wehrle PF, Posch J, Richter KH, Henderson DA. An airborne oubreak of smallpox in a German hospital and its significance with respect to other recent outbreaks in Europe. *Bull World Health Organ.* 1970;43:669–679.

64. Henderson DA, Moss B. Smallpox and vaccinia. In: Plotkin SA, Orenstein WA, eds. *Vaccines.* 3rd ed. Philadelphia: WB Saunders; 1999: 74–97.

65. Gill DM. Bacterial toxins: a table of lethal amounts. *Microbiol Rev.* 1982;46:86–94.

66. Simpson LL. Peripheral actions of the botulinum toxins. In: Simpson LL, ed. *Botulinum Neurotoxin and Tetanus Toxin.* New York: Academic Press Inc; 1989: 153–178.

67. Franz DR, Pitt LM, Clayton MA, Hanes MA, Rose KJ. Efficacy of prophylactic and therapeutic administration of antitoxin for inhalation botulism. In: Das Gupta B, ed. *Botulinum and Tetanus Neurotoxins and Biomedical Aspects.* New York: Plenum Press; 1993: 473–476.

68. Chin J, ed. *Control of Communicable Diseases Manual.* 17th ed. Washington, DC: American Public Health Association; 2000: 70–75.

69. Middlebrook JL. Contributions of the U.S. Army to botulinum toxin research. In: Das Gupta B, ed. *Botulinum and Tetanus Neurotoxins and Biomedical Aspects.* New York: Plenum Press; 1993: 515–519.

70. Kappler J, Kotzin B, Herron L, et al. V beta-specific stimulation of human T cells by staphylococcal toxins. *Science.* 1989;244:811–813.

71. Stiles BG, Bavari S, Krakauer T, Ulrich RG. Toxicity of staphylococcal enterotoxins potentiated by lipopolysaccharide. *Infect Immun.* 1993;61:5333–5338.

72. Bavari S, Olson MA, Ulrich RG. Engineered bacterial superantigen vaccines. In: Brown F, Norrby E, Burton D, Mekalonos J. *Vaccines 96.* Cold Spring Harbor, NY: Cold Spring Harbor Laboratory Press; 1996:135–141.

73. Brugsch HG. Toxic hazards: The castor bean. *Mass Med Soc.* 1960;262:1039–1040.

74. Wilhelmsen C, Pitt L. Lesions of acute inhaled lethal ricin intoxication in rhesus monkeys. *Vet Pathol.* 1996;33:296–302.

75. Association for Professionals in Infection Control and Epidemiology (APIC) Bioterrorism Task Force, CDC Hospital Infections Program Bioterrorism Working Group. *Bioterrorism Readiness Plan: A Template for Healthcare Facilities.* APIC: 1999. Available at www.apic.org/html/educ/readinow.html.

76. Holloway HC, Norwood AE, Fullerton CS, Engel CC, Ursano RJ. The threat of biological weapons: prophylaxis and mitigation of psychological and social consequences. *JAMA*. 1997;278:428–430.

77. Ezzell J. Acting Chief, Special Pathogens Branch, Diagnostics Systems Division, US Army Medical Research Institute of Infectious Diseases, Fort Detrick, Md. Personal communication, November 1995.

Chapter 29

MEDICAL RESPONSE TO INJURY FROM IONIZING RADIATION

DORIS BROWNE, MD, MPH

D. Browne, Colonel, Medical Corps, US Army (Retired); President and Chief Executive Officer, Browne and Associates, Inc., Washington, DC; formerly, Director, Medical Research and Development, US Army Medical Research and Materiel Command, Fort Detrick, Frederick, Maryland 21702

INTRODUCTION

Military medical health care providers need to be familiar with the health effects of radiation exposure and the other devastating effects of a nuclear explosion or accident. At the same time that superpowers are dismantling nuclear bombs, smaller powers are building nuclear arsenals, and radiation exposure scenarios include those involving low-yield nuclear devices deployed by terrorists and accidents during transportation or dismantlement of weapons. Even without bombs, there is an increasing chance of radiation exposure from sources such as nuclear power plants, research facilities, and hospitals. The potential also exists for exposure from depleted uranium munitions; industrial, hospital, and research waste sites; and directed energy devices. Military medical preparedness is important to meet the operational challenges presented by these scenarios. Since the late 1940s, nuclear weapon proliferation has continued to pose a global threat and one for which military medical personnel must train and plan. This new operational environment requires a review of the US military's medical policies, equipment, and research requirements.

HISTORY OF NUCLEAR WEAPONS

In the United States, the development of nuclear weapons grew out of concern in the 1930s that Germany was developing a nuclear weapon. The start of World War II, with the Japanese attack on Pearl Harbor and the German and Italian declaration of war on the United States in December 1941, increased the impetus for the United States to develop its own nuclear weapon. The program to develop a bomb was under way by the fall of 1942. To supply the materials needed, the US government secretly started a massive project to manufacture uranium in three plants and plutonium in a fourth. The first three nuclear weapons were detonated in 1945,[1] the first in a test in the New Mexico desert and the second and third over the Japanese cities of Hiroshima and Nagasaki. The devastation from these detonations brought an end to the war and a realization of the overwhelming challenges that nuclear detonations or accidents present to medical providers. The single detonation in Hiroshima caused about 45,000 deaths and more than 90,000 casualties during the first 24 hours. The medical system could not handle the massive number of casualties because most medical treatment facilities and personnel were destroyed in the detonation.[2]

In subsequent years, the nuclear capability of the superpowers became overwhelming. As the years passed and the threat of a nuclear confrontation grew, efforts to restrain the use of nuclear weapons also grew. A nuclear nonproliferation agreement was signed[3] and included most, but not all, countries with nuclear capabilities. At the end of the Cold War, the United States and the Union of Soviet Socialist Republics initiated a disarmament program to decrease the stockpile of nuclear weapons. While nuclear weapons detonation from a theater or strategic nuclear confrontation is now much less likely to occur, the threat of a detonation from a terrorist group or an accident in one of the many industries that uses radioactive material is a growing concern.

BIOLOGICAL EFFECTS OF NUCLEAR WEAPONS

The radiation referred to in this chapter is ionizing radiation. Ionizing radiation can be divided into two categories, particulate and nonparticulate radiation. The most important types of particulate radiation are alpha, beta, and neutron; the nonparticulate types would be gamma rays and roentgen rays (Table 29-1).[4]

Alpha particles are helium atoms without their electrons. They are unable to penetrate the outer layer of the skin. Alpha radiation poses no external hazard but becomes hazardous if it enters wounds or body orifices. Internal contamination with alpha radiation is a significant long-term health hazard.

Beta particles are similar to electrons but come from the nucleus of the atom. They travel several meters in air and are capable of penetrating several centimeters into the skin. They represent a cutaneous radiation hazard and internal contamination hazard if deposited into deep-lying organs.

Neutrons are one of the uncharged particles in the nucleus of the atom. They are not directly ionizing but can penetrate the body and interact with body water, producing recoil protons that release energy by excitation and ionization. Neutrons are effectively shielded by hydrogenous material such as water and plastics.

Gamma rays are photons that travel great distances at the speed of light and can penetrate deeply into body tissues. The acute radiation syndrome is

TABLE 29-1

CHARACTERISTICS OF NUCLEAR RADIATIONS

Name	Emitted By	Range in Air	Tissue Penetration	Radiation Stopped By
Alpha	Unfissioned uranium and plutonium	5 cm	First layer of skin	Clothing, paper
Beta	Fission products	12 m	Several layers of skin	Clothing
Gamma	Fission products	100 m	Total body	Several feet of concrete, earth, water, or plastic
Neutron	Emitted only during fission	100 m	Total body	Several feet of concrete, earth, water, or plastic

Adapted from: Luckett LW, Vesper BE. Radiological considerations in medical operations. In: Walker RI, Cerveny TJ, eds. *Medical Consequences of Nuclear Warfare*. In: *Textbook of Military Medicine*. Washington, DC: Department of the Army, Office of the Surgeon General, Borden Institute; 1989: Table 10-1, p 229.

largely a result of significant exposure to gamma and roentgen rays. Shields for gamma rays are made of high-density concrete or lead.

The two major radioisotopes used in nuclear weapons are plutonium-239 and uranium-235. Plutonium emits alpha, beta, and gamma radiation. The type of radioactive exposure in a nonexplosive weapons accident is likely to be alpha radiation. The quantity present does not usually cause a significant external radiation hazard; contamination through intact skin results in little, if any, absorption. Internal exposure is another matter. The two major routes of internal exposure are through inhalation and wound contamination. The critical organs for systemic contamination are the bones and the lungs. Whole-body retention of internalized plutonium is detectable in body tissues for about 200 years, in the skeleton for 100 years, and in liver tissue for 40 years.

The primary physical effects associated with a nuclear detonation are blast, thermal radiation, and nuclear radiation. Each of these can cause injury and death. Burn injuries may occur alone or in combination with blast and radiation injuries. The production of blast and thermal injuries depends on the distance from ground zero of the casualty and the yield of the weapon. In a nuclear theater, the yield of a nuclear weapon is likely to be between 10 and 100 kilotons; the ranges for blast, thermal, and radiation injuries are likely to be similar.[4] The distance from ground zero for production of injuries that are fatal to half of those exposed is given in Table 29-2.

Blast Injuries

Blast injuries are either direct or indirect. Direct injuries result from high pressures of the blast wave (also called static overpressure), and indirect injuries result from missiles and displacement of the body by the blast winds (called dynamic overpressure). Following a nuclear weapon detonation, energy will be generated from the blast effects of the detonation and becomes the blast wave as it moves out from the blast center. A nuclear detonation also has a relatively long pressure pulse, which is more effective in causing blast injuries than a conventional weapon detonation. This blast wave produces

TABLE 29-2

THE DISTANCE (m) FROM DIFFERING SIZES OF NUCLEAR EXPLOSIONS THAT WILL PRODUCE INJURIES THAT KILL HALF THE PERSONS EXPOSED

Injuries	Weapon Yield (kilotons)			
	0.5	10	100	1,000
Static overpressure: 6 psi*	380	1,000	2,200	4,600
Thermal: 2 degree burns	580	2,100	5,500	14,500
Radiation: 500 cGy†	700	1,200	1,700	2,400

*pounds per square inch
†centigray
Source: Giambarresi L. Nuclear weapons: Medical effects and operational considerations. *7th MEDCOM Med Bull.* 1986;43(7):7–10.

injuries by exerting a crushing effect that engulfs the human body. The rate of increase of pressure is too rapid for the body to compensate, leading to large pressure differentials and resulting injuries. These static overpressure injuries include eardrum rupture, lacerations in alveoli and pulmonary vessels leading to pulmonary edema, superficial peritoneal hematomas, rupture of the liver and spleen, and intestinal perforations. Abdominal injuries resulting from static overpressure can occur in conjunction with thoracic injuries or by themselves. In the ileum, cecum, and colon there may be segmental perforations of the intestinal wall that result in peritonitis. This type of intestinal injury is more commonly seen in underwater blast injuries.

Indirect blast injuries from a nuclear detonation are similar to those of conventional weapons. The missile and displacement injuries from the blast wind of a nuclear detonation are products of lower overpressures than injuries from the blast wave. Injuries resulting from dynamic overpressures may be caused by the physical displacement of persons by winds and by impact injuries.[4] The relationship between static overpressure and dynamic overpressure wind velocities is shown in Exhibit 29-1.

Thermal Injuries

Of the wide spectrum of energies resulting from a detonation of a nuclear weapon, 35% is thermal energy. Thermal radiation causes direct burn injuries (ie, radiant energy absorbed by the skin) and indirect burn injuries (ie, ignition or heating of clothing by fires started by the radiation). The energies that cause these injuries are infrared radiation and visible light. Burns from infrared radiation are the most frequently seen injury. The burns are classified as flash burns or flame burns. Flash burns are caused by the direct effect of short pulses of thermal energy being absorbed by the skin, causing intense burns and charring of the skin. Because the skin is a poor heat conductor and the exposure is quick, though, flash burns are most often only superficial. Flame burns are caused by secondary fires (eg, burning buildings, tents, or clothing) ignited by radiation. Burn injuries add significantly to the patient load of the medical units. They occur alone or, what is more likely, in combination with blast and radiation injuries. The complications and logistical requirements for treating warfighters with burn injuries would place great demands on the battlefield medical units. It is predicted that at least two thirds of the radiation casualties will have com-

---

EXHIBIT 29-1

WIND VELOCITIES CORRESPONDING TO PEAK OVERPRESSURES: THE RELATIONSHIP OF STATIC TO DYNAMIC OVERPRESSURES

Static Peak Overpressure (psi[*])	Dynamic Overpressure Wind Velocity (mph[†])
30	670
10	290
5	160
2	70

A nuclear weapon likely to be used during warfare would likely be in the 10 to 100 kiloton range and would produce 5 to 6 psi and roughly 160 to 200 mph winds. Distance from ground zero also has an effect, as does whether the detonation occurs in the air, underground, underwater, or on the surface. For a 1 megaton detonation, 6 psi would occur at about 4 km, lethal burns at about 14 km, and 5 Gy radiation levels at 2 km.

---

[*]pounds per square inch
[†]miles per hour
Source: Giambarresi L. Nuclear weapons: Medical effects and operational considerations. *7th MEDCOM Med Bull.* 1986;43(7):7–10.

---

bined injuries, that is, burns and other radiation exposure or wounds and radiation exposure. Burns produced the most significant synergistic effect on mortality in the combined injury model.[5]

Visible light energy will cause eye injuries, such as flash blindness and retinal burns. Flash blindness is caused by the initial flash of light produced by the nuclear detonation and results in transient blindness due to bleaching of the visual pigments in the retinal photoreceptors. The retina cannot receive the energy as rapidly as it is sent. This causes reversible blindness lasting from a fraction of a second to about 3 seconds and an after-image lasting several minutes if the detonation occurs during the day. If the detonation occurs at night, the flash blindness will be prolonged about 3-fold, with resulting inability to adapt to darkness for about 30 minutes. Retinal burns are caused by the thermal energy focused directly on the retina when the fireball is in the direct line of vision. Retinal burns usually cause permanent deficits in the visual field. Both types of thermal radiation (infrared and visible) travel at the speed of light so there is no chance of warning the affected population once a device has been detonated.

Radiation Injuries and Acute Radiation Syndrome

Neutrons and gamma rays are emitted in the fission process of a weapons detonation. They are referred to as "prompt" nuclear radiations because they are produced simultaneously with the nuclear explosion. Some neutrons may also undergo a scatter collision. Alpha and beta particles are quickly absorbed and only reach a few feet from the detonation. Radiation may produce injuries as a result of a single acute exposure to prompt neutrons and gamma rays from a nuclear detonation or from continual or intermittent exposure to residual radiation or fallout. The characteristic manifestations of radiation injury are dose and dose-rate related and called acute radiation syndrome (ARS).[6] ARS is a combination of relatively well-characterized clinical syndromes that occur in stages over a period of hours to weeks following exposure to radiation. The severity of symptoms depends on the dose, dose rate, dose distribution, duration of exposure, sensitivity of the cells to radiation, and cellular replication time. Cells that are more immature or undifferentiated are more sensitive to radiation. As cells mature or become more differentiated, they become less sensitive to radiation.

The clinical syndromes that make up ARS are hematopoietic syndrome, gastrointestinal syndrome, and central nervous system syndrome (sometimes called the cardiovascular/central nervous system syndrome or the neurovascular syndrome). Each of these syndromes follows a clinical course manifested in four stages that differ in intensity and duration based on the radiation dose. The first stage is the prodromal or initial stage, which occurs minutes to several days after exposure. Symptoms include acute incapacitation by nausea, vomiting, diarrhea, hyperthermia, erythema, hypotension, and central nervous system manifestations.[7] The latency stage, which follows the prodromal stage, is a period during which the patient is symptom-free and appears to have recovered from the radiation exposure. Next is the manifest illness stage, which is difficult to manage therapeutically because it is the period of maximum immunosuppression. Patient survival depends on the rapidity and aggressiveness of clinical therapy. The final stage is recovery, which depends on early treatment immediately after exposure and during the first several weeks following exposure coupled with individual sensitivities and preexisting conditions.[8]

The Hematopoietic Syndrome

The hematopoietic syndrome is seen after acute whole body exposure in the range of 1.5 to 8 gray (Gy, a measure of absorbed radiation dose equivalent to 100 rads). Doses less than 1 Gy of gamma radiation (in cases of exposure from a radiation accident, the radiation is likely to be primarily gamma radiation and some limited neutron radiation that cause ARS) usually produce few or no symptoms in humans. Higher doses may cause significant symptoms, and doses greater than 2.5 Gy may be life-threatening without therapeutic intervention. The prodromal stage, with its symptoms of transient nausea, vomiting, and diarrhea, occurs about 2 hours following exposure and may persist for several days. The latency stage may last for 2 to 3 weeks, at which time the manifest illness stage becomes evident. Significant symptoms occur at this time and may include fever, diarrhea, malaise, petechiae, epilation lymphopenia, and sepsis. The characteristic pathology of pancytopenia and death will result from hemorrhage and infection at doses of greater than 2.5 Gy without medical support. Half the humans exposed to a mid-lethal radiation dose of approximately 4.5 Gy will die if they do not receive medical intervention.[9] Though survival is still possible after acute whole-body exposures of around 8 Gy, exposures greater than 8 Gy usually result in 100% mortality, especially if there has been no medical intervention.[10]

The Gastrointestinal Syndrome

The gastrointestinal syndrome occurs after acute whole-body exposure to a wide range of doses (8 to 20 Gy). It is manifested earlier than the hematopoietic syndrome, usually occurring within 1 week of exposure. As early as 2 hours following exposure, the onset of prodromal symptoms will begin, and the latency stage can be as short as several days to about a week or even absent at the higher end of the dose range. Radiation interferes with the turnover of the mucosal cells lining the digestive tract.[11] The gastrointestinal mucosa lines the glandular structures in the submucosal space of the crypt epithelium. The columnar stem cells within the crypt regions are one of three less-differentiated cells. The intestinal stem cells are extremely radiosensitive, consequently leading to severe gastrointestinal symptoms from radiation damage. The damaged mucosa allows bacteria to enter the bloodstream. Patients present with vomiting, diarrhea, denudation of the small bowel mucosa, and sepsis. Early mortality is likely and is due to volume depletion and electrolyte imbalance with the characteristic symptoms of crampy abdominal pain and watery diarrhea that becomes bloody. This is followed by shock and death. While the gastrointestinal syndrome has a grave prognosis, those with lower-dose exposures may recover with medical management.

Central Nervous System Syndrome

The central nervous system syndrome is the least well characterized of the ARS syndromes. It is believed that doses of above 10 Gy may result in direct toxic damage to the nervous system,[12] but this syndrome occurs after doses of radiation of 20 to 30 Gy or greater.[9] Prodromal symptoms usually occur within minutes of exposure and persist for about 2 days. Laboratory animal data are relied on for this syndrome as there is little human information available on exposures in this range. It is known that death occurs relatively quickly following exposure. The presenting symptoms are lethargy, hypotension, hyperexcitability, disorientation, confusion, ataxia, respiratory distress, and convulsive seizures; these can quickly develop into coma and death. Pathological changes are evident and include microvascular damage (vasculitis) and increased intracranial pressure, cerebral edema, and cerebral anoxia. Radiation doses in this range are universally fatal even with medical intervention.

Combined Injury

Combined injury is the association of radiation injury with thermal burns, traumatic or other mechanical wounds, or both. The mortality rate for combined injuries increases significantly in the absence of medical care. An otherwise benign traumatic or burn injury may become lethal when combined with radiation exposure in excess of 2 Gy. Radiation and conventional injury seem to act in a synergistic manner and result in increased mortality. The biological effect of combined injuries will significantly increase the casualty's burn injuries and affect his or her ability to recover from a nuclear detonation.[13,14]

CASUALTY MANAGEMENT

Traditionally, military medical readiness for nuclear warfare has been focused on the management of large numbers of casualties resulting from a massive nuclear exchange between major powers. Modeling of nuclear scenarios for today's medical preparedness requires readiness training and understanding of medical operations in a nuclear environment or a radioactively contaminated environment.[15–17] With increasing use of nuclear materials, there is an increased probability of accidental radiation exposure or contamination of individuals working with or around such nuclear material. Examples include the release of radiation in Chernobyl, Ukraine (1986)[18]; Brazil (1987)[19]; and Tokaimura, Japan (1999).[20] A person's external or internal exposure to radiation or radioactive material does not, however, constitute a medical emergency. Contamination, whether internal or external, must be minimized as soon as possible to prevent further exposure to the individual and decrease the possibility of spreading contamination to the general public.

Triage

Triage is a mechanism of rapid evaluation of casualties based on their clinical condition and the prioritization of their treatment based on that evaluation. It is a process of sorting at the accident or detonation site. Triage priority should be given to victims with a good likelihood of recovery. The two keys to effectiveness and efficiency in the triage system are speed of assessing and categorizing patients and coordination of resources. Patient flow and response to care are integral parts of triage. They must be continually reassessed and reevaluated. The designated triage officer must have a well-trained response team. Good clinical judgment, intuitive clinical acumen, ability to handle stress, and awareness of available resources are but a few of the required characteristics of a good triage officer.

The health and safety of the general public in a nuclear exposure, whether from nuclear weapons detonation or power plant accidents, is a critical concern for the first emergency management responders to arrive at the accident scene (the response team) and depends on the exposure rate, the quantity of radioactive material present, and the public's perception of radiation exposure.[21] A nuclear weapons accident may result in immediate nonradiological threat from toxic or explosive hazards to the general public. The radiological contamination can also create a long-term concern of risk to the public's health. In a weapons accident, it is likely to be alpha particles that are the primary radiological hazard, not beta or gamma radiation. Dose effects from given exposures and dose rates of external and internal contamination provide data for the prediction of clinical response in the contaminated patient.

Contamination: External and Internal

Fallout causes an external hazard from gamma and high-energy beta emitters. Significant reduction in this exposure can be achieved through timely decontamination or prevention of external contamination. To keep the exposure to a minimum, the principles of time, distance, and shielding should be applied. Shielding is simply using protective clothing or placing dense material between the person and the radiation source. Surgical attire such as gowns, caps, shoe covers, and gloves will provide protection from beta radiation. Minimizing the time spent in the contaminated environment will reduce the radiation dose, and maintaining a significant distance from the radiation source can reduce the exposure. From ground zero or the point source of radiation, the level of radiation falls off by the square of the distance away from the source. This is similar to the seven-ten rule, which indicates that at any given time after exposure the radiation reading seven times later will decrease by a factor of ten from the original reading[22] (Table 29-3).

Most radiation does damage only after entering the body. Cursory decontamination, such as brushing off radioactive fallout dust or washing exposed skin, will reduce the radioactive exposure and minimize the risk that radioactive material will be internalized. Radiation injuries from internal contamination occur through various routes, such as inhalation, ingestion, and absorption from contamination on the skin or in wounds. The number of radionuclides with potential for internal contamination are many, but they are rarely encountered or represent only minor hazards to humans. The human body rarely incorporates enough radioactivity to cause ARS or to become acutely life-threatening. The late consequences of internal contamination, however, pose a greater potential risk. Whenever an unusually large dose of radionuclide is internalized, it is important to treat the individual as if he or she had ARS while also attempting to decorporate, mobilize, or block the radionuclide. The hematopoietic system, gastrointestinal system, and lungs should be given special attention. Radioactive isotopes of an element can behave differently when internalized into a biological system. Some isotopes preferentially taken up via gastrointestinal absorption are cesium (^{137}Cs), iodine (^{131}I), phosphorus (^{32}P), strontium (^{90}Sr), and tritium (^{3}H).[23]

Some actinides (eg, plutonium, americium, uranium, curium) and other radionuclides (eg, polonium, radium, iodine) of medical significance enter the body primarily via inhalation. Inhalation of

TABLE 29-3

SEVEN-TEN RULE FOR RESIDUAL RADIATION DECAY

Time Passed (h)	Fraction of Original Reading Remaining
1	1.0
7	0.1
49	0.01
343	0.001

Source: Vesper BE. External decontamination. *7th MEDCOM Med Bull.* 1986;43(7):30–31.

radionuclides into the bronchial tree and alveoli and transport across the alveoli into the bloodstream depend on the particle size and solubility. Of the radioactive isotopes inhaled, about 25% are deposited in the nasal passage and upper bronchial tree; cilia move them to the nasopharynx where they are swallowed and enter the gastrointestinal tract. The remaining particles are deposited in the airways, trachea, and pulmonary lymph nodes and deep in the lungs. Highly insoluble oxide forms of compounds are retained in the lungs for a longer period of time before being translocated to the tracheobronchial and pulmonary nodes and finally to the liver years after exposure.[24]

Treatment

For treatment purposes, patients with radiation injury are classified according to the severity of radiation exposure. The categories are mild, moderate, severe, and lethal. Treatment should be based on the injury, not the radiation dose estimated from a film badge or other measuring device (Figure 29-1). The most reliable guides are changes in levels of blood cells and cytogenetics resulting from bone marrow injury. Hematopoietic growth factors, such as granulocyte colony-stimulating factor (G-CSF), are potent stimulators of hematopoiesis and when administered early following radiation exposure may induce effective granulocytosis and prevent the consequences of severe neutropenia. Marrow transplantation may also be indicated in some cases.[25]

Management of those with internal contamination depends on the ability of the provider to decrease internal absorption and deposition or to increase excretion and elimination of the absorbed radionuclide. Early care is the most effective.[26] Lung contamination may quickly spread to the blood and target organs if the material is soluble and smaller than 5 µm. Larger soluble particles will likely remain in the lung, resulting in direct damage to lung tissue. Treatment for soluble material is dilutional (eg, blocking, chelating, mobilizing) to enhance excretion. Lung lavage may be useful for insoluble radionuclides but should only be used as a last resort because of associated complications of the procedure and the need for an experienced provider to perform it.

Infections

Infectious complications are another consequence of radiation exposure. For those exposed to

sublethal levels of radiation, infections can be prevented with the use of immunomodulators to enhance nonspecific resistance to infection. Initial medical care of patients with moderate (2-5 Gy) and severe (5-10 Gy) radiation doses should include early measures to reduce pathogen acquisition, such as emphasis on food with low microbial content, frequent hand washings or the wearing of gloves, and air filtration. Prophylactic selective gut decontamination with oral antibiotics is recommended. Antiemetic agents, such as the H2 blockers, are required to control nausea and vomiting.

The management of existing or suspected infection (eg, neutropenia, fever) in irradiated persons is similar to care provided to other immunocompromised, febrile, neutropenic patients. First, a regimen of

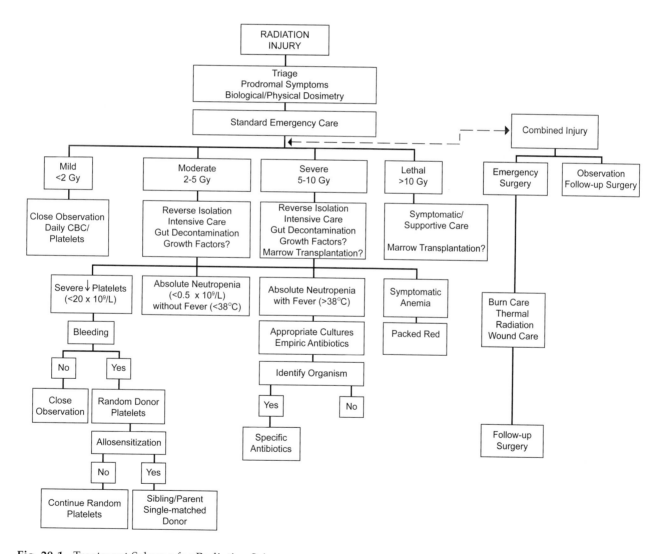

Fig. 29-1. Treatment Schema for Radiation Injury
Reproduced with permission from Browne D, Weiss JF, MacVittie TJ, Pillar MV, eds. *Treatment of Radiation Injuries.* New York: Plenum Press; 1990.

empiric antibiotics should be selected based on the pattern of bacterial susceptibility, nosocomial infections in the care facility, and the degree of neutropenia. Combination antibiotic regimens (eg, broad spectrum beta-lactam penicillin or cephalosporin plus aminoglycoside with or without vancomycin) are recommended for initial therapy for patients with profound neutropenia. Monotherapy, using drugs such as imipenem or ceftazidime, is appropriate for patients with less intense neutropenia. Antifungal drugs such as amphotericin B or fluconazole should be added, if indicated, for patients who remain febrile for 7 days or more while on or after 7 days of antibiotic therapy. If the fever and neutropenia persist for more than 48 hours after the start of antibiotic and antifungal therapy, viral titers should be obtained and antiviral therapy (eg, acyclovir) added. In cases where there is resistant gram-positive infection, vancomycin should be added. Cultures may be useful for monitoring acquisition of resistant bacteria and the emergence of fungal infections.[25]

Combined Injuries

Because the prognosis for combined injuries is worse than for either traumatic injury or radiation injury alone, it is important that comprehensive medical care is initiated to reduce mortality, especially if a total-body radiation exposure of sublethal or medium-lethal levels is combined with various types of conventional insults (eg, trauma, burns). Emergency and definitive care for combined injuries include early surgical interventions. Management of burns and soft tissue injuries is more difficult in combined injured casualties due to loss of skin and muscle, damage to vasculature, and necrotic tissue. It is recommended that surgical management for combined injury wounds and thermal burns be initiated as soon as possible but at least within 36 to 48 hours of radiation exposure. Elective surgical procedures should not be done until the patient is showing signs of recovery from the hematopoietic injury or is responding to cytokine therapy.

The Skin

Skin damage from radiation exposure occurs in varying degrees and is related to radiation quality and absorption of the radiation dose. Radiation burns may require repeated therapy and prolonged rehabilitation. Initial management is conservative; analgesic support, antibiotics, and surgical intervention may become necessary as the tissue becomes necrotic, painful, and infected. Good clinical judgment and management expertise in local radiation injury is necessary to prevent unnecessary suffering by the patient. Magnetic resonance imaging, radioactive isotope scanning, and thermography can help assess the extent of tissue damage, sufficiency of local microcirculation, and viability of the remaining tissue.[27]

PROTECTION FROM RADIATION

Every effort must be made to minimize radiation exposure and contamination in a radiation environment. Time, distance, shielding, and contamination control are the basic factors to consider in controlling or minimizing radiation exposure. After a nuclear detonation, fallout can be expected to contaminate equipment and personnel. The radiation dose received is directly proportional to the time of exposure. The shorter exposure, the less radiation received, so minimizing the time spent in the contaminated area will reduce radiation exposure. The radiation dose can be estimated by multiplying the dose rate at a specified point by the time the person remains at that location. To minimize exposure, tasks that must be performed in a contaminated area must be planned in advance and a stay-time established so as not to exceed a certain dose of radiation. Exposed personnel should decontaminate as quickly as possible to lower their total radiation exposure. Time can be used to allow the radiation to decay naturally. The seven-ten rule is a good general rule (see Table 29-3).

Respiratory protection and contamination control during the weapons recovery phase (the period when the weapon is being located and it is determined if the nuclear component has detonated) is a priority task for a nuclear accident response team. The first responders, such as the firefighters and the explosive ordnance personnel, will not usually have enough radiation survey equipment to assess the situation properly because of the urgent need to reduce the serious hazards of fire and potential explosion. These personnel rely on well-rehearsed standard operating procedures and well-designed protective equipment. Following the initial operations, the response force will establish a contamination control station near but upwind from the accident location. At the accident site, there may be extremely high levels of contamination on equipment and debris and resuspension of fine particulate, which will make respiratory protection necessary. There may also be physical and toxic hazards.

Respiratory protection criteria are based on the conditions at the accident site. Less respiratory protection may be needed in locations where the contamination is no longer airborne than in areas with high resuspension rates or during periods of high winds. Workers' exposure to airborne particles should be limited, but this must be done within the imperatives of the operations being performed. To quantify the contamination level, a target protective action guide (PAG) is established. If the averaged air concentration of radioactive particles is above this PAG, the situation should be evaluated and respiratory protection considered. For most work, the PAG is an averaged air concentration of 1.5 Bq/m². This approximates an

exposure of 2×10^{-4} Sv for each hour of exposure. For the initial phase, 250 hours of work can be performed before the annual dose limit of 0.05 Sv is attained.[28] If the air concentration is well documented, a person can be allowed to enter an area of higher activity for a shorter period of time, as long as the whole-body exposure is well documented. Decontamination is necessary for all persons and equipment after leaving the contaminated area, and qualified technicians must monitor the level of radioactivity before granting access to noncontaminated areas.

The isolation gowns or surgical scrub garments used when universal precautions are being followed for communicable disease control are suitable for protection from external radiation contamination. There is also specially made anti-contamination protective clothing.

SUMMARY

It is an increasing probability that military forces will be faced with situations of radiation exposure in operational environments other than war. This risk can occur as a result of weapons dispersal, damaged nuclear reactors, medical and research facilities' sources, industrial waste dumps, depleted uranium munitions, and terrorist attacks. With the increased nuclear capabilities in the world today there is an ever-present likelihood of radiation accidents occurring. Health care providers must be prepared to handle the medical aftermath of an accidental nuclear exposure. While much of the medical management will be based on clinical judgement and astute evaluation, it is necessary to have a plan of medical management available to deal with the contingency of an unforeseen nuclear event. The casualty must be assessed for the presence of a combined injury, the type and level of radiation exposure must be calculated, and the treatment and decontamination begun as rapidly as safely possible. In a massive casualty situation the success

of the medical operations will depend on the adequacy of the planning, training, and pre-positioning.

Based on past massive casualty situations, a significant disparity may exist between the available medical resources and the casualties needing therapeutic management. The establishment of policies and doctrines along with a rigorous plan for training and implementation must be instituted before a contingency looms. Past experiences and wartime consequences have shown that it is imperative to be prepared for any nuclear contingency and include mechanisms to handle the psychological stresses that follow radiation exposure and its potential late effects.

A better understanding of the effects of radiation and trauma will result in improved management of radiation casualties and a decrease in the logistical drain on limited medical resources. A multidisciplinary approach is needed to manage life-threatening outcomes resulting from accidental exposure to radiation.

REFERENCES

1. Walker RI, Conklin JJ. Military radiobiology: A perspective. In: Conklin JJ, Walker RI, eds. *Military Radiobiology*. Orlando, Fla: Academic Press; 1987: Chap 1.

2. Glasstone S, Donlon PJ, eds. *The Effects of Nuclear Weapons*. Washington, DC: Department of Defense and Department of Energy; 1977.

3. United Nations. Treaty on the Nonproliferation of Nuclear Weapons. 1 July 1968.

4. Giambarresi L. Nuclear weapons: Medical effects and operational considerations. *7th MEDCOM Med Bull.* 1986;43(7):7–10.

5. Alt LA, Forcino DC, Walder RI. Nuclear events and their consequences. In: Walker RI, Cerveny TJ, eds. *Medical Consequences of Nuclear Warfare*. Part I, Vol 2. *Textbook of Military Medicine*. Falls Church, Va: TMM Publications, Office of the Surgeon General; 1989

6. Cerveny TJ, MacVittie TJ, Young RW. Acute radiation syndrome in humans. In: Walker RI, Cerveny TJ, eds. *Medical Consequences of Nuclear Warfare*. Part I, Vol 2. *Textbook of Military Medicine*. Falls Church, Va: TMM Publications, Office of the Surgeon General; 1989.

7. Anno GH, Baum SJ, Withers HR, Young RW. Symptomatology of acute radiation effects in humans after exposure to doses of 0.5–3.0 Gy. *Health Phys*. 1989;56:821–838.

8. Young RW. Acute radiation syndrome. In: Conklin JJ, Walker RI, eds. *Military Radiobiology*. Orlando, Fla: Academic Press; 1987: 165–190.

9. Wald N. Acute radiation injuries and their medical management. In: *The Biological Basis of Radiation Protection Practice*. Baltimore: Williams and Wilkins; 1992: Chap 12.

10. Browne D, Weiss JF, MacVittie TJ, Pillai MV, eds. *Treatment of Radiation Injuries*. New York: Plenum Press; 1990.

11. Gunter-Smith PJ. Effect of ionizing radiation on gastrointestinal physiology. In: Conklin JJ, Walker RI, eds. *Military Radiobiology*. Orlando, Fla: Academic Press; 1987: 135–151.

12. Medical Effects of Nuclear Weapons Course Lecture Notes. Bethesda, Md: Armed Forces Radiobiology Research Institute; 1993.

13. Bowers GJ. The combined injury syndrome. In: Conklin JJ, Walker RI, eds. *Military Radiobiology*. Orlando, Fla: Academic Press; 1987: 192–214.

14. Hirsch EF, Burke JF. Combination of thermal burns and whole-body irradiation. In: Walker RI, Gruber DF, MacVittie TJ, Conklin JJ, eds. *The Pathophysiology of Combined Injury and Trauma: Radiation, Burn, and Trauma*. Baltimore: University Park Press; 1985.

15. North Atlantic Treaty Organization. *NATO Handbook on the Concept of Medical Support in NBC Environments*. AMedP-7(A). Brussels: NATO: 1993.

16. Conklin JJ, Monroy RL. Management of radiation accidents. In: Conklin JJ, Walker RI, eds. *Military Radiobiology*. Orlando, Fla: Academic Press; 1987: 347–363.

17. Dons RF, Cerveny TJ. Triage and treatment of radiation injured mass casualties. In: Walker RI, Cerveny TJ, eds. *Medical Consequences of Nuclear Warfare*. In: *Textbook of Military Medicine*. Washington, DC: Department of the Army, Office of the Surgeon General, Borden Institute; 1989: 37–53.

18. United Nations Scientific Committee on the Effects of Atomic Radiation. *1988 Report to the General Assembly: Annex G: Early Effects in Man of High Doses of Radiation*. New York: UN; 1988: 545–647.

19. Valverde NJ, Cordeiro JM, Oliveira AR, Brandao-Mello CE. The acute radiation syndrome in the cesium-137 Brazilian accident, 1978. In: Ricks RC, Fry SA, eds. *The Medical Basis for Radiation Accident Preparedness II*. New York: Elsevier; 1990: 89–107.

20. International Atomic Energy Agency. *Report on the Preliminary Fact Finding Mission Following the Accident at the Nuclear Fuel Processing Facility in Tokaimura, Japan*. Vienna: IAEA; 1999.

21. Defense Nuclear Agency. *Nuclear Weapon Accident Response Procedures (NARP) Manual*. Washington, DC: DNA; 1984. DNA Publication 5100.1.

22. Vesper BE. External decontamination. *7th MEDCOM Med Bull*. 1986;43(7):30–31.

23. National Council on Radiation Protection and Measurements. *Management of Persons Accidentally Contaminated With Radionuclides*. Bethesda, Md: NCRPM; 1980. NCRP Report 65.

24. National Academy of Sciences, National Research Council. *Effects of Inhaled Radioactive Particles*. Washington, DC: NAS, NRC: 1961. Publication 848.

25. MacVittie TJ, Weiss JF, Browne D, eds. *Advances in Treatment of Radiation Injuries*. In: *Advances in Bioscience*. Vol 94. New York: Pergamon; 1996: 341.

26. Mettler FA, Kelsey CA, Ricks RC. *Medical Management of Radiation Accidents*. Boca Raton, Fla: CRC Press; 1990.

27. International Atomic Energy Agency. *What the General Practitioner Should Know About Medical Handling of Over-exposed Individuals*. Vienna: IAEA; 1986. IAEA-TECDOC-366.

28. Browne D. Clinical management of radiation injuries. In: Bushberg J, Browne D, Metler F. *Radiological Emergency Medical Management*. Orlando, Fla: Academic Press (in press).

Chapter 30

THE ROLE OF VETERINARY PUBLIC HEALTH AND PREVENTIVE MEDICINE DURING MOBILIZATION AND DEPLOYMENT

VICKY L. FOGELMAN, DVM, MPH; JOANNE BROWN, DVM; GEORGE E. MOORE, DVM; W. DAVID GOOLSBY, DVM, MPH; RANDALL THOMPSON, DVM; AND PAUL L. BARROWS, DVM, PhD

V. L. Fogelman; Colonel, US Air Force, BSC; Academic Director, International Health Program, US Air Force Radiobiology Research Institute, 8901 Wisconsin Avenue, Bethesda, MD 20889-5603

J. Brown; Colonel, Veterinary Corps, US Army (Retired); Rt 2 Box 152B, Monticello FL 32344; formerly, DoD Veterinary Laboratory, 2472 Schofield Road, Bldg 2632, Fort Sam Houston, TX 78234-6232

G. E. Moore; Colonel, Veterinary Corps, US Army; Chief, Department of Veterinary Sciences, Army Medical Department Center and School, Bldg 2840, Suite 248, 2250 Stanley Road, Fort Sam Houston, TX 78234-6145

W. David Goolsby; Lieutenant Colonel, Veterinary Corps, US Army (Retired); 1247 Shadowood Drive, Spartanburg, SC 29301; formerly, Chief, Plans and Programs, DoD Veterinary Service Activity, 5109 Leesburg Pike, Falls Church, VA 22041

R. Thompson; Major, Veterinary Corps, US Army; Attn: Commander, EAMC-VS (Korea), Unit 15252, APO AP 96205-0025; formerly, Chief, Field Services Branch, Department of Veterinary Science, AMEDD Center and School, 2840 Stanley Rd, Fort Sam Houston, TX 78234

P. L. Barrows; Colonel, Veterinary Corps, US Army (Retired); 56 Crazy Cross Road, Wimberly, TX 78676; formerly, Director, DoD Veterinary Service Activity, Chief, US Army Veterinary Corps, Department of Veterinary Sciences, Army Medical Department Center and School, Bldg 2840, 2250 Stanley Road, Fort Sam Houston, TX 78234-6145

HISTORICAL PERSPECTIVE

The US military recognized the need for veterinarians as early as the mid-1800s. Horses and mules were a critical component of the fighting force during the Civil War, as they had been in previous conflicts, but they often received little or no medical care. Meat procured for the troops was also frequently unwholesome, resulting in significant morbidity and even death among US fighting forces.[1] Although the US Army Quartermaster General appealed to Congress for creation of a veterinary corps in 1853, his request was denied; as a result, more than 1.2 million horses and mules died during the Civil War due to lack of sufficient veterinary care.[2]

After the Civil War, public attention was drawn to the inhumane and indifferent care of horses and the failure to protect military forces from unsafe food and zoonotic diseases. Generals Grant and Sherman became proponents of an organized military veterinary corps after witnessing the inhumane treatment of animals during the war and recognizing the positive impact that a well-trained veterinary corps had on the British and German armies. The formation of the American Veterinary Medical Association and the Bureau of Animal Industry also contributed to the effort to establish an organized veterinary service in the US military. Both organizations represented organized veterinary medicine, understood the relationship between public health and preventive medicine, and made appreciable gains against many animal diseases.[3] These factors, plus increased Congressional interest after hearing of the US casualties from beef "embalmed" in formaldehyde during the Spanish-American War, resulted in the formation of a military veterinary service under the National Defense Act of 1916.[4]

The original mission of the Army Veterinary Service was to treat horses and mules and to inspect meat for the Quartermaster Corps. In 1917, the role of veterinary medicine in human health was recognized as the Veterinary Corps was integrated into the Army Medical Department. More than 2,000 veterinarians served in the world wars, more than 1,100 in the Korean War, and more than 1,200 in the Vietnam War.[3,5] There were more than 1,330 Army veterinarians and veterinary specialists assigned to the Army veterinary service and 900 more in the Reserve Component in 1999. The mission of today's military veterinary service is to provide food safety and inspection services, zoonotic disease prevention and control, laboratory and medical research support, and clinical veterinary services for government-owned animals.

The US Air Force also formed a veterinary service after it became a separate entity in 1947. This service, while similar in function to the US Army Veterinary Service, included the additional mission of overseeing base food service sanitation programs and performing foodborne illness outbreak investigations. In 1980, by Congressional mandate, all clinically related veterinary activities were placed under the auspices of the Army Veterinary Corps; veterinarians and veterinary technicians who chose to remain in the Air Force became public health officers or technicians with the function of managing all food safety, communicable disease, occupational health, medical entomology, epidemiology, and public health education programs for the base or command to which they were assigned. The Air Force still recruits veterinarians as public health officers.

VETERINARY MOBILIZATION FORCE STRUCTURE

The veterinary deployment force is transitioning to a flexible structure, which consists of specialized detachments that can be assembled into a tailored veterinary support package based on mission needs. The initial deployment element is a team from the Veterinary Surveillance Detachment, which provides the initial food inspection and food microbiological laboratory support, sets up zoonosis control programs, and provides primary and preventive care for military working dogs in-theater.

A Veterinary Food Procurement Detachment is also available to support local procurement of such foodstuffs as red meats, poultry, eggs, dairy products, ice, and bottled water. Finally, an Animal Medical Detachment provides full-service medical and surgical care to deployed military working dogs. This detachment also supports zoonosis control programs and civic action animal health programs as directed.

The US Army Civil Affairs and Psychological Command, which is part of Special Operations Command, has veterinary staff officers at the battalion and brigade levels and as part of their deployable teams. These staff officers establish liaison with the host-nation government, coordinate in-country support, and define potential humanitarian civic action projects for US forces within the mission. Civil Affairs veterinarians are often deployed in support of conventional military units that lack veterinary assets.

Veterinarians are also assigned in support of Special Forces operations. During deployments, the Special Forces Group (SFG) veterinarian may serve with the Environmental Science Officer as the SFG's preventive medicine team. This team focuses on the prevention of disease and nonbattle injury in Special Forces personnel. The preventive medicine team's mission includes food and water safety, field sanitation and hygiene, pest control, and prevention and control of zoonotic diseases. During deployments with a primary medical mission, such as humanitarian civic action, the veterinarian works with the host nation to improve the lives of the local human population primarily by improving the health and welfare of their animals. The Special Forces veterinarian is also involved in sustainment training of the Special Forces medic. This training

includes a range of topics from zoonotic and foreign animal disease recognition to local procurement of food, including field slaughter and carcass evaluation. The SFG veterinarian serves as a member of the Group Surgeon's office and a special staff officer to the SFG commander on all veterinary matters.

The US Army Veterinary Corps, as the Department of Defense (DoD) Executive Agent for Veterinary Services, provides equitable veterinary support to all the military services. Veterinary Staff Officers identify resourcing requirements in the operational plans of the warfighting Commanders in Chief (CINCs) and individual military services. Examples of veterinary support across military service lines include food inspection support of Navy supply ships at sea; support of Marines during the training exercise Operation Ocean Venture, and support of US Central Command and the Air Force in Southwest Asia.

PUBLIC HEALTH AND PREVENTIVE MEDICINE RESPONSIBILITIES

Food Safety and Quality Assurance

Food service in the field must provide nutritious, wholesome food to military personnel. Veterinary services, logistics, food service, and preventive medicine are all involved in ensuring that wholesome food reaches the force. Veterinary Service personnel ensure that all food entering, stored in, procured in, or issued in a theater of operations meets wholesomeness and quality assurance standards through a series of inspections beginning before food enters the theater and ending at the point of issue to personnel. Deployed veterinary personnel inspect food intended for military local purchase in foreign countries, approve sanitation levels at local food production facilities, inspect food transport vehicles, and perform in-storage surveillance inspections of all foods, including operational rations. Veterinarians may also on occasion perform antemortem and postmortem inspection of food animals intended for consumption by military forces. Veterinary personnel also provide recommendations and support to commanders on disposition of contaminated food, foodborne illness outbreak investigations, and food decontamination. Veterinarians are also trained to inspect, monitor, and test food and food-producing animals suspected of being contaminated with nuclear, biological, and chemical (NBC) agents.

During contingency operations, Army veterinary food inspection personnel are usually located at the theater surgeon's office, with area support teams assigned to support the food supply system. In multinational operations, the responsibility for food procurement, preparation, and delivery, as well as food

safety, may be shared among the participating nations. Differences in standards may exist, but the underlying principles of sanitation and food safety remain.

Food safety involves control of physical, chemical, and microbiological threats. A potentially hazardous food (PHF) is a food that is capable of supporting either the rapid and progressive growth of infectious or toxigenic microorganisms or the relatively slower growth and toxin production of organisms such as *Clostridium botulinum*. It is the PHFs that are the biggest concern in food safety. An additional concern is contamination of generally safe foods (or non-PHFs) with a significant dose of an infectious agent, such as the contamination of salad with *Salmonella*. Exhibit 30-1 shows examples of PHFs and of generally safe foods.

Procurement

Assuring the safety of the food supply begins with procuring wholesome subsistence. Within the continental United States, numerous government agencies contribute to the maintenance of a safe food supply, including state and local public health agencies, the US Department of Agriculture (USDA), the US Department of Commerce, and the US Food and Drug Administration, as well as the Army Veterinary Service. In most overseas areas of operation, the Army Veterinary Service and the US Air Force Public Health Service are charged with performing all of the food safety functions of these agencies.

All local food production sources must be approved by the US Army Veterinary Service or the

EXHIBIT 30-1

POTENTIALLY HAZARDOUS FOODS

Potentially Hazardous Food is food that is natural or synthetic and that requires temperature control because it is in a form capable of supporting

1. The rapid and progressive growth of infectious or toxigenic microorganisms,

2. The growth and toxin production of *Clostridium botulinum*, and

3. In raw shell eggs, the growth of *Salmonella enteriditis*.

Examples include:

- Food of animal origin that is raw or heat-treated

- Food of plant origin that is raw (eg, raw seed sprouts) or heat-treated

- Garlic and oil mixtures that have not been modified to stop growth of infectious or toxigenic microorganisms

This definition does not include:

- Food in an unopened, hermetically sealed container commercially processed to achieve and maintain commercial sterility under conditions of nonrefrigerated storage and distribution

- Food for which laboratory evidence demonstrates that the rapid and progressive growth of infectious or toxigenic microorganisms or the growth of *S enteriditis* in eggs or *C botulinum* cannot occur (It may contain a preservative, another barrier to the growth of microorganisms, or a combination of barriers that inhibit the growth of microorganisms.)

US Air Force Public Health Service personnel before the military purchases foods from these sources. These approvals vary greatly in their complexity, depending on the food being procured (Table 30-1). In

TABLE 30-1

COMPLEXITY OF APPROVAL FOR VARIOUS FOODS

Food	Complexity of Approval	Reason
Dairy/ice cream	Very complex	Herd health, plant sanitation, equipment standards, no final consumer safety process
Processed dairy	Complex	Herd health, plant sanitation
Beef, pork, lamb, veal	Complex	Herd health, plant sanitation, items cooked before consumption
Poultry	Complex	Flock health, plant sanitation, items cooked before consumption
Ice and water	Moderately complex	Plant sanitation, water source, filtration systems
Fresh fruits and vegetables (whole)	Less complex	Usually not potentially hazardous but may be a problem if feces (night soil) are used in the growing area
Bakery	Less complex	Cooked product, usually not potentially hazardous
Shell eggs	Moderately complex	Flock health, plant sanitation
Sandwich, salad, and prepared foods	Moderately complex	Plant sanitation, food handler risks, no final and prepared foods consumer safety process
Minimally processed fresh fruit and vegetable juice	Moderately complex	Agricultural practices, plant sanitation, water treatment

some parts of the world, sanitary practices may make approval difficult, so some products readily available in the United States may not be easily obtained overseas. For example, milk production plants in some countries do not meet US pasteurization standards and thus provide potential for transmission of zoonotic diseases, such as tuberculosis, through milk. The US Army Veterinary Service maintains a directory that lists the establishments that have been inspected and have met sanitary standards.[6] Food establishments providing certain nonhazardous foods need not be approved or listed in the directory. This information can be obtained from the Veterinary Service or through the Armed Forces Medical Intelligence Center in Frederick, Md.

Transportation

Food procured from an approved source must be transported to the consumer. Whether civilian or military, the transportation system presents many risks to food safety. Good vehicle sanitation is important to ensure a minimal risk of contamination. The vehicle should be clean and covered, and the food storage compartment kept in good repair. The vehicle must have the ability to maintain the proper temperatures, and consideration must be given to the time it takes to convey perishable products. Extended delivery distances increase the risk of in-transit damage or refrigeration breakdowns, which in turn increase the potential for food spoilage and contamination.

Similar attention must be paid to the transport and distribution of food items from a centrally located military supply point in an area of operations to the final destination at the unit. Limitations on availability of transportation may lead to attempts to mix loads. While the efficient use of transportation is good, food stocks should not be mixed with incompatible cargo (eg, petroleum products, chemicals, cleaning compounds, other potential contaminants). Refrigerated conveyances should be used when possible to transport perishable goods. If refrigerated vehicles are not available, insulated containers may be used, after due consideration is given to time and temperature factors. If chill or freeze temperatures will not deviate significantly and there is a short time between transit, preparation, and serving, use of nonrefrigerated vehicles may be feasible. Coordination with veterinary and preventive medicine personnel must be conducted before employing this method of transit. An additional concern in the tactical environment is the physical damage that can occur when food is transported in heavy-duty trucks over rough terrain with improper packing and strapping.

In-storage Protection

The primary protection factors to be considered when storing subsistence are proper temperature control and protection from contamination, infestation, and the elements. If possible, storage sites should include enclosed buildings that offer protection from the elements and reduce insect and rodent contamination. Food storage sites should not be placed adjacent to petroleum product points, highly trafficked dirt roads, areas subject to flooding, or other obvious sources of contamination. The goal is to use a site that will minimize damage, contamination, and deterioration of the products. At a field site, pallets and tarps or plastic coverings may be used. Storing food products in direct sunlight may significantly reduce their quality and shelf life. At no time should chilled or frozen food items be stored without proper refrigeration (Table 30-2).

Operational rations are of particular interest. They are often stressed by storage in adverse environmental conditions (eg, extreme heat) and may become contaminated by chemicals (eg, petroleum) or by NBC agents during wartime operations. Foods that have been held under improper storage conditions for excessive periods of time may also be hazardous to human health. Army Veterinary Service and Air Force Public Health Service personnel perform periodic surveillance inspections of food items in storage. This mission is primarily performed by enlisted food inspectors under the direction of a veterinarian or public health officer. These individuals can advise commanders as to the condition, identity, quality, and wholesomeness of food products within the system, as well as make recommendations on proper storage. After Hurricane Andrew

TABLE 30-2

APPROPRIATE TEMPERATURES FOR THE STORAGE OF FOODS

Food	Proper Storage Temperature
Frozen goods	–18°C (0°F) or below
Chilled items	–2°C to 4°C (28°F to 40°F)
Fresh fruits and vegetables	2°C to 13°C (35°F to 55°F), depending on the commodity
Semi-perishables*	Refrigerated storage not required but items must be protected from the elements in a cool, clean, dry area on pallets or shelving units

*For example: rice, beans, flour

hit Florida in 1992, military food inspectors assisted local community leaders and military commanders in determining which foods stored in facilities without electricity were fit for consumption.

Food Service

Food service in the field focuses on several key concerns. Increased likelihood of contamination from the environment, limited resources, potentially stressed food supplies, and extended transport of finished, cooked food all contribute to an increased potential for foodborne illness. Food service personnel must strive to maintain food facilities at the highest level of sanitation to minimize sources of contamination within the facility. Training of transport personnel who deliver prepared food to field sites is also extremely important. Veterinary personnel can also provide recommendations and support to commanders on appropriate site selection for food distribution points and field kitchens.

The single most important concept for food safety is the time and temperature relationship: the time a food is held at a temperature where microbial growth can occur must be kept to a minimum. Foods must be held at a temperature that is either too hot or too cold for extensive microbial growth. This includes the time during storage of the uncooked food, preparation, cooking, cooling, storage of the cooked food, transportation of the cooked food, holding on the serving line, and reheating of leftovers. The most common single cause of foodborne illness outbreaks is improper cooling following preparation of food (Exhibit 30-2).

Operational Rations

Operational rations are those foods that are used to support service members in the field and include a number of options. They are discussed more fully in chapter 17, Nutritional Considerations in Military Deployment. One of the safest food items procured by the military is the Meal, Ready-to-Eat (MRE) ration. Commercial retort technology is used when making the main course of the ration. Additional safety factors are built into the process to ensure a wholesome product. Inspections throughout the process by in-plant quality control personnel and the USDA provide added safety assurance. Army Veterinary Service personnel are stationed at assembly plants to make final inspections before MREs are distributed. Like any other subsistence item, the MRE can develop problems if it is abused. Extremes of temperature can lead to breakdown of either the packaging or the product. Exposure to chemicals or petroleum products can cause chemical contamination of the food, and saving portions for reuse after opening can result in bacterial contamination.

Disease Prevention and Control

Zoonotic Diseases

One of the most important responsibilities of veterinary personnel in the field is to prevent unnecessary lost duty time for military personnel caused by zoonotic diseases. The Army Veterinary Service is responsible for establishing appropriate zoonotic dis-

---

EXHIBIT 30-2

FACTORS MOST OFTEN NAMED IN FOODBORNE OUTBREAKS

Reported cases of foodborne illness usually involve more than one of these factors:

- Failure to properly cool food (the leading cause of foodborne outbreaks)
- Failure to thoroughly heat or cook food
- Infected employees who practice poor personal hygiene at home and at work
- Preparing food a day or more in advance of being served
- Adding raw, contaminated ingredients to food that receives no further cooking
- Allowing foods to stay for too long at temperatures favorable to bacterial growth
- Failure to reheat cooked foods to temperatures that kill bacteria
- Cross-contamination of cooked food by raw food, improperly cleaned and sanitized equipment, or employee mishandling of food

Reprinted with permission from: The Educational Foundation of the National Restaurant Association. *Serving Safe Food Certification Coursebook*. TEFNRA; 1995.

ease prevention and control programs. A portion of this function is accomplished by ensuring that effective food safety programs are in place. For example, inspection of dairy plants in foreign countries to ensure that proper pasteurization procedures are being performed contributes to prevention of milk-borne diseases, such as brucellosis and bovine tuberculosis.

Animal control programs and commander and service member education are also important elements of zoonotic disease control in the field. Because of the risks of disease transmission and personal injury, wild, feral, and domestic animals may pose serious threats to deployed personnel. Animals adopted as unit mascots pose some of the greatest threats. Puppies can develop rabies at as early as 6 weeks of age and can be heavily infected with endoparasites and infested with ectoparasites transmissible to humans. Animals such as lizards are potential sources of salmonella infection, and wild rodents and mammals are often attracted to camp sites by accumulation of trash, improper food storage, and other unsanitary practices. Animal bites can be a frequent occurrence in deployment settings if effective animal control measures are not in place. Veterinarians play a key role in advising commanders on animal control, field sanitation, and other practices that if implemented early and consistently will greatly reduce the likelihood of transmission of zoonotic diseases.

Rabies is often one of the most important zoonotic disease threats during contingency operations. Rabies is enzootic in the dog in many parts of the world, including numerous countries in Africa, Asia, and Central America. Feral dogs are quite common in these areas. Because of the close relationship between humans and dogs and most people's lack of understanding of the rabies threat, deployed personnel often put themselves at risk for rabies exposure. Military veterinarians assigned or deployed to foreign countries can provide information on the prevalence of rabies and other zoonotic diseases of interest to commanders, health care providers, and deployed personnel. Veterinarians also serve as the quarantine authority for animal bite cases involving humans and serve as members of the Rabies Advisory Committee, which makes recommendations for postexposure rabies prophylaxis in animal bite patients. It is very important that all animal bites are reported to the assigned veterinarian as soon as they occur so that efforts can be made to locate the animal for quarantine or other appropriate action.[7]

Government-owned animals, such as military working dogs, may act as sentinels for diseases of importance to humans. For example, during Operation Joint Endeavor in Bosnia, 5 of 14 military working dogs developed babesiosis, a tickborne disease, in March of the first deployment year.[8] This outbreak served as a sentinel event for tick activity in the theater and allowed early notification of commanders to reinforce their units' use of personal protection measures against ticks. Military veterinarians should be included in discussions of the prevalence and risk of transmission of zoonotic diseases to military personnel in deployment areas.

Public Health Laboratory Support

Veterinary laboratory support for the US military is provided by three laboratories, each of which serves a specific region. The laboratory at Fort Sam Houston, Tex, supports military personnel stationed in the continental United States, the Caribbean islands, Central America, and the Pacific Rim. The laboratory at Schofield Barracks, Hawaii, supports Hawaii and parts of Southeast Asia; and the laboratory at Landstuhl, Germany, serves Europe, the Middle East, and Africa.

A major mission of the veterinary laboratories is to provide microbiological, chemical, toxicological, and radiological analysis of food items, bottled water, nonprescription drugs, and cosmetics for safety, wholesomeness, and contractual compliance. The laboratories have food analysis capabilities that include more than 100 microbiological and chemical tests, in addition to numerous specific toxicological and radiological tests. Microbiological testing capability ranges from simple plate counts to specific pathogen identification. Chemical and toxicological testing capabilities are quite varied and can be used to determine both safety and quality of tested products. Examples of such tests include the milk phosphatase test for the adequacy of pasteurization, specific drug residue tests, and tests for pesticides, heavy metals, histamines, and aflatoxins. Food and water can also be tested for radiological contamination, and veterinarians serve as part of incident response teams for radiological emergencies.

These veterinary laboratories play a vital role in determining the causative agent in foodborne disease outbreaks. Specific testing can be conducted for the following food pathogens: *Staphylococcus aureus* (both organism and toxin), *Escherichia coli* (including O157:H7), *Campylobacter jejuni, Clostridium perfringens*, *Cl botulinum*, *Listeria monocytogenes*, *Bacillus cereus*, *Shigella* species, *Vibrio parahemolyticus*, *Yersinia enterocolitica*, and *Aeromonas hydrophila*.

In addition, the regional veterinary laboratories provide some diagnostic testing capabilities for animal diseases. Animal brain tissue can be tested for rabies, and specific serologic tests can be performed for the causative agents of rabies, ehrlichiosis, babesiosis, Lyme disease, equine infectious anemia, bluetongue, toxoplasmosis, leptospirosis, brucellosis, and Rocky Mountain spotted fever. Additional information on veterinary laboratory capabilities can be obtained in Army Regulation 40-28, *DoD Veterinary/Medical Laboratory Food Safety and Quality Assurance Program*,[9] or by contacting the appropriate support laboratory.

Veterinarians provide laboratory support in the field in another capacity as well—as members of the Theater Area Medical Laboratory (TAML). Veterinary support to the TAML includes a veterinary pathologist and a veterinary laboratory animal specialist with training in public health. These officers provide the capability for rapid field diagnosis of zoonotic diseases and identification of potential biological warfare agents using technology based on enzyme-linked immunosorbent assay and polymerase chain reaction technology adapted for field use. These individuals can also survey endemic animal populations, perform epidemiologic investigations, and identify potential disease reservoir hosts that can affect the health of deployed personnel. Typical diagnostic capabilities include tests for agents that cause such diseases as plague; anthrax; brucellosis; rabies; eastern, western, and Venezuelan equine encephalitis; and numerous hemorrhagic fevers.[10]

Disaster Operations and Military Operations Other Than War

Military veterinary units play a very important role in disaster response and humanitarian assistance operations.[11] Their primary responsibilities are much the same as during regular deployments, plus assisting civil authorities in animal disaster relief efforts as necessary. During wartime operations or civilian disasters involving potential NBC contamination of foods, veterinary personnel are responsible for the operation of detection equipment used to determine the extent of contamination of foods and food animals. They also provide commanders with recommendations on whether or not to decontaminate foods.[12] Military veterinar-

ians involved in disaster situations, both in the United States and overseas, may be asked to assess the impact of animal loss on a local population and to provide recommendations concerning the care and feeding of live animals.

Although the US Public Health Service is the lead agency in providing veterinary response to natural disasters in the United States, US Forces Command (FORSCOM) supplies assets to supplement civilian resources on request. After Hurricane Andrew, when the governor of Florida determined that the state alone could not handle the emergency, military veterinary personnel were deployed to the area to provide assistance in food inspection, treat sick and debilitated animals, assess veterinary capabilities in the area, and assist the community in returning to its predisaster status.[11,13]

Military veterinarians also assist with evacuations of military-owned pets and government-owned animals from disaster locations overseas. Both Army and Air Force veterinarians supported the evacuation of more than 2,000 pets from the Philippines following the eruption of Mount Pinatubo in 1991. In the summer of 1996, US Army veterinary personnel assisted in the evacuation of 85 pets from Riyadh, Saudi Arabia, after the bombing of a US military housing complex there. The human-animal bond is very strong, and this intervention by veterinary personnel during times of extreme stress helps to relieve the anxiety felt by service members concerned about their pets' welfare during a disaster.

Military veterinary personnel have long been integral to military operations other than war. There are many recent examples of veterinary support in conjunction with DoD humanitarian operations. In November 1995 during Joint Operation Balikatan, US Army veterinary personnel visited the Philippines to work and train with Philippine military veterinarians. During the exercise, US and Philippine military veterinary personnel provided veterinary preventive medicine interventions, including more than 6,000 rabies vaccinations to dogs located around Olongapao City. This preventive measure provided a protective barrier against human rabies in a country that reported more than 340 human rabies deaths and more than 60,000 treatments for dog bites in 1995.[14]

FORSCOM and Special Operations Command veterinary personnel supported US military operations in Haiti from 1994 to 1996. In an example of military veterinarians providing assistance to other countries in identifying and controlling potentially

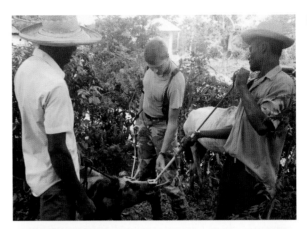

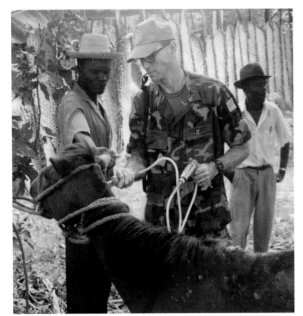

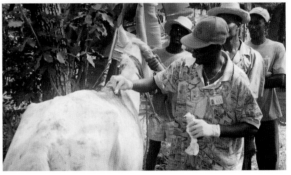

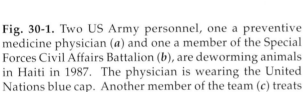

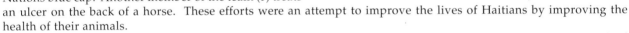

Fig. 30-1. Two US Army personnel, one a preventive medicine physician (*a*) and one a member of the Special Forces Civil Affairs Battalion (*b*), are deworming animals in Haiti in 1987. The physician is wearing the United Nations blue cap. Another member of the team (*c*) treats an ulcer on the back of a horse. These efforts were an attempt to improve the lives of Haitians by improving the health of their animals.
Photographs: Courtesy of Lieutenant Colonel Jeffrey M. Gambel, Medical Corps, US Army, Walter Reed Army Medical Center, Washington, DC.

devastating animal diseases within their countries, a veterinary support team operating with the US Joint Task Force in Haiti identified the first confirmed cases of hog cholera in Haiti. They worked closely with the USDA and Haitian government personnel to vaccinate hogs and develop a control program for this economically devastating disease[15] (Figure 30-1). Veterinary civic action projects often focus on food safety as well as animal health.

Foreign Animal Disease Threats

The United States has been described as an island surrounded by a sea of animal disease. Because of quarantine procedures and animal disease eradication programs, the United States is relatively free of many of the most serious animal diseases. Deployed personnel are at risk of inadvertently introducing foreign animal diseases (FADs), such as foot and mouth disease, into the United States via contaminated food, clothing, and equipment. Primary responsibility for preventing the introduction of FADs belongs to the USDA. Introduction of livestock or poultry diseases into the United States

could ultimately cost US citizens billions of dollars. Preventing the introduction of FADs and remaining aware of the risks involved is a responsibility that should be emphasized to personnel deploying to and returning from foreign nations. Military veterinarians are the primary source of information and guidance during deployment regarding FADs.

FORSCOM acts as executive agent for the DoD in the implementation of contingency plans to support the Regional Emergency Animal Disease Eradication Organization, which is part of the USDA. Under the FORSCOM plan, military veterinary assets are made available to support the USDA in efforts to control FADs entering the United States. Military veterinarians have assisted the USDA in controlling outbreaks of exotic Newcastle disease in California poultry, Venezuelan equine encephalitis in Texas horses, and avian influenza in Pennsylvania birds.[16]

One excellent example of the veterinary role in preventing introduction of a FAD into the United States was the Ebola Reston outbreak. In December 1989, a commercial nonhuman primate importer in Reston, Va, began to experience unusual losses of laboratory monkeys recently arrived from the Philippines to an apparent hemorrhagic fever syndrome. The animals, in addition to being infected with simian hemorrhagic fever, were also infected with Ebola virus. Military veterinary personnel were deployed to mount a week-long emergency biosafety-level-4 operation to help contain and manage the potential public health crisis. Fortunately, the Reston strain of Ebola virus is apparently not pathogenic to humans. The Reston Ebola incident has served as a useful model for the study of complex issues and management of highly hazardous emerging disease outbreaks.[17]

Research Support

Military veterinarians play an important role in force protection as research pathologists, physiologists, toxicologists, and laboratory animal specialists, assisting in development of effective preventive measures against infectious diseases such as Ebola virus infection and Venezuelan equine encephalitis and against potential NBC threats such as botulinum toxin, ionizing radiation, and various chemical agents.

Veterinary pathologists at the US Army Medical Research Institute for Infectious Diseases, Fort Detrick, Md, and the Walter Reed Army Institute of Research, Silver Spring, Md, collaborate with investigators to provide detailed anatomic pathology evaluation of animal tissues at both gross and microscopic levels. They also develop and apply immunologic, cytochemical, and genomic technologies to diagnose and describe the pathogenesis of militarily significant diseases such as Ebola virus. In 1996, a USAMRIID veterinary pathologist traveled to the Ivory Coast of Africa as part of a World Health Organization sponsored collaborative team trying to identify the primary animal reservoir for Ebola virus.[18]

Military laboratory animal veterinarians also support research applicable to contingencies. Laboratory animal veterinarians assigned to USAMRIID, the Walter Reed Army Institute of Research, and the US Army Medical Research Institute for Chemical Defense (USAMRICD) provide procurement, medical care, and maintenance support for animal colonies used in military research. Military laboratory animal veterinarians were the first to develop large, disease-free animal colonies, a critical component in performing infectious disease research. Veterinary toxicologists help to determine the effects of biological toxins and chemical agents on animals. Research performed by veterinarians at USAMRICD in conjunction with other investigators to determine the effects of low-level chemical exposure on animal models has

been used to help estimate possible effects on humans of potential low-level exposure to chemical agents during the Persian Gulf War.

Military veterinarians with advanced degrees in food technology help develop safer and more durable field rations for use in many different operational settings. Veterinarians at Natick Laboratories, Natick, Mass, have been intensely involved in developing new techniques for preserving foods, improving methods of performing field food analysis and inspection, and developing safer, more durable, and more palatable operational field rations.

Military Working Dogs

Traditionally, military working dogs (MWDs) have been used by all the military services as force multipliers in missions such as scouting, tracking, mine or explosives detection, narcotic detection, and sentry or base defense work. On deployment, MWDs are often sentinels for exposure to environmental hazards that might affect military personnel. Effective preventive medicine measures in keeping these valuable dogs on the job are necessary not only during procurement and training but also during deployments and while the animals are at their home stations.

Military working dogs have been used by the United States since World War I, in which their use was limited but their effectiveness was acknowledged. In World War II, there was again a recognized need for the use of dogs to support military forces. The Dogs for Defense program did not become viable until 1943, yet during the remaining 2 years of World War II more than 15,000 dogs were used in government service. These dogs were employed by the Army and the Marine Corps in both the European and Pacific theaters, and by the Coast Guard for shore patrols along US waters. MWDs have been used in each major conflict since World War II, including the Persian Gulf War.[19] After the Persian Gulf War, the MWD program was downsized in the four military services.

Veterinarians oversee training and treatment of the dogs and ensure that the environmental stresses of a particular deployed area, heat in particular, are not harmful to the dogs. Veterinary personnel must also control infectious diseases, pests, and parasites in the dogs. A veterinary officer must examine and certify each dog before it is deployed.

The Veterinary Pathology Division at the Armed Forces Institute of Pathology, Washington, DC, acts as the pathology referral laboratory for military working dog tissue and clinical specimens submitted for analysis. This division also maintains a military dog tissue repository, samples from which can be used for studies on diseases prevalent in MWDs during contingency operations and for studies on MWDs as sentinels for disease among military service members deployed worldwide. Effective and aggressive preventive veterinary medicine is required to keep these "four-footed service members" fit to accomplish their missions.

SUMMARY

Veterinary personnel provide a valuable force multiplier for mobilization and deployment operations. From protection of the military food supply and care of government-owned animals to vital laboratory support, military veterinarians and their enlisted staffs provide a wide range of services that contribute to the health and well-being not only of animals but also of US fighting forces. Military veterinarians are extremely knowledgeable about the natural history and biology of diseases carried by animals and foods and can provide commanders with critical information for preventing such diseases in the field. It is important to include veterinarians in the medical aspects of contingency planning and operations.

Acknowledgment

The authors would like to thank the following individuals for their assistance in this chapter: Colonel Ron Dutton, US Army, VC, Office of the Command Surgeon, FORSCOM; Colonel Gerald Jaax, US Army, VC, US Army Medical Research Institute of Infectious Diseases; Colonel Nancy N. Jaax, US Army, VC, Chief, Pathology Division, US Army Medical Research Institute of Infectious Diseases; Lieutenant Colonel Fred Lyons, US Army Reserve, VC; Lieutenant Colonel Irving W. McConnell, US Army Reserve, VC; and Colonel Stephanie Sherman, US Army, VC.

REFERENCES

1. *Veterinary Service in Wartime.* Chicago: Veterinary Magazine Corporation; 1942.

2. Steward MJ. Too little, too late; the Veterinary Service of the Civil War. *Modern Veterinary Practice.* 1983;894–895.

3. Merillat LA, Campbell DM. *Veterinary Military History of the United States.* 2 vol. Kansas City: Haver-Glover Laboratories; 1935.

4. Office of the Surgeon General, US Department of the Army. *U.S. Army Veterinary Corps: A Half Century of Progress.* Washington, DC: OTSG, DA; 1966.

5. *US Army Veterinary Service in World War II.* Washington, DC: Office of the Surgeon General, Department of the Army; 1961.

6. US Department of the Army, US Veterinary Command. *Directory of Sanitarily Approved Food Establishments for Armed Forces Procurement.* Fort Sam Houston, Tex: DA, VETCOM; updated annually. VETCOM Circular 40-1.

7. US Departments of the Army, Navy, and Air Force. *Veterinary Health Services.* Washington, DC: DA, DN, DAF; 1994. Army Regulation 40-905, SECNAVINST 6401.1A, ARI 48-131.

8. Office of the Chief, Army Veterinary Corps. *Veterinary Service News.* June 1996. Memorandum.

9. US Department of Defense. *DoD Veterinary/Medical Laboratory Food Safety and Quality Assurance Program.* Washington, DC: DoD; 1995. Army Regulation 40-70, NAVSUPINST 4355.6A.

10. Jaax N, COL, VC, Chief, Pathology Division, US Army Medical Research Institute of Infectious Diseases. Personal communication, 1996.

11. Zuziak P. Military veterinarians assist in hurricane relief effort. *J Am Vet Med Assoc.* 1993;202:712–714.

12. US Department of the Army. *Veterinary Service: Tactics, Techniques, and Procedures.* Washington, DC: DA; 1997. Field Manual 8-10-18.

13. Stamp GL. Hurricane Andrew: The importance of coordinated response. *J Am Vet Med Assoc.* 1993;203:989–992.

14. Heil JR. Army veterinarians do battle against disease. *J Am Vet Med Assoc.* 1996;209:1682.

15. Dutton R, COL, VC. Office of the Command Surgeon, US Forces Command. Personal communication, 1996.

16. Huxsoll DL, Patrick WC 3rd, Parrott CD. Veterinary services in biological disasters. *J Am Vet Med Assoc.* 1987:190:714–722.

17. Jaax G, COL, VC. US Army Institute of Infectious Diseases. Personal communication, 1996.

18. Woolen N, US Army Medical Research Institute of Infectious Diseases. Personal communication, 1996.

19. US Lemish MG. *War Dogs: Canines in Combat.* Washington, DC: Brassey's; 1996.

ABBREVIATIONS AND ACRONYMS

A

A/C/Y/W-135: the tetravalent vaccine

A2LA: American Association for Laboratory Accreditation

AAFMS: Army Aviation Fighter Management System

ABCA's QSTAG: American, British, Canadian, and Australian's Quadripartite Standardization Agreement

AC: active component of the US Armed Forces

AC: alternating current

AC: hydrogen cyanide (hydrocyanic acid)

ACGIH: American Conference of Governmental Industrial Hygienists

ACLS: Advanced Cardiac Life Support

AFEB: Armed Forces Epidemiological Board

AFMIC: Armed Forces Medical Intelligence Center

AGE: arterial gas embolism

AMAL: Authorized Medical Allowance List

AMS: acute mountain sickness

ANG: Air National Guard

AOR: area of responsibility

AR: Army regulation

ARCENT: US Army component, US Central Command

ARD: acute respiratory disease

ARNG: Army National Guard

ARS: acute radiation syndrome

ASD(HA): Assistant Secretary of Defense (Health Affairs)

ASHRAE: American Society of Heating, Refrigerating, and Air-Conditioning Engineers

ASMB: area support medical battalion

ASVAB: Armed Services Vocational Aptitude Battery

ata: atmosphere-absolute

ATC: Air Transportable Clinic

ATH: Air Transportable Hospital

B

BAL: British anti-Lewisite

BCG: bacille Calmette-Guerin

BI: battle injury

BMI: body mass index

BOD: biochemical oxygen demand

BOD_5: biochemical oxygen demand measured after 5 days

BPG: benzathine penicillin G

BUMED: Bureau of Medicine and Surgery

BW: biological warfare

BW: biological weapon

C

C and R: Construction and Repair

CA: civil affairs

CAM: Chemical Agent Monitor

CBI: China–Burma–India theater, World War II

CCP: critical control point

CDC: US Centers for Disease Control and Prevention

CENTAF: US Air Force component, US Central Command

CENTCOM: US Central Command

CERCLA: Comprehensive Environmental Response, Compensation, and Liability Act

CFR: case fatality rate

CFR: Code of Federal Regulations

CFU: colony-forming unit

CG: phosgene (carbonyl chloride)

CHCS II: Composite Health Care System II

CHO: carbohydrate

CHO-E: carbohydrate-electrolyte

CHPPM: Center for Health Promotion and Preventive Medicine

CINC: Commander-in-Chief

CINCCENT: Commander in Chief, US Central Command

CIVD: cold-induced vasodilation

CK: cyanogen chloride

CN: Mace

CNS: central nervous system

CO: carbon monoxide

COA: course of action

COD: chemical oxygen demand

CONPLAN: concept plan

C-P: chloroquine plus primaquine

CPAP: continuous positive airway pressure

CPE: chemical protective ensemble

CS: Clinical Services

CSC: combat stress casualty

CSC: Combat Stress Control

CSR: Combat Stress Reaction

CW: chemical warfare

D

DACOWITS: Defense Advisory Committee on Women in the Services

DALY: disability adjusted life years

DAN: Diver Alert Network

dapsone: 4,4'diaminodiphenylsulfone

DASD: Deputy Assistant Secretary of Defense

dBP: decibel peak

DC: direct current

DCI: decompression illness

DCS: decompression sickness

DDT: dichlorodiphenyltrichloroethane

DEET: N,N-diethyl-1,3-methylbenzamide

DIA: Defense Intelligence Agency

DMO: Diving Medical Officer

DMT: Diving Medical Technicians

DNBI: disease and nonbattle injury

DoD: Department of Defense

DODMERB: Department of Defense Medical Evaluation Review Board

DOEHRS-HC: Defense Occupational and Environmental Health Readiness System in Hearing Conservation

DP: displaced person

DPMIAC: Defense Pest Management Information Analysis Center

DPRK: Democratic Peoples Republic of Korea

E

EEE: eastern equine encephalitis

EFMP: Exceptional Family Member Program

EOD: explosive ordnance disposal

EPA: US Environmental Protection Agency

EPW: enemy prisoner of war

ER: emergency room

F

FAD: foreign animal disease

FDA: Federal Drug Administration

FDA: Food and Drug Administration

FDL: Forward Deployed Laboratory

FDME: Flying Duty Medical Examination

FEMA: Federal Emergency Management Agency

FID: Foreign Internal Defense

FIFRA: Federal Insecticide, Fungicide, and Rodenticide Act
FORSCOM: US Forces Command
FRAGORD: fragmentary order
FRP: Federal Response Plan
FST: Field Sanitation Team
FST: Field Sanitation Team
fsw: feet of seawater
FTX: field training exercise

G

G1: Personnel
G3: Operations
G4: Logistics
GA: tabun
GB: sarin
G-CSF: granulocyte colony-stimulating factor
GD: soman
GF: no expansion, no common name
GI: gastrointestinal
GLOC: G force–induced loss of consciousness
GTMO: US Naval Base at Guantanamo Bay, Cuba

H

HACCP: Hazard Analysis Critical Control Point
HACE: high altitude cerebral edema
HAPE: high altitude pulmonary edema
HARH: high altitude retinal hemorrhage
HAZMIN: hazard minimization
HCA: humanitarian civic assistance
heliox: helium-oxygen mixture
HIV: human immunodeficiency virus
HMMWV: High Mobility Multipurpose Wheeled Vehicle
HSO&R: Health Services Operations and Readiness

I

ICU/CCU: intensive care unit/cardiac care unit
IDA: Individual Dynamic Absorption
IDC: Independent Duty Corpsman
IMA: Individual Mobilization Augmentee
IND: investigational new drug
IRR: Individual Ready Reserve
IUD: intrauterine device
IV: intravenous

J

JCS: Joint Chiefs of Staff
JE: Japanese encephalitis
JTF: Joint Task Force

L

LD$_{50}$: the dose that is lethal to 50% of those exposed
LIC: low-intensity conflict
LITE: low-intensity training and exercise
LRP II: Food Packet, Long Range Patrol II

M

MACV: Military Assistance Command, Vietnam
MAST: military anti-shock trousers
MCA: Medical Civic Action
MCLG: maximum contaminant level goal
MCRD: Marine Corps Recruit Depot
MEDCAP: Medical Civic Action Program
MEDIC: Medical Environmental Disease Intelligence and Countermeasures

MEDRETE: Medical Readiness Training Exercise
MEF: Marine Expeditionary Force
MEPCOM: US Military Entrance Processing Command
MEPS: Military Entrance Processing Stations
MEPSCAT: Military Enlistment Physical Strength Capacity Test
MHS: Military Health System
MOPP: mission-oriented protective posture
MOS: Military Occupational Specialty
MOUT: military operations in urbanized terrain
MRC: major regional conflict
MRDA: Military Recommended Daily Requirement
MRE: Meal, Ready-to-Eat
MSDS: Material Safety Data Sheet
MWD: military working dog

N

NAMRU: Naval Medical Research Unit
NAVCENT: US Navy component, US Central Command
NBC: nuclear, biological, and chemical
NCA: National Command Authority
NCO: noncommissioned officer
NDMS: National Disaster Medical System
NEISS: National Electronic Injury Surveillance System
NEPMU: US Navy Environmental and Preventive Medicine Unit
NER: Near East Relief
NFCI: nonfreezing cold injury
nitrox: nitrogen-oxygen mixture
NOE: nap-of-the-earth
NPDES: National Pollutant Discharge Elimination System
NSC: Naval Safety Center
NSN: National Stock Number
NTU: nephalometric turbidity unit

O

OCONUS: outside the continental United States
OCP: oral contraceptive pill
OCS: Officer Candidate School
OOTW: operations other than war
OPLAN: operational plan
OPORD: operation order
OPSEC: operational security
OSHA: Occupational Safety and Health Administration
otempo: operational tempo

P

P: peak
PAG: protective action guide
2-PAM Cl: pralidoxime chloride
Pap: Papanicolaou
PEEP: positive end-expiratory pressure
PEL: permissible exposure limit
PFIB: perfluoroisobutylene
PH DART: Public Health Disaster Assistance Response Team
PHF: potentially hazardous food
PM: preventive medicine
PMO: Preventive Medicine Officer
PMT: Preventive Medicine Technician
PO$_2$: partial pressure of oxygen
POIS: pulmonary over-inflation syndrome
PPM: personal protection measure
ProMED: Program for Monitoring Emerging Diseases
PSRC: Presidential Selected Reserve call-up
PT: physical training
PTSD: posttraumatic stress disorder

PULHES: *p*hysical capacity, *u*pper extremities, *l*ower extremities, *h*earing, *e*yes, overall p*s*ychiatric impression

R

RC: reserve component of the US Armed Forces
RCRA: Resource Conservation and Recovery Act
RCW: Ration, Cold Weather
RDIC: Resuscitation Device, Individual, Chemical
ROWPU: Reverse Osmosis Water Purification Unit
RR: relative risk
RTC: Navy Recruit Training Command
RVF: Rift Valley fever

S

SARA Title III: Superfund Amendment and Reauthorization Act Title III
sarin: GB; O-isopropyl methylphosphonofluoridate
SASO: Security and Support Operations
SCAP: Supreme Commander for the Allied Powers
scuba: self-contained underwater breathing apparatus
SEAL: US Navy *Se*a, *A*ir, and *L*and
SEB: staphylococcal enterotoxin B
SF: US Special Forces
SFG: Special Forces Group
SMS: Sleep Management System
SOF: Special Operations Forces
soman: GD
SPF: sun protection factor
SPRINT: Special Psychiatric Rapid Intervention team
STANAG: standardization agreement
STD: sexually transmitted disease

T

tabun: GA
TAIHOD: Total Army Injury and Health Outcomes Database
TAML: Theater Area Medical Lab
TB: tuberculosis
TOC: total organic carbon
TSCA: Toxic Substances Control Act

U

USACHPPM: US Army Center for Health Promotion and Preventive Medicine
USAFR: Air Force Reserve
USAFR: US Air Force Reserve
USAID: US Agency for International Development
USAMRICD: US Army Medical Research Institute of Chemical Defense
USAMRIID: US Army Medical Research Institute of Infectious Diseases
USAR: US Army Reserve
USARV: US Army, Vietnam
USASOC: US Army Special Operations Command
USCGR: US Coast Guard Reserve
USDA: US Department of Agriculture
USEPA: US Environmental Protection Agency
USMCR: US Marine Corps Reserve
USNR: US Naval Reserve
USSOCOM: US Special Operations Command
UTI: urinary tract infection

V

V̇o$_2$max: maximum oxygen consumption
VA: Department of Veterans Affairs
VAERS: Vaccine Adverse Events Reporting System

VECTOR: Soviet Institute of Microbiology and Virology, now named Russian State Research Center of Virology and Biotechnology
VEE: Venezuelan equine encephalitis
VX: no expansion, no common name

W

WBGT: Wet Bulb Globe Temperature
WEE: western equine encephalitis
WHO: World Health Organization
WNF: west Nile fever
WRAIR: Walter Reed Army Institute of Research

INDEX

A

AAFMS. *See* Army Aviation Fighter Management System

ABCA Standardization Agreement, 433–434

AC. *See* Active component

Accession Medical Standards Analysis and Research Activity, 155–156

Accession standards
  DoD physical standard goals, 147
  evidence-based, 154–156
  history of, 148–152
  implementation of, 152–154
  purpose of medical standards, 147–148

Acclimatization
  hot environments and, 368–369, 374

Acetazolamide
  high-altitude illness prophylaxis, 399

ACGIH. *See* American Conference of Governmental Industrial Hygienists

ACLS. *See* Advanced Cardiac Life Support

Active component, 131, 132, 140–142

Acute mountain sickness, 399–400

Acute radiation syndrome, 657–658, 660–661

Acute respiratory disease. *See also* Respiratory diseases
  modes of transmission, 180
  surveillance program, 182–183

Adenovirus infections, 186

Advanced Cardiac Life Support, 604–605

Advisory boards, 149

Aedes aegypti, 38, 40, 63, 84, 475–476, 478–479

Aedes albopictus, 480

Aedes spp., 475–476, 482

Aeromedical evacuation, 571–572

AFEB. *See* Armed Forces Epidemiological Board

AGE. *See* Arterial gas embolism

Age factors
  musculoskeletal injuries and, 200

Air Force. *See* United States Air Force

Air Force Academy
  DODMERB evaluation, 153

Air Force Special Operations Command, 240–241

Air National Guard, 133, 138, 140, 239–240

Air quality
  carbon monoxide, 456–457
  contaminants, 457
  controls, 457
  health concerns, 454–455
  indoor air, 463
  military considerations, 458
  monitoring, 457–458
  ozone, 456
  particulate matter, 456
  policy issues, 458
  standards, 457
  sulfur dioxide, 456

Air Quality Act of 1967, 457

Air Transportable Clinics, 237

Air Transportable Hospitals, 237

Airborne disease transmission, 177–179

Akers, Colonel William A., 49

A2LA. *See* American Association for Laboratory Accreditation

Alaska
  cold injuries suffered by US Army during World War II, 31–35
  earthquake of 1964, 97

Alaskan Indians
  relief efforts of preventive medicine professionals, 84

Alcohol consumption
  cold environments and, 397

Alexander, Dr. M.S., 84

Allen, Captain Alfred M., 48–49, 111

Allied Expeditionary Force, 69

Allied Military Government of Occupied Territory, 66

Alphavirus, 478, 482

Altitudes. *See* High-altitude environments

Alving, Dr. Alf, 119, 120

AMAL. *See* Authorized Medical Allowance List

Ambien, 293

Ambient air quality, 454–458

American, British, Canadian, Australian Standardization Agreement, 433–434

American Association for Laboratory Accreditation, 428–429

American Conference of Governmental Industrial Hygienists, 463

American Department of the Inter-Allied Rhineland Commission, 66

American Forces Germany, 65–66

American Polish Relief Expedition, 86–87

American Red Cross Commission, 86

American Relief Administration, 87

American Society of Heating, Refrigerating, and Air-Conditioning Engineers, 179

American trypanosomiasis, 490

American Typhus Commission, 70

AMS. *See* Acute mountain sickness

Anatomic factors
  musculoskeletal injuries and, 200–202

Anemia, hookworm, 108–109

ANG. *See* Air National Guard

Anhidrotic heat exhaustion, 382

Animal bites
  diving and, 588

Anopheles spp., 28, 84, 475–477

Anthrax
  outbreak in Sverdlovsk, USSR, 631

Antimalarial Drug Development Program, 120

Anxiety. *See also* Combat Stress Control; Psychological stress
  development of, 304–305

AORs. *See* Areas of Responsibility

ARD. *See* Acute respiratory disease

Area support medical battalions, 233–234

Areas of Responsibility, 255–256

Armed Forces Epidemiological Board, 45, 48, 110

Armed Forces Medical Intelligence Center, 217, 280

Armed Forces Preventive Medicine Recommendations, 280

Armed Services Vocational Aptitude Battery, 152

Armenia
  relief efforts of preventive medicine professionals following World War I, 86

Army. *See* United States Army

Army Aviation Fighter Management System, 294–298

Army General Classification Test, 150

Army Injury Pyramid, 199